PRACTICAL PAEDIATRICS

Commissioning Editor: Ellen Green
Project Development Manager: Janice Urquhart
Project Manager: Nancy Arnott
Designer: Erik Bigland
Illustrator: Richard Tibbitts

PRACTICAL PAEDIATRICS

EDITED BY

M. J. Robinson MD FRACP
Formerly Reader and Associate Professor of Paediatrics, University of Melbourne, Australia;
Emeritus Professor of Paediatrics, University of Malaya, Kuala Lumpur, Malaysia

D. M. Roberton MD FRACP FRCPA
McGregor-Reid Professor of Paediatrics, University of Adelaide,
Adelaide, Australia

FIFTH EDITION

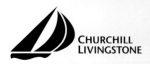

CHURCHILL LIVINGSTONE

EDINBURGH LONDON NEW YORK PHILADELPHIA ST LOUIS SYDNEY TORONTO 2003

CHURCHILL LIVINGSTONE
An imprint of Elsevier Science Limited

First edition 1986
Second edition 1990
Third edition 1994
Fourth edition 1998
Fifth edition 2003

ISBN 0 443 07139 X

British Library Cataloguing in Publication Data
A catalogue record for this book is available from the British
Library

Library of Congress Cataloging in Publication Data
A catalog record for this book is available from the Library of
Congress

Note
Medical knowledge is constantly changing. As new information
becomes available, changes in treatment, procedures, equipment
and the use of drugs become necessary. The editors, contributors
and the publishers have taken care to ensure that the information
given in this text is accurate and up to date. However, readers are
strongly advised to confirm that the information, especially with
regard to drug usage, complies with the latest legislation and
standards of practice.

 your source for books,
journals and multimedia
in the health sciences
www.elsevierhealth.com

The
publisher's
policy is to use
**paper manufactured
from sustainable forests**

Printed in China

Preface

We are pleased to be able to publish a further edition of *Practical Paediatrics*. Previous editions have been used widely and have proved very useful to medical students at all stages of their medical school courses. It has been gratifying to learn also of the popularity of the textbook with nursing and allied health trainees, as well as its usefulness for graduates, trainees in specialties, and general practitioners.

This edition continues the problem-based practical approach to learning, but differs significantly from previous editions in a number of aspects. The content of chapters has been presented, where possible, in a format that includes important points as bullet point lists. The text in many chapters has been reduced and the layout has been carefully designed to allow for easier reading and learning. Tables have been highlighted, and the quality of the illustrations has been improved.

As in the 4th edition, each section concludes with self-assessment questions, followed by the answers and relevant commentaries. Almost all of the multiple choice questions in this edition are new, and we sincerely thank our contributors for undertaking this invaluable exercise. The further reading for each section has been totally revised, with an emphasis on material from the literature that provides clear evidence for the basis of medical practice in child health. The further reading material has been complemented by the addition of web references for each section, making the book even more up to date. These web sites contain useful medical information, but also information in lay terms that can be useful in aiding the understanding of parents, children and young people. Clinical examples again have been included in each chapter to emphasize the practical aspects of the clinical information, and almost all are new in this edition.

More than one-third of the authors for this edition are new to *Practical Paediatrics,* and we are grateful for the fresh perspective provided in the chapters that they have contributed. We also thank again those contributors who have written for us in the past.

There are several chapters on entirely new topics in this edition. A few 4th edition chapters have been omitted, but in most instances the material they contained has been incorporated in other chapters in this new edition. New chapters include electronic learning resources, indigenous culture and health, and life events of normal children. The section entitled paediatric emergencies has been expanded, and a chapter entitled drugs used in paediatrics is another addition. There is new material on sudden infant death syndrome and unexpected death in infancy, on developmental screening, HIV infection, vitamin D and calcium metabolism, and gastro-oesophageal reflux and *Helicobacter pylori* infections. All chapters have been reviewed carefully, and almost all have been extensively rewritten.

We thank all of our 79 contributors who have met deadlines despite their heavy day-to-day workloads. We have been very fortunate in the assistance provided by our secretary in Adelaide (Carol Sandison) and we thank her for her invaluable input. Janice Urquhart, our in-house editor, has been superb in encouraging us, helping us meet deadlines and for the many helpful suggestions relating to the book's presentation and design. She has been patience personified; we cannot thank her enough. We also thank Ellen Green of Elsevier, who has been such a strong advocate for *Practical Paediatrics* throughout.

While this book has the undergraduate medical student as its primary aim, we also see it as continuing to be useful to post-graduate nurse educators, other health professionals, graduates preparing for the early components of their post-graduate paediatric examinations, and general practitioners.

Again we remind medical students that by reading one chapter of this book each day during their paediatric attachments, together with the appropriate self-assessment section, they will cover the entire text and should develop a comprehensive understanding of the practical provision of health care for children and their parents. We hope our readers will find the 5th edition of *Practical Paediatrics* as useful as we believe it to be.

Max Robinson
Melbourne
Don Roberton
Adelaide 2003

Contributors

Jennifer Batch MD FRACP
Royal Children's Hospital Foundation Variety Professor of Paediatrics, and Director of Endocrinology and Diabetes, Royal Children's Hospital, Herston, Queensland, Australia

Spencer W. Beasley MB ChB MS FRACS
Professor of Paediatric Surgery, Christchurch School of Medicine, University of Otago, New Zealand; Clinical Director, Department of Paediatric Surgery, Christchurch Hospital, Christchurch, New Zealand

Bruce Benjamin OBE DLO FRACS FAAP
Clinical Professor, Sydney University, Sydney; Consultant ENT Surgeon, Royal North Shore Hospital and Royal Alexandra Hospital for Children, New South Wales, Australia

David L. Bennett MB BS FRACP
Adolescent Health Physician; Head, Department of Adolescent Medicine, The Children's Hospital, Westmead, New South Wales; Associate Professor, University of Sydney, New South Wales, Australia

David R. Brewster BA MD MPH FRACP PhD
Clinical Dean, Northern Territory Clinical School, Flinders University, Darwin; Head of Paediatrics, Royal Darwin Hospital, Northern Territories, Australia

Leo Buchanan MB ChB FRACP
Te Atiawa and Taranaki iwi; Paediatrician, Lower Hutt Hospital, Lower Hutt, New Zealand

John R. Burke FRACP
Nephrologist, Mater Misericordiae, Royal Children's and Princess Alexandra Hospitals, Brisbane, Queensland, Australia

Fergus Cameron FRACP DipRACOG MD
Endocrinologist, Royal Children's Hospital, Parkville, Victoria, Australia

Neil Campbell MB BS FRACP
Consultant Neonatologist, Royal Children's Hospital, Melbourne, Victoria, Australia

Allan Carmichael MD FRACP
Professor of Paediatrics and Child Health; Dean, Faculty of Health Science, University of Tasmania; State Adviser, Child Health Services, Tasmania, Australia

Anne B. Chang MB BS PhD MPHTM FRACP
Paediatric Respiratory Consultant, Department of Respiratory Medicine, Royal Children's Hospital, Brisbane and Department of Paediatrics and Child Health, University of Queensland, Australia

Kevin Collins MB BS FRACP
Neurologist, Department of Neurology and Department of Child Development and Rehabilitation, Royal Children's Hospital, Melbourne, Victoria; Senior Paediatric Neurologist, Monash Medical Centre, Melbourne, Victoria, Australia

Jennifer Couper MB ChB MD FRACP
Paediatric Endocrinologist, Women's and Children's Hospital, Adelaide, South Australia; Associate Professor, University of Adelaide, South Australia, Australia

Richard T. L. Couper FRACP MB ChB
Senior Paediatric Gastroenterologist, Department of Paediatrics, Women's and Children's Hospital, Adelaide, South Australia, Australia

Peter Cundy MB BS FRACS
Senior Visiting Orthopaedic Surgeon, Women's and Children's Hospital, Adelaide, South Australia, Australia

Geoff Davidson MB BS MD FRACP
Director, Centre for Paediatric and Adolescent Gastroenterology, Women's and Children's Hospital, Adelaide, South Australia; Clinical Professor, Department of Paediatrics, University of Adelaide, Adelaide, South Australia, Australia

Martin B. Delatycki MB BS PhD FRACP
Medical Geneticist Genetic Health Services Victoria, Royal Children's Hospital, Melbourne, Victoria; Honorary Senior Lecturer, University of Melbourne; Honarary Lecturer, Monash University, Melbourne, Australia

Richard Doherty FRACP DipObs RCOG
Professor of Paediatrics and Head, Department of Paediatrics, Monash University; Head of Infectious Diseases Unit, Monash Medical Centre, Melbourne, Victoria, Australia

James E. Elder MB BS FRACS FRACO
Director, Department of Ophthalmology, Royal Children's Hospital, Melbourne, Victoria, Australia

Peter Flett MB BS FRACP FAFRM MRACMA
Director, Paediatric Rehabilitation; Unit Head,
Rehabilitation Service, Department of Child and
Adolescent Development and Rehabilitation,
Women's and Children's Hospital, Adelaide,
South Australia, Australia

David Forbes MB BS FRACP
Paediatric Gastroenterologist, Princess Margaret
Hospital for Children, Perth, Western Australia;
Associate Professor, Department of Paediatrics,
University of Western Australia, Australia

Kevin Forsyth MD PhD FRACP FRCPA
Head of Paediatrics and Child Health, Flinders
University and Flinders Medical Centre, Bedford Park,
South Australia, Australia

Vicki Gallard BSc DipNut&Diet
Chief Dietician, Women's and Children's Hospital,
Adelaide, South Australia; Lecturer, Nutrition and
Dietetics, Flinders University, South Australia, Australia

Lyn Gilbert MB BS MD FRACP FRCPA
Director, Centre for Infectious Disease and
Microbiology Laboratory, Institute of Clinical
Pathology and Medical Research Services, Westmead
Hospital, New South Wales; Clinical Professor in
Infectious Diseases and Medicine, University of Sydney,
Sydney, New South Wales, Australia

Mike Gold MB ChB MD FRACP FCP
Paediatric Allergist, Department of Paediatrics,
University of Adelaide; Women's and Children's
Hospital, Adelaide, South Australia, Australia

Brian Graetz BA(Hons) MPsych DipT
Clinical Psychologist, Women's and Children's
Hospital, Adelaide, South Australia, Australia

H. Kerr Graham MD FRCS FRACS
Professor of Orthopaedic Surgery, University of
Melbourne, Melbourne; Consultant Orthopaedic
Surgeon, Royal Children's Hospital, Melbourne,
Victoria, Australia

Philip Graves MB BS MPH DCH MRCP FRACP
Senior Lecturer, Department of Paediatrics, Monash
University, Victoria, Australia

Keith Grimwood MD FRACP
Professor and Head, Department of Paediatrics and Child
Health, Wellington School of Medicine, University of
Otago; General and Infectious Diseases Physician,
Capital Coast Health, Wellington, New Zealand

Roger K. Hall OAM MDSc FRACDS FICD
Senior Dental Surgeon, Royal Children's Hospital,
Melbourne; Associate Professor, University of
Melbourne, Victoria, Australia

Jane Harding MB ChB DPhil FRACP
Professor of Neonatology, University of Auckland;
Specialist Neonatologist, National Women's Hospital,
Auckland, New Zealand

A. Simon Harvey MD FRACP
Paediatric Epileptologist, Children's Epilepsy Program,
Royal Children's Hospital and Austin Repatriation
Medical Centre, Melbourne, Victoria, Australia

Richard Henry MB BS MD DipClinEpi FRACP
Deputy Dean and Head, School of Women's and
Children's Health, University of New South Wales,
Australia

Harriet Hiscock MB BS FRACP GradDipEpi
Paediatrician and Research Officer, Centre for
Community Child Health, Royal Children's Hospital,
Melbourne, Victoria, Australia

Neil J. Hotham BPharm
Specialist Drug Information Pharmacist, Women's and
Children's Hospital, Adelaide, South Australia, Australia

David Isaacs MB BChir MD FRACP FRCPCH
Senior Staff Specialist, Paediatric Infectious Diseases,
Children's Hospital, Westmead, New South
Wales, Australia

Christine Jeffries-Stokes MB BS BMedSci MPH
FRACP
Paediatrician, Kalgoorlie-Boulder, Western Australia,
Australia

Diana Jolly MB BS BMedSci DCCH MPH FAFPHM
Fellow in Child Psychiatry, Women's and Children's
Hospital, Adelaide, South Australia, Australia

Colin Jones MB BS PhD FRACP
Director, Department of Nephrology, Royal Children's
Hospital, Parkville, Victoria, Australia

Andrew Kornberg MB BS FRACP
Director of Neurology, Royal Children's Hospital,
Parkville, Victoria; Deputy Director, Melbourne
Neuromuscular Research Institute, St Vincent's
Hospital, Melbourne, Victoria, Australia

Ursula Kuhnle MD
Consultant Paediatrician and Paediatric Endocrinologist,
Division of Paediatric Endocrine Research, University
Children's Hospital, Munich, Germany

Peter N. LeSouëf MD MRCP FRACP
Respiratory Physician, Department of Respiratory
Medicine, Princess Margaret Hospital, Perth, Western
Australia; Professor of Paediatrics, University of West
Australia, Australia

Jan Liebelt MB BS MSc FRACP HGSA
Clinical Geneticist, Women's and Children's Hospital,
Adelaide, South Australia, Australia

Joseph Macdessi MB BS
Paediatric Registrar, The Children's Hospital,
Westmead, New South Wales, Australia

James McGill MB BS FRACP
Paediatric Metabolic Diseases Physician and Geneticist,
Department of Metabolic Medicine, Royal Children's
Hospital, Herston, Queensland, Australia

Craig Mellis MB BS MPH MD FRACP
Professor of Paediatrics, Paediatric Chest Physician and
Head of Department of Paediatrics and Child Health,
University of Sydney, Sydney, New South Wales,
Australia

Jerry Moller BSocAdmin MPolAdmin
Principal Consultant, New Directions in Health and
Safety, Flagstaff Hill, South Australia, Australia

Barry Nurcombe MD FRACP FRANZCP DPM
Director, Child and Adolescent Psychiatry,
The University of Queensland, Queensland, Australia

Frank Oberklaid AOM FRACP DCH MD
Director, Centre for Community Health, Royal
Children's Hospital, University of Melbourne,
Melbourne, Victoria, Australia

Mark Oliver MB BS MD FRACP
Senior Fellow, Department of Paediatrics, University of
Melbourne, Murdoch Research Institute, Victoria,
Australia

Edward O'Loughlin MD FRACP
Paediatric Gastroenterologist, The Children's Hospital,
Westmead, New South Wales, Australia

Rod Phillips MB BS PhD FRACP
Consultant in Paediatric Skin Disease, Department of
Paediatrics, Royal Children's Hospital, Parkville,
Victoria, Australia

Jeremy Raftos MB BS(Hons) FRACP
Director, Paediatric Emergency Department, Women's
and Children's Hospital, Adelaide, South
Australia, Australia

Dinah Reddihough BSc MD FRACP FAFRM
Director, Department of Child Development and
Rehabilitation, Royal Children's Hospital, Melbourne,
Victoria, Australia

Don M. Roberton MD FRACP FRCPA
McGregor-Reid Professor of Paediatrics, University of
Adelaide; Head, Department of Paediatrics, Women's
and Children's Hospital, Adelaide, South Australia,
Australia

Maxwell J. Robinson MD FRACP
Formerly Reader and Associate Professor of Paediatrics,
University of Melbourne; Emeritus Professor of
Paediatrics, University of Malaya, Kuala Lumpur,
Malaysia

Maureen Rogers MB BS FACD
Head of Department of Dermatology, The Children's
Hospital at Westmead, New South Wales, Australia

Remo Russo MB BS FRACP FAFRM·
Senior Consultant, Department of Child and Adolescent
Development and Rehabilitation, Women's and
Children's Hospital, Adelaide, South Australia,
Australia

Michael Sawyer MB BS PhD DipChildPsych FRCPC
FRANZCP
Head, Research and Evaluation Unit, Women's and
Children's Hospital; Professor of Child and Adolescent
Psychiatry, University of Adelaide, Adelaide, South
Australia, Australia

Susan M. Sawyer MB BS MD FRACP
Respiratory Physician, Department of Respiratory
Medicine, Royal Children's Hospital, Melbourne,
Victoria; Deputy Director and Head, Clinical Services,
Centre for Adolescent Health; Associate Professor,
Department of Paediatrics, University of Melbourne,
Melbourne, Victoria, Australia

Ben Saxon MB BS FRACP FRCPA
Paediatric Haematologist and Oncologist, Department of
Haematology, Women's and Children's Hospital,
Adelaide, South Australia, Australia

Jill Sewell MB BS FRACP
Deputy Director, Centre for Community Child Health,
Royal Children's Hospital, Melbourne, Victoria,
Australia

Frank Shann MB BS MD FRACP FJFICM
Director of Intensive Care, Royal Children's Hospital,
Melbourne, Victoria; Professor of Critical Care
Medicine, University of Melbourne, Victoria, Australia

Peter D. Sly MD FRACP
Head of Division of Clinical Sciences, TVW Telethon
Institute for Child Health Research, Perth; Director,
Clinical Research and Education, Princess Margaret
Hospital, Perth, Western Australia, Australia

Peter Smith FRACP MD FRCPA
Dean, School of Medicine, University of Auckland,
Auckland, New Zealand

Michael South MB BS DCH FRACP MRCP MD
Director, Department of General Medicine, Royal
Children's Hospital, Melbourne, Victoria; Associate
Professor, University of Melbourne, Victoria, Australia

David Starte MB BS MRCP FRACP
Senior Staff Specialist in Developmental Paediatrics,
Chatswood Assessment Centre, Royal North Shore
Hospital, Chatswood, New South Wales, Australia

Geoffrey D. Stokes
Chairperson, Wonguthua Birni, Aboriginal Corp.,
Western Australia; Executive Member, Goldfields Land
Council, Kalgoorlie-Boulder, Western Australia,
Australia

Graeme Suthers MB BS PhD FRCACP
Head, Familial Cancer Unit, South Australia Clinical
Genetics Service, Women's and Children's Hospital,
Adelaide, South Australia, Australia

Geoff Tauro MB BS FRACP FRCPA
Formerly Senior Specialist Haematologist, Royal
Children's Hospital, Melbourne, Victoria, Australia

Barry J. Taylor MB ChB FRACP
Professor of Paediatrics and Child Health, Dunedin
School of Medicine, University of Otago, New Zealand

Rita Teele MD FRANZCR
Radiologist, Starship Children's Hospital and National
Women's Hospital, Auckland; Honorary Professor of
Anatomy, Auckland Medical School, Auckland,
New Zealand

Elizabeth Thompson MD FRACP
Clinical Geneticist, South Australian Clinical Genetics
Service, Women's and Children's Hospital, Adelaide,
South Australia, Australia

James Tibballs BMedSci MB BS MEd MBA MD
FANZCA FFICANZCA FACTM
Deputy Director, Intensive Care Unit, Royal Children's
Hospital, Melbourne, Victoria; Medical Consultant,
Poisons Information Centre, Royal Children's Hospital,
Melbourne, Victoria; Principal Fellow, Australian
Venom Research Unit, Department of Pharmacology,
University of Melbourne, Victoria, Australia

Karen Tiedemann MB BS FRACP
Clinical Haematologist and Oncologist, Royal
Children's Hospital, Melbourne, Victoria, Australia

David Tudehope AM MB BS MRACP FRACP
Director of Neonatology, Mater Mothers Hospital,
Brisbane, Queensland; Professor of Neonatal
Paediatrics, Department of Paediatrics and Child
Health, University of Queensland, Queensland,
Australia

Graham Vimpani PhD FRACP FAFPHM
Professor of Paediatrics and Child Health; Director,
Child Adolescent and Family Health Service, Child and
Youth Health Network, Wallsend, New South Wales,
Australia

Keith Waters MB BS FRACP
Clinical Director, Department of Clinical Haematology
and Oncology, Royal Children's Hospital, Melbourne,
Victoria, Australia

Neil Wigg MB BS FRACP MPolAdmin
Executive Director, Community Child Health Service,
Royal Children's Hospital and Health Service District,
Brisbane; Adjunct Associate Professor, Department of
Paediatrics and Child Health, University of Queensland,
Queensland, Australia

Ian Wilkinson MB BS FRACP
Paediatric Neurologist, Director of Paediatric and
Adolescent Medicine, John Hunter Children's Hospital,
Newcastle, New South Wales, Australia

James Wilkinson FRACP MCRP FRCP FACC
FRCPCH
Director of Cardiology, Royal Children's Hospital,
Melbourne, Victoria, Australia

Contents

Part 23
Paediatrics in the future

CURRENT PAEDIATRICS

1 Child health and disease

G. Vimpani

Australian children

Statistics concerning Australian children

- 20.7% of the Australian population is aged 0–14 years.
- 14.2% of the Australian population is aged 15–24 years.
- 4% of Australian children are indigenous.
- 86% live in southeastern mainland States.
- 6% were born overseas — 38% in Asia; 36% have at least one overseas-born parent.
- 29% births are ex-nuptial; 12% children live in single parent families.
- 1:5 children will experience divorce of their parents before their 16th birthday.
- 22% of under-twos participate in formal child care.
- 12.6% of children under 14 years live in relative poverty.
- Australia ranks comparatively poorly, coming 15th out of 23 rich countries in proportion of children living below 50% of the national median income.

Australia is a highly urbanised nation with a total estimated population in 1999 of 18.9 million, of whom 1.27 million (6.7%) are children aged less than 5 years, 2.65 million (14.0%) are children aged 5–14 years, and 2.69 million (14.2%) are young people aged 15–24 years (Table 1.1). Following colonisation in the 18th century, the proportion of children declined to a low of 24% in 1943, but increased steadily with the baby boom of the 1950s, levelling out at about 30%. Since then, although the actual number of children aged 0–14 years has increased, the proportion has decreased to a record low of 20.5%. This decline is due mainly to a drop in fertility, from 3.4 children per woman in the baby boom years to the current level of 1.75 children per woman. The projected child population proportion (aged 0–14 years) in the year 2031 is 17.7%, or 4.2 million. The majority (85.9%) of Australian children live in the southeastern mainland states. There are 68% who live in urban centres with populations greater than 100 000, with 28% living in rural areas (most in centres with populations under 10 000) and less than 5% living in remote areas. Children living in rural and remote areas comprise a larger proportion of the total population in those areas.

About 6% of Australia's children were born overseas: 14% of these are from the UK and Ireland, 12% come from European countries, 38% from Asia and 13% from New Zealand. Reflecting the cosmopolitan nature of Australia today, at least 36% of all Australian children have at least one parent who was born in a country other than Australia. Over 154 000 or about 3.95% of the child population are indigenous and these account for around 40% of all indigenous Australians.

Between 1950 and 1998 the proportion of ex-nuptial births rose from around 5% to 29% — about half of these were to women in de facto relationships. Couple families (two parents or carers, married or de facto) include 88% of children, while 12% live in one parent families. For children living in single parent families, 70% live with a parent who is separated or divorced, 20% with a parent who never married, and 10% with a widowed parent. Of 978 000 children living with only one natural parent in 1997, most (88%) lived with their mother in either a one parent (68%) or in step or blended families (20%). Of all divorced couples, 53% involve at least one child. About one in five will experience parent divorce before their 16th birthday. Children in single parent families fare less well socially,

Age (years)	State/Territory								Australia	% of Australian population
	NSW	Vic	Qld	SA	WA	Tas	NT	ACT		
0–4	432 457	307 498	241 753	94 167	127 176	31 582	17 565	21 159	1 273 589	6.72
5–9	445 762	323 526	255 400	99 276	133 223	34 151	17 412	21 797	1 330 883	7.03
10–14	437 248	317 100	251 154	100 627	137 028	34 791	15 495	21 918	1 315 727	6.95
15–19	439 958	322 372	258 370	100 700	135 854	34 517	14 582	24 396	1 330 972	7.03
20–24	444 561	342 394	254 096	99 714	139 690	29 913	16 760	27 308	1 354 582	7.15

Table 1.1 Estimated Australian population of children and young people (age, State), 1999

educationally and physically than children in two parent families, often because of the accompanying socio-economic disadvantage these families experience.

During the period between 1986 and 1996, the labour force participation rate of women with children who were aged under 15 years increased from 49% to 59%, with much higher rates in 1996 noted for women of older children and those in couple families compared with single parent families (56% compared with 10%). Between 1984 and 1996 the proportion of under 2 year olds in formal child care increased from 8% to 22%; for 3–4 year olds the proportion rose from 41% to 59% (and if one excludes preschools this proportion doubled from 12% to 24%). The type of care involved largely depends on the age of the child. Half of the children under 2 years in formal care are in long day care centres, with around 6% in family day care. A further 39% are involved in informal care from friends and relatives. Seventy six per cent of all 3 and 4 year olds experience non parental care — 36% in preschools, 17% in long day care, and 5% in family day care, with 41% experiencing informal care with or without other forms of non parental care.

Poverty is a well known determinant of population health. The term 'poverty' means different things to different people. There are three different approaches to defining poverty:

- *absolute poverty* — where a family's income does not pay for basic necessities such as shelter and food
- *relative poverty* — where a family's income is low in comparison to the income of other families
- *subjective poverty* — where a poor family is defined as one that believes its income is inadequate for its needs.

Most developed countries, including Australia, adopt the relative approach. UNICEF estimates that one in six children in industrialised countries live in relative poverty; Australia ranks behind many European countries, coming 15th of 23 wealthy countries, with 581 000 or 12.6% of its children aged under 14 years living in households with incomes lower than 50% of the national median. The overall rate of relative poverty amongst indigenous children is three times higher than that for non indigenous children.

Changes in disease patterns

The health status of children has always reflected an interaction between biological susceptibility and their experience of the physical, chemical and psychosocial environment. Paediatrics has changed dramatically during the last 50 years as mortality for all life threatening conditions, and infectious disease incidence in particular, has declined substantially (Fig. 1.1). Although improved levels of education, housing, hygiene, immunisation and antibiotics have far from eliminated

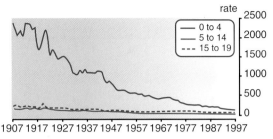

Rate per 100,000 population.
Source: AIHW Mortality Monitoring System

Fig. 1.1   Death due to all causes, by age of child. Source: AIHW (Australian Institute of Health and Welfare) Mortality Monitoring System.

infectious disease (witness the emergence of AIDS), the morbidity and mortality due to infection, particularly for those 14 years and younger, has been reduced markedly in developed societies.

Examples of the declining incidence of infectious disease are many, but of particular importance is the greatly reduced incidence of tuberculosis; chronic suppuration of chest, bone and ear; rheumatic fever and rheumatic heart disease, and streptococcal infections of all types. It should be noted that the incidence of all infections was falling well before the advent of antibiotic and chemotherapeutic drugs, which, incorrectly, have often been given the major credit for control of infection.

In contrast, some other childhood diseases have shown a rising prevalence, for which the causes are unclear. There has been an increase in the prevalence of asthma symptoms (present in around 20% of children in community surveys) and hospital admissions, with asthma now the leading cause of admission of children to hospital. In addition, new challenges have been posed by the emergence of what have been termed 'problems of developmental health and wellbeing' that are related to the pace of social and family change during the past 30 years. Examples are child maltreatment, behaviour and learning problems, youth suicide, eating disorders, substance misuse, and early onset criminal behaviour.

Child health

In evaluating disease incidence and the health status of a community, mortality and morbidity figures are used. There has been a centuries old traditional focus on mortality, partly because of compulsory reporting of death. However, mortality is a very crude index of health and is of limited value in assessing the health status and health needs of a community. A strict disease focus cannot describe the full spectrum of child health. An important difference between child and adolescent health compared with adult health is that the young person is developing

Table 1.2   Domains of child health. (After Starfield B 1987 Journal of Chronic Diseases 40 (Suppl. 1) 109s–115s)

Health domain	Description
1. Longevity	Projected life expectancy
2. Activity	Functional status, ability/disability
3. Comfort	Symptoms
4. Satisfaction	Satisfaction with own health
5. Disease	Presence and progression of defined disease states
6. Achievement	Social and emotional development
7. Resilience	Ability to resist threats to health

rapidly, a process in which genetic and environmental influences are critical. In this transactional process 'goodness of fit' between young people and their environments is a determinant of good outcomes, including the impact of disease and disorder on functional capacity. The 1946 World Health Organization (WHO) definition defines health as 'a state of complete physical, mental, and social well-being and not merely the absence of disease or infirmity'. A more practical and complete way of thinking about child health involves the seven categories shown in Table 1.2.

Describing health therefore requires more than a consideration of morbidity and mortality. It is similarly important to understand risk and protective factors and behaviours that may have positive and negative impacts on health. From a practical point of view, complete paediatric clinical assessment requires a consideration of all of the above domains. This applies equally to the child with leukaemia, cystic fibrosis, acute bacterial meningitis, developmental delay, child maltreatment, behaviour problem or even a child who presents for a well child review.

Mortality

Changing patterns of mortality

- Increasing life expectancy — but indigenous population about 20 years less.
- Improved neonatal mortality associated with better perinatal care.
- Improved postneonatal mortality associated with declining rate of sudden infant death syndrome (SIDS).
- Indigenous infant mortality (16.0) three times higher than non indigenous (5.0).
- 40% deaths in 1–14 year olds due to unintentional injury, despite 59% fall since 1979.
- Cancer accounts for 60% of deaths due to acquired disease.
- Declining infectious disease mortality consolidated by immunisation.
- Substantial decline in traffic accident mortality in adolescents (52% males, 21% females since 1961).
- 40% increase in adolescent male suicide deaths since 1979.
- 7.4% of youth deaths in 1998 related to drug dependence.

The WHO and Australian Bureau of Statistics (ABS) definitions shown in Table 1.3 are important in collecting data on mortality. Many countries do not use the WHO definitions, and the ABS alternatives in relevant categories are detailed. Caution should, therefore, always be exercised in comparing published mortality rates internationally.

Life expectancy at birth in Australia increased substantially throughout the course of the 20th century, largely as a result of improved infant and child mortality, and is amongst the highest in the world. Life expectancy

Table 1.3   Definitions of mortality and mortality rates

	Description	WHO		Australian Bureau of Statistics (ABS)	
		Birth weight (g)	Gestation (weeks)	Birth weight (g)	Gestation (weeks)
Stillbirth	Stillborn infant	≥1000	≥28	≥500	≥22
Neonatal death	Death within 7 days of birth (ABS within 28 days)	≥1000	≥28	≥500	≥22
Infant death	Death within 1 year of birth	≥1000		≥500	
Liver birth	Any birth which shows signs of life after being born				
Perinatal mortality rate	Stillbirths plus neonatal deaths per 1000 births, live and still				
Infant mortality	Infant deaths per 1000 live births				
Postneonatal mortality rate	Infant deaths between 28 days and 1 year per 1000 live births				

in Australia in 1998 was 75.9 years for males and 81.5 years for females. Regrettably, indigenous children can expect to live about 20 years less than the rest of the Australian population.

Infant mortality rates are important indicators of child health, particularly when analysed as component neonatal and postneonatal rates. Neonatal mortality has always been influenced by pregnancy complications and fetal growth and development, including the presence of congenital anomalies, whereas postneonatal mortality rates are related more commonly to social and environmental conditions. Since the 1920s in Australia, when both these rates were very high, there has been a rapid decline, especially in postneonatal mortality, as social and environmental conditions improved and infectious disease was progressively controlled (Fig. 1.2). With the advent of neonatal intensive care in the late 1960s, the neonatal mortality rate declined even further, to the point where, today, neonatal and postneonatal rates are again at similar, albeit much lower, levels. Despite these improvements in neonatal mortality rates, it is disconcerting to note that there has not been any improvement in the proportion of low birth weight infants (6.6% overall, but 13.1% in indigenous births), and morbidity rates in the smallest surviving infants have increased.

In Australia, Aboriginal mortality rates are substantially higher at all ages. Although there have been major gains for all Australians in infant and perinatal mortality, from a rate of approximately 100 per 1000 live births at the turn of the twentieth century to the 1998 figure of 5.0, the rates are still 2–3 times higher for indigenous (16.0) than for non indigenous Australians (Fig. 1.3).

Figure 1.4 shows the comparative neonatal, postneonatal, and infant mortality rates for a number of developed countries. A reduction in the indigenous infant mortality rate would significantly improve the Australian figure. An excess of male over female infant deaths is observed worldwide.

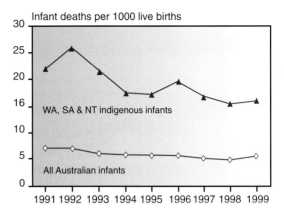

Fig. 1.3 Indigenous infant mortality rate. Source: Both indigenous and total Australian rates are based on data derived from the AIHW National Mortality Database.

Causes of death

Neonatal deaths

Table 1.4 shows the major causes of death in the neonatal period in one State (Victoria) in Australia. Causes generally are similar in other parts of Australia. Sixty per cent of these deaths occur on the day of birth, with most being due to extreme prematurity or poor fetal growth, congenital malformations or pregnancy complications. Forty four per cent of neonatal deaths result from a malformation, although only 18% of these deaths involve a known chromosomal abnormality. Further reductions in the incidence of neural tube defects (NTDs) will occur with use of the now proven preventive effect of periconceptional folate supplementation in mothers of both high risk (previous NTD affected conception) and low risk (no previous NTD affected conception) infants.

There remains major scope for further improvement in neonatal mortality, particularly with the development of an understanding of the determinants of premature labour, intrauterine growth restriction, developmental anomalies and other perinatal conditions. As shown in Figure 1.5, very little is known about the causes of prematurity, and even less about its prevention. Progress has been hampered by research which has not distinguished between placental insufficiency (leading to intrauterine growth retardation) and preterm labour as causes of low birth weight.

It is not surprising, therefore, that there has been little change in the incidence of low birth weight in recent generations. Indeed, there has been a slight rise in its incidence in the last decade (from 6.3% to 6.6%), which is partly explained by a higher proportion of older mothers giving birth. In 1998 the birth rate in women over 35 years of age exceeded that in those under 19 years for the first time. Fortunately, however, the perinatal mortality rate is now similar for major birth weight groups. This has only come about during the last 20 years when newborn inten-

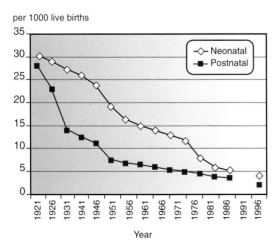

Fig. 1.2 Neonatal and postneonatal mortality rates 1921–1996.

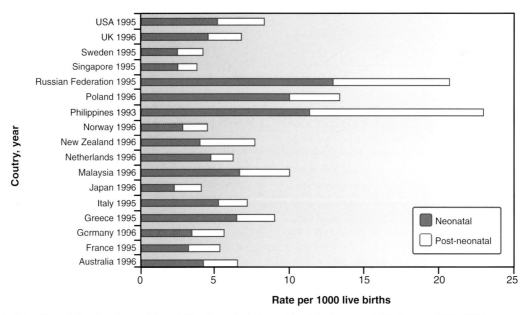

Fig. 1.4 Neonatal and postneonatal mortality rates, selected countries, latest year available. Source: AIHW, 2000.

Table 1.4 Causes of neonatal deaths in Victoria, Australia, 1997. (Source: Consultative Council on Obstetric and Paediatric Mortality and Morbidity, Annual report for 1997, with permission)

Cause of death	Number	%
Non malformations		
Multiple pregnancy	16	
Birth asphyxia and intrapartum hypoxia	10	
Premature rupture of membranes	9	
Infection	9	
Extreme prematurity	7	
Antepartum haemorrhage	6	
Preeclampsia	4	
SIDS	4	
Fetal haemorrhage	3	
Other	21	
Subtotal	89	56
Malformations		
Multiple abnormalities	15	
Congenital heart disease	11	
Neural tube defects	7	
Urinary anomalies	4	
Trisomy 21	1	
Other chromosomal anomalies	10	
Other	23	
Subtotal	71	44
Total	160	100

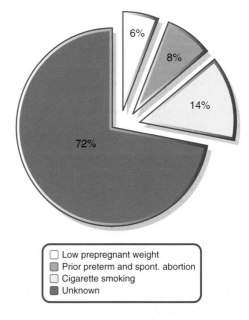

Fig. 1.5 Determinants of preterm labour in a developed country. After Kramer MS 1987 Pediatrics 80: 502–511.

Postneonatal and child deaths

Table 1.5 shows that, for the State of Victoria, Australia, 28% of deaths in the postneonatal period are sudden and unexpected (SIDS), and occur in an infant who is apparently well — a marked fall from the 48% noted from this cause only 3 years earlier.

Recent case–control and cohort studies have provided strong evidence for an association of the prone sleeping position with risk of SIDS (Ch. 13). Other risk factors

sive care has improved survival for high risk neonates dramatically. During this time, the reduction in mortality has been greatest for the 1000–2499 g group.

Table 1.5 Causes of postneonatal infant and child deaths in Victoria, Australia, 1997. (Source: Victorian Council on Paediatric and Maternal Mortality, with permission)

Cause of death	Postneonatal 1–11 months		Child 1–14 years	
	No	%	No	%
Determined at birth				
Birth asphyxia	2		4	
Malformation/birth defect	29		34	
Prematurity	12		1	
Other	2		6	
Subtotal	45	52	45	29
Sudden infant death syndrome (SIDS)	24	28	1	1
Injury (unintentional)				
Motor vehicle	1		22	
Drowning	1		7	
Burns	1		4	
Asphyxia	3		4	
Other			8	
Subtotal	6	7	45	29
Acquired disease				
Infection	6		9	
Malignancy	3		37	
Other	2		10	
Subtotal	11	13	56	37
Intentional injury	1	1	5	3
Suicide	0		1	1
Total	87		153	

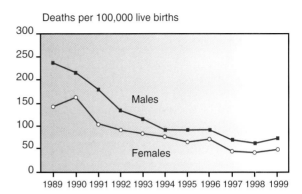

Fig. 1.6 Sudden infant death syndrome rate. Estimates based on data from AIHW National Mortality Database.

also have been identified consistently from epidemiological studies: these include maternal cigarette smoking, lack of breastfeeding, overheating of the baby, and a parental history of illicit drug use. Concomitant with reductions in prone sleeping practice, dramatic reductions in the rate of SIDS have been observed in both Australia and New Zealand. In 1998, the SIDS rate for males was less than a quarter of the 1987 rate (the peak year), and for females the rate in 1998 was one third of that in 1987 (Fig. 1.6). This breakthrough with an astonishingly simple intervention seems now to be confirmed, although its precise mechanism is not yet fully explained. However, the rate of SIDS in indigenous infants remains higher than in Caucasians.

Causes of death between 1 and 14 years

More than 98% of children survive from birth to 15 years of age. The mortality rates for children aged 1–14 years

declined by 45% for males and 44% for females between 1979 and 1998. Unintentional injuries, poisoning and violence account for over 40% of deaths despite a 59% fall since 1979, with male rates about 1.6 times higher than in girls. Motor vehicle accidents (involving occupants, pedestrians and cyclists) accounted for half the injury deaths, and drowning (domestic pools, dams and drains, rivers and sea, and domestic buckets) for a further quarter of the deaths. These were the commonest causes of unintentional injury deaths, with the remainder being attributed to burns, asphyxiation and a number of rarer causes (Table 1.5). Other major causes include malignancy and congenital abnormalities.

The decline in injury mortality has been due to a number of preventive actions, including child resistant packaging of medication (poisoning deaths are now rare, although hospital admission remains relatively common), traffic and driver control measures (infant and child seat restraints, improved vehicle design, traffic control through speed cameras, random breath testing, local area traffic control, and cyclist helmets), and domestic pool isolation fencing (Ch. 9). Added to these measures has been an increase in public awareness of child safety through targeted and mass media education campaigns. As with disease, the challenge to reduce injury morbidity now follows these important gains in saved lives.

Of the one quarter in this age group who die from disease, 60% succumb to cancer despite important advances in long term survival from surgery (for example, Wilms tumour), chemotherapy and radiotherapy (for example, acute lymphocyctic leukaemia and lymphomas).

Another important cause of preventable infectious disease mortality in children is *Haemophilus influenzae* type b (Hib) meningitis. Following the introduction of Hib conjugate vaccines in Australia, a more than 80% reduction in invasive Hib disease incidence has occurred (Fig. 1.7).

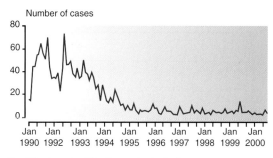

Fig. 1.7 Invasive Hib disease in Australia.
Source: Communicable Diseases Network — Australia New Zealand — National Notifiable Diseases Surveillance System.

Causes of death between 15 and 19 years

Mortality rates in this age group are about five times higher than in children aged 5–14 years, although substantially lower than rates in the 0–4 year group (Fig. 1.1). The principal causes of death in adolescents are injury (50%), particularly traffic related causes (where alcohol use is an important contributor to mortality), suicide (20%) and cancer (10%). The mortality rate for males is twice that of females in this age group. While death rates for females have declined by 21% since 1961, in males the corresponding decline is 52%, largely as a result of a substantial reduction in traffic injury mortality, despite an increasing number of vehicles and young drivers and passengers (Table 1.6). However, there has been a disturbing increase in adolescent male suicide, with the rate increasing by 40% between 1979 and 1998 — currently four times higher than the female rate. Drug dependence accounted for 7.4% of youth deaths in 1998 and has risen sharply in recent years, especially among males.

Morbidity

Changing patterns of morbidity

- Rising prevalence of asthma in children and young people (12.3–19.2%).
- Increasing concern about problems of developmental health and wellbeing — 35% of paediatric consultations for behaviour problems, 13% for learning problems.
- 14% of children have mental health problems — higher rates associated with low income, coercive parenting, family conflict, blended/single families and in children with chronic illness.
- 29% and 24%, respectively, of children exposed to coercive and inconsistent parenting styles had mental health morbidity compared with 11% exposed to encouraging styles.
- Disability affects 7% of 0–14 year olds, but chronic illness and disability account for 50% of all paediatric consultations.
- Rising incidence of cerebral palsy in births under 1500 g (from 10 to 70 per 1000 live births in last 25 years).
- 10% of all hospital admissions involve children under 15 years.

Information about child health can be obtained from cross sectional community prevalence surveys or longitudinal cohort studies, health service provider records (for example, community nurses, school health services, general practitioners, paediatricians and hospitals), and from national health insurance data.

Children and adolescents presenting to general practitioners

From an ongoing national survey of general practice statistics, it is known that 15.8% of total general practice

Table 1.6 Mortality rates for major causes of deaths in young persons aged 15–19 years, Australia, 1961–1999. (Source: Australian Bureau of Statistics, with permission)

Cause of death	Deaths per 100 000 15–19 years old				
	1961	1971	1981	1990	1999
Injury (all causes)	57.2	88.2	65.5	49.0	51.3
Motor vehicle	36.6	63.4	47.3	26.5	24.0
Drowning	2.2	2.6	1.5	1.0	1.7
Suicide	3.8	9.3	6.7	11.5	12.5
Cancers	6.4	7.6	6.1	4.7	7.2
Infectious disease	1.6	1.0	0.9	0.9	1.1
Drug related					8.8
All causes	**85.9**	**114.2**	**85.3**	**67.0**	**76.9**

encounters in Australia are for children aged 0–14 years, with a further 9.8% for young persons aged 15–24. The top five reasons for consulting a doctor (including but not limited to general practitioners) in children aged under 15 years was for a respiratory condition (upper respiratory infection including tonsillitis, asthma and acute bronchitis) and immunisation.

Children and adolescents presenting to specialised paediatric services

In the Australian health care system, children may be referred to a consultant or specialist paediatrician by a general (or primary care) practitioner for consultation on difficult problems, or for management of rare or difficult to treat chronic illnesses. Paediatricians work in the community and/or in general hospitals with paediatric facilities (secondary paediatric services) or children's hospitals with extensive subspecialty services (tertiary hospitals). In addition, public and private hospitals provide accident and emergency services for children. The pattern of injuries and acute and chronic illnesses seen in these settings varies according to the mix of private and public paediatric hospitals servicing urban and rural communities. The case mix (pattern of clinical problems) differs for outpatient clinic attendances, emergency department presentations and hospital admissions.

A 12 month survey of the practice profile of paediatricians in the Barwon region of Victoria in 1996–1997 found that 10% of the childhood population had consulted a paediatrician practising in the community during this period: 68.9% of consultations concerned medical problems, with CNS/disability and the respiratory system each accounting for 16% and gastrointestinal problems a further 14%. Nearly 35% of children seen had behavioural problems, with 76% of these relating to attention deficit hyperactivity disorder (ADHD), which was the most common diagnosis overall. A further 14.5% of consultations concerned children with epilepsy or another disability, 13% were for children with learning problems and 10% were for asthma. Just over 4% of all consultations involved children with significant social problems. At least 50% of these paediatric medical consultations involved children with a chronic illness.

Attendances at an accident and emergency department provide a further component of the picture of child injury and acute illness. Gastroenteritis, asthma and injuries dominate the mix of clinical conditions treated in this setting.

Around 10% of hospital admissions in Australia are for children under 15 years. The reasons for hospital admission of children vary according to the type of hospital (secondary versus tertiary) and, therefore, the types of surgical and medical treatments that are provided. The admission case mix is also changing as the pattern of clinical management evolves; for example, the average length of stay for asthma has been reduced from 6 days to just over 2 days during the past 20 years. Table 1.7 shows how minor surgical procedures account for a large proportion of hospital admissions, and also that asthma is by far the single leading reason for hospital admission in children.

The prevalence of asthma in Australia is one of the highest in the world, with more than two million Australians estimated to be affected by the disease. Asthma is more prevalent in young people, with 12.3% of 1–4 year olds, 19.2% of 5–9 year olds and 18.7% of 10–14 year olds reporting asthma as a long term condition in the 1995 Australian Health Survey. Rates are slightly higher in males, and Queenslanders report a higher prevalence than Tasmanians.

Health behaviours

- Increased immunisation uptake has followed Australian Childhood Immunisation Register (ACIR) — 87% fully immunised at 1 year.
- Plateau in rates of adolescent smoking with higher rates among girls (32% versus 28%).

Table 1.7 Hospitalisations for the ten most frequent AN-DRGS (Australian Diagnosis Related Groupings) in 0–14 year olds by State and territory, 1996–97 (Source: AIHW Hospital Morbidity Database 1999, with permission)

AN-DRG	Condition	Rank	NSW	Vic	Qld	WA	SA	Tas	ACT	NT	Total
187	Bronchitis and asthma	1	10 469	6411	5329	3304	3881	501	332	263	30 496
122	Tonsillectomy and/or adenoidectomy	2	8854	7824	6737	2775	2850	572	502	91	30 215
727	Neonate, adm weight <2499 g	3	8302	6540	5245	2314	2518	765	2083	360	28 235
124	Myringotomy with tube insertion	4	6346	8084	3616	2578	3664	640	461	125	25 514
350	Gastroenteritis aged <10	5	7796	2997	3918	1876	2078	360	455	547	20 048
128	Dental extractions and restorations	6	3871	4572	3934	2352	1689	576	238	163	17 033
473	Fracture, sprain, strain and dislocation of upper arm or lower leg	7	5235	2792	3895	1346	1090	332	245	165	15 103
135	Otitis media and upper respiratory tract infection	8	5236	2216	3630	1649	1508	292	201	178	14 921
188	Whooping cough and acute bronchiolitis	9	4385	2474	1583	1320	1389	200	139	268	11 766
726	Neonate, adm weight >2499 g	10	3608	2705	1991	741	405	229	206	182	10 085

• Rising rates of obesity — 25% of Sydney and Melbourne 7–18 year olds overweight.

A number of factors that rely on public participation have a profound impact on child health, and on future good health as an adult. In traditional societies, parenting was a responsibility of the clan, not just the biological parents. The quality of parenting provided in developed countries is now arguably one of the major determinants of public health, being implicated in the high prevalence of academic failure, disruptive behaviour and other mental health problems, intentional and unintentional injuries, substance misuse and juvenile crime. Other health behaviours may also have benefits or adverse effects; for example, high rates of breastfeeding and immunisation, child restraint use in motor vehicles, sun exposure protection using clothing and sun screen creams, healthy nutrition, active life styles, pool fences and swimming competence, and bicycle helmets all have an impact on disease and injury prevention. Harmful behaviours, such as cigarette smoking, may result in the smoker's exposure, or passive exposure of the fetus or infant, to the hundreds of potential carcinogens in cigarette smoke and its other toxic effects on the respiratory and cardiovascular systems. The physician who cares for children has a crucial role in contributing to parent and child awareness of the real opportunities the individual has in making healthy life style decisions that will benefit all members of the family.

Immunisation

Immunisation is one of the most effective disease prevention tools. Australia has a strong tradition of successful mass immunisation through local government, community nurses and general practitioners. Immunisation schedules in the states are modelled on the National Health and Medical Research Council (NHMRC) recommendations (Ch. 8), and the Commonwealth is responsible for providing schedule vaccines free of charge to all Australian children.

The Australian Childhood Immunisation Register, which is managed through the national health insurance scheme (Medicare) was established as part of the National Childhood Immunisation Program begun in 1996. It provides a reminder and recall system direct to parents, and also makes available a mechanism to monitor vaccine uptake within the community. Doctors are paid to notify the ACIR each time they immunise a child. Since the implementation of the register and a range of incentives directed at parents and health care providers to promote immunisation, there has been a progressive increase in the proportion of children immunised (Table 1.8).

Epidemiological evidence suggests that failure to be immunised is due to a number of factors, including parent apathy linked with lack of awareness of the importance of

Table 1.8 Proportion of 1 year old children in Australia who are fully immunised. (Adapted from data from ABS, ACIR and the Communicable Diseases Network Australia, with permission).

Data source	DTP (%)	OPV (%)	Hib (%)	All (%)
ABS, April 1995	86.2	86.3	62.3	51.4
ACIR, March 1997	77.4	77.2	77.2	74.9
ACIR, March 2001	91.5	91.4	94.6	91.2

ABS, Australian Bureau of Statistics; ACIR, Australian Immunisation Register; DTP, diphtheria, tetanus and pertussis vaccine; OPV, oral polio vaccine; Hib, *Haemophilus influenzae* type b conjugate vaccine.
Note
ABS April 1995 value for DTP is for pertussis only. Immunisation coverage for diphtheria and tetanus at that time was 88.5%. The proportion fully immunised in 1995 (51.4%) includes Hib, which was added to the immunisation schedule in April 1993. The proportion fully immunised in 1995 excluding Hib was 70.8%.

immunisation, its safety and its effectiveness, and health professionals' poor performance in delivering age appropriate immunisation.

Smoking and sun exposure

The massive increase in the incidence of lung cancer in men over the age of 50 years preceding the1980s and in more recent years the rise in women, along with the increase in melanoma in both sexes, stands in stark contrast to the relatively stable incidence of most other cancers. What have these outcomes got to do with paediatrics? The answer is that the behaviours associated with an increased risk of these diseases commence in childhood and adolescence.

Smoking related disorders

The current patterns of lung cancer incidence and mortality in men (a 2% per year decline) and women (a 1.6% per year increase) probably reflect smoking behaviour patterns 20 years ago. Most smokers commence smoking in adolescence, and this behaviour, once established, may be difficult to change. In addition, the number of pack years of smoke exposure is directly related to the risk of smoking related cancers, cardiovascular disease and numerous other health problems. The relationship between media exposure to cigarette promotion and the likelihood of young people becoming smokers is strong and well established. With increasing awareness of the profound and irrefutable causal relationship between cigarette smoking and disease, and with new laws restricting the way in which cigarettes may be advertised, the prevalence of adolescent smokers in Australia has

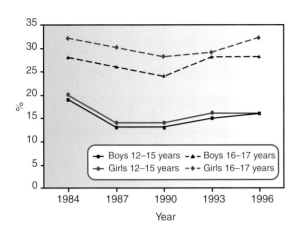

Fig. 1.8 Proportion of adolescents (12–17 years) who are current smokers, 1984–1996. Source: Hill, White and Letcher, 1999.

finally started to decline during the past 15 years but, disturbingly, rates are higher in 16–17 year old girls (32%) compared with boys (28%) (Fig. 1.8). Furthermore, the recent widespread recognition of the harmful effects of both prenatal and postnatal passive smoke exposure in children (low birth weight and prematurity and all their consequences, respiratory infections, asthma, otitis media, impaired lung growth) has led to rapid changes in public policy, laws and community practices aimed at reducing environmental tobacco smoke exposure, especially for children. The clinician's role is to assist in the education of young parents, to provide access to professional quit programmes, and to encourage smokers in the meantime to smoke only outside the family home, and never in the family vehicle or in the company of children.

Melanoma

In the case of melanoma, the incidence rates have increased markedly since 1983, especially for males. Australian melanoma rates are among the highest in the world, with a tenfold difference in incidence between Australia and England and Wales. Melanoma risk is related to UV radiation exposure and the incidence is higher in individuals with many moles, fair sun-sensitive skin, and those who have intermittent high recreational exposure. It is thought that exposure in childhood may be particularly important. It is therefore disconcerting to note that surveys have found that between 9% and 12% of children and young people in all age groups who have been exposed to the sun have not used sun protection.

Obesity and physical fitness

There has been growing concern about the increasing levels of obesity and lack of physical fitness in children and young people in Australia (Ch. 7). In 1985, 4% of boys and 6% of girls where classified according to their

body mass index (BMI, a measure of weight for height) as being overweight. A more recent study (2000) found that about 25% of children aged 7–18 years in Sydney and Melbourne were overweight, practising sedentary lifestyles and consuming a diet high in fat and low in the intake of fruit and vegetables. It is of some concern that around one third of children under 12 years do not eat any fruit or fruit products and more than one in five do not eat any vegetables or vegetable products.

Disability

In addition to acute problems, modern child health care is very much concerned with the long term management of a number of disorders associated with physical and intellectual disability (Chs 11, 59). Many of these disorders are determined genetically, and until comparatively recently were fatal in early life. Examples include cystic fibrosis, thalassaemia major, spina bifida, phenylketonuria, haemophilia and various malignancies.

In 1993, the overall prevalence of disability in children 0–14 years was estimated to be about 70 per 1000. Forty four children per 1000 in the 0–4 year age group, 88 per 1000 in the 5–9 year group and 78 per 1000 in the 10–14 year age group were reported to have one or more disabilities. In all age groups boys had higher rates of disability than girls.

An increasingly important cause of disability is very low birth weight (less than 1000 g). With modern technology approximately two thirds of very low birth weight infants will survive, although significant disability will remain in up to 25% of survivors. Indeed, there has been a steady rise in the incidence of cerebral palsy over the past 20 years in infants weighing less than 1500 g at birth (Fig. 1.9). Other disabilities include intellectual disability,

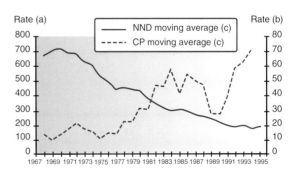

Fig. 1.9 Very low birth weight (less than 1500 g), neonatal death (NND) and cerebral palsy (CP) rates in Western Australia 1987–1996. (a) Neonatal death rate per 1000 live births. (b) CP rates per 1000 live births. (c) 3 year moving averages; note that CP moving average rate for 1994 is derived from 2 years data only. Source: Cerebral Palsy Register, Institute for Child Research, Perth, Australia (unpublished data).

auditory and visual problems, and epilepsy, alone or in combination. It should be remembered, however, that the vast majority of cases of cerebral palsy and of intellectual disability are not related to birth asphyxia or other perinatal events.

Emotional and behavioural problems

The management of emotional and behavioural problems of childhood is an important challenge in a large proportion of paediatric consultations (Chs 16–18). A national survey of child and adolescent mental health in 1999 found that 14% of children and young people had mental health problems, with higher rates being noted in boys, and children living in low income, step/blended and sole parent families. Although one in five teenagers have mental health problems, most will not seek or receive treatment. Children with chronic illness have a doubled risk of emotional maladjustment, and those with chronic physical disorders that affect the brain, notably spina bifida, epilepsy and cerebral palsy, have the highest risk.

Conversely, paediatric disorders which are still poorly understood have frequently been attributed to emotional causes, when there has been good evidence that psychological factors may also be a consequence of the disorder. Maternal mood disorder is common in infancy and in later childhood and is associated with a range of adverse outcomes such as infant cry–fuss behaviour (colic), feeding and sleep problems and cognitive or behavioural problems in older children. Other conditions, such as recurrent abdominal pain, encopresis, enuresis, headache, school refusal and school failure may be associated with emotional problems in the children themselves, but again caution needs to be exercised about the direction of causality. The role of the child's doctor is to recognise that emotional factors may be both a contributor to and a consequence of the child's physical symptoms, and there is a duty especially not to diagnose a psychological cause in the absence of overt and specific evidence of psychological dysfunction. Recognising the emotional as well as the physical consequences of children's diseases is crucial to effective paediatric care.

Social and family factors

It is now recognised that family and social factors significantly modify disease and must be taken into account if total care is to be provided. These factors include family size and financial status, physical characteristics of the home, behaviour and way of life of parents, their education, attitudes, habits, and the family's capacity to select and use the various types of care available. Poverty is, in particular, a well established risk factor for a large number of health problems. Often this is compounded in recent migrants where isolation and acculturation difficulties confer additional stress on young families. Maternal depression in this situation has been shown to be an important accompaniment of child development and adjustment difficulty.

Parenting

The ability of children to self-regulate their behaviour is influenced by the nature of the relationship between children and their caregivers in early life. The risks of disruptive behaviour disorders, such as oppositional defiant disorder and conduct disorder and later criminality are greatly increased in children where there is insecure attachment between infants and their caregivers in the early years of life, and where parental disciplinary styles are coercive or inconsistent. The West Australian Child Health Survey found a substantially increased rate of mental health morbidity in children exposed to these parenting styles (29% and 24%, respectively) compared to encouraging styles (11%).

Future directions

There is widespread recognition that social, environmental, family and technological changes during the past 30 years have contributed to the changing pattern of child health mortality and morbidity. There is also increasing awareness that patterns of behaviour, health and wellbeing that are established in fetal life and childhood become to some extent biologically embedded, affecting neuroendocrine and neuroimmunological functioning, and, as such, have lifelong implications for physical and mental health, coping and competence. The health and wellbeing experience of children is thus increasingly being seen as having wide ramifications for the competence, coping and adaptability of human populations undergoing massive social changes associated with their transformation from industrial to globalised, information based economies. Child health, as it was at the turn of the twentieth century, but for very different reasons, is once more at centre stage in the grand vision of improving the health and wellbeing of human populations.

Electronic learning resources 2

K. Forsyth

The greatest information store is no longer our libraries. Information is now held in a non existent physical place — the internet. Information is stored in binary code in servers throughout the world but is hidden from our view. When words are entered in a search engine, a list is provided; however, we have no idea of the validity or robustness of this information, and probably no concept of the authority or integrity of the author. In the area of professional information for instruction, there are many hazards for the unwary.

Although there are extensive databanks of information available electronically, some of which are of great merit as instructional aids, the process of learning requires that information to be taken through a process where it becomes knowledge gained by the learner. There are available to us enormous technical developments in information technology and developments in education where the process of learning and construction of learning, which has been known within educational circles for some time, is being applied to teaching that occurs within medical education. This can be linked with the ability to deliver educational materials using information technology. These educational approaches have been well articulated by Houle (1974) with a move from a teacher focus to a learning focus. The educational process then becomes one of developing student competencies. The teacher's role is not to provide detailed information but to enable learning to occur by the students. This allows an interactive and individualised learning experience for students. One of the educational challenges is to provide learning that is active and self-directed rather than passive. Such self-directed learning enables those learning to absorb information, connect between different ideas and to use multiple means to glean information and gain a linked, connected, integrated and cohesive understanding of the topic.

Self-directed integrated learning may be assisted using information technology. Information technology can enable learners actively to construct their world of learning and the knowledge that they are gaining. Active learning includes the ability for a learner to represent a construct in multiple modalities. The recognition by Gardner *'if you only know it one way it's a very fragile knowing'* is an articulate way of stating the need for learners to come to an understanding of a concept through a number of different routes. Properly developed educational resource material utilising information technology enables such construction and the ability to represent concepts in multiple ways.

Increasingly, as computers become more powerful and sophisticated, it will be easier to construct 'virtual learning worlds'. In competency based disciplines such as medicine, creating virtual worlds will be, in some situations, more effective and much cheaper than providing concrete experimental learning experiences for students. An example is the management of the fitting child. From informal surveys of final year medical students, it has been estimated that only 10% of graduating students have witnessed a convulsion. At Flinders University in South Australia, a CD-ROM has been developed that contains videos of all the major seizure types. In addition, there is a virtual emergency room with a 'fitting child' scenario. The student is required to manage this situation. The advantage of this type of learning is apparent from the observation of a medical student that *'it is better for the computer, rather than the coroner, to tell you that you have mismanaged the child'*. This type of learning is becoming an important component of curricula in medical schools.

In parallel with these developments, new modes of educational research needs are needed. Computer based learning is essentially a new discipline. New tools to evaluate the effectiveness of computers as an instructional strategy are required. Ehrmann (1996) encapsulates this with his comment that *'few educators, evaluators and researchers have paid much attention to educational strategies for using technologies, too often they have been victims of rapture of technology'*.

Electronic leaning resources are readily available on the internet. In addition, there are many CD-ROM products which deal with specific areas; the better ones provide an interactive approach that enhances the learning experience.

The following is a list of internet resources that students of paediatrics are likely to find helpful.

Paediatric web sites

Key: A, applications/programs; CE, Windows CE PDA; I, still images; ML, multilingual; P, Palm PDA; Ps, Psion (EPOC) PDA; Q, online quiz; T, text; V, video images.

Core paediatric sites

1. **Medic.Com Paediatric medicine:**
   http://www.medic8.com/Paediatrics.htm [T, I, V]
   (UK)
   An excellent site with a comprehensive selection of relevant paediatric links including paediatric medicine organisations, journals, databases, online textbooks and educational sites.

2. **General Pediatrics:**
   http://www.generalpediatrics.com/ [T, I] (USA)
   A large site with extensive coverage of paediatric medical conditions and many links to other useful paediatric web pages. Compiled by Dr D. D'Alessandro, University of Iowa College of Medicine.

3. **Harriet Lane Links:** http://www.med.jhu.edu/peds/ neonatology/poi.html [T, I] (USA)
   The Harriet Lane Links (formerly Pediatric Points of Interest) provides an edited collection of paediatric resources (5225 links). Maintained and edited by physicians at the Johns Hopkins University, this site attempts to catalogue, review and score existing links to paediatric information on the internet.

4. **COMSEP:** http://www.unmc.edu/Community/ comsep/ main.html [T] (USA)
   The Council on Medical Student Education in Pediatrics (COMSEP) home page provides a multitude of links to paediatric educational resources, clinical cases sites and paediatric departments. It also provides the common core paediatric curriculum for US medical schools.

5. **PEDINFO; An Index of the Pediatric Internet:**
   http://www.pedinfo.org/ [T] (USA)
   An extensive index of general and specialist paediatric resources on the internet.

6. **PEDIATRIC linx:** http://www.pediatriclinx.com/ [T] (USA)
   Regular reviews and updates in the paediatric specialties.

7. **PEDBASE:** http://www.icondata.com/health/ pedbase/pedlynx.htm [T] (Canada)
   This paediatric database (PEDBASE) contains brief descriptions of over 550 childhood illnesses.

8. **BUBL LINK:** http://link.bubl.ac.uk/paediatrics [T] (UK)
   A collection of selected and peer reviewed internet resources in paediatrics.

9. **Omni Paediatrics**: http://omni.ac.uk/subject-listing/ WS100.html [T] (UK)
   A gateway for reviewed paediatric sites and some directed community education. Mostly UK content.

10. **Virtual Children's Hospital**: http://www.vh.org/ VCH/ [T] (USA)
    This site, maintained by the Children's Hospital of Iowa and the University of Iowa, has an extensive collection of links to useful paediatric sites worldwide.

11. **The Merck Manual Pediatric Section:**
    http://www.merck.com/pubs/mmanual/section19/ sec19.htm [T] (USA)
    A full text searchable version of the paediatric section of the Merck Manual of Diagnosis and Therapy (17th edn, 2000). A valuable and up to date resource with links to other medical specialties.

12. **Paediatric Sites For Medical Students:**
    http://www.health.adelaide.edu.au/paediatrics/ paedsite.htm [T, I] (Australia)
    A collection of links to web based paediatric resources for medical students.

13. **Subspecialty Collection from the American Academy of Pediatrics:**
    http://www.pediatrics.org/collections/ [T] (USA)
    A topic specific archive of specialist paediatric studies published in the journal Pediatrics from January 1997 to the present. Within each category, further links and automated eSearches of Medline have been included to extend exploration of the topic areas.

14. **Martindale's Health Science Guide; Obstetrics, Pediatrics and Gynecology:**
    http://www-sci.lib.uci.edu/HSG/MedicalPed.html [T, I] (USA)
    A wide ranging site covering dictionaries and glossaries, an interactive anatomy browser, interactive patient cases, literature searches and useful links. Developed under the auspices of the University of California Library, USA.

15. **eMedicine Online Medical Textbooks:**
    http://www.emedicine.com/ [T, I] (USA)
    A collaborative peer reviewed site containing hundreds of online textbook chapters in many subject areas including paediatrics. A very valuable resource, and the whole site is updated and extended frequently.

16. **Paediatric Resources from the University of Iowa Family Practice Handbook, 3rd edition** [T, I] (USA)
    a. Online handbook of treatment and therapy for the most common paediatric conditions:
       http://vh.radiology.uiowa.edu/Providers/ClinRef /FPHandbook/10.html
    b. Common paediatric drugs:
       http://vh.radiology.uiowa.edu/Providers/ClinRef /FPHandbook/20.html
    c. Tabulated preventive care guidelines:
       http://vh.radiology.uiowa.edu/Providers/ClinRef /FPHandbook/Misc/FrontCover.html

17. **Medscape Pediatric Resource Centers:**
    http://pediatrics.medscape.com/Home/Topics/ pediatrics/pediatrics.html [T] (USA)
    Extensive collection of resources for various paediatric diseases including paediatric oncology, group B

streptococcal disease, asthma, growth and development and new variant Creutzfeldt–Jakob disease.

18. **Children's Medical Centre of the National University Hospital:**
http://www.nuh.com.sg/Cmc/Useful%20sites%20 small%20frame.htm [T] (Singapore)
Scores of useful paediatric links for medical students and paediatricians. Subjects covered include inborn errors of metabolism/metabolic diseases, neonatology, endocrinology and metabolism and neurology. There are also many useful links to patient support organisations for sick children and their parents.

19. **Band-Aides and Blackboards:**
http://funrsc.fairfield.edu/~jfleitas/sitemap.html [T] (USA)
Stories of paediatric chronic illness written by children and adolescents with these conditions. Although provided primarily as a service for patients, it is a wonderful resource for medical students hoping to gain some understanding of the effect of chronic illness on the lives of young people.

General medical sites with paediatric content or relevance

1. **Medscape:** http://www.medscape.com/ [T, I] (USA)
Medscape contains news, reviews, medline searching, online *Harrisons' Internal Medicine* and links to hundreds of valuable medical sites. The site can be tailored to provide targeted information and automatic weekly update emails for paediatrics or most other specialties. Membership is required but registration is free.

2. **AusDoctors:** http://www.ausdoctors.net/ [T, I] (Australia)
Doctors net UK: http://www.doctors.net.uk [T, I] (UK)
Both these sites provide free online access to the *Textbook of Pediatrics,* 5th edition, by Forfar and Arneil. Registration for both sites is free for medical students and doctors.

3. **Doctors Guide:** http://www.docguide.com/ [T, I, ML] (USA)
A free registration medical site that provides access to online clinical updates and paediatric clinical cases.

4. **PubMed Central:**
http://www.pubmedcentral.nih.gov/ [T, I] (USA)
A growing web based archive of journal literature for the life sciences being developed by the National Center for Biotechnology Information (NCBI) at the US National Library of Medicine (NLM). It includes free online access to the British Medical Journal, Arthritis Research, and Critical Care.

5. **Free On-line Medical Journals:**
http://www.freemedicaljournals.com/ [T, I] (USA)
Link page to over 500 free online medical journals.

6. **British Medical Journal:** http://www.bmj.com/ [T, I] (UK)
The 'collected resources' link contains an archive of paediatrics papers published in the BMJ.

7. **Student British Medical Journal:**
http://www.studentbmj.com/ [T, I] (UK)
Paediatric news and articles are presented in a format specifically tailored to medical students.

8. **British National Formulary (BNF) Online:**
http://bnf.vhn.net/home/ [T, I] (UK)
The online BNF is published jointly by the British Medical Association and the Royal Pharmaceutical Society of Great Britain. It is a very concise and accurate drug reference and is updated twice yearly.

9. **Drug Interactions:**
http://www.georgetown.edu/departments/ pharmacology/davetab.html [T, I] (USA)
An online medline linked guide to drug metabolism by the cytochrome P_{450} (CYP) enzyme family by Dr D.A. Flockhart, Georgetown University. These tables allow prediction of drug interactions based on racial expression of CYP subtypes and known inducers and inhibitors of these enzymes.

10. **National Organisation for Rare Diseases:**
http://www.rarediseases.org/lof/lof.html [T, I] (USA)
Search pages provide brief information on rare paediatric diseases.

11. **Genetic and Rare Conditions Site:**
http://www.kumc.edu/gec/support/ [T] (USA)
Medical Genetics, University of Kansas Medical Center.

12. **OMIM™:** http://www3.ncbi.nlm.nih.gov/omim/ [T] (USA)
Online Mendelian Inheritance in Man (OMIM). A very useful and authoritative site for information on paediatric genetic syndromes.

13. **The CDC Prevention Guidelines Database:**
http://aepo-xdv-www.epo.cdc.gov/wonder/ prevguid/prevguid.htm [T] (USA)
This site offers a comprehensive compendium of the official guidelines and recommendations published by the US Centers for Disease Control and Prevention (CDC) for the prevention of diseases (immunisation), injuries and disabilities.

14. **National Cancer Institute's Database:**
http://cancernet.nci.nih.gov/pdqfull.html [T] (USA)
The National Cancer Institute's (NCI) comprehensive information database contains screening, prevention, treatment and supportive summaries for health care professionals. The main site links to the NCI's pediatric oncology branch.

Search databases

National Library of Medicine, USA: The National Library of Medicine (NLM) offers *'PubMed'* and

'*Internet Grateful Med*', which are two free systems to search MEDLINE: http://www.nlm.nih.gov/databases/freemedl.html [T] (USA)

Free access to medline is also available from the home pages of Medscape, the British Medical Journal, AusDoctors, Doctor's net UK and from many other medical sites. An online tutorial in the use of PubMed is available at: http://www.library.health.ufl.edu/pubmed/pubmed2/ [T] (USA)

Evidence based medicine

1. **Cochrane Colloboration:**
    http://www.update-software.com/ccweb/cochrane/revabstr/mainindex.htm [T] (UK)
    A core site for EBM information and links to EBM resources on the web.
2. **Washington Pediatric EBM:**
    http://depts.washington.edu/pedebm/ [T] (USA)
    The University of Washington School of Medicine paediatric EBM resources with CATS (critically appraised topics).
3. **National Guidelines Clearinghouse:**
    http://www.guideline.gov/index.asp [T] (USA)
    A public resource for evidence based clinical practice guidelines.

Clinical teaching and clinical cases

1. **The Virtual Pediatric Patient:**
    http://www.vh.org/Providers/Simulations/VirtualPedsPatients/PedsVPHome.html [T, I] (USA)
    A useful case based teaching resource for common paediatric problems compiled by Donna M. D'Alessandro and Tamra E. Takle, University of Iowa College of Medicine.
2. **Asthma Management:** Guidelines for the Primary Care Physician: http://www.vh.org/Providers/ClinGuide/Asthma/Asthma.html [T] (USA)
    American guidelines. Dr Miles Weinberger, University of Iowa College of Medicine.
3. **Paediatric Critical Care Resource:**
    http://pedsccm.wustl.edu/All-Net/main.html [T, V, I, ML]
    Associated with the picuBook project (http://picuBOOK.net) supported by the European Commission.
    Excellent peer reviewed articles on a wide range of paediatric emergency and critical care subjects (European Union).
4. **Correlapaedia** — a Correlative Encyclopedia of Pediatric Imaging, Surgery, and Pathology: http://www.vh.org/Providers/TeachingFiles/CAP/CAPHome.html [T, I, CS, Q]
    Edited by Michael P. D'Alessandro, University of

Iowa College of Medicine, Steven J. Fishman, MD, Harvard Medical School, and Deborah E. Schofield, Children's Hospital of Los Angeles (USA)
* 1997 winner of the American Academy of Pediatrics '*Best of the Pediatric Internet Award*'.

5. **COMSEP Clinical Cases:**
    http://www.unmc.edu/Community/comsep/cases/int.html;
    http://www.unmc.edu/Community/comsep/cases/non-int.html and
    http://www.unmc.edu/Pediatrics/educ/quiz.htm
    (USA), [T, I, Q]
    A collection of non interactive and interactive paediatric clinical cases and a self-study online test.
6. **University of Virginia Pediatric Cases:**
    http://hsc.virginia.edu/medicine/clinical/pediatrics/CMC/casemenu.html (USA) [T, I]
    Several short and long clinical cases in paediatrics compiled by Stephen M. Borowitz, University of Virginia.
7. **University of Kansas Pediatric Cardiology Cases:** http://www.kumc.edu/kumcpeds/cardiology/cardiology.html [T, I] (USA)
    Online lectures, images and case studies in paediatric cardiology.
8. **OnLine Pediatric Surgery Handbook** for Residents and Medical Students:
    http://home.coqui.net/titolugo/handbook.htm [T] (USA)
    A valuable text resource which can be downloaded as a PDF file. A branch of the parent website
    Pediatric Surgery Update:
    http://home.coqui.net/titolugo/index.htm#psu
    Edited by Doctor Lugo-Vicente, University of Puerto Rico School of Medicine, with independent teams of international contributors and reviewers.
9. **UAB Pediatric Surgery:**
    http://pedsurg.surgery.uab.edu/ [T, I] (USA)
    A growing collection of well constructed paediatric surgery multimedia tutorials on topics including spinal dysraphism and laryngotracheal reconstruction. Compiled by Drs W. Hardin and M. Wulkan at the Division of Pediatric Surgery, University of Alabama, Birmingham.
10. **Pediatric Critical Care Medicine (PedsCCM):**
    http://PedsCCM.wustl.edu/ [T] (USA)
    A peer reviewed, collaborative information site for health professionals, this site helps disseminate information to promote quality care for critically ill and injured infants and children. The site also offers free AvantGo updates of the latest paediatric critical care evidence based treatment available for automatic palm OS download.
11. **American Academy of Pediatrics Policy Statements and Clinical Practice Guidelines:**
    http://www.aap.org/policy/pcyhome.cfm [T] (USA)

12. **University of Virginia Pediatric Pharmacotherapy**:
    http://hsc.virginia.edu/cmc/pedpharm/
    pedpharm.html [T] (USA)
    A monthly online review of new paediatric drugs and drug use in the USA.

13. **Great Ormond Street Library Paediatric Resources**:
    http://www.ich.ucl.ac.uk/library/noframes/
    paeds.htm [T] (UK)
    A collection of paediatric websites particularly relevant to practice in the UK.

14. **HIV Manual:**
    http://www.mcg.edu/PedsOnL/ForHealthProf/
    PedAids/INDEX.HTM [T] (USA)
    'A Manual for the Management of HIV Infections in Infants, Children and Adolescents' by Dr W. S. Foshee MD, The Medical College of Georgia/ Children's Medical Center.

15. **Medical Connect:** http://www.medconnect.com/ [T] (USA)
    An online CME/CE centre with weekly paediatric cases.

16. **Paediatric ALS:**
    http://www.mja.com.au/public/issues/aug19/arcg/
    arcg.html [T] (Australia)
    Paediatric advanced life support guidelines from the Australian Resuscitation Council Guidelines.

17. **Vanderbilt Pediatric Digital Library:**
    http://www.mc.vanderbilt.edu/peds/pidl/ [T] (USA)
    The Vanderbilt Medical Center Pediatric interactive digital library is an extensive online reference for the paediatric specialties.

18. **Pediatric Dermatology:**
    http://162.129.72.40/derm/cd_lists.cfm [T, I] (USA)
    A very simple, but comprehensive online paediatric dermatology atlas by Dr B.A. Cohen and Dr C.U. Lehmann of Johns Hopkins University School of Medicine.

19. **Paediatric Lung and Heart Sounds:**
    http://www.rale.ca/ [T, S] (Canada)
    RALE: Repository of lung and heart sounds from the University of Manitoba. Requires RealPlayer™ which can be downloaded free at: http://www.real.com.

20. **Pediatric Pulmonology Sites:**
    http://www.peds.umn.edu/divisions/pccm/default.ht ml [T] (USA)
    Links to paediatric respiratory medicine and critical care sites from the University of Minnesota.

21. **Infectious Diseases in Children**:
    http://www.slackinc.com/child/idc/idchome.htm [T] (USA)
    The monthly newsletter's online version offers original journal articles, news, specialty forums and chat rooms.

22. **Dr Steve's Guide to the Pediatric Internet:**
    http://fammed.crozer.org/peds/steve.htm [T] (USA)
    An extensive collection of paediatric links to specialty paediatric sites, academic and clinical departments (mostly USA), paediatric organisations and medical journals. Compiled and maintained by Dr S. Morgan, Crozer Chester Medical Center, USA.

23. **OncoLink-Pediatrics**:
    http://www.oncolink.upenn.edu/specialty/ped_onc/ [T, I] (USA)
    A collection of paediatric oncology resources with a 'case of the month' and other educational material aimed at medical students, doctors, parents and sick children. Compiled by the haematology and oncology specialists at the Children's Hospital of Philadelphia, USA.

Anatomy and imaging resources

1. **Paediatric Imaging and Radiology Site Collection** edited by Dr M. D'Alessandro, University of Iowa College of Medicine [T, I] (USA)
   a. **General Pediatric Imaging:**
      http://www.pediatricradiology.com/ [T, I]
   b. **Thoracopedia** — Paediatric respiratory medicine images:
      http://www.vh.org/Providers/TeachingFiles/TAP /Thoracopedia.html [T, I]
   c. **Paediapaedia** — an encyclopedia of paediatric disease with brief text notes, radiological images and differential diagnoses:
      http://www.vh.org/Providers/TeachingFiles/PAP /PAPHome.html [T, I]

2. **MedicalStudent.com:**
   http://www.medicalstudent.com/[T, I]
   A digital library of authoritative medical information for all students of medicine.

3. **Radiology Cases In Pediatric Emergency Medicine and Neonatology:**
   http://www2.hawaii.edu/medicine/pediatrics/
   pemxray/pemxray.html and
   http://www2.hawaii.edu/medicine/pediatrics/
   neoxray/neoxray.html (USA) [T, I]
   An extensive collection of radiological images of paediatric emergencies and neonatology. The contents of the site can be downloaded and run on a PC. Compiled by Drs Yamamoto, Inaba and DiMauro, University of Hawaii John A. Burns School of Medicine. This site was awarded the 1996 Professional Medical Education Award by the American Academy of Pediatrics.

4. **Fetal Echocardiography Homepage:**
   http://www.med.upenn.edu/fetus/ [T, I] (USA)
   An extensive library of still fetal echocardiograph images.

5. **Pediatric Imaging and Pathology:**
http://WWW.UAB.EDU/pedradpath/cases.html
[T, I] (USA)
A useful collection of teaching files from the Departments of Pediatric Imaging and Pathology, Children's Hospital, Alabama.

6. **The Whole Brain Atlas:**
http://www.med.harvard.edu/AANLIB/home.html
[T, I, V] (USA)
An excellent online neuroanatomy resource consisting of both still and video images of clinical cases with correlated neuroimaging (CT, MRI and PET scans). Compiled by Drs K. A. Johnson and J. A. Becker of Harvard Medical School.

National paediatric organisations

1. **The Royal Australasian College of Physicians:**
http://www.racp.edu.au/

2. **American Academy of Pediatrics:**
http://www.aap.org/

3. **Royal College of Paediatrics and Child Health:**
http://www.rcpch.ac.uk/

4. **Canadian Paediatric Society:** http://www.cps.ca/

5. **Society for Adolescent Medicine (SAM):**
http://www.adolescenthealth.org/ [T] (USA)
A multidisciplinary organisation of professionals committed to improving the physical and psychosocial health and wellbeing of adolescents. The site includes access to online publications such as position papers on a range of adolescent health related issues and an extensive and annotated list of links to web sites of interest.

Handheld/PDA resources for paediatrics

The quality and quantity of applications for handheld computers, also known as palmtop computers or personal digital assistants (PDAs), has improved significantly in recent years. There are now three major PDA operating systems (OSs): Palm OS, EPOC and Windows CE. Currently Palm OS is the most popular PDA OS worldwide; it is fast, intuitive, memory efficient and requires very little hardware. The Palm OS is used in Palm, IBM, Handspring visor and TRG-pro PDAs. These PDAs use touch screen handwriting recognition or a screen based keyboard for manual data entry, but keyboards can be attached. The Palm OS has by far the largest amount of medically related software and much of it is regularly updated and improved.

The Epoc OS is very popular in Europe and is utilised by the Psion series 3 and series 5 PDAs. The Psion-Epoc combination is a powerful stand alone system with excellent integrated software and technologically advanced hardware. Psions have the advantage of a large screen and use quality integrated keyboards for manual data entry. Currently Epoc medical software is quite limited in scope and quality compared with that available for the Palm OS system.

The Windows CE OS is fast gaining popularity, especially in North America. It is essentially a miniaturised version of Windows 95/98 and, like the palm top, usually utilises touch screen handwriting recognition or a screen based keyboard for manual data entry. The newer Windows CE version 3 is quicker and more memory efficient than previous versions and many Palm OS medical software programs are becoming available in Windows CE format.

1. **The 2000 Guide to Handheld and Palmtop Computing Resources for Health Care Professionals, 2nd edition:** http://themedical-guide.hypermart.net/ [P, Ps, CE, T, A] (Aust)
The essential guide for medical resources for Palm OS, Windows CE, Psion 3/5, and Newton OS handheld computers compiled by Ralph La Tella. Explanatory notes accompany each product and are often accompanied by actual screen shots of the application. It contains an extensive collection of paediatric software (Australia).

2. **PDAs for Health Care Providers:**
http://educ.ahsl.arizona.edu/pda/index.htm
[P, CE, T, A] (USA)
A valuable web page providing links to health related resources for Palm OS and Windows CE PDAs from the Arizona health services library.

3. **Medical Pocket PC:** http://MedicalPocketPC.com/
[CE, T, A] (USA)
Core site for health related resources for the Windows CE platform.

4. **Useful sites containing medical reviews, discussion forum and downloads of freeware, shareware and commercial medical softwares for PDAs** [T, A] (USA)
- Handango: http://www.handango.com/
- Palm Gear: http://www.palmgear.com/
- TuCows PDA:
http://pda.tucows.com/index.html
- Handheldmed.com:
http://www.handheldmed.com/
- Washington University Medical Palm Initiative:
http://medicine.wustl.edu/~wumpi/
- PDAMD:
http://www.pdamd.com/vertical/home.xml
- Healthy Palm Pilot: http://www.healthypalmpilot.com/
- Peripheral Brain: http://pbrain.hypermart.net/
- The Medical Piloteer: http://www.medicalpiloteer.com/
- Doctor's palm:
http://www.doctorspalm.com/index.htm
- Physics Palm pilot pages:
http://www.geocities.com/HotSprings/Spa/6134/doctor.html

- Burdie's medical palm site: http://www.geocities.com/HotSprings/Spa/6134/doctor.html

5. **AvantGo.com Peds:**
   http://avantgo.com/channels/detail.html?cha_id=1487&cat_id=&type=search_result&data=pediatrics [P, T] (USA)
   This AvantGo link allows automatic download of contemporary paediatric abstracts and news items.

6. **Paediatric pharmacopoeias**
   a. Epocrates: http://www.epocrates.com/ [P, T] (USA)
      The Epocrates package consists of the **qRx 4.0** drug reference guide and the **qID 1.0**, the infectious disease treatment guide for the Palm OS. Adult and paediatric doses, drug interactions and adverse effects are readily assessed. Available free online, where it is revised and peer reviewed monthly.
   b. **Tarascon ePharmacopoeia:**
      http://www.medscape.com/ [P, T] (USA)
      Tarascon ePharmacopoeia is a PDA drug reference guide based on the popular pocket Tarascon drug booklet and similar to Epocrates qRx 4.0. It is available for free download but only within the USA from the medscape site.
      No equivalent PDA pharmacopoeias comprehensively covering paediatric medications used in the UK, Europe or Australasia are currently available.

7. **The Pediatric Pilot Page:** http://www.keepkidshealthy.com/pedipilot.html [P, T] (USA)
   Has links to numerous Palm OS paediatric software sites.

8. **Pediatrics on Hand:** http://pediatricsonhand.com/ [P, T] (USA)
   Compiled by Dr Stockwell, contains several useful handheld paediatric applications written for Palm OS.

9. Handheld hospital patient clinical management applications:
   a. **Palm OS**
      — PatientKeeper: http://www.patientkeeper.com
      — WardWatch: http://www.watch.aust.com/pilot/wardwatch
   b. **Psion**
      — Client_L: http://www.palmaris.com
      — MediKit: http://www.palmaris.com
   c. **Windows CE**
      — Patient Tracker: http://www.handheldmed.com (Under Software)

10. **Memoware:** http://www.memoware.com/ [P, Ps, CE, T, A] (USA)
    Memoware is an extensive repository of PDA documents and applications for the Palm, EPOC and Windows CE operating systems. The medical section has a host of useful paediatric documents such as immunisation regimens, specialised paediatric pharmacopoeias and developmental milestone references. Many of the documents require industry standard PDA document readers of databases such as Doc, SmartDoc, HanDbase, iSolo, Jfile 4, List, TealDoc, TealInfo or WordSmith. These are all inexpensive (less than $25) and can be obtained via PDA software sites like Handango, TuCows PDA and Palm Gear (see above). The HanDbase website also has many medically relevant documents available for free download: http://www.ddhsoftware.com/ [P, Ps, CE, T, A] (USA).

Acknowledgements

The assistance of Dr R. Wilcox, who undertook the initial internet searching and web site analyses, is gratefully acknowledged.

PART 1 FURTHER READING

Australian Institute of Health and Welfare 1998 Australia's children: their health and wellbeing. AIHW, Australian Government Printing Service, Canberra

Australian Institute of Health and Welfare 1999 Australia's young people: their health and wellbeing. AIHW, Australian Government Printing Service, Canberra

Australian Institute of Health and Welfare 2000 Australia's Health 2000. Australian Government Printing Service, Canberra

Houle C O 1974 The design of education. Jossey, Bass, San Francisco

Keating D, Hertzman C 1999 Developmental health and the wealth of nations. Guilford, London

Knupfer N N 1993 Teachers and educational computing, changing roles and changing pedagogy. In: Muffoletto R, Knupfer N N, (eds) Computers in education: social, political and historical perspectives. Hampton Press, Cresskill NJ

Lynn M C 1996. Cognition and distant learning. Journal of the American Society of Information Science 47(11): 82–84

Useful links

http://www.aaat.org/elephant.htm (Ehrmann S C 1996 The flashlight project: spotting an elephant in the dark)

19

CLINICAL ASSESSMENT

3 Clinical consultation: history taking and examination

D. M. Roberton, M. South

History taking and physical examination are essential components of the diagnostic process, and this is especially so in the area of child health. In most presentations, the majority of the information required to formulate a diagnosis comes from the history, with a smaller amount coming from the physical examination. In many cases, no investigations are required. A common paediatric scenario is one in which a case of diagnostic difficulty is solved by an experienced clinician who simply takes a thorough history.

Clinical consultations in paediatrics are different from those in adult medicine

The approach to clinical history taking and physical examination of children is different from that used for adults in several respects:

- It is much more common in paediatrics for the history to be given by a third party such as the parent or another caregiver. Be aware that the description of symptoms may be modified by the parent's perceptions or interpretations, and by factors such as anxiety. First time parents sometimes do not know that what they perceive as a problem is in fact part of the normal range of variation for children.
- There are many extra components of the history and examination that are important in children and require special emphasis according to the age and presenting problem. Examples include: the pregnancy and birth, feeding history in infancy, immunisations, growth, developmental milestones, behaviour and schooling.
- The approach to establishing rapport with the patient and how the examination is conducted will both need to be modified according to the age and development of the patient. There are differences in the techniques of physical examination and in expected findings at different ages.

Differences from adult consultation will be emphasised in the sections that follow.

Clinical example

Louise, a 4 month old girl, was the first baby in her family. She was taken to the general practitioner by her mother Mary, who was very anxious because she felt that her baby was constipated, having a bowel action only once every 3 days. Mary was worried that this was because she was not producing enough breast milk. She had been advised by a relative to give Louise laxative drops and to switch to bottle feeding. Careful history taking revealed that Louise was feeding well and was passing a partly formed stool every third day without difficulty. There were no abnormalities on examination. Her growth chart showed that she was putting on weight well and was following just above the 50th centile for her age. Mary was shown the chart to reassure her that her baby was thriving. It was explained that Louise's stool frequency was within the normal range for breastfed babies. Mary was encouraged to continue breastfeeding.

Planning your approach to the consultation

A number of factors will modify the way you should set about the consultation:

- *The age and developmental status of the child.* Your approach will be quite different for a newborn baby, a preschool age child, an older child, and an adolescent.
- *The urgency and nature of the presenting problem.* In an emergency presentation, urgent treatment will obviously take priority over obtaining a complete history. It is, however, usually appropriate to return to aspects of the history at another time. It is clearly not necessary that a complete past history and developmental assessment be performed if a 4 year old presents with acute diarrhoea and vomiting; however, it would be essential if the presentation were because of parental concern over the child's speech.
- *The possibility of splitting the consultation into more than one session.* This is often appropriate for the assessment of more complex problems. Young children will often become bored, tired, hungry or irritable if a consultation lasts more than about 30 minutes. This can limit their ability to concentrate or cooperate with the assessment.

Establishing rapport with the child and family

Your success in obtaining valuable information from the history and physical examination will depend partly on your knowledge of what information to seek, and greatly on how you go about the task. Establishing a good relationship with the child and family is essential. The parents need to know who you are, and to understand the purpose and likely outcome of the consultation. The child needs to feel comfortable in the environment and with you, particularly as you move on to the physical examination. Stranger anxiety, especially in children from about 8 months to 5 years of age, can be a significant obstacle. Experience and understanding help to overcome this.

The physical environment makes a big difference to how children feel. An adult may tolerate undressing in a cold room to be examined, but a 2 year old will probably cry. A bright, colourful room with pictures on the wall and toys on the floor is much more conducive than a 'sterile' clinical environment. A good range of toys, drawing materials, puzzles and other activities for all ages will be helpful.

Introduce yourself to the parents and, if of an appropriate age, to the child. Explain who you are, and your role in the child's care. A common complaint from parents of recently hospitalised children or children attending clinics is that they met many doctors, not really knowing who they were or who was 'in charge'.

Ask what the child likes to be called. Just how much you should talk directly to the child at this stage will vary with the age of the child, and with your assessment of how relaxed the child is. Some children respond well to questions and comments about their favourite sports team, school or a toy they have brought with them, while others will be shy and anxious if you address them directly. Learn to read children's responses and adapt accordingly.

Children's behaviour will often reflect how their parents are feeling. It is common for parents to feel anxious when attending a medical consultation. If you can form a good relationship with the parents, they will feel more at ease during the consultation, and you will have a better relationship with the child.

Key learning point

- To obtain the trust of a child, you also need to gain the trust of the parent/s.

Sometimes it is appropriate to reassure the child at the start that nothing unpleasant is going to happen during the consultation (e.g. no blood tests or 'needles'). The child may associate visits to the doctor with memories of past uncomfortable experiences. Never hesitate to explain why you are asking a certain question or performing a particular part of the examination.

Details of appropriate techniques for history taking and physical examination for adolescents are given in Chapter 14.

Taking the history

The current problem

Start by asking the parent (and/or child), about the current problem. It is important to find out what they perceive to be wrong, and why they have chosen to seek medical attention at this time. A referral letter from another practitioner may have provided you with some information but it is essential to understand the problem from the parent's and child's perspective.

Questions such as: 'Why have you come to the hospital?' or 'What is worrying you about James?' may be good ways to begin. If there is more than one problem, ask the parents to list them. Then approach the problems in order of perceived importance. Leave some space in your written record to add additional problems as they come to light during the history. Let the parent tell the story of the presenting problem/s without interruption. You may need to prompt them to go right back to the onset of the symptoms as parents sometimes commence their description part way into an illness (e.g. from the time they last saw the family doctor). Questions like 'When was she last completely well?' can be very helpful here.

> ### Clinical example
>
> William, a 5 year old boy, was brought by his parents because they noticed that he was tired each day in the late afternoon. He would lie on the sofa and be uninterested in playing. This had been going on for nearly a year, since he started school. The rest of the history and examination were unremarkable. The parents' concerns seemed out of proportion to what is fairly common behaviour in early school age children. When asked why they had chosen to seek a medical opinion now, they revealed that a child of one of the mother's work colleagues had recently been diagnosed with leukaemia, and tiredness had been one of the features of her illness. The parents were secretly very anxious that William might have the same diagnosis.

Understanding the sequence and evolution of symptoms can be just as important as listing the symptoms themselves. The pattern of evolution will often reveal the diagnosis (e.g. central abdominal pain, later moving to the right iliac fossa in appendicitis).

When seeking extra detail or clarification, ensure your questions are open (e.g. 'Did he have any vomiting or diarrhoea?') rather than leading (e.g. 'He had no vomiting or diarrhoea?'). Be sure that the parent understands the terminology you use and always avoid medical jargon. Asking if the child has a symptom using a word the parents have never heard of, such as dyspnoea, will nearly always elicit a negative response, whereas an enquiry about breathing difficulties may result in a more accurate answer. Terms that you use every day, such as 'wheezing', may not mean the same thing to the lay person, so try to obtain a clear description. Sometimes it helps to ask parents to mimic the symptoms themselves, such as a cough or type of gait.

Older children can usually provide many of the details themselves. They can be asked if they agree with the description given by the parent or have anything to add.

Key learning points

- Do not use abbreviations or medical jargon during discussion with the family (say 'blue' rather than 'cyanosed' and 'breathing difficulty' rather than 'dyspnoea').
- When the family use descriptions such as 'wheezing' or 'croupy' make sure that these words mean the same to them as they do to you.

You will then explore the symptoms in more detail (e.g. if the presenting symptom is cough, you will want to learn its character, if it is repetitive, if it occurs under certain circumstances, and if it is moist or dry). You will want to enquire about appropriate epidemiological features such as whether anyone else in the family or other contacts had similar symptoms, or if anyone at home is a smoker.

Learn to listen carefully and to distinguish which comments represent direct observation (e.g. 'he kept crying and pulling up his legs') from those which represent parental inference (e.g. 'he kept having spasms of tummy pain').

Past history

This should be kept relevant to the current problem and the age of the child. It is important to ask if the current problem has ever occurred in the past and about past illness which might relate to the current presentation (e.g. a past history of meningitis will be very relevant for a 2 year old who now presents with a seizure disorder).

In infants, it is important to obtain a history of the mother's pregnancy (her health, nutrition, use of medications, alcohol intake and smoking during the pregnancy, etc.), details of the birth (gestation, problems during labour, breech delivery, use of forceps or caesarean section), and the condition of the infant at birth (including the Apgar score if known, and the need for any medical interventions such as oxygen therapy). What were the birth weight and other measurements? Ask about the

infant's course in the first few weeks, including any illness and details of feeding and weight gain. Parents may have the child health record, which will provide many of these details. Simple questions such as 'Was the mother allowed to hold her baby immediately after birth?', and 'How soon was the baby discharged from hospital after birth?' can probe for problems. In young children, the early feeding history is also important.

Details of the pregnancy, birth and early course of postnatal life are usually of less significance for an older child presenting with an acute illness. They will be important, however, in an older child if the presenting problem is neurological or if there is a concern about developmental progress.

Family and social history

The young child's world is the family and it is very important to obtain an understanding of the familial and social contexts of the child's illness and management. Ask about the age and health of the child's parents and siblings. Who else lives in the same household, and who provides most of the child's care? Does the child live in more than one household, as is often the case when parents are separated? Does the child attend day care, kindergarten, or school? Is there a family history relevant to the child's presenting problems?

> ### Clinical example
>
> Annie, an 11 year old girl, had been suffering from recurrent headaches in the last 6 months. These seemed to occur mostly in the evening and more frequently when she was tired or stressed in any way. They were sometimes associated with vomiting. The family history revealed that her mother had a long history of migraine headaches and that the onset of these was at a similar age to Annie.

Find out about the family's housing and economic situation. Are the parents employed? Do they receive any financial allowances or community services? Look for factors that might adversely affect the child's health (e.g. smoking by household members), or that may influence management decisions (e.g. if the family live a long way from hospital and don't have a car).

It is usually useful to draw a brief family tree (Fig 3.1).

Systems review

A brief check for other symptoms should be undertaken, using the usual organ systems approach. Again, learn to ask your questions in a non leading way. Questions should be relevant to the current problem and the age of

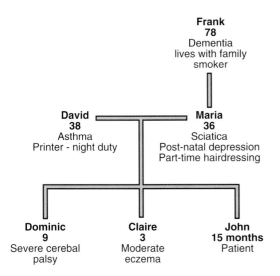

Fig. 3.1 This brief family tree reveals a lot about the genetic and environmental factors that affect John, who now presents with recurrent cough and wheeze.

the child, rather than a long list of routine items. Ask about recent travel or potential environmental exposures if they are relevant to the presenting problem.

Growth and development

One of the aspects of children that clearly differentiates them from adults is that they are growing physically and acquiring new developmental skills. The achievement of a child's full growth and developmental potential is a central component of childhood and it follows that progress in this area requires careful assessment during the clinical consultation.

In infancy, growth is mainly assessed by checking for adequate weight gain, while in older children linear growth and appropriate body weight are both assessed. Where possible, birth measurements and any other previous growth measurement should be plotted on appropriate length/height, weight and head circumference centile charts. This provides two types of information: an estimate of growth achievement in comparison with that expected for the 'normal' population; and also growth progression with time in relation to expected genetic potential by observing 'tracking' along centile channels. Measurements are recorded most commonly in the parent held child health record. Linear growth can also be plotted on growth velocity charts. An appropriate nutritional intake is an obvious and important prerequisite for normal growth: you should find out the usual daily pattern of food intake (breastfeeding in early childhood, type of formula feeds, and intake pattern in later childhood) (Ch. 7).

You should also ask questions to ascertain whether developmental progress is within normal expectations.

This can be done for young children by asking specific 'screening' questions which determine developmental progress at hallmark ages for each of the four major areas of development: gross motor, fine motor/adaptive, language and special senses, and personal–social. This assessment has its greatest importance in the early years of life to enable early detection of developmental difficulties (e.g. hearing impairment, motor difficulties due to cerebral palsy) and allow early intervention.

For older children, ask about progress at kindergarten or school, including parents' assessment as to motor skills and cognitive abilities in comparison with siblings and peers. For school age children, enquire as to special abilities that their child exhibits both in learning and in skills in sports or other activities. Ask children what they enjoy most in their learning activities ('What things are really fun to do?'), and in what activities they see themselves as having special abilities ('What are you really good at?').

More details of developmental assessment can be found in Chapter 4.

Behaviour

A brief history of the child's general behaviour is appropriate. Sometimes a perceived behavioural difficulty will be the presenting problem and a more detailed history will be necessary (Chs 15, 16).

Medications

Enquire about current and past medications including any adverse reactions and suspected drug allergies. Ask specifically about prescription medications, and over the counter items. Complementary or alternative therapies are now frequently used in children but parents often forget or are reluctant to mention their use.

Key learning point

- Remember to ask about all types of therapy used. Specifically enquire about complementary or alternative medications and other therapies.

Immunisation status

Full details of past immunisations should always be obtained. Don't just ask 'Is she up to date with immunisations?', or 'Has he had all his needles?'. The answer you get will often be 'yes' and may be incorrect. Take time to go through what has been administered and compare this to the recommended schedule. Again, the child health record will be useful if available. Remember that unless there is a specific contraindication, every clinical consultation should be seen as an opportunity to check immunisation status, and to offer immunisations that are due or have been missed (Ch. 8).

Closing questions

Complete the history taking by providing the parent or child with the opportunity to add extra information that may have been left out, and to air their own concerns about causes for the presenting problem. The following closing questions will sometimes bring out very important information:

- Is there anything else that is worrying you?
- Is there anything else I should know or anything I have forgotten to ask you?
- Do you have any ideas of your own about what may be causing your child's symptoms?

Key learning point

- The closing questions will often be the ones to bring out the parent's deepest concerns regarding their child's problem. Don't omit this important opportunity, and leave yourself enough time to ask.

Throughout the history taking, you will have the opportunity to observe the child. Remain observant so that you notice symptoms such as coughing or tachypnoea, developmental features of the child's play, and the interaction of the parent and child. This is a part of the physical assessment which is just as important as the more formal physical examination that follows.

The physical examination

Introduction

The purpose of the physical examination is to provide additional information to aid in the diagnosis, assessment of the response to therapy, clues to comorbidities, and to provide important screening data on growth and development.

Young children will not understand why they are being physically handled by a stranger. Shyness and stranger anxiety may limit their cooperation and some will simply refuse any physical contact. This is particularly the case for children between approximately 9 months and 3 years of age. Obtaining cooperation and a successful examination requires skill, understanding and practice. Don't be surprised or concerned if you are unsuccessful sometimes, as this also happens to experienced paediatricians. Try coming back to the examination at a different time or with a different approach. Establishing good rapport with the parent and child during the introduction and history taking as described above will facilitate the physical examination.

Privacy during physical examination is just as important to children as to adults. You need to be friendly, relaxed, with a quiet and calm voice, and use gentle, unhurried physical movements. Undertake the examination by gentle opportunity, and vary the order in which you perform the components of the examination according to the child's cooperation. It is often the case with young children that you are not able to undertake all aspects of the examination at one time because it is tiring or frightening for the child. This means coming back at a later stage to continue.

You need to be prepared to examine the child in the position in which he or she is most relaxed. This might be on the examination couch, but for young children is more likely to be on the mother's lap, cuddled over the father's shoulder, or even lying on the floor! Undressing a young child completely will often upset him or her, and you should consider what it is necessary to expose according to the clinical situation.

Useful data can be obtained by careful observation from a distance and this is a very important technique for examination of small children.

Clinical example

Ravi, an 18 month old boy, presented to hospital with a history of cough and noisy breathing. His elder sibling had recently had a cold. Ravi was obviously frightened and upset when placed on the couch for the physical examination. He cried and clung to his mother's blouse when the Emergency Department Resident tried to undress him.

David, the Paediatric Registrar, suggested that Ravi be sat on his mother's lap while he observed him from a short distance. The nurse handed Ravi a brightly coloured toy. He stopped crying and started to examine the toy. David was able to note that Ravi was well grown, did not look seriously unwell, and he was alert. He was pink in room air, there was a clear nasal discharge, and he had an obvious barking cough and mild stridor when resting. David asked that Ravi's mother lift his upper clothing to expose most of his chest. Ravi looked apprehensive but did not cry. David was able to observe good symmetrical chest movements with a respiratory rate of 22 per minute, and there was minimal indrawing of the intercostal soft tissues. David approached with his stethoscope but again Ravi looked as if he was about to cry. David knew that auscultation of the chest would not add much additional useful diagnostic information in this setting and so he desisted.

Ravi was diagnosed as having viral croup of mild to moderate severity.

In situations where you think the child's tolerance of the examination may be limited, ask yourself what are the most important items that you need to examine. It is often useful to do these first, rather than adopting the more traditional sequence of examination used in adults and older children. Usually it is best to leave any potentially distressing components until last (e.g. examination of ears and throat).

You will become a skilled examiner of patients of any age if you learn to be a careful observer, and this is particularly so in the case of children. Teach yourself to really listen to what you hear, to look at what you see, and to feel what you touch.

Most paediatricians develop their own techniques or 'tricks' for obtaining a child's cooperation with aspects of the examination. Some techniques rely on distraction (e.g. producing a previously unseen toy just prior to auscultation of the precordium). Some may use an incremental approach to obtaining the child's confidence. For example, in an anxious child, one might commence auscultation of the lungs by placing the stethoscope on a less threatening area than the chest, such as the child's thigh, then moving it onto the chest once the child has learned it is not uncomfortable. Alternatively one might auscultate the father's chest first so the child can see that nothing unpleasant is involved. The details of these techniques is not as important as the principle of learning methods which suit your own style of interacting with children.

As described for taking the history, physical examination of children needs to be adapted according to the presenting problem and the working differential diagnoses as they are formulated during the consultation. It is important to emphasise that successful physical examination of children is not about ticking the boxes in a checklist. Knowing exactly what to examine in any given situation, how to do it in a child of this age, and how to interpret the results are much more important and only come from experience in caring for children. The appendix to this chapter includes a list of the items that are commonly included during the physical examination as a guide only — don't use it as a checklist for every child.

General observation and behaviour

What are your first impressions of the child? Is she happy and relaxed, or does she seem tense and uncomfortable? Is she in pain? Is she of normal appearance or different from what you expect? Is she normally grown or small/large/obese/malnourished? Does she respond normally and in an age appropriate way to her parents and siblings? How does she respond to you and to the surroundings? Are her understanding and language or other communication age appropriate? Does she appear to hear and see normally? Is there anything obvious such as noisy breathing, bruising, abnormality of limb movement, skin rashes or abnormal pigmentation? Does she move/crawl/walk/run/climb normally? Are her fine motor movements while playing, drawing, or getting undressed and dressed normal?

These initial impressions can be of great importance and provide useful clues for your overall assessment of the nature of the child's health problems and their impact.

Measurements

Except in emergencies, measurement of weight and height and plotting these variables on centile charts should be a routine part of the examination for all children. Children are ideally weighed in only light undergarments, and in babies the nappy should be removed. Height should be measured accurately using purpose made equipment (Ch. 63).

Specific examination

It is assumed that the reader already has a good understanding of normal examination technique and expected findings for adult patients. There are many differences in the techniques and expected findings in children and these are emphasised below.

Vital signs

Normal ranges for heart rate, respiratory rate and blood pressure vary with age. Table 3.1 gives approximate values for children at rest. Note that blood pressure upper normal values can be different in boys and girls. If hypertension is suspected, consult age and gender specific graphs.

Table 3.1 Some normal ranges for vital signs at different ages in childhood			
Age	Respiratory rate (breaths/min)	Heart rate (beats/min)	Systolic blood pressure (mmHg)
Newborn	40–60	100–160	50–75
1 week to 3 months	30–50	80–160	50–85
3 months to 2 years	20–40	80–140	60–100
2 years to 10 years	14–24	60–100	70–110
>10 years	12–20	50–100	85–120

Respiratory system

The pattern of respiration in young infants often has a large abdominal component. The chest wall is compliant so that conditions which cause reduced lung compliance or airway obstruction will more readily be manifest by indrawing of the soft tissues of the chest wall, and in more serious disease the rib cage itself may be drawn in during inspiration. The breath sounds in infants are more readily heard because of the thin chest wall, and they often sound harsher on auscultation than in older children and adults. These normal differences in auscultation findings are even more pronounced in the upper parts of the right lung, sometimes leading inexperienced examiners to suspect pathology in this area.

Cardiovascular system

A thorough description will be found in Chapter 51. Selection of an appropriate sized cuff is important for accurate measurement of blood pressure.

Abdomen

Compared with older children, the abdomen of a young infant appears protuberant, and the umbilicus may be everted. The liver is normally palpable up to 2 cm below the right costal margin, and it is sometimes possible to feel the tip of a normal spleen and the lower pole of the right kidney.

Rectal examination should not be performed routinely. If indicated by the presenting problem, it should be undertaken once only and by the person who will be making management decisions based on the findings (e.g. a surgical registrar in the case of suspected appendicitis).

Genitalia

In infant boys, assessment of the penis and scrotum should be considered part of the normal routine examination, as unsuspected inguinal hernia, undescended testes and urethral abnormalities may be detected. It is normal for the prepuce to be non retractile and adherent to the glans up to around 4 years of age.

In girls, examination of the genitalia is usually undertaken only when indicated.

Central nervous system

Formal examination of the nervous system is time consuming and many aspects require cooperation from the patient. In young children, observation of movement and behaviour can provide most of the necessary information, with specific neurological examination being reserved for children where the primary concern is the nervous system. Routine sensory examination is necessary only rarely.

Skin

Examination of the skin is important not only in dermatological problems: congenital skin lesions may give diagnostic clues to other conditions. For example, the characteristic pale patches of tuberous sclerosis may give the diagnosis in a child who is being assessed for developmental delay and seizures (Ch. 74).

Musculoskeletal system

Examination for congenital hip disease should be routine in young infants (Ch. 25).

Special senses

From the history and general observation, you should be able to assess that the child can see and hear adequately. Screening examination for hearing and vision must be age appropriate (Chs 75, 76) and formal assessment by an audiologist or optometrist may be required.

Development

A brief screen of developmental achievements and progress should be undertaken. Detailed assessment is not routine unless indicated by the clinical problem (Ch. 4).

Head and neck

In babies, examine the head size and plot it on the centile chart. Check the head shape, the fontanelles and the sutures (Ch. 32). The posterior fontanelle is often closed by 2 months of age and the anterior fontanelle closes some time between 12 and 24 months.

Examine the teeth if present, for their number, pattern of eruption and the presence of caries or abnormalities (Ch. 77). Take this opportunity to remind parents of the importance of good dental care and of regular attendance with a dentist.

Examination of the mouth, throat and ears requires good cooperation or appropriate restraint of the child. Observation of experienced practitioners is the best way to learn these techniques.

Concluding the examination

As mentioned in the section on taking the history, it can be helpful to ask the parent or child if there is anything else they would like you to check at this point. Your examination may also have revealed findings that prompt you to return and take further details in the history.

Note taking

It is important that you produce an accurate and clear record of the history and examination findings. This will be needed to help you later and as a record for future staff involved in the child's care. A few items will need to be jotted down briefly as you go along but the rest of the record should be written after the consultation is completed. You will not develop a good rapport with the family if you are constantly gazing at your papers and writing notes.

In younger children, you will have adapted the order of the physical examination to fit the clinical problem and their tolerance of the examination process. Whatever the sequence in which you obtain your information, it is still important to record your findings in a logical and structured format.

The consultation as part of the therapy

Doctors often think of the management of a clinical problem as a chronological sequence commencing with history taking and examination, followed by formulation of a differential diagnosis, appropriate investigations, final diagnosis, treatment, assessment of response, and outcome. Most families who have an ill child will not arrive at your consultation with that same perspective. They will have come because they perceive their child has a problem, and they will often be anxious that it might turn out to be serious. They will be in a foreign environment and one that may have frightening associations for them. They may not know who exactly you are, nor if you are the best person to help them with their child's problem.

You will be in a position to help ease at least some of the family's anxieties long before you have even arrived at a diagnosis. You can achieve this by being friendly, by explaining who you are, conveying that you are genuinely interested in their concerns and that you value their time and opinions as much as your own. Use language they understand, give them time and opportunities to express their concerns fully, be gentle and caring during your examination, and give a clear explanation of what you think the problem might be and the nature and purpose of any investigations or treatment that you recommend. In this way, you will help to obtain the family's confidence and trust, which in turn will improve their willingness to cooperate with the plan of investigation and treatment that is required.

You will not acquire all these skills overnight, but learning them is rewarding and fun, and you will be a much more effective doctor for children and their families at the end of the process.

Key learning points

- Skills in history taking and examination cannot be acquired adequately by reading a textbook — make sure you get lots of practice with children of all ages and in different clinical settings.
- Learn to appreciate what constitutes normal growth, development and physical findings on examination. Take every opportunity you can to observe normal children (who might be visiting the hospital, in the cafeteria, or even travelling on public transport). Try and guess their ages from your observations (based on size, development and behaviour) and then ask how old they really are.
- Adapt the content and techniques of history taking and examination to fit the age of the child and the urgency of the medical problem.
- Learn to be flexible in your approach — some patients will need to be examined on the floor!

Appendix

Items that are commonly included in the physical examination

Those items marked (#) are usually included, while others will be noted in selected situations only.

❑ Height (#)	❑ Weight (#)	❑ Head circumference
❑ Pulse rate (#)	❑ Respiratory rate (#)	❑ Blood pressure (#)

General appearance
- ❑ looks well / unwell / sick / very sick (#)
- ❑ alertness (#)
- ❑ distressed / cooperative
- ❑ general body build
- ❑ overall development including speech
- ❑ facial appearance / dysmorphism (#)
- ❑ posture, movement
- ❑ interaction with parents (#)

Skin
- ❑ colour / pigmentation / jaundice / cyanosis / pallor (#)
- ❑ bruising / petechiae / rashes / scars
- ❑ turgor
- ❑ visible blood vessels
- ❑ subcutaneous fat

Nails / hair
- ❏ cyanosis / pallor / clubbing
- ❏ haemorrhages
- ❏ distribution and colour of hair

Lymph nodes
- ❏ size / mobility / tenderness of nodes in each group (cervical, occipital, axillary, inguinal, etc.)

Head
- ❏ size / shape / posture
- ❏ fontanelles: presence / shape / tension
- ❏ bruit / percussion

Eyes
- ❏ appearance / blinking / ptosis / nystagmus
- ❏ visual acuity / fields
- ❏ ocular movements / squint
- ❏ lids / discharge
- ❏ fundoscopic appearance
- ❏ light and corneal reflex

Ears
- ❏ position / shape
- ❏ discharge
- ❏ hearing (#)
- ❏ appearance of tympanic membranes

Nose
- ❏ shape / flaring with respiration / discharge / bleeding
- ❏ patency of airway / mucosal appearance / polyps

Mouth / lips / teeth / gums/ palate / pharynx
- ❏ colour of lips, tongue and buccal mucosa
- ❏ presence of exudates / coating / ulcers
- ❏ lip swelling or scaling / fissuring
- ❏ number of teeth and presence of caries
- ❏ breath odour / salivation
- ❏ petechiae / bleeding
- ❏ colour of pharyngeal mucosa
- ❏ size, colour and presence of exudate on tonsils

Chest / lungs
- ❏ shape / symmetry / deformities (including Harrison's sulcus, rickety rosary)
- ❏ expansion of chest and pattern of breathing
- ❏ soft tissue indrawing with respiration
- ❏ pattern and rate of breathing
- ❏ cough / stridor / wheezing
- ❏ percussion note
- ❏ breath sounds / added sounds

Breasts
- ❏ development (Tanner stage)

Heart
- ❏ appearance of precordium: deformity / activity
- ❏ pulse: rate / rhythm / strength / nature
- ❏ blood pressure
- ❏ apex beat / cardiac impulse / thrills
- ❏ percussion of cardiac dullness
- ❏ heart sounds / added sounds
- ❏ features of cardiac failure

Abdomen
- ❏ shape / distension / visible mass / movement with respiration
- ❏ visible veins / peristalsis
- ❏ percussion / ascites
- ❏ tenderness on palpation
- ❏ enlarged organs / palpable mass
- ❏ anus / rectum (avoid examination in children unless specifically indicated)

Genitalia
- ❏ development (Tanner stage)
- ❏ presence of testis in scrotum
- ❏ scrotal swellings / hernia
- ❏ urethral / vaginal discharge
- ❏ evidence of injury

Spine
- ❏ posture / deformity / hair / dimples/ tenderness

Limbs
- ❏ deformity / contractures
- ❏ muscle development
- ❏ hip dislocation (Ch. 25)
- ❏ joints: tenderness / swelling / range of movement / temperature / colour

Nervous system
- ❏ alertness / responsiveness / general ability
- ❏ abnormal movements / gait / posture
- ❏ tone / power / coordination / symmetry of movement
- ❏ reflexes / primitive reflexes
- ❏ special sensory examination
- ❏ sensation
- ❏ cranial nerves

Developmental assessment
See Chapter 4

Developmental screening and assessment

D. Starte, J. Macdessi

We continue to develop new skills throughout life but it is in childhood that this process is most dramatic. As with physical growth, the rate of developmental growth is a defining distinction of paediatric medicine. There are major developmental changes in primary and high school children but it is the first 5 years of life, during which the majority of basic skills are acquired, that is a predominant focus for developmental paediatrics. Doctors learning about child development often wish to memorise lists of milestones but fail to appreciate the diversity of normal variation. Adults are not expected to have an even distribution of talents themselves, in their families or in their colleagues; yet when we consider children we often assume they will all walk at 12 months, talk in phrases at 2 years and draw faces at 4 years. It is the variability in normal patterns of development that makes the area fascinating and creates complex challenges in screening and diagnosis.

Screening is the process of detecting presymptomatic disorders in order to intervene and change their natural history. Screening uses tests of known accuracy in healthy or at risk populations to uncover those with the target problem before symptoms arise. Further diagnostic testing can then be performed, before appropriate intervention is carried out. In the developmental context, some tests are used commonly to formalise the process. Examples are:

- the Denver II
- the Australian Developmental Screening Test (ADST).

Developmental surveillance is a routine part of all paediatric interactions. This requires the doctor to have a working knowledge of normal development in all of its forms and to be able to detect variations which may be indicative of significant disorders.

Assessing normal development (developmental surveillance)

Child development progresses in many areas simultaneously. It is as necessary to know the various developmental systems, as it is to know the physical systems. Each will have its component parts, and the rate of progress in all of these components may be similar (when delayed, this is described as a global delay) or discrepant (described as specific or selective delay). The process of determining a child's developmental progress is no dif-

Clinical example

Sinclair, a 3 year old child of English speaking parents, only had a vocabulary of 20 words. His medical history was normal. The parents were reassured by his normal hearing assessment, as well as by the father's own history of initial poor speech development as a child. However, the preschool staff became concerned about the degree of his language difficulty and whether it was part of a global developmental delay. The words he knew were used singly, were clearly articulated and were used in their appropriate context, but to indicate his needs, he resorted to leading an adult by the hand. No phrases or small sentences were heard. He understood two step commands and used facial expressions, hand gesturing and eye to eye contact appropriately. At preschool, he was interested in the other children, but they often excluded him in play when he couldn't talk properly. He showed examples of imaginative, constructive and cooperative motor play. There were no behavioural concerns and he was an affectionate child.

Assessment with the Griffiths Mental Developmental Scales showed that his abilities tested within the average range for his age, other than a mild delay in speech and language skills. During the assessment, he was cooperative and persevered with the tasks at hand. Sinclair therefore had an isolated expressive language disorder of presumed familial origin, and was referred to a speech pathologist for assessment, therapy and liaison with the preschool teacher to modify his preschool curriculum.

ferent from any other system and starts with a good history. Parents are often remarkably accurate at recalling recent developmental changes, but more distant events may require prior notice so that sources such as relatives and baby books can be reviewed. A simple structured questionnaire filled in before the interview, such as the Parent's Evaluation of Developmental Status, can allow parents to consider the details in the waiting room or at home. Most developmental interactions are best scheduled for a well child visit or review.

Key learning points: needs for developmental surveillance

- Adequate time and privacy.
- Good communication skills.
- Knowledge of normal developmental ranges.

Table 4.1 Areas of development (input requires sensation; output requires motor control)

Gross motor control	Movement sensation — kinaesthesia, vision and vestibular input Large muscle coordination produces agility
Vision and fine motor	Vision and visual perception guidance Small muscle coordination produces dexterity and clear speech
Language and hearing	Hearing and auditory processing distinguish speech sounds Receptive language encodes words and sentences into ideas Expressive language encodes ideas as words and sentences leading to speech Pragmatic language enables socially interactive conversation
Social and daily living skills	Watching and listening inform imitation Fine and gross motor skills enable imitative actions Feeding, dressing and household tasks lead to self-care Nurturing fosters self-confidence and independence Temperament moderates emotional regulation

- History of family patterns of behaviour and development.
- Examination for neurological and syndromic features.
- Attention to sensory functions, e.g. vision and hearing.
- Belief in parents' reporting accuracy.

A good history starts with the pregnancy and delivery and progresses through the neonatal, infancy, toddler and preschool years. The areas to consider are covered in Table 4.1, and parents should be asked open ended questions about their child's progress, such as 'Tell me how she is getting around?', which would be more likely elicit revealing answers than 'Is she walking now?' This process is time consuming and parents need to feel relaxed and unhurried if they are to give their best information. Some of the information may well be sensitive,

especially when there are problems, and a private setting without interruptions is important. The key is to look for areas of development delayed beyond the normal range and not to compare the child with 'normal milestones', which are merely the average age of achievement. Half of the population will not meet modal milestones by definition, and their use can worry many parents unnecessarily. It is preferable to use the normal ranges in Table 4.2. Many developmental patterns are familial, and so are many developmental disorders. Do not accept delay as a normal variation because an uncle did not talk until he was 4, as the uncle may also have had a developmental language disorder or deafness. Other 'causes' such as being a twin, bilingualism or tongue tie should not be accepted, and actual delays need to be excluded by more formal diagnostic assessment. Assuming the child

Table 4.2 Normal ranges (approximately 25th centile to 90th centile)

Age	Gross motor control	Vision and fine motor	Language and hearing	Social and daily living skills
2–4 months	Head steady in sitting	Follows object through 180°	Squeals with pleasure	Smiles
5–8 months	Sits without support	Passes cube hand to hand	Turns to soft voice Baba/Gaga babble (up to 10 months)	Feeds self biscuit
9–14 months	Stands with support	Neat pincer grasp of raisin	Mama or Dada specifically	Indicates needs by gesture
12–16 months	Walks well alone	Stack of two cubes (up to 21 months)	Three words (up to 21 months)	Drinks from a cup
15–24 months	Walks up steps	Scribbles spontaneously	Points to one body part	Removes garment
21–36 months	Jumps on the spot	Draws vertical line in imitation	Uses plurals and phrases	Puts on clothing Plays tag with other children
3–4½ years	Balances on one foot for 5 s	Copies a ladder Draws a face	Understands cold, tired and hungry Asks 'Wh' questions	Separates from mother

Table 4.3   Developmental equipment

Gross motor control	Steps, for walking up and down
	Tennis ball, for kicking, throwing and catching
	Tricycle, for riding and pedalling
Vision and fine motor	Raisins, for pincer grasp and self feeding
	2.5 cm blocks, for simple stacks, counting and colour matching
	Simple inset puzzles, for matching and sorting shapes
	Small crayon/pencil, for scribbling and drawing
	Paper, for above and folding and cutting
Language and hearing	Doll, for identifying body parts and pretend play
	Simple picture book, for pointing out items/describing the action
	Telephone or dictaphone, for encouraging spontaneous speech
Social and daily living skills	Eyes and ears, for listening to parents and observing interactions
	Mirror, for watching baby's responses to self
	Toy cup, plate and cutlery, for demonstrating feeding self or doll

is delayed because of these is a common source of late diagnosis and delayed effective intervention.

As each area is reviewed through the different stages of childhood, any apparent delays or unusual features can be clarified with the family. This allows the developmental examination to be targeted. While many children are shy and perhaps fearful, a quiet patient approach will often bring out the showoff in children, especially for tasks about which they are confident. For this reason it is best to start looking at non verbal areas (blocks, puzzles, drawing, etc.), and having appropriate furniture at the child's height will enable you to get down to the child's eye level. Simple equipment (Table 4.3) can be used to elicit a range of skills and the session should remain a

play activity. Remember that too much direct eye contact, especially from above, can be threatening, and a relaxed tangential approach across the child may be more successful. Refusal to cooperate is a regular occurrence and it is better to reschedule than to persist and teach the child that your sessions are going to be unpleasant.

The most important conclusion that needs to be drawn from this exercise is to ensure that there are no warning signs of a potential problem (Table 4.4). Should doubt exist, it is always better to seek a second opinion and to arrange some simple therapy or intervention than to provide false reassurance. It may make you feel better to reassure, but families who waste months finding help for their child will often feel very angry.

Table 4.4   Warning signs to worry about; be concerned if the child is not doing this (items marked * are a worry if they <u>are</u> present)

Age[†] (months)	Gross motor control	Vision and fine motor	Language and hearing	Social and daily living skills
3	Complete head lag*	Following with eyes	Searching for sounds with eyes	Smiling
6	Preference for one hand Persistent Moro*	Squint*	Head turn to soft voice	Interest in people
9	Sitting with support	Persistent hand regard*	Ba-ba-ba babble	Awareness of strangers
12	Pulling to stand Standing with support	Pincer grasp	Trying one or two words	Constant* mouthing
18	Walking alone	Constructive play with blocks Casting toys*	Six words Constant dribbling*	Pointing at items Finger feeding
24	Running	Turning book pages	Fifty single words	Interested in other children Helps in dressing
36	Kicking a ball	Drawing lines	2–3 word phrases Echolalia*	Active play with peers
48	Pedalling and hopping	Drawing a face	Sentences and 'Wh' questions	Imaginative play Toilet trained — day

†Or at any age if there is parental concern (parents are usually right) or regression in skills.

Diagnosing the problem (developmental assessment)

While this process is broadly a more detailed version of simple surveillance, it is common for doctors with particular experience in the area to be involved in teams with other professionals with specific expertise. These professionals may be:

- social workers or community nurses, who are highly skilled in family support and interactions
- psychologists, skilled in intelligence testing and behavioural interventions
- physiotherapists, with skills in movement and coordination
- speech pathologists, with language and oromotor skills
- occupational therapists, with daily living skills, seating and manual dexterity.

However, in good teams all players learn from each other and considerable role release can occur. Some specialised teams will need specific expertise from orthoptists, audiologists and orthotists as well as technical support personnel to help with specific equipment.

The history taking, which often includes parental questionnaires, will be very detailed about the nature of the concerns raised as well as the medical, developmental and family history. It is most important to be clear about the family's expectations of the assessment, so that their agenda is covered fully. It may be helpful to arrange a home visit by one of the team initially to break the ice with the family and to see the child in more natural surroundings. Most families are understandably anxious about a formal developmental assessment, as it may lead to bad news. Anything done to reduce the family's apprehension will also be likely to reduce the child's fears and improve the reliability of the assessment as a sample of the child's development. To this end, the venue for the assessment should not be overly clinical and the staff should be understanding and welcoming.

Key learning points: needs for developmental assessment

- Multidisciplinary team approach.
- Colleagues working as equals.
- Good information gathering.
- Standardised tests of development and intelligence.
- Complementary standardised behavioural questionnaires.
- Ample time to discuss the findings with the family.
- Written reports to the family with a plan of action.
- Follow up on any recommendations made.

Information can also be gained from people who know the child, such as teachers, therapists and doctors. This requires consent from the family to approach them, but can be very useful if done in advance, so that the developmental assessment can be interpreted in the light of the child's wider world. Sufficient time needs to be allocated at the assessment for all of the issues to be covered and this can take several hours. A choice of professionals to see the family can be made based on the concerns expressed and the information gathered. During the assessment, each professional will need some time to work with the child and also to talk with the parents to clarify history details particular to their involvement.

Most teams will attempt some form of formal test of developmental status, often performed by the psychologist, to assess the degree and distribution of any developmental delay or disability. This is not just to gain a score, but provides a structured way of reviewing all aspects of cognitive development in an age appropriate framework. In young children, this may be a developmental test such as the Griffiths or Gesell Scales, and in older children a standard intelligence test is often used such as the Weschler tests (WPPSI or WISC), the Stanford-Binet or the Differential Ability Scales.

A developmental quotient (DQ or GQ) derived from the former tests includes aspects of self-care and motor development and is a broader concept than intelligence quotient (IQ), which relates more specifically to cognitive capacity. It is usual to talk about a delay in development when the child is young (say under 3 years) and the prognosis uncertain. When it seems that the child has a permanent developmental disorder it is better to call it a disability, as many parents assume that any delay will eventually resolve. In addition, specific behavioural questionnaires may be used to assess the severity of symptoms suggestive of autism, attention deficit hyperactivity disorder (ADHD) or other behavioural disorders such as oppositional defiant disorder or anxiety disorders.

Key learning points: possible investigations for developmental presentations

- Low average to borderline delay alone: consider variation from family norms.
- Mild/moderate delay or above with language delay/dysmorphisms: chromosomes, DNA for fragile X, thyroid.
- Boys with above: creatinine kinase.
- Severe intellectual deficit: lactate/pyruvate, amino and organic acids.
- Large head, CNS or skin signs: CT/MRI; watch for family history of large head.
- Small head: TORCH titres; mild maternal PKU; MRI.
- Loss of speech skills: sleeping EEG; neurometabolic tests.

- Old houses, renovations, pica: blood lead.
- Syndromic or dysmorphic features: genetics opinion before specific DNA studies.

Note

Remember to *offer* investigations: not all families are as focused on aetiology as medical staff.

The medical examination (Ch. 3) will ensure that growth parameters are measured, especially head circumference, and signs of dysmorphism and neurocutaneous disorders are sought. The aim is to detect any condition that might be causing the developmental delay, or indeed any general medical problem that may be exacerbating it. While a thorough physical examination is desirable, particular attention needs to be paid to the neurological system, looking for signs of cerebral palsy and other neuromotor disorders (Ch. 57). Some ingenuity may be needed after a long developmental session to engage the child in play again. Indeed much can be learned from observing the developmental testing (preferably through a one way screen) or working with the physiotherapist or occupational therapist to dovetail the necessary observations. Special attention is often paid to vision and hearing screening at this time, and much has been written about this. However, a note of warning is necessary, as these senses are vital for children's learning. For intervention to be as efficient as possible, these senses need to be acute. It may therefore be more of a service to the child to ensure that he or she is seen by a vision or hearing professional than to perform some rough screening test, especially when the developmental concerns are specific to that sense (i.e. hearing to language or vision to motor skills). Again, false reassurance needs to be avoided at all costs.

Many children coming to developmental teams will already have a diagnosis such as Down syndrome or cerebral palsy, but some conditions are less obvious and need particular vigilance, e.g. velocardiofacial syndrome, fragile X syndrome (Ch. 29), the mucopolysaccharide storage disorders, thyroid deficiency or lead excess and in boys muscular dystrophy. Investigations or further opinions should be recommended to families as needed, to help exclude any conditions that appear likely. Chromosome analysis or specific DNA tests have the highest positive yield in most developmental presentations. Imaging and EEG testing are less rewarding unless specific signs or symptoms of neurological disorder are present.

Once all members of the team have had their chance to interact with the child and family, it is time to bring everything together. This fusion of professional opinions should occur before further discussions with the family so that they can be presented with a cohesive view for their child. The feedback session can be scheduled on the same day or later; it is always helpful to have both parents present and any close family supports that

Clinical example

Max is a 3 year old boy with an unremarkable past medical or family history. However, from the age of 2 years there were concerns about his development, in particular his language and gross motor skills. Four months ago, a speech pathology assessment revealed a mild receptive and expressive language delay. Despite progress with speech therapy, a review of his general development was requested because of concerns that he was also stumbling when running. Compared to his sister he was slightly later in sitting (8 months) and walking (15 months) and he initially had difficulties in climbing frames but he still cannot jump or kick a ball well, and walks up and down stairs one step at a time.

Max was examined using the Griffiths Mental Developmental Scales, which showed age appropriate puzzle skills, low average range fine motor and language skills and slightly more delayed gross motor skills. On examination he had a lordotic posture, a waddling gait, only slightly overdeveloped calf muscles, and mild difficulty getting up from a sitting position on the ground. A proximal myopathy was suspected in association with his very mild developmental delay. The initial CK was 33 000 units/litre and a dystrophin gene analysis was arranged. Max went on to have a muscle biopsy, which showed the typical changes of Duchenne muscular dystrophy.

they request, e.g. grandparents. Once the team's view has been clearly stated, it is normal to ask for the family's reaction and to discuss this. This will hopefully lead to discussions covering investigation, aetiology, prognosis, genetic advice and a plan of action. Recommendations can be formulated with the family as to what needs to be done by whom, where and when. This all needs to be recorded carefully and copies given to the family on the day, as much of what is said may be forgotten, especially when the news is shocking. However, the manner in which it is imparted is likely to be remembered for all time and care taken with the time available, privacy and if necessary the use of interpreter services will help optimise a potentially traumatic session.

All parents need copies of all reports generated; further copies can be sent to all those involved with the child if the family are agreeable. Follow up can be arranged to review any investigations or to help establish intervention services. Many parents feel a sense of grief if the child has a serious developmental problem and it may be necessary to provide written material and counselling to help then understand that this is a normal reaction. Failure to resolve the grief reaction can lead to ongoing anger, depression or marital conflict and may delay important remedial action for the child.

Clinical example

When Jesse was 2 years 1 month old, he was referred for assessment of his development because of speech and language delays. On the developmental assessment he displayed a mild developmental delay overall, with an age equivalent level of 1 year 5 months. His weaknesses were in the areas of personal–social, language and fine motor skills, which were moderately delayed (1 year age equivalent level). His strength was in gross motor skills, which were normal (2 year 4 month age equivalent level). Speech therapy and occupational therapy were arranged and when he started preschool an individualised educational programme was established for him.

Jesse was reviewed again at the age of 3 years 11 months and still showed an overall mild delay (2 years and 7 months). Gross motor skills remained his personal strength, being within normal limits, and his puzzle solving skills had improved to a borderline level. However, his weakest areas continued to be language and fine motor skills, which were still moderately delayed. Speech therapy and occupational therapy programmes continued, and a special needs teacher was arranged to provide further educational support at preschool.

At the age of 5 years and 2 months a reassessment was arranged to plan for school placement based on his general learning progress and support needs. He was assessed using the Differential Ability Scales (an IQ test), which demonstrated a general conceptual ability around the 1st percentile (IQ = 63), in the mild deficit range. When considered together with parental, teacher and therapist reports and his two previous developmental assessments, it was clear Jesse had a long term intellectual disability of mild degree. Mainstream kindergarten placement with integration support was arranged, with possible progression to an appropriate smaller support class at primary school age.

that control resource allocation find such a subtle approach too hard and may resort to headline diagnostic labels as an entry ticket to funding support. Also, some families need a clear label to work with, but they also need to understand that any human individual is far more subtle and complex than a single label or even a list of comorbid disorders.

Clinical example

At 4 years 3 months, Adrian has only three recognisable words. He avoids eye to eye contact, and pays little attention to what is asked of him, preferring to play alone. He makes sounds as he wanders around a room, laughing and giggling for no apparent reason, looking at himself in the mirror and often flapping his fingers close to his face. He is quiet, only becoming upset with the sound of a vacuum cleaner or a passing police car siren. He appears distant, not spontaneously giving or accepting affection. He is toilet trained and can undress completely but needs assistance to get dressed. He cannot pedal a tricycle, has poor ball playing skills, and an immature pencil grip with only circular scribbling. At preschool he needs constant direction and encouragement by the staff, and he has not developed any friendships.

Assessment with the Griffiths Mental Developmental Scales indicated a moderate intellectual disability with non verbal skills at around 2–2.5 years, but his verbal skills are further delayed at 12–18 months. His behaviour is consistent with a diagnosis of autistic disorder, as he has a specific impairment in forming social relationships, in communicating and in playing imaginatively in addition to his developmental disability. Adrian has high support needs and requires intensive educational programming and behaviour modification to develop to his optimum potential.

Areas of diagnostic dilemma

Many children do not fit neatly into a diagnostic box, and the widely used DSM-IV and ICD-10 classifications cannot always be relied on to describe a particular child's developmental profile and difficulties adequately. There may be a range of overlapping problems of varying degree that need to be acknowledged. Having moved from simple categorical classification (boxes) to a linear spectrum model (a line), it is clear that even this is inadequate. One way of viewing the child's diagnosis is as a series of linear spectra, which can be set at various levels rather like a sound mixing board. It is then possible to have a child who has a mild intellectual disability with a lot of attentional and impulse control problems, minor sensory oversensitivities and obsessional features with good gross motor skills. This model allows the intervention plan to be tailored to the child's and family's specific needs very closely. Unfortunately, many bureaucracies

Autism

Since Leo Kanner's original description, the definition of this disorder has expanded considerably. The core diagnosis of autistic disorder has clear criteria involving:
- delayed language and nonverbal communication
- little interest in socialisation, with repetitive unimaginative play
- reliance on routines and rituals, repetitive motor mannerisms and unusual sensory sensitivities.

However, there are many children who have some but not all of these features. It is now usual to reserve the diagnosis of autistic disorder for children who fulfil the DSM-IV criteria, and to use the term 'autistic spectrum disorder' for children who have a basic lack of social empathy or interest in communication, especially with their own peers or siblings. These children will have some of the features of autistic disorder but not all. Indeed those with more language disorder and less social difficulty may be labelled as having 'semantic–pragmatic language disorder', and those with better language function but poor social interactions, clumsy motor skills and perhaps an unusual speech pattern can be described as having Asperger disorder. This constellation of pervasive developmental disorders is being recognised with increasing frequency and may indeed be increasing in actual prevalence (Ch. 18).

Attention deficit hyperactivity disorder

This disorder is very common on its own or with specific areas of developmental weakness, especially language. However, the core deficit of delayed impulse inhibition can occur to an extent in children with intellectual disability or autism. Recognition of this can lead to including additional treatment possibilities in the child's plan of management (Ch. 17).

Intellectual disability

By definition, over 2% of the population will have an IQ that is more than 2 SD below the mean or below 70. This is 1 in 50 children, making it by far the most common major disability. The delay occurs in all areas of development fairly evenly, and is described as mild, moderate, severe or profound, depending on the deviation from the mean on testing. It is usual to make the diagnosis from assessment of cognitive function and adaptive function; this latter is the ability of the child to perform everyday tasks in the real world and is sometimes assessed with specific inventories such as the Vineland Adaptive Behaviour Scales. Children with significant discrepancies between their verbal and nonverbal cognitive or reasoning skills are more likely to have a specific learning disability than an intellectual disability and full scale scores should be viewed with caution (Ch. 11).

PART 2   SELF-ASSESSMENT

Questions

1. A 2 year old girl becomes distressed when you attempt to palpate her abdomen. You know the abdominal findings are important to your ability to establish a diagnosis in this case. You should:
   (A) Enlist the assistance of a parent or nurse to restrain her for the examination
   (B) Omit the abdominal examination
   (C) Sedate her to enable an adequate examination
   (D) Explain the purpose of the examination and obtain her cooperation
   (E) Return to examine the abdomen later

2. Which of the following would be considered within the age appropriate normal ranges?
   (A) A foreskin which is adherent to the glans in a 2 year old boy
   (B) A systolic blood pressure of 45 mmHg in a 3 year old child
   (C) A liver edge palpable 2 cm beneath the right costal margin in a 6 month old baby
   (D) A reluctance to allow examination of the abdomen in an 18 month old girl
   (E) An anterior fontanelle that is closed in a 2 month old baby

3. Which of the following developmental observations are age appropriate?
   (A) Partial head lag noted when pulled up from a lying position at 2 months
   (B) No bisyllabic babbling at the age of 8 months
   (C) At 10 months, picking up a raisin with the thumb opposed to the side of the index finger
   (D) At 15 months, not being able to walk independently
   (E) Three recognisable words at the age of 2 years

4. Which of the following developmental findings would be of concern in a 3 year old child?
   (A) Parents reporting fewer words than 6 months ago
   (B) Not yet kicking a ball
   (C) Limited imaginative or 'make believe' play
   (D) An expressive vocabulary of 80 words
   (E) Poor representational drawing of people and faces

5. Jason is a 2 year 5 month old boy for whom a Griffiths Mental Development Scale assessment revealed scores indicating a significant delay in language and motor skills of mild to borderline degree (GQ=70). Which of the following comments are definitely true?
   (A) He has a developmental delay
   (B) He has an intellectual disability
   (C) From this one can plan appropriate school placement
   (D) He should be thoroughly investigated for a specific medical cause
   (E) This assessment would exclude or confirm a pervasive developmental disorder, e.g. autism

6. With psychometric testing which of the following are true?
   (A) Over 2% of the population will have a standard score more than 2 standard deviations from the

mean with a mean GQ or IQ below 70 on the Griffiths or Weschler scales, respectively

(B) Those with a borderline intellectual disability have a standard IQ score between 1 and 2 standard deviations from the mean, and comprise about 14% of the population

(C) Those with a mild intellectual disability have a standard score between 2 and 3 standard deviations from the mean and comprise about 2% of the population

(D) Those with a moderate to severe intellectual disability have a standard score beyond 3 standard deviations from the mean and comprise about 0.13% of the population

(E) Approximately 68% of the population have an IQ within average range

Answers and explanations

1. The correct answer is **(E)**. If she is restrained (A), she will cry and you will feel nothing more than a rigid abdominal wall. Omitting the abdominal examination (B) is not reasonable in this case if you think the findings will be important. Examination under sedation (C) is sometimes appropriate where important diagnostic information cannot be obtained any other way but it would not be the next approach in this situation. A 2 year old will not have the developmental abilities to understand an explanation of why her abdomen needs to be palpated (D). This is especially so if she is already upset. Returning to examine the abdomen later is usually the best approach. This might be done during the same consultation but in a different way, e.g. with her cuddled over her father's shoulder, or if in hospital it might work to examine her later while she is asleep.

2. The correct answers are **(A)**, **(C)** and **(D)**. It is normal for the prepuce to be non retractile and adherent to the glans (A) up to around 4 years of age. A systolic blood pressure of 45 mmHg in a 3 year old child (B) would be very low (normal range 70–110). In the absence of other signs of liver or cardiac disease, a liver edge palpable 2 cm beneath the right costal margin would be considered normal in a 6 month old baby (C). Stranger anxiety is often very pronounced in children of 18 months of age (D). It often requires considerable skill and patience to overcome the child's natural reluctance to allow physical examination. The anterior fontanelle usually closes sometime between 12 and 24 months of age. If it is found to be closed in a baby of 2 months of age (E), then this

should prompt a search for associated abnormalities such as microcephaly.

3. The correct answers are **(A)**, **(B)**, **(C)** and **(D)**. Except for (E) these are all within the normal range of development. By 14 months there should be proper words emerging that have a specific meaning such as 'MaMa', 'No' or 'Up'.

4. The correct answers are **(A)**, **(B)** and **(D)**. (A) Whenever a parent reports a loss of a previously attained skill, this warrants careful attention. (B) The stability on one leg to allow the other foot to kick a tennis ball should be present by 30 months. (D) At the age of 3 years an expressive vocabulary range of over 200 words is appropriate. (C) and (E) Representational drawing and imaginative play should be present by at least 4 years.

5. (A) False. A psychometric assessment is a 'snap shot' perspective of a child's development and can be affected by performance on the day. Confirming a developmental delay, global or specific, requires consensus, with reports from the parents and other professionals involved (e.g. teacher, speech pathologist, occupational therapist). (B) and (C) Both are false. It is usual to talk about a delay in development when the child is under 3 years and the prognosis is uncertain. With early intervention there may be potential catch up in the delay. A repeat assessment prior to school entry (either an IQ psychometric assessment or a specific language/motor skills assessment) may demonstrate such progress. However, if the delay has not resolved, the child may well have a permanent developmental disorder; this can then be referred to as an intellectual or specific learning disability. This will have implications for the child's learning, and school placement may need to be modified depending on the degree. (D) False. Investigations should be guided by the entire assessment including medical history (e.g. EEG if there is a suspicion of epileptic events), social and family history (has he had normal developmental stimulation?) and examination (e.g. DNA analysis for fragile X if there is relevant dysmorphology). (E) False. A history of a child's behaviour as well as play and social skills would be important to consider when concluding whether this child has a pervasive developmental disorder such as autism.

6. **All are true**. But in gauging the severity of a child's developmental or intellectual disability, the details of behaviour, socialisation and activities of daily living should also be taken into consideration before the impact on academic performance can be predicted.

PART 2 FURTHER READING

Batshaw M L 1997 Children with disabilities, 4th edn. Maclennan and Petty, Sydney

Burdon B 1993 Australian developmental screening test. The Psychological Corporation, Harcourt Brace Jovanovich, Sydney

Frankenburg W K, Dodds J S, Archer P, Shapiro H, Bresnick B 1992 The Denver II: A major revision and restandardisation of the Denver Developmental Screening Test. Journal of Pediatrics 89:91–97

Glascoe F P 2001 Are over referrals on developmental screening tests really a problem? Archives of Pediatric Adolescent Medicine 155:54–59

Goldbloom R B 1992 Pediatric clinical skills. Churchill Livingstone, Edinburgh

Illingworth R 1980 The development of the infant and young child — abnormal and normal. Churchill Livingstone, Edinburgh

Lord C et al 2000 The Autism Diagnostic Observation Schedule-Generic: a standard measure of social and communication deficits associated with the spectrum of autism. Journal of Autism Development and Disorders 30:205–223

Pollack M 1993 Textbook of developmental paediatrics. Churchill Livingstone, Edinburgh

Rudolph M, Levine M 1999 Developmental problems in paediatrics and child health. Blackwell Science, Oxford, Ch.7

Shah B 2000 Atlas of pediatric clinical diagnosis. WB Saunders, Philadelphia

Skellern C, Rogers Y, O'Callaghan M 2001 A parent-completed developmental questionnaire: follow up of ex-premature infants. Journal of Paediatric Child Health, 37:125–129

Useful links

http://www.jrnldbp.com (Journal of Developmental and Behavioral Pediatrics)

http://www.nichcy.org (The National Information Centre for Children and Youth with Disabilities)

http://www.pedsexam.mc.duke.edu (Assessment of normal child development)

http://www.pedstest.com (Parent's evaluation of developmental status)

PART 3

SOCIAL AND PREVENTIVE PAEDIATRICS

5 The child and the family

N. Wigg and M. J. Robinson

> Virtually all aspects of early human development, from the brain's evolving circuitry to the child's capacity for empathy, are affected by environments and experiences that are encountered in a cumulative fashion, beginning early in the prenatal period and extending throughout the early childhood years.
>
> *(Shonkoff and Phillips 2000)*

A healthy child is one who is physically well, whose emotional needs are met and who is socially adjusted.

The physical needs of the child

- Care and protection from violence.
- An adequate diet to provide for nutritional needs.
- Protection against heat and cold in early life, and protection against physical dangers, e.g. fire, electricity, water, poisons, motor vehicles.
- Prevention of illness through good living standards, education, health surveillance, immunisation and other public health measures.

Children grow and thrive in the context of close and dependable relationships that provide love and nurturance, security, responsive interaction and encouragement of exploration. Without at least one such relationship development is disrupted and the consequences can be severe and longlasting.

The emotional and social needs of the child

- The opportunity to grow up in a family context with close and dependable relationships with one or more adults (parents).
- Consistent, positive caregiving.
- Reasonable limits to be set on the child's behaviour.
- Feelings of being worthwhile, concern for the wellbeing of others.
- The development of self-help skills and a sense of achievement.
- Opportunities for play, recreation and companionship.
- Opportunities to learn and explore.
- Sensitive responses to emotional needs during illness, particularly in chronic illness.
- Recognition of each child's individuality.
- Recognition of the basic rights of every child as outlined by the United Nations Declaration of the Rights of the Child.

To meet the physical, social and emotional needs of their children, parents, and others in a caring role must fulfil their own needs. These caregiver needs include:

- adequate housing and transport
- freedom from unnecessary economic stress
- freedom from community and domestic violence
- easy access to family support and early childhood services, such as child care, health and education services
- knowledge of how to access community supports and services
- social networks and extended family supports
- an understanding of child development and behaviour.

The growth and development of a child in the family and community context are determined by the interplay of genetic, physical, social and emotional factors and experience. The balance of risk and resilience factors influences a child's developmental pathway.

Risk factors preventing optimal progress might include:

- family conflict and disintegration
- economic disadvantage (low household income)
- parental mental health disorders
- individual child factors, such as low intellectual ability or difficult temperament
- external factors, such as unsafe neighbourhoods, environmental threats, war, etc.

Balanced against these are *resilience* factors, which are protective and promote wellbeing:

- safe, nurturing home environment
- consistent, supportive caregiving
- individual factors, e.g. normal intellectual ability
- sense/experience of success, self-determination and achievement.

The building blocks for intellectual development

- A loving and nurturing caregiving/family environment.
- Child rearing beliefs and practices designed to promote healthy adaptation.
- The opportunity to play, learn, explore and communicate.
- The growth of self-regulation of physiological systems, emotions, behaviours and social interactions.
- Positive and consistent human relationships.

- Access to developmentally appropriate educational settings: children are active participants in their own development and learning.
- Good physical health.

As a child grows from a newborn infant to an independent young adult, his or her social environment expands and diversifies. A young infant has all its needs met within the immediate family. Contact with other young children is important for the social and emotional development of the preschooler. A young teenager may spend more time with peers than with her or his family. The structure of the family, the style of parenting and the capacity to support the growing child's progressive independence, are all important determinants of the health and well-being of children.

The Australian family

Australian society is multicultural, with pluralistic values and child rearing practices. Child and family centred health care of children and young people should be carried out within the cultural and values framework relevant to the child.

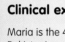

Clinical example

Maria is the 4 year old daughter of professional Pakistani parents. Her behaviour is demanding, overly active and often aggressive. Her communication skills are delayed. Both parents state that in their families of origin children are not disciplined until school age, and are cared for by the extended family.

Behavioural intervention needed to include these views of parenting.

Traditionally Australian families have been made up of mother (usually at home), father and two or more children. This picture of the 'nuclear' family no longer represents the Australian family.

Many families in Australia do not contain dependent children. The Australian Bureau of Statistics (ABS) reports that, in 1997, for families with dependent children:
- Seventy-four per cent of children aged 0–14 years lived in intact families (where all children lived with both natural parents).
- Eighteen per cent of children lived in one parent families.
- Of children living in one parent families, 89% lived with the mother and 11% with the father.
- Of all children living in couple families, 92% of children lived with married couples while the remainder lived with a couple in a de facto relationship.
- Over the last 10 years, the proportion of couple families with children has declined, while the proportion of one parent families has increased.

Three demographic trends have altered the structure of Australian families with children:
- the rate of divorce
- the age of marriage and having the first child
- the decision of women not to have children.

Over the last 20 years marriage rates have fallen, and the age at first marriage and age of first birth have increased dramatically. The median age of first marriage for women is now almost 27 and the median age of first birth is over 28 years. Consequently family size is smaller. In contrast, divorce rates rose in the 1970s, stabilised in the 1980s and increased slightly again in the 1990s; however, the rate of divorces involving children declined from 61% in 1986 to 54% in 1997.

There has been an increase in de facto relationships, which have become more socially acceptable in the last 20 years, including those in which children are involved. The proportion of ex-nuptial births (mothers not married) had risen to 29% in 1998, and at least half of these births were to women in de facto relationships.

Increasingly, women are deciding to remain childless. In the 1990s 27% of women did not have any children. Family size and fertility rate for indigenous women are also falling. During the 1960s indigenous women had a total fertility rate of around six babies per woman, which fell during the 1970s to about three and in the 1990s to 2.4. Indigenous women are more often younger at the time of first birth.

Families at work

- Forty-two per cent of children aged 0–14 years live in families where both parents are employed (full- or part-time).
- Eighteen per cent of children live in a family where the parent(s) are not employed.
- Nearly 21% of 0–2 year olds live in a family without an employed parent.
- Of children in one parent families, less than half of these parents are employed.
- A higher proportion of couple families have both parents employed, compared with one parent families that have the parent employed.

For many Australian families with children it is essential financially for both parents to have paid employment.

Clinical example

Casey, age 4, was brought to the emergency department of a busy metropolitan hospital, with a temperature of 38°C. Both his parents work full-time, and Casey had spent his day at the neighbourhood child care centre. After a 2 h wait, Casey was seen and sent home with antibiotics for a 'cold'. After-hours suburban medical services were not available.

'Mum at home, and Dad at work' is not the reality for many children. Accessible and affordable child care, family day care or other informal child caring/minding arrangements are needed.

Coincident with these changes in families and communities, the incidence of child abuse (physical, emotional and sexual) is thought to have risen over the last three decades; however, data about the rates of abuse are incomplete and much goes unrecorded.

Children of families in distress

Economic disadvantage/poverty

Poor people are more likely to have poor health. There is a gradient of socioeconomic effects on health: the more affluent you are, the more likely you are to experience good health; the poorer you are, the worse your health is likely to be. There is no magical cut-off point above which your health is protected.

Low household income is associated with lower purchasing power, material deprivation and reduced ability to participate in everyday community activities.

Low income households tend to occur in neighbourhoods that have fewer communal resources and where the social and physical environments are hazardous. Being poor is also often associated with much greater stress, feelings of lowered self-worth, powerlessness and helplessness. Mental and physical health problems follow.

International standards define poverty as a household income of less than 50% of the median income for that nation or State. In 1999, 12.5% (1 in 8) Australian children lived in poverty.

Single parent families are much more likely to live in poverty. The resultant inadequate diet, lack of opportunities, emotional stress, etc. may be coupled with the emotional turmoil both children and parents experience in separation and divorce. In general terms, children in one parent families have poorer mental and physical health than their peers in two parent families. However, much of this difference can be explained by lower household income and the stress of financial hardship. The majority of children in one parent families experience good health.

Low family income may affect the health of the children in many ways, for example:
- lower birth weight
- lower rates of breastfeeding
- poorer vaccination rates
- poorer growth
- higher rates of infectious diseases.

Socially marginalized families/groups

Indigenous Australians (Aboriginal and Torres Strait Islander peoples) have poorer health than other Australians. Indigenous children have poorer nutrition and growth, higher rates of infectious disease, higher injury rates and high rates of infant and child mortality.

The reasons for the persistence of relatively poor health of indigenous children are complex. Certainly living conditions, fewer educational opportunities and poor access to goods and services all contribute. So do cultural disruption, high levels of poverty, lack of access to culturally acceptable health care, and racism.

Clinical example

Taliah is the third child of a 21 year old Aboriginal mother. The family lives in a small town in the Northern Territory. Taliah is 6 months old, is growing and developing well, is breastfed and is free of illness. Her older brother and sister have much poorer health. Before her birth Taliah's mother joined the local 'strong women, strong babies' programme.

Multicultural Australia includes many immigrant groups whose children are at greater health risk. Many families come to Australia to escape persecution and civil disruption, and bring the legacy of trauma and loss.

The major problems experienced by ethnic minority groups include lack of employment opportunity (and associated low household income), social isolation, non familiarity with health care and other social services, and barriers due to communication problems and cultural differences.

Culturally sensitive health care services that include bilingual workers and interpreter services are essential. Doctors and other child health workers should recognise the vast range of child rearing and health care practices of ethnic groups in Australia.

Families affected by mental health problems and drug abuse

Children's early development and health depends on the health and wellbeing of their parents. Postnatal depression is relatively common, affecting about 15% of mothers. Severe postnatal depression impacts on the establishment of infant–mother relationships (attachment). Disorders of attachment result in infant health problems, such as sleep problems, failure to thrive, disturbed behaviour such as excessive crying, and subsequent emotional and behavioural problems.

Children who grow up in families where one or both parents have a mental health problem frequently experience inconsistent parenting and disturbed relationships within the family. The scene is set for such children to develop behavioural, emotional and mental health problems.

The Western Australian Child Health Survey identified that 20% of 12–16 year olds had a significant mental health problem (Zubrick et al 1995). Thus one in five teenage school children will have a mental health problem and most will not seek or receive treatment (Ch. 16).

Alcohol is by far the most widely used and abused drug in our society. Drinking alcohol is not only accepted, but expected, behaviour in Australia. Approximately two out of three men and one in two women drink alcohol at least once a week. Of those who drink, about 10% of men and 6% of women are in the medium to high risk groups. The abuse of alcohol by one or both parents has a profound effect on the family.

Clinical example

Trent, a 9 year old boy, was noted to be performing poorly at school by his teacher. He was a bright student but had become inattentive and frequently disrupted other children in the classroom. His writing had deteriorated. When the family was contacted, it was discovered that Trent's father had recently left the family after months of disharmony due to his excessive drinking.

Social worker assistance was obtained and Trent received counselling. Trent is now involved in Scouts and his school performance is improving.

Children of alcohol dependent parents suffer anxiety and unhappiness and may be exposed to violence and argument. In many cases this leads to the child becoming antisocial, engaging in alcohol/drug use and developing mental health problems, such as depression. Alcohol and drug (e.g. heroin) addiction frequently leads to financial stress in a family, together with deterioration in family relationships and parental separation. The consequences on children are severe.

Family violence

Sixteen per cent of Australian couples experience violence in the relationship. For 4% of couples the level of physical violence is such that physical harm is a likely outcome.

Our society tolerates high levels of violence in the media, in sport and in the community generally. However, violence in the family context has a profound effect on children. Violence between parents is frequently associated with violence towards their children.

Children who witness violence as a 'problem solving' technique at home may adopt similar patterns of behaviour, particularly when they themselves become parents.

Services for the child and family

General practitioners (family doctors) provide the mainstay of health services for children and families. Their primary health care services are complemented by a range of Government funded community health and social services. It is beyond the scope of this chapter to detail these services, and the following are given as examples only.

For families with young infants

- Well-child care in child health centres.
- Home visiting programmes, for families with additional needs, e.g. Family CARE Program, Good Beginnings.
- Residential services.
- Parent help lines, child health lines (24 h, 7 day telephone advice lines).
- Printed and online information services.

For families with preschoolers

- Health surveillance, including immunisation and health promotion.
- Injury prevention and safety promotion.
- Health service component to child care and preschool services.
- Telephone and other information services.
- Health screening prior to school entry — provided by child health nurses.
- Developmental assessment clinics and early intervention services.

For families with school aged children

- Support services provided by education departments, e.g. guidance officers, counsellors.
- Assessments of children by child health nurses.
- Health education.
- Community mental health services.
- School oral health (dental) services.

The Federal Government provides a number of pensions or benefits administered by Carelink and the Department of Family and Community Services. These include the family allowance, child care supplements, supporting parents and carer benefits.

State Governments and non Government agencies (often Church affiliated) provide many family and community support services.

The field of family support services is complex and accessing the 'right service at the right time' is frequently a major problem for families experiencing distress. Family doctors and other child health workers need to know about the child and family services available in their area, and about Government benefits for families.

6 Indigenous culture and health

G. D. Stokes, C. Jeffries-Stokes

PART 1: AUSTRALIAN INDIGENOUS CULTURE AND HEALTH

Definition

The definition of an Aboriginal or Torres Strait Islander commonly used in Australia requires three criteria be satisfied. The definition is a person who is of Aboriginal or Torres Strait Islander descent, who identifies as an Aboriginal or Torres Strait Islander and who is recognised as an Aboriginal or Torres Strait Islander within the community in which they live.

Population statistics

The number of Aboriginal and Torres Strait Islander people living in Australia at the time of white settlement will never be known accurately but it was probably at least 300 000 and possibly as many as one million people. By the 1920s, this number had plummeted to about 60 000 due to the introduction of new diseases, brutal treatment and the effects of rapid social and cultural change. Data from the 1991 Australian Bureau of Statistics (ABS) census show that almost 265 000 people identified themselves as Aboriginal or Torres Strait Islander. By the year 2000 this was estimated to have grown to almost 500 000 people, or 2.5% of the population of Australia.

The age structure of the Aboriginal and Torres Strait Islander population of Australia is markedly different from that of the rest of the population. High fertility rates and short life expectancy combine to result in a very young population. Forty per cent of the indigenous population is under the age of 15 years compared with 21% of the non indigenous population, with only 2.5 of the indigenous population over the age of 65 years compared with 12% of the non indigenous population.

The history of Aboriginal people in Australia

No one knows for sure when Aboriginal people first came to Australia — the Dreamtime stories describe the creation of Aboriginal people, the land, plants and animals as occurring at the same time and Aboriginal people believe that they have always been here in Australia. Scientific evidence suggests that Aboriginal people have been here for at least 50 000 years.

Settlement by non Aboriginal people in Australia has been relatively recent in historical terms. For example, the official British settlement of Western Australia began in Albany in 1826, and from here non Aboriginal people spread out across the state. This took some time. The Goldfields were first explored by non Aboriginal people just over 100 years ago; in the northern Goldfields white settlement began only about 80 years ago, and in some places as recently as 60 years ago. This represents white settlement of the Goldfields in living memory — there are elderly Aboriginal people who can still recall seeing the first white person who came to their area. This is similar to many areas throughout Australia.

There is ample evidence that the first settlers thought of the Aboriginal people as savages and had very little understanding of Aboriginal culture and way of life. Aboriginal people were shot, poisoned, imprisoned and pushed off their land into camps or reserves on the outskirts of settlements. They had little immunity from the diseases brought by the settlers and hundreds died from infections such as measles, leprosy and influenza. Aboriginal people infected with sexually transmitted diseases or leprosy were arrested and were transported to remote isolation camps.

In 1905 in Western Australia the Aborigines Act was passed and remained in force until 1963. This meant that the Chief Protector of Aborigines became the legal guardian of all mixed race children and Aboriginal people lost all rights of citizenship in their own country. They could not marry, get work, move about, or go to school or to hospital without permission from the Chief Protector. They could not be in town after 6 p.m. and had to carry a 'dog licence' or identification papers all the time. Their children were forcibly removed and put into missions where they were deliberately separated from their families and culture. Many were also subjected to emotional, physical and sexual abuse. Many never saw their parents again and some still have not been able to even find out who their families are. The missions operated under the 1905 Act until 1963 and then continued until the mid 1970s in many areas as, even though the legislation had changed, community attitudes had not.

In 1967 a referendum was conducted and Aboriginal people were finally given equal rights under the law as citizens of Australia. In practice enormous inequality still exists.

Health status

One area where inequality is most evident is in the health status of indigenous Australians compared to non indigenous Australians. The life expectancy of indigenous men and women is 18–20 years less than that of their non indigenous counterparts and the infant mortality rate is about three times higher for infants of indigenous parents.

Indigenous Australians suffer higher rates of disease in almost all categories than non indigenous Australians and are admitted to hospital almost twice as often.

Infant and child mortality rates are 2–3 times higher for Aboriginal and Torres Strait children than for other Australian children. They are more likely to be of low birth weight (less than 2.5 kg). Aboriginal and Torres Strait Islander children suffer higher rates of:
- upper and lower respiratory tract illness
- gastrointestinal illness
- skin infestation.

Many also suffer from diseases that are more common in developing countries, such as rheumatic fever and chronic otitis media. The higher rates of many of these illnesses are probably due to the substandard conditions in which many Aboriginal and Torres Strait Islander people live.

The skin system and family relationships

Many of Australia's Aboriginal people believe that all people in the world belong to a 'skin group'. Most people, however, have long ago lost the tradition of passing on and identifying their skin groups. Aboriginal people all over Australia maintain the skin groups and the customs of relationships defined by the skin groups. Some Aboriginal people have lost contact with their culture and may not know the name of their skin group but they still conduct their relationships within the family and within the wider community according to the customs handed down in their families. These customs have their origins in the skin group system.

In the Eastern Goldfields and Central Desert areas of Western Australia there are four major skin groups, although in some areas these are further subdivided. The names of the skin groups in the Wongutha language of the Eastern Goldfields are Gurrimurra, Boorungu, Panaka and Tjarru.

Each family will have members of all four skin groups. For example a Gurrimurra man marries a Boorungu woman. Their children will be Panaka. A Panaka man marries a Tjarru woman and their children will be Gurrimurra. A child will always be the same skin group as the paternal grandfather.

The four skin groups define all relationships in the Aboriginal community. All members of the same skin groups will be brothers (goorda) and sisters (gaggu) or grandfather and grandchild (dhamu) or grandmother and grandchild (guburli). The members of other skin groups will in turn be father, mother, spouse or in laws. This is regardless of whether any blood relationships exist or not. Marriage is only allowed between people who have the appropriate skin relationship: a member of one skin group can only marry someone from one other, strictly defined skin group. Blood relationships are also considered and marriage between people who are closely related by blood, even if their skin groups are compatible, may not be allowed.

The skin groups define how people will relate to each other — grandparents must be treated with respect. Members of the same skin group (brothers and sisters and grandparents) are responsible for each other's social and moral education and conduct. Parents are responsible for the love and nurturing of their children. In many areas punishment should not be meted out by the parents — it is the responsibility of the older members of the same skin group. This is particularly important in the medical setting because the parents alone may not be allowed to make major decisions, give consent for procedures or make a child submit to treatment. In many cases these issues should be dealt with by the grandparents and the whole family needs to be involved.

The skin groups also define important spiritual and ceremonial roles in communities that still practise traditional culture and ceremonies. These are usually secret and are not discussed outside the skin group.

Aboriginal people are able to determine the skin group of a newcomer by recognising spiritual characteristics and by knowing the newcomer's family and kin relationships. The skin groups have nothing at all to do with physical appearance and do not relate to skin colour.

Non Aboriginal people also have skin groups. Once they have become familiar to Aboriginal people they will be able to work out their skin groups by observation of the types of relationships that they form with Aboriginal people. Until the skin group of a newcomer is determined it may be very difficult to communicate with Aboriginal people but, once a skin group is recognised, that person will be accepted as part of the Aboriginal community and extended family.

A different way of thinking

Australian Aboriginal people do not think of themselves as individuals; they see things from the perspective of the tribe or community. Nothing is owned by an individual: everything, including children, belong to the group.

Because of this sense of community, the family, cultural and spiritual responsibilities come before all other responsibilities. Providing for the family today may be much more important than saving for something that may never happen.

Many Aboriginal people do not think of time in the same way as non Aboriginal people; they rarely keep watches or clocks, and things happen when the time is right rather than at the right time.

People are valued not for their achievements but for the people that they are; this is particularly true of strangers and non Aboriginal people — titles and academic achievement mean very little. Age, experience and personal qualities are much more important.

Health, illness and spirituality: an Aboriginal perspective

All aspects of life have a deep spiritual dimension for Aboriginal people. The concepts of health and illness cannot be separated from this, and good physical health is not possible without consideration of family, land and spirit.

Many Aboriginal people believe that illness occurs when spiritual health is compromised as a result of wrongdoing or perhaps magic. Because of the concept of family and community, illness may strike because of transgressions by another person, usually a family member, and may be seen as a form of payback. Whatever the cause, it may be necessary to take steps to address the spiritual causes of illness before good health can be restored.

Issues surrounding childbirth and gynaecology are seen as strictly women's business and anything to do with the male genitalia, urinary system or body markings is considered to be men's business. This is highly secret for many Aboriginal people and should not even be discussed where a person of the opposite sex might overhear the conversation. Such issues need to be addressed very sensitively and privately.

Death

When an Aboriginal person dies, many believe that their spirit must make the journey to the spirit world. This journey must not be interrupted so the name of the person who has died is not spoken. This is because the spirit may feel that it is being called back to the world of the living and not be able to rest. Even people who have the same or a similar name as the dead person will take another name or use a nickname for a time so that there is no confusion for the spirit. Often a special name ('Gunbina' in the Wongutha language) is used by people with the same or a similar name. This usually continues for at least a year or until after the spring rains that wash the earth and renew it.

Stories about the person who has died will be told and their life celebrated using a special term ('Rubagee' in the Wongutha language) to refer to them, or terms such as my brother, your father, etc. instead of naming them.

The cause of death needs to be explained and any people who may have contributed to or caused the death need to be identified and appropriate punishment delivered. It is important for any medical staff involved in the care of the person who has died to talk to the family and, if possible, explain the cause of death.

Mourning ('sorry business') is an important part of the ceremonies surrounding death. Many Aboriginal people will feel the need to mourn loudly and even injure themselves as a demonstration of their grief. This may be in part to ensure that the spirit feels suitably appreciated. There is a large public display of grief by the family and the funeral arrangements are usually taken care of by the 'in laws' to allow the family to grieve properly.

The funeral and burial take place when the family is all assembled and people will often travel great distances to attend. This is very important and is often considered more important than any other responsibilities (including work). Another ceremony is held a year later to complete the burial and mourning.

Approaching Aboriginal people

Many people are unsure of how to approach Aboriginal people and particularly wish to avoid causing offence. This frequently results in missed opportunities for meeting and getting to know Aboriginal people. Here are some simple guidelines to assist in these situations. They are by no means complete and Aboriginal people from different areas will have different customs but these hints should help to establish relationships so that these differences and customs can be explored.

Eye contact

Most Aboriginal people consider it extremely rude to establish direct eye contact. For some people it will indicate a lack of manners, while for others it is considered highly offensive and a breach of traditional law. It is therefore not usual for Aboriginal people to sit or stand opposite another person, and it is better to sit beside or at right angles to the other person so that you both look at the same view rather than at each other.

Introductions

It is usual to introduce yourself by name — first name and surname. This helps to establish who you are and who your family is. This also helps in working out your skin group. Names for some groups also have great power and if you know an Aboriginal person's name but they do not know your name they may feel very uncomfortable and in a position of weakness in the relationship. To establish that you are all on an equal footing it is advisable to introduce yourself properly.

Shaking hands

When Aboriginal people meet they usually touch each other, often hugging each other but at least shaking hands. They do not usually expect a non Aboriginal person to want to touch them so they may not offer their hand to a stranger to shake but you should offer your hand. This establishes that you have no fear of touching them and that you meet as equals. Sometimes it may be awkward to shake hands, and in this case a light touch on the shoulder is acceptable and will not cause offence with Aboriginal people of either sex.

Conversation

It is important to give an opportunity for the Aboriginal person to get to know you, to know what you are like and to work out your skin group. If you already know other Aboriginal people it is particularly helpful to mention them as you may find you have friends or acquaintances in common. It is also very reassuring for Aboriginal people if you have visited their country — so ask where they are from and mention it if you have visited the area. It is equally important to show some of your own personality. All Aboriginal people consider themselves related to each other, so they are usually quite informal with each other and, although this will depend on the circumstances of the meeting, it is usually best to just relax and be yourself.

The right words

The word Aborigine came from the Latin *ab origine* and means from the beginning. It is used to describe the original inhabitants of Australia. This implies that they are a single group but in fact they are many diverse and different groups with different names, languages, traditions and culture, although the groups have strong links with each other. Wherever possible tribal names should be used: Koori, Yamatji, Wongutha, Ngoongar and so on.

When the term Aboriginal is used it is always spelt with a capital A. Prior to 1967 Aboriginal people were classified as part of the native fauna or animals of Australia. After 1967 they were given citizenship in their own country. Therefore a capital 'A' is always used in recognition of their humanity, unlike cats, dogs and other animals who are referred to with lower case. In general the term 'Aboriginal people' is preferred, rather than 'Aborigines'. Although Aboriginal people may use other terms to refer to themselves, such as Blackfella or Blacks, these terms should not be used by non Aboriginal people and may cause great offence.

PART 2: MAORI VIEW OF CHILD HEALTH AND ILLNESS
L. Buchanan

Children in the New Zealand population

Children under the age of 15 currently make up 23% of New Zealand's population. The ethnic breakdown of these 830 000 children contains four major groupings:

- European: (60%)
- Maori: (24%)
- Pacific Islands: (7%)
- Asian: (5%).

Who is Maori?

Until the 1980s, the official census definition of this question was based on a child having 'half or more' Maori origin. Now, however, census data and common usage define Maori as a person of Maori ancestry who chooses to identify as Maori. It is important to be aware that the unifying term Maori really dates from the time of European occupation of New Zealand.

Historically, tribal divisions were quite marked. Informed observers as recently as the 1930s referred to Aotearoa (New Zealand) as a series of islands joined by narrow strips of land!

What are the traditional features of the culture in which a Maori child might be raised?

The shared understandings of the Maori would see the child as offering a hope for the future, a continuity of the inheritance lines (whakapapa). Moreover, the child could not be seen as separate from the extended family (whanau). The child's grandparents would be expected to play an important supportive role. Maori has been described as a culture that puts people before self so that the young child would be expected to receive considerable arohatanga (warmth and love) and awhinatanga (help and assistance).

The truth of course is that modern Maori live in diverse cultural worlds. There is no one definition that will cover the range of lifestyles currently practised by Maori. Some tamariki (children) will be raised in relatively isolated communities in frequent contact with the activities carried out on the marae (special meeting place for a subtribe) for their families. Others will be raised in a city, with perhaps only occasional contact with an urban marae or no contact whatsoever. Moreover, globalisation has hit Maoridom, with increasing numbers of Maori children now living in the larger Australian cities.

What are the particular features defining health for Maori?

Traditionally, health was seen as the responsibility of the whole community. The development of health had to include manaaki (care for others), whaanaungatanga (maintaining the family) and wairua (spiritual values). Much of the regulation of health was related to very ancient concepts of tapu and noa. A tapu situation which might apply to a person (for example, a woman who had just had a baby), a place or an object would be off limits with restricted contact. Items classified as noa would have relaxed access. Sickness or illness coming to an individual would be viewed as the result of a breach of tapu.

For Maori the Eurocentric notions of a mind and body split or equivalent theories in approaching health would be seen as incomprehensible. Wholeness or wellness for Maori was summarised brilliantly by Mason Durie as needing to involve the four walls of a house, each supporting the others. These four pillars are:

1. taha hinengaro (thoughts and feelings)
2. wairua (spiritual side)
3. taha tinana (physical side)
4. taha whanau (family).

In this context it is not surprising that the traditional healing activities placed a heavy emphasis on karakia — prayers and incantations. Massage, water and occasionally surgical interventions also played their part. Medicinal infusions, poultices or lotions also were used but to some extent the increased development and interest in this type of remedy has accelerated since European contact.

Historical issues of relevance to Maori health

The document servicing a partnership for the English Crown with Maori and thus forming the basis for the modern New Zealand nation was the Treaty of Waitangi. Maori far outnumbered Europeans in the New Zealand of 1840. If Maori concepts of health are firmly based in Maori culture, then a founding document promising recognition and protection of that culture is seen as highly relevant to Maori health. Debate on these points has been particularly intense during the last 20 years. In the health debate on the Treaty, Maori have placed particular importance on the second article promising protection of their treasures (health is seen as one of these) and on the third article promising the same rights (taken to include health rights) as their new English brothers and sisters.

It is a matter of speculation now how sincere Lord Normanby might have been in the language he suggested should be used in the Treaty, when he was contemporaneously dealing with British interests in the opium war in Hong Kong and in diplomatic difficulties with the Russian Court at St Petersburg.

Further to this, a fourth clause, read only at the important first signings at Waitangi, has certainly provoked significant comment in discussions on Maori health: 'The Governor says the several faiths of England, of the Wesleyans, of Rome and also the Maori custom, shall alike be protected by him.'

Current social and economic circumstances in which Maori children are being raised

Care needs to be taken in either overcalling or undercalling available total population data that measure the social and economic circumstances of a people. One frustration for Maori is that the items that can be measured more readily are external forces that may shape a person's wellbeing (for example, house ownership, income level, formal educational attainment). Even where apparent or implied deprivation seems to exist it should be clear that not all people will see themselves as deprived. Internal forces that may be just as crucial to a person's wellbeing are much harder to measure (for example, loss of knowledge about what it is to be Maori or loss of contact with extended family or loss of traditional tribal land).

While acknowledging these limitations, the New Zealand Ministry of Health's 1999 document on social inequalities in health has stark data on the deprivation profiles of European and other ethnic groups versus the Maori ethnic group. The profiles of 'advantage' are very unfavourable to Maori. Maori unemployment rates are high. Likewise, comparisons of Maori and non Maori household income distribution in 1997 show Maori over-represented in the lowest two quintiles and very under-represented in the highest economic quintile. A significant reliance on Government grants for many Maori is the background for the view that some Maori elders put that one of the biggest challenges ahead for Maori is to be weaned off the breast of Government welfare.

If one moves more to the current ethos of the circumstances in which Maori children are raised, two additional points stand out:

- It is a myth that Maori have big families. The huge drop in the Maori fertility rate between 1960 and 1990 means that, with the exception of adolescent fertility rates, Maori fertility rates are very similar to the rates for non Maori.

- Nearly 40% of Maori children are living in one parent families, compared with around 15% of children of European ethnicity.

Working with the Maori child and family

Welcoming every member of the supporting family (whanau) or just an individual parent needs to be undertaken with courtesy and respect. Some general enquiries about what is happening in the family and where they are from are advisable before taking a formal history of the concerns about the child. Direct eye contact from an older child or some of the whanau might not occur at first and should not be interpreted as rudeness or diffidence. If the family are running late or have missed previous appointments, remember that people other than doctors can also have busy lives. Consultants on teaching ward rounds or in multidisciplinary clinic sessions might like to introduce or refer to the others present with them as their supporting whanau. If the doctor has some familiarity with Maori greetings and enquiries, this knowledge should first perhaps be used in an exchange with the child rather than the adults present. Maori can feel embarrassed if the non Maori professional launches into te reo (the language) and they are non speakers.

It is important tactfully to consider what the special significance of a child's symptoms might be to that family. A carefully taken family history is therefore essential. An alertness to the normal Maori view that matters of a psychological nature can cause physical symptoms and that the life of the child has a spiritual and sacred component should not be overlooked.

When it comes to the clinical examination of the child it should be remembered that the head, the breasts and the genitalia are customarily tapu areas, so the usual sensitivities about these parts of the examination should be respected.

A doctor should tend towards formality in dress code in working with Maori — especially if a younger person. One needs to remember that the doctor is a kind of Western medicine equivalent of the tohunga (person with special training and responsibilities to guard those things sacred and special). Certainly, if invited to a special function on a marae the doctor needs to find out in advance what the protocol requirements are for that marae and observe them.

Should a Maori child in one's care die then there is a real sense of urgency within the extended family for the child's body to be given over to the family as soon as is feasible. This is partly to facilitate grieving but also to recognise the special spiritual nature of the child and the child's membership of the extended family.

Some specific problem areas for Maori children and how these might be overcome

Mortality and hospitalisation rate

Compared with non Maori children, tamariki Maori are significantly more likely to die before reaching the age of 15 years (Fig. 6.1).

The leading contributors to this differential mortality are:

- sudden infant death syndrome
- injuries and poisonings
- road traffic accidents.
- respiratory conditions.

Paralleling this increased mortality risk is a significantly increased hospitalisation rate, especially in children under the age of 5 years (Fig. 6.2). Respiratory conditions, injuries and poisonings are the main contributors to this.

Specific challenges

Sudden infant death syndrome (Ch. 13)

The rate for this continues to be 3–4 times higher in Maori compared to non Maori. Decreasing maternal smoking in pregnancy and after the child's birth, more culturally focused promotion of breastfeeding, and pointing out the risks of bedsharing with the baby in situations involving smoking and the taking of either cannabis or alcohol should help reduce this risk.

Respiratory problems in childhood

Much of the morbidity and mortality from infections and/or asthma is concentrated in the preschool years. Continued campaigns to reduce the high incidence of cigarette smoking amongst Maori women should help here. In addition, the promotion of substantial breastfeeding until at least the child's first birthday should

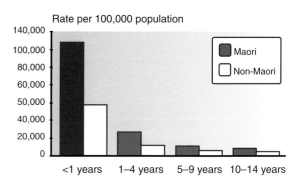

Rate per 100,000 population

Fig. 6.2 Hospitalisation rates from all causes, Maori and non Maori 0–14 year olds, by age group, 1995. Source: Ministry of Health 1998.

assist. In asthma, compliance issues with recommended programmes appear to be helped by having services delivered by Maori service providers.

Child abuse

Compared with non Maori children, tamariki are four times more likely to be hospitalised for injuries sustained as a result of deliberately inflicted physical harm. Notifications to the statutory authority for investigating child abuse in New Zealand have likewise been found to be higher for Maori.

This is a complex challenge for Maoridom. Promoting traditional cultural beliefs about the importance of children, what it is to be Maori, and keeping people in touch with their whanau, should help. The pressures on single parents needs more open discussion among Maori.

Injuries and poisonings

Injury hospitalisation data for children aged less than 15 years mirrors injury death trends. The areas not reflected in this are drowning and suffocation. Both these problems are also unfortunately overrepresented among Maori.

To some extent these problems must represent issues relating to the child's supervision by the whanau. Their prevalence suggests dysfunctional whanaus or situations in which parents have lost contact with what it is to be Maori and have children.

Behavioural problems in schools

The suspension and expulsion rate from schools might be taken as a marker of more serious behavioural difficulties in children. Comparative data on this question have been analysed for the years 1992–1997 and show higher rates for Maori. Some of these data might reflect inappropriate management techniques of Maori children by a predominantly non Maori teaching force. On the other hand, adverse behaviour by children has been shown to be linked with socioeconomic disadvantage and family adversity.

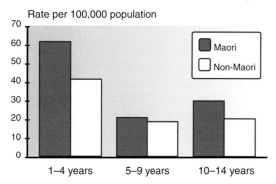

Rate per 100,000 population

Fig. 6.1 Mortality from all causes, Maori and non Maori 1–14 year olds, by age group, 1995. Source: Ministry of Health 1998.

The demonstration that attention deficit hyperactivity disorder (ADHD) is an important contributor to difficult childhood behaviours, and that undetected or inadequately treated ADHD is associated with poor judgement and risk taking behaviour in adult life, calls for alertness to this possibility needing consideration when seeing a Maori child with difficult behaviour. ADHD certainly exists among Maori families, in line with the demonstration that this problem occurs in many cultures.

Glue ear

This has been a challenge known to be overrepresented among Maori children for many years. Hospitalisation rates for this problem between 1980 and 1997 show higher rates for Maori children.

A marked reduction in this condition could be achieved by promoting more prolonged breastfeeding, reducing cigarette smoking in the child's environment and in high risk families, and perhaps delaying the start of the child's attendance in a kohanga reo (language nest) or other preschool facility until age 2 years.

Rheumatic fever

This is now almost exclusively a Polynesian disease in New Zealand. The discharge rate from New Zealand hospitals for acute rheumatic fever is seven times higher for Maori than non Maori. In some parts of New Zealand with a higher Maori population, incidence figures for this problem are as high as reported anywhere in the world.

While it may be true that some genetic predisposition plays a part in this high incidence, it is also likely that overcrowding in houses contributes. Primary prevention by obtaining compliance with 10 day antibiotic courses for streptococcal throat infections would help. Earlier rather than later recognition of the signs of acute rheumatic fever and effective surveillance of appropriate secondary prevention programmes is required.

Immunisation rates

The accurate collection of data on this question has vexed many paediatricians in New Zealand during the last 30 years. What has been a nearly uniform finding, however, is that immunisation uptake rates in Maori are only about 70% of those seen in non Maori. Progress in reducing this discrepancy has been associated with programmes particularly targeting Maori, such as hepatitis B immunisation, or in having Maori health providers take over the task as part of a core package.

Making contact with the Maori community

Doctors working with children should be as familiar with the specific local Maori health initiatives that relate to

Clinical example

Rangi, a 7 year old Maori boy, had a slightly sore throat 10 days before his acute presentation. This was treated at home with paracetamol and settled. Then, over a 36 hour period, he developed back pains followed by a swollen tender left ankle. The ankle pain woke him at night and he had difficulty weight bearing.

He had a low grade fever of 38.2°C; his left ankle was hot, tender and swollen and he complained of right knee pain. Other joints were not involved. On cardiac examination there was a soft mid diastolic murmur near the apex. Rangi's Hb was 112 g/l, total WBC 25 000/mm^3 and ESR 105 mm/h. There was no growth from a throat swab but his ASOT titre was elevated at 1:1860.

A presumptive diagnosis of acute rheumatic fever gained further support from an echocardiogram showing changes in the mitral valve. His acute symptoms settled within 24 hours of commencing aspirin. No further cardiac signs developed and he was discharged home after 5 days. Arrangements were made with a public health nurse for him to receive injections of benzathine penicillin every 3 weeks. Compliance was high because an uncle also had rheumatic heart disease and had had further severe valvular heart damage because of repeated episodes of rheumatic fever.

children as they should be with organisations providing well child care or supporting specific chronic illnesses. Most public hospitals have a definite Maori liaison service, while marae based health clinics are becoming more common.

The way forward

Back to the future! The first step must be to put the house in order. Durie's idea of the four walls of the house needing to be in harmony cannot be overemphasised. Maori do need to rediscover what it is to be Maori. Strengthening the whanau has to be the first step in any 'closing the gaps' policy for tamariki. With whanau and broader tribal support for the child, sensible gains can be made from the Maori desire for health services for Maori to be given by Maori. The wise use of any monies becoming available from Government compensation for previous land acquisitions or settlements could help this process.

In the 1996 census, only 2.5% of New Zealand medical practitioners identified themselves as Maori, while the total Maori population was 14.5%; therefore, in the short to medium term non Maori medical practitioners of good will — sensitive to Maori nuances — are going to continue to be needed to support Maori children and their families.

Kia kaha! Kia manawanui! Tihei Mauriora!

7 Nutrition

R. T. L. Couper, V. Gallard

Children require a healthy diet for normal day to day activity and for growth and development. Nutrient and energy requirements change markedly during infancy, childhood and adolescence. Life events, such as school and job performance, and the development of lifestyle related diseases, such as hypertension, obesity, hyperlipidaemia and some cancers, may be influenced by childhood diet.

Nutrients

Nutrients are food components required for optimal growth, development and body function. Macronutrients (protein, fat and carbohydrate) are energy sources and are essential for cellular homeostasis. Micronutrients, which include vitamins, minerals and trace elements, are required in much smaller amounts.

Individual nutrient requirements vary with age, size, growth and health status. Recommended dietary intakes (RDIs) are the levels of essential nutrients considered to be adequate to meet the known nutritional needs of virtually all healthy people. The RDIs are derived from estimates of requirements for different ages and sex and include a wide safety margin to allow for variation in absorption and metabolism. The RDIs are population standards and do not account for specific individual needs, which may vary due to illness, injury or activity. They do, however, exceed the nutrient requirements of most individuals and should be used only as a guide. The Australian RDIs for infants and children are provided in the National Health and Medical Research Council (NHMRC) *Recommended Dietary Intakes for Use in Australia* (1992).

Dietary Guidelines for Australians

The Australian NHMRC released 'Dietary Guidelines for Children and Adolescents' in 1995 (Table 7.1). The guidelines apply to healthy children from birth to 18 years of age; they focus on the development of healthy eating patterns, and apply to the total diet. The dietary guidelines, in conjunction with the RDIs, assist in the provision of complete nutritional advice.

Table 7.1 Dietary Guidelines for Children and Adolescents, National Health and Medical Research Council, Australia, 1995

- Encourage and support breastfeeding
- Children need appropriate food and physical activity to grow and develop normally. Growth should be checked regularly
- Enjoy a wide variety of nutritious foods
- Eat plenty of breads and cereals, vegetables (including legumes) and fruits
- Low fat diets are not suitable for young children. For older children, a diet low in fat, and in particular low in saturated fat, is appropriate
- Encourage water as a drink. Alcohol is not recommended for children
- Eat only a moderate amount of sugars and foods containing added sugars
- Choose low salt foods

Guidelines on specific nutrients
- Eat foods containing calcium
- Eat foods containing iron

Energy

Energy from food is released during metabolism and is required by the body for:
- growth and synthesis of new tissue
- metabolic processes
- physiological functions
- activity.

Fat, protein, carbohydrate and alcohol provide energy which is measured in kilojoules (kJ) or kilocalories (kcal), 1 kcal providing 4.182 kJ. Fat provides a concentrated source of energy, contributing 37 kJ/g, approximately twice that provided by an equivalent weight of protein or carbohydrate. Fat contributes 50% of total energy in breast milk or standard infant formula. The average diet of older children provides 30–40% of total energy from fat, 45–55% from carbohydrate and about 15% from protein. Most of the energy intake in children is used for growth and development. Recommendations for energy intake are difficult to determine, even for individuals of similar age, sex and size, because requirements vary. The NHMRC recommended energy intakes for Australian infants and children (1991) are based on FAO/WHO/UNU estimates of energy requirements (1985).

Nutritional assessment

Nutritional assessment should combine physical examination and laboratory tests with an adequate assessment of feeding practice and dietary intake. If children do not receive adequate nutrition, they do not grow. Childhood growth is best assessed by auxological measurements, particularly weight and height. When a child fails to grow because of poor nutritional intake, he or she loses weight before linear growth declines, and usually stunting occurs before circumferential growth of the head declines. Serial measurements are much more useful than single measurements. Interpretation of trends may allow the genesis of a problem to be pinpointed. Psychosocial deprivation may result in growth failure in the absence of other illnesses and despite seemingly adequate intake.

Many countries have their own growth standards which are adaptable for their ethnocultural mix. A child's growth status is usually expressed as a percentile of normal. However, the weight or height at a point in time is expressed more accurately as a standard deviation score or Z score. In the developing world, WHO charts allow weight to be expressed as a percentage of ideal body weight. More sophisticated measurements such as the body mass index (BMI: weight(kg)/height (m^2)) are more useful in adults than in growing children and adolescents. Recently (2000) good age related international standards for BMI in children have been developed from age cross sectional studies in various countries.

Physical examination is valuable but is not particularly sensitive for detecting subtle signs of malnutrition. Children should be inspected for muscle wasting, which is usually most prominent in the femoral quadriceps and gluteal muscles. The integument, teeth, bones and eyes should be inspected for signs of vitamin and trace element deficiency.

Laboratory parameters are not particularly useful. A decline in serum proteins, particularly albumin, occurs late in malnutrition. Prealbumin and retinol binding globulin are better indices of early malnutrition than serum albumin. A full blood examination, and in particular the mean cell volume, may serve to indicate iron, folate and vitamin B$_{12}$ deficiency. Other trace elements and vitamins can be measured in plasma. However, red blood cell or buccal mucosal cell measurements more accurately reflect cellular deficiencies.

Basal metabolic rate and resting energy expenditure can be assessed using indirect calorimetry. Cell mass can be determined by measuring total body potassium-40 (^{40}K) which is a naturally occurring stable isotope. Total body water can be measured by bromide dilution, deuterium labelled water and bioelectrical impedance. Total body nitrogen can be measured by neutron capture. These expensive methods are available only as research tools.

Assessment of dietary intake

The adequacy of children's dietary intake should be determined by asking:

- what they eat
- how much they eat
- when and where they eat
- who feeds them
- what they like to eat.

The parent or primary caregiver should be asked what the child usually eats during a typical day. It is necessary to ask specific structured questions to ensure accurate and detailed information. For example, do not ask what is eaten for breakfast, but rather what is the first thing that the child eats or drinks in the morning, so that any food consumed prior to breakfast is included. Work through each meal and mid meal period. Specific questions about food quantities, methods of food preparation, snacks, drinks and eating away from home should be asked. The last is particularly important for children in daycare, for latchkey children and in certain cultural situations where children may be fed by grandparents. Budget limitations and food preparation skills will influence the type of foods consumed, and should be identified tactfully.

A checklist of commonly eaten foods is useful to ensure that significant foods are not forgotten, and as a means of checking quantities and frequency of consumption. The information obtained can be checked against the Food Guide to Healthy Eating or the Healthy Diet Pyramid and the Dietary Guidelines for Children and Adolescents. If the initial assessment raises concerns a referral to a dietitian should be made.

Dietitians are skilled in elucidating details of food intake in order to determine adequacy of energy and nutrient consumption. Retrospective methods of intake assessment such as diet histories and 24 h recall require an accurate history from the caregiver or child. Some people desire to please, and report what they think the child should be eating. If detailed information regarding specific nutrients is required, the dietitian may utilise a food record, which involves detailed recording of measured food intake over a number of days. Careful and detailed instruction is necessary, particularly as to the size of food portions and food preparation techniques. Computer analysis provides a comprehensive assessment of energy and nutrient intake, which can be compared to the reference values for the child's age and sex. Apart from the provision, quality and acceptability of food, there are many factors influencing dietary intake. Social, family, environmental and cultural influences should be considered. If children are unhappy, they may eat poorly or take solace in food and eat to excess.

Inadequate dietary intake generally occurs because children cannot eat, or simply do not eat. Children who cannot eat include those with short bowel syndrome, dysphagia or other gastrointestinal anomalies. Alternative feeding methods such as nasogastric or gastrostomy feeding may be necessary to assist these children to meet their nutritional needs. Behavioural, psychological and family issues need to be addressed in order to manage those who refuse to eat.

If uncertainty exists as to the adequacy of intake or growth, or a more complex problem is identified, it may be necessary to admit the child to hospital for further observation, assessment and management. This involves an assessment of intake and weight gain during the provision of a nutritionally adequate diet. If poor weight gain and intake is observed, further assessment following adequate energy and nutrient provision through the use of a nasogastric tube may be required.

Nutrition in utero

Fetal nutrition is currently of intense interest to epidemiologists, particularly as it appears that fetal events programme health outcomes in later life. In utero growth restriction has been associated with an increased risk of hypertension and non insulin dependent diabetes mellitus in adult life. This phenomenon has been termed the 'Barker hypothesis' after the idea's progenitor. Although a nutritious diet in pregnancy may be of long term benefit to the fetus, most in utero malnutrition in Western societies results from placental insufficiency. A specific nutrition provision both prior to and from the time of conception may be of help; for example, supplementary folic acid or increased dietary folate markedly reduces the incidence of neural tube defects (Ch. 27).

Breastfeeding

Australia is a signatory to the 1991 WHO/UNICEF Baby Friendly Hospital Initiative and is committed to the elimination of practices interfering with the successful initiation and maintenance of breastfeeding. Hospitals are encouraged to adopt the 'ten steps to successful breastfeeding' (Table 7.2).

Table 7.2   Ten steps to successful breastfeeding. (From *Protecting, promoting and supporting breastfeeding: the special role of maternity services*, a joint WHO/UICEF statement, Geneva, 1989, World Health Organization)

Every facility providing maternity services and care for newborn infants should:

1. Have a written breastfeeding policy that is routinely communicated to all health care staff
2. Train all health care staff in skills necessary to implement this policy
3. Inform all pregnant women about the benefits and management of breastfeeding
4. Help mothers initiate breastfeeding within half an hour of birth
5. Show mothers how to breastfeed, and how to maintain lactation even if they are separated from their infants
6. Give newborn infants no food or drink other than breastmilk, unless medically indicated
7. Practise rooming-in (allow mothers and infants to remain together), 24 hours a day
8. Encourage breastfeeding on demand
9. Give no artificial teats or pacifiers (also called dummies or soothers) to breastfeeding infants
10. Foster the establishment of breastfeeding support groups and refer mothers to them on discharge from hospital or clinic

---

Advantages of breastfeeding

Breastfeeding has many benefits for both the infant and the mother. Breast milk is precisely tailored for the infant's needs and contains many factors protective against infection (see Infant formulae below) and growth factors. The low sodium content of human breast milk is important, given the immaturity of the human infant's renal concentrating mechanisms. Breastfed babies benefit through the reduction of risk or severity for a number of diseases, including gastro-oesophageal reflux, pyloric stenosis, respiratory illness (especially in smoking households), infantile infectious diarrhoea, inflammatory bowel disease, some childhood cancers, later onset of coeliac disease and insulin dependent diabetes mellitus, otitis media, urinary tract infections, meningitis, sudden infant death syndrome and necrotising enterocolitis. Although there is some evidence that breastfeeding may protect against allergic disease in atopic families, the evidence for a population wide protective effect is inconclusive. The long chain polyunsaturated fatty acids present in breast milk may enhance cognitive and visual development in the infant.

Breastfeeding assists with bonding between mother and infant, and most women find it to be pleasurable and interactive. Breastfeeding may partially protect women against premenopausal breast cancer, ovarian cancer and osteoporosis. Lactational amenorrhoea may act as a contraceptive adjunct, especially in the developing world.

Contraindications to breastfeeding

There are few contraindications to breastfeeding. Mothers with active untreated tuberculosis, brucellosis or recently acquired maternal syphilis should not breastfeed. In developed countries, HIV positive mothers should not breastfeed as the risk to the infant outweighs the benefits of breastfeeding. Pooled breast milk banking is not currently acceptable in the developed world, due to the risk of exposure to pathogens, particularly HIV. In the developing world the protective effect of breast milk outweighs the risk of HIV infection. Hepatitis B antigen positive mothers can breastfeed once the infant has been immunised. Infants with metabolic disorders such as galactosaemia and maple syrup urine disease cannot breastfeed. Partial breastfeeding is possible for infants with phenylketonuria.

Breastfeeding initiation and persistence

Approximately 85% of mothers in Australia and other Western countries breastfeed at hospital discharge. The prevalence of breastfeeding falls to 50% at 3 months and 25–30% at 6 months after delivery. Women of higher socioeconomic and educational status generally breastfeed longer than the less privileged. Information about the advantages and management of breastfeeding, including where to obtain advice and support, if needed, should be made available to all new mothers.

Breastfeeding is promoted by placing the infant on the breast as soon as practical after delivery. The oxytocin released by this process contracts uterine vessels and reduces uterine haemorrhage. Breastfeeding should not be restricted, and the mother needs to be aware that this is a key factor in establishing feeding and promoting milk production. Care needs to be taken to ensure frequent feeding of infants in certain situations; examples are the mother who has had a lower segment caesarean section, or the infant who requires phototherapy for physiological jaundice. Some infants are unduly sleepy and this can be a problem with the initiation of lactation, but usually resolves. An infant who does not wake to feed, and sleeps more than 6–8 h overnight, should be woken for feeds. Rooming in with the mother should occur. Supplementary feeds should be avoided, as the infant has a relatively low fluid and caloric requirement during the first 48 h of life. The use of a dummy (pacifier) should be discouraged as it may interfere with normal breastfeeding. Preliminary information suggests that children who use a dummy routinely suffer a small but detectable disadvantage on psychometric testing. Twins, and triplets, can successfully breastfeed, with the provision of appropriate education, support and encouragement.

Reasons given by mothers for stopping breastfeeding include:
- pain and discomfort (for example, sore nipples, mastitis, thrush)
- anxiety regarding the adequacy of milk supply
- return to work.

It is essential for these mothers to have access to appropriate support and advice, particularly when feeding is still being established. The current policy of early discharge from maternity hospitals may be counterproductive to breastfeeding.

Home visiting by midwives, hospital breastfeeding support units, lactation consultants, Nursing Mothers Association of Australia (NMAA) and maternal and child health nurses can provide support for mothers. Some workplaces provide daycare facilities which will promote breastfeeding persistence and are flexible in their arrangements for nursing mothers. The use of handheld or mechanical breast pumps to express breast milk while at work may also facilitate ongoing breastfeeding. Community attitudes to public breastfeeding may also deter mothers from persisting with it.

Common problems with breastfeeding

Problems may exist with both maternal technique and anatomy, as well as with the infant's suck and oropharyngeal anatomy. In addition, insufficient milk supply is often perceived to be a major problem, which may lead to unnecessary cessation of breastfeeding. Most women are physiologically able to produce sufficient milk. Appropriate education, encouragement and support may be all that is needed. Mothers frequently complain of nipple pain or cracked nipples, the most common cause of this being incorrect positioning and attachment. The infant may have an incorrect sucking action. Attention to maternal technique, including positioning and nipple placement, should correct this problem. Ideally, the baby should engulf the nipple and areolus. This places the nipple posteriorly in the mouth and prevents abrasion on sucking. If the baby is positioned, attached and sucking correctly the mother should not experience nipple pain.

Cracked nipples are the usual cause for blood in breast milk. Cracked nipples will heal if breastfeeding persists. Eczema and dermatitis can be caused by nipple creams, soaps, shampoo and perfumes. Rather than nipple creams, it is preferable to use a few drops of expressed hind milk on the nipple to promote healing. Breast thrush (*Candida* infection) requires treatment of both mother and infant.

Feeds should be commenced on alternate sides. It is important to ensure that the infant empties the first breast before offering the second breast. This reduces engorge-

Arabella was born at term following an uneventful pregnancy and delivery. Her mother was very keen to feed her first baby, but experienced considerable pain from sore, cracked nipples soon after discharge from hospital. She returned to the hospital to seek advice from a lactation consultant who noted that Arabella was incorrectly positioned and attached.

Correct positioning and attachment, which is vital for successful breastfeeding, resolved the problem of sore nipples, enabling Arabella's mother to continue to breastfeed without discomfort.

Arabella breastfed on demand, approximately 3 hourly. At 4 weeks of age she started sleeping longer between feeds and suckled less vigorously. Her mother became very anxious and was concerned that her milk supply was inadequate, particularly as it became apparent that Arabella had not gained weight when weighed at a clinic visit. It was evident that the feeding difficulty was the result of infrequent feeding and maternal anxiety. She was encouraged to feed her baby more frequently, including during the night, and to ensure that Arabella drained the first side before offering the second. Her husband was encouraged to bring her Arabella during the night. As a result, the milk supply increased and Arabella gained weight appropriately.

Simple advice and encouragement prevented this mother from ceasing breastfeeding unnecessarily.

ment and the risk of mastitis. Additionally, hind milk has a higher fat content than foremilk and may promote satiety. Both breasts should be offered at each feed, particularly when establishing feeding, although a satisfied infant may not always feed from the second breast. Engorgement usually occurs early in lactation or if breastfeeding has been suspended. Again, appropriate positioning and attachment, with unrestricted feeding, ensuring emptying of breasts will help. Mastitis may occur as a result of a blocked milk duct. Correct positioning and attachment along with frequent feeding helps clear the duct. Infective mastitis usually requires antibiotic treatment and mothers may be systemically unwell.

Infants with palatal anomalies such as cleft palate may not be able to breastfeed. However, expressed breast milk should be provided through the use of spatulate teats or squeeze bottles. This may reduce the risk of middle ear disease in these infants. Other problems include lactose intolerance due to lactase immaturity. Frequent watery stools in a thriving infant secondary to lactase immaturity should not result in a change of feeding practice. Breast milk jaundice may occur, and is not detrimental to the baby. This improves with persisting breastfeeding, and there is no need to stop breastfeeding.

Infant formulae

Health professionals and caregivers are faced with a bewildering array of infant formulae for non breastfed infants. Health professionals who give advice about formulae should be familiar with the different types and understand when particular formulae should be used. Manufacturers and importers of infant formulae in Australia have agreed to a Code of Practice (1992) in accordance with the WHO Code of Marketing of Breastmilk Substitutes. The primary aim of the WHO Code is to protect and promote breastfeeding, and to ensure proper use of infant formulae, if required, through the provision of adequate information and appropriate marketing and distribution. The Australia New Zealand Food Standard Code includes a standard for Infant Formula, which is currently under revision. The new standard 2.9.1 will specify the requirements for composition, quality and labeling for infant formulae sold in Australia and New Zealand, and will be more prescriptive than the existing R7 Infant Formula Standard. (ANZFA, Australia New Zealand Food Authority, 2002).

While the nutritional composition of infant formulae resembles that of human milk, it is not possible to incorporate the many immunological factors that have been identified in human milk. These include specific immune factors such as IgA, maternal lymphocytes and macrophages, and other non specific protective factors such as lactoferrin, lysozyme and bifidus factor. Additionally, there are many other factors in human milk, including nucleotides, specific long chain polyunsaturated fatty acids, bile salt stimulated lipase, cholesterol, free amino acids, oligosaccharides and growth factors, that cannot be simply added to formulae. Manufacturers frequently modify formulae in an attempt to mimic human milk, but cannot make modifications unless the factor to be added has been proven safe, stable and beneficial.

Requirements of formula fed infants

The infant's appetite determines the volume and number of feeds required. Demand feeding for bottle fed infants is appropriate. Term infants require approximately 120–160 ml/kg/day to meet their fluid and nutrient needs during the first 4–6 months of life when milk feeds provide the sole source of nutrition. The number of feeds per day changes as the infant grows, and the number of feeds per day decreases with increased feed volumes.

Establishment of a feeding pattern is often easier for mothers of breastfed infants, as they respond to the infant's demands and do not focus on the volume consumed at each feed. The actual number and volume of feeds taken by bottle fed infants causes considerable anxiety for some parents. Reassurance should be given that the infant's appetite is the best guide, and as long as the infant gains weight consistently, but not excessively, and is thriving and active, progress is satisfactory.

Standard infant formulae

Standard infant formulae are recommended for healthy term infants who are not breastfed. The nutrient compositions of these standard formulae are very similar, with minor variations in the protein, fat and carbohydrate content.

- *Protein.* All standard infant formulae have cow's milk protein as a basis, which is modified in order to produce a protein composition more like that of human milk. The cow's milk protein is modified through heat treatment processes, with the addition of whey in order to modify the casein:whey ratio so that it is similar to that of human milk. Despite this, the amino acid profiles of infant formulae remain different from those of human milk.
- *Fat.* The fat sources in standard infant formulae are a mixture of vegetable oils with or without butterfat. It is possible to achieve ratios of saturated to unsaturated fatty acids that are similar but not identical to those of human milk. Although the degree of saturation may be similar the structure of the fats is not the same, resulting in differences in digestion and absorption. The fatty acid composition of human milk also varies with the maternal diet, and can be modified favourably by substituting some of the saturated fats in the diet with appropriate mono- and polyunsaturated fatty acids. Some manufacturers now add long chain polyunsaturated fatty acids to formulae, as there is evidence that these play an important role in infant development, with advanced visual pathway maturation and a postulated benefit for intelligence. The fat composition in formulae may also promote the formation of soaps in stools, contributing to constipation in some infants.
- *Carbohydrate.* The carbohydrate source in standard infant formulae is lactose.

All formulae are supplemented with vitamins and minerals. These standard infant formulae are suitable for the first 12 months of life and are labelled 'suitable from birth'. The common practice in the community, and with some medical practitioners, of changing from one formula to another because an infant is irritable or unsettled should be strongly discouraged. Changing brands on a frequent basis does not help settle the infant and can lead to mistakes in reconstitution, as scoop size and methods of preparation vary.

Preparation of formula

Having selected an appropriate formula, it is essential that it is prepared correctly and hygienically, using safe water and sterilised utensils and equipment. Formula should be prepared according to the manufacturer's directions, using the scoop provided to measure the powder carefully. Studies have highlighted significant inaccuracies in measuring the amount of powder for formula reconstitution, and other mistakes in preparation of formula. Health professionals need to ensure that parents understand how to prepare formula, and should never assume that they can readily follow the instructions. Parents can be tempted to use less formula powder to save money, resulting in an underfed infant, or to overfeed by adding extra powder in an attempt to achieve more rapid growth if a 'chubby' baby is desired.

Modified formulae and other milks

Preterm formulae

Breast milk may not be available for preterm infants, and if available may not provide sufficient energy. However, it is preferable, if possible, to supplement breast milk with a human breast milk fortifier, glucose polymer or fat supplement than totally to provide requirements with a preterm formula. Even though incremental growth may be initially less impressive, preterm infants who have received breast milk appear to have a developmental advantage over those who have received commercial formulae.

'Follow on' formulae

'Follow on' formulae are promoted as 'suitable only for babies over 6 months'. These formulae have a higher protein content, higher renal solute load, and increased levels of some minerals, including iron and calcium, compared with standard infant formulae. Although safe, there is little rationale for the use of these formulae in place of the standard infant formula.

Cow's milk

Breast milk or an appropriate formula are recommended as the major source of milk during the first 12 months of life. Cow's milk is not recommended as the primary milk source during this time. The reasons for this include:
- low iron content and poor availability of iron
- higher levels of protein, sodium, potassium, phosphorus and calcium compared with human milk or formula
- high renal solute load
- lack of vitamin C and essential fatty acids
- potential gastrointestinal tract blood loss, secondary to cow's milk colitis.

It is appropriate to introduce cow's milk into the infant's diet during the second 6 months of life in the form of foods such as custard, yoghurt and cheese. Full cream cow's milk can be introduced as the main milk source from 12 months of age. The fat in milk is an important source of energy, fat soluble vitamins and fatty acids for young children. Reduced fat milk should not be introduced into the diets of young children before 2 years of age, and skim milk should not be used before 5 years of age, unless there is a specific medical condition, such as hypercholesterolaemia.

Goat's milk

The macronutrient composition of goat's milk is similar to that of cow's milk. Goat's milk is not recommended for infant feeding. If parents insist on goat's milk, a goat's milk infant formula fully supplemented with vitamins and minerals should be used because goat's milk is markedly deficient in folate and other vitamins. If fresh goat's milk is used, it must be pasteurised or boiled and supplemented with folic acid, vitamins B_{12}, B_6, A and C. A child with a true cow's milk protein intolerance will almost certainly be intolerant to goat's milk protein. Goat's milk is also unlikely to reduce atopy.

Soy formulae

The widespread use of soy formulae for infant feeding in the community is not justified. Soy formulae are commonly and usually inappropriately used for suspected cow's milk protein intolerance, lactose intolerance, colic, and in an attempt to prevent allergies. Up to 50% of children with cow's milk protein intolerance will also be allergic to soy protein, and it is preferable for these children to be given a formula with hydrolysed protein. There is no evidence that soy formulae protect against allergies. Soy formula is not required for lactose intolerance as there is no need to eliminate milk protein.

The presence of phytates in soy formulae may inhibit absorption of minerals, particularly calcium. Soy formulae have a higher aluminium content than other formulae. This places preterm infants or infants with poor renal function at risk of toxicity, especially renal osteodystrophy. More recently it has been noted that these formulae contain high levels of soy phyto-oestrogens, which theoretically may be harmful to infants. Currently available evidence, however, suggests that these appear to have a low affinity for human oestrogen receptors, and do not appear to have any adverse effects on growth and development. A major concern is the potential for these phyto-oestrogens to contribute to infertility. Reassuringly, high rates of infertility have not been reported in human populations ingesting significant quantities of soy.

Soy formulae should only be used in galactosaemic infants, and for infants of vegetarian families reluctant to use cow's milk. Soy beverages, or soy drinks available in supermarkets and health food stores, should not be used for children under 2 years of age. Calcium supplemented brands should be chosen if used for older children.

Lactose modified formulae

Low lactose or lactose free formulae are the feeds of choice for formula fed infants with true lactose intolerance (Ch. 69). The nutrient composition is similar to that of standard formulae with the exception of the carbohydrate, which is either predigested lactose (glucose, galactose) or glucose polymers. In older children with lactose intolerance, enzymatic drops containing lactase may be used with cow's milk.

Semi-elemental formulae

Semi-elemental formulae are designed to meet the needs of infants who are intolerant of intact protein, who maldigest protein and fat (Ch. 70), or who have problems with severe diarrhoea, food intolerance or allergy. The protein in these formulae is partially hydrolysed to peptides and free amino acids. The fat in some formulae contains varying amounts of medium chain triglyceride. The formulae are expensive and should only be used with medical guidance.

Other fluids

Milk, either breast or formula, provides sufficient food and fluid for the first 5–6 months of life. Breastfed babies do not require other fluids, even in hot weather, if they are fed frequently. Formula fed infants may be offered small amounts of cooled, boiled water between feeds during very hot weather.

Gastro-oesophageal reflux (Ch. 71)

If an infant is happy and thriving, frequent spilling of feeds is of little consequence. Indeed, some spilling of feeds arguably is physiological and is very prevalent. Most parents can be reassured that gastro-oesophageal reflux is essentially innocuous. None of the medical therapies available for reflux, such as formula thickeners, cornstarch or prokinetic agents, is likely to help a breastfed infant. Rice cereal should not be used in infants under 3 months of age, due to reduced salivary and pancreatic amylase production in early infancy. Food thickeners which increase the consistency of formula can be tried in formula fed infants. However, thickened feeds may retard gastric emptying and the results may be disappointing.

Introducing solid foods

Timing of introduction of solids

Breast milk or an appropriate formula will be sufficient to meet the needs of the healthy, growing infant until 4–6 months of age. At this time solid foods can be introduced safely, supplementing the milk intake, which remains the major source of nutrition until about 12 months of age. The World Health Organization has undertaken a systematic review in order to determine the optimal duration of exclusive breastfeeding (that is, no other fluids or foods). As a result, the WHO Expert Consultation Group has recommended exclusive breastfeeding for 6 months (2001).

The 'introduction of solids' refers to the process of introducing different foods, new food textures, and methods of feeding. 'Weaning' is a term that has been used previously to describe this process, but is not appropriate as it implies cessation of breastfeeding. Solid foods may also be referred to as 'transitional foods' or 'beikost'.

By 4–6 months of age infants have lost the tongue thrust or extrusion reflex, have head control, and are able to sit without support, allowing them to manipulate solid foods. The digestive system has also matured, with pancreatic amylase levels sufficient for digestion of starches. Most infants at this age are showing an interest in the world around them and are receptive to trying new foods. Healthy fullterm infants are born with iron stores that are sufficient for the first 4–6 months of life, after which these become depleted and milk feeds need to be supplemented with other dietary sources of iron, particularly haem derived iron.

Introduction of solids before 4 months of age can displace breast milk or formula, but the solids do not necessarily supply sufficient energy and nutrients for the rapidly growing infant. Solids can also result in decreased breast milk supply, as a result of reduced frequency and intensity of sucking. Early solids may also result in food allergy. Delaying the introduction of solids until later during the second 6 months of life may compromise growth and nutritional status.

The first foods

The introduction of a variety of foods is often referred to as the 'educational diet' as it begins the child's lifetime experience of food. The first foods to be introduced should be soft and smooth, although the infant quickly learns to manage foods of different textures, with the 'chewing reflex' using the gums developing around 7–9 months. Iron fortified infant cereals are usually introduced first, as these can be mixed to the desired consistency with breast milk or formula. Fruit and vegetables are introduced gradually. Sources of haem iron such as meat and poultry are recommended at about 7 months of age. Custard, yoghurt and cheese can also be introduced. Egg yolk is suitable from this time, but it is advisable to leave egg white until around 12 months of age, because ovalbumin is one of the more common causes of allergic reaction in infants.

A wide variety of commercial baby foods is available and useful as convenience foods. Food standards ensure that these have suitable nutritional content. The foods are, however, generally limited in flavour and texture, with all ingredients being mixed together, resulting in somewhat limited educational value. It is preferable to offer a modified version of family foods. Most infants will be eating a variety of modified family meals by 12 months of age.

Techniques for introducing solids

A relaxed and flexible approach is essential because the environment in which the child is introduced to new foods will affect the child's attitude to food. The principles of introducing solid food are as follows:
- Introduce only one food at a time, never rush.
- New foods should be offered several days apart, avoiding confusion and allowing food allergy/intolerance to be identified.
- Offer each new food separately.
- Do not add sugar, fat or salt.
- Avoid extremes of food temperature.
- Do not forcefeed.

Parents should not be discouraged if the infant rejects foods. Variation in appetite from day to day is both common and normal, and all infants will progress at different rates. Fluids other than breast milk or formula, such as water or diluted juice, are best offered in a cup to avoid reliance on the bottle and the tendency to suck for comfort, which can be a difficult habit to reverse. Infants should not be settled in bed with a bottle, as this can cause nursing bottle caries (Ch. 77).

Cultural traditions influence the timing of solid introduction and the types of foods that are introduced. If nutritionally adequate, culturally appropriate foods and preparation methods should be fostered. Some cultural traditions, such as chewing food for the infant, should be discouraged. Social and medical factors also influence the introduction of solid foods; for example, prolonged hospitalisation may impede the establishment of a normal diet.

Feeding the toddler

Between 1 and 3 years of age, growth and appetite slow markedly. The child displays independent thought and action. Young children have limited control over their food choices and rely on caregivers to provide a variety of foods. Caregivers should understand normal behaviour and eating patterns of toddlers, as unrealistic expectations may create feeding problems.

A variety of simple, nutritious foods should be offered at regular intervals, as toddlers are rarely able to meet their needs with three meals alone. Snacks should be nutritious, supervised and not offered immediately before meals. Considerable variation in the amount of food eaten at different meal and snack times is common, but total daily energy intake tends to be relatively constant.

Parents often perceive young children to be 'difficult' eaters if they eat a limited variety or quantity of food, refuse to eat at specific meal times, or exhibit erratic eating patterns. These traits are typical of toddlers, given their limited attention span, variable appetite, constant activity and increasing independence. Threats, scolding, bribery and use of food as a reward are likely to create rather than resolve problems. Food fads are relatively common at this age, and may develop for no apparent reason or following illness or a traumatic event. Such fads disappear as quickly as they start and are rarely a danger to health.

Excessive intake of milk or fruit juice

Excessive intake of milk or fruit juice may reduce appetite and, as a result, limit the variety of food intake. This is more likely to be a problem for toddlers who are bottle fed, as children are less likely to drink excessively from a cup. Bottle feeding should be avoided beyond 18 months of age. Excessive milk intake may result in iron deficiency.

Excessive fruit juice consumption, particularly apple and pear juice, can result in toddler diarrhoea due to saturation of the facilitated diffusion of fructose. It can also result in poor growth. Frequent sucking or going to sleep with a bottle of fluid containing sugar, including milk and fruit juice, also can result in tooth decay or nursing bottle caries.

Safe feeding practices for young children

Upper airway obstruction due to food inhalation is a particular problem for young children, particularly those aged 1–3 years. Almost 90% of choking deaths occur before the age of 5 years. There are a number of reasons why young children can choke:
- Toddlers are mobile and have a tendency to place all small objects in their mouths.
- Incisor teeth erupt 10 months to 2 years before the molars: for a significant period of time children are able to bite off portions of food without being able to grind or chew them properly.
- Swallowing coordination takes time to develop in young children.
- Food is more likely to impact in small airways.

Safe eating practices for children under 4 years of age include avoidance of hard foods such as raw carrot, celery sticks and apple pieces. These foods need to be cooked or grated. Other foods, such as nuts, popcorn, corn chips and hard sweets, are unsuitable for young children. Caution also needs to be exercised with non friable foods such as sausages, chicken and other meats, which need to be cut into small pieces that are easily manageable. Tough skins on sausages and hot dogs should be removed. The eating environment is a key factor in preventing choking. Children should not be forcefed, should be sitting quietly while eating, and must be supervised.

Problems with feeding

Most long term problems with feeding stem from infancy and early childhood. Young children can be frustratingly picky, but over a period of time most children achieve a balanced intake. Some children may persistently choose only one food (such as custard) or may avoid foods of certain textures (lumps). If a very limited diet is consumed, a dietitian should be consulted in order to assess the adequacy of energy and nutrient intake. Speech pathologists can assist with oral stimulation and the introduction of different tastes and textures.

If a child refuses to feed, a medical reason should be sought. Very occasionally, no reason will be found and the child may require long term supplemental feeding either through a nasogastric tube or a gastrostomy tube. For protracted feeding a gastrostomy is preferable; accidental dislodgment of the tube rarely occurs and the concealment of the gastrostomy allows the child freedom of movement and less unwanted attention. This form of supplemental feeding is also useful in chronic illness or neurological compromise, such as cystic fibrosis or cerebral palsy.

In children without an underlying chronic illness, this form of feeding should not be adopted lightly. Feeding is a learned response and the prolonged avoidance of food provision in itself may result in difficulties when attempting to re-establish oral intake at a later time.

Specific nutritional concerns during childhood

Medical practitioners are often faced with problems involving feeding toddlers and young children. Many of these problems originate from parental beliefs about diet. Commonly encountered problems include the provision of restricted vegetarian diets, non allergenic diets, and diets which are believed by parents to ameliorate the effect of attention deficit disorder. Occasionally diets that have excessive amounts of vitamins and minerals are used in an attempt to ameliorate the effects of disorders such as Down syndrome. Usually children have no choice in these diets, which may be limited in variety and interest. This in itself can lead to poor intake. There is usually no scientific evidence available to validate the

effects of these diets. Despite this, they are often promoted enthusiastically by alternative health therapists.
Parents who provide these diets for their children may
have difficulty responding to medical advice. Others are
unaware that the diet may not, contrary to their best
intentions, be nutritionally sound. Considerable patience
and encouragement may result in the institution of a more
nutritionally appropriate diet.

Low fat diets during childhood

Limiting fat in young children's diets may restrict energy
intake and compromise growth and development. There
is controversy, however, as to whether a low fat diet will
lower serum cholesterol effectively during childhood and
at the same time allow optimal growth and development.
Studies which have demonstrated lowered serum lipid
profiles and appropriate growth on low fat diets have not
examined specifically the possible adverse effects of low
fat diets on central nervous system development.
Although no adverse effects have been displayed, the
NHMRC currently advises against the use of low fat
diets, specifically reduced fat milk, for young children.
High fat, low nutrient foods such as crisps and take away
fried foods should be discouraged. These foods also tend
to be high in salt and low in fibre content.

It is recommended that for Australian children from
6 months to 2 years of age, approximately 40% of total
energy should be derived from fat. A gradual reduction in
the proportion of energy from fat, to 35–40% of total
energy intake, is recommended from age 2 to 5 years,
with a corresponding increase in complex carbohydrate
intake, including breads and cereals. Approximately 35%
of total energy as fat is recommended from 5 to 14 years
of age, reducing to 30% of energy from 15 years of age.
Equal proportions of monounsaturated fat, polyunsaturated fat and saturated fat are desirable.

Vegetarian diets

Vegetarian diets may be chosen for many different
reasons, often based on nutrition beliefs, or on religious
or moral grounds. 'Vegetarian' can refer to a variety of
different types of vegetarian eating, including non red
meat eaters, lacto vegetarians who eat milk and dairy
products, lacto ovo vegetarians who include eggs in addition to milk products, and vegans whose diets consist
only of plant foods, excluding all meat, eggs and milk
products. Vegetarianism during the period of life when
growth is occurring may present particular problems
because infants, children and adolescents have specific
nutrient needs that must be met in order to support
optimal growth and development.

The lower energy and higher fibre content of vegetarian diets can limit children's total energy intake, as

Clinical example

Zoe presented with a respiratory infection at
4 years of age. Her mother reported that Zoe
constantly had a cold and was always tired,
but she had attributed this to the fact that she had
recently started kindergarten. Relatives and her
kindergarten teacher, however, had indicated that they
thought Zoe looked very pale and unwell, and lacked
energy. Her height was 96 cm (10th percentile) and she
weighed 11 kg (below 3rd percentile). Her mother
remarked that she was surprised that Zoe was unwell
with inadequate weight gain as she thought that the
family's vegetarian diet was 'very healthy'.

Further questioning revealed that Zoe drank 300 ml
soy milk daily, ate no meat or fish, no dairy products or
eggs. Her mother was happy to consult a dietitian.
Analysis of Zoe's daily intake revealed an inadequate
energy intake, providing about 75% of her estimated daily
energy requirement. Her intake of calcium, iron, zinc and
other nutrients were below the RDI.

The dietitian explained to Zoe's mother that despite her
efforts to provide a healthy diet, the high fibre, low fat
intake with a limited variety of foods was not providing
sufficient energy (kJ/cal) and nutrients to meet Zoe's
needs. While happy to make some changes, her mother
was reluctant to give Zoe dairy products, so was advised
to ensure that Zoe was offered at least 600 ml calcium
fortified soy milk daily. The dietitian also discussed ways
in which to achieve a nutritionally adequate vegetarian
diet, and provided practical ideas for increasing energy
intake. Iron deficiency anaemia was identified and Zoe
was started on iron supplements.

Any form of dietary modification is a potential concern
in children, and it is important to ensure that the type and
quantity of foods eaten is adequate to provide the energy
and nutrients essential for growth and development.

they may not consume sufficient volume to meet their
needs. Close monitoring of growth and development of
vegan children, in particular, is necessary. Careful attention to the planning of vegetarian diets for children is
essential. The assistance of a dietitian should be sought
in planning these diets, to ensure the provision of sound
nutritional advice. Energy, protein, iron, calcium and
zinc and vitamin B_{12} are also of concern if a vegan diet
is being followed.

Infants

Providing that the mother is consuming an adequate vegetarian diet, infants can be successfully breastfed. Strictly
vegan mothers who are not receiving vitamin B_{12} place
their child at considerable risk of profound neurodevelopmental delay. Vegetarian mothers who formula feed often
prefer not to use formulae based on cow's milk. An appropriately fortified infant soy formula may be used. Solid
introduction should commence in the usual way, between
4 and 6 months of age, but particular attention needs to be

given to iron, if haem iron containing foods are being avoided. Infants placed on vegan diets are most at risk of nutritional deficiencies. Children who develop iron deficiency anaemia may be at risk of a persistent small neurocognitive impairment, even with iron repletion.

Children and adolescents

Children on well planned semi-vegetarian, lacto or lacto ovo vegetarian diets are adequately nourished if appropriate attention is given to selection of suitable iron sources, and sufficient vitamin C is consumed to maximise iron absorption. Vegan diets place children at risk of iron deficiency anaemia. Children on vegan diets require calcium fortified soy milk to ensure adequate calcium intake. The risks of vegetarian diets for adolescents, particularly vegans, are significant, due to the rapid growth that occurs during puberty. Sufficient energy and an adequate intake of iron, calcium, zinc and, if vegan, vitamin B_{12} must be ensured.

Hypoallergenic diets

Hypoallergenic diets are usually adopted for atopic eczema, allergic rhinitis and asthma. They are often implemented without medical advice and are seldom effective. Alternative health practitioners sometimes promote these diets. Food contains myriad potential allergens. The chances of identifying the correct allergen are small. With the exception of immediate hypersensitivity responses to food where a single food allergen can be clearly identified, there is little prospect of success. What usually results is the progressive introduction of an increasingly restricted diet and a corresponding reduction in nutrient intake, including energy, protein and calcium. Referral to a recognised paediatric allergist may result in a sensible examination of the issues, and determine whether or not any dietary restrictions are necessary. If so, the advice of a dietitian should be sought. Occasionally, the elimination of salicylates and food additives such as tartrazines, sulphites and monosodium glutamate may benefit the patient with asthma (Ch. 42).

Diets for attention deficit hyperactivity disorder (ADHD)

These diets are usually adopted without medical advice. Two forms exist. Firstly, food colours and additives are avoided. There is some evidence in double blind placebo trials that this withdrawal may benefit the occasional child. If this form of diet is to be used, some form of placebo controlled trial should be undertaken. Diets low in bioamines also have been promoted as beneficial for children with attention deficit disorder.

The second form of diet involves the avoidance of refined sugar. There is no reputable proof that this type of

diet is of any benefit. The provision of adequate energy intake beyond the first 6 months of life is very difficult with this type in a developed society. A meaningful examination of the effect of diet in this condition is possibly only if the children strictly meet the DSM IV criteria for attention ADHD (Ch. 17).

Nutrition issues for adolescents

Adolescence is a time of rapid growth and physical development associated with high nutrient needs (Ch. 14). There are, however, barriers to healthy eating for teenagers that influence food choice and result in many teenagers having unhealthy diets. These include:

- susceptibility to advertising
- inappropriate food preferences
- peer group pressure
- lack of interest in/knowledge of nutrition, no cooking skills
- increasing independence, own money, and eating away from home
- concerns about body shape and size, and associated dieting.

Common features of teenage eating include skipping meals, consumption of a limited variety of foods, frequent consumption of high fat, high sugar, low nutrient foods, a lack of fibre, and fad dieting. Fast food which is usually high in fat, refined carbohydrate and salt is promoted during peak television viewing hours. Fast food consumption may contribute to the increasing prevalence of adult obesity in Western society, particularly when combined with a sedentary lifestyle.

Poor and sometimes inappropriate body image may account for the fad diets that are quite common among teenage girls and boys. Girls in particular will often modify their diets to avoid food which they see as high in fat and energy, such as meat or milk, which may result in an entire food group being omitted from their diet. The avoidance of milk and milk products during the time of peak accumulation of bone mass and calcium accretion may play a role in osteoporosis later in life. Cola drinks which are high in phosphoric acid may interfere with calcium accretion. Limiting sources of iron, such as red meat, can lead to iron deficiency.

Appropriate nutrition education and role modelling needs to be provided both at home and in the school setting.

Problems of over- and undernutrition

Obesity

The prevalence of obesity is increasing. Australia is now the second 'fattest' nation on earth. Obese children will often have obese parents or siblings. Most adult obesity has its origin in childhood.

Obesity related morbidity is physical, psychological and socioeconomic. Morbid effects of obesity include:
- hypertension
- non insulin dependent diabetes mellitus
- hyperlipidaemia
- ischaemic heart disease
- cerebrovascular disease
- oesteoarthritis
- slipped femoral epiphyses and Blount disease (tibia vara)
- non alcoholic steatohepatitis and cirrhosis
- nephropathy
- teasing and social ostracism
- poor employment prospects
- marital difficulties.

Obesity may equate to the societal norm for beauty in some Pacific Island communities. The parents of obese children, and often the children themselves, have a distorted body image and frequently believe the child to be much closer to societal norms for body habitus than the child actually is. There are also racial differences in the utilisation of foods. Black American females have lower resting energy expenditure than their white counterparts and the adoption of a sedentary lifestyle and a high fat diet may promote obesity.

Obesity can be regarded as being of either infantile or later childhood onset. Historically this classification was explained by increased adipocyte number in infantile onset obesity and increased adipocyte size in the later onset type. This explanation is now regarded as erroneous. Babies often are very chubby with a maximum adiposity being obtained in normal subjects between 5 and 6 months of age. Most fat babies are of normal size by school age. Those who remain obese often have an accelerated rate of growth for both length and weight. This has been attributed to relative hyperinsulinism, as insulin may serve as a growth factor in early childhood. An accelerated bone age and early puberty results. Ultimately these children are no taller and may even be shorter than their non obese peers. However, a child who is both very obese and short early in life should be investigated for an endocrine cause of obesity. Because of the capacity for linear growth these children have a better prognosis than late onset obesity.

Obesity in later childhood often coincides with an emotionally traumatic event such as marital separation. Possibly because of the pyschosocial concomitants children with late onset obesity have a poor prognosis for weight control. Rapid increases in weight may occur. Linear growth usually is not accelerated. These children are often miserable at school. Attendance to their psychological needs may be beneficial. Females in particular may adopt nutritionally inappropriate diets with little success.

Management of obesity

An ounce of prevention is worth a pound of cure. Early education programmes aimed at parents are probably the most effective means of promoting public awareness of the risks of obesity. Once a person is fat, long term success with weight reduction is limited, which can be disappointing for both the patient and the physician. Physicians who manage obesity require patience and should set modest and attainable goals. Restrictive diets to achieve weight loss may be unrealistic, especially in younger growing children. It is necessary to provide sufficient energy to keep the weight stable while allowing linear growth to continue, and this will result in a reduction in obesity over time. The most important ingredient for success is motivation on the part of the child and parents. The whole family should be involved in the weight reduction process.

A healthy diet for the obese child is also a healthy diet for the entire family. Crash diets are not appropriate. Apart from being nutritionally inadequate, the child will become disillusioned and compliance will be poor. The parents need guidance in the provision of a healthy and balanced diet with a reduction in total fat and sugar, and an increase in fibre containing foods. High energy, low

Clinical example

Albert presented to his family doctor at 13 years because he was being teased at school about his weight. He weighed 74 kg (8 kg more than the 97th percentile), measuring 167 cm in height (90th percentile). He was 112% of ideal body weight (IBW); BMI was 26.5.

His history revealed that he bought his lunch at school daily (usually a pie, crisps and soft drink), and was home by himself for several hours after school each day as both parents worked. During this time he would watch television using the channel controller and play computer games while snacking on biscuits and crisps, and drinking fruit juice. His mother had also bought muesli bars for him, thinking that these were healthier and being unaware that they actually had a high fat and sugar content. Albert did not play any sport.

The doctor's advice was to take a sandwich from home for lunch with a piece of fruit, to limit fruit juice to 1–2 glasses per day and to substitute the high energy, low nutrient snacks (crisps, biscuits, muesli bars, chocolate, etc.) with fruit, vegetables and low fat dairy products. Albert was encouraged to try activities such as walking, bike riding, swimming or other recreational activity on a daily basis. He was limited to one television programme each day. The family was referred to a dietitian for comprehensive dietary advice.

Twelve months later Albert's weight was 76 kg (now 3 kg greater than the 97th percentile) and his height 174 cm (90th percentile). He had received a new bike for Christmas, which he now rode to school each day with his friends.

nutrient snacks between meals should be avoided, and replaced with foods such as fruit, bread and cereals and low fat dairy products. Practical ideas regarding food preparation are often beneficial. 'Skipping meals' is of no advantage as this will only result in compensatory intake at some other time. Providers of extra food, such as grandparents, should be included in any plans to modify the child's intake, to ensure that they understand and are familiar with the changes that need to be made.

Exercise should be encouraged, keeping in mind that a considerable amount of exercise is required to burn off even a kilogram of fat. Exercise is unlikely to be maintained if the child does not enjoy the chosen activity. Setting a good example and ensuring that exercise is enjoyable provides a template for success and the entire family should be encouraged to participate in additional recreational activities. If practical, children should walk to school. After-school activities which limit exercise, such as television and computer games, should be curtailed.

Support groups and programmes may be very useful. Encouragement and praise for goals attained will engender a desire to attain future targets. International Weight Watchers, which emphasises a healthy diet in a situation where improvements are met with approval, may work well with some adolescents, particularly if another family member attends. Commercial diet programmes are expensive and limited. It is very difficult for the extremely morbidly obese to lose weight. Pharmacological therapies are usually ineffective. However, the lipase inhibitor orlistat may have a role in starting weight loss prior to the effective institution of exercise and dietary programmes. Occasionally weight reduction surgery such as gastroplasty may have a role in life threatening obesity. Approaches which combine healthy eating with exercise are most realistic and more likely to result in long term improvement in weight.

Malnutrition

Malnutrition is the leading cause of childhood morbidity and mortality worldwide. The root causes of malnutrition vary between the industrial and the developing world. Ample food is currently produced to feed the world's population but social and political forces, such as war, lack of transport infrastructure, degradation of arable land with slash and burn agriculture and the market based economy, currently conspire to keep food from the most needy. The world's burgeoning population and the ravages of diseases, particularly HIV infection in areas such as subSaharan Africa and drug resistant malaria in Africa and Asia threaten to dismantle the good work achieved by agencies such as the FAO in developing disease resistant crops and encouraging sustainable agriculture patterns.

A malnourished child is a child whose weight is less than 80% of standard weight for age, using WHO growth charts. Generalised reduction of food intake or starvation results in protein-energy malnutrition. The ultimate result of protein calorie malnutrition is *marasmus* (from the Greek 'to waste away') or weight reduction below 60% of standard weight for age. Children who have a proportionately greater deprivation of protein than energy may develop *kwashiorkor* (from the Ghanaian 'deprived child'). These children are malnourished and oedematous. Children who are both oedematous and have a weight below 60% of normal body weight for age suffer from marasmic kwashiorkor. If malnutrition has occurred relatively acutely, height and weight discrepancies may result. If malnutrition has been severe and protracted, stunting may occur and often future growth is compromised, even after adequate energy provision. The issues pertaining to malnutrition and appropriate corrective strategies are quite different between industrial and developing world countries.

Malnutrition in the developed world

Poverty plays a role in malnutrition in the developed world. However, other factors such as ignorance, food faddism and psychopathology also contribute. Some factors such as maternal concern about obesity, which may engender concern in children quite inappropriately, are seldom seen in the developing world.

In Australia marasmus rarely develops in a malnourished child, usually because of intervention from social agencies or because medical intervention occurs. Kwashiorkor is virtually never seen, even in the indigenous population where protein-energy malnutrition often occurs. Both food intake and increased metabolic demands secondary to infectious disease burden contribute to protein-energy malnutrition. In the top end of the Northern Territory, up to 20% of hospitalised Aboriginal children are estimated to be malnourished; 12% are wasted; 5% are stunted and 3% are both wasted and stunted. Apart from substantially increasing the risk of infant mortality, long term somatic growth and neurocognitive function may be compromised.

Nutritional repletion of significantly malnourished children in developed countries should be undertaken in hospital. Marasmic children are at an increased risk of Gram negative sepsis. Appropriate cultures for microbiological agents should be taken in the event of a fever and the child started on antibiotics. Children should be graded up on feeds rather than started immediately on full feeds. The energy requirements should be calculated using the ideal body weight rather than the actual body weight. Enteral feeds should be high energy and close to isotonic in osmolarity. Electrolyte shifts may result if feeding is too vigorous, and the resultant hypokalaemia and hypophosphataemia may be life threatening; this is more likely if feeds are hypertonic. Refeeding oedema may also occur, and while not problematic, may be disconcerting to parents.

Malnourished children may also have specific vitamin and trace element deficiencies. These should be assessed and corrected. By far the most common deficiencies in developed societies are in iron and folate. In deprivation situations the children also may suffer from rickets and occasionally scurvy. The patterns of vitamin and trace element deficiencies in the developing world are quite different. Detailed discussions of vitamin and trace element deficiencies can be found in most major textbooks on nutrition (see Further Reading).

Intervention of social agencies, psychosocial help for disturbed parents and budgeting help for parents on the poverty line may be required upon discharge from hospital. Dietary supplements may be provided through hospital pharmacies. Regular follow up by both a paediatrician and a dietitian will allow prompt intervention if adequate weight gain is not sustained.

Malnutrition in the developing world

Malnutrition is endemic in the developing world. Children often receive insufficient energy. Malnutrition and kwashiorkor frequently date from the cessation of breastfeeding and the arrival of a new infant. In some parts of the developing world, high quality protein, particularly meat, poultry and fish, is in short supply. The cessation of breast feeding also predisposes the child to respiratory and diarrhoeal disease. The increased metabolic demands of infection may result in further nutritional deficits. Both humoral and cell mediated immunity may be compromised and this may result in further infection. Immunisation may not be freely available and sanitation may be rudimentary. Water is frequently contaminated. Infection with HIV is a major contributor to malnutrition, particularly in Africa. All these factors combine to contribute to a spiral of malnutrition and disease that can be very difficult to break.

Children with kwashiorkor have a typical appearance consisting of a protuberant belly, muscle wasting, dependent oedema, flaking skin with depigmentation ('flaky paint' dermatitis), glossitis and angular cheilitis. These children often have other vitamin deficiencies, especially B vitamin deficiencies such as thiamine leading to beriberi, and niacin leading to pellagra. Vitamin A deficiency can result in blindness and may significantly worsen mortality from diarrhoea and measles. Long term consequences include insulin dependent diabetes mellitus secondary to tropical pancreatitis, and also a significant reduction in IQ and school performance. Endemic iodine deficiency in some Asian countries may result in reduced intellectual performance.

Hospitalisation should be reserved for the most malnourished. Limited health resources may render this a reality. For the less severely malnourished the risk of nosocomial infection outweighs the benefit of hospital refeeding. Community refeeding clinics may be highly successful. Eating can be observed and a healthy local diet with high energy supplements should be supplied. The malnourished gut may display partial villous atrophy and a functional hypolactasia, which may take a long time to recover. Milk and milk solids may be poorly tolerated initially. Vitamins and iron should be supplied in deficiency states. The intestinal parasite load, which may be considerable, should be reduced by using an appropriate anthelmintic.

Prevention of malnutrition should be a primary concern of health planners. The causes of malnutrition are multiple, and hard to correct. The utopian goal, espoused by the United Nations sponsored World Summit for Children in 1990, of enabling children to maximise their genetic potential through the provision of adequate food for their growing minds and bodies is still elusive.

Eating disorders: anorexia nervosa and bulimia

The diagnostic criteria for these disorders are discussed in Chapter 18. These conditions are common, with prevalence rates for anorexia nervosa alone of 0.5–1.0% being reported in Australia and New Zealand. They contribute disproportionately to hospital costs and bed stay statistics.

Therapy consists principally of nutritional rehabilitation and emotional support (Ch. 18). The paediatrician should not underestimate the semistarved state of these patients and should cautiously but vigorously renourish them. This should be the initial and primary aim. Nasogastric tube feeding is required if the patient shows significant cardiovascular slowdown, bradycardia postural hypotension and hypothermia. Particular care is needed to avoid electrolyte imbalance and potassium and phosphate supplementation may be required. The patient will often cajole lower targets and attempt to subvert therapy. This is potentially upsetting for the person assuming responsibility. Accepting that this will occur and being sympathetic and encouraging may help the patient through a difficult time. Compromise is not a good thing in the initial management and may lead to later problems with setting limits. Involving the family in care and in psychological rehabilitation is essential for long term success. The best results are obtained in specialised eating disorder clinics where psychiatric and nutritional expertise are provided using a team approach.

Implications for adult life of a healthy diet

A balanced and healthy diet prolongs life and reduces the risk of development of many diseases. Reducing obesity may reduce the prevalence of non insulin dependent diabetes. A reduction in obesity and salt intake lowers the risk of hypertension and associated cerebrovascular and cardiovascular diseases. Reducing saturated fat intake may reduce the prevalence of atheroma and some cancers, especially breast cancer. Eating overcooked red meat may increase the risk of colon cancer.

High fibre diets may reduce the risk of diverticulosis and colon cancer. Fruit and vegetables are rich in complex carbohydrates, and vitamins that may serve as antioxidants. A diet that is rich in these substances, is relatively low in total fat, but includes monounsaturated and polyunsaturated fats, as well as complex phenols, may prolong life. There is increasing evidence that dietary ingestion of biological amines may affect mood. Patients with chronic illnesses such as renal or liver failure, or patients with metabolic disease such as phenylketonuria or galactosaemia may require specific lifelong modifications to their diet as a therapeutic adjunct.

Immunisation 8

D. M. Roberton

Immunisation provides protection against specific infectious diseases. It is the right of every child to be protected against vaccine preventable diseases: parents, caregivers and health professionals need to ensure that immunisation is available to all children.

Protection against subsequent infection after surviving the initial challenge has been recognised for many centuries for some infections. The use of material from smallpox lesions for vaccination was practised in early dynasties in China. Edward Jenner has been credited with the recognition that vaccination with cowpox virus could protect against challenge with smallpox. Smallpox was declared eradicated worldwide in 1979.

Diphtheria immunisation began in Australia in the 1920s, and immunisation campaigns against pertussis (whooping cough) were initiated in the 1940s. Triple antigen vaccine (DTP: diphtheria, tetanus and pertussis) has been used in Australia since 1953. Endemic poliomyelitis began to decline after the introduction of immunisation in the early 1950s, and now has been eradicated in the developed world. It is likely that poliomyelitis will be the second vaccine preventable disease which will be eradicated worldwide. Measles immunisation has been available in Australia for nearly 30 years.

Immunisation remains one of the most important public health priorities in developed and developing countries. In the developing world, many millions of childhood deaths occur each year from vaccine preventable diseases such as tetanus and measles because of lack of access to vaccines and vaccine provider services. Thus immunisation and its promotion remains one of the major activities of the World Health Organization, with the aim of achieving universal immunisation for children.

Principles of immunisation

Immunisation may be passive or active.

Passive immunity

Passive immunity refers to the acquisition of preformed antibody. The fetus receives maternal IgG antibodies during the later weeks of pregnancy, and breastfeeding supplies IgA antibody at the mucosal surfaces of the gastrointestinal tract.

Passive immunisation as a means of disease prevention is used in the form of:
- normal human immunoglobulin for protection against measles and hepatitis A, and as
- specific high titre preparations against cytomegalovirus (CMV), varicella, tetanus, rabies, hepatitis B and diphtheria.

Passively acquired immunoglobulin has a relatively short half-life and does not lead to active immunity.

Active immunisation

Active immunisation involves administering antigen so that an immune response develops that is similar to that occurring after naturally acquired infection. This immune response should be one that entails the development of lifelong immunological memory, and lifelong prevention from the disease which results from infection with that infecting agent.

Active immunisation to prevent infection or the effects of infection may be performed using:
- whole organisms (live or killed)
- components of organisms (subunit vaccines, polysaccharide vaccines)
- modified products of the infecting organisms (toxoid vaccines)
- manufactured components of organisms (recombinant vaccines).

Requirements of vaccines

Ideally, a vaccine should:
- give complete protection from the disease caused by the infection
- give lifelong protection
- cause no adverse effects
- need to be given once only
- be able to be given in combination with other vaccines
- be able to be administered easily and without discomfort
- be stable under a wide range of storage conditions
- have a long storage life
- be easy and cheap to manufacture.

Principles of vaccine selection

Diseases and the vaccine types used for prevention of these diseases are listed in Table 8.1. The immunisation strategies used for these diseases have been developed to take account of the following factors:

- *The nature of the disease process.* For example, toxoid vaccines are used to prevent diseases in which exotoxins are responsible for the disease. Examples are diphtheria and tetanus.
- *The route of infection.* For example, oral poliovirus vaccines are used to provide mucosal immune responses to polioviruses, which infect via the gastrointestinal tract.
- *Variations in the characteristics of the organisms causing disease.* For example, influenza vaccines need

modification regularly to provide protection from currently prevalent strains; poliovirus vaccine contains three strains of live attenuated vaccine virus to encompass the three strains of poliovirus likely to cause disease, and pneumococcal polysaccharide vaccine contains polysaccharide from the 23 most prevalent of the more than 80 strains of pneumococci causing disease.

- *The nature of the immune response.* For example, *Haemophilus influenzae* b (Hib) vaccines and pneumococcal vaccines are much more effective in children under the age of 2 years when given as protein conjugated vaccines rather than as polysaccharide vaccines because of the nature of the immune response at this age; measles immunisation is not undertaken until the age of 9–12 months in most countries because passively acquired maternal antibody remains in sufficiently high concentration to be able to neutralise the administered live attenuated vaccine virus strain prior to this age.
- *The effects of infection on the host.* For example, rubella immunisation is provided for all children at age 1 year and again at preschool age to provide immunity before their childbearing years for girls, and to decrease the prevalence of rubella in the community, thereby decreasing the risk of exposure of pregnant women to rubella. These strategies have resulted in a dramatic decrease in the incidence of intrauterine fetal rubella infection and the subsequent malformations resulting from fetal rubella infection in early pregnancy (congenital rubella embryopathy) (Ch. 27).

Immunisation schedule for routine childhood immunisation

The immunisation schedule recommended in Australia by the National Health and Medical Research Council (NHMRC) is presented in Table 8.2. There are minor differences in the schedule in individual States because of the contract prices for supply of different types of combination vaccines.

Vaccines are provided to registered immunisation providers and generally are free of charge. Immunisation providers are general practitioners, local authority immunisation services, some hospital services, particularly in children's hospitals, and some maternal and child health agencies. All immunisation providers must be familiar with:

- the immunisation schedule
- vaccine storage and handling requirements
- requirements for informed consent for vaccine administration
- adverse effects of immunisation
- potential contraindications to immunisation.

Table 8.1 Vaccine types for schedule vaccines and other commonly available vaccines

Disease	Vaccine type
Schedule vaccines	
Hepatitis B	Yeast recombinant DNA subunit vaccine
Diphtheria	Toxoid (formaldehyde treated toxin)
Tetanus	Toxoid (formaldehyde treated toxin)
Pertussis	Acellular vaccine containing 2–5 purified or recombinant antigens from *Bordetella pertussis*, (killed whole cell *B. pertussis*, still used in some countries)
H. influenzae b (Hib)	Polysaccharide (PRP-OMP) protein conjugate
Poliomyelitis	OPV: attenuated live poliovirus, given orally (types 1, 2 and 3) (Sabin vaccine) IPV: inactivated poliovirus vaccine, used in some countries
Measles	Attenuated live virus (freeze dried)
Mumps	Attenuated live virus (freeze dried)
Rubella	Attenuated live virus (freeze dried)
Other commonly used vaccines	
Hepatitis A	Inactivated hepatitis A strain
BCG	Live attenuated bacteria
Influenza	Subunit vaccine derived from inactivated virus
Varicella	Attenuated live virus (freeze dried)
Pneumococcal infections	Conjugate vaccine containing seven serotypes, and also multivalent vaccine containing 23 pneumococcal polysaccharides (not conjugated)
Meningococcal infections	Conjugate meningococcal C vaccine, and also multivalent vaccine containing polysaccharides from types A, C, w135 and Y (not conjugated)

Table 8.2   The NHMRC Standard Immunisation Schedule for immunisation for Australian children born after May 1, 2000

Age	Vaccine	Route	Milestone
Birth	HBV	i.m.	
2 months	DTPa	i.m.	
	Hib	i.m.	
	OPV	oral	
	HBV	i.m.	
4 months	DTPa	i.m.	
	Hib	i.m.	
	OPV	oral	
	HBV	i.m.	
6 months	DTPa	i.m	
	OPV	oral	
	[HBV*	i.m]	Milestone 1
12 months	MMR	s.c.	
	Hib	im	
	[HBV*	i.m]	Milestone 2
18 months	DTPa	i.m.	Milestone 3
4 years	DTPa	i.m.	
	OPV	oral	
	MMR	s.c.	
10–13 years^	HBV 1	i.m.	
1 month later	HBV 2	i.m.	
5 months later	HBV 3	i.m.	
Prior to leaving school (15–19 years)	Td (ADT)	i.m.	
50 years	Td (ADT)	i.m.	

HBV   Recombinant hepatitis B vaccine.
[HBV*]   HBV is given in one of two forms of combination vaccine in different States in Australia, leading to minor differences in the schedule. In New South Wales, Queensland, South Australia, the ACT and the Northern Territory, a DTPa-HBV combination is used at 2, 4 and 6 months. In Victoria, Tasmania and West Australia, an Hib-HBV combination vaccine is used at 2, 4 and 12 months. Therefore by age 12 months all infants will have received four doses of HBV in total.
DTPa   Acellular diphtheria, tetanus and pertussis vaccine.
OPV   Oral poliovirus vaccine.
Hib   *Haemophilus influenzae* b conjugate vaccine (PRP-OMP — this particular Hib conjugate vaccine is used because it gives high level antibody responses after the 2 and 4 month immunisations, and therefore gives improved protection in early infancy in comparison with other conjugate Hib vaccines).
MMR   Measles, mumps and rubella vaccine.
HBV^   This course of HBV is only for those children born before 1 May 2000, who did not receive HBV in infancy as it was not part of the routine schedule for infants at that time. This part of the immunisation schedule will only continue until 2010, when the HBV immunised 2000 birth cohort will have reached the age of 10 years.
Td   Tetanus and diphtheria vaccine for adults (also known as ADT).

These details are provided in Australia at approximately 2 yearly intervals by the NHMRC Immunisation Working Party as *The Australian Immunisation Handbook*, which is made available to all immunisation providers and to other health care providers who have a role in immunisation services.

Administration of vaccines

Storage of vaccines

Most vaccines need to be stored in a temperature range between 2 and 8°C. Maintenance of the cold chain is required from the time of manufacture until the time of administration. Vaccine storage temperature conditions must be monitored continuously, using thermometers capable of recording maximum and minimum temperatures.

Consent for immunisation

Parents or guardians must be given adequate information that will allow them to make an informed decision about immunisation for their child. The information given should include:
- the benefits and risks of immunisation
- the common side effects of the various vaccines.

This information preferably should be available in written form, and is provided in a form suitable for parents and guardians in *The Australian Immunisation Handbook*. Valid consent is necessary prior to each immunisation episode.

Preimmunisation questionnaire

In some circumstances, the risk of adverse reactions to immunisation is increased in the presence of some conditions. A standardised questionnaire should be used routinely prior to each immunisation episode. The questionnaire should enquire whether the child:
- has had any previous severe reactions to any vaccine
- has any condition which may lower immunity (for example, treatment with systemically absorbed steroid medications, chemotherapy, pre-existing immune deficiency disorder or disorder affecting immunity, such as leukaemia)
- lives with someone with lowered immunity
- might be pregnant (for girls of childbearing age)
- has had a vaccine containing live viruses within the last month.

Children should be assessed to ensure that they are well enough to have vaccine administered: immunisation should be deferred only rarely but may be delayed temporarily if there is a temperature over 38.5°C, if the child has diarrhoea or vomiting, or if he or she is obviously unwell for other reasons.

Sites of vaccine administration

Intramuscular vaccine administration in infants under the age of 1 year should be at the junction of the upper and middle one thirds of the anterolateral thigh. If two separate intramuscular vaccines are being given, one vaccine is given in one thigh and the other vaccine in the other thigh.

In children over the age of 1 year, intramuscular vaccines are given into the mid deltoid region of the upper arm.

Adverse effects of immunisation

Immunisation promotes an immune response. As part of this there is often some evidence of minor inflammation in association with parenterally administered vaccines. The most common side effects in the past in Australia were with whole cell pertussis vaccines: local swelling, crying and irritability, and fever. These occur very much less frequently with the acellular pertussis vaccines (DTPa). Vaccines containing Hib cause minor local swelling and erythema in about 1:20 infants. Measles immunisation may be followed by a mild and transient measles-like illness, with a slight fever and a brief rash, about 7–10 days after immunisation.

Rarely, there may be major events in association with immunisation procedures. Anaphylaxis is very rare, but every immunisation provider must have the appropriate equipment and training for dealing with anaphylaxis. The most important components of management of anaphylaxis are maintenance of the airway and the administration of adrenaline (Ch. 20).

Convulsions sometimes are seen in association with immunisation procedures. Simple febrile convulsions may occur in conjunction with febrile responses to DTP or measles immunisations in children predisposed to febrile convulsions; however, these are not contraindications to further immunisation. Immunisation is not associated with sudden or unexpected infant death syndrome (SIDS). Several studies, including a recent well controlled study in New Zealand, have shown that the relative risk for SIDS is decreased in immunised children.

Disorders that are not contraindications to immunisation

Immunisation is not contraindicated in children:
- with minor upper respiratory tract illness (colds, cough, sore throat) at the time immunisation is due
- using inhaled steroid medications for control of asthma
- with atopic disorders
- receiving antibiotics

- with controlled epilepsy, a history of febrile convulsions, a family history of epilepsy, or stable neurological disorders
- who have been premature or who are growing poorly.

Clinical example

Joshua, aged 6 months, was brought to the community health centre by his 18 year old mother to see a doctor for advice about a rash on his cheeks, behind his ears and over his upper trunk. The rash was due to infantile eczema. On questioning, it was found that he had not yet received any of his childhood immunisations. His mother said that this was because he always seemed to have a runny nose when due for immunisation, and she had been concerned that immunisation might make his rash worse.

She was reassured that immunisation was not contraindicated in the presence of rhinitis or eczema and that immunisation was important in infancy. Advice on the management of eczema was given. Joshua received his first DTPa, Hib, hepatitis B, and OPV (oral poliovirus vaccine) immunisations that day from the health centre's immunisation clinic. The immunisations were recorded in his health record and in the Childhood Immunisation Register, and appointments were made for further DTPa, Hib, hepatitis B and OPV immunisations at ages 8 and 10 months. He achieved his second immunisation 'milestone' by receiving MMR and HBV on his first birthday.

Children who appear to have allergic reactions to eggs can be immunised, as egg components are not contained in vaccines in the routine childhood immunisation schedule. However, where children have anaphylactoid reactions to egg components advice should be given about immunisation by specialty immunisation clinics before these children receive MMR (measles, mumps and rubella vaccine), and they generally should not have influenza and yellow fever vaccines.

Specific immunisation considerations

Prematurity

Premature infants should receive their immunisations at the appropriate age after birth, regardless of their gestational age. For example, an infant born 8 weeks prematurely should commence the immunisation schedule at the age of 2 months, even though the gestational age would only be at 'term' if not born prematurely. Because of a slight risk of reversion of the live virus vaccine strains if passaged repeatedly within neonatal units, OPV is not commenced until the time of discharge from hospital for low birth weight and premature infants.

Clinical example

Jake was born at 26 weeks gestation after his mother unexpectedly went into premature labour. He had significant respiratory distress in the first 3 weeks after birth, requiring surfactant, and he was ventilated for 2 weeks. He then needed supplementary oxygen for 4 weeks. He needed parenteral nutrition for the first 4 weeks of life, then nasogastric tube feeding for 4 weeks, before he was able to suck and be fed expressed milk from a bottle.

The day he was born, he received his first dose of hepatitis B vaccine as part of the routine schedule of vaccines. At 8 weeks after birth, when he was still equivalent to 34 weeks gestation, he received DTPa vaccine, Hib vaccine and his second dose of hepatitis B vaccine as part of the routine immunisation schedule. The DTPa vaccine and hepatitis B vaccine were given as a combination vaccine, DTPa-HBV, into his lateral thigh, and the Hib vaccine was given at the same time into the other thigh. In the normal schedule, oral poliovirus vaccine (OPV) would also be given at this time, but as he was still in the neonatal intensive care unit, the OPV was delayed until the day he was discharged to his home, at the age of 12 weeks. His equivalent gestation when he was discharged was 38 weeks.

At the time of discharge, arrangements were made for Jake to have his 4 month schedule immunisations (DTPa-HBV, Hib) and OPV 4 weeks after discharge, when he was 4 months old. This was followed by DTPa-HBV and OPV at the age of 6 months, and MMR and Hib on his first birthday.

Missed or delayed immunisations

If a child has not received immunisation at the appropriate ages, 'catch up' immunisation schedules are used. The immunisation schedule does not have to be recommended nor are additional doses of vaccine needed. Schedules for catch up immunisation for DTP, hepatitis B virus (HBV) and Hib immunisation are available in *The Australian Immunisation Handbook*.

Live virus vaccines

Live virus vaccines such as MMR and OPV can be given on the same day if necessary, for example for catch up immunisation; however, if different live virus vaccines cannot be given on the same day they should be given at least 4 weeks apart.

Comparison of effects of diseases and vaccines

The benefits of immunisation greatly outweigh the risks of any adverse events associated with administration of vaccines used in the childhood immunisation schedule. Table 8.3 lists some comparisons for vaccine preventable diseases and effects which may be associated with the corresponding vaccines. A more complete listing is available in *The Australian Immunisation Handbook*.

Recording of immunisation administration

Accurate recording of vaccine administration is essential. This must include:

- the vaccine administered
- the vaccine batch number and any other appropriate identifying information
- identification of the immunisation service provider
- the date at which the next immunisation is due.

This information should be recorded in a parent held Child Health Record, and in the records of the immunisation service provider. It should also be entered in nationwide immunisation databases. The Australian Childhood Immunisation Register (ACIR) was commenced in January 1996 for this purpose. The register is used for providing a reminder system to inform parents and caregivers when the next immunisation is due for their child. Within Australia, uptake of immunisation is encouraged by using financial incentives within the Family Allowance funding programme for immunisation completed according to the 'immunisation milestones', and by payment of immunisation providers for high rates of immunisation and for notification to the ACIR.

Other vaccines

Other vaccines are available that are not part of the routine childhood immunisation schedule.

Bacillus Calmette–Guérin (BCG)

Immunisation with BCG is no longer provided for all children in Australia nor in many other countries where the overall prevalence of tuberculosis is low. However, it may be recommended for:

- neonates in Aboriginal and Torres Strait Islander communities in regions of high incidence
- neonates or young children in households containing immigrants or recent arrivals from countries of high incidence, for example from some South East Asian and Indian subcontinent countries
- children who will be travelling to live in countries of high tuberculosis prevalence.

Varicella vaccine

Varicella vaccine normally is given at 12–18 months of age as a single dose vaccine, and can be given at the same

Table 8.3 Benefits and side effects of childhood immunisations. (Source: Modified from *The Australian Immunisation Handbook*, NHMRC, 2002)

Infection	Effects of infection	Side effects of immunisation
Hepatitis B	Persistent carrier state common after infection. Long term risk of chronic hepatitis and primary liver cancer	Minor fever in 2–3%, local inflammation in 5–15%.
Diphtheria	Toxin causes nerve and heart damage. Mortality 1 in 15	DTPa may cause minor local reactions such as swelling, redness and discomfort in approximately 15% of recipients
Tetanus	Toxin causes nerve and muscle changes resulting in paralysis, convulsions. Mortality 1 in 10.	As under diphtheria above
Pertussis	Whooping cough. Mortality and morbidity highest in infants. Mortality 1 in 200 if infected in first 6 months of life	As under diphtheria above
Poliomyelitis	Febrile illness, followed by paralysis in many. Mortality 1 in 20 hospitalised patients. Permanent paralysis in many	Paralysis related to vaccine strain virus in 1 in 2.5–5 million recipients or close contacts
Haemophilus influenzae b	Systemic infections such as meningitis, epiglottitis, bone and joint infections. Meningitis mortality 1 in 20, long lasting morbidity 1 in 4	Discomfort or local inflammation in 5%. Fever in 2%
Measles, mumps and rubella	Measles encephalitis in 1 in 1000–2000. Mumps encephalitis in 1 in 200. Congenital rubella syndrome if infected in first trimester of pregnancy	Minor fever, local inflammation in up to 10%. 1 in 1 million may develop measles vaccine strain encephalitis; 1 in 3 million may develop mumps vaccine strain encephalitis

time as MMR vaccine. It is recommended for all children, but is not yet provided free of charge in Australia. Older children and adults who do not have a history of clinical varicella infection should also have varicella vaccine. A single dose provides excellent protection under the age of 13 years; over the age of 13 years two doses of varicella vaccine are recommended.

Pneumococcal vaccine

Conjugate pneumococcal vaccine, containing polysaccharide antigens from the seven most prevalent disease causing pneumococcal serotypes, is provided for infants and children of Aboriginal and Torres Strait Island origin in Australia because of their high susceptibility to infection. The antigens are conjugated to a protein carrier to provide a longlasting immune response. Pneumococcal immunisation also is important in individuals at high risk, such as those with asplenia or sickle cell disease. Adults over the age of 65 years should receive pneumococcal vaccine (over 50 years for Aboriginal and Torres Strait Islander people).

Meningococcal vaccine

This is used for the control of outbreaks of meningococcal disease, in those with complement deficiency disorders, in those with asplenia or splenic dysfunction, and is required for pilgrims attending the Hajj. Polysaccharide vaccine is used in most countries. A conjugate meningococcal C vaccine is available which is thought to provide longlasting protection against meningococcal C disease, including in infants, and a conjugate meningococcal A and C vaccine is recommended for use in subSaharan Africa.

Influenza vaccine

Annual immunisation with influenza vaccine is recommended for:
- children and adults receiving immunosuppressive therapy
- children with cyanotic congenital heart disease
- children with chronic severe renal and pulmonary diseases
- adults over 65 years of age.

Hepatitis A vaccine

Hepatitis A vaccine currently is not recommended for general use in children; however, a combination hepatitis A and B vaccine is available.

Immunisation in special circumstances

HIV infection

Infected or potentially infected infants and children should receive the standard immunisation schedule, although it is recommended that inactivated poliovirus vaccine (IPV) be given in place of OPV (Ch. 41). BCG should not be given to children with HIV in areas where the risk of tuberculosis is low. Conjugate pneumococcal vaccine is recommended for all HIV infected individuals.

Asplenia

Children with asplenia (congenital; after splenectomy, for example for hereditary spherocytosis, or splenectomy in the treatment of malignancy) should have pneumo-

> ### Clinical example
>
> Jessica had a blood test performed when she was admitted to hospital with a high fever at the age of 3 years. The fever was due to a viral lower respiratory tract infection, and the fever and infection resolved without any need for specific treatment. However, the blood film showed red cells which were reported as containing Howell–Jolly bodies, suggestive of asplenia. An abdominal ultrasound was not able to identify any splenic tissue. She did not have any cardiac murmurs, and an echocardiogram did not show any associated cardiac murmurs.
>
> She had had all her scheduled immunisations up to the age of 18 months, including Hib vaccine. Her parents had also arranged for her to have varicella vaccine at the age of 18 months on the advice of their family doctor. However, her asplenia placed her at increased risk for bacterial infections, particularly those due to organisms with polysaccharide outer capsules. She therefore received pneumococcal conjugate vaccine and meningococcal C conjugate vaccine. It was also recommended that she receive meningococcal polysaccharide vaccine, as this contained additional antigens for the meningococcal A, w135 and Y serotypes. She was commenced on penicillin prophylaxis and her parents were advised that this would be needed for life. Her parents were told that she would need a repeat dose of the meningococcal polysaccharide vaccine in about 5 years' time, as immunity in response to polysaccharide vaccines tends to wane with time, whereas that from conjugate vaccines is thought to be longlasting.

coccal and meningococcal vaccines. Conjugate Hib vaccine should be given if it has not been received in infancy.

Sickle cell disease

Children with sickle cell anaemia should be given Hib vaccine as part of the routine schedule, and also should receive pneumococcal vaccine.

Travel

Advice for specific vaccines to protect against infection while travelling in other countries depends on the nature of endemic infections in those countries. Information can be obtained in Australia from the Commonwealth Department of Health, Australia, or from offices of the World Health Organization. It is important for travellers also to have up to date immunisation for diphtheria, tetanus and poliomyelitis, and to be aware of simple hygiene and protective measures for preventing infection.

Primary immunodeficiency disorders

Live virus vaccines and BCG should not be used in children with primary immunodeficiency disorders (Ch. 43).

Passive immunisation

Passive immunisation entails the use of normal human immunoglobulin preparations or hyperimmune (high titre) immunoglobulin. Passive immunisation may be used in children in the circumstances described below.

Normal human immunoglobulin

- Immunoglobulin replacement in primary or acquired immunodeficiency disorders.
- Measles prophylaxis.
- Hepatitis A exposure.

High titre immunoglobulin

- Cytomegalovirus infection or prophylaxis in immuno-compromised individuals.
- Varicella prophylaxis (zoster immune globulin).
- Tetanus or tetanus prone wounds.
- Rabies exposure.
- Hepatitis B exposure, including babies born to hepatitis B carrier mothers.
- Diphtheria antitoxin (horse serum derived).
- RSV prophylaxis in very high risk ex premature infants with severe ongoing pulmonary disease.

Future vaccines and vaccine development

Potential changes to immunisation strategies for children in the near future in Australia and many other countries include:

- availability of efficacious multivalent vaccines such as DTPa-Hib-hepatitis B and MMR-varicella, leading to a significant reduction in injections, especially in the first year of life
- booster immunisations for pertussis in older children and adults
- change from OPV to IPV (using IPV in combination vaccines such as DTPa-HBV-IPV) to avoid the remote risk of vaccine associated paralytic poliomyelitis-like illness after OPV immunisation.

Other developments in immunisation during the next 5–10 years are likely to lead to the availability of rotavirus vaccines, and serotype independent pneumococcal and meningococcal vaccines. Prototype vaccines against respiratory syncytial virus (RSV) and parainfluenza viruses are undergoing clinical trials, as are liquid intranasal vaccines against influenza. There is a great need for vaccines against malaria and other parasitic diseases causing widespread morbidity globally, and for vaccines with greater efficacy against tuberculosis. Public health strategies will have as their primary focus procedures and community campaigns to ensure the highest possible uptake, in both developing and developed countries, of the highly effective vaccines already available.

Child injury 9

D. Jolly, J. Moller

Injury is the leading cause of death for children and young adults in the developed world. It is also a major reason for admission to hospital. Most such injuries are preventable. The science of injury prevention is well developed, but is not widely applied. Doctors need to be well informed and to be community leaders in this field.

Trends in child injury over time

Time trends are only available for mortality data. Figure 9.1 shows the child injury death rates for children aged 0–4, 5–9, 10–14 years for the period 1979–1998. A clear downward trend can be observed, with the greatest advances being for younger children where changes in transport related deaths and poisoning have made a major contribution. The cause of the reduction of injury related death varies by age group. An exception to this trend is deaths from fire and flame injuries, which have not declined. Figure 9.2 and Table 9.1 show the current distribution of child injury mortality by cause and by age group. One disturbing feature is the emergence of self-inflicted death among children age 10–14 years.

It is encouraging to note that increased knowledge and action in injury prevention have been associated with the downward trend, but much remains to be done. This chapter aims to enhance knowledge of patterns of injury by age group and setting, and introduces principles of prevention. Armed with this knowledge, doctors will be in a good position to be community leaders in child injury prevention.

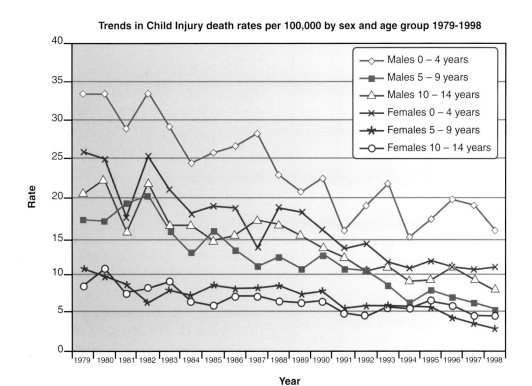

Fig. 9.1 Trends in child injury death rates per 100 000 by sex and age group, 1979–1998.

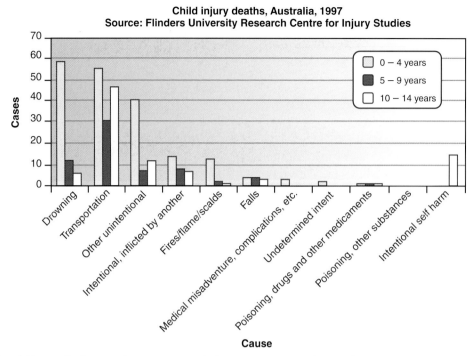

Fig. 9.2 Child injury deaths, Australia, 1997. Source: Flinders University Research Centre for Injury Studies.

Table 9.1 Summary of child injury death rates, Australia, 1997: rates per 100 000 by 5 year age group. (Source: Flinders Research Centre for Injury Studies)

Type of injury	0–4 years	5–9 years	10–14 years
Transportation	4.33	2.36	3.58
Drowning	4.57	0.91	0.46
Falls	0.31	0.3	*
Fires/flame/scalds	1.01	*	*
Other unintentional	3.17	0.53	0.91
Intentional self-harm	*	*	1.14
Intentional, inflicted by another	1.08	0.61	0.53
All causes	14.94	4.94	7.01

* Counts < 3 are too low to calculate meaningful rates.

Prioritising injury prevention efforts

This process is essential in planning programmes. Usual ways of prioritising efforts take into account leading causes of death in each age group and leading causes of hospitalisation, or give special consideration to those rare injuries which nevertheless cause a great deal of morbidity. Motor vehicle traffic injuries are much more important in terms of bed days (i.e. more severe injuries) than they are in terms of rates of hospitalisation. Relatively rare injuries, such as water transport accidents, firearm injuries and flame burns, rank high in terms of average length of stay.

Clinical example

Ryan, aged 2 years, is the youngest in a family of three children. On a Saturday morning, Ryan's father was getting ready to take Brett, his older son, to football, and his mother was at the same time hurrying her daughter as she was late for her violin lesson. The family had recently bought a large 4WD vehicle. In the rush and confusion, Ryan wandered out of the open front door and began to explore around the driveway. Unaware of Ryan's presence, his father got into the car and began to back it down the driveway, at the same time yelling quite loudly to his older son to 'get a move on'. Just then, Brett emerged from the front door and screamed for his father to 'stop!' From his vantage point he could see that his father was about to back the car over Ryan.

Four wheel drive vehicles are usually higher than conventional cars, and this makes it very difficult to see behind the vehicle. Note that the near injury also occurred at a time of family distraction and high levels of activity.

Principles of injury prevention in children and adolescents

The principles of injury prevention need to take the following into consideration:

- interplay between child development and injury
- perceptions of preventability
- host–agent–environment model
- active versus passive methods of prevention.

Interplay between child development and injury

The abilities and activities of a child change rapidly from year to year of age, and sometimes even from month to month. The environment for each stage is different, and so are the risks to which the child is exposed. For example, a 2 year old has developed considerable mobility and speed of movement but this is in no way matched by development of the ability to understand and negotiate traffic on a road. Older children have developed greater motor and conceptual skills, and are beginning to negotiate their way around a neighbourhood; however, with these new skills comes exposure to a new hazard, that of cycles. The developmental framework draws attention to the fact that development is an ongoing process. The sequence is as follows:

- skill development
- consequent exposure to new hazards
- mastery of these hazards and further skill development
- exposure to new hazards.

This process continues until adulthood.

It is important to limit strategically the hazards to which a child is exposed. It would be unrealistic to suggest that all cuts and abrasions received in exploring the world could be prevented, but exposure to an unfenced pool or an open road will not result in a minor

injury. Doctors need to have a good understanding of child development, and the skills and hazards of each age group, and to advise parents accordingly.

Perceptions of preventability

It is now recognised that injuries are predictable events, and are therefore preventable. It is no longer acceptable to talk of such events as 'accidents' or 'acts of God'. Social perceptions of the potential for injury control have changed during the last 25 years. Injuries that were once thought of as not being preventable, for example injury of an infant in a car crash, are now realised to be almost completely preventable, for example by the use of an appropriate infant restraint.

Host–agent–environment model of prevention

Some of the first studies to describe patterns, and therefore predictability, of injury likened injury to infectious disease, with 'host', 'agent' and 'environment' factors all determining whether an individual became ill. Host factors which are relevant have been discussed in the developmental framework. Generally, motor skills which are in advance of judgement skills make children vulnerable. It is not feasible to modify these childhood features, but it is important to be aware of them. Agent factors are modified more easily. An example of this is the temperature of hot water. Lowering the temperature of household hot water systems to below 55°C will mean that inadvertent exposure of a child to hot water is less likely to result in a significant burn. Environment factors include, for example, fencing a swimming pool or fencing a child's play space.

Active versus passive methods of prevention

This refers to the actions that need to be taken on every occasion in order to prevent an injury, compared with once only actions which will prevent most future injuries. For example, 'active' prevention of electrocution by a toddler poking scissors into a power point would be constant vigilance by the carer when the child is crawling around on the floor. 'Passive' prevention would be insertion of covers into the power points and/or installation of an earth leakage circuit breaker. Generally, passive prevention is more effective, although it may involve a greater expense initially. However, not all injuries can be controlled with passive measures. For example, parents need to be aware that young children can be scalded by hot coffee or tea, and that to hold a child and drink coffee at the same time is potentially hazardous. Active awareness each time the parent has coffee is needed to prevent this injury. Active strategies focus on behaviour, and passive strategies focus on the environment.

Clinical example

Louise, aged 6 years, was playing in the school playground with her new friend Melissa. Louise had been reluctant to start school and had tended to stay in the background at playtime. Now, after a whole year at school, she was much more confident and with the arrival of Melissa at the school she really enjoyed playtime. They climbed all over the climbing towers, and went down the slippery dip. Then Louise began to make her way across the 'monkey bars'. This equipment is like a horizontal ladder, often five feet or more off the ground. Not having acquired sufficient skill, she fell after two rungs, sustaining a greenstick fracture of her radius. Although the surface of the playground had been covered with tan bark, which should have provided a soft fall, this had been scattered by the many children playing there, and the soft surface had not been maintained.

Many believe that monkey bars are unsuitable play equipment for young children, who do not have sufficient skill to negotiate them safely. Height of play equipment off the ground remains an issue. Maintenance of a soft surface is very important.

Clinical example

Hamish, aged 10 years, and his friend Nick were starting to get bored with the school holidays. Looking for something different to do, they climbed into the boat that was on a trailer in the back yard. Stowed in the front of the boat was a can of fuel. Between them, they decided that they would make a bomb and test it out in the field across the road. They gathered several unmarked chemicals and other substances from the garden shed, mixed them up with the fuel and then poured it back into the can. They carefully carried the can to the field, avoiding being seen by Hamish's mother, who was entertaining several friends for lunch. Over in the field, they put a piece of rag in the top of the can, gave it a really good shake and then lit it. The resultant explosion was certainly very effective, but they were of course far too close themselves to the flames and both sustained serious burns to the face and hands. The dry grass of the field was set alight, and the flames spread rapidly across the ground. The boy's screams quickly brought the ladies from their lunch; the ambulance and the fire brigade then arrived.

Supervision is still important at this age, and parent distraction with another task was a factor in the injury. Despite education about the dangers of petrol, many children will still experiment with it, usually with very unpleasant results. It is helpful to limit access to this and other chemicals.

Strategies for prevention

Strategies for prevention can be considered under the following headings:
- time related
- legislative
- educational.

Time related

Road crash injuries have been studied and preventive strategies have been designed with a time related framework.

Before the injury

- Prevent the creation of the hazard.
- Reduce the amount of hazard.

During the injury

- Modify the rate of release of the hazard.
- Separate in time or space the hazard and that which is to be protected.

After the injury

- Begin to counter the damage.
- Stabilise, repair and rehabilitate.

Legislative approach

Examples of this are the introduction of compulsory seat belt use, compulsory child restraints in cars, the use of child resistant containers for certain medications, and compulsory fencing of backyard swimming pools. Legislation, which conforms more closely to the passive model of injury prevention, has been shown to be very effective.

Educational approach

An example of this is the anticipatory guidance that child health nurses incorporate into their child health surveillance programmes, and the community education campaigns about particular injuries. This approach is more familiar to health professionals. It is a necessary prerequisite to behaviour change in the community, but unless there are some legislative or other types of structural changes, education alone is unlikely to change injury rates. This means that the two approaches, legislative and educational, are interdependent.

Important injuries and their settings

Prevention of injuries in childhood incorporates active, passive, legislative and environmental approaches. These approaches can be applied to the three broad age groups mentioned earlier. As discussed above, the settings and patterns of the injuries change for each age group.

Birth to 4 years

Important setting

- The home.

Major injuries

- Drowning
- Motor vehicle injury
- Falls
- Poisoning
- Scalds.

Ages 5–9 years

Important settings

- Home
- School
- Community and recreation venues.

Major injuries

- Motor vehicle injury
- Burns from flame injuries
- Falls.

Ages 10–14 years

Important settings

- Roads
- School
- Community, sporting and recreational venues.

Important injuries

- Motor vehicle injury
- Burns from flame injuries
- Pedal cycle and scooter related injuries.

Summary

Child injury control is important. Injury is the leading cause of death and is a major reason for hospital admission and long term disability in this age group. It is known that almost all of these injuries are preventable. Concern about injury and action to enhance its control need to operate at several levels in the community. Injury prevention must be seen to be relevant to everyone and to be of concern to the individual family, local government, schools and the broader community. Doctors in all branches of the profession have a key role in the community in identifying hazards and providing leadership for change.

Failure to thrive

M. J. Robinson

'Failure to thrive' is the term used to describe failure of somatic growth. It implies failure to gain weight normally. When there is concomitant failure of linear growth the problem is usually a longstanding one. Severe reduction in head circumference suggests there has been intrauterine growth retardation.

Growth is a complex process and is discussed in detail in Chapter 63. For normal growth, the following conditions are necessary:

- a proper physical and emotional environment
- adequate nutrition
- correct tissue utilisation
- an appropriate genotype; that is, one compatible with normal growth.

When these conditions are not met, normal growth does not occur and the child fails to thrive. Standards for normal growth (growth charts) are available for most Western societies and many developing countries. It is of the greatest importance that doctors caring for children have ready access to growth charts and that they use them.

Growth charts plot weight, length and head circumference from birth to the end of adolescence; one such set is illustrated in Chapter 63. All children should have their weight and length recorded from birth and serially thereafter at child health clinics, so that deviations from the normal will soon become apparent. Growth failure may occur from birth, as in cystic fibrosis, whereas in coeliac disease, for example, growth fails after a period of normal growth.

Doctors are often consulted by anxious parents who believe that their child is not growing to their expectations. In the second year of life appetite deteriorates and activity increases. Weight gains are slower at this time and, unless parents fully understand this phenomenon, unsatisfactory feeding practices will develop, with all the behavioural problems that these bring. Reference to growth charts will rapidly define a growth problem and will provide reassurance to those parents who mistakenly believe that their child is not thriving.

Properly kept growth charts also identify the child whose height and weight are below the 3rd percentile and who require further investigation. However, it should be recognized that while the 3rd percentile is taken as an indication for further investigation, 3% of 'normal' children will fall below these limits.

Despite reference to growth charts and much reassurance, some parents will continue to worry about their child's physical development. The doctor will need great patience in managing this situation; in some cases there will be an underlying psychosocial problem within the family which will need to be identified and treated.

There are a large number of reasons why an infant may fail to thrive. Most can be identified by the basic methods of clinical paediatrics: a complete history, observation of the interaction between mother and baby and a thorough physical examination. A few simple laboratory tests will often be necessary. Extensive investigation of failure to thrive is usually not required in Australian society, but when necessary it will be indicated on the basis of obvious dysfunction of one or more of the body systems; for example, bowel disturbance and abdominal distension will suggest investigation for malabsorption, whereas dehydration in the absence of bowel losses may suggest renal or adrenal disease.

Non organic failure to thrive

In Australian society the commonest cause of failure to thrive does not have an organic basis but is the result of inadequate parenting and poor nutrition. Many of these children feed well and gain weight when admitted to hospital for investigation. When the investigations do not provide an organic basis for the growth failure, closer

---

Clinical example

Charlie, aged 2 years, presented with his mother to the family doctor. He had not gained weight for the past 4 months. In addition, his appetite for solid foods had deteriorated, but on further questioning he was taking at least 500 ml of milk each day.

He was active and alert and his height and weight were in the 50th percentile for age. No abnormality could be found after a careful physical examination. Because of maternal anxiety, a chest X ray, blood count and urine microscopy were ordered. These were also normal and his mother was reassured, shown his normal growth chart and informed that it was very common for toddlers to exhibit this eating behaviour. His mother was advised against further investigations, forcefeeding and appetite stimulants.

Clinical example

Sally was seen at the request of the child health nurse for poor weight gains. When seen it was noted that she was not very clean and had a nasty napkin rash which was ulcerated in some areas. Apart from this there was no abnormality to be found. She was alert and was constantly sucking her fingers. A chest X ray, blood count and microscopy of urine were also normal. Concern over the quality of care of this infant prompted referral to the Children's Protection Agency. Suspicions were confirmed with the finding that Sally was left at home alone and unattended at times. Both parents confessed to alcohol and substance abuse. Sally was placed in foster care where she thrived normally. The parents accepted counselling before Sally was returned to them.

inquiry will usually reveal a number of psychosocial problems; for example:

- It is common for the family to be in the lower socio-economic group.
- The pregnancy may have been unplanned and unwanted.
- The infant was born within 18 months of a sibling.
- The mother is often young, single or deserted and frequently depressed.
- Obstetric complications are not infrequent.
- A satisfactory bond between mother and baby has never been established.
- These infants are almost always bottle fed, with formulae often poorly prepared.
- Immunisation schedules are incomplete.
- Minor infections are very frequent.

The causes of the growth failure in these infants are multiple. Poor physical care due to ignorance or indifference is an important factor. Poor care may be associated with stress within the home. Neglect may be of sufficient degree to constitute frank child abuse (Ch. 12). Some babies are difficult behaviourally, and when this is added to the socioeconomic and psychological difficulties the problem is compounded.

The diagnosis of non organic failure to thrive can be made only after a thorough enquiry into the psychosocial background. The physical examination must be thorough and a few simple tests such as microscopy and culture of urine, chest X ray and blood count are advisable.

Management is difficult because of the multiple factors involved and the inadequate facilities within our society for the care of these families. Long term studies indicate that these children grow up with significant psychosocial problems in adulthood. It is not surprising to find that the non organic failure to thrive syndrome is perpetuated in the next generation. Management is supportive, involving much reassurance, home help, and other support

services such as community nurses, infant and maternal welfare personnel and medical social workers (Ch. 5).

Organic causes of failure to thrive

Organic causes are many. The following classification is essentially a clinical one:

- *failure of intake* from:
  underfeeding
  congenital abnormalities
  dyspnoea
  neurological disease
  behavioural factors

- *Abnormal losses* through:
  vomiting
  stools
  urine

- *Failure of utilisation* from:
  chronic infection
  metabolic disorders
  endocrine disorders
  constitutional, genetic, chromosomal abnormalities and intrauterine lesions.

Failure of intake

Underfeeding

This may occur in the breastfed baby if the breasts are large and engorged and particularly if the nipples are inverted. Regular weighing will detect inadequate intake. In the bottle fed infant the teat may be defective, the baby may be too sleepy or irritable to feed or the milk mixture may be too weak or insufficient in amount. It is a simple matter to calculate the total daily milk intake required for the bottle fed infant and relate it to the weight of the infant (Ch. 7). This fundamental calculation is all too often omitted in assessing infants who are failing to thrive.

Congenital abnormalities

Those interfering with feeding include:
- cleft palate
- Pierre Robin syndrome (micrognathia, cleft palate, glossoptosis)
- bilateral facial palsy (Möbius syndrome).

Dyspnoea

If severe, intake will be reduced. Failure to thrive is a common component of:
- severe congenital heart disease

- chronic heart failure
- chronic asthma — if poorly controlled
- cystic fibrosis — if poorly controlled.

Neurological disease

Those lesions associated with feeding difficulties include:
- severe cerebral palsy with pseudobulbar palsy
- pharyngeal incoordination
- hypoxic–ischaemic lesions associated with very low birth weight and cerebral birth injuries
- some rare cerebral degenerative disorders (Ch. 57)
- Werdnig–Hoffman spinal muscular dystrophy through severe muscle weakness
- following severe meningitis, encephalitis and uncontrolled hypoglycaemia.

Clinical example

Peter, aged 6 months, presented because of poor weight gains and difficulty with feeding. If forcefed he would extend his head, arch his back and extend all four limbs (exaggerated Moro reflex). On examination, his weight, length and head circumference were all below the 3rd percentile. There was increase of extensor tone in all four limbs, persistence of primitive reflexes and exaggeration of all tendon reflexes. When feeding, sucking and swallowing were poorly coordinated, with choking and much distress.

He had been born by emergency caesarean section because of cord prolapse during labour. The clinical picture was of spastic quadriplegia with pseudobulbar palsy leading to significant difficulties with feeding. Sometimes nasogastric tube feeding or gastrostomy is required in these infants to allow for adequate nutritional intake and to reduce the risk of aspiration lung disease.

Behavioural factors

Some infants are excessively alert, restless, feed poorly, sleep fitfully and do not suck steadily or contentedly. The reasons for this behaviour are obscure but genetic factors, maternal anxiety and inadequate parenting may play a part.

Abnormal losses

Vomiting

The causes of vomiting are discussed in Chapter 68. For vomiting to be associated with failure to thrive it must be severe and persistent. Vomiting may be the result of a mechanical problem or the result of toxic or infective factors.

Gastrointestinal disorders
These include:
- gastro-oesophageal reflux
- hypertrophic pyloric stenosis
- coeliac disease (Ch. 70)
- incomplete/recurrent intestinal obstruction, e.g. Hirschsprung disease, midgut volvulus
- Some oesophageal lesions, e.g. stricture, duplication, achalasia.

Renal lesions
- Urinary tract infection.
- Renal insufficiency.
- Renal tubular lesions — rare, but may need to be considered (Ch. 62).

The index of suspicion for renal disease must be high in any infant or child who is vomiting and failing to thrive.

Clinical example

Anne, aged 3 months, was born after a normal pregnancy and labour. Her birth weight was 2.1 kg. She was breastfed but her weight gains did not exceed 50 g/week. The following results were obtained from urinalysis:
- WBCs 25 000/mm^3
- RBCs 1000/mm^3
- Culture *Escherichia coli* >10^5 organisms/ml, sensitive to trimethroprim, ampicillin, gentamicin, cephotaxime and nitrofurantoin.

Following a course of ampicillin, she fed well and started to gain weight. A renal ultrasound demonstrated dilated pelvicalyceal systems bilaterally; a micturating cystogram revealed grade 4 vesicoureteric reflux. She continued to thrive on prophylactic trimethoprim.

Metabolic disorders   There are a number of metabolic disorders that present with vomiting and failure to thrive. All are rare and are discussed in Chapter 31.

Toxic agents   These include the fetal alcohol syndrome and lead poisoning; the latter used to be an important cause but is now rarely seen, although lesser degrees of lead exposure have significant implications for intellectual handicap.

Stools

Failure to thrive may be associated with persistent diarrhoea or steatorrhoea. When taking a history the nature of the stools needs to be defined (Chs 69,70).

Urine

Losses from urine which may result in failure to thrive may involve, alone or in combination, glucose, water, salt and base; the following disorders need to be considered:
- diabetes mellitus (Ch. 66)
- chronic renal failure (Ch. 62)
- adrenal insufficiency (Ch. 65)
- diabetes insipidus: large volumes of very dilute urine characteristic; response to pitressin differentiates from renal diabetes insipidus
- renal tubular defects (rare).

Failure of utilisation

Chronic infection

In this situation, anorexia and an increase in metabolic rate are responsible for failure to thrive. The disorder is usually obvious but this may not always be the case, for example in tuberculous infection and Still's disease. Other chronic infections that need to be considered include chronic asthma, cystic fibrosis (Ch. 50) and immune deficiency disease (including HIV infection).

Metabolic disorders

There are a number of metabolic defects that present because of failure to grow. These are discussed in Chapter 31. Should one be suspected, gas chromatography and mass spectrometry of urine are the key investigations.

Endocrine disorders

Hypothyroidism, formerly a common cause of growth failure, is now rarely seen in countries where neonatal screening is practised. Pituitary deficiency, and in particular isolated growth hormone deficiency, is unusual in infancy.

Constitutional, genetic, chromosomal and intrauterine abnormalities

- Some infants have a *genotype of small stature and slow growth*. Some in this group, which is usually familial, have low levels of somatomedin and often respond to large doses of human growth hormone.
- *Intrauterine growth retardation*: these infants are referred to as primordial dwarfs.
- *Chromosomal abnormalities*: the commonest is Down syndrome (trisomy 21); less common chromosomal abnormalities are trisomy 13 and trisomy 18.
- *Intrauterine infections*: intrauterine rubella, cytomegalovirus and toxoplasmosis may alter potential for growth and may present in infancy.
- *Bone dysplasias*: growth failure is a feature. More than 300 have been described. They are separated on the basis of their physical appearance, their radiology and the mode of inheritance (Ch. 29).

There is a group of children who fail to thrive and grow but remain undiagnosed despite extensive investigation. Some remain small while others, for no known reason and quite suddenly, grow normally.

11 The child with a developmental disability

P. Graves

Developmental disabilities

Definition

There are, amongst all children, differences in the way they think, learn, move, speak, read, relate to other people, and respond to what is going on around them. These are neurologically based functions that develop in each child as a result of interaction between inborn capacity and the environment. When those differences are such that the child is placed at a disadvantage compared to his or her age peers we talk in terms of a disability. Developmental disabilities are differences in neurologically based functions that have their onset before birth or during childhood and are associated with significant long term difficulties.

The concept embraces groups of conditions at the severe end of the spectrum (such as intellectual disabilities, cerebral palsies, autism spectrum disorders, blindness and deafness) as well as groups of conditions at the mild end of the spectrum (such as learning disorders, clumsiness and disorders of attention). These latter conditions, although relatively mild, may have quite severe consequences for the affected individual and family. There is substantial overlap between the mild and severe groups and between the mild group and normal children.

Most of these conditions result from a static brain insult or maldevelopment and are associated with a permanent, but not unchanging, disability pattern. These children improve in all areas of function with age, but their differences relative to the general population remain. A few result from conditions in which there is ongoing pathology. For these children there is subsequent failure to develop new skills and ultimately loss of previously acquired skills.

Disabilities tend to be multiple; that is, it is common for neurologically based disabilities, such as intellectual disability, cerebral palsy, epilepsy, vision impairments and hearing impairments, to coexist. More than half the children with a developmental disability can be expected to have one or more additional disabilities.

Terminology

Many terms are used to refer to these children and these conditions. Some are inaccurate and many are, intention-

ally or unintentionally, hurtful. The World Health Organization recommends distinguishing between the disease or disorder and the impairment, disability and handicap which may result from it. The *disease* or *disorder* is the underlying pathology (for instance, Down syndrome or congenital rubella). The *impairment* is the consequent functional limitation at organ level (for example, intellectual impairment or vision impairment). The *disability* is the inability of the person to perform tasks (such as reading and mobility) that results from an impairment. The World Health Organization also recommends referring to the person first and the disease, impairment or disability second. So we should refer to a child with Down syndrome or a child with an intellectual disability rather than to a Down syndrome child or an intellectually disabled child. The differences may appear minor but they are extremely important to people with disabilities and their families. *Handicap* refers to the outcome of interaction between a person with a disease, impairment or disability and society. These may be attitudinal, as in the case of a child with epilepsy being denied the opportunity to go on a school camp or any child who is teased because he or she is different. They may include access difficulties for children in wheelchairs or the diverse difficulties faced by children who cannot read. This classification is currently undergoing revision. The revised system, ICDIH-2 (International Classification of Disabilities, Impairments and Handicaps 2), is being developed to include greater consideration of environmental factors and a greater emphasis on opportunities for participation.

Prevalence

Prevalence estimates of children with disabilities vary: estimates are usually between around 3% and around 10–20%. The lower figure is appropriate for those children at the severe end of the spectrum and the higher figure incorporates those at the milder end. Differences in stated prevalence of specific disabilities more frequently reflect differences in definition and ascertainment methods than they do real differences in occurrence.

Management

Developmental disabilities are not curable. There are, however, medical, educational and social interventions that can make a substantial contribution to the care of children with disabilities. The future quality of life for children with disabilities and their families is as much a measure of the society in which they live as it is dependent on the nature and severity of their disability. Most societies, through their governments, acknowledge a responsibility to provide decent standards of medical care, family support, education, shelter, recreation and vocation options for children and adults with disabilities. National laws (for example, disability service, equal opportunity and antidiscrimination legislation) and international agreements, such as the United Nations Standard Rules on the Equalization of Opportunities for Persons with Disabilities, reflect an approach which goes beyond basic services to the basic rights and equality of all people, regardless of their abilities. All societies are different in the services they provide and all vary in the extent to which they approach the ideals of full acceptance, inclusion and equality. There are, however, core services to which most children with disabilities and their families can expect access:

- *Health care.* Detection, assessment and aetiological diagnosis of the underlying disorder. Diagnosis, assessment and treatment of associated health problems.
- *Information.* Information about the child's condition, including prognosis and recurrence risk, entitlements and the services that are available.
- *Consumer groups.* These provide mutual support, information about specific conditions and advocacy.
- *Financial assistance.* To compensate for extra costs and loss of income.
- *Habilitation and equipment.* To enable children with disabilities to overcome their impairments to the greatest extent possible; for example, physiotherapy and wheelchairs for children with motor impairments, speech therapy and assisted communication for children with communication impairments.
- *Family support.* To enable parents and other members of the family to fulfil their potential in life; for example, childcare, practical assistance in the home with dressing, bathing and feeding, and periods of residential care outside the family home.
- *Education.* Equal access to a broad educational curriculum at primary, secondary and tertiary level. Increasingly the emphasis is on providing this within mainstream schools. This frequently involves a modified curriculum and extra assistance within the classroom.
- *Transport.* Access to transport, which, through subsidy, modification or relaxation of parking restrictions, enables families and children to overcome disadvantages related to the children's disabilities.
- *Recreation.* Services such as 'buddy' programmes, attendants, facilitated access to mainstream recreational activities, and special clubs and sporting groups.
- *Environmental modification.* Ramps, wider doorways, wheelchair accessible toilets, simplified written instructions, opportunities to take examinations orally, self-opening doors, auditory signals at traffic lights, lower shop counters and lift buttons.
- *Vocational training.* Young people with disabilities can expect to have access to a range of training programmes specifically designed to provide them with the opportunity for gainful and satisfying employment.

Intellectual disabilities

Definition

Children with intellectual disabilities have diffuse cognitive impairments which affect their capacity to learn, communicate, care for themselves and live in our complex society. Standardized tests of intellectual function (IQ tests) are designed to produce a normal, bell-shaped frequency distribution curve. The lower limit of normal is arbitrarily set at 2 standard deviations below the mean. On most tests the mean is standardised at 100 and 1 standard deviation is 15. Thus the lower limit of normal on most tests is 70. IQ tests are an attempt to measure basic intellectual ability, as opposed to acquired knowledge. They are not perfect and have been misused in the past to reinforce racial and gender prejudices and to further disadvantage already marginalised social groups. Used properly, however, they produce results that, in children of school age, are reproducible and consistent over time. They generally reflect the child's basic capacity and provide detailed information on the child's pattern of abilities and how he or she might best be assisted to learn. Definitions of disability also include the concept of early onset, usually defined as before birth or during childhood, and day to day functioning, such as difficulties in self-care and interpersonal skills.

The World Health Organization divides intellectual disabilities into mild (IQ 50–69), moderate (IQ 35–49), severe (IQ 20–34) and profound (IQ < 20). For preschool children the term 'global developmental delay' tends to be used in preference to intellectual disability. This reflects the relative variability of assessments of developmental function in young children (although ability patterns are fairly stable from the age of 2 years) and a desire to use a gentler term in the early stages of diagnosis.

Prevalence

Estimates vary from 1 to 7%, with most estimates being in the range 0.67–3% (Table 11.1). The variation is due to differences in definition, methodology and true differences in prevalence.

Table 11.1   Prevalence estimates for children with intellectual disabilities

Source	Location	Age (years)	Prevalence (%)	
			IQ 50–69	IQ <50
Rutter, 1970	Isle of Wight, UK	5–14	2.53	0.34
Hagberg, 1984	Gothenburg, Sweden	8–12	0.37	0.30
Wellesley, 1992	Western Australia	6	0.30	0.39
Matilainen, 1995	Central Finland	8–9	0.56	0.63
Strømme, 2000	Akershus County, Norway	8–13	0.35	0.62

Presentation

- At birth, with features known to be associated with cognitive disability such as a recognisable dysmorphic syndrome, e.g. Down syndrome, or a single major malformation, such as microcephaly.
- With concerns about development. Children with more severe intellectual disabilities will usually present in the first 2–3 years of life with developmental delays. Sometimes the concern will be about one area of development (often speech), although all areas are usually affected. Children with milder intellectual disabilities will frequently present later.
- As a result of follow up of children at increased risk, such as a child who was small for gestational age or a child with a past history of meningitis.
- With another problem which may be the result of an underlying intellectual disability, such as a feeding, sleep or behavioural disturbance, or due to the same underlying pathology that has caused the intellectual disability, such as epilepsy.

Assessment

For parents, the possibility that there may be something wrong with their child is a major stress. Many undergo further hardship as a result of inappropriate reassurance. The evaluation of a child presenting with possible developmental delay requires an open mind, careful listening, a thorough history and examination, developmental assessment, and investigations to find the cause (Table 11.2). Assessment of development involves a quantitative assessment of skills in all areas of development. As in the assessment of growth, the results must then be compared with results for normal children of the same age. Typically a screening test such as the Denver II Developmental Screening Test (Ch. 4) is used. Once suspected, an abnormality will need to be confirmed by further, more detailed testing.

Differential diagnosis of intellectual disability

- *Slow development in a normal child*. Often this consideration can only be resolved by repeated assess-

Table 11.2   Assessment of a child with a suspected intellectual disability

History
Family pedigree
Pregnancy, birth, neonatal details, including birth weight, length, head circumference
Early feeding
Developmental milestones
Specific illnesses
Psychosocial environment

Examination
Growth, including head circumference
General responsiveness
Dysmorphic features
Skin pigment abnormalities
Neurological examination, including assessment of vision and hearing
General physical examination

Investigations
Depending on the history and physical examination findings, these may include:
Karyotype, including DNA testing for fragile X syndrome and any suspected microdeletion
Cranial imaging study, magnetic resonance imaging (MRI) or computerised tomography (CT)
EEG
Urine metabolic screening
Thyroid function
Mucopolysaccharide screening test
Serology for congenital infections
Creatine phosphokinase
Maternal Guthrie test

ments over time. It helps to consider the history: ask about family history of slow development and about recent developmental progress. During what may be quite a prolonged period of uncertainty, it helps to involve a developmental therapist (physiotherapist, occupational therapist, speech pathologist) who will be able to provide a more detailed assessment and some practical assistance.

- *Specific impairments*. Isolated impairments of vision, hearing, motor function, language and social communication may all present with global delay. The differentiation is made by specific evaluation of these areas. All children presenting with developmental delay warrant formal assessment of vision and hearing.

- *Environmental deprivation.* This is not a common cause of severe developmental delay, although it may exacerbate existing delays. If considered, it should be confirmed by demonstrating an improved rate of development after a change of environment.
- *Ongoing neural pathology.* Children with ongoing neural pathology may present initially with developmental delay that may mimic that due to a static insult. There will frequently be a slowing of development, followed by a period where there is little or no developmental progress, and finally a period of regression with loss of previously acquired skills. It is thus important to consider *rate* of development as well as current level — a parameter that is easier to measure if the developmental assessments are precise. Conditions in which there is ongoing neural pathology include intracranial tumours, storage disorders and demyelinating disorders.
- *Undetected or poorly treated epileptic seizures* may also cause developmental slowing or regression. In particular Landau–Kleffner syndrome and subclinical electrical status during slow wave sleep are two conditions in which epilepsy, which may not be apparent clinically, is associated with developmental regression.

Aetiology

Doctors have been criticised in the past for their pessimism in seeking the aetiology of intellectual disability. The cause of intellectual disability provides important information on the nature of the underlying disorder, likely complications and natural history. It helps parents deal with the grief associated with the discovery that their child has a disability.

Epidemiological studies since the 1970s have found that the cause of intellectual disability can be identified in 25–57% of cases of mild intellectual disability and in 70–90% of cases of moderate, severe and profound intellectual disability. Prenatal factors generally account for the majority of known causes: chromosome abnormalities, of which Down syndrome is the most common, form the largest group of these (Table 11.3).

An alternative approach to aetiology is through the analysis of risk factors. Poor nutrition, low social class and low maternal education are all known to be associated with intellectual disability. Iodine deficiency is considered to be the greatest cause of intellectual disability worldwide. These approaches also have important management implications, particularly at population and global levels.

Table 11.3   Causes of intellectual disability. (Source: Strømme P and Hagberg G, 2000)

Time of onset	IQ 50–69 (%)	IQ < 50 (%)
Prenatal		
Genetic		
Chromosomal	4	22
Specific syndromes	12	13
Neurodegenerative/ developmental	0	8
Familial	9	6
Acquired	5	4
Unknown		
Dysmorphic, unspecified syndromes	13	9
Brain anomaly	7	9
Subtotal	50	71
Perinatal	5	4
Postnatal	1	5
Unknown	44	20
Total	100	100

Some specific conditions

Down syndrome

Down syndrome is the most common abnormality associated with intellectual disability and accounts for approximately 25% of children with an IQ of less than 50. The incidence in Australia is approximately 1 in 1000 births. This is lower than in the past because of the reduced number of older women having children and the increased availability of intrauterine diagnosis. Intrauterine diagnosis was formerly offered to women at increased risk because of increased maternal age. It is now possible to identify high risk pregnancies in women of all ages through a variety of maternal blood and ultrasound examinations. Increasingly these are being offered to all pregnant women within a population. These tests have the potential to identify approximately 60% of cases of Down syndrome.

Approximately 95% of children with Down syndrome have standard trisomy 21; the remainder have additional chromosome 21 material as translocation D/G or G/G, or trisomy/normal mosaicism. The extra chromosome may be of maternal (in approximately two thirds) or paternal origin. The incidence of Down syndrome increases with maternal age, rising to 1% in women over 40 years of age and 2% in those over 45 years. Despite the higher incidence in older women, the vast majority of children with Down syndrome are born to mothers aged 20–30 years.

The spectrum of intellectual disability in Down syndrome varies from mild to profound, with most children being in the moderate and severely disabled range. With active early educational intervention, some children will be functioning at age appropriate level. Despite this, the vast majority of children with Down syndrome will have a significant intellectual disability. The common neonatal characteristics are shown in Table 11.4.

Children with Down syndrome have increased susceptibility to infection. Congenital heart disease occurs in 60%, one third of whom have an atrioventricular canal and one third a ventricular septal defect. Conductive deafness occurs in 60–80%, and many benefit from hearing aids in early life. Vision impairments, hypothyroidism due to autoimmune thyroiditis, ligamentous laxity and duodenal atresia are common. Haematological abnormalities, including leukaemia, which is approximately 20 times more common in those with Down syndrome than in the general population, and Hirschsprung disease are occasionally present. Estimates of life expectancy at birth vary from 30 to 45 years, although children who survive the infectious and cardiac hazards of infancy can be expected to live longer than this.

Fragile X syndrome

Fragile X syndrome is the second most common condition associated with intellectual disability. It is inherited as an X linked recessive abnormality. Prevalence studies in Australia and the United Kingdom suggest that 0.03–0.05% of all males and 0.05% of all females are affected. The fragile site on the X chromosome, at Xq27.3, is associated with abnormal CGG trinucleotide repeats. When the number of abnormal repeats exceeds 200 there is deactivation of the FMR-1 gene with failure to produce FMR protein. The role of FMR protein is unknown.

Boys with fragile X syndrome have above average height, increased ear size, large broad heads and, from the age of 6–8 years, orchidomegaly. There are connective tissue abnormalities with mitral valve prolapse, aortic root dilatation and hyperextensibility of the joints. Intellectual disability may be mild to severe. Many have features of attention deficit/hyperactivity disorder, with poor concentration, increased activity and fidgetiness. Features of autism (hand flapping, reduced eye contact and intolerance to change) are also common, although generally not severe enough to justify a diagnosis of autism. Similar features are present to a lesser extent in affected girls.

Diagnosis of fragile X syndrome is made using a specific DNA probe on peripheral blood leucocytes.

Other fragile sites occur on the X chromosome, resulting in fragile X syndrome B (or FRAXB), FRAXC, FRAXD, FRAXE and FRAXF. FRAXB, C and D are not clinically significant. FRAXE is associated with mild intellectual disabilities, and FRAXF may occasionally be associated with mild intellectual disabilities.

Clinical example

Peter has an older sister and a younger brother. His mother is a teacher and his father an engineer. Peter presented with language delay at the age of 3 years. His sister was said to be having learning problems at school. Peter was born after an uneventful pregnancy and delivery. He said his first words at 18 months and by 3 years had about six single words of speech. He tended to be quite active and distractible. Physical examination was unremarkable and developmental testing suggested he was performing at a 15–18 month level. Fragile X DNA testing for Peter, his mother and his older sister was positive. His younger brother will be tested only if he develops symptoms or if he requests it. His sister has had further cognitive assessment and has a mild intellectual disability. Both she and Peter are now receiving additional educational assistance.

Prader–Willi and Angelman syndromes

These conditions, which are clinically quite dissimilar, are both due to microdeletions on chromosome 15 (subregion q11–q13). In Prader–Willi syndrome, the deletion is of the paternally derived segment; in Angelman syndrome, the deletion is of the maternally derived segment. The cytogenetics are complex with a range of abnormalities, including microdeletion and uniparental disomy, being found in both conditions. Precision in diagnosis is justified as the recurrence risk is different in each case.

Children with Prader–Willi syndrome are frequently below average birth weight. As infants they are hypotonic and fail to thrive. Later they develop voracious

Table 11.4 Common neonatal characteristics of Down syndrome. (Source: Hall B 1966 Mongolism in newborn infants. Clinical Pediatrics 5:4)

Clinical features	Incidence (%)
Hypotonia	80
Poor Moro reflex	85
Joint hyperextensibility	80
Excess skin at the back of the neck	80
Flat facial profile	90
Slanted palpebral fissures	80
Anomalous auricles	60
Dysplasia of midphalanx of fifth finger	60
Single palmar crease	45

appetites and will often steal food and raid pantries and refrigerators. They become obese, are generally short, have small external genitalia, and small hands and feet. Their intelligence ranges from moderately severe intellectual disability to low normal. Firm measures to control dietary intake are the basis of management.

Children with Angelman syndrome are usually of lower birth weight than their siblings. They have feeding problems and an unusual cry in infancy. They walk with a stiff legged gait, have a tremor, and tend to hold their hands up and flap. They are generally happy and love water. They have subtle dysmorphic features which become more prominent over time. There is a wide smiling mouth, long face, prominent chin, and they are usually fairer than their siblings. Seizures occur in 82%.

Rett syndrome

> **Clinical example**
>
> Helen presented at the age of 2 years with delayed motor and language development. She was born after a normal pregnancy and delivery and had three healthy older siblings. There was no family history of disability. There were no concerns in her first year. At presentation she was walking well; she had no speech; she was not making eye contact when spoken to; and she had some repetitive hand mannerisms. A diagnosis of autism was made. On review 3 months later she had lost a number of hand skills and her walking had deteriorated. She was wringing her hands and it became clear that she was developing the classical features of Rett syndrome. The MECP2 gene test was positive. She subsequently developed seizures which have proved difficult to control and, at the age of 6 years, scoliosis, which required surgery. She is now confined to a wheelchair, and has no speech (but appears very alert and interested in her surroundings).

Rett syndrome is a severe condition that affects only girls. Prevalence estimates range from 0.44 to 0.96 per 10 000 females. Pathologically there is evidence of arrested neuronal development with deficient neuronal arborization and migration. The basal ganglia and midbrain are particularly involved. Rett syndrome is associated with a gene on the X chromosome, called MECP2, in a proportion of affected girls.

Four clinical stages are described. In stage I, from around 6 months to 4 years, there is developmental stagnation. In stage II, from 1 to 4 years, there is rapid regression with loss of hand skills and speech. In stage III, from 3 to 14 years, the girls appear reasonably stationary. Most have no speech and many do not walk. In stage IV, there is slowly progressive immobility and weakness. Severe scoliosis and seizures are common.

Velocardiofacial syndrome

Children with velocardiofacial syndrome and the related conditions of DiGeorge and conotruncal anomaly face syndrome have a microdeletion of chromosome 22q11.2. Clinical expression is often variable and may include cardiac anomalies, craniofacial features (including low set abnormally formed ears, hypertelorism, microcephaly, and palatal anomalies). Delayed speech, learning difficulties (the mean IQ is in the low normal range), behavioural difficulties and disorders of attention are common.

Duchenne muscular dystrophy

Although principally a neuromuscular degenerative disorder, this condition may also cause cognitive delays and present with cognitive, particularly language, difficulties. Duchenne muscular dystrophy needs to be considered in any boy with delayed motor development (Ch. 58).

Multiple minor malformations and dysmorphic syndromes

Multiple minor congenital anomalies, that is, those that do not affect function, usually suggest the presence of a major anomaly. In the presence of developmental delay they suggest that the delays are due to an intracranial malformation. When particular groups of malformations coexist frequently they are recognised as a *dysmorphic syndrome*. Increasing numbers of dysmorphic syndromes, such as Rubinstein–Taybi syndrome, Smith–Magenis syndrome and Williams syndrome, are now known to be due to chromosomal microdeletions (Ch. 29).

Iodine deficiency

Iodine deficiency is reported to occur in 130 countries worldwide. Clinical manifestations result from thyroxine deficiency. They include goitre, sleepiness and loss of energy, which are common; mild degrees of brain damage; and cretinism, which may affect between 1 and 10 per cent of children in affected areas. Prevention is through the use of iodised salt combined with effective monitoring programmes. While most cases occur in the developing world, there is concern that this disorder is re-emerging in the developed world, including the United States, New Zealand, Europe and Australia.

The effects of intellectual disability on the child, family and community

For the affected child there will be delays in acquiring new skills. Children with *mild intellectual disability* often do not present until school age, when they have problems learning to read and write. All academic learning will be difficult. As adults they can be expected to be capable of living independently and maintaining a job in open employment. Problems with reading, writing, handling money and interpersonal relationships are likely to persist.

Children with *moderate intellectual disabilities* usually present with developmental delays in the preschool years. They can be expected to have greater difficulties with educational learning and will require specific teaching to master basic social skills, such as dressing, feeding, preparing food, using public transport and living independently. As adults they will be capable of productive employment and independent living, although some ongoing support is likely to be needed.

Children with *severe and profound intellectual disabilities* will often have little or no speech and may require assistance with dressing and feeding. They are capable of mastering new skills but progress will be very slow.

For the family the realisation that their child has a disability is a major source of grief. The pain of mourning for the loss of the anticipated normal child is frequently associated with feelings of guilt, denial and anger. Families generally find anniversaries, major life events, such as starting school, and contact with other non disabled children difficult because these remind them of their loss. However, it is a mistake to attribute all family stress to grief. In a United Kingdom study of 1000 families the key areas of parental need were listed as follows:

- material support: finance, housing, transport, and equipment
- social and practical support: information, advice and counselling, support for their children, and respite care
- recognition by professionals of the parents' role and expertise.

The parents expressed their frustration with service providers' negative attitudes towards their children and with deficiencies in services.

For the community, a prevalence rate of 1–3% and the move away from segregated services means that most people will have some contact with a person with an intellectual disability. Current community approaches to disability aim to include people with intellectual disabilities as an integral part of society and to seek ways (for example, modified education curriculum, equal opportunities legislation) to facilitate their acceptance. Community services such as childcare, kindergartens, schools, transport, libraries and recreation facilities are available to all children, including those with intellectual disabilities.

Management

An overview of services which should be available is provided at the beginning of this chapter.

The doctor's role

Many professionals have useful contributions to make to the care of children with intellectual disabilities. Doctors, who are usually the pivotal figures in the early diagnostic phases, should be well informed about child and family services in order to advise the families. They will need to be aware of potential associated conditions, such as impairments of vision and hearing, epilepsy and cardiac anomalies, and ensure that these are detected early. As the child grows older the doctor's role will become more peripheral. However, there will still be a need to review the aetiological diagnosis, treat associated conditions and intercurrent illnesses, and provide advice for families and others involved in the child's care.

Disclosure

Parents prefer to be told of their child's disability as soon as possible. They prefer to be told together and in private. The person telling them should be sensitive to their situation and allow sufficient time for adequate explanations. It is also recommended that there be a follow up discussion, provision of written material to the family and early referral to services.

Parent self-help groups

Many parents indicate that their greatest source of support is from other parents in similar situations. Self-help groups for specific conditions and groups for broader disability categories are to be found in most communities.

Preschool services

Early intervention services for children with developmental delays have been becoming more widespread since the 1970s. Initially these focused on educational interventions for the children. Review of the latter indicates that developmental gains for the children are small and tend to be short lived. The literature now supports an approach which is more directed at enhancing an understanding of the child's ability pattern, assisting the child in areas of disability, and providing practical family support from the time of diagnosis. Most children with disabilities can attend services used by all other children in their community, with their needs supplemented by developmental and educational consultants and practical family support.

School

There has been a major revolution in special education over the past three decades. Most children who now receive special education do so in mainstream schools. With changes in school organisation, teacher training and curriculum, it is now possible to educate all children with disabilities in mainstream schools. Full inclusion of children with disabilities is advocated in the United Nations Standard Rules (1994). Most countries, however, still maintain special schools and offer parents a choice of inclusive or non inclusive education. The important issue for those advising families is how the child should be educated, that is, considering the child's pattern of abilities and its implications for learning, rather than where the education takes place.

12 Child abuse

A. Carmichael

While abuse, neglect and exploitation of children have been recognised throughout history and continue in the form of child labour and prostitution in parts of the developing world today, the prevalence of child abuse in industrialised societies has been acknowledged only since the mid 20th century. In 1946 and 1953 two American radiologists, Caffey and Silverman, raised the possibility of non accidental injury to children, but it was 1962 before Henry Kempe coined the term 'battered child syndrome' and forced reluctant professionals and communities to acknowledge the problem. The earliest Australian reports of physical child abuse were from Birrell and Birrell in 1966. Also in 1966 Bialestock reported the neglect of children resulting in non organic failure to thrive, and in 1971 Oates and Yu reported non organic failure to thrive in children admitted to hospital and the sequelae in the form of emotional and learning difficulties in teenagers. Since the 1970s, child sexual abuse has become increasingly recognised, as has emotional abuse. In the last decade, the long term effects of abuse and neglect, mediated through both biomedical and environmental influences on the developing brains of young children have been documented with sequelae of behavioural and developmental problems, school failure and criminality.

Definition

Child abuse may be defined as involving physical injury, sexual abuse or deprivation of nutrition, care and affection in circumstances which indicate that injury or deprivation may not be accidental or may have occurred through neglect.

Prevalence

During the past decade the Australian Institute of Health and Welfare has collated prevalence data from the States and Territories which indicate that reported cases (notifications) have increased from 45 468 in 1988–1989 to 107 134 cases in 1999–2000. This number of notifications approximates 20 per 1000 children aged 0–16 years. Approximately 45% of notifications are substantiated. There is substantial interstate variation largely related to differing legislative and reporting approaches.

However, of substantiated cases, overall physical abuse, emotional abuse and neglect each comprise approximately 25–30%, with sexual abuse comprising 10–25%.

National data on mortality, injury and harm due to child abuse are not available, but in New South Wales in 1999–2000, six deaths were reported. Serious injuries amongst a series of 3451 substantiated cases of physical abuse included 41 fractures, 22 burns and scalds and 100 lacerations and welts. From these, some 50–100 cases of permanent disability would be expected, although these data are not collected currently. Recent Australian statistics are consistent with present estimates of the incidence of child abuse in other developed countries, ranging between 10 and 20 cases per 1000 live births.

Current understanding acknowledges that child abuse and neglect exist as a spectrum of conditions, as shown in Figure 12.1. Abnormalities in the child may range from death through physical injuries, failure to thrive, developmental, emotional and behavioural problems to normality. Corresponding labels that relate to these disorders are indicated in the diagram. Sexual abuse (described in detail below) may be added, with features ranging from normality to emotional and behavioural disorders and, in rare cases, injury. The concept of a spectrum is useful in that it recognises overlap between various types of abuse. For example, developmental and behavioural disturbances due to emotional abuse or neglect will often be present in children who are physically abused. Furthermore, it indicates that in some families there is a progression of abuse from minor degrees of abnormality to more serious injury, thus emphasising the importance of early identification and intervention. The diagnosis of child abuse may be clear cut towards the more severe end of the spectrum (failure to thrive and physical injury), while at the other end firm categorisation is difficult. This is especially so in differentiating 'at risk' situations from extremes of normal child rearing practices, which are particularly complex in a multicultural society such as Australia.

Clinical presentation of abused or 'at risk' children

The clinical approach to children who may be abused or neglected requires, like other problems presenting

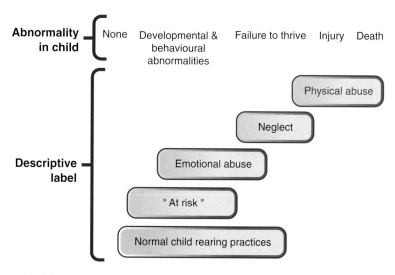

Fig. 12.1 Spectrum of child abuse.

medically, a thorough history and examination followed by appropriate investigations.

Features of history suggestive of child abuse

- *Inappropriate parental concern.* This may relate to late presentation for an injury or other problem. It may also alert to an 'at risk' situation, in which the child is presented repeatedly for what may be seen as a minor medical problem, or 'overanxiety' in the face of medical reassurance that no serious illness exists. This circumstance may represent a cry for help on the part of the parent and be a point of early identification and intervention.
- *Frequent accidents.* While some children, due to their different temperament and personalities, seem more accident prone than others, the child presenting with frequent accidents should be carefully evaluated for potential non accidental injury. Consideration should be given to the quality of care and supervision exercised within the home, as studies of children presenting with frequent accidents have shown overlap between accidental and non accidental injury.
- *Previous injury or abuse in other siblings.* It has been established that within some families only one child of a number may be subject to abuse, perhaps by virtue of temperament, personality or parental expectation. However, in other families, particularly those where there is violence, alcoholism or multiple problems, abuse may affect all children.
- *Inconsistent histories.* The explanation of an event or incident causing the injury or presentation may vary when histories are taken at different times or when two caregivers give different explanations in relation to the same event. It is important not to overlook the history

given by the child, as even children of 3 or 4 years of age may give a very straightforward account of what has happened to them.
- *Acute disturbance or crisis in the social situation.* While this is not a necessary or consistent feature in child abuse, it may indicate a precipitating or exacerbating factor leading to the abuse. It also acknowledges that physical abuse and neglect are more often found in families from socioeconomic groups where stress factors such as unemployment, poverty and limited access to resources are more prevalent.

Features on examination indicative of child abuse

- *Injuries inconsistent with events described or with the child's developmental level.* The presence of a skull fracture in a 6 week infant who is alleged to have rolled off a bed represents a classic example in this category. The gross motor development of a 6 week infant is such that rolling is not yet achieved (Ch. 4). Similarly, a toddler presenting with a transverse fracture through the shaft of the humerus, allegedly resulting from a fall, would lead to suspicion that an injury of much greater force has occurred.
- *Bruising or other injuries at unusual sites.* The normal toddler or preschool child often sustains bruises over the anterior tibiae, extensor surfaces of the forearms or even on the forehead from normal activity and minor accidents. However, bruises over flexor surfaces of arms or legs, face or on the back should raise concern about non accidental injury. Bruising around the mouth or a torn frenulum in a young infant suggests the use of undue force when the child was fed.

- *Burns and scalds.* In recent years, large paediatric burns units have reported that 5–10% of their admissions are a result of child abuse. Small burns at unusual sites without adequate explanation, especially cigarette burns, are pathognomonic of child abuse.
- *Non organic failure to thrive, developmental delay, emotional and behavioural disturbances.* These findings may be manifestations of child abuse and neglect and may present alone as the main problem leading to the diagnosis (Ch. 10).
- *Fear or apathy in a child.* The toddler who seems unduly wary of parents or strangers may be exhibiting a sign of past abuse. Kempe coined the term 'frozen awareness' for this apprehensive response in toddlers.
- *Subdural haematoma and retinal haemorrhages.* These central nervous system signs should be regarded as pathognomonic of child abuse unless proved otherwise. Subdural haematomas in small children may be caused by direct trauma, but when present with retinal haemorrhages they are indicative of vigorous shaking.

Documentation of history and examination

Precise documentation of history and examination findings in children suspected of being abused is essential. Detailed descriptions, together with clearly marked diagrams and photographs are recommended to record the extent and evolution of physical injury including bruising.

Investigations when child abuse is suspected

Investigations are required to confirm or extend diagnosis and in some instances for medicolegal purposes. When physical injury is present, a skeletal survey is required to seek current and past evidence of bony injury. Initial imaging is best done by skull X ray and a total radionuclide bone scan of body and long bones to detect recent injury. Further X rays may be taken to define 'hot spots' on the bone scan and to detect old fractures (Fig. 12.2). In addition, X rays will also exclude rare conditions such as osteogenesis imperfecta as a cause for frequent or early fractures.

A full blood examination, including platelet count and clotting studies, is more relevant for medicolegal purposes than for clinical diagnosis, as bleeding and bruising resulting from bleeding or coagulation disorders should be suspected on the basis of clinical findings and then confirmed by investigation.

The specific organic causes for failure to thrive should be excluded by appropriate investigation when indicated

> ## Clinical example
>
> Christine was a previously well 6 week infant brought to hospital by her parents after she had 'coughed up' some bright red blood. On examination, she had a torn frenulum of her upper lip, a small bruise over the left temporal region and three old bruises around her right eye. Her parents did not know how these injuries had occurred. A diagnosis of suspected child abuse resulted in her admission to hospital, where a bone scan revealed 'hot spots' in the midshaft of the left tibia, at the left knee and right chest. Subsequent X rays were performed (Figs 12.2 and 12.3).
>
> The clinical features of torn frenulum, bruising of different ages without adequate explanation, and unexplained fractures confirmed the diagnosis of child abuse. Protective Services were involved and following investigation and a Children's Court hearing, she was placed in the care of her grandmother under a Supervision Order.

by the clinical findings (Ch. 10). A confirmatory finding in children with non organic failure to thrive due to abuse and neglect is their documented weight gain with normal feeding in a hospital or out of home care environment.

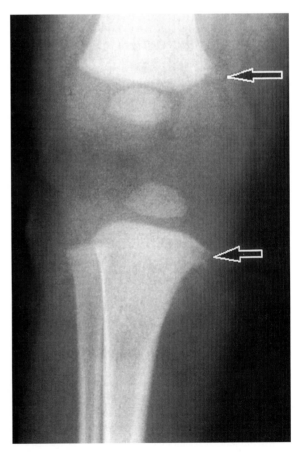

Fig. 12.2 X ray of left knee of Christine showing chip metaphyseal fractures to lower femur and upper tibia.

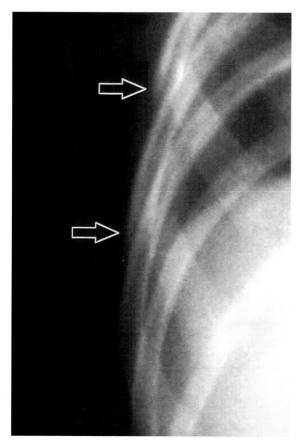

Fig. 12.3 Radiograph of chest of Christine showing fractures of right 5th, 6th and 7th ribs in the axillary region.

Table 12.1 Indicators of sexual abuse
1. Direct reports from children
2. Pregnancy in adolescents
3. Prepubescent venereal disease
4. Genital or rectal trauma
5. Precocious sexual interest or preoccupation
6. Indiscreet masturbatory activity
7. Sexual abuse of other family members
8. Repeated absconding from home in adolescent girls
9. Social withdrawal and isolation
10. Fear and distrust of authorities
11. Negative self-esteem, depression, suicidal behaviour, substance abuse
12. Somatic complaints including abdominal and pelvic pain

Child sexual abuse (CSA)

Kempe (1978) has defined this as the 'involvement of dependent, developmentally immature children and adolescents in sexual activities that they do not fully comprehend, to which they are unable to give informed consent, or that violate the social taboos or family roles'. Centres dealing with CSA report that, while almost all perpetrators are male, 20–30% of victims are also male. In contrast to adult sexual assault, 80% of cases involve chronic incest, with only approximately 20% resulting from a single episode of sexual assault or rape by a stranger. Further, the mean age of presentation in many CSA centres is 7 years or less, with the likelihood of penetration or intercourse increasing with increasing age of the victim. In many incestuous families, sexual abuse of all children, especially girls, may occur. Those commonly involved are the stepfather, de facto father, grandfather or other male relative.

Based on history and examination and having regard to the epidemiology of reported cases, it is again possible to list indicators, as shown in Table 12.1. These may be con-

sidered presumptive evidence of sexual abuse (1–4), possible indicators (5–9) and other conditions (10–12) which may occasionally be manifestations of CSA.

The following comments elaborate on some of the listed indicators. The numbers in the headings relate to Table 12.1.

Direct reports from children (1). The child's report should be believed unless it can be proved inaccurate. Previous teaching and overemphasis on the early work of Freud and others, which attributed children's reports of sexual activities to fantasy, has now been refuted. This has resulted in the slow acceptance of the validity of most incidents reported by children.

Adolescent pregnancy (2). Here it is important to rule out premature but peer appropriate sexual activity.

Prepubescent venereal disease (3). Prepubescent venereal disease, when discovered, is pathognomonic of CSA. However, non specific vaginal discharge may also be a presentation of CSA. The child with recurrent vaginal discharge or genital warts requires careful evaluation.

Genital or rectal trauma (4). A thorough genital examination, in particular close inspection of the external genitalia and anus, is important in all cases of suspected CSA. This examination should be undertaken by an experienced practitioner, preferably with access to a colposcope for magnification and photography if necessary. Pelvic examinations are rarely indicated in prepubertal girls and it should be noted that the absence of abnormal findings does not exclude CSA, especially in the young child. Conversely, abnormal examination findings alone should not be relied on for diagnosis.

Possible indicators (5–9). Should any of the possible indicators (5–9) be present, CSA should be considered seriously as a cause and an appropriate history and examination performed.

Non specific behaviour (10–12). Non specific behaviour and other clinical associations (10–12) are less

Clinical example

Ruth presented at the age of 13 years because of physical and behavioural problems. For the past 6 months she had been listless, uninterested in school and had broken off several friendships at school. During the last month she had complained of recurrent abdominal pain, urinary frequency and dysuria. On physical examination she was withdrawn, with some tenderness over the suprapubic region. Her pubertal status was Tanner stage 4 for breast and pubic hair development. She denied sexual activity.

Microscopy of her urine revealed numerous white cells and there was a mixed growth on culture. Because of problems in obtaining an appropriate urine sample for further culture and because of the lower abdominal pain and tenderness she was referred for a gynaecological opinion. Pelvic examination was performed in the presence of a chaperone. There was pain in the region of the cervix and there was a purulent vaginal discharge, culture of which resulted in a mixed growth of Gram positive and Gram negative cocci and bacilli. Specific antigen for **Chlamydia trachomatis** was detected by enzyme immunoassay.

When told of the diagnosis of a sexually transmitted vaginitis and a pelvic infection, Ruth admitted sexual intercourse. After further discussion she tearfully told of sexual abuse by her stepfather during the last 6 months. Notification was made to the Child Protection Services, and the police charged the stepfather. A care order from the court prevented any further contact between Ruth and her stepfather. Sexual abuse had been the cause of her altered mood and behaviour, as well as causing the recurrent abdominal pain.

frequently manifestations of CSA than the preceding indicators, but CSA should always be considered in the differential diagnosis. It should also be noted that CSA can present in children who exhibit normal peer appropriate behaviour and achievement; many children may conceal carefully any sign of sexual victimisation, which may only be revealed when the child or young adolescent leaves home.

Management of abused and neglected children

When child abuse is suspected, the safety and protection of the child is of paramount importance. In the first instance, for cases of physical abuse and neglect, this often involves admission to hospital for treatment of the presenting problem, such as reduction of fractures, repair of lacerations, observation and management of head injuries, or appropriate feeding if non organic failure to thrive is suspected. Investigations also will be facilitated by hospital admission. These aspects are usually dealt with under the guidance of an experienced paediatrician, with consultation from an orthopaedic surgeon, neurosurgeon, ophthalmologist and paediatric gynaecologist when appropriate.

Admission also allows for a thorough assessment of the child and family. For this to be achieved properly a multidisciplinary team is required, as the initial assessment and later therapeutic intervention must involve professionals, such as social workers, psychologists and child psychiatrists, who are competent in the emotional and social assessment of children and families. Expertise also is required in the areas of physical development and behavioural problems of children, as these areas must be assessed in any child with evidence of physical or sexual abuse or neglect.

Once child abuse is suspected on initial assessment, protective intervention must be undertaken. Doctors in all States and Territories of Australia (except Western Australia) are required by legislation to report suspected child abuse to a protective authority, namely a government social welfare or community services department, or the police. Notification, whether mandatory or not, is usually followed by further assessment, culminating in a multidisciplinary case conference at which a plan for ongoing management is formulated. Decisions will be influenced by the nature of the abuse, the family circumstances and in particular the continuing risk to the child. There are usually two main options:

1. The parents may agree voluntarily that they need help and enter into a counselling, supportive or therapeutic programme.
2. The case may be brought before a Children's Court for safe custody through a Care and Protection application. If this is granted, the case will usually be adjourned for further hearing within a matter of weeks, during which more detailed assessment occurs. A number of options are available to the Children's Court:
   a. The case may dismissed.
   b. The child may be allowed to return home with the parents, but under the supervision of an officer of the Social Welfare or Community Services Department. Under these circumstances, the parents often will be required to accept counselling and support.
   c. The child may be removed from the parents' care and placed in the care of the State as long as he or she remains at risk of significant harm. An obvious prerequisite for return to the parental home will be change in the home environment after counselling and social support for the parents.

Child sexual abuse

Child sexual abuse is best managed by referral to hospital or to community based sexual assault centres with the ability to manage child victims. Protection of the child in these cases often involves removal of the perpetrator from the home rather than admission of the child to hospital.

Principles of assessment of the ability of the family to protect and care for the child similar to those outlined above for physical abuse and neglect will apply. Additionally, in CSA, specific therapy for the child victim is required, together with support and counselling for other family members. Treatment of the perpetrator is essential to the reconstitution of the family and in some States pretrial diversion treatment options are being developed, following their successful use in overseas centres.

Difficulties in the management of child abuse

The management of child abuse is not easy. Parents almost invariably deny accusations of child abuse, so that anger and hostility are often present, particularly when a safe custody order is granted. Often facilities for parent counselling are inadequate and many abused children are returned home before the situation is a safe one and parents have been supported adequately. Follow up of families who have abused their children is difficult, because such families move often and leave no forwarding addresses. This makes appraisal of therapeutic techniques difficult, but long term studies confirm that even when abuse ceases, many children are at risk of emotional, educational and behavioural problems in later years. Despite this, there are a proportion of families who are rehabilitated and subsequently care for their children in an appropriate manner.

Prevention of child abuse

Although the larger part of this discussion has been devoted to the management of abused children, it is generally agreed that the most effective strategy for management is prevention. A number of overseas studies have documented the merit of identification of high risk families in the antenatal and perinatal period, followed by selected home visiting by support workers. Similar programmes, such as Good Beginnings, are now established in Australia. Maternal and child health nurses in Australia maintain contact with approximately 90% of infants during the first year of life, providing preventive and supportive programmes. Therefore, this service, especially where linked with general practitioners and other community health services, is well placed to play a primary preventive role in child abuse.

Further preventive strategies include education for parenthood within schools, in premarital counselling and during pregnancy. The use of programmes such as 'protective behaviours' have been developed to assist prevention of child sexual abuse. These programmes encourage children to accept that they have a right to feel safe at all times, and that if they do not feel safe they are able to seek help from supportive adults.

Finally, measures which reduce stresses on families, such as those caused by unemployment and poverty, together with positive family support and child care programmes are likely to reduce the incidence of child abuse.

These and other measures have recently been highlighted in Australia through the National Strategies for Prevention of Child Abuse and Neglect, coordinated by the National Child Protection Council (1993), the National Council for the Prevention of Child Abuse (1997) and currently the National Children's and Families Council.

13 Sudden infant death syndrome and sudden unexpected death in infancy

B. J. Taylor

Until 1991, the following was true of sudden infant death syndrome(SIDS):

> When theories compete in profusion
> Then the experts conclude, in confusion,
> There'll be flaws in all laws
> Of this unexplained cause
> Till the problem is solved by exclusion.
>
> *Lady Limerick, 1976*

The discipline of epidemiology has now given us some useful facts that have led to an increased understanding of infant physiology, and population intervention has reduced the number of SIDS deaths dramatically. This chapter examines the prevention and potential causes of sudden unexpected death in infancy and looks at the follow up care needed when it does occur.

Definitions

Infant (0–1 year) mortality has declined consistently during the last 70 years and New Zealand data are used to illustrate this (Fig. 13.1). The majority of this decline has been through falls in neonatal (0–1 month) mortality; postneonatal (1–12 month) mortality declined at a much slower rate until the early 1990s, when most countries, led by New Zealand and the Netherlands, introduced focused public health campaigns to change infant care practice. All areas that have introduced these changes have had dramatic decreases in postneonatal mortality rates. In both Australia and New Zealand, as well as the UK and USA, between 40 and 60% of deaths in the postneonatal period are unexpected and usually occur outside the hospital in the infant's own home.

In 1970, Beckwith defined the sudden infant death syndrome as 'The sudden death of an infant or young child which is unexpected by history, and in which a full postmortem examination fails to demonstrate an adequate cause of death.' There has been an important addition to this definition: namely, including an on site investigation of the death as being just as important as the postmortem in making the diagnosis. This definition remains widely accepted and for most purposes is synonymous with the terms 'cot death' (NZ and UK) and 'crib death' (USA), although these terms should not be used because many of the deaths occur outside the 'cot'.

In 1979, the World Health Organization (WHO) assigned International Classification of Diseases (ICD) code 798.0 to SIDS. It is important to note that any other condition noted on the death certificate takes priority over SIDS in the coding rules, such that if the pathologist believes the death is due to SIDS and puts this as the first diagnosis, but as a secondary diagnosis puts down 'pneumonitis', then the latter takes precedence and national statistics will not include this case as SIDS. Thus, comparing SIDS rates between countries is very difficult and it is generally better to compare total mortality rates within a tightly specified age group.

There are three characteristic postmortem findings in most babies who are labelled as having SIDS. These are:
- multiple intrathoracic pleural, pericardial and thymic petechiae (found in 80–90% of SIDS and thought to suggest the occurrence of obstructive apnoea before death)
- congested heavy lungs with marked pulmonary oedema (present in any asphyxial death)
- liquid blood in the heart (cause totally unknown).

Historically, until early in the twentieth century, SIDS would have been labelled as 'overlaying' (as in Solomon's judgement — 1 Kings 3: 16–22). Subsequent labelling has included the terms below, and many others since:
- 1890s: 'capillary bronchitis or suffocating catarrh of children'

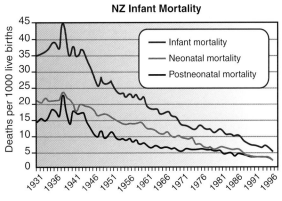

Fig. 13.1 New Zealand infant mortality.

- 1900–1945: 'status thymico-lymphaticus' (pressure on trachea, lungs, and great vessels by an enlarged thymus)
- 1940s: 'accidental mechanical suffocation'
- 1950s: 'fulminating respiratory infection'.

Incidence and geographical variation

There are many difficulties in making any comparisons between countries, as there are important differences in labelling and in postmortem rates. Of some use is the comparison of postneonatal mortality rates or 1–5 month mortality rates. Comparison of deaths from congenital defects suggests no major differences between countries, but there are major differences in postneonatal death rates because of differences in the numbers of deaths labelled as SIDS. Because of specific campaigns in different countries, there have been some dramatic changes in SIDS and postneonatal mortality. Thus, until the early 1990s, the highest rates of SIDS were found in New Zealand and Tasmania (~4 per 1000 live births); an intermediate incidence in Australia, the USA and the UK (~2 per 1000); and low rates in Scandinavia (~1.2 per 1000), Singapore, Hong Kong and Japan (~0.5 per 1000). Most Pacific Island communities have low rates.

Since 1989, major campaigns promoting:

- supine sleeping
- avoidance of smoking in pregnancy
- breastfeeding
- avoidance of overheating

have been associated with at least a 50% decline in the number of SIDS deaths. Further analysis suggests that this is almost entirely due to change in infant sleep position, with no significant changes in smoking behaviour or other factors. Thus, in the UK SIDS rates are down to <0.5 per 1000, and in New Zealand have fallen to <2 per 1000.

In most countries with significant minority indigenous populations, their rates of SIDS are higher than in other ethnic groups. In New Zealand, the rates for Maori infants remain approximately three times the non Maori rate and there have not been the same decreases in SIDS deaths that have been seen in other groups.

Demography

For babies who die of SIDS, the distribution of the age of death is typical (Fig. 13.2) and is replicated in almost every study of SIDS from all countries. This is one of the main epidemiological facts that all theories of SIDS must take into account or explain.

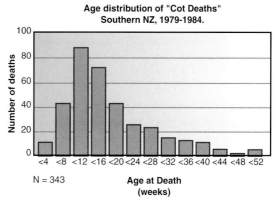

Fig. 13.2 Age distribution of 'cot deaths' (*n* = 343), southern New Zealand, 1979–1984.

Until the change in sleep position, there was a marked seasonal variation, with a winter excess in most countries. With most babies now sleeping on their backs there is now only a minor increase in the number of SIDS in winter. There is an overrepresentation of infants who die in those born to young mothers (aged <20 years), mothers who are smokers and those in lower socioeconomic groups.

Aetiology of sudden death in infancy

Because SIDS is a diagnosis of exclusion (no obvious cause at postmortem examination or on investigation of the site of death), the investigating team must think of the known causes of sudden and unexpected death in infancy before allocating the label SIDS. The medical causes that must be considered are the following.

Cardiac. Cardiac arrhythmias can cause sudden death, and the most obvious of these is a genetic disorder called the prolonged QT syndrome. Thus, a family history of sudden death, deafness and/or epilepsy may be relevant and could lead to other family members having an ECG or 24 hour Holter monitoring in order to make this diagnosis. Genetic studies are possible on a child who has died but this is still not a routine procedure.

Metabolic. A small percentage (<1% in the UK) of babies dying of SIDS probably die as a result of *medium-chain acetylcoenzyme A deficiency (MCAD)*. MCAD should be suspected if the baby was starved before death or if there was any unusual smell about the baby. The cause of death in these babies is hypoglycaemia, as they are unable to use medium chain fatty acids for energy. At postmortem, the clue may be extreme fat droplet deposition in the liver.

Homicide. This must always be kept in mind, and especially in the situation where there have been other siblings who have apparently died of SIDS. In general, it is thought that around 10% of SIDS cases may in fact be homicide. There is a helpful statement about these issues from the American Academy of Pediatrics.

Infection. Sudden and overwhelming infection is a possible cause of sudden death. Pneumococcal or meningococcal septicaemia or meningitis are often of particularly sudden onset but it should usually be possible to detect them at postmortem examination.

Seizure causing apnoea. This is theoretically possible but impossible to be sure about without a clear history. There are no pathological markers of this in infancy.

Usually it is not possible to make a clear diagnosis of a medical condition, and the death is then labelled as SIDS. Our current understanding of SIDS is based to a large degree on the interaction of three factors, as illustrated in Figure 13.3.

The vulnerable baby

Many studies have reported an association with low birth weight and the presence of other factors that suggest the baby is not as responsive as others, either generally or in the hours before death. There is some evidence that 40–50% of SIDS victims demonstrate poor weight gain prior to death, but this is not a very helpful predictor as ~35% of control infants will show similar growth patterns.

Necropsy data have shown that more SIDS babies (but not the majority) than controls (which are hard to find) have some evidence of chronic hypoxia, acute hypoxia (elevated hypoxanthine levels in the vitreous humor), small scars in the respiratory centre of the brainstem, and increased fetal haemoglobin levels and alterations in brainstem kainate receptors and serotinergic networks. Microbiological studies have suggested the presence of toxin producing staphylococcal species more often in the nasopharynx or stools and it has been shown that the presence of nicotine increases the toxicity of these staphylococcal toxins manyfold. Finally, it has been suggested recently that babies that have died of SIDS may have a genetically determined different cytokine response to infection.

The environment

The main contribution of epidemiology to solving some of the mysteries of SIDS started with the description of large differences in the incidence of SIDS between different countries; these were confirmed by similar large differences in postneonatal mortality rates. This strongly suggested that some environmental variables were influencing SIDS and led to many case–control studies of infant care practices which identified prone and side sleeping as increasing the risk of SIDS. The risk of dying when placed to sleep prone compared to supine is approximately five times higher in countries where babies tend to sleep on soft surfaces, and somewhat lower in countries where babies sleep on very firm surfaces.

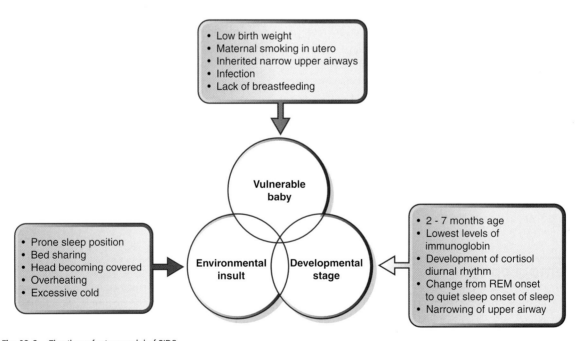

Fig. 13.3 The three factor model of SIDS.

There is now convincing evidence that side sleeping is also dangerous, but mainly because it increases the risk of the baby turning to the prone position while asleep. It is also most dangerous the first time the baby turns or is put to sleep prone.

Other environmental factors that may contribute appear to be the baby being either too hot or too cold, being found with the head covered by bedding, or sharing the sleeping surface with adults who are smokers. The interaction of bed sharing and maternal smoking is particularly important. Bed sharing with non smokers minimally increases the risk of SIDS, while the combination is associated with a very high risk (odds ratio of 4.55). This interaction perhaps explains the high rate of SIDS in indigenous peoples where the bed sharing/maternal smoking combination is particularly common.

More recently, there has been increasing evidence that having the head completely covered is a particularly dangerous risk factor. Practices parents can initiate to avoid this risk appear to be the avoidance of using blankets and sheets, using a sleeping bag arrangement instead. Recent European case–control data suggest a decreased risk with use of sleeping bag arrangements. Some recommend placing babies to sleep with their feet at the base of the cot so that they are unable to move further under the bedding, but this is unproven and babies can still move sideways under the bedding.

Finally, there is some evidence to suggest that babies that are either excessively insulated, or are in excessively hot rooms, or are underinsulated in cold rooms have a higher risk of SIDS. Because of the many different thermal environments in which a baby may sleep, it is hard to recommend any particular room temperature. Instead, it is wise to recommend that mothers check the temperature of their babies' hands and feet and compare this with the core temperature. The hands and feet should be slightly cooler than core (by about 2°C). If they are cold, either more insulation (bedding or clothing) or a warmer room is needed. If the peripheries are the same temperature as core, the room is either too hot or less bedding and clothing are needed. Obviously infection could interfere with this assessment and parents should be told not to increase the amount of clothing or bedding of a baby with an infection.

Some environmental factors appear to be protective. These are:
- the use of a dummy (pacifier) during sleep
- the sharing of the sleeping room (but not the bed) with adults (but not children)
- breastfeeding, although this factor is more controversial.

There is now also convincing evidence that immunisation in infancy decreases the risk of SIDS.

Multiple hypotheses and SIDS

There is a long list of popular and not so popular theories as to the cause of SIDS. These range from the 'ammonia theory' (where the increased risk in male babies is attributed to the fact that they are more likely to pass urine closer to the face), to other theories which have had many millions of dollars spent on research disproving them (for example, the central apnoea theory). Current theories with considerable evidence backing them are the following.

1. Obstructive apnoea

The relative dimensions of the upper airway appear to be a strongly inherited feature. It appears that babies' upper airway dimensions actually get smaller during the first 6 weeks of life, and this supports the idea that infants are at more risk of significant obstruction at 6 weeks of age than in the first few weeks of life. At the clinical level it is important to remember this if a baby is seen in the newborn period with signs of upper airway obstruction or significant indrawing. Remember that if these features are seen awake they could be much worse when asleep and overnight oximetry may be needed to document this.

2. Decreased arousal responses

It is now clear that many babies encounter various environmental insults that require them to wake from sleep and attract their caregiver's attention. Many of these stresses appear to be respiratory in nature; in particular, babies, especially those who put their face into bedding, need to able to move the face away, or increase ventilation dramatically, or finally arouse and cry for help. The causes of poor arousal are being sought but already it is clear from physiological studies that babies do not arouse so well to a variety of stimuli when sleeping in the prone position. It is thought that maternal smoking in pregnancy may specifically affect the baby's ability to arouse from pure hypoxia and it is clear that some sedatives decrease the ability to arouse. More controversial and unproven in human infants are the effects of overtiredness, hyperthermia or hypothermia and certain stages of viral infections.

3. Abnormal immunological responses in the lung

4. Prolonged QT syndrome

The evidence supporting this theory was recently boosted considerably by the publication of a large prospective study of ECGs in the first few days of life in many thousands of Italian babies. This suggested that, in their population, many babies who subsequently died of SIDS had a prolonged neonatal QT. As the risk of death in the prolonged QT syndrome can be decreased by the use of beta blockers, this study must be taken seriously. However, there have been many criticisms of the study and most authorities do not believe that the evidence is strong enough for screening of the newborn population. In practice, an ECG should, however, be done where siblings are born to families who have a strong family history of SIDS and in infants presenting with apparent life threatening events (ALTEs).

Parent support after an unexpected infant death

Following the unexpected death of a baby, parents feel a profound sense of loss, guilt and depression. This may be complicated if a babysitter, relative or sibling was looking after the child at the time that the death occurred. For young parents, this is often their first experience of a death in the family. Because of the need for an on site investigation, parents should meet either the paediatrician or pathologist involved and this places some significant obligations on these practitioners. Initially, a somewhat abbreviated medical history is taken and this needs to be followed up with further meetings and history taking once a postmortem has been carried out. Some parents value support at this early stage from someone who has been through the same trauma, but many do not appreciate this until later. Initially, simply offering such contact is sufficient. If parents wish this support, it can usually be organised with the local SIDS parent support organisation.

During the first few days, parents need to be given the result of the postmortem examination and very practical advice on where their baby is, what happens next, and who they can turn to for help. They also need to be given some understanding of the syndrome. This is very important in helping them to understand what has happened, and to come to terms with the reality of their baby's death.

Although this is a distressing time, and decisions will be difficult to make, both the parents and other family members should be encouraged to be involved in making decisions; 'taking over' by professionals is equally disabling. When the baby is certified dead at home, parents should be consulted about when the baby leaves the house to go to the mortuary.

Over the next few weeks and months, parents will hear, read, and experience a whole range of reactions and theories from others which may often compound their guilt, anger and distress. Unexpected infant deaths have a profound effect on relationships. Some couples will share the experience and become closer, but, more commonly, the stress shows up differences that may be hard for individuals to reconcile.

Every parent will experience the process of grieving in his or her own different way. Some will re-experience from the past; others will protect themselves from the pain by denial. With time, most parents come to terms with their baby's death; some continue searching for answers for themselves, while others turn to helping others. The time of the anniversary of either the birth or the death often rekindles some of the emotions.

The effects on other children, grandparents and the extended family need to be considered, and advice offered on how best to involve other children in the family with the process of grieving. Siblings need to be told clearly that the death was not because of anything they did or thought, as the 'magical' thinking of younger children can leave them feeling responsible for the death.

Eventually, many parents think of having more children. At this time, preventable factors and support after the birth should be discussed. If it is done before this time, it may compound the guilt they are feeling.

Checklist for dealing with the sudden death of a baby

1. Read and take a copy of 'Information for Parents' (available from local SIDS associations).
2. Sympathetically interview the parents about their baby's past health.
3. Examine the baby, and confirm death.
4. Record the history and examination, including recent consultations, family illness and any physical signs.
5. Clothe and wrap the baby, and take him or her to the parents to see and hold as long as they desire.
6. Explain what you think is the cause of death.
7. Explain to the parents that the police and coroner have a duty to investigate all sudden and unexpected deaths, and that they will have to make a statement to the police, who may want to examine the baby's room and bedding.
8. Offer support. Often very practical advice about the postmortem examination, funeral arrangements, cremations, registration of death and other details will be needed during the next few days. It is important that this information is given in written form because parents of children in this age group often have no experience of making funeral arrangements.
9. Check care needs of dependent relatives and other children.

10. Inform the on call paediatrician at the local hospital.
11. Ask whether the parents would like to see a chaplain or minister, or have their baby blessed.
12. If the mother is breastfeeding, offer advice on suppression of lactation and expression of milk.
13. Inform the coroner of the death.
14. Suggest that the parents might like to photograph the baby and/or take a lock of hair.
15. Leave an 'Information for Parents' leaflet and local support contact telephone number.
16. Explain that a paediatrician will contact them in the next few days with the preliminary results of the postmortem.
17. Inform the Community Child Health Department or equivalent to cancel surveillance and immunisation appointments.

Care of the adolescent

D. L. Bennett

Using traditional outcome measures, the health status of adolescents appears to be good and their use of the health care system usually is low. Nevertheless, many of the problems causing disadvantage, disability and death in this age group are not related to disease, but to preventable high risk behaviours. This poses a considerable challenge to the medical profession, which traditionally is more comfortable dealing with threats to health in children or adults.

Young people often are too self-conscious to initiate a discussion of their personal concerns or problems. Doctors need to be aware of adolescent health issues, including common medical disorders, willing to discuss sensitive issues, able to create a trusting relationship that can lead to anticipatory guidance, and possess the skills to encourage a young person to make informed lifestyle decisions.

What is adolescence?

Adolescence is defined as the developmental period between childhood and adulthood, beginning with the changes associated with puberty and culminating in the assumption of adult roles and responsibilities. The complex interactions between physical, mental, emotional and social development and the rapid pace of change mark this period as a unique and critical phase of life. The gradual development of an autonomous sense of self and a coherent sexual identity, coping with parental, family and peer relationships, and making educational, career, religious and lifestyle choices are some of the important issues facing the adolescent. The process of growing up generally involves experimentation, risk taking and, at times, denial of consequences.

The World Health Organization defines adolescence in terms of the arbitrary age range 10–19 years and refers to the 10–24 years age grouping as 'young people'.

Developmental issues

Although one will always be dealing with a unique and special individual, three substages of adolescence are recognised. They provide a useful framework for assessing the stage of development of a young person:

- Early adolescence (10–13 years): the predominant issues are the new bodily sensations and changes of puberty and a preoccupation with normality. Same sex peers become all important and the struggle for self-determination begins. High levels of physical activity and mood swings are common.
- Mid adolescence (14–16 years): the major focus is on achieving independence, particularly from parents, and establishing oneself among peers as a worthwhile individual. There is enjoyment of new intellectual powers, and relationships have a narcissistic quality.
- Late adolescence (17–20 years): the orientation is towards the future with an emphasis on defining one's functional role in terms of work, lifestyle and relationship plans. A degree of psychological autonomy, a realistic body image and a more comfortable sense of one's sexual identity will have been established. Relationships increasingly involve mutual caring and responsibility.

Puberty

The events of puberty, that is, the time when one becomes able to conceive children, follow a predictable sequence, although the time of onset, velocity of change and age of completion are extremely variable. The average duration of puberty is about 3 years. Height and weight increase and peak during the adolescent growth spurt, with 25% of final height and 50% of final weight being achieved during this time.

The *Tanner staging system* of pubertal development is based on breast, genital and pubic hair changes, with stage 1 being prepubertal and stage 5 the adult developmental stage (Tables 14.1 and 14.2). As well as indicating the biological stage of development, Tanner staging correlates with special events and therefore is useful in clinical assessment:

- in girls, peak height velocity (PHV) occurs early (Tanner stage 2 or 3), while menarche is a late event (Tanner stage 4) and is usually preceded by at least 2 years of breast development.
- in boys, peak height velocity is achieved later than in girls (Tanner stage 4), while the first ejaculation (semenarche) normally occurs around mid puberty (Tanner stage 3).

Table 14.1 Classification of genitalia maturity stages in boys (After Tanner JM 1962 Growth at adolescence, 2nd edn. Blackwell Scientific, Oxford)

Stage	Pubic hair	Penis	Testes
1	None	Preadolescent	(< 3 ml)
2	Scanty, long, slightly pigmented	Slight enlargement	Enlarged scrotum, pink, texture altered
3	Darker, starts to curl, small amount	Longer	Larger
4	Resembles adult type, but less in quantity, coarse, curly	Larger, glans and breadth increase in size	Larger, scrotum dark
5	Adult distribution, spread to medial surface of thighs	Adult	Adult

The experience of puberty is to have a changing body which feels out of control. Feelings of helplessness and persecution are common and may not abate until about 12 months after the growth spurt has ended. The typical aggressiveness, sexual arousal and unpredictability of the early adolescent are due largely to hormonal changes.

Approach to the adolescent patient

Medical problems of adolescence cluster in four major categories: concerns and conditions related to pubertal growth and development; pre-existing conditions complicated by adolescence; concerns related to mental health, lifestyle and risk taking behaviour; and conditions associated with adult morbidity.

Adolescent patients have neither the naivety of the child nor the awareness or experience of the adult, and usually they are nervous about seeing a doctor. An average consultation takes more time. The following suggestions about conducting an interview will help the adolescent feel comfortable and establish a relationship of trust:

- Be warm, sincere and non judgemental, but be careful not to condone risky behaviour.
- See the adolescent alone, at least for part of the visit, as this avoids appearing to be aligned with parents and invites a more mature response.
- Assure confidentiality, but be mindful that disclosure of suicidal intent or abuse must be reported and, if the adolescent appears to be at significant risk, explain the need to involve parents and/or authorities.
- Respond openly to the adolescent's initial reactions (that is, acknowledge and reflect back), particularly if there is apparent discomfort or hostility.
- Clarify the reasons for the interview and fully explore the chief complaint, as the young person's view may be at variance to that of others.
- Be yourself, while maintaining a professional manner; adolescents are quick to detect and reject phoniness.
- Request permission to ask sensitive questions, for example, 'Is it all right if I ask you some personal questions?'; young people are surprisingly candid if approached in an open and accepting way.
- Explore the young person's agenda, listen carefully and provide non verbal support, for example, eye contact, head nods.
- Use an interactive rather than an interrogative style; progress from neutral to more sensitive topics, using a third person approach for delicate subjects, for example, 'Are there drugs in your school? Are any of your friends involved? Do you use drugs?'
- Answer the young person's questions simply and honestly.

Important aspects of the history

The history, the most important aspect of the screening evaluation, involves obtaining an inventory of the

Table 14.2 Classification of sex maturity stages in girls. (After Tanner JM 1962 Growth at adolescence, 2nd edn. Blackwell Scientific, Oxford)

Stage	Pubic hair	Breasts
1	Preadolescent	Preadolescent
2	Sparse, lightly pigmented, straight, medial border of labia	Breast and papilla elevated as small mound, areola diameter increased
3	Darker, starts to curl, increased amount	Breast and areola enlarged, no contour separation
4	Coarse, curly, abundant but less than in adult	Areola and papilla form secondary mound
5	Adult feminine triangle, spread to medial surface of thighs	Mature, nipple projects, areola part of general breast contour

Table 14.3	Sexual behaviour risk assessment
No risk	No sexual contact
Low risk	No penetration, penetration with consistent condom use
Moderate risk	Unprotected oral sex
High risk	Unprotected vaginal/rectal intercourse

Table 14.4	Sexually transmitted disease (STD) risk assessment. (After Remafedi G 1990 Adolescent Medicine: State of the Art Reviews 1: 565–582)
No risk	No sexual contact
Moderate risk	Low/moderate risk sex, few partners, asymptomatic
High risk	Moderate/high risk sex, multiple partners, past STD/pregnancy, substance use, STD contact

adolescent's background, current circumstances, behaviour and feelings. The key elements are as follows:

- Past medical history from both adolescent and parent: a description of mother's pregnancy; the adolescent's birth size; immunisations; childhood illnesses and allergies; developmental milestones and general behaviour; accidents, hospitalisations and surgery; current medications.
- Family history, mostly obtained from parents: the age and health status of family members; chronic illness in the family (especially cardiovascular disease in a relative aged under 55 years); recent bereavement; vocational status of the parents.
- Review of systems: weight patterns and dietary habits; physical activity; physical symptoms related to any organ system; dental and eye care; menstrual history, including date of occurrence of menarche.
- Medicosocial history: sexual experiences: onset of sexual intercourse, partners' gender and number of partners, relationship duration, contraception, pregnancy, sexually transmitted diseases, sexual abuse; use of tobacco, alcohol or other drugs (Tables 14.3 and 14.4).
- Psychosocial history: family relationships (parents and siblings); peer relationships; school and career performance and goals; special interests, hobbies and skills; evidence of depression and suicidality.

The Children's Hospital of Los Angeles *Health Risk Profile Assessment*, the HEADSS exam (H, Home environment; E, Education and employment; A, peer Activities; D, Drugs; S, Sexuality; S, Suicide/depression), provides 'a psychosocial biopsy' and serves as a useful aide memoire.

The physical examination

This should be thorough, gentle and thoughtful, with precautions to protect the young person's modesty and privacy. Much of the examination can be performed in the sitting position, with an easy progression from head to toe. Ongoing dialogue and reassurance will lessen anxiety. Take the opportunity to provide information about developmental and health matters.

Particular note should be taken of the physical changes and conditions that are related to pubertal growth and development; height and weight and percentiles, Tanner stage of sexual development, breast examination, testicle examination (Fig. 14.1)

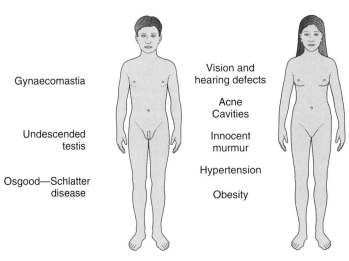

Gynaecomastia

Vision and hearing defects

Acne
Cavities

Undescended testis

Innocent murmur

Osgood—Schlatter disease

Hypertension

Obesity

Thyroid enlargment

Fibroadenomas

Scoliosis

Record height, weight and sex maturity rating

Fig. 14.1 What to look for on physical examination.

A vaginal examination is rarely indicated for pubescent and early adolescent girls if considered not to be sexually active but, for the sexually active adolescent, may be indicated (Committee of Presidents of Medical Colleges, Vaginal Examination in Children and Young Women, 1998) for:

- sexually transmitted diseases — screening or diagnostic
- pregnancy
- pelvic pain or other gynaecological symptoms
- sexual assault
- Pap smears, commencing 1 or 2 years after first sexual intercourse.

Other elements of the examination include: blood pressure (although hypertension is rare in this age group, there is a higher incidence of secondary causes); skin; teeth and gums; vision and hearing; lymph glands and thyroid gland (enlargement is indicative of dysfunction and requires investigation); chest; abdomen; posture; skeletal/spinal examination; and central nervous system (of special importance in the presence of clumsiness, poor school performance, personality change or unprovoked emotional outbursts).

Laboratory tests

Laboratory tests should be kept to a minimum in the asymptomatic adolescent. The following tests would be performed if indicated:

- electrolytes, blood count and ESR with eating disorders
- liver function tests and serology for hepatitis B or HIV in drug users
- thyroid function tests in the presence of goitre, a short or tall young person, menstrual irregularities or general performance concerns, weight loss
- bone age, hormone levels and karyotype with problems of growth and development
- cholesterol and triglycerides with a high risk cardiovascular history
- STD screen and HIV testing in sexually active adolescents at risk or if requested; Pap smear in sexually active girls
- virology titres and immunoglobulins with chronic fatigue/postviral syndromes.

An elevated serum alkaline phosphatase level is generally related to accelerated bone growth and correlates with the time of peak height velocity, i.e. Tanner 2 in girls, Tanner 3 in boys (Fig. 14.2).

Wrapping up

At the end of the assessment:

- Summarise your assessment and define the main concerns.
- Review options and outline management plan.

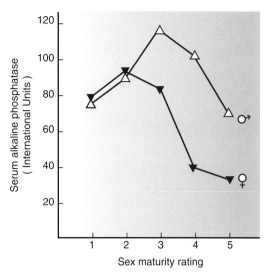

Fig. 14.2 The relationship of serum alkaline phosphatase concentrations to sex maturity ratings in adolescents. After Bennett et al, 1976.

- Invite questions or comments.
- Discuss 'what to tell Mum and/or Dad' and then include them in the feedback session.
- Consider other adolescent resources to call upon if necessary.

Problems of growth and development

In our society, media stereotypes have created physical standards that are impossible to meet. As well as having a heightened awareness of bodily change, adolescents are normally narcissistic and are preoccupied with issues of adequacy. Young adolescents are often concerned that their growth and development are not progressing normally. For boys, in particular, the psychological effects of being slow to develop, too short or too thin in comparison with one's peers can be profound, while excessive tallness may provide particular difficulties for girls.

Delayed puberty occurs in approximately 2% of the adolescent population and is defined as the absence of any signs of pubertal development by the age of 13 years in girls and 13.5 years in boys, or the failure of developmental progression during a 2 year period (Ch. 63).

Constitutional delay of puberty accounts for 90% of cases, and is a diagnosis of exclusion. Details of parental growth at adolescence, family photographs and the prediction of ultimate adult height from bone age X rays are important aspects of assessment. The treatment of choice is to allow nature to run its course, with the provision of ongoing reassurance and support as necessary.

Constitutional tall stature accounts for approximately 90% of cases of tall stature. In general, the use of high dose oestrogen therapy to close the epiphyses should be reserved for adolescent females with a predicted adult height greater than 183 cm (6 ft) and with indications of psychological adjustment difficulties. In rare circumstances, high dose testosterone treatment can be used to curtail linear growth in extremely tall boys.

> **Clinical example**
>
> Adam presented at age 14 years 1 month because he was worried that he had not yet entered puberty. He had no significant past medical history. His father was also a 'late developer' but his older brother started puberty at 12 years. On examination, he measured 150 cm (10th centile) and weighed 43 kg (10–25th centile). He had no pubic hair development and both testes measured 3 ml in volume. Full physical examination revealed no abnormalities. Gonadotrophins and serum testosterone were at prepubertal levels. DHAS and serum cortisol were within normal limits. Thyroid function, full blood count and biochemistry were all normal. His bone age was 11 years 6 months. Adam was thought likely to have constitutionally delayed puberty. He was reassured that he would grow significantly taller and should progress through puberty normally. He was reviewed at 6 monthly intervals and there was evidence of pubertal development by his 15th birthday. Adam's anxiety and the effect on his peer relationships were also addressed: this helped him to be confident about attaining full pubertal development and growth.

Breast problems

Some adolescent girls are particularly sensitive about their breasts, which may be too large, too small or unequal in size. Benign breast masses are common in this age group and include:

- benign fibroadenomas: firm, usually painless lesions that tend to persist
- fibrocystic lesions: often multiple and may vary in size and tenderness with the menstrual cycle.

Gynaecomastia is a common finding in boys, occurring in up to 70% of 14 year old boys, with a falling prevalence thereafter. Although it is usually transitory, the presence of visible breast enlargement almost invariably causes concern and embarrassment. Several kinds of gynaecomastia are recognized:

- Benign adolescent hypertrophy with firm, somewhat tender breast tissue immediately beneath the areola is by far the most common and tends to resolve spontaneously within 12–18 months.
- Gynaecomastia (Fig. 14.3) resembling normal female breast development may require surgical management if there is enduring psychological distress.

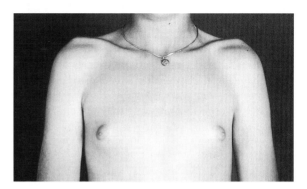

Fig. 14.3 Boy with gynaecomastia.

- Gynaecomastias associated with an endocrine disorder, Klinefelter syndrome or drug ingestion are all rare.

Menstrual disorders of adolescence

Menstrual disorders require of the practitioner an understanding of basic menstrual physiology and a gentle and reassuring approach. Following menarche, usually at age 12 or 13 years, the menstrual cycles are often irregular and anovulatory for 2 years. Common pubescent menstrual problems include premenstrual syndrome, failure to menstruate (amenorrhoea), excessive menstrual bleeding (menorrhagia) and painful menstrual periods (dysmenorrhoea).

Premenstrual syndrome

Premenstrual syndrome is often unrecognised in adolescents, and has complex dynamics and a difficult history. Management consists of validating the patient's symptoms, reassurance, education, eliminating contributing factors and attempting prevention. Medical therapies are usually symptomatic or aim to induce anovulation (oral contraceptive pill (OCP) or progesterone).

Amenorrhoea (absent menses)

In secondary amenorrhoea, the most common menstrual abnormality in adolescents, the cause is usually hypothalamic, although pregnancy must be excluded. Primary amenorrhoea (no menses by 16 years), which is rare, can be due to delayed menarche related to undernutrition and/or strenuous exercise or to congenital abnormalities such as an imperforate hymen.

Repeated heavy menstrual bleeding

This is relatively uncommon in adolescents and requires detailed investigation at an appropriate gynaecological service. It is important to exclude pregnancy, infection and blood dyscrasias, although the majority of cases result from hormonal imbalance (anovulatory dysfunctional bleeding) and respond to cyclical progestogens or combined oestrogen–progesterone pills and iron replacement.

Dysmenorrhoea

This is very common in adolescents and can be severe and disabling. Detailed investigation usually is not indicated. Explanation, reassurance and simple methods are generally sufficient, otherwise a prostaglandin inhibitor or oral contraceptive pill can be prescribed.

Problems of eating and nutrition

Adolescents have relatively high nutritional requirements due to increases in growth rate and physical activity. In general terms, if the kilojoule intake is adequate, the intake of other nutrients will be satisfactory, with the exception of iron in females. Snacks are accepted as contributing to a well rounded diet, although most fast food is excessively high in fat and salt.

Obesity

Obesity is a common problem in adolescence and is likely to endure into adulthood. There may be aetiological contributions from familial, environmental, societal and psychological factors. With personal motivation and family support as important prerequisites to change, management involves a realistic appraisal of lifestyle, in particular eating habits and exercise. An appropriate goal is maintenance of weight while the growth spurt proceeds. Anorectic drugs have no place in management. Obese adolescents generally feel unattractive and may be unhappy and isolated. In younger adolescents, supervised peer group activities can enhance self-esteem and provide encouragement and support.

Anorexia nervosa

Anorexia nervosa is a primary psychological disorder which peaks in the early teens and again around 18 years. It affects approximately one in 200 girls aged 15 to 19 years, irrespective of geography, ethnic origin or socioeconomic status. The ratio of girls to boys affected is approximately 30:1. The clinical features, diagnosis and management are discussed in Chapters 7 and 18.

It is generally accepted that around 40% of those affected recover fully and 30% improve significantly, while 20% remain unimproved or experience repeated episodes of weight loss, bulimia and vomiting. The overall mortality for anorexia nervosa is 5–10%, including a considerable number from suicides in the slightly older population. For those who recover, future problems may include rebound obesity, osteoporosis, prolonged amenorrhoea or relapse of the eating disorder.

Clinical example

Sally, aged 14 years, had been restricting her food intake for 10 months in order to lose weight. She began to skip breakfast and lunch and drank only water. Although Sally had lost 10 kg, she believed she was still overweight and she wanted to lose a further 4–5 kg. She was particularly unhappy with her 'flabby' thighs and stomach and admitted to being extremely anxious about gaining weight. She had been jogging every morning for the past 3 months and would do 150 sit ups in her room every night. Jenny denied vomiting, laxative or diuretic use. Having had 1 monthly to 2 monthly periods since her menarche at age 12, she had not had a period for the past 4 months.

Sally was in year 9 and was a very bright student. She lived at home with both parents and an older brother and described her family as 'extremely close'. She had several good friends at school but felt she did not fit in because they were all 'tall, thin and pretty'. Sally felt quite sad and tearful most of the time but denied any suicidal ideation.

On examination, Sally weighed 42.1 kg (10th centile) and measured 168 cm (90th centile). Her pulse rate was 48/min and her blood pressure was 90/60 without a postural drop. Her hair felt dry and brittle and her skin was dry with some lanugo hair present. Apart from being very thin, there were no other abnormal findings. Her ESR was <1. Full blood count, biochemistry, thyroid function tests, prolactin and gonadotrophins were all within normal limits.

Sally met the criteria for anorexia nervosa. Outpatient management included intensive medical and dietary review in the first instance. She would have needed inpatient care if she had continued to lose weight, but after several visits her weight stabilised. Psychosocial and family assessments took place once she stopped losing weight and was medically more stable. Psychiatric review was considered appropriate if her depression persisted or worsened.

Skin conditions

Acne

Acne is virtually universal in adolescence. It is a multifactorial disease with contributions from adult levels of circulating androgens and sebum output, *Corynebacterium acne*, liberation of free fatty acids in the skin, and heredity. Prevalence peaks between the ages of 14 and 16 years in females, and 16 and 19 years in males. In girls it will often increase premenstrually. Clinically, acne is manifest by comedones, papules, pustules and nodules (Fig. 14.4). The psychological impact can be enormous.

Drying agents and antibiotics remain the mainstays of treatment in mild to moderate cases. Vaginal moniliasis is a problem for girls on tetracycline unless the dosage is kept low. The treatment of severe, cystic acne has been revolutionised by the availability of isotretinoin, a derivative of vitamin A, although there are significant

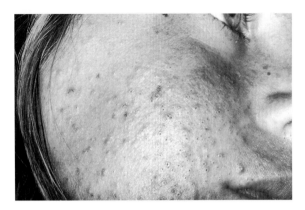

Fig. 14.4 Multiple comedones and blackheads.

side effects and pregnancy must be avoided while on treatment.

Other skin conditions occurring frequently in adolescents include warts, atopic eczema, seborrhoea, tinea pedis and cruris, and scabies.

Orthopaedic conditions

During early adolescence, a number of orthopaedic conditions are found that rarely occur in other age groups.

Idiopathic scoliosis

Idiopathic scoliosis of adolescence is probably a genetic disorder, with 85% of cases occurring in girls (Fig. 14.5). It is asymptomatic and has a tendency to progress with the growth spurt. Of every 1000 adolescent girls, 2–3 will develop scoliosis of sufficient severity to require treatment. The simply performed forward bending test reveals a posterior chest prominence (rib hump) resulting from rotation of the thorax. Radiological evaluation enables estimation of the degree of curvature, while a bone age (wrist X ray) helps determine potential growth.

Minor curves detected early may only need observation with serial X rays. When needed, treatment involves wearing a body brace, for 23 hours per day, to stop progression. Surgery, involving the placement of Harrington

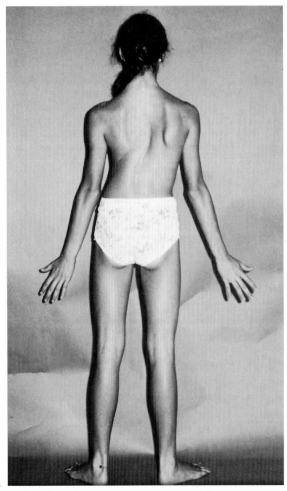

A

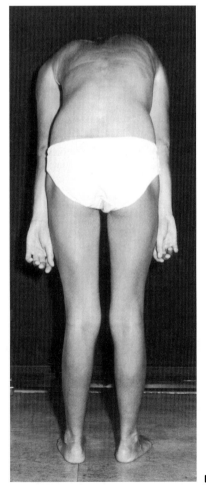

B

Fig. 14.5 **A** Girl with severe scoliosis, showing **B** chest hump on trunk flexion.

rods and spinal fusion, is reserved for curves too severe for bracing (Ch. 25).

Adolescent kyphosis

Adolescent kyphosis is also known as adolescent round back, Scheuermann disease and vertebral epiphysitis. Clinical manifestations include a round deformity of the back and, in over one half of patients, persistent pain localised in the involved area. X ray findings confirm the diagnosis. For mild cases, a bed board, sleeping without a pillow, limited activity and postural activities are usually sufficient. More severe cases require orthopaedic consultation for a back support or a hyperextension cast or brace.

Osgood–Schlatter disease

Osgood–Schlatter disease is the most common knee disorder of adolescence, occurs predominantly in active males and is usually unilateral. There is painful enlargement of the tibial tuberosity at the insertion of the patellar tendon. Treatment includes explanation of the condition, restriction of activity for several weeks or longer or, if symptoms are severe and unresponsive, a cylinder cast for a few weeks. The prognosis is excellent but there may be recurrence with excessive activity.

Slipped capital femoral epiphysis

Slipped capital femoral epiphysis involves the femoral head slipping on the femoral metaphysis. The condition, which is both chronic and gradual in 80% of cases, is more prevalent in males than females (1.5:1.0) and usually occurs during the pubertal growth spurt. It is often associated with obesity and delayed skeletal maturation and occurs bilaterally in 25–40% of cases. Symptoms include hip or knee pain (from obturator nerve referral) and the patient walks with a limp with the hip externally rotated and the foot pointing to the side. Signs include decreased flexion, adduction and internal rotation of the hip. X ray changes and bone scan findings (increased uptake at the involved epiphyseal plate) are characteristic. Orthopaedic referral is required, as surgery is the only reliable treatment.

Chronic illness and disability

The prevalence of chronic illness in adolescents, that is, of a permanent condition with residual disability, is estimated at between 10 and 20%. For many, the origins will have been during childhood, with medical and surgical advances continually improving survival. Approximately 80% of children with chronic illness survive into adulthood.

Serious conditions or injuries, particularly those related to accidents, can also be acquired during adolescence. It is estimated that approximately 200 young people become paraplegic in Australia each year. During adolescence, common disease states may exhibit different characteristics: epilepsy may commence or worsen; asthma may worsen with the impact of stress, non compliance or smoking; and diabetes mellitus frequently becomes more brittle and difficult to control.

Characteristic responses to illness have been described in adolescents and may be viewed as important ways to diffuse or diminish anxiety. Responses such as denial, intellectualisation, compensation and regression are viewed as generally adaptive, while extreme hostility, panic, withdrawal or suicidal behaviour are clearly maladaptive and require more active psychological intervention. The general effects of chronic illness are best appreciated within the framework of the developmental tasks and substages of adolescence (Table 14.5).

Issues related to the condition itself are also important:
- Age: the early adolescent going through puberty appears to be most vulnerable.
- Visibility of the condition: the more visible the disability, the less the stress and psychological suffering and vice versa.
- The degree of functional impairment: impaired mobility is demoralising and socially handicapping for the adolescent, with mild gait disturbances causing more emotional difficulties than more severe limitation.
- Prognosis: the stress of uncertainty is greater than when the course is known, even when the clinical trajectory leads to death.
- Course of the illness: a stable or predictable course is less distressing than a fluctuating and unpredictable one.

Table 14.5 Impact of serious illness and disability. (After Bennett DL 1984 Adolescent health in Australia: an overview of needs and approaches to care. Australian Medical Association, Sydney)

Early adolescence	Mid adolescence	Late adolescence
Distortion of body image	Enforced dependency	Effects upon educational and vocational goals
Isolation from peers	Decreased acceptance by peers	Concerns about relationships, future marriage and children

Key issues in management are:

- Acknowledging that the chronically ill adolescent has the same developmental needs as all other young people. One is treating an 'adolescent with diabetes', rather than a 'diabetic adolescent'.
- Encouraging responsibility for self-care, self-reliance and the development of creativity in the young person.
- Limiting intrusive medical examinations or procedures.
- Providing honest and understandable information about the condition and its consequences, but do not focus only on negative consequences.
- Helping parents to reduce overanxiety, overattention and overprotectiveness.
- Avoiding the conspiracy of silence with the dying adolescent, who will generally be well aware of the seriousness of the situation anyway.

Psychosomatic disorders

The term 'somatisation' has been introduced in recent years to describe patients with somatic complaints that do not have an organic basis. Increased sensitivity to biological change makes adolescents particularly vulnerable in this regard and they may attribute significance to physical symptoms well beyond their medical importance. Given the well recognised association between psychological distress and physical discomfort, the more problems an adolescent faces growing up, the greater the likelihood of there being an illness related response. Recurrent abdominal pain, chest pain, headache and fatigue are symptoms commonly associated with stress in adolescents. If there is a discrepancy between symptomatic complaints and the physical findings in an unwell adolescent, the following approach should be taken:

- Enquire as to what was happening at the time of onset, especially with regard to family, school and peers.
- Explore the possible origin of the symptom, that is, is it borrowed from the young person's own medical history or from someone else's?
- Accept the legitimacy of the complaint(s) and keep an open mind on diagnosis. Indicate, however, that symptomatic illness and stress are commonly associated phenomena, especially in adolescents, and that all potentially relevant issues need to be explored.
- Resist the almost inevitable pressure to provide a medical label, as this can lead to excessive and inappropriate organic 'work up'.
- Arrange a family interview, as this may provide clues to the underlying meaning of the illness; for example, the young person's 'being sick' may mask or reflect family distress or dysfunction (a depressed parent, serious illness in the family, a disturbed marriage or bereavement).

Clinical example

Lisa, aged 15 years, had been unwell for about 8 months with recurrent sore throat, fatigue, headaches and generalised muscle aches. Her illness began with an acute episode of glandular fever which was documented by seroconversion. Lisa missed almost 4 weeks of school during her acute illness and, since returning, had found it difficult to concentrate and keep up with her school work and extracurricular activities. She continued to miss several days a term due to her symptoms. She had been to three different doctors and had multiple investigations including full blood count, biochemistry, thyroid function and immunoglobulins, all of which were normal. She was referred to an ear, nose and throat surgeon for an opinion about tonsillectomy. A diagnosis of depression had been made 1 month previously and she was commenced on antidepressants. Another doctor had diagnosed chronic fatigue syndrome. Lisa was an only child, had been achieving well at school and had competed in long distance running at State level. Her parents had spent most of their weekend time taking her to training and competitions and were very concerned about her illness.

Gentle exploration of psychosocial and family issues, with ongoing medical review to monitor physical symptoms, provided opportunities for each family member to express their anxieties about Lisa growing up and becoming independent. Lisa also worried that she might not reach the goals she set for herself at school and sport. After 3 months of working with a broad based and family oriented approach, Lisa's symptoms subsided and she returned to school and training with more realistic expectations.

Depression and suicide

Emotional swings are to be expected in adolescents. Also, given the need to reconcile inner drives with outside expectations, stress is inevitable. Certain groups of young people are especially vulnerable and more likely to show negative effects in mood and behaviour. They include:

- Teenagers who are different: chronically ill; minority groups in terms of ethnicity, culture, religion or sexuality.
- Teenagers who experience serious losses or other traumas: parental death or 'separation', rejection, abuse.
- Teenagers in difficult external circumstances: homeless, unemployed, poor, in institutions, in isolated rural areas.

Australia has one of the highest rates for youth suicide in the Western world, with over 400 young people in the 15–24 age group committing suicide each year. As a result of using more lethal methods, boys outnumber girls for successful suicide by around 4:1. However, girls are four times more likely to attempt suicide. And for every completed suicide, there may be 50 or more attempts. Risk factors include a previous suicide attempt, a suicide in the family, depression and psychotic illness. Other important factors are alcohol and drug abuse, conduct disorder, eating disorder, significant losses and family problems. Precipitating events include: sudden alienation from parents in the absence of other supportive relationships; rejection by a peer whose relationship has been highly valued; a significant and often public failure, usually academic or athletic; and family disruption or dissolution, especially if the young person experiences self-blame. Another high risk group for suicide are young gays and lesbians. Estimates suggest these young people are three times more likely to attempt suicide and may account for 30% of all adolescent suicides.

With all troubled adolescents, it is important to identify signs of depression (Table 14.6) and critical to ask explicit, direct questions about suicidal thoughts and plans. Depressed young people are not always aware of the finality of death, may be seeking an escape from an intolerable problem and may view suicide as the only solution ('tunnel vision'). The principles of intervention are: always take consideration of suicide seriously; alert parents or guardians; address safety issues; assess available supports; ascertain further information; ask for help and consider referral (Ch. 18).

Indications for referral of a depressed adolescent:
- serious risk of self-harm
- unsupportive environment
- failure to respond to initial treatment
- bipolar disorder or other psychiatric condition.

Risky behaviours

Young people are growing up within a complex, generally permissive, future oriented and materialistic society in which ongoing changes in social norms create uncertainty about appropriate behaviour. The youth subculture permits increasing access to the opposite sex, money, cars, motorcycles, alcohol and drugs. Adolescents experiment with new activities, testing their limits, exploring

---

Table 14.6 Typical features of adolescent depression

Persistent sadness or volatile mood
Feelings of helplessness and hopelessness
Irritability, withdrawal, persistent boredom
Low energy, poor concentration
Changes in eating or sleep patterns
Deteriorating school performance
Increased risk taking; alcohol and drug abuse
Frequent complaints of physical illness

---

new skills and enjoying the often exhilarating sense of freedom involved. Difficulties arise in the context of:
- ignorance (lack of prior experience or adequate information)
- impulsiveness and thrill seeking
- cognitive immaturity (strong denial mechanisms, a sense of omnipotence and an ability to comprehend long term consequences)
- feelings of inadequacy and poor self-worth.

A large body of evidence indicates that risky behaviours are interrelated and that the factors that put a young person or peer group at risk are cumulative. There are positive correlations, for example, between the use of alcohol and the use of drugs, such as tobacco and marijuana. The greater the use of drugs, the more likely the involvement in other risk behaviours, such as sexual activity, aggression and delinquency. There is also considerable continuity of health risk behaviour from adolescence into adulthood.

Motor vehicle accidents are the leading cause of adolescent deaths, with many such deaths involving alcohol or other drugs (Chs 1, 9). Young people need help to anticipate and avoid drink driving and joy riding situations and to handle peer pressure to participate in these risky situations.

Cigarette smoking is dangerous to health. Although young people know this, they often believe they can quit easily at a later date. As virtually all smokers develop the addiction during adolescence, effective primary prevention at this time theoretically would avert more premature deaths than all other measures combined. Counselling focused on the negative social effects of smoking (bad breath, stained fingers and teeth, expense) is likely to be more effective with young people than emphasising long term consequences.

Alcohol use by adolescents varies in extent and context. In addition to exploring these factors, an attempt should be made to distinguish the potentially dependent drinker from the larger recreational group, with additional questions regarding family history of alcoholism (signifying four times the risk of becoming a dependent drinker), drinking during the week, blackouts, drinking alone, and secrecy and guilt feelings surrounding alcohol use.

Illicit drug use also challenges the doctor to attempt to separate from the larger recreational group both the reckless, irresponsible user and the potentially dependent young person who uses chemicals for the anxiety relieving effect. Solitary use is highly significant. It is important to enquire about drug use over the previous months, including:
- over the counter preparations: cough syrups, analgesics
- prescribed medications: tranquillisers, pain killers
- household products: glue, aerosols, petrol

- street drugs: cannabis (most widely used illicit substance), cocaine, LSD and others, including heroin.

Reproductive health problems

The acquisition of reproductive capability, the emergence of sexual feelings and thoughts, and the development of sexual identity are all fundamental tasks of adolescence. In the Western world, sexual activity in adolescents occurs at an early age, the mean age of first intercourse being 16 years. Approximately 50% of teenagers have had intercourse by year 12 of education. Initiation of sex for most adolescents is unplanned and remains a sporadic occurrence, although around 20% are sexually active on a frequent basis. While many young people are knowledgeable about safe sex practices, and condom use appears to be increasing, relatively few actually take consistent precautions. Concerns about sexual orientation are not uncommon in adolescents, with overseas research suggesting that as many as 25% of adolescents have homosexual experiences.

Risk factors for teenage pregnancy include low family income, being the child of a teenage parent, marital problems between parents, low self-esteem, poor school performance and attendance, and psychological and emotional problems. A significant number of teenage pregnancies (approximately half) are terminated by therapeutic abortion. The majority of young women who opt to continue a pregnancy decide to keep their baby. A higher risk of obstetric complications is related to late presentation and poor attendance for antenatal care. Young mothers face many adjustment problems.

Adolescents are more vulnerable to sexually transmitted diseases (STDs) than adults because they have sex more often, with greater numbers of partners (usually serial monogamy) and are less likely to use condoms. The serious consequences include:
- Lifelong recurring infections and infectiousness: herpes simplex virus (HSV) with vulval blisters and commonly endocervicitis.

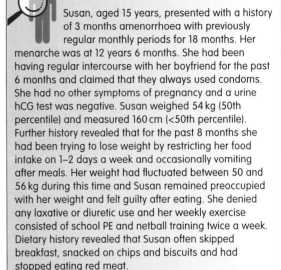

Clinical example

Susan, aged 15 years, presented with a history of 3 months amenorrhoea with previously regular monthly periods for 18 months. Her menarche was at 12 years 6 months. She had been having regular intercourse with her boyfriend for the past 6 months and claimed that they always used condoms. She had no other symptoms of pregnancy and a urine hCG test was negative. Susan weighed 54 kg (50th percentile) and measured 160 cm (<50th percentile). Further history revealed that for the past 8 months she had been trying to lose weight by restricting her food intake on 1–2 days a week and occasionally vomiting after meals. Her weight had fluctuated between 50 and 56 kg during this time and Susan remained preoccupied with her weight and felt guilty after eating. She denied any laxative or diuretic use and her weekly exercise consisted of school PE and netball training twice a week. Dietary history revealed that Susan often skipped breakfast, snacked on chips and biscuits and had stopped eating red meat.

Susan had a subclinical eating disorder. Secondary amenorrhoea can be associated with disordered eating in the absence of weight loss. Full blood count, ESR, electrolytes, thyroid function tests, prolactin and gonadotrophins were performed. Management involved dietary counselling and physical monitoring as well as exploration of the psychosocial issues. Safe sex, contraception and the possible need for STD screening also were addressed.

- higher incidence of cervical dysplasia: human papilloma virus (HPV) with condylomata acuminata (vulval warts).
- pelvic inflammatory disease (PID), ectopic pregnancy and sterility: *Chlamydia trachomatis* and *Neisseria gonorrhoeae*.
- disabling illness and death: human immunodeficiency virus (HIV) and acquired immune deficiency syndrome (AIDS).

Doctors must stress the importance of both birth control and STD prevention, which means recommending and explaining condom use in conjunction with other contraceptives.

PART 3 SELF-ASSESSMENT

Questions

1. **Which of the following are correct?**
   (A) At least 15% of Australian families with dependent children are one parent families
   (B) Children of one parent families are at risk of emotional and/or intellectual deprivation
   (C) Aboriginal child health is now at a similar level to that of other Australian children
   (D) The Commonwealth government through its Department of Ethnic Affairs is responsible for the health of migrant children
   (E) A de facto parent is not eligible for the family allowance

2. **Which of the following statements are true or false?**
   (A) Preschool education is compulsory
   (B) All children should be given a complete physical examination on commencing school
   (C) All young children of working mothers are at risk of emotional deprivation
   (D) Infant welfare clinics provide health surveillance for 90% of children in the first year of life
   (E) Child health nurses are very useful in assessing physical growth but are not helpful in assessing development

3. **Tjitji is a 6 month old male Aboriginal child who has a tight foreskin which balloons when he passes urine (phimosis). Which of the following are correct?**
   (A) Circumcision should be avoided if at all possible
   (B) The parents may need to consult other family members before consent is given if any surgery is contemplated
   (C) Treatment is not indicated
   (D) He is at risk of urinary tract infection
   (E) Treatment options should be discussed privately and where the conversation cannot be overheard

4. **Nunurfa is a 2 year old Aboriginal child who presents with a purulent discharge from her ears and on examination she has perforated ear drums. Which of the following are correct?**
   (A) This is an uncommon condition
   (B) Treatment is not indicated
   (C) This condition can be associated with long term sequelae, such as deafness
   (D) This condition can become chronic and require surgical treatment
   (E) Streptococcal infection is a common aetiological factor in this condition

5. **You are a young male doctor, new to the area, and an Aboriginal mother brings her child for immunisation at the clinic. However, she does not make eye contact with you, she does not speak to you and refuses to hold the child for the immunisation. She leaves as soon as the immunisation is given. What are the implications of this?**
   (A) She does not like you
   (B) She does not want her child to be immunised
   (C) She does not care about the child
   (D) She should have been encouraged to bring a family member with her
   (E) You are not known to her or her community so cultural considerations prevent her from talking to you

6. **A 5 month old formula fed infant has been diagnosed with lactose intolerance following gastroenteritis. His mother has asked you which formula she should be using. You would recommend:**
   (A) Lactose free formula
   (B) Soy formula
   (C) Low lactose formula
   (D) Low lactose or lactose free formula
   (E) Goat's milk based formula

7. **There are many factors which may contribute to iron deficiency in children, including prematurity, gastrointestinal disease, blood loss and dietary factors. Which of the following may cause iron deficiency?**
   (A) Cow's milk as the primary milk source during the first 12 months of life
   (B) Inadequate total food intake
   (C) Excessive milk intake
   (D) Delayed solid introduction
   (E) All of the above

8. **Ms B is 6 months pregnant and visits you, her general practitioner, because she is unsure if she should breastfeed. She has heard a number of things about breastfeeding and wants to know if they are true or false. She has heard:**
   (A) Breastfeeding makes you lose your figure
   (B) Breast milk provides the best nutrition for a baby
   (C) You cannot tell if a baby has had enough milk from the breast, but with bottle feeding you can see the empty bottle
   (D) You can go back to work and breastfeed
   (E) Breastfeeding helps prevent a baby catching infections

   Which of the above are correct?

9. A 14 year old girl, Sarah, comes to see you with her mother. Sarah appears to be a healthy weight but has started to avoid foods such as milk and meats as friends have told her that these foods will cause her to become overweight. Her mother is keen for Sarah to learn more about healthy eating and appropriate weight control. What would you advise her to eat?
   (A) Milk and dairy products
   (B) Bread and cereals
   (C) Fruit and vegetables
   (D) Meat, fish, poultry, eggs, legumes, nuts
   (E) All of the above

10. Alicia is aged 13 months and should have had Hib vaccine and measles/mumps/rubella (MMR) vaccine at the age of 12 months. However, Alicia had had a rash 4 weeks ago, which a doctor at a 24 hour medical centre had said looked like 'baby measles'. Her mother was concerned that immunising her against measles might be harmful if she had already had measles, and sought further advice. Which of the following would be appropriate?
    (A) Take a blood sample for measurement of measles antibody titres
    (B) Give mumps and rubella vaccine only
    (C) Give Hib vaccine only
    (D) Delay MMR vaccine for 3 months to avoid the immunosuppression induced by measles
    (E) Proceed with MMR and Hib immunisation

11. Cain is due to have his scheduled OPV, MMR and DTPa immunisations at the age of 4 years. He had a febrile illness at the age of 19 months which was also associated with a brief generalised convulsion. There was a family history of febrile convulsions in that his father had had three brief convulsions in association with fevers in early childhood. Cain also had been admitted to hospital twice in the last year with asthma, and was on inhaled corticosteroid medication (100 μg twice daily) as preventive treatment for his asthma. He had mild eczema which had not required treatment. Which of the following are correct?
    (A) He should receive the recommended schedule vaccines
    (B) Immunisation should be delayed because he is on inhaled corticosteroid medication
    (C) His inhaled steroid medications should be ceased for 4 weeks to allow a better immune response to his vaccines
    (D) He has no significant risk of a febrile convulsion after this immunisation
    (E) He has a higher risk of a vaccine associated paralytic poliomyelitis-like illness because he has had febrile convulsions previously

12. Maurice, a 6 year old boy, migrates to Australia from Europe. He had cystic fibrosis and is taking antibiotics because of purulent sputum. He had DTPw vaccine, Hib vaccine and OPV vaccine at the age of 3, 4 and 5 months, MMR vaccine at 12 months, and DTPw and Hib vaccines at age 18 months. When his parents approach their local primary school they are told that he will need further immunisation. As his family doctor, you would:
    (A) Recommend a primary course of DTPa vaccine, as he has received DTPw vaccine previously in a schedule that differs from the Australian schedule
    (B) Wait until the course of antibiotics is completed before giving any vaccines
    (C) Recommend yearly influenza vaccine
    (D) Recommend varicella vaccine
    (E) Recommend conjugate pneumococcal vaccine and a course of hepatitis B vaccine

13. Sam, aged 3 years, was sitting on the couch in front of the television with his 5 year old brother Nick. Their mother prepared them some instant noodles and handed them to each boy. She then went to attend to her baby daughter, who had been crying for several minutes. It was the end of the day and both boys were tired and irritable. Nick decided he wanted to watch another channel, grabbed the remote control and began channel surfing. Sam screamed for him to stop and also made a grab for the remote control. Unfortunately he could not balance the noodles at the same time, and the boiling liquid spilled all over him. He sustained superficial but significant burns to his abdomen and legs. Which of the following statements are true?
    (A) Many injuries occur when a parent is distracted from the usual level of supervision
    (B) The mother must have made the noodles too hot as they would not usually cause a burn
    (C) Sitting at a table and being supervised would have prevented this injury
    (D) This behaviour sounds very disturbed and both children should have a psychological assessment

14. Three and a half year old Emily was exploring her grandparents' garden. She was visiting with her parents. All the adults were inside the house chatting, and thought that Emily would be safe in the small enclosed yard. However, they had forgotten about the garden shed. Emily, in her explorations, went into the shed and chose to taste the interesting greenish granules, which unfortunately were rat poison. Her parents at this time thought they should check on her and found her with a mouthful. Which of the following are correct?

(A) Children of this age can be taught not to attempt to taste substances

(B) The mother should be aware of Emily's actions at all times

(C) Drugs, household chemicals and garden chemicals should be locked away

(D) In the event of an injury, the nearest poison information centre should be contacted

15. **Marcus, aged 8 years, had received a new scooter for his birthday. He was the last of his group of friends to get one, and had been pressuring his parents for some time. He had felt left out, as his friends were now using their scooters to get to school and he had been walking. He zoomed all over the neighbourhood, delighted with his gift. Although he was quite well coordinated, he was thrown off balance by an unexpected bump in the footpath, and swerved into the path of an oncoming car. The car managed to miss him, but the fall to the asphalt resulted in concussion and a fractured skull. Which of the following are correct?**

(A) A helmet would have most likely prevented the fractured skull

(B) Scooters are not suitable means of road transport for children under 12 years of age

(C) Children should have lessons in use of scooters, and then be able to go anywhere with them

(D) Supervision and suitable venues for use of scooters are important

16. **In an infant who fails to gain weight and grow normally and in whom no physical abnormality can be detected, it is important to:**

(A) Check the urine for a possible urinary tract infection

(B) Perform a sweat test

(C) Check the karyotype

(D) Consult with the Children's Protection Agency

(E) Admit the infant to hospital for investigation and to observe the infant feeding

17. **The following may be indications that an infant who is failing to thrive may not have an organic lesion:**

(A) An alert, but irritable infant constantly sucking his or her fingers

(B) Maternal illness following delivery

(C) Poor attendance at the Child Health Centre and incomplete immunisation for age

(D) A young single mother

(E) An infant showing signs of poor care, for example soiled clothing, wet napkin with an obvious napkin dermatitis

18. **Which of the following is/are true?**

(A) The rate of growth (length and weight) is greater in the first year of life than at any other time

(B) Girls with Turner syndrome invariably have associated physical abnormalities

(C) Infants whose weight and length are below the 10th centile require hospitalisation for investigation

(D) Growth failure and anorexia may be the presenting signs of renal failure in infancy

(E) Congenital HIV infection may present as a problem of failure to thrive in infancy

19. **In which of the following disorders is failure to thrive due to failure of oral intake?**

(A) Werdnig–Hoffmann disease

(B) Pierre Robin syndrome

(C) Spastic quadriplegia

(D) Behavioural disorder

(E) Giardiasis

20. **The concept of developmental disability implies:**

(A) A disability that is long term

(B) Onset before birth or during childhood

(C) A static encephalopathy

(D) A disability based on neurological dysfunction

(E) Most affected children are unlikely to lead independent lives as adults

21. **In intellectual disability:**

(A) Diagnosis is solely dependent on IQ testing

(B) The IQ must be more than 2 standard deviations below the mean

(C) World Health Organization criteria define severe intellectual disability as an IQ less than 70

(D) Most recent prevalence estimates are below 2%

(E) The disability must be diagnosed during childhood

22. **Children with intellectual disabilities:**

(A) May present at or soon after birth with malformation syndromes

(B) May present in the preschool years with sleep disturbance or behaviour problems

(C) Are generally easy to differentiate from children with low normal abilities

(D) Are generally easy to differentiate from children with degenerative disorders

(E) Will usually be delayed in all areas of development

23. **Concerning the causes of intellectual disabilities:**

(A) The cause is more likely to be known in cases of moderate and severe intellectual disability than in mild intellectual disability

(B) A specific cause can be identified in most cases of severe intellectual disability

(C) Iodine deficiency is a major cause in Australia and New Zealand

(D) Most known causes are of prenatal origin

(E) Fragile X syndrome affects males and females equally

119

24. **A 2 year old boy presents with concern about development. Recent assessment suggests that his developmental skills are at a 1 year old level. Appropriate management is to:**
    - (A) Advise the family that he is too young to make a diagnosis and that we should wait another year before doing anything
    - (B) Reassure the parents that he will probably catch up
    - (C) Arrange testing of vision and hearing
    - (D) Order a wide range of investigations, including MRI scan, karyotype and fragile X DNA tests
    - (E) Refer the family to a multidisciplinary early intervention programme

25. **You are asked to see a 6 year old girl with Down syndrome, who has recently moved into your area, to complete a form for review of her disability allowance. The family say she has always been healthy and has not needed medical care. You should:**
    - (A) Complete the form and leave further review up to the family
    - (B) Organise a limited range of assessments, including vision, hearing, thyroid function and cardiology review
    - (C) Organise all the assessments listed in (B) plus barium swallow, cervical spine X ray and full blood examination
    - (D) Recommend the local special school for her education
    - (E) Provide the family with information about the local Down syndrome association

26. **Which of the following features would arouse suspicion of child abuse in young (preschool) children?**
    - (A) Scalding of the upper back
    - (B) Scalds to both hands, with demarcation of the burn at the wrists
    - (C) Bilateral subdural haematoma in an infant
    - (D) Fundal haemorrhages
    - (E) Bruising of varying ages to forehead and anterior tibiae

27. **Which of the following statements is/are true of suspected child sexual abuse?**
    - (A) Fewer than 10% of victims are male
    - (B) The majority of perpetrators are strangers to the child
    - (C) Examination under anaesthesia is required if the history suggests sexual abuse with vaginal intercourse
    - (D) A vaginal introitus with horizontal diameter measuring 1 cm in a conscious prepubertal girl is suggestive of child sexual abuse
    - (E) Child sexual abuse is excluded if an intact hymen is found on examination

28. **Which of the following statements is/are true with respect to investigation of preschool children in whom child abuse is suspected?**
    - (A) X ray of the skull is preferred to a bone scan where head trauma is suspected
    - (B) A bone scan will detect skeletal trauma of long bones earlier than an X ray
    - (C) A clotting profile, including platelet count, is required in the investigating of bruising
    - (D) Developmental screening is required in the assessment of the young child
    - (E) The results of clinical findings and investigations are sufficient to determine management of abused children

29. **Melanie, a 13 year old gymnast, presents with right wrist pain following a hyperextension injury sustained during practice. Examination of the hand, wrist and elbow reveals full range of motion with no swelling, bruising or point tenderness. X rays of the wrist show no evidence of fracture or dislocation. She is treated with a wrist splint and NSAIDs, briefly improves, but returns 5 days later with recurrent right wrist pain. The most likely diagnosis is:**
    - (A) Wrist sprain
    - (B) Missed stress fracture of distal radius
    - (C) Persisting with gymnastics training
    - (D) Scaphoid fracture
    - (E) Non compliance with medication

30. **Andrew, an adolescent male aged 14 years, is seen with a complaint of chest pain. On examination he is noticed to have mild gynaecomastia (firm somewhat tender swelling beneath the nipple), more prominent on the left side, but is otherwise normal. Pubic hair and genitalia are at Tanner stage 3. Would you:**
    - (A) Ignore the finding completely because you know it will go away in time
    - (B) Comment upon it, find out how he feels about it and reassure him accordingly
    - (C) Biopsy it with a view to excluding malignancy
    - (D) Recommend surgery for cosmetic reasons
    - (E) Treat it light heartedly as a joke

31. **A 16 year old girl complains of vaginal discharge. She has not had sexual intercourse. Findings on pelvic examination are normal. Among the following, the organism most likely to be recovered from the vagina is:**
    - (A) *Chlamydia trachomatis*
    - (B) *Gardnerella vaginalis*
    - (C) *Trichomonas vaginalis*
    - (D) *Escherichia coli*
    - (E) *Neisseria gonorrhoeae*

32. Which of the following statements about adolescent sexuality are true?

(A) Approximately 25% of adolescents have homosexual experiences

(B) Condom use among adolescents has decreased in recent years

(C) Pregnant teenagers who continue with their pregnancy are more likely to keep their baby than give it up for adoption

(D) Adolescents are less vulnerable than adults to sexually transmitted diseases

(E) Pelvic inflammatory disease (PID) is a major cause of infertility

33. Which of the following statements are true?

(A) Concrete thought is typical of mid adolescence

(B) Girls have an earlier growth spurt than boys

(C) The average duration of puberty is about 5 years

(D) Gynaecomastia is a relatively rare condition in adolescent boys

(E) Menarche is preceded by at least 2 years of breast development

Answers and explanations

1. At least 15% of Australian families with dependent children are one parent families, but that figure may be low as marriage breakup is increasing (**A**). Many marriage breakups are, however, childless. Although many single parents are able to meet their children's physical, emotional and intellectual needs very well, the majority of single parents are at a significant disadvantage because of financial difficulty, inadequate housing, isolation and in many cases depression, perhaps through death of the partner, inability to cope alone and disapproving community attitudes, to name but a few reasons (**B**). Aboriginal children suffer many more infections of almost any type than other Australian children. Infant mortality rates are also greatly increased (C). The health of aboriginal children is a sad reflection of the concern the community has for their welfare. Migrant children are eligible for exactly the same health benefits that are available to other Australian children, namely, via family doctors, child health clinics, public hospitals and community health centres (**D**). They are also eligible for the same government health benefits. Couples in a de facto relationship have similar rights to those available to married couples (E).

2. (A) False. While preschool education is not compulsory, over 90% of 4 year old children attend. Because of current economic conditions, government sponsored 3 year old kindergartens are not available. The preschool year is important in preparing the child for school. (B) False. This is no longer necessary as physical disorders (particularly congenital) are almost always identified earlier. Tests of vision and hearing are routinely performed on entering school. Tests of vision are routinely repeated at year 8. Screening for scoliosis in girls is also done at this time. (C) False. Provided working mothers have adequate support, for example, from spouse, relatives, creche and so on, their children will not suffer emotional deprivation. (**D**) True. (E) False. Child health nurses are trained in applying tests of developmental screening, e.g. the Denver Developmental Screening Test. One of the more important functions of the child health nurse is to identify infants at risk for developmental delay.

3. (A) True. Circumcision for many Aboriginal people is an issue of great cultural and spiritual significance. It is not usually necessary for the treatment of phimosis as steroid cream may be an effective non surgical treatment in some cases. When surgical treatment is required, an alternative to full circumcision is to split the edge of the foreskin to enlarge the meatus without removing the foreskin. (**B**) True. The family will need to be consulted regarding any surgical procedure as the parents share responsibility for the child with the family. This is particularly true in situations that have additional cultural significance. (C) False. Phimosis can be associated with an increased risk of urinary tract infection and, if severe, can cause significant obstruction to the urinary tract. (**D**) True. (**E**) True. Any discussions about the genitalia involve issues of a culturally sensitive nature and should be approached sensitively.

4. (A) False. Unfortunately this is a common condition in Aboriginal children, although relatively uncommon in non Aboriginal children. (B) False. Treatment is indicated and needs to be continued until the perforation is healed. (**C**) True. This condition is commonly associated with deafness or partial hearing loss, which can contribute to poor school performance and educational outcomes. This in turn reduces employment prospects and can have lifelong effects both physically and socially. (**D**) True. This condition can be an ongoing problem and surgical intervention to patch the eardrum is often required. (**E**) True. Upper respiratory tract infection is more common in Aboriginal children than non Aboriginal children and infection with this organism contributes to chronic ear disease.

5. (A) This may be true or false, depending on whether or not you took time to introduce yourself and whether you treated her with respect and consideration for her culture. (B) This may be true or false but as she has presented for immunisation it is likely that

she does want her child to be immunised. However, she may not entirely trust that immunisation will be beneficial and not harm the child. It is important to provide accurate information about immunisation for all patients. (C) False. She clearly cares enough to bring her child for immunisation even though it is obviously difficult for her. (D) True. It is not the role of the mother to allow her child to be hurt in any way, even for the good of the child. She should have been encouraged to bring her mother or another family member who would be able to hold the child for the immunisation while she comforts the child. (E) True. Without knowing your skin group it may be taboo or not permitted for her to speak to you or even look at you.

6. The correct answer is (D), although it would be appropriate to advise (A) or (C). These formulae have a composition similar to standard infant formulae with the exception of lactose. Lactose free formula contains glucose polymers as the carbohydrate source, while low lactose formula contains predigested lactose (glucose and galactose), with a very small amount of residual lactose; this is almost always well tolerated. Soy formula (B) does not contain lactose but should not be recommended for lactose intolerance as there is absolutely no need to change the source of protein in the formula. Goat's milk based formula (E) is not appropriate.

7. The correct answer is (E). (A) Cow's milk is not recommended as the main milk source during the first 12 months of life: breast milk or formula should be used during this time. Cow's milk is a poor source of iron (low iron content and the iron present is poorly absorbed), and may cause gastrointestinal blood loss in infants under 12 months of age if used as the primary milk source. It may be introduced in foods such as cheese, custard and yoghurt as part of solid introduction. Inadequate total food intake (B) may be the result of food refusal, illness, dieting, eating disorders, poverty or other factors and may well result in a deficiency in the intake of many nutrients, including iron. Excessive milk intake (C) may cause iron deficiency in toddlers, as the over-consumption of milk tends to displace other foods. This is most commonly seen in children from non English speaking backgrounds living in Western societies, whose parents are not familiar with the Western foods available and tend to rely on milk, rather than introduce a variety of new foods as the child gets older. Delaying the introduction of solid foods (D) after 6 months can lead to iron deficiency, as iron stores from birth are depleted, growth is rapid, and iron rich foods are needed to supplement breast milk or formula. Vegetarian diets must also be carefully planned for children as these can lead to inadequate iron intake, along with inhibited iron absorption due to the presence of a high concentration of phytates in many of the foods frequently included in these diets.

8. The correct statements are (B), (D) and (E).

9. The correct answer is (E). Adolescents should be encouraged to eat a wide variety of foods, in accordance with the Australian Dietary Guidelines. Fruit, vegetables, bread and cereals provide energy and nutrients, such as complex carbohydrates and vitamins A, B, and C, and are the major sources of fibre in the diet. Milk and dairy products are vital sources of calcium, and choosing low fat products will assist with weight control. Lean meats are an invaluable source of nutrients, such as iron and zinc, in the diet of teenagers, and avoidance of iron rich foods can lead to iron deficiency. This is a particular problem for teenage girls with poor dietary intake, given their increased needs for iron during a time of rapid growth and development and iron loss resulting from menstruation. It is important to highlight the role of physical activity in achieving and maintaining a healthy weight, preventing osteoporosis, and forming the basis for a healthy adult lifestyle (although this often is not a major concern for teenagers, who tend to focus on the present). Emphasis should also be placed on the need for the whole family to be involved. Sarah's mother needs encouragement and support too: parents are key role models and can significantly influence both eating habits and the level of physical activity undertaken by their children. A referral to a dietitian would be appropriate.

10. The correct answer is (E). True measles infection is very uncommon in developed countries in the first year of life, and many other types of infection, such as enteroviral infections, are associated with rashes during this period (A). She should have MMR vaccine and Hib immunisation as indicated by the schedule (E), and it is not appropriate to delay (D) or alter (B), (C) the schedule.

11. The correct answers are (A) and (D). Although a fever may occur in some children after immunisation, the risk of a febrile convulsion is very small, particularly at this age (D). It would be appropriate for him to have paracetamol if any fever were to occur. There is no increased risk of adverse events related to these immunisations while he is on inhaled corticosteroids (B), and inhaled corticosteroids will not interfere with the immune response to vaccines (B), (C). There is no association known between vaccine associated paralytic poliomyelitis-like illness (which is very rare) and the previous occurrence of convulsions of any type (E).

12. The correct answers are **(C)**, **(D)** and **(E)**. (A) He does not need to restart his DTP schedule: DTPw is a very effective vaccine, and many countries overseas use a 3, 4 and 5 months of age schedule for the primary course with very good efficacy. Use of antibiotics is not a contraindication to immunisation and antibiotics will not interfere with the immune responses to vaccines (B). He should proceed with the usual schedule vaccines for preschool age (DTPa, MMR, OPV). He should also be given pneumococcal conjugate vaccine because of his risk of increased morbidity from pneumococcal lower respiratory tract infection as a result of his cystic fibrosis (E). For the same reason, he should have yearly influenza vaccine with inactivated influenza subunit vaccine, and he should have varicella vaccine as a single dose.

13. **(A)** and **(C)** are correct. Instant noodles are a convenient food but a newly recognised cause of scalds in children (B). They are made with boiling water and accordingly will cause scalds if spilt on the skin. Such foods should be given when children are sitting at a table and supervised. Note this injury occurred at a time of distraction of the parent. The behaviour of the boys is normal (D). Sibling conflict, particularly at the end of the day, is a usual part of family life.

14. **(C)** and **(D)** are correct. Brightly coloured tablets and chemicals look like sweets to children, who are not very discriminating about taste (A). Ideally, Emily's mother or father would be aware of her actions at all times, but it is because this represents an ideal rather than reality that the 'passive' measures of locking drugs and poisons away is so important (B). Parents are usually, with instruction and coaching, able to make their own homes safe for children by removing or locking away obvious hazards (C). Not all of the houses they visit will have made the same provision, and extra vigilance is required. Extending the child proofing to houses which are frequently visited, for example, grandparents, is also useful. Awareness of a poison information centre and phone number is very important (D).

15. The correct answers are **(A)**, **(B)** and **(D)**. The answer C is only partially correct, as explained below. Scooters are very popular and have caused many injuries without an appropriate strategy for their safe use being developed. As they resemble bicycles in being means of transport, similar safety measures should be adopted. Helmets will prevent many head injuries, and children under 12 should not be near a road with scooters. Lessons in use could be useful, but a child under 12 would not have the required eye–hand coordination to avoid motor traffic safely.

16. The correct answer is **(A)**. In infancy, a urinary infection may be symptomless. Failure to thrive may be the result of the infection alone or it may be associated with renal insufficiency (A). It is unusual for cystic fibrosis to present without evidence of abnormal stools, chest infection or a positive family history (B). In this era, many centres screen for cystic fibrosis. A chromosomal abnormality could be the cause, but a karyotype analysis would not usually be done as a first line investigation of failure to thrive in the absence of distinctive phenotypic features of a syndrome, such as Turner syndrome, in a female child (webbed neck, widely spaced nipples, oedema of hands and feet in early life) (C). A Child Protection Agency would not be consulted in relation to a child failing to thrive unless there was a suspicion of poor care or suggestion of family dysfunction (D). It is preferable to observe the infant–mother interaction, provide feeding advice and check urine and blood and perhaps X ray the chest before considering admission to hospital (E).

17. **All are correct**. (A) suggests the infant is hungry and the feeding needs are not being met. Maternal illness may have meant that there was not the opportunity for mother–infant bonding (B). The mother may have been suffering postnatal depression. However, many mothers who have had a postnatal illness care for their baby properly. Poor attendance for health care and for immunisations for an infant suggest family dysfunction (C). Many single mothers have few family or financial supports. Some have been deserted by the father or have parents who refuse to provide assistance or support when needed (D). Depression is far from rare in this situation. Poor physical care of the infant suggests lack of interest, ability, or financial and physical resources (E).

18. The correct answers are **(A)**, **(D)** and **(E)**. Weight triples in the first year of life and length increases by at least 12 cm per year. This is even greater than that achieved at puberty. Girls with Turner syndrome may present solely because of short stature (B), and may have few if any other phenotypic abnormalities, especially if they have marked XO mosaicism. If (C) were the case we would be investigating 10% of all children, an unnecessarily high number. Growth is considered normal if it falls within the ranges between the 5th and 95th centiles. Chronic renal failure may present with growth failure in infancy (D). In addition there is usually a metabolic acidosis and a normochromic and normocytic anaemia and there may also be associated bone abnormalities (renal rickets). HIV infection is common in Africa and in the United States, and is becoming common in some parts of Asia. It is seen less often in Australia and New Zealand.

19. The correct answers are **(A)**, **(B)**, **(C)** and **(D)**. Werdnig–Hoffmann disease is a neuromuscular

123

disorder of infancy and is usually fatal before 1 year of age. The muscular weakness prevents adequate sucking and hence intake (A). In Pierre Robin syndrome, the tongue tends to prolapse into the pharynx, obstruct the airway and thus prevent sucking (B). Spastic quadriplegia is frequently associated with pseudobulbar palsy, resulting in pharyngeal incoordination and choking during feeding (C). Hence intake is compromised. Some infants, for reasons that are not clear, become upset when feeding is attempted. In addition they often sleep poorly, cry frequently and are excessively restless. No cause is found and intake is reduced (D). Giardia infects the small bowel, resulting in diarrhoea and malabsorption. Intake is usually adequate and often is excessive because of hunger (E).

20. **(A)**, **(B)**, **(C)** and **(D)** are true. Some would debate (C) and (D) and include slowly progressive disorders and neuromuscular disorders. Clearly also disorders of onset in late childhood, such as acquired brain injury, have more in common with similar disorders of adult onset than with, say, the cerebral palsies. The definitions tend to be a little inconsistent. The basic principles, as outlined, remain. (E) is false. Disabilities at the mild end of the spectrum, such as clumsiness, specific learning disabilities, and even degrees of intellectual disability, are quite compatible with normal productive lives, although the individual differences do tend to persist.

21. **(B)** and **(D)** are true. (A), (C) and (E) are false. IQ testing is important and generally reliable, but there are problems, including cultural bias. Tests of day to day functioning must also be included. The WHO criteria for severe intellectual disability are IQ 20–34. The onset must be in childhood; detection and diagnosis could be later.

22. **(A)**, **(B)**, and **(E)** are true. (C) is false. The dividing line between normal and abnormal is not clearcut and in borderline children may vary from day to day. (D) is also false. Degenerative disorders may be slow in onset and may present with slow development.

23. **(A)**, **(B)** and **(D)** are true. (C) is false, although there are concerns at the re-emergence of iodine deficiency in these and other developed countries. (E) is also false. Affected females tend to be less severely disabled than affected males.

24. (A) and (B) are false. From the age of 2 years onwards ability patterns are quite stable and catchup is unlikely. This boy's delays are serious and the family need to be informed of this — openly and with sensitivity. **(C)**, **(D)** and **(E)** are true. Associated disorders of vision and hearing are common; aetiological investigation should be vigorous — you might

also consider urine metabolic tests and referral to a geneticist; early intervention programmes provide a range of helpful services.

25. There are no definite right and wrong answers here. (A) is perhaps a little irresponsible — you should at least discuss the advantages of health monitoring with the family. (B) is appropriate, but should be done after discussion with the family. Problems in these areas are all common in Down syndrome and may not be obvious clinically. (C) is excessive, but the risk of atlantoaxial dislocation is worth discussion. (D) Most children with Down syndrome attend regular schools: the parents should be told of the options in your area and make their own choice. (E) is always a good idea.

26. **(B)**, **(C)** and **(D)** are correct. (A) While scalding to the upper back can occur to a young child in a bath under the hot tap, uniform burns to the hands (B) suggest that they have been forcibly immersed and held in hot water. (C) Subdural haematoma and fundal haemorrhages (D) both result from shaking injuries to infants and young children, with haemorrhaging from small ruptured vessels. (E) Bruising to the forehead and anterior tibiae are extremely common in young children, resulting from falls and bumps sustained during normal activity.

27. **(D)** is correct. (A) While most child sexual assault victims are female, most centres report 20–25% of victims are male. (B) There is also a misconception that perpetrators are often strangers, but this applies in approximately 20% of cases only; most are family members, close friends or associates of the family. (C) Genital examination is required as part of the evaluation of suspected child sexual abuse. An experienced examiner should conduct the examination, and photographs at colposcopy are now used routinely. Only in rare cases, such as with severe injury, is examination under anaesthesia required. (D) A normal examination does not exclude child sexual abuse. It has been reported that if the introital opening is greater than 4 mm in a conscious child there is a high correlation with child sexual abuse. However this finding alone is not diagnostic of child sexual abuse. (E) Hymenal tags, clefts and scars are indicative of abuse.

28. **(A)**, **(B)**, **(C)** and **(D)** are correct. (A) Both bone scans and X rays are used in determining the presence and extent of skeletal trauma. A bone scan of the head is not a useful examination, and a skull X ray is required. (B) Bone scans of limbs will often detect early trauma, including periosteal haematoma and metaphyseal damage. Skeletal survey by X rays can be used to examine further suspicious areas and to detect past fractures. (C) Clotting studies and platelet

counts are required only rarely for diagnosis, but are usually obtained for medicolegal purposes. (D) A number of young children who sustain physical abuse also suffer environmental deprivation and neglect, with consequent delayed development. Developmental screening is an essential part of the assessment. (E) Case management of child abuse requires multidisciplinary assessment. A psychosocial assessment of the child and family is essential in addition to the medical findings. This multidisciplinary management is facilitated by a case conference.

29. The correct answer is (D). Scaphoid fracture is the most common fracture of the carpal bones, representing 70% of all wrist fractures. It is a commonly missed orthopaedic injury (others being anterior cruciate ligament tear, slipped capital femoral epiphysis, femoral neck stress fracture, ulnar collateral ligament tear, posterior tibial tendon rupture and Achilles tendon rupture). Scaphoid fracture typically presents as distal radial wrist pain after a fall on an outstretched hand. On examination, there is tenderness in the anatomical snuff box. Diagnosis is aided by an anteroposterior wrist film with 30° supination and ulnar deviation. Poor blood supply to the scaphoid constitutes a risk of non union, the risk of which increases with delayed diagnosis. Treatment varies with the location of the fracture but generally involves immobilisation with a short arm cast for 6–8 weeks.

30. The correct answer is (B). Body conscious teenagers are very sensitive about changes which they often view a gross abnormalities. Often it is too threatening to bring up and they may present a symptom which will direct the doctor's attention to the area of concern. It is important to explain that pubertal gynaecomastia is a normal finding and relieve anxiety. Offer a follow up visit to discuss it further.

31. The correct answer is (B). In evaluating the results of bacteriological culture of the vagina or cervix, it is important to know which organisms are predominantly acquired as a result of sexual activity. Studies comparing the vaginal flora of sexually active and virginal adolescents suggest that some agents are almost exclusively associated with vaginal or oral sexual intercourse. For example, *Neisseria gonorrhoeae* and *Trichomonas vaginalis* are found in the genital tract of only those females who have had some genital contact. Certain other organisms are found more commonly, or in greater numbers, in the vaginal flora of sexually active females. These organisms include *Ureaplasma urealyticum*, *Mycoplasma hominis* and *Chlamydia trachomatis*. Although Chlamydia has been recovered on occasions from adolescent girls who are virginal by history and on physical examination, it is most likely to have been acquired by sexual transmission.

32. (A), (C) and (E) are correct. (A) While not uncommon during adolescence, homosexual experiences do not necessarily herald the beginnings of a homosexual orientation. A sensitive exploration of this issue by a doctor can lessen anxiety in the young person with such uncertainty. (B) Surveys of sexual behaviour indicate that, overall, condom use has increased in adolescents in recent years. The AIDS scare and improved sex education are considered probable reasons for the trend. (C) Putting a baby up for adoption is now extremely rare. Teenagers who opt to continue with their pregnancy almost invariably end up keeping their baby. (D) The vulnerability of young people to STDs is related to their having sex more often than adults, having more partners and being less likely to use condoms. For girls, there are additional biological factors, including: increased zone of ectopy (columnar cells are less resistant to infection); increased penetrability of the cervical mucous plug to STD agents; decreased prevalence of protective antibodies in comparison to adults. (E) PID is not only a common cause of ectopic pregnancy but also a major cause of infertility in women.

33. The correct answers are (B) and (E). Answers (A), (C) and (D) are false. (A) While cognitive development is not quite as predictable as earlier thought, most adolescents will have moved beyond concrete thought processes (formal operations) by the mid teens. (B) Girls experience accelerated growth with the onset of puberty, while for boys the growth spurt is a late pubertal event. (C) The duration of puberty can be a little as 2 years or less or as long as 5 years or more; 3 years is about average. (D) Pubertal breast development (gynaecomastia), thought to be caused by transient hormonal imbalance favouring oestrogen, occurs in approximately 70% of boys around mid puberty. (E) Breast budding (Tanner rating 2) precedes menarche by at least 2 years; for girls who enter puberty, this is a reassuring piece of information.

PART 3   FURTHER READING

American Academy of Pediatrics 2001 Committee on Child A and neglect: distinguishing sudden infant death syndrome from child abuse fatalities. Pediatrics 107: 437–441 (Erratum appears in Pediatrics 108: 512; 108: 812

Angus G, Hall G 1996 Child abuse and neglect Australia 1994–1995. Child Welfare Series Number 16. Australian Institute of Health and Welfare. Australian Government Publishing Service, Canberra

Australian Bureau of Statistics 1994 Australia Now. Special article — Statistics on the indigenous people of Australia, Year Book Australia. ABS, Canberra

Australian Institute of Health and Welfare 1998 Australia's children. Their health and wellbeing. AIHW, Canberra

Ballas M T, Tytko J, Mannarino F 1998 Commonly missed orthopaedic problems. American Family Physician 57: 267–274

Barratt T M, Avner E D, Harman W E 1999 Pediatric nephrology. Lippincott Williams and Wilkins, Baltimore

Becker A E, Grinspoon S K, Klibanski A, Herzog D B 1999 Eating disorders. New England Journal of Medicine 340: 1092–1098

Bedford H, Elliman D 2000 Parental objections to immunisation and responses. BMJ 320: 240–243

Bennett D L 1995 Growing pains: what to do when your children turn into teenagers. Doubleday Australia, Sydney

Bennett D L, Ward M S, Daniel W A Jr 1976 The relationship of serum alkaline phosphatase concentrations to sex maturity ratings in adolescents. Journal of Pediatrics 88: 633–636

Beresford B 1996 Expert opinions. Policy Press, Bristol

Bhati K, Anderson P 1995 An overview of Aboriginal and Torres Strait Islander health: present status and future trends. Australian Government Publishing Service, Canberra

Blackwell C C, Weir D M 1999 The role of infection in sudden infant death syndrome. FEMS Immunology and Medical Microbiology 25: 1–6

Byard R W, Gallard V, Johnson A, Barbour J, Bonython-Wright D 1996 Safe feeding practices for infants and young children. Journal of Paediatric Child Health 32: 327–329

Carmichael A 1983 The needs of the abused child in the community. Australian Paediatric Journal 19: 143–146

Capute A J, Accardo P J 1996 Developmental disabilities in infancy and childhood, 2nd edn. Paul H Brookes, Baltimore

CARPA Standard Treatment Manual 1994. Central Australian Rural Practitioners Association, Alice Springs

Casey K 1994 Teaching children with special needs. Social Science Press, Wentworth Falls, New South Wales

Cassidy S B, Schwartz S 1998 Prader–Willi and Angelman syndromes. Disorders of genomic imprinting. Medicine 77: 140–151

Cole T J, Bellizzi M C, Flegel K M, Dietz W H 2000 Establishing a standard definition for child overweight and obesity worldwide. International survey. BMJ 320: 1–6

Comerci G D, Schwebel R 2000 Substance abuse: an overview. State of the Art Reviews: Adolescent Medicine 11: 79–102

Commonwealth Department of Human Services and Health 1996 Proposed plan of action for the prevention of abuse and neglect of children from non-English speaking background. Australian Government Publishing Service, Canberra

Couper R T L, Couper J J 2000 Prader–Willi syndrome. Lancet 356: 673–675

Decker MD 2001 Principles of pediatric combination vaccines and practical issues related to use in clinical practice. Pediatric Infectious Diseases Journal 20(11 Supplement): S10–18

Donaghy B 1997 Leaving early: youth suicide: the horror, the heartbreak, the hope. Harper Collins, New York

Donaghy B 1999 Unzipped: everything teenagers want to know about love, sex and each other. Harper Collins, New York

Durie M 1994 Whaiora — Maori health development. Oxford University Press, Oxford

Durie M H 1989 The treaty of Waitangi and health care. New Zealand Medical Journal 102: 283–285

Eastman C J 1999 Where has all our iodine gone? Medical Journal of Australia 171: 455–456

Essery S D et al 1999 The protective effect of immunisation against diphtheria, pertussis and tetanus (DPT) in relation to sudden infant death syndrome. FEMS Immunology and Medical Microbiology 25: 183–192

Filiano J J, Kinney H C 1992 Arcuate nucleus hypoplasia in the sudden infant death syndrome. Journal of Neuropathology and Experimental Neurology 51: 394–403

Fleming P J et al 1999 Pacifier use and sudden infant death syndrome: results from the CESDI/SUDI case control study. CESDI SUDI research team. Archives of Disease in Childhood 81: 112–116

Ford R P et al 1993 Breastfeeding and the risk of sudden infant death syndrome. International Journal of Epidemiology 22: 885–890

Gilbert R E et al 1995 Bottle feeding and the sudden infant death syndrome. BMJ 310: 88–90

Gohlke B C, Khaldikar V V, Skuse D, Stanhope R 1998 Recognition of children with psychosocial short stature: a spectrum of presentation. Journal of Pediatric Endocrinology and Metabolism 11: 509–517

Gordon A E et al 1999 The protective effect of breast feeding in relation to sudden infant death syndrome (SIDS): III detection of IgA antibodies in human milk that bind to bacterial toxins implicated in SIDS. FEMS Immunology and Medical Microbiology 25: 175–182

Grossman D C 2000 The history of injury control and the epidemiology of child and adolescent injuries. Future of Children 10: 23–52

Gunn T R, Tonkin S L 1989 Upper airway measurements during inspiration and expiration in infants. Pediatrics 84: 1

Helweg-Larsen K et al 1999 Interactions of infectious symptoms and modifiable risk factors in sudden infant death syndrome. The Nordic Epidemiological SIDS study. Acta Paediatrica 88: 521–527

Henson R, Hadfield J M, Cooper S 1999 Injury control strategies: extending the quality and quantity of data relating to road traffic accidents in children. Journal of Accident and Emergency Medicine 16: 87–90

Huppke P, Laccone F, Kramer N, Engel W, Hanefield F 2000 Rett syndrome: analysis of MECP2 and clinical characterization of 31 patients. Human Molecular Genetics 9: 1369–1375

Kang M 2000 Sex files: exploring sexuality through Dolly magazine. Youth Studies 1928–1933

Kemp J S et al 2000 Unsafe sleep practices and an analysis of bedsharing among infants dying suddenly and unexpectedly: results of a four-year, population-based, death-scene investigation study of sudden infant death syndrome and related deaths. Pediatrics 106: E41

Kempe C H, Silverman F N, Steele B F, Droegmueller W, Silver H K 1962 Battered child syndrome. JAMA 181: 17

Kinney H C et al 1983 'Reactive gliosis' in the medulla oblongata of victims of the sudden death syndrome. Pediatrics 72: 181–187

Kinney H C, Filiano J J, White W F 1997 Muscarinic cholinergic receptor binding in SIDS brain stems: a review. Pediatric Pulmonology 23: 136–138

Kinney H C, Filiano J J, White W F 2001 Medullary serotonergic network deficiency in the sudden infant death syndrome: review of a 15-year study of a single dataset. Journal of Neuropathology and Experimental Neurology 60: 228–247

Kousham E K, Gracey M 1997 Persistent growth faltering among Aboriginal infants and young children in north-west Australia: a retrospective study from 1969–1993. Acta Paediatrica 86: 46–50

Lazarus R, Baur L, Webb K, Blyth F, Gliksman M 1995 Recommended body mass cut off values for overweight screening programmes in Australian children and adolescents: comparisons with North American values. Journal of Paediatric Child Health 31: 143–147

L'Hoir M P et al 1999 Dummy use, thumb sucking, mouth breathing and cot death. European Journal of Pediatrics 158: 896–901

Loder R T 1998 Slipped capital femoral epiphysis. American Family Physician 57: 2135–2142

Lucas A, Morley R, Cole T J, Gore S M 1994 A randomised multi-centre study of human milk vs formula and later development in preterm infants. Archives of Disease in Childhood. Fetal and Neonatal Edition 70: 141–146

MacFarlane K, Waterman J, Connerly S et al 1986 Sexual abuse of young children: evaluation and treatment. Guilford Press, New York

Matilainen R, Airaksinen E, Mononen T, Launiala K, Kaarianen R 1995 A population-based study of mild and severe mental retardation. Acta Paediatrica 84: 261–266

Ministry of Health 1998 Our children's health. Ministry of Health, New Zealand

Mitchell E A 1990 International trends in postneonatal mortality. Archives of Disease in Childhood 65: 607–609

Mitchell E A 1999 Changing infants' sleep position increases risk of sudden infant death syndrome. New Zealand Cot Death Study. Archives of Pediatrics and Adolescent Medicine 153: 1136–1141

Mitchell E A et al 1992 Four modifiable and other major risk factors for cot death: the New Zealand study. Journal of Paediatric Child Health 28: S3–8

Mitchell E A et al 1993 Dummies and the sudden infant death syndrome. Archives of Disease in Childhood 68: 501–504

Mitchell E A et al 1995 Immunisation and the sudden infant death syndrome. Archives of Disease in Childhood 73: 498–501

National Health and Medical Research Council 1992 Recommended dietary intakes for use in Australia. Australian Government Publishing Service, Canberra

National Health and Medical Research Council 1995 Dietary guidelines for children and adolescents. Australian Government Publishing Service, Canberra

National Health and Medical Research Council 1996 Infant feeding guidelines for healthcare workers. Australian Government Publishing Service, Canberra

National Health and Medical Research Council 2002 Australian immunisation handbook, 8th edn. Australian Government Publishing Service, Canberra

National Inquiry into the Separation of Aboriginal and Torres Strait Islander children from their Families 1997 Bringing them home. Commonwealth of Australia, Canberra

Ngata P, Pomare E 1992 Cultural factors in medicine taking — a Maori perspective. New Ethical June: 43–50 (IHC)

Oates R K 1990 Understanding and managing child sexual abuse. Harcourt Brace Jovanovitch, Sydney

Panigrahy A et al 1997 Decreased kainite receptor binding in the arcuate nucleus of the sudden infant death syndrome. Journal of Neuropathology and Experimental Neurology 56: 1253–1261

Pimental M M 1999 Fragile X syndrome (review). International Journal of Medicine 3: 639–645

Plitponkarnpim A, Andersson R, Jansson B, Svanstrom L 1999 Unintentional injury mortality in children: a priority for middle income countries in the advanced stage of epidemiological transition. Injury Prevention 5: 98–103

Plotkin S A, Orenstien W A 1999 Vaccines, 3rd edn. WB Saunders, Philadelphia

Recommendations for nutrition and physical activity for Australian children 2000 Medical Journal of Australia 173: 51–56

Reed D B, Claunch D T 2000 Nonfatal farm injury incidence and disability to children: a systematic review. American Journal of Preventive Medicine 18(4 Supplement): 70–89

Rivara F P, Aitken M 1998 Prevention of injuries to children and adolescents. Advances in Pediatrics 45: 37–72

Royal Commission into Aboriginal Deaths in Custody 1991 Australian Government Publishing Service, Canberra

Rutter M, Tizard J, Whitmore K 1970 Education health and behaviour. Longman, London

Schwartz I D 2000 Failure to thrive: an old nemesis in the new millennium. Pediatrics in Review 21: 257–264

Schwartz P J et al 1998 Prolongation of the QT interval and the sudden infant death syndrome. New England Journal of Medicine 338: 1709–1714

Scragg R K et al 1996 Infant room-sharing and prone sleep position in sudden infant death syndrome. New Zealand Cot Death Study Group. Lancet 347: 7–12

Selikowitz M 1990 Down syndrome: the facts. Oxford University Press, Oxford

Shils M E, Olson J A, Shike M, Ross A C 1999 Modern nutrition in health and disease. Lippincott, Williams and Wilkins, Philadelphia

Shonkoff J P, Phillips D A 2000 From neurons to neighborhoods. The science of early childhood development. National Academy Press, Washington, DC

Stanley FJ 2001 Centenary article — child health since federation. In Year Book Australia 2001. Australian Bureau of Statistics, Canberra

Strasburger V C, Greydanus D E 2000 At-risk adolescents: an update for the new century. State of the Art Reviews: Adolescent Medicine 11: 1–210

Strømme P, Hagberg G 2000 Aetiology in severe and mild mental retardation: a population-based study of Norwegian children. Developmental Medicine and Child Neurology 42: 76–86

Summers A M et al 2000 Association of IL-10 genotype with sudden infant death syndrome. Human Immunology 61: 1270–1273

Suskind R M, Lewinter-Suskind L 1993 Textbook of paediatric nutrition, 2nd edn. Raven Press, New York

Taylor B J, Williams S M, Mitchell E A, Ford R P 1996 Symptoms, sweating and reactivity of infants who die of SIDS compared with community controls. New Zealand National Cot Death Study Group. Journal of Paediatrics and Child Heath 32: 316–322

UNICEF 1997 The state of the world's children. Oxford University Press, Oxford

UNICEF 2000 A league table of child poverty in rich nations. Florence, Italy

United Nations 1994 The standard rules on the equalization of opportunities for persons with disabilities. United Nations, New York

Veit F, Schwarz M 1995 Adolescent suicide attempts: a general practice perspective. Australian Family Physician 24: 2042–2044

Wellesley D G, Hockey K A, Montgomery P D, Stanley F J 1992 Prevalence of intellectual handicap in Western Australia: a community study. Medical Journal of Australia 156: 94–102

White J L, Malcolm R, Roper K, Westphal M C Jr, Smith C 1981 Psychosocial and developmental factors in failure to thrive: one to three year follow up. Journal of Developmental and Behavioral Pediatrics 2: 112–114

White P C, Spenser P W 2000 Congenital adrenal hyperplasia due to 21 hydroxylase deficiency. Endocrine Reviews 21: 245–291

Willinger M, James L S, Catz C 1991 Defining the sudden infant death syndrome (SIDS): deliberations of an expert panel convened by the National Institute of Child Health and Human Development. Pediatric Pathology 11: 677–684

Willinger M, Hoffman H J, Hartford R B 1994 Infant sleep position and risk for sudden infant death syndrome: report of meeting held January 13 and 14 1994, National Institutes of Health, Bethesda. Pediatrics 93: 814–819

Wilson C A et al 1994 Clothing and bedding and its relevance to sudden infant death syndrome: further results from the New Zealand Cot Death Study. Journal of Paediatrics and Child Health 30: 506–512

Wilson M E 2001 Travel related vaccines. Infectious Disease Clinics of North America 15: 231–251

World Health Organization 1980 International classification of impairments, disabilities, and handicaps. WHO, Geneva

Zubrick SR, Silburn SR et al 1997 Western Australia Child Health Survey: developing health and wellbeing in the nineties. ABS Cat. No. 4303.5. Australian Bureau of Statistics and the Institute for Child Health Research, Perth

Zupancic J A et al 2000 Cost-effectiveness and implications of newborn screening for prolongation of QT interval for the prevention of sudden infant death syndrome. Journal of Pediatrics 136: 481–489

Useful links

http://www.aifs.org.au (The Australian Institute of Family Studies publishes widely on all aspects of Australian family life. It is also a clearing house for published work on child abuse and neglect)

http://www.aihw.gov.au (To access data about the health of Australia's children and young people)

http://www.anad.org (National Association of Anorexia Nervosa and Associated Disorders)

http://www.cdc.gov/travel (CDC site for information on vaccines for travellers)

http://www.cps.ca/english/publications/InfectiousDiseases.htm (Canadian Pediatric Society website on infectious diseases and immunisation)

http://www.cyh.com (Excellent site with extensive information on parenting and child health issues, with information presented for children, young people and parents)

http://www.ext.vt.edu (Virginia Tech and State University: educational programs and resources)

http://www.fns.usda.gov (Food, nutrition and consumer services)

www.health.gov.au/pubhlth/publicat/immu.htm (Site for Department of Health and Aged Care in Australia, with links to pages for the Australian Immunisation Handbook, and Australian Immunisation Schedules)

http://www.healthinfonet.ecu.edu.au (Information on the health of Australia's indigenous people)

http://www.healthinsite.gov.au (Up-to-date information on important health topics such as diabetes, cancer, mental health, asthma)

http://www.immunisation.org.uk/ (An NHS/Health Promotion England website which gives information for providers, and the public, on vaccine preventable disorders and immunisation issues)

http://kidsafe.greenweb.com.au (Kidsafe Australia)

http://www.kidsourcc.com (In depth education and healthcare information for parents)

http://www.nisu.flinders.edu.au (National Injury Surveillance Unit)

http://www.nlm.nih.gov/medlineplus/childhoodimmunization.html (Medline Plus site on childhood immunisations, with very useful links to NIH, CDC and American Academy of Pediatrics and other position papers)

http://www.nutd.homestead.com/home.html (Nutrition advice)

http://www.NutritionAustralia.org (Aims to provide scientifically based nutrition advice)

http://www.racp.edu.au/indig/atsih.htm (Aboriginal and Torres Strait Islander health)

http://www.reachout.asn.au (for adolescent health)

http://www.sidsaustralia.org.au/ (SIDS Australia on line)

http://www.sidsfamilies.com/email.shtml (SIDS families email support groups)

http://www.sids.org/ (American SIDS Institute)

http://www.sids.org.uk/ (The Foundation for the Study of Infant Deaths)

http;//www.traveldoctor.com.au (Commercial Australian site for travel vaccine information)

http://www.travelvax.com.au (Commercial Australian site for travel vaccine information)

http://www.unicef.org (The latest news from Unicef)

http://www.unicef-icdc.org (UNICEF 2000 A league table of child poverty in rich nations. Florence, Italy)

http://www.update-software.com/cochrane/default.HTM (Cochrane library home page: explore abstracts (search term Vaccines) for listing of Cochrane reviews on evidence base for use of particular vaccine strategies)

http://www.usda.gov (United States Department of Agriculture)

http://www.who.int/inf-pr-2001/en/note2001-07.html (Results of a WHO review of exclusive breastfeeding)

http://www.who.intl/ith/ (WHO site for information on vaccines for travellers)

http://www.youthealth.com (An interactive site for young people)

BEHAVIOUR AND MENTAL HEALTH NEEDS IN CHILDHOOD

Life events of normal children

H. Hiscock, F. Oberklaid

Child development, from conception through to adolescence and on to adulthood, proceeds in ways that generally are predictable. Children achieve developmental milestones at certain ages (Ch. 4) and these anticipated milestones provide an important yardstick against which to assess the individual child's development. A departure from these predictable developmental milestones, usually in the form of delay or unusual and unexpected behaviours, provides the first sign that development is not proceeding normally.

The development of infants and young children is greatly dependent on their interaction with the environment. In the early years it is the parents, most often the mother, who shape the infant's environment. Research in recent years has served to re-emphasise the importance of the caretaking environment on the developing brain; the sort of environment that a young child is exposed to has a major impact on functioning later in life.

A key requirement for optimal child development is secure attachment to a trusted caregiver, usually the mother, with consistent affection and caring in the first few years. A child's and subsequently an adult's emotional health are significantly influenced by these early relationships between the young child and his or her caretakers.

Assessment of the development of behaviour of a child is therefore never undertaken in isolation — the environmental context is a critical part of the assessment. The child's behaviour and development are always the result of a complex series of transactions between the child and the environment and assessment always considers both.

Risk and resilience

There are well documented risk factors that make the child vulnerable to a less than optimal outcome. Similarly, there are protective factors that increase the resilience of the child and increase the likelihood of a good outcome. Some of the risk and protective factors can be:
- biological (prematurity, chronic health problems)
- temperamental (difficult versus easy temperament)
- parental (level of education, genetics); familial (family cohesion); socioeconomic (level of income, poverty)
- community (type of neighbourhood, facilities).

Appropriate caretaking by the parents provides some of the most important protective factors in promoting optimal development. Recent research suggests that this caretaking environment actually influences the structure of the brain, with the development of neural pathways that are determined largely by environmental inputs.

Risk and protective factors are not inevitable in individual children, operate differently at different ages, and tend to be cumulative, so that combinations of risk or protective factors are more powerful than individual factors.

Developmental stages

In the course of the child's development there are certain periods which can be viewed as important transition points. Each of these transitions is associated with predictable developmental events and behaviours, stresses and potential problems. The negotiation of each of these transitions is an important milestone that allows the child and the family to proceed to the next level of development. Stresses and problems encountered during these transitions may result in the child progressing down developmental pathways that lead to later problems.

A number of important transitions are considered below.

Birth

The goal is to produce a healthy, fullterm infant, together with a healthy mother who can cope with the inevitable stresses and change in lifestyle that come with a newborn baby.

Risk factors include maternal physical and mental illness, substance abuse, smoking, adolescence/single pregnancy and poverty. Infant risk factors include genetic defects, birth trauma and prematurity.

Professional interventions. Regular antenatal care enables early detection and intervention for many maternal and fetal complications. During labour the presence of a supportive partner or trusted friend has been shown to decrease time in labour and reduce complications. Early mother–baby contact facilitates breastfeeding and sets the stage for a positive mother–infant relationship. While in hospital it is important to establish linkages with postnatal services such as maternal and child health nurses, general practitioners, home visiting, and other community services.

Home with the new baby

This is often a challenging time for the family. Parents and family aim to establish a routine incorporating the needs and demands of the new infant. Parents bring to this trans-action their own beliefs and experiences, with varying levels of confidence and competence and skills at handling stress, uncertainty and fatigue. Parents begin to understand their baby's visual, motor and verbal cues and respond appropriately. This is the beginning of a reciprocal rela-tionship or 'dance'. This relationship shapes the baby's brain, especially during the first 3 years of life. If things do not go smoothly, and the mother perceives the infant as difficult and demanding, the long term mother–child relationship can be compromised, setting the stage for possible future parenting and behaviour difficulties.

Establishing appropriate feeding patterns, preferably breastfeeding as this has many advantages, is another crucial task.

Risk factors include an unwanted child, prenatal compli-cations, problems with bonding and attachment, maternal depression, social isolation, few or no identified supports and a stressful family situation.

Professional intervention. Providing support to parents through what is inevitably a stressful time, even in well functioning families, is essential. Assisting parents with realistic expectations and understanding of their baby's developmental needs and linking them up with a network of family and professional supports are crucial interven-tions. Sometimes there are early clues as to serious dys-function, such as maternal depression or major difficulties in the mother–child relationship, so that more intensive intervention may be required.

Early infancy (first 6 months)

All parents need to learn how to manage the following inevitable issues:

- *Crying.* All infants cry. This is now understood to be a normal part of development. However, some infants are difficult to console and the crying causes major stress for their parents. About 10% of infants cry more than 3 hours per day, 3 or more days per week for 3 or more weeks. These infants are often labelled 'colicky'. Underlying medical causes for crying are uncommon (<5%) and include cow's milk protein allergy, lactose intolerance and possibly gastro-oesophageal reflux.
- *Feeding.* Most mothers want to breastfeed their infant but not all mothers find it easy. Problems with incorrect attachment to the breast are common and may lead to difficult and painful breastfeeding and ultimately early weaning.

- *Sleeping issues.* Most infants establish a sleep pattern after 3 months of age, although they do not begin to sleep through the night until 6 months. Common parental complaints include difficulties settling their infant and frequent night waking.

> ### Clinical example
>
> A mother presents with her 7 week old baby boy. She says the baby is crying 2–3 hours a day and appears hungry. She is breastfeeding her baby every $1\frac{1}{2}$ hours, and says she has no milk so she wants to wean to formula. Her baby vomits a small amount after most feeds and her general practitioner has prescribed a medication for reflux. After a careful examination to exclude a physical cause of the crying, you explain that all babies cry, and that crying reaches a peak around 6–7 weeks of age and then decreases by age 3–4 months. You encourage her to keep breastfeeding and to space the feeds to every 2–3 hours so that the baby has a good feed and is not snack feeding. You discuss tiredness signs in babies and explain how to settle her baby when he is tired. You ask her to keep a feed/cry diary and to stop the reflux medication. Two weeks later, her baby is crying less and settling to sleep better. He is feeding every 3 hours and seems content.

If issues of crying, feeding and sleeping are not addressed, parents may become tired, frustrated, incon-sistent and even potentially abusive. A secure attachment may not form between the infant and caregiver and infants may miss out on the consistent and affectionate caretaking environment that has been shown to have such a major impact on brain development and function throughout childhood and beyond.

Another important task is the introduction of solids, with many mothers beginning to think about weaning towards the end of this period.

Risk factors include postnatal depression, parental conflict, inappropriate maternal expectations, and stress and fatigue. Infant risk factors include difficult tempera-ment, excessive crying and irritability, sleep problems and difficulty feeding.

Professional intervention. Providing support and appro-priate information so that parents have realistic expecta-tions and adequate coping strategies is important. Parenting needs to be consistent and caring, and a 'good-ness of fit' needs to be established between parenting style and infant needs and behaviours. Medication and frequent formula changes are usually inappropriate for sleeping and crying problems. Rather, parents need reas-surance that their infant is healthy and does not have any underlying medical condition. They should aim to settle their infant with a consistent approach that enables the infant fall to asleep on their own rather than being held, rocked or fed to sleep. Mothers experiencing problems with breastfeeding should be managed by someone experienced in the area, such as a community nurse or lactation consultant.

Late infancy (6 to 12 months)

This is a time of rapidly emerging cognitive, developmental and social competencies in the infant. He or she is interested in the environment, and will very often initiate interaction with caregivers, wanting to play and to be stimulated in appropriate ways. Paradoxically, during this time period the first signs of stranger anxiety and separation protest become evident. The infant becomes anxious around strangers and is no longer willing to be picked up by an unfamiliar person. The infant also may begin to become distressed when the parent is out of sight, for example at bed time or if left in the care of a babysitter or in childcare.

During this time, food issues become increasingly important, with most mothers completing weaning during this time and moving towards a varied diet with regular meals.

Risk factors include maternal and family stress, inappropriate responses to increasing infant needs for stimulation and social interaction, difficulty changing from breast/bottle feeding to educational diet, sleep difficulties and irritability.

Professional intervention. Continued support for parents, provision of accurate information about developmental and other needs of their rapidly developing infant, and ensuring that there is a 'goodness of fit' between the infant and parents are essential. Parents should realise that much of their infant's behaviour is exploratory and the infant is not being deliberately naughty. Sleep problems can be managed with behavioural interventions such as 'controlled crying', where parents leave their infant for increasing periods of time to enable them to fall asleep on their own. Good eating habits can be established with regular mealtimes of a short duration (typically 20 minutes or less) and encouraging the older infant to finger feed. Parents should offer a variety of foods, understanding that their infant may try a food many times before finally accepting it.

Toddler period (1 to 3 years)

This is a very major transition time, as the child moves from being an infant, who still is almost totally dependent, towards an active, curious toddler with an increasingly complex set of developmental competencies, including language. One of the normal developmental tasks in this age group is to develop autonomy, and this often challenges the parents as the toddler is oppositional, stubborn, seems always to be testing boundaries and likes to get his or her own way. Temper tantrums are common when the child is frustrated at being unable to master a task or restrictions are placed on his or her autonomy by parents saying 'no'. Sleep problems and problems around mealtime also are very common. They are more common in children with a difficult temperament and are made worse by inconsistent parenting.

Most children will begin, and some will complete, toilet training during this time period and this sometimes becomes a symbol of the struggle between the parents and the child regarding the child's autonomy. Signs of developmental delay, including language problems, also become evident during this time period.

Risk factors include difficult temperament, difficult behaviours (tantrums, overactivity, eating and sleeping problems, difficulty with socialisation) and developmental delay. Family factors include inconsistent parenting and inappropriate responses, poor social support and family stress.

Professional intervention. Parents need to know what is normal and how to effectively manage common problems. For example, when a child has a temper tantrum, parents should:
- stay calm
- walk away
- ignore the behaviour until the tantrum stops
- praise the child when appropriate behaviour begins again.

Most tantrum behaviour will escalate initially and then decline with this approach. For more aggressive behaviour, 'time out' may be used. This involves placing a child in a quiet room or corner for a maximum of 1 minute per year of age whenever the undesired behaviour occurs. This is effective in children over 18 months of age and its use should be limited initially to only the two or three most problematic behaviours.

Preschool period (3 to 5 years)

During this period, there continues to be a rapid explosion in language, cognitive ability and social skills. While the young child may have been left in childcare or in other child minding situations, the child now begins to participate in a more structured learning environment. This is an enriching experience in which the child's natural curiosity is stimulated by systematic input from trained preschool teachers, and by exposure to other children of the same age. Language continues to develop rapidly, as does the child's cognitive ability.

At the end of this period the child makes the very important and symbolic transition to school, so issues of school readiness become apparent. To undertake a successful transition to school, children need to master a range of motor, cognitive and social skills. They need to:

- be toilet trained
- be able to use a pencil
- be able to focus and maintain attention on a task
- have sufficient language skills
- be able to understand instructions and to make their needs understood
- have the social skills that enable them to interact with peers and with adults
- have the developmental competencies to function in a much more structured learning environment.

Rate of maturation during the preschool period may be uneven, and is certainly not linear. The child who appears 'immature' at the age of 4 years, for example, may mature rapidly during the following 6 months. Generally, girls are more mature than boys when they start school.

Risk factors in children include language or other developmental delay, poor social skills, difficulty focusing attention, separation difficulties from parents, behaviour problems (especially aggression). Family risk factors include low maternal educational levels, bilingual background, poverty and being a single parent.

Professional intervention. Parents of preschool children often seek professional help for concerns about language or developmental delay, behaviour problems, delayed toilet training, or questions about school readiness. Assessment at this age needs to be cautious because of the variability in maturation rates. Providing parents with information about realistic expectations in this age group, and teaching them basic skills in behaviour modification, is often very helpful. Many problems are minor and often transient, and simple short term interventions are often effective. However, in some children there are emerging signs of more serious problems, including developmental delay, communication problems, attentional difficulties and more serious behaviour problems. These children may require vision and hearing testing, a speech assessment, and, where an autism spectrum disorder is suspected, a multidisciplinary assessment.

Most children are toilet trained by 4 years of age. A delay in training may be due to a global developmental delay or may reflect a toddler's 'battle' with parents as the toddler tries to establish autonomy. A programme of regular toileting together with frequent praise and rewards (for example, stickers) will often achieve continence.

A number of tests assess school readiness but none is sufficient in isolation. The decision to send a child to school should be made by the parents, with input from those involved with the child, especially the preschool and primary teachers.

School years (over 5 years)

School is an important formative experience for all children. Children who have difficulty functioning at school, because of learning difficulties, attentional or behaviour problems or social difficulties, will almost always experience their impact beyond school. The child's experience at school can be either a protective or a risk factor for adjustment in childhood and for functioning later in life. Children who struggle academically or socially have been shown to be at major risk in adolescence and later life for poor outcomes, including delinquency, unemployment and depression.

The early years of school are particularly important. Children who have difficulty reading from the outset, and who are not established readers by the end of grade 2, are likely to continue to have problems throughout their school career.

Risk factors include chronic health problems, vision and hearing deficits, problems with concentration, and subtle developmental weaknesses in the areas of motor function, visuomotor integration, temporal sequential organisation (problems remembering the order of information) and language. Risk factors in the family include low parental education, low expectations of school achievement, parenting difficulties and other family dysfunction. Other risk factors include a poor match between the child's temperament and preferred style of learning and classroom placement or teacher expectations and teaching style, etc.

Professional intervention. It is important to identify school learning and behavioural difficulties as soon as possible so that appropriate interventions can be put in place. The longer this is delayed, the greater the chance of a poor outcome. Assessment should involve close evaluation of biological, developmental, behavioural and environmental factors that may be contributing to problems. Hearing and vision should be assessed. Often in this age

---

Clinical example

A mother presents with her 8 year old son Ed. His teachers have complained that he is 'mucking around' in class and disruptive. He has problems with spelling and writing. His father had similar problems at school and left in year 10. His mother says that Ed is fine at home and tends to play computer games or ride his bike. You note that he is quiet during the consultation and he says he has few friends at school. You arrange for his vision and hearing to be assessed and they are normal. You conduct a neurodevelopmental assessment, which reveals weaknesses in auditory sequencing and language processing. The school psychologist performs a cognitive assessment, which reveals Ed has normal intelligence but a specific learning difficulty involving reading, writing and spelling. You discuss this with his teachers who arrange remedial teaching and more computer time for Ed's class work.

group a multidisciplinary evaluation that includes a special educational assessment is the most appropriate. Where possible, a child should be referred to an educational psychologist for formal cognitive testing, including tests of intelligence. A detailed and comprehensive assessment will often point to the need for specific developmental and educational interventions that address the individual needs of the child. These may include remedial classes at school and/or tutoring outside school.

Adolescence

Adolescence is a time of immense change (Ch. 14). The young person needs to adjust to physical and emotional change, acquire an appropriate gender role, join peer groups, become emotionally independent of parents and other adults, and prepare for career and relationships in life. While most adolescents negotiate this period successfully, up to one in five will experience significant physical or emotional problems. Adolescents often experiment with drugs, alcohol and cigarettes and nicotine addiction usually begins in adolescence.

Risk factors include chronic health problems, learning disability, social isolation, parent physical or mental illness and family dysfunction.

Professional intervention. Health professionals need to address the concerns of the young person as well as the parents. Clarifying the professional obligation of confidentiality at the start of a consultation will reassure and facilitate rapport. In addition to addressing specific problems, screening questionnaires that encompass home, school, recreation, drug use, sexual activity and suicide/depression issues enable a full picture of the adolescent to emerge. Parents need to know what is normal during adolescence and be given effective strategies for both communicating with their adolescent and managing common problems.

Common problems presenting in the preschool and school environment

Preschool

Hitting and biting are common in the preschool setting. Occasional biting is usually experimental. Repeated hitting or biting may occur when a child is frustrated, stressed or feels powerless. The key to management is identifying the cause of the frustration or stress (for example, not wanting to share a toy), then removing, redirecting or distracting the child away from the cause. Parents should respond promptly and calmly, telling their child not to hit or bite when they remove the child from the situation.

Tantrums are very common (see Toddler section above). Where possible they should be ignored, as any form of attention tends to increase their frequency.

Language delay affects around 10% of preschool children (Ch. 4). Causes include simple language delay (expressive and/or receptive), deafness, autism spectrum disorder, global developmental delay and social–emotional deprivation. Referral for a speech therapy assessment is recommended if a child uses less than 20 words at 2 years of age, or does not understand simple instructions without gesture, or has no two word combinations at $2^1/_2$ years. Any child with a language delay needs to be referred for audiology testing to exclude hearing problems.

School

Attention difficulties manifest in many ways, including:
- poor concentration
- 'daydreaming'
- quiet withdrawal
- disruptive behaviour.

Causes include attention deficit hyperactivity disorder (ADHD), learning difficulties, intellectual disability, language delay, absence seizures, hearing and vision problems and depression/anxiety. Each of these can affect a child's learning. Treatment depends on the underlying cause and health professionals need to liaise with the child's teacher to ensure that the teacher understands the child's difficulties and how they may affect learning (Ch. 17).

Learning difficulties occur when a child of normal intellect performs at least one standard deviation below their potential ability in one or more areas of reading, spelling, writing or mathematics. Learning difficulties affect 10–15% of school children. Early recognition, diagnosis and remedial teaching are vital to ensure that the child does not lose confidence and become angry, depressed or frustrated. Children with learning difficulties should also have their vision (Ch. 76) and hearing (Ch. 75) assessed and any problems treated so that their ability to learn in the classroom is optimised. Children with learning difficulties will not, in all likelihood, grow out of their problems, so reassurances that the child will improve with maturity are usually ill founded and inappropriate.

Bullying is the deliberate desire to hurt someone with words or actions. Children who are bullied may refuse to go to school, be very tense and unhappy after school, or may show other signs of unhappiness such as difficulty sleeping. Children who bully may be physically punished at home and are more likely to grow up to hit their own partners and children. Managing bullying involves the whole school, with increased awareness, teaching students about conflict resolution and assertiveness training, peer counselling and improved adult supervision.

Common child and adolescent mental health problems

16

M. Sawyer, B. Graetz

Child and adolescent mental health problems are common in the community. They have a significant impact on the lives of children and parents and also impose a substantial financial burden on families and communities. In Australia, a recent national survey estimated that 14% of children and adolescents experience significant mental health problems. Adolescents with mental health problems frequently exhibit a range of other health risk behaviours, including smoking, drinking and drug abuse. They also report much higher rates of suicidal ideation and behaviour than other adolescents in the community. Only a minority of children and adolescents with mental health problems receive professional help.

This chapter describes common mental health problems experienced by children (for brevity, the term 'children' will be used to refer to children and adolescents). It also describes practical steps that can be taken to help children, parents and families. The chapter is divided into three sections. The first section describes the features of common mental health problems, the second describes general approaches to the assessment and management of these problems, and the final section provides information about some specific problems experienced by children.

Features of mental health problems

Two approaches are used to describe childhood mental health problems. One approach views childhood problems as lying on a continuum from those with very few problems to those with a large number of problems. Children identified as having a very large number of problems are considered to fall in the 'clinical range' of the continuum and to be in need of help. Typically, problems are divided into two broad groups called *externalising problems* and *internalising problems*. The former includes problems such as overactivity, aggressive or antisocial behaviour. The latter includes problems such as anxiety, depression or shyness. Questionnaires completed by children, parents and teachers are used to identify those children in need of help. When a continuum approach is used it is possible

to compare the number of problems reported for an individual child with the number typically reported for others of the same age and sex in the community. It is also possible to assess the effectiveness of treatment by evaluating whether there is a reduction in the number of children's problems.

The second approach divides childhood mental health problems into a range of different mental disorders. Each mental disorder consists of a different group of symptoms. There are two main classification systems that identify these symptom groups. One is the International Classification of Diseases developed by the World Health Organization (ICD-10), and the other is the Diagnostic and Statistical Manual developed by the American Psychiatric Association (DSM-IV). This categorical approach is used widely in mental health services to describe children's problems. A common feature of both approaches is their focus on observable features of children's problems rather than on the presumed aetiology of these problems. This has encouraged a broad investigation of the aetiology of children's problems during the last three decades.

Features of internalising problems

Many children experience anxiety or sadness; however, when these problems are severe or persist over time, they may indicate the presence of a mental disorder and the need for professional help. In particular, children with high levels of internalising problems should be assessed for the presence of depressive disorders or anxiety disorders.

Children with depressive disorders feel sad, lack interest in activities they previously enjoyed, criticise themselves, and are pessimistic or hopeless about the future. DSM-IV identifies two types of depressive disorder. Major depressive disorder consists of acute episodes of depressed mood, loss of interest and pleasure in activities, appetite and sleeping disturbance, low energy, low self-esteem, poor concentration and feelings of hopelessness. Children with dysthymic disorder experience similar problems but their symptoms are less severe. The main feature of dysthymic disorder is the persistence of symptoms over a very long period of time. Children with both disorders may think that life is not worth living and they may contemplate suicide. It is essential that all children with depressive disorders be carefully evaluated for suicidal risk (Ch. 18).

While fear and anxiety are common to the human condition, some children experience anxiety that is well beyond that which occurs during normal development. These children suffer personal distress and their anxiety interferes with their daily functioning. Children with anxiety disorders exhibit physiological symptoms (for example, tremors, sweating and palpitations), maladaptive behaviours (for example, avoidance of feared situations) and maladaptive thinking (for example, 'I cannot talk in front of the class because people will think I'm stupid').

DSM IV identifies a number of different types of anxiety disorder. One of the most common among children is separation anxiety disorder, which is defined as excessive and developmentally inappropriate anxiety regarding separation from home or from major attachment figures. Separation anxiety disorder is a common cause of persistent school refusal. Obsessive compulsive disorder is characterised by obsessions (persistent thoughts, impulses or images that are intrusive and distressing) and compulsions (repetitive behaviours or mental acts utilised to reduce anxiety or distress). This disorder causes considerable distress for children and parents. It is important for medical practitioners to be familiar with the typical symptoms of this disorder as effective interventions are available to provide help. These include both psychotropic medications and behavioural treatments. Social phobia, which typically begins during the teenage years, is comprised of fear of social or performance situations in which embarrassment can occur. This condition can adversely affect the development of social skills and can also hinder academic progress at school. Adolescents with this disorder may be reluctant to attend professional services because of their insecurity and fear of social embarrassment.

Features of externalising problems

Externalising problems refer to problems such as temper tantrums, aggressive behaviour, stealing and truancy. Boys are more frequently identified as having externalising problems than girls. Problems in this area, particularly those involving aggressive behaviour, can persist over long periods of time. For example, infants with a difficult temperament may develop oppositional and defiant behaviour as preschoolers and subsequently a conduct disorder during later primary school or high school.

Two common mental disorders in this area are conduct disorder and attention deficit hyperactivity disorder (ADHD). The typical behaviour of those with conduct disorder include bullying, frequent physical fights, deliberate destruction of other people's property, breaking into houses or cars, staying out late at night despite parental prohibitions, running away from home, or frequent truancy from school. ADHD is defined as a persistent pattern of inattentive behaviour and/or hyperactivity/ impulsivity that is more frequent and severe than is typically observed in individuals of the same age. Children with inattentive behaviour problems make careless mistakes with school work, find it hard to persist with tasks and are distracted easily. Those with problems in the area of hyperactivity/impulsivity often fidget and talk excessively, interrupt others, and are described as constantly being 'on the go'.

Assessment and management of mental health problems

Assessment

A careful assessment of children's problems is an essential prerequisite to effective treatment. This should include information about the child's current problems, a developmental history and relevant information about the child's family and social environment. It is important to develop a clear understanding of the nature of a child's presenting problems and the factors that have given rise to these problems. One way of organising these factors is shown below:
- predisposing factors
- precipitating factors
- perpetuating factors
- protecting factors.

In each area, consideration should be given to the possible influence of biological, psychological and social factors.

Information about children's problems should be obtained from children, parents and teachers. Children are the key source of information about their internal state, including their experience of subjective feelings such as anxiety and depression. Parents can provide information about more readily observed behaviour such as sibling conflict or school refusal. Parents are also an important source of information about the early development of children and the chronicity and severity of current problems. Teachers are the best source of information about children's academic progress and they can provide important information about the quality of children's peer relationships. The assessment and treatment of ADHD relies heavily on reports from teachers.

An example of a child with a mental health problem, and factors that may be contributing to this problem, is given in the clinical example.

Clinical example

Peter is a 12 year old boy who lives with his single mother. Peter's mother has a history of depression and his father has been treated for alcohol abuse. Peter's mother is seeking advice about how to manage his defiant and aggressive behaviour. She said that from the time he was born she has struggled to cope with Peter's difficult temperament and behaviour. This problem has greatly worsened since she divorced Peter's father last year. Since the divorce Peter has had little recent contact with his father and he was suspended from school on one occasion after damaging property in the school science centre. Peter's teacher described him as being easily distracted and impulsive during the last year. Despite these problems, Peter has continued to maintain satisfactory academic progress and his teacher believes that Peter's intelligence is above average.

The following factors are important in this problem:
- predisposing factor: family history of psychiatric disorder
- precipitating factor: divorce of parents
- perpetuating factor: rejection by father
- protecting factor: child's intelligence.

Management

The management of childhood mental disorders is complex. Many disorders persist over long periods of time (e.g. ADHD) or tend to recur (e.g. major depressive disorder). In light of this, the development of long term management plans is often necessary. The development of such plans requires consideration of several key issues. First, it is important to recognise that specific interventions are now available for many disorders. It is important to be familiar with these interventions and to avoid 'one size fits all' methods of counselling. Second, the management of children's problems often involves the use of a combination of biological (for example, psychotropic medications), psychological (for example, behaviour modification programmes) and social (for example school based programmes) interventions. Finally, the management of children's problems requires the cooperation of children, parents and teachers. Medical practitioners responsible for the treatment of children with mental disorders must involve all of these groups in the care of children.

A range of psychological interventions is available to help those with mental disorders. These include:
- individual psychotherapy which focuses on helping children
- family therapy which focuses on relationships between all family members
- behaviour modification which focuses on the antecedents and consequences of children's behaviour
- cognitive therapy which focuses on maladaptive thinking styles.

Recent reviews have drawn attention to the importance of correctly implementing these interventions. It appears that a failure to do this may explain why their effectiveness when delivered in clinic settings is less than that achieved in the university or research environments where they were developed.

A wide range of medications are used to treat children with mental disorders. However, an ongoing concern is that, while many of these medications have the potential to provide help, evidence of their efficacy is largely based on studies of adults. With the exception of psychostimulant medications used to treat ADHD, there is a paucity of evidence to guide clinicians in the appropriate use of medications for the treatment of childhood mental disorders. As a result, when psychotropic medications are used to help children, very clear treatment goals should be identified, along with careful monitoring of effectiveness and adverse effects. Pharmacological treatment should always be used as part of a broader management plan developed in conjunction with children and parents. Only one psychotropic medication should be prescribed at a time to manage a child with a mental disorder. After an appropriate trial, if one medication is ineffective an alternative may be selected. Only after consultation with a child psychiatrist or paediatrician experienced in paediatric psychopharmacology should multiple psychotropic medications be used concurrently to treat a child with a mental disorder.

Special issues

Suicidal behaviour

All suicide attempts should be treated seriously. Although suicidal ideation and behaviour are very rare before the age of 12 years, they become more frequent during adolescence. Approximately 2% of schoolchildren attempt suicide and attempts are often associated with serious mental health problems. Completed suicide is less common. Completed suicide occurs more frequently among boys (2–3 per 10 000 adolescents per year) who tend to choose more lethal methods than girls.

Suicidal ideation and behaviour are often associated with symptoms of a depressive disorder along with a history of abuse of alcohol or other drugs. Many young people who attempt suicide live in families where there is a high level of interpersonal conflict and where parents have a history of mental disorder or drug and alcohol abuse. As well as a history of chronic adversity, many young people report an immediate precipitant to their suicide attempt. This may involve an argument over parental or school discipline, or a difficulty in a relationship with a friend.

All children who report thoughts of suicide or who attempt suicide should be assessed carefully. This should include assessment of the mental state of the child and the seriousness of the suicidal attempt. Characteristics which suggest that a suicide attempt was serious include:

- family history of suicide attempts
- previous history of suicide attempts
- presence of a mental disorder (e.g. major depressive disorder)
- evidence of premeditation and planning
- an expectation by the young person that the attempt would result in death
- a suicide attempt made while alone or isolated
- precautions were taken to make discovery unlikely during or after the suicide attempt.

During the period of time that a young person remains at high risk for suicide, it is important that they be in a safe environment where their behaviour can be monitored. During this time their mental status should be assessed and help provided to address personal or family problems. In some circumstances, such as when a young person has a serious mental disorder or where they have no secure place of residence, it is necessary to arrange hospital admission.

It is important to provide appropriate treatment for depressive disorders experienced by young people who make suicide attempts. This should include the use of specific counselling techniques such as cognitive behavioural therapy and the use of antidepressant medication. Every effort should be made to reduce the impact of ongoing stressors, such as family conflict, that may precipitate further suicide attempts. When appropriate treatment methods are employed, a high rate of recovery can be achieved. However, major depressive disorder often recurs and it is important that young people and their parents are advised of this continuing risk of further episodes and the symptoms which may signal the onset of a recurrence.

Attention deficit hyperactivity disorder

ADHD is one of the most common mental disorders experienced by children. The core symptoms of the disorder are inattentiveness, impulsivity and hyperactivity. It is important to recognise that this behaviour may not be evident in the structured office environment of a medical practice. In light of this, it is essential to obtain reports from parents and teachers about the child's home and school behaviour. Many children with ADHD have other comorbid mental disorders such as anxiety or conduct disorders. Furthermore, they may be experiencing learning difficulties, family conflict, peer relationship problems and low self-esteem.

The management of ADHD requires the use of a range of different interventions, including:

- medication
- parent training
- classroom behaviour management
- remedial education
- family support.

It is important to explain the basis of the child's behaviour to children, parents and teachers. Stimulant medication is an effective treatment for children with this condition. However, to achieve maximum effect, careful titration of medication dosage is necessary, using reports from parents and teachers to identify the effectiveness of different dosage regimens. Even when good effect is achieved, however, children's inattentiveness and impulsivity may be more problematic than that of other children. For this reason, parents will need ongoing help with effective management strategies. It is also important to ensure that children receive appropriate remedial education when a learning problem is identified. One of the disappointing findings from studies that have evaluated the effectiveness of stimulant medication in the longer term is evidence that the academic progress of many children with ADHD continues to lag behind that of their peers.

School refusal

Children who refuse to attend school can be divided into two broad groups. In the first group, the most common reason for school refusal is excessive anxiety related to school attendance. Less commonly, other mental disorders may disrupt school attendance. Children in the second group refuse to attend school as part of a general pattern of rule breaking and defiance of authority. The term 'truancy' is used to describe the behaviour of this latter group.

Anxiety and depression

A small number of children exhibit high levels of distress when they first commence school and this may be associated with temper tantrums, excessive fearfulness and complaints of somatic symptoms (for example, stomach aches or headaches) for which no biological cause can be identified. In some children this pattern persists and it may give rise to a situation where children do not attend school for long periods of time. School refusal adversely affects these children in two areas. First, the children are at greatly increased risk of receiving an inadequate education. Second, they miss out on important socialising experiences. As a result, they may enter later life lacking important social skills. For these reasons, school refusal is a very serious problem that requires urgent and effective management. It will often be necessary to provide help to children and parents over long periods of time.

Among younger children who refuse to attend school there may be a history of separation anxiety disorder. Children with this disorder have a history of anxiety when separated from their primary caregiver, may insist on sleeping in their parents' bedroom at night and may refuse to stay overnight with friends. In primary school, the children will describe their fear of separation from parents, describe worrying about their parents at school and may be excessively anxious if their parents are late to collect them from school. They may also express fear of punishment from teachers or concern about bullying by peers. Adolescents who refuse to attend school may be suffering from social phobia. Adolescents with this condition experience marked fear of social or performance situations. As a result, they are reluctant to attend school, where they have to mix socially with peers and demonstrate adequate academic progress. Children with depressive disorders may become reluctant to attend school as they withdraw from social activities and struggle to cope with their sadness, low self-esteem and loss of concentration.

Assessment should be initially broad based and aimed at understanding the cause of children's problems. A developmental history should be obtained, with a particular focus on symptoms of anxiety or depression. Information should be obtained about the child's environment both at home and at school. This should include information about family functioning, the classroom and school environment, and peer relationships. It is essential that contact be made with children's teachers to obtain information about these latter issues. Information should also be obtained about the severity, duration and pervasiveness of school non attendance, noting possible antecedents of the problem and consequences which may be responsible for maintaining the behaviour.

There are a number of specific approaches that can be used to help children with school refusal due to anxiety disorders. Implementing these requires the combined efforts of children, parents and teachers. Children need help to better manage their anxiety. This should include the use of techniques such as:

- relaxation training
- systematic desensitisation
- cognitive restructuring
- shaping and contingency management.

Parents need to be taught how they can manage children's temper tantrums and how to help children who report somatic complaints. In two parent families, it is important that both parents participate in treatment programmes. In situations of chronic school refusal, assessing the significance of children's somatic complaints can be helped by close liaison with a general practitioner who can quickly assess a child and advise parents whether the presence of a physical illness precludes school attendance. This support can reduce the pressure on parents who must decide whether or not to allow their child to miss further schooling. Where there is no evidence of a physical illness, every effort should be made to ensure that children return to school at the earliest possible opportunity. Teachers can play a vital role in supporting children's return to school after an absence and helping to reduce anxiety at school due to bullying or performance pressure.

Truancy

In contrast to children with anxiety disorders, children who are truant from school do not tend to return home, they often exhibit other antisocial behaviour, and their parents may be unaware that children are failing to attend school regularly. Among these children, school refusal is part of a general pattern of rule violation, defiance of authority and aggressive behaviour. It is difficult to help these children because many will refuse to cooperate with treatment and will identify the school system as being irrelevant to their needs. There is a high rate of learning difficulties among this group of children, which further alienates them from school culture and learning. There may be conflict between parents and school staff about who should take responsibility for the child's behaviour. Some children may be suspended from school when they violate school rules. This simply perpetuates an existing problem of non attendance at school.

Enuresis and encopresis

Nocturnal enuresis

While most children have achieved bladder control by the age of 5 years, a significant number continue to have problems with nocturnal enuresis. This is embarrassing for children and a burden for their parents.

In the absence of physical causes, such as a urinary tract infection, nocturnal enuresis is generally not a serious problem. Indeed, it may simply reflect normal variation in the development of bladder control where there is a familial tendency to later maturation of bladder control. Discussing this familial pattern with parents may help them better understand the nature of their child's problem. Exposure to stressful events may also induce children with previously good bladder control to recommence bed wetting. For younger children, management consists of reassurance and the establishment of a convenient pattern of hygienic care of bed and clothing. Simple procedures such as fluid restriction at night or getting children to empty their bladder when the parents are ready to retire may help. Incentive systems can be put in place to assist children's motivation to remain dry. One method is to reward children for achieving a given number of consecutive dry nights, with the number of nights gradually extended over time.

For more persistent cases of bed wetting an enuresis alarm is an effective treatment. The alarm consists of a detector mat placed on a child's mattress. The mat is connected to an alarm and when the child begins to urinate during sleep, a circuit is completed and the alarm sounds. The procedure (often called a 'bell and pad') uses simple conditioning rules to train children to achieve better bladder control. Many children's hospitals or chemists have such devices available for hire. However, it is important to ensure that both the mat and alarm function properly or they will not condition children to achieve better bladder control. In recent years, desmopressin nasal spray has also been used as a short term treatment for children with nocturnal enuresis. Tricyclic antidepressants, such as imipramine, should no longer be used to treat bed wetting due to high relapse rates, the possibility of adverse cardiac side effects, and the risks of severe morbidity or even mortality if taken in significant overdose.

Encopresis

Encopresis affects between 2 and 8% of primary school children. It is more common among boys, and a high proportion of children with encopresis have concomitant constipation. The problem is distressing for children and may be associated with parent–child conflict. Several types of encopresis have been described:
- constipation with overflow
- failed toilet training
- toilet phobia
- stress induced loss of control
- provocative soiling.

Considerable overlap may occur between these different types of encopresis. However, the descriptions provide a general indication of the types of issues that must be considered when assessing children with encopresis. Before treatment is commenced, it is important to identify the causes of the child's encopresis. This should include a physical examination to identify whether a child has constipation.

There are three elements to the treatment of encopresis. First, it is important to treat constipation when this is present. This can generally be achieved through the use of laxatives or microenemas. Less commonly, it will be necessary to employ a bowel washout. Second, it is important to ensure that the diet contains adequate fibre to reduce the likelihood of future constipation. Third, it is important to establish a routine of regular toilet use. Establishing a new pattern of regular toilet use can be difficult with children. There may be a history of conflict between parents and children about toilet use. Children may also be unclear about the linkage between irregular toilet use and encopresis, particularly if previous interventions have focused largely on punishing children who soil their clothes. Finally, children may be upset or embarrassed about their problem and may refuse to participate in treatment programmes.

It is important to ensure that children understand why they are experiencing constipation and soiling. A simple schematic diagram showing the key features of the gastrointestinal system can be used to help children understand the nature of their problem. Children need to understand that constipation occurs when there is a build up of faeces because of a failure to empty the bowel regularly. Once they understand this, it is easier to work with them to plan a programme of regular toilet use. Small rewards given after each use of the toilet can be helpful with young children. In children with toilet phobia, rewards may be given initially for simply sitting on the toilet for a few minutes and then progress to rewards provided when the child empties the bowel in the toilet. To achieve maximum effect, rewards need to be given immediately after children use the toilet, they need to be inexpensive (because of the need to reward each use of the toilet) and they must be given consistently when the child uses the toilet. Jointly identifying appropriate rewards can be used to build a therapeutic alliance with children and encourage their cooperation with the treatment programme. Seeking children's active involvement in treatment planning can also be used to reduce the conflict between children and their parents, with the latter taking on a more supportive and advisory role.

Problems of infancy

Infant mental health is a rapidly developing field. Debates about nature versus nurture have been abandoned in favour of interactional models that link the styles of parenting to an infant's physical health, developmental maturity and evolving personality. This is set in a cultural and extended family context. Attachment theory describes the relationships thus produced between infant and parent. There is increasing evidence that these interactional styles, already measurable by 12 months of age, predict children's interactional patterns later in life.

Recent work has shown that early experiences have a measurable effect on infants' brains. It is believed that tract and synapse development is significantly conditioned by the style of parenting; that is, an infant's brain has the potential to develop and mature, and this potential can best be achieved by parenting which is tuned to the needs of the infant. Thus, appropriate parenting in which love and limits are evident, along with a focus on helping with developmental stages, is likely to promote tract development.

It is known that a wide range of parent and infant issues can interfere with optimal parenting. These include, for instance, postnatal depression and anxiety, troubled marital relationships and compromised role models of parenting and prematurity. Physical or emotional abuse has particular and long lasting consequences. There are a growing number of interventions being developed to address these problems in the early years. There is also a growing body of knowledge about the benefits of early (for example, antenatal) identification of parent risk factors and the potential for health promotion and early intervention at this early stage of an infant's development.

Hyperactive and inattentive children

17

J. Sewell

Hyperactive and inattentive behaviours are common in children, ranging in a continuum from normal behaviours, especially in young children, to developmentally inappropriate behaviours that impair daily activities at home and at school.

Developmentally inappropriate levels of hyperactivity and inattention may be the result of many factors, often in combination. These risk factors (Table 17.1) must all be considered in the assessment of children with difficult behaviour, especially when considering the diagnosis of attention deficit hyperactivity disorder (ADHD).

Definition of attention deficit hyperactivity disorder

ADHD is considered to be a developmental disorder, characterised by inattention and hyperactivity/impulsivity. The underlying neurobiological pathway involves the frontal–striatal–cerebellar networks, with deficits occurring in response inhibition and in executive functioning; that is, working memory, organisation, interference control and emotional regulation.

The diagnosis of ADHD is made using DSM-IV criteria. It is a descriptive diagnosis, without implying cause, as it is not a discrete entity, and has multiple causes. There must be developmentally inappropriate symptoms of inattention (Table 17.2) and/or hyperactivity/impulsivity (Table 17.3) with onset before 7 years of age, impairing social, academic or occupational functioning across multiple settings, and not as a result of pervasive developmental disorder, psychosis or severe emotional disorders. Subtypes include mainly inattentive, mainly hyperactive or combined.

ADHD is common. The prevalence in the school aged population generally is considered to be 3–5%, although a recent community survey of childhood mental health in Australia found a prevalence of 11%. Males are affected more commonly, particularly with hyperactivity. There is a higher incidence in disrupted families and in those with low incomes, again particularly with hyperactivity. There is a strong genetic factor, with about 30% of siblings, 20–25% of parents and 80% of identical twins affected. Molecular genetic studies have focused on chromosomes that regulate dopamine, the neurotransmitter most associated with attention, motivation and movement. Two candidate genes, the dopamine transporter and dopamine receptor genes, are reported to be associated with ADHD.

Table 17.1   Risk factors for hyperactivity and inattention

Difficult temperament
Poor parenting skills
Family dysfunction
Child abuse
Developmental delay
Language disorders
Learning difficulties
Anxiety/mood disorders
Sleep disorders
Medical conditions, for example:
　very low birth weight or small for gestational age
　fetal alcohol syndrome
　lead poisoning
　acquired brain syndrome (head injury)
　chromosomal abnormalities, e.g. fragile X
　food intolerance (rare)

Table 17.2   DSM-IV: Symptoms of inattention

Careless mistakes
Difficulty sustaining attention
Seems not to listen
Poor task completion
Difficulty with organisation
Avoids tasks requiring sustained attention
Loses things
Easily distracted
Forgetful

Table 17.3   DSM-IV: Symptoms of hyperactivity/impulsivity

Fidgeting
Often leaves seat
Overactive, restless
Difficulty playing quietly
'On the go'
Talking excessively
Blurting out answers
Difficulty awaiting turn
Interrupts others

141

Many children with ADHD have associated neuro-developmental or mental health problems (comorbidities) (Table 17.4). Because of overlapping features, separation into these diagnostic categories is complex and somewhat artificial; however, it is helpful in completing a descriptive assessment and recommending specific management guidelines.

Table 17.4   Comorbidities with ADHD

Learning difficulties (LD; 10–30%)
Language disorder (30–50%)
Oppositional defiant disorder (ODD; 30–50%)
Conduct disorder (CD; 16–20%)
Mood disorders
Developmental coordination disorder
Tics, Tourette syndrome

Clinical example

Christopher, aged 6 years, is in his second year of school. His teacher complains that he never sits still, does not complete tasks, talks too much, interrupts and is well behind with reading. His mother recalls that he has been 'on the go' since about 2 years of age, always prefers playing outdoors rather than settling to games inside, never seems to remember instructions or the house rules, and acts without thinking about the consequences. He hates homework and 'forgets' to bring home his school reader.

Christopher's problems are consistent with a diagnosis of ADHD and learning difficulties. Stimulant medication and consistent structure at home and at school help his behavioural symptoms, but he also requires remedial reading support in the classroom.

Clinical example

Miranda, aged 3$\frac{1}{2}$ years, is extremely active, aggressive and oppositional, and has a mild language delay. Recently her mother separated from Miranda's father and is now in a new relationship. The family have moved several times, and have been involved with a number of family support agencies. Her parents want her to go on stimulant medication like her older half brother. They are committed to the care of their children.

Miranda is diagnosed with oppositional defiant disorder and language delay, in the context of a dysfunctional but committed family. She could also be diagnosed with ADHD on DSM-IV criteria, but such a diagnosis at this age may be misleading and shift focus away from the critical issue of effective family support.

community context. Thorough physical examination helps to exclude the rare associated medical conditions. Neurodevelopmental assessment provides information on motor skills and auditory and visual processing. Many children require formal assessment of auditory, cognitive, language and educational function. Neuroimaging, quantitative EEGs and psychophysiological tests (for example, of continuous performance) are research tools only at this stage, and not yet ready for use in clinical diagnosis.

The diagnosis of ADHD can only be made against a thorough understanding of normal patterns of development and behaviour. This is particularly important when considering the diagnosis in a preschool aged child, with wide variations expected in normal behaviour, development and temperament, and vulnerability to adverse family and social circumstances.

Assessment

The assessment of children for ADHD with its multiple risk factors and comorbidities requires skilled interpretation of information from the child, family and teachers. Relevant factors are:
- medical
- developmental
- family history
- family and social environment
- the school setting
- academic progress
- socialisation skills.

Behavioural patterns over time, antecedents and consequences of behaviours, and family and school management of behaviours must be understood. Standardised behavioural rating scales completed by parents, teachers and adolescents help to put the behaviours into a normal

Management

ADHD is a chronic condition requiring long term management based on partnership with the child, the family and the child's teachers from year to year. Counselling on the nature, causes, risk factors and course of ADHD, setting realistic expectations in the light of such understanding, and making accommodations at home and at school will help the child maintain confidence and self esteem.

Multimodal management includes:
- stimulant medication
- parent behaviour management
- classroom behaviour management
- management of comorbidities, for example:
  — special education support for learning difficulties
  — treatment of anxiety, depression
- family support, parent support groups.

Stimulant medication

Stimulant medication (methylphenidate and dexamphetamine) is the most effective treatment for ADHD and improves target symptoms in about 75% of children with the condition. Improved concentration and decreased hyperactivity, impulsivity and distractibility lead to enhanced task completion, academic progress and social interaction sustained over time.

Both medications are short acting, safe and have a low profile of adverse effects that either subside spontaneously within the first 2 or 3 weeks of treatment, or can be managed by altering the dose or timing of medication. Insomnia, appetite suppression and headache can be troublesome in some children.

Clinical example

Andrew, aged 13 years, is in year 8. Although he coped academically in primary school, he is having difficulty with organising himself, working through assignments and getting homework completed on time. His written work is messy, he is distracted easily and he daydreams in the classroom. He is worried he will not do well enough at school to go to university.

Andrew's assessment indicates long term problems with attention, distractibility and impulsivity. He commences stimulant medication for his ADHD and develops better organisation, task completion, interest in work and neater handwriting. He now feels he is much closer to reaching his academic potential.

There is considerable community concern that too many children are taking stimulants and other psychotropic drugs, with overdiagnosis and medicalisation of social problems, and risk of psychological dependence on drugs instead of developing self-responsibility. The reality is that ADHD is a developmental disorder with significant long term risk factors in educational, social and vocational outcome. Currently only 2% of school aged children in Australia have been prescribed stimulant medication, despite the prevalence of ADHD of at least 3–5%. There is very good scientific evidence for the long term safety of these drugs. Medication treatment is only one of the treatment modalities for ADHD. It is critically important for health professionals to advocate community services and family support for children who are at risk for adverse developmental, behavioural and social outcomes, whether or not they have ADHD.

Behaviour management

Behaviour management programmes use a structured setting to promote behavioural control, reinforcing

Table 17.5   Behavioural strategies

To reinforce: 'catch 'em being good'; use verbal praise and concrete rewards
- Teach listening skills
- Teach problem solving skills, i.e. 'game plan'

To reduce: ignore unwanted behaviours
- 'Act don't speak', i.e. clear discipline with minimal reprimands and discussion
- Logical consequences

appropriate behaviours and reducing negative behaviours with specific strategies. Emphasis should be on antecedent support and control, rather than on consequences; that is, anticipation of the difficulties and plan/teach to avoid (Table 17.5).

In the classroom, additional techniques include seating the child close to the teacher, breaking tasks down into small units, frequent exercise breaks (preferably productive and responsible, for example, taking a message to the office), structured teaching materials adapted to the child's needs, and unrelenting positive encouragement.

Alternative/complementary therapies

A small number of children react to synthetic food colours with severe irritability and restlessness. These children, who are very few in number, are helped by dietary restriction. There is no evidence that a sugar free diet, megavitamins, sensory integration training or biofeedback are of therapeutic benefit.

Outcome

Hyperactivity tends to diminish in adolescence, although physical restlessness may continue. Inattention, impulsivity and distractibility can continue into adulthood, although self-understanding and self-regulation improve with developmental, cognitive and emotional maturation. Comorbidities, such as learning difficulties, subtle language disorders and conduct disorders, and associated risk factors, such as family dysfunction and poor educational opportunity, can contribute to adverse outcomes, such as poor school retention, limited vocational outlook and risk taking behaviours in adolescence and early adulthood.

Summary

There are many reasons why children have hyperactive and inattentive behaviours. These behaviours must be interpreted with an understanding of what is normal development and behaviour, and how these interact with family and community function. When such behaviours are excessive and pervasive, a diagnosis of ADHD may be made, paying attention to causes, risk factors and comorbidities.

Treatment of ADHD is multimodal, with stimulant medications being safe and most effective, but adjunctive behavioural management and family support are essential. Understanding and adjustment in the school setting, with appropriate educational support, are paramount for the child's long term psychological health.

Key learning points

- Not all children with hyperactivity and inattention have ADHD.
- ADHD is common; seen in 3–5% of children.
- There are multiple causes — a continuum of normal behaviours plus risk factors.
- Assessment is complex — consider risk factors and comorbidities.
- Stimulant medication is safe and effective.
- Long term behavioural and family support is required.
- Adverse outcomes in adolescence and early adulthood are common, particularly in association with reading difficulty and aggressive behaviour.

Major psychiatric disorders

B. Nurcombe

The major psychiatric disorders are characterised by relatively specific symptomatology and severe impairment of social, educational and recreational functioning. The primary care physician's role in the management of these disorders is to recognise them as early as possible, assess the patient for risk of harm, refer the family for psychiatric evaluation, collaborate in shared care treatment, and ensure that the patient's general health is maintained. The following symptoms should alert the primary physician to the possibility of a serious psychiatric disorder:

- Infancy and early childhood:
    failure to thrive without physical cause
    rumination (that is, regurgitation, chewing and spillage of gastric contents)
    delay in spoken language
    failure to respond normally to parental physical contact or voice
    stereotyped, repetitive movements (for example, hand flapping)
- Middle childhood:
    severe, persistent oppositional behaviour, aggressiveness, or impulsive temper
    persistent stealing
    developmentally inappropriate sexual behaviour
    persistent fire setting
    cruelty to animals
    truancy
    unexplained absences from school
    severe, persistent separation anxiety (for example, on leaving home to go to school)
    failure to speak outside the home
    obsessions and compulsions
    persistent depressive or irritable mood
    deterioration in school performance
    failure to make friends, solitary interests
- Adolescence:
    unexplained loss of weight, uncontrolled dieting
    secretive bingeing and vomiting
    deterioration in school performance
    social withdrawal and cessation of sporting/recreational activities
    disorganized thought processes, hallucinations, delusions
    persistent or recurrent depressive mood
    suicidal ideation or attempted suicide
    panic attacks

excessive risk taking, running away from home, sexual promiscuity
recent gravitation toward 'bad companions'
unexplained school absences/truancy
frequent fighting/explosive rage
persistent unexplained physical symptoms.

Infancy and early childhood

Reactive attachment disorder

This group of disorders is associated with deficiency in the infant's capacity to elicit care, or impairment in the caregiver's emotional responsiveness, or a combination of both. Typically, the infant fails to initiate or respond appropriately to social interaction, exhibiting social withdrawal, inhibition, avoidance, or heedlessness and a superficial, undiscriminating sociability. Often, as a result of depression, psychosis, personality disorder or severe psychosocial stress, the parent has failed to attend to the infant's basic needs for affection, contact comfort and stimulation, or there have been so many changes of caregiver that the infant has not been able to develop a stable attachment. In severe reactive attachment disorder, the infant's physical development (height, weight, head circumference) slows or stops, a condition known as non organic failure to thrive (Ch. 10). Attachment disorder should be distinguished from pervasive developmental disorder, intellectual retardation and developmental language disorder. Non organic failure to thrive should be differentiated from physical causes of failure to thrive (Ch. 10).

Psychosocial dwarfism is usually encountered in children from 18 months to 7 years of age. It is associated with physical and intellectual growth failure, reversible neuroendocrine dysfunction and bizarre eating patterns (for example, polyphagia, food hoarding). Typically, after hospitalisation, the child gains weight dramatically only to stall after returning home. The prognosis for intellectual and social development is poor unless adequate surrogate care is provided or the primary caregiver's parental capacity can be addressed.

Rumination involves the persistent, repeated regurgitation, chewing and spilling of gastric contents, not due to a gastrointestinal or other medical condition. In infants it is associated with emotional neglect. In older, intellectually retarded children it used to be encountered in circumstances of gross institutional neglect. Rumination may be so severe as to lead to inanition and death. In infants, the treatment is to provide consistent contact comfort, with holding, rocking, eye contact and soothing vocalisations. In older children, behavioural treatment is required.

Pervasive developmental disorders

This group of conditions is characterised by delay and deviance in intellectual, communicative and social development, together with stereotyped behaviour and circumscribed interests.

> ### Clinical example
>
> Jerry, aged 4 years, has been referred by his mother because his preschool teacher is concerned about his poor language and lack of interest in other children. His mother says that Jerry has always been 'different'. He doesn't seek or give affection. He doesn't play properly with his toys, but prefers to line them up or watch them falling, one by one, off a table. If anyone interrupts this game, he screams. He is fascinated with light switches and electric fans, and likes to parrot television commercials. Jerry avoids looking at you by averting his gaze to one side. He does not respond to your questions. At one point, he suddenly becomes upset and begins to run around your office on tiptoes, flicking his fingertips. You refer him to a developmental paediatrician for full diagnostic workup.

Autistic disorder is characterised by the following clinical features:
- marked impairment of eye to eye gaze and communicative gestures
- failure to develop peer relationships
- lack of socioemotional reciprocity
- impaired capacity for joint attention
- incapacity for make believe play
- failure to imitate others
- delay of language development
- unusual use of language (for example, for self-enchantment rather than communication)
- stereotyped, restricted interests and rituals
- motor mannerisms (for example, finger flicking or hand flapping).

Autistic disorder occurs in about 1 out of 1000 children, with a male to female ratio of 3:1. In a minority of autistic children, usually the most severely retarded, a physical cause can be diagnosed (e.g. congenital rubella, fragile X syndrome, herpes encephalitis, neurofibromatosis, phenylketonuria, tuberose sclerosis). For other autistic children there is evidence for a genetic causation,

probably involving several genes; however, the precise method of transmission is unclear.

The child should be assessed as follows:
- physical examination
- dental examination
- assessment of hearing and vision
- psychological testing for cognitive level and pattern of intellectual abilities
- speech and language assessment
- laboratory testing and chromosomal examination to exclude known physical causes of the autistic syndrome
- electroencephalography.

Autistic disorder should be differentiated from the following conditions:
- developmental language disorder
- intellectual retardation
- sensory impairment (e.g. deafness)
- selective mutism (see below)
- severe psychosocial deprivation
- childhood schizophrenia
- other types of pervasive developmental disorder (see below).

Although many parents become concerned that their child is abnormal by the time he or she is 6–12 months of age, autistic disorder is often not diagnosed until much later. This is regrettable because the earlier the diagnosis, the sooner effective treatment can be provided. In a minority of cases, the child is described as developing normally at first, only to regress into an autistic state when 2 or 3 years old.

The best predictors of outcome are IQ and the presence of functional speech at 5 years of age. Epilepsy occurs in about 20%, usually in adolescence. Treatment is multidisciplinary and involves habit training, social reinforcement, the alleviation of avoidant, stereotyped behaviour and the promotion of communicative development. There is evidence that early intervention, commencing in the second or third year of life, can be effective in promoting language and social development. Pharmacotherapy has a limited role, and is of use mainly in children who exhibit severe hyperactivity, aggressiveness, or self-harm.

Parents are not usually concerned about children with *Asperger disorder* until the child is 2–4 years old. By middle childhood, the child exhibits the following characteristics:
- impairment of non verbal communication (for example, impaired eye contact, lack of facial expression and gesture, and monotonous vocal intonation but intact language development otherwise)
- average intelligence or above
- lack of interest in peer relationships
- lack of social reciprocity, shared enjoyment and humour

- circumscribed interests (for example, computer games) and inflexible routines
- mannerisms (e.g. hand flapping) and motor clumsiness.

It is unclear whether Asperger disorder is a variant of, or different from, autistic disorder and whether it is distinct from non verbal language disability, semantic pragmatic processing disorder and schizoid personality disorder. Because of uncertainty about the boundaries of this condition, its prevalence is unclear, perhaps 4 per 10 000, with a 10:1 ratio in favour of males. By adolescence, many children with this condition become frustrated by their lack of friends and the teasing or social rejection to which they are prone. Treatment involves social–cognitive language programming in the educational mainstream. As adults, people with Asperger disorder are more effective in jobs that make few social demands.

Middle childhood

Disruptive behaviour disorder

Oppositional defiant disorder and *attention deficit disorder* are described in Chapters 16 and 17. *Conduct disorder* refers to a group of children characterised by some or all of the following:
- persistently aggressive behaviour (bullying, intimidation, frequent fighting, cruelty, coercive sexual behaviour, use of a weapon)
- destructiveness (fire setting, vandalism)
- deceitfulness (breaking and entering, stealing, lying, trickery)
- rule violation (truancy, staying out late at night, running away from home, refusal to accept rules at home or school).

This condition can emerge first in adolescence, but the more serious kinds of conduct disorder evolve in middle childhood from earlier oppositional defiant behaviour. A recent study has found a prevalence of 3% in Australian children and adolescents, with a male-to-female ratio of about 3:1. Conduct disorder is commonly associated with other problems, particularly attention deficit disorder (Ch. 17), alcohol and substance use disorder, mood disorder, post-traumatic stress disorder and learning disorder.

The genetic background of conduct disorder is unclear, but twin and adoption studies suggest that there is an inherited component. Other risk factors form a sequential developmental cascade, as follows:
- maternal smoking during pregnancy
- difficult infant temperament
- early parental neglect with disruption of infant attachment

- coercive, inconsistent parental discipline
- exposure to parental antisocial behaviour, domestic violence or substance abuse
- coaching by parents who promote violent behaviour
- exposure to physical or sexual abuse
- growing up in a marginalised, socially disadvantaged environment
- minority group status
- relatively impaired verbal intelligence
- learning problems
- the mindset that other people will be hostile, rejecting or unfair to one
- gravitation toward like minded antiauthoritarian companions
- truancy
- early initiation into smoking, sexual activity and alcohol or drug taking.

If conduct problems do not first appear until adolescence, and few of the above risk factors are operative, the individual will probably not go on to become antisocial as an adult. When behaviour problems begin at an early age and many of the cumulative risk factors apply, it is more likely that the individual will become an adult criminal.

Children with conduct problems are usually referred for evaluation during late childhood or adolescence. It would be preferable if this serious disorder could be detected and treated earlier. The combination of early educational intervention with parenting programmes (for example, triple-P) designed to alter coercive child rearing holds promise. Until the last 10 years, no intervention programmes had been found to be effective for older children. Recently, multisystemic therapy involving goal directed strategic/behavioural family therapy aimed to promote effective parenting, along with individual counselling and environmental intervention, has produced good results. The placement of offenders in therapeutic foster homes has also shown promise. In foster home programmes, the house parents are trained to be firm and consistent in their discipline, and to ensure that the adolescent does not mix with antisocial peers. It is ineffective to treat children who have conduct disorder in community or institutional groups composed of like minded peers.

Anxiety disorders

Separation anxiety disorder is described in Chapter 16. *Generalised anxiety disorder* is characterised by persistent, excessive worrying about life events (for example, school performance, clothes, dating) accompanied by physical symptoms (for example, abdominal pains, headaches, fatigue, diarrhoea, urinary frequency). Children with this disorder are likely to have been behaviourally inhibited as preschoolers. Generalised anxiety disorder overlaps with *social phobia*, in which the child is particularly fearful of performance situations that incur the scrutiny of others (for example, reading in front of the class, going to the toilet away from home, athletic competition). *Panic disorder* involves repeated attacks of sudden, disabling anxiety, often without any apparent precipitant, associated with the physiological concomitants of anxiety (for example, hyperventilation, racing heart, cold sweaty hands, choking sensations, dizziness, fainting, fear of dying). The onset of panic disorder is most often in mid adolescence, although it can occur in middle childhood. *Selective mutism* is probably a variant of social phobia. In this condition, the child, usually a girl, fails to speak in social situations outside the home or to strangers. The average age of onset is 2 to 3 years. In about 30% of cases there has been a premorbid speech or language problem. Selective mutism should be differentiated from deafness, intellectual disability, developmental language disorder, aphonia, and the inability of a migrant child to understand English.

Anxiety disorders frequently coincide with attention deficit disorder and depressive disorder. Anxiety disorders are often familial, but without specificity as to type. Whereas behavioural inhibition (which may precede anxiety disorder) has a genetic component, parental anxiety (especially separation or social anxiety) is highly contagious. Treatment, therefore, must involve the parents.

🔍 Clinical example

Barbara's mother tells you that she is worried because Barbara, who is 10 years old, has begun to behave in an odd manner. She touches doorknobs again and again, and spends ages getting to bed because she must arrange her teddy bears just so around her pillows and at the foot of the bed. She has reluctantly admitted to her mother that she arranges the teddy bears in that way in order to ward off aliens who might abduct her at night. She wriggles her toes and clenches her jaw in a special way but does not know why she does so. When she tries to resist wriggling her toes, she becomes very anxious and has to give in and do it. You refer Barbara to a psychiatrist who confirms your impression that Barbara has obsessive compulsive disorder. She is started on sertraline and referred to a clinical psychologist for behaviour therapy.

Obsessive compulsive disorder is characterised by the following:
- Recurrent, distressing thoughts about such matters as germs, contamination, or harming the self or others, or preoccupation with excessive moralization or religiosity (obsessions).

- Recurrent distressing rituals involving excessive washing, repeating, checking, touching, counting or ordering (compulsions).
- These thoughts or actions are regarded by the patient as abnormal and are resisted, but the patient is forced to continue to think thus, or to continue the actions.
- Symptom exacerbation in times of stress (for example, starting at a new school).
- Impairment of functioning (for example, completing chores, getting ready for bed, finishing schoolwork, relating to other family members).

This condition has a 6 month prevalence of 0.5–1%. The onset is usually between 6 and 11 years, with bimodal peaks. The male to female ratio is probably equal, although males predominate in the younger age group. Neuroimaging, neuropsychological and genetic studies support the concept that the disorder is neuropsychiatric in nature, and possibly related to a single major gene superimposed on multiple genes of minor effect. A subgroup of patients may have sustained an autoimmune reaction between caudate nucleus neurones and antibodies to β-haemolytic streptococci. Obsessive compulsive disorder should be distinguished from:
- transient benign habits and rituals such as 'not stepping on the crack' (no impairment)
- the worries associated with generalized anxiety disorder (in which the worries are about daily events)
- Tourette disorder (associated with tics)
- Pervasive developmental disorder (in which the rituals are not distressing, and there is marked social impairment).

Obsessive compulsive disorder is commonly comorbid with other anxiety disorders, mood disorder, tic disorder and disruptive behaviour disorders. Obsessive compulsive disorder often persists into adulthood.

Anxiolytic drugs (e.g. benzodiazepines) should be avoided in the treatment of anxiety disorders because there is no evidence that they are effective, and they have addictive and sedative potential. The most effective treatment is a combination of relaxation training, systematic desensitisation and cognitive behaviour therapy. Since parental anxiety is commonly associated with childhood anxiety disorder, family therapy is always indicated.

In obsessive compulsive disorder, cognitive behaviour therapy involving exposure to anxiety provoking situations, systematic desensitisation and the prevention of compulsive responses to anxiety provoking stimuli has been found to be effective. Behavioural treatment is the treatment of choice in this disorder, although clomipramine (a tricyclic antidepressant) and serotonin specific reuptake inhibitors are effective and well tolerated. Family therapy is aimed to educate the family and to disentangle the parents from the child's rituals.

Adolescence

Major depressive disorder

> ### Clinical example
>
> Bill, aged 14 years, was referred by his mother because the school had become concerned about his surliness, rebelliousness and tendency to submit class assignments with macabre content. His mother says that he does nothing to help her at home and that he spends most of his time in his bedroom listening to 'heavy metal' rock music. Bill's father left her and the four children several years ago, to live in a distant city and start a new family. Bill presents as a slim adolescent, dressed all in black, with close cropped hair and a nose ring. After initially sparring verbally, he admits that he hates his life. He sleeps poorly and is too tired to concentrate in school He has recently begun to smoke marijuana. He has no friends he can rely on except, maybe, 'potheads'. He thinks often about committing suicide, probably by jumping from a bridge. You diagnose mood disorder and refer him for psychiatric evaluation.

Although there is no doubt that children can feel depressed, it is not clear that they can develop a true major depressive disorder. There is better evidence for the validity of this diagnosis in adolescence. The characteristic symptoms of major depressive disorder are as follows:

- persistent depressed or irritable mood
- feelings of worthlessness and hopelessness
- suicidal ideation
- loss of pleasure in activities which were enjoyed previously
- social withdrawal and cessation of sporting and recreational activities
- insomnia or hypersomnia
- loss or gain of weight
- loss of concentration and deterioration in school performance
- lack of energy, ready fatigue.

Depressive symptoms are commonly associated with anxiety, conduct problems, post-traumatic symptomatology, eating disorder, learning disability, substance abuse and school refusal. A recent Australian population survey found the 6 month prevalence of depression to be 3% in childhood and adolescence. Typically, there is an increased prevalence of depression in the families of depressed children. However, the genetic background of the disorder is still unclear, as is the nature of the interaction between genetic propensity and the adverse life events that often precede depressive episodes. The clinician should be alerted to the possibility of depression whenever school performance inexplicably drops or there is a change in mood, control of temper, social involvement or sleep patterns. Information is needed from both parent and child with regard to the clinical features of the case and the psychosocial stressors that have affected and are affecting the patient. In less serious cases, individual and family counselling can be effective. In more serious cases, the child should be assessed for risk of suicide (Ch. 16) and, if appropriate, admitted to hospital.

Treatment should be individualised and goal directed. Cognitive behavioural therapy, psychodynamic therapy, interpersonal psychotherapy and family therapy may be required separately, or in various combinations. There is no evidence that tricyclic or heterocyclic antidepressant drugs are effective in child/adolescent major depression. Furthermore, they can have serious side effects and may be lethal in suicide attempts. There is evidence for the efficacy and greater safety of serotonin specific reuptake inhibitors. Although most depressed adolescents recover from depression within a year, many relapse, and the risk of subsequent episodes continues into adulthood.

Bipolar disorder

There is controversy over the validity of the diagnosis of bipolar disorder in childhood, and its prevalence. It is not clear whether some cases of apparent attention deficit hyperactivity disorder are really suffering from a form of mania, or whether attention deficit hyperactivity disorder can be a precursor of bipolar disorder. It is clear, on the other hand, that bipolar disorder is underdiagnosed in adolescence, and that it is often confused with schizophrenia at that time.

In bipolar I disorder, the patient has experienced at least one manic or mixed manic–depressive episode. In bipolar II disorder the patient has experienced at least one episode of both major depression and hypomania, but no manic or mixed episodes. Mania is characterised by the following symptoms:

- abnormally elevated or irritable mood persisting for at least 1 week
- grandiose thinking
- pressured speech, racing thoughts and distractibility
- increased activity and recklessness
- marked deterioration in functioning at school, with peers and at home.

Hypomania is characterised by similar but less intense symptoms and less functional deterioration. In a mixed episode, manic and major depressive symptoms coincide. Adolescents with mania often have hallucinations, paranoid ideas and marked lability of mood, causing the aforementioned diagnostic confusion with schizophrenia. The risk of suicide is increased in bipolar disorder, especially during depressive phases.

Bipolar disorder is familial, but the mode of genetic transmission has not been elucidated. Bipolar disorder should be differentiated from schizophrenia, major depression with agitation, post-traumatic stress disorder, disruptive behaviour disorder, and disorder of mood or delirium secondary to a medical condition (for example, hyperthyroidism, porphyria) or intoxication with illicit or prescribed drugs (for example, amphetamines, phencyclidine). The treatment of bipolar disorder is primarily pharmacological. The drug of choice is lithium, the blood levels and side effects of which must be monitored closely. Valproate and carbamazepine may be preferred if the patient's family is chaotic or unreliable. The relapse rate may be reduced if the patient remains on lithium throughout adolescence.

Schizophrenia

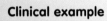

> ### Clinical example
>
> Annabelle, aged 15 years, was always an emotionally fragile child who tended to have intense, dependent relationships with her peers. However, recently she has become withdrawn and self-absorbed, telling her mother that she wants to drop out of school and pursue religious studies. At interview, she is fearful and apparently distracted. She asks you whether the interview is being videotaped. After some time she reveals that she has been 'chosen' to do something very important in the world. She became aware of this as a result of a revelation, one day recently, when the earth shone and she 'knew' her destiny. Her conversation meanders and is often difficult to follow. Several times in the interview she stops talking and smiles to herself. Physical examination is normal. You refer her to a psychiatrist who confirms your diagnosis of schizophrenia, admits Annabelle to hospital and commences antipsychotic medication. After Annabelle's discharge, you monitor her medication and she sees the psychiatrist every 6 weeks.

Although schizophrenia can occur in preadolescence, it is rare at that time. It is predominantly a disorder of late adolescence and early adulthood. Schizophrenia is a neurodevelopmental disease, foreshadowed, in many cases, by delayed developmental milestones and impaired development of language and cognition. Common prodromal symptoms are:

- social isolation or withdrawal
- deterioration in functioning at home, at school, and in grooming and personal hygiene
- lack of energy
- hypersomnia
- inappropriate or dulled affect
- unexplained panic

- disorganised, vague conversation with poverty of content
- odd, overvalued beliefs (for example, of telepathy), rituals or magical thinking
- unusual perceptual experiences (for example, that the body or face is changing, feelings of unreality, fear of losing control).

The following symptoms are typical after the onset of schizophrenia:

- hallucinations (most commonly auditory)
- delusions (for example, of persecution, thought insertion, thought loss)
- thought disorder with disorganised or incoherent conversation
- disorganised behaviour (for example, posturing, catatonic stiffness, agitation)
- flattening of affect, poverty of speech, anergia.

Schizophrenia is a familial disorder with a complex mode of genetic transmission and variable expressivity, operating according to a multifactorial threshold or mixed model of transmission. Schizophrenia should be differentiated from:

- mood disorder (especially bipolar I disorder)
- psychosis due to medical disease (for example, epilepsy, brain tumour, porphyria, AIDS) or substance abuse (for example, stimulants, cocaine, hallucinogens, phencyclidine)
- other psychoses (complex post-traumatic stress disorder, with dissociative hallucinations, schizophreniform disorder).

Acute schizophrenia conveys a risk of suicide or self-endangerment. Acute cases should be hospitalised for diagnosis and stabilisation. Patients are usually treated initially with a rapidly acting neuroleptic such as haloperidol. Most patients do not respond to medication until 2–4 weeks have elapsed. The newer ('atypical') antipsychotic drugs (such as clozapine, risperidone, olanzapine and quetiapine) are associated with relatively few side effects other than weight gain, sedation and, in some cases, sexual dysfunction. Psychoeducation for parents is essential in order to foster compliance and independent living skills and to counteract the high levels of emotional expression between family members that increase the likelihood of relapse. Liaison with the school is necessary. A poor prognosis is associated with early or insidious onset, low socioeconomic status, family history of schizophrenia, absence of precipitating stress and many negative symptoms.

Post-traumatic stress disorder

Post-traumatic stress disorder occurs in response to the personal experience of overwhelming, terrifying, potentially lethal stress directed toward oneself or someone with whom the child has a close attachment. In childhood and adolescence, the commonest kinds of threat causing post-traumatic stress disorder are motor vehicle accidents, burn injury, natural or manmade disasters, animal attack, criminal assault, observation of parental homicide or suicide, and war. A particularly pathogenic stress or threat involves repeated exposure to coercive intrafamilial physical or sexual abuse when the child is unable to disclose or escape the abuse and when, after disclosure, the non abusive caregiver fails to provide adequate support. The clinical features of post-traumatic stress disorder in childhood are very similar to those in adulthood:

- persistent intrusive imagery concerning the traumatic event
- repetitious play representing the event
- generalised nightmares and trauma nightmares
- the conviction that one is destined for an early death and that there were omens before the trauma
- avoidance of things, people or situations that remind one of the event
- persistent autonomic arousal with an exaggerated startle response.

When post-traumatic stress disorder is caused by repeated physical or sexual abuse, dissociative symptoms are likely to be manifested, for example:

- amnesia for all or part of the event or events
- vagueness, daydreaming and the sense of being estranged from others
- trance like states
- audiovisual hallucinations that represent fragmentary memories of the abuse
- bodily symptoms such as pseudoseizures and pelvic pain that represent somatic memories of the abuse.

Post-traumatic stress disorder is likely to be comorbid with, or to be succeeded by:

- mood disorder
- anxiety disorder
- hyperactivity
- alcohol/drug use
- dissociative and somatoform disorders
- intermittent explosive disorder
- borderline personality disorder.

Recent clinical research suggests that children under the age at which sequential, narrative, autobiographical memory can be encoded and recounted (that is, below 3 years of age) can manifest a form of post-traumatic stress disorder. The outcome of acute stress is affected adversely if the child is separated from parents, if the parents die, if the parents develop psychiatric symptoms (especially post-traumatic stress disorder), or if there is a contagion of symptoms between children. After civilian catastrophes, family reunification and assistance with shelter and physical needs take precedence. Group debriefing of affected children has been recommended,

but its efficacy is uncertain. Only those children who continue to manifest symptoms after 1 month should be referred for individual treatment. In post-traumatic stress disorder associated with child maltreatment, cognitive behaviour therapy and family therapy have proven helpful. If medication is required, serotonin specific reuptake inhibitors such as sertraline may be useful in reducing hyperarousal.

Somatoform disorders

This group of disorders is characterised by physical symptoms that suggest an underlying physical disease but for which either no such basis can be found, or the symptoms are disproportionate in intensity or duration to a known physical disorder. *Somatisation disorder* and *hypochondriasis* involve the conviction that physical symptoms have a physical cause and the tendency to present repeatedly for medical care even though no physical cause can be found. The commonest presentations are of abdominal pain, headaches or fatigue and muscle weakness. This kind of problem is generally associated with other family psychopathology such as parental anxiety, depression or somatisation, and may be based on the parent's conviction that the child has a physical disease such as chronic fatigue syndrome. It is frequently encountered in sexually abused children. In *conversion disorder* the dramatic symptoms suggest a physical disease but no such disease can be found and the symptoms are distributed or displayed in accordance with a naive view of bodily functioning (for example, glove and stocking anaesthesia). The commonest conversion symptoms are paralysis, paresis, anaesthesia, paraesthesia, vomiting, aphonia, headaches, blindness and deafness. Conversion disorder typically follows or accompanies a severe psychosocial stress such as sexual abuse, bereavement or family conflict.

The prevalence of somatoform disorders is probably high. They are closely related to the emotional climate of the family and to parental psychopathology. The primary physician should investigate thoroughly to rule out organic pathology, avoiding interminable testing lest the symptom become chronic and irreversible. Psychiatric consultation should be sought as early as possible. In conversion disorder, once the hidden stressor is disclosed, symptoms usually dissipate with suggestive therapy such as graduated exercises. In somatisation syndromes the family can be helped to interpret the symptoms as signs of stress and to manage stress, for example with relaxation exercises.

Eating disorders

Anorexia nervosa is characterised by:
- an intense fear of becoming fat or losing control of eating

- a relentless pursuit of thinness
- secretive food refusal, dieting and exercise causing marked loss of weight (below 85% of weight expected)
- the perception of being overweight despite extreme thinness
- amenorrhoea.

Bulimia nervosa is characterised by:
- binge eating with a sense of loss of control
- self-induced vomiting
- the use of dieting, laxatives, diuretics, enemas and exercise to control or reverse weight gain.

Both eating disorders are much more common in girls than in boys; ballet dancers, gymnasts and fashion models are particularly at risk. The prevalence of these conditions has greatly increased during the last 30 years, possibly due to the publicity given in the media to tall, slim fashion models. In the 15–25 year old group, bulimia is more common than anorexia nervosa. The onset of anorexia occurs in two peaks: early and late adolescence. Bulimia usually begins in late adolescence and may be a sequel of earlier anorexia nervosa.

The adolescent who develops anorexia nervosa is likely to have been a compliant, conscientious child who had an enmeshed relationship with her mother. Secretive dieting and exercise often begin after a minor precipitant, such as being told that one is overweight. The child hides the amount of weight loss from her parents. Menses cease. The child becomes moody, irritable and withdrawn. Eventually, the physical signs of starvation appear:
- emaciated facies and body
- fine body hair growth
- dry hair
- cold hands
- slow pulse
- low blood pressure.

The child resists medical help and is unable to appreciate how emaciated she has become. The adolescent with bulimia nervosa has dramatic weight fluctuations and develops swollen salivary glands, abraded knuckles and dental caries. Eventually, due to chronic metabolic alkalosis, kidney function may be compromised.

Eating disorders are best conceptualised as the product of family psychopathology expressed as eating disorder in one family member. Excessive dieting may represent the pursuit of an idealised body image and self-control by a child who perceives herself as helpless to direct her own life. The retching of the bulimic adolescent reflects the self-loathing and self-harm associated with chronic depression and guilt.

Eating disorders must be differentiated from other disorders that can cause weight loss; for example, malabsorption disorders, chronic infection, occult malignancy, substance abuse, chronic depression, paranoid schizophrenia and psychogenic vomiting.

Hospitalisation and paediatric/psychiatric collaboration are required if the patient is metabolically unstable, as evidenced by dehydration, inanition, electrolyte imbalance, bradycardia, and low blood pressure, if she resists treatment, or if outpatient treatment has failed. Nasogastric feeding is required in extreme cases. The patient is not discharged from hospital until a reasonable target weight is attained. Treatment plans should be individualised and goal directed. Anorectic patients respond best to a combination of family therapy and psychodynamic psychotherapy. Bulimic patients, who are usually older, generally respond best to cognitive behaviour therapy. Long term follow up studies have revealed that about 50% of anorectics recover, 25% have chronic anorexia nervosa and 25% have other psychiatric disorders. There is a significant mortality. Recovery is uncommon after 12 years of anorexia nervosa. The outcome of bulimia nervosa has not been studied.

PART 4   SELF-ASSESSMENT

Questions

1. **A 2 year old girl screams and kicks every time she does not get what she wants. You tell her mother that:**
   (A) She must punish her daughter for this otherwise the tantrums will continue
   (B) Temper tantrums are part of normal development and occur because her daughter has limited language to express her frustration
   (C) She should stay calm and walk away from her daughter when a tantrum begins
   (D) She should put her daughter in 'time out' for 2 minutes when she has a tantrum
   (E) She should discuss how to manage the tantrums with her husband so that their approach is consistent

2. **A 2½ year old boy uses a few single words but does not put two words together. He tends to grunt when he wants something and does not point or use gestures. He does not understand simple instructions or gestures.**
   (A) He is likely to have expressive language delay only
   (B) He should be referred for a speech assessment
   (C) His language development is within normal limits
   (D) A full developmental assessment should be undertaken to exclude global developmental delay
   (E) He should be referred for audiology testing

3. **Worried parents present with their 14 year old son. They are concerned that he is spending a lot of time in his room, that his school work is deteriorating and that he has problems sleeping and eating. You should:**
   (A) Tell the parents that their son may be taking marijuana and because this is common in adolescence they should not worry about it
   (B) Talk with the adolescent about his home and school life, recreation, drug use, sexual activity and depression issues
   (C) Assure the adolescent that even if he tells you he is taking drugs, everything he says to you is confidential
   (D) Talk with the adolescent's teachers about his school performance

4. **Which of the following disorders are more common in boys?**
   (A) Enuresis
   (B) Autistic disorder
   (C) Conduct disorder
   (D) Delayed speech and language

5. **At what age is separation anxiety usually first evidenced?**
   (A) School commencement (4–5 years)
   (B) 7 years
   (C) Second 6 months of life
   (D) 12–14 years

6. **Encopresis:**
   (A) Is an important diagnostic sign in Hirschsprung disease
   (B) May be the result of punitive toilet training methods
   (C) Frequently is associated with significant emotional and/or family disturbance
   (D) May present with apparent diarrhoea
   (E) Most children with soiling have normal anal sphincter control

7. **What advice would you give the mother of a 3 year old who sucks his thumb?**
   (A) Paint both thumbs with a foul tasting potion
   (B) Reassure her that this is a common behaviour which will usually stop of its own accord
   (C) Smack or punish him each time until he stops
   (D) Refer the parents for marital therapy

8. **Oswald, a 4 year old boy, presents with tantrums, low frustration tolerance, high activity level and very difficult behaviour when out shopping or visiting. He was born following a normal pregnancy, labour and delivery. His motor development was normal, but by 2 years of age he had six words and by 3 years he had started to combine words. He had a limited vocabulary and his speech was difficult to understand. Which of the following would be part of your initial management plan?**
   (A) Send the parents to a 'parenting' course
   (B) Examine the ears and refer for an audiological assessment
   (C) Commence a trial of stimulant medication
   (D) Refer for a developmental assessment
   (E) Refer for a speech pathology assessment

9. **Magda, a 7 year old girl, is in trouble at school for poor attention, daydreaming, not trying, being disruptive and doing careless work. There had been no problems with behaviour at home until the last few months. Her mother says that she is moody and uncooperative. She is not keen on sport. Which of the following options are appropriate?**

(A) It would be important to assess her educational level, with particular reference to reading skills

(B) Family disruption or abuse may be the underlying problem

(C) A detailed assessment regarding auditory and visual perception may be necessary

(D) She should be taken aside and encouraged to try harder

(E) Fine and gross motor coordination should also be assessed

10. **Lois, a 3 year old, presents with excessive activity, poor concentration, tantrums and poor sleeping of 6 months duration. Should you:**

(A) Do a trial of exclusion of milk, egg, wheat, yeast products and synthetic colours and preservatives from the diet

(B) Commence on methylphenidate

(C) Obtain more information regarding development and family circumstances

(D) Implement a behavioural management programme

(E) Refer the child to a child psychiatrist

11. **Which of the following statements are true regarding ADHD:**

(A) ADHD is caused by chaotic family circumstances

(B) In dysfunctional families, children with ADHD should not be treated with stimulant medication

(C) Significant aggressive behaviour in the preschool period worsens the outlook for ADHD

(D) ADHD is more common in children with unemployed parents

(E) ADHD should not be diagnosed when difficult behaviours are only noticed at school

12. **Which of the following statements are true regarding ADHD:**

(A) Most children with ADHD have associated learning problems

(B) If the child does not display overactive or inattentive behaviour under assessment in the doctor's office, the diagnosis of ADHD is dismissed

(C) Excessive sugar consumption does not cause hyperactive behaviour

(D) Behaviour consistent with ADHD usually commences prior to school age

(E) Special EEG and brain imaging studies are required to make a diagnosis of ADHD

13. **In Sally's mid year report in grade 2, the teacher comments on vagueness and careless work, and the grades for various aspects of literacy and maths skills are mostly B (Beginning). She complains to her mother that the kids in her grade won't let her play with them. What is the appropriate management?**

(A) Assume Sally has ADHD, and commence on stimulant treatment

(B) Arrange audiology assessment to ensure Sally can hear normally

(C) Encourage the parents to spend 1 or 2 hours with Sally each evening, going over her school readers and teaching the times tables

(D) Take a careful history of early development, behaviour and social functioning

(E) Plan for Sally to repeat grade 2, so that reading can 'click in' as she gets more mature

14. **Which of the following statements is/are true in relation to autistic disorder?**

(A) Occurs with equal frequency in males and females

(B) Is associated with severe language impairment

(C) The autistic child sees people as objects rather than human beings

(D) May be associated with overt brain damage

(E) Responds well to specific medication

15. **Which of the following statements is/are true in relation to conduct disorder?**

(A) Conduct disorder occurs more commonly among males

(B) Antisocial behaviour which violates social norms and the rights of others is characteristic

(C) Conduct disorder has no serious prognostic implications

(D) Learning disorders and hyperactivity are commonly associated with conduct disorder

(E) Multisystemic therapy has produced favourable results

16. **Anorexia nervosa is:**

(A) More common among females

(B) Due to a pituitary tumour

(C) Caused by the pursuit of thinness and the fear of obesity rather than a true loss of appetite

(D) Associated with significantly increased mortality

(E) Best treated with antidepressants

17. **A 12 month old infant, when not being nursed, frequently puts his fist into his mouth, regurgitates stomach contents, rolls it around his mouth, and allows the vomitus to spill out of his mouth. Which of the following statements is/are true about this condition?**

(A) More common in females

(B) Can be an outcome of lack of stimulation

(C) Is a sign of high levels of psychic arousal

(D) Is best treated with a low dose sedation

(E) Can be related to maternal depression and withdrawal

Answers and explanations

1. The correct answers are **(B)**, **(C)**, **(D)** and **(E)**. Punishment (A) is inappropriate as this will not alter

the behaviour and may make it worse. Tantrums are common at this age (B) and should not be reacted to (C). Time out for 1 minute for each year of age may be useful as negative reinforcement (D), and consistency of approach for both parents (and other caregivers) is important (E).

2. The correct answers are **(B)**, **(D)** and **(E)**. Although isolated expressive language delay is common, his lack of understanding could represent hearing impairment (E) and his lack of use of gestures could represent global delay (D). Certainly his language is not within normal limits for his age (C).

3. The correct answers are **(B)** and **(C)**. You will need to spend time taking a careful and sympathetic history from the adolescent by himself (B). Your responsibilities are to him, and therefore you must maintain confidentiality (C) unless he agrees with you that his parents may be informed, in which case you would have these discussions with his parents, ideally in his presence. You should not tell his parents without his consent (A). It may be helpful to talk with his teachers (D), but again this needs to be with his agreement. Informing his teachers about drug use would not be appropriate.

4. **All answers are correct**. Prepubertal boys are referred to child psychiatric clinics 2–3 times more frequently than girls. This male predominance is greatest in externalising disorders and developmental disorders.

5. The correct answer is **(C)**. Separation anxiety is a normal developmental phenomenon usually appearing in the second 6 months of life. It is quite different from separation anxiety disorder, which has peaks at 5–7 and 12–13 years of age.

6. The correct answers are **(B)**, **(C)**, **(D)** and **(E)**. Hirschsprung disease almost always presents with an incomplete large bowel obstruction in the neonatal period, well before toilet training is contemplated. It is a very uncommon undiagnosed cause of later encopresis (A). Poor or punitive toilet training by anxious or frustrated parents can cause severe anxiety in some children, with later encopresis (B). Some, but by no means all, children with encopresis may come from disturbed homes or may have significant other emotional difficulties (C). In some children with severe constipation, there may be overflow of fluid bowel contents from higher in the colon, past the areas of retained faeces, with involuntary leakage per rectum of foul smelling faecal material. This may be thought erroneously to be diarrhoea (D). Most children with encopresis have normal sphincter control (E), although longstanding preceding constipation may have caused rectal and sigmoid dilation, with loss of rectal sensation to distension.

7. The correct answer is **(B)**. Thumbsucking is common in toddlers and occurs more often if the child is tired or anxious. It almost always stops spontaneously but addressing the cause of the child's anxiety, for example, marital conflict, may be helpful in the minority of cases where this is a contributing factor.

8. Correct answers are **(B)**, **(D)** and **(E)**. It is common for children with language delay to have behavioural problems related to frustration. (A) Referring for a parent training course initially may be ignoring the underlying problem. (B) It is important to exclude a hearing loss as the cause for language delay and to have a speech pathology assessment. (C) Stimulant medication is inappropriate. (D) A developmental assessment would be helpful to identify whether any other areas are delayed. (E) To identify, among other things, whether there is a receptive, expressive or an articulation difficulty. Maternal depression or other family problems may contribute to language delay.

9. **(D)** is not helpful but **all of the others should be investigated**.

10. The correct answers are **(C)** and **(D)**. (A) Although commonly advocated throughout the community, young children should not be placed on restrictive diets without dietetic and medical supervision, and an effort made to establish on a firm clinical basis that it is necessary and significant. The ingestion of synthetic colours does affect a very small proportion of children and these substances can be avoided without any restriction of foods required for good nutrition. (B) The use of stimulant medication is not appropriate unless a careful diagnosis of significant attentional difficulties is made. This can be very difficult in a 3 year old and it would be very rare for an experienced physician or psychiatrist to be prescribing it for a child before attending preschool. (C) Clearly more information is required before an assessment can be complete and a management programme implemented. (D) Guidelines regarding management of tantrums and setting limits consistently and firmly may be helpful. (E) Referral to a child psychiatrist would only be necessary if the problems were severe and intransigent.

11. **(C)**, **(D)** and **(E)** are correct. (A) is incorrect. Although ADHD is diagnosed more commonly in these families, the family circumstances are a risk factor exacerbating neurobiological vulnerabilities rather than a true cause. (B) is also incorrect, and a child with diagnosed ADHD should be offered a trial of stimulant medication. Improved behaviour may also help overall family function. Close monitoring of treatment is required, as well as family support. (C) is correct. Aggressive behaviour in the young child is a high risk factor for continued

155

antisocial behaviour, and in combination with ADHD makes the future successful negotiation of the developmental tasks of adolescence problematic. (D) is also correct. Socioeconomic risk factors of family disruption, poverty and unemployment all contribute to increased prevalence of ADHD. (E) is correct: the behavioural traits of ADHD are pervasive across settings. If only seen at school, consider learning problems, social interaction difficulties and bullying.

12. **(A)**, **(C)** and **(D)** are correct. Although figures vary between studies, over half have learning and language disorders significantly affecting academic progress (A). Children with ADHD can display more contained behaviour in unfamiliar and relatively overwhelming settings such as the doctor's office (B). (C) is true. Despite the common lay concern that high sugar intake causes difficult behaviour in some children, controlled studies have shown there is no association. (D) also is true. Although the clear diagnosis of ADHD is often difficult in preschool children, retrospective history usually reveals consistent behavioural patterns from early childhood. At the time of presentation of a younger child, it may be difficult to distinguish from the normal range of behaviour, but patterns persisting into school years make the diagnosis clearer. Although many research groups are studying the significance of measures of brain function (E), such tests are not yet sufficiently robust for diagnostic purposes in individual children.

13. **(B)** and **(D)** are correct. Although Sally may have the inattentive type of ADHD, much more assessment of behaviours at home and at school is required before making this diagnosis (A). Although Sally's hearing acuity is unlikely to be the significant factor, a mild hearing loss must be excluded (B). Measurement of auditory perception, e.g. short term auditory memory and figure–ground perception is essential, as auditory processing problems are common in children and could be a cause of Sally's presenting problems. Excessive homework for a child who does not understand the underlying learning concepts leads to pressure, unrealistic expectations, frustration and reactive behaviours, which may include inattention and distractibility (C). (D) is correct. The combination of poor academic and social functioning indicates possible mild developmental delay/borderline intellectual disability. Sally's inattention may be related to her inability to understand what is required. An educational psychology assessment would be indi-

cated to measure learning and overall cognitive ability. However, it cannot be assumed that Sally's problems are due to immaturity (E). Further assessment is required. If she has ADHD, appropriate management including remedial education should enable her to stay with her peers. If she has developmental delay/borderline intellectual disability, a modified education programme and special needs support will be required in the long term.

14. The correct answers are **(B)**, **(C)** and **(D)**. Autistic disorders occur approximately three times more commonly in boys than in girls (A). Autism is associated with severe language impairment. If the autistic child has not acquired language by the age of 5 years, adequate speech development is unlikely ever to occur. (B) The autistic child has major difficulty forming any meaningful interpersonal relationships. (C) Some children with cerebral palsy and other CNS disorders may exhibit features of autism. (D) There are no medications which have a specific effect on autism. (E) Some medications may modify some of the behavioural symptoms of autism, but they do not alter the central features of the disorder.

15. The correct answers are **(A)**, **(B)**, **(D)** and **(E)**, all of which are characteristic of conduct disorder. (C) A history of behaviour problems sufficient to make a diagnosis of conduct disorder is associated with a morbidly increased risk of delinquency and antisocial personality disorder. (E) Multisystemic therapy is a recently introduced form of therapy which has proven effective in controlled studies.

16. The correct answers are **(A)**, **(C)** and **(D)**. (B) Although a pituitary tumour may rarely present with an anorexia nervosa-like picture, no CNS pathology is regularly found in anorexia nervosa. (C) Patients with anorexia nervosa are typically fearful of being fat, not anorectic. (D) Mortality rates from starvation and suicide of up to 10% have been reported in follow up studies. (E) The indication for prescription of antidepressants in anorexia nervosa is the presence of depression or obsessive compulsive disorder, not anorexia nervosa itself.

17. The correct answers are **(B)** and **(E)**. The condition is rumination, of which is due to lack of contact stimulation, usually due to severe maternal depression or to institutional neglect. The condition is due to low rather than high levels of psychological arousal. (A) There is no sex difference. (C) These children self-stimulate because they lack sufficient external stimulation. (D) Sedation is ineffective and is contraindicated.

PART 4 FURTHER READING

American Academy of Pediatrics 2000 Clinical practice guideline: diagnosis and evaluation of the child with Attention-Deficit/Hyperactivity Disorder. Pediatrics 105: 1158–1170

American Academy of Pediatrics 2001 Clinical practice guideline: Treatment of the school-aged child with Attention-Deficit/Hyperactivity Disorder. Pediatric 108: 1033–1044

American Psychiatric Association 2000 Diagnostic and statistical manual of mental disorders, 4th edn. American Psychiatric Association, Washington, DC

Bernstein G A et al 1999 Practice parameters for the assessment and treatment of children and adolescents with anxiety disorders. Journal of the American Academy of Child and Adolescent Psychiatry 36 (10 Supplement): 69S–84S

Birmaher B, Ryan ND, Williamson DC et al 1996 Childhood and adolescent depression: a review of the past 10 years. Parts I and II. Journal of the American Academy of Child and Adolescent Psychiatry 35: 1427–1439, 1575–1583

Dixon S, Stein M 2000 Encounters with children: pediatric behavior and development, 3rd edn. Mosby, St Louis

Fritz G K, Fritsch S, Hagino O 1997 Somatoform disorders in children and adolescents: a review of the past 10 years. Journal of the American Academy of Child and Adolescent Psychiatry 36: 1329–1338

Goodman R, Scott S 1997 Child psychiatry. Blackwell Sciencè, London

Greydanus D E, Wolraich M L 1992 Behavioral pediatrics. Springer-Verlag, New York

Herbert M 1999 Clinical child psychology, 2nd edn. Wiley, Chichester

Jensen P, Hinshaw S, Swanson J et al 2001 Findings from the NIMH multimodal treatment study for ADHD (MTA): implications and applications for primary care providers. Journal of Developmental and Behavioral Pediatrics 22: 60–73

Kaminsky L, Oberklaid F 1999 Your child's health. Random House, Sydney

Levine M D, Carey W B, Crocker A C 1999 Developmental–behavioral pediatrics, 3rd edn. WB Saunders, Philadelphia

Lucas A R 1996 Anorexia nervosa and bulimia nervosa. In: Lewis M (ed.) Child and adolescent psychiatry: a comprehensive textbook, 2nd edn. Williams & Wilkins, Baltimore, Ch. 53

National Health and Medical Research Council 1996 Attention deficit hyperactivity disorder (ADHD). National Health and Medical Research Council, Canberra

Nurcombe B 2000 Developmental disorders of attachment, feeding, elimination, and sleeping. In: Ebert M H, Loosen P T, Nurcombe B (eds) Current diagnosis and treatment in psychiatry. McGraw Hill, New York, 533–539

Piacenti J, Bergman R L 2000 Obsessive compulsive disorder in children. Psychiatric Clinics of North America 23: 519–533

Reddy Y C J, Srinath S 2000 Juvenile bipolar disorder. Acta Psychiatrica Scandinavica 102: 162–170

Sawyer et al 2000 The mental health of young people in Australia. Mental Health and Special Programs Branch, Commonwealth Department of Health and Aged Care, Canberra

Schmitt B D 1987 Seven deadly sins of childhood: advising parents about difficult developmental phases. Child Abuse and Neglect 11:421–432

Steinhausen H-C, Juzi C 1996 Elective mutism: an analysis of 100 cases. Journal of the American Academy of Child and Adolescent Psychiatry 35: 606–614

Tanguay P E 2000 Pervasive developmental disorders: a 10-year review. Journal of the American Academy of Child and Adolescent Psychiatry 39: 1079–1095

Therapeutic Guidelines: Psychotropic 2000 Version 4. Therapeutic Guidelines Limited, Melbourne

Volkmar F R 1996 Childhood and adolescent pyschosis: a review of the past 10 years. Journal of the American Academy of Child and Adolescent Psychiatry 35: 843–851

World Health Organization 1992 The ICD-10 classification of mental and behavioural disorders. Clinical descriptions and diagnostic guidelines. WHO, Geneva

Zeanah C H 1999 The handbook of infant mental health, 2nd edn. Guilford Press, New York

Useful links

http://www.aacap.org (American Academy of Child and Adolescent Psychiatry)

http://www.adders.org/ausmap.htm (Australian support for ADH)

http://www.apa.org (American Psychology Association)

http://www.chadd.org (USA parent support group, many links, pamphlets for download)

http://www.growinghealthykids.com (Epidemiology and management of problems occurring during infancy, preschool, adolescent and young adult transitions)

http://www.nimh.nih.gov (United States National Institute of Mental Health)

http://www.nlm.nih.gov (United States National Library of Medicine)

http://www.parenting.sa.gov.au/pegs (Parenting advice for common problems; guide no. 55 for ADD)

PART 5

PAEDIATRIC EMERGENCIES

19 Paediatric emergencies: causes and assessment

J. Raftos

There are many causes of collapse leading to the need for emergency medical intervention in the child. Table 19.1 lists some of the common paediatric emergencies. In approaching the critically ill child, the diagnosis is however of secondary importance to:
- the structured **primary assessment**, and
- **timely resuscitation procedures**, as required.

The **primary assessment** follows a stepwise progression through:
- **A**irway
- **B**reathing
- **C**irculation
- **D**isability (deficiency of cerebral function), with attention to

- **E**xposure.

This structured approach is based on the knowledge that the brain requires a continual supply of its two main metabolites: oxygen and glucose. An airway problem, by depriving oxygen supply, will most rapidly lead to death and therefore must be corrected first. A breathing problem preventing oxygen moving into the lung and carbon dioxide out of the lung is the next priority. A circulatory problem preventing the oxygen being carried to the brain is next, and so on.

The resuscitation measures required and management of the collapsed child are described in detail in Chapter 20.

Table 19.1   Causes of paediatric emergencies

Airway	Breathing	Circulation	Disability	Exposure
Croup	Asthma	Congenital heart disease	Seizure	Hypothermia
Epiglottitis	Bronchiolitis	Duct dependent lesions	Meningitis	Hyperthermia
Laryngeal foreign body	Pneumonia	critical aortic stenosis	Encephalitis	Inflicted injury
Bacterial tracheitis	Foreign body	hypoplastic left heart	Head injury	
Trauma	Congestive heart failure	coarctation	Raised intracranial pressure	
Angioneurotic oedema	Neuromuscular diseases	Dysrhythmias	Hypoglycaemia	
Retropharyngeal abscess	Trauma	bradycardia	Metabolic disorder	
	pneumothorax	tachycardia	Poisoning	
	haemothorax	supraventricular	Envenomation	
	lung contusion	ventricular		
	flail chest	torsades de pointes		
	Near drowning	fibrillation		
	Smoke inhalation	Pulseless electrical activity		
	Metabolic acidosis	Shock		
	diabetic ketoacidosis	cardiogenic		
	Poisoning	cardiomyopathy		
	Salicylates	heart failure		
	Methanol	myocardial contusion		
		hypovolaemic		
		haemorrhage		
		vomiting/diarrhoea		
		burns		
		distributive		
		septicaemia		
		anaphylaxis		
		spinal cord injury		
		obstructive		
		cardiac tamponade		
		hypertension		
		dissociative		

The primary assessment

Airway

The child and infant airway, compared with that of the adult, presents particular anatomical and physiological differences that increase its susceptibility to compromise. Infants are obligate nose breathers. Infants and small children have smaller airways and a smaller mandible, proportionately larger tongue and more floppy epiglottis and soft palate. The narrowest portion of their airway is below the cords at the level of the cricoid ring, in contrast to adults, where the narrowest portion is at the level of the vocal cords. The trachea is short and soft and hyperextension or flexion of the neck may cause obstruction.

Ensuring that the patient has a patent airway is of the highest priority. In evaluating the airway a look, listen and feel approach is used.

Movement of the chest wall and the abdomen should be carefully looked for. The degree to which intercostal and other accessory muscles are being used to overcome obstruction should be noted. Paradoxical movement of the abdomen may be noted if there is upper airway obstruction.

Listening over the mouth and nose for air movement should follow. Particular note should be made of inspiratory stridor, which is a sign of tracheal, laryngeal or other upper airway obstruction. In severe obstruction, expiratory sounds may also be heard but inspiratory noises predominate. A stethoscope should be used to listen over the trachea and in the axillae for air movement.

Finally the examiner, by placing his or her face close to the child's mouth, may feel evidence of air movement.

Breathing

In childhood, conditions that result in respiratory compromise are the most common reason for emergency intervention and are the major cause for poor outcome.

As with the airway, there are important differences between the child and the adult. Children have a higher metabolic requirement. They have more immature musculature with easy fatigability of the diaphragm, which is the major muscle of respiration. The chest wall is more compliant and the ribs are horizontal, decreasing the efficiency of the bellows effect.

The airways in the child are proportionately smaller, and therefore produce an increased resistance to air flow, especially when traumatised or inflamed. Resistance across an airway is inversely proportional to the fourth power of the radius:

$$R = 1/r^4$$

Thus, halving the radius increases the resistance very significantly.

Having established patency of the airway, evaluation for the presence and adequacy of breathing should follow. It is helpful to divide this into three aspects:

- effort of breathing
- efficacy of breathing
- effects of respiratory inadequacy on other organs.

Effort of breathing

Respiratory rate is age dependent (Table 19.2). Tachypnoea is an early response to respiratory failure. Increased depth of respiration may occur later. Tachypnoea does not always have a respiratory cause and may occur in response, for example, to metabolic acidosis. As the intercostal muscles and diaphragm increase their contraction, intercostal and subcostal recession develop. In the infant, sternal retraction may also occur.

The ribs are horizontal in young children; therefore, the sternomastoid muscles must be recruited to further raise the ribs to increase ventilation.

In infants and small children flaring of the alae nasi may be seen. It must be remembered that in this age group 50% of airway resistance occurs in the upper airway, and this is an attempt to reduce this resistance.

The effort of breathing is diminished in three clinical circumstances. These must be recognised, as urgent intervention may be required. Firstly, exhaustion may develop as a result of the increased respiratory demands. The younger child is even more prone to this due to more immature musculature. Secondly, respiration requires an intact central respiratory drive centre. Conditions such as trauma, meningitis and poisoning may depress this centre. Thirdly, neuromuscular conditions that cause paralysis, such as muscular dystrophy and Guillain–Barré syndrome, may result in respiratory failure without increased effort.

Symmetrical movement of the chest should be confirmed. In the younger child the diaphragm is the main muscle of respiration; therefore, one should also look for movement of the upper abdomen.

Table 19.2	Vital signs by age		
Age (years)	Respiratory rate (breaths/min)	Heart rate (beats/min)	Systolic blood pressure (mmHg)
<1	30–40	110–160	70–90
1–2	25–35	100–150	80–95
2–5	25–30	95–140	80–100
5–12	20–25	80–120	90–110
>12	15–20	60–100	100–120

Inspiratory and expiratory noises should be noted. Wheezing is heard with lower airway narrowing, as in asthma, often with a prolonged expiratory phase. Crepitations may be heard with pneumonia and heart failure.

Efficacy of breathing

Auscultation of both sides of the chest will confirm air movement. Beware the silent chest! Oximetry is useful for providing a measure of arterial oxygen saturation (SaO_2), which reflects the efficacy of breathing; however, oximetry may be difficult to obtain in the cold or shocked child and is less accurate when the SaO_2 is less than 70%.

Effects of respiratory inadequacy on other organs

The impact of hypoxia on the cardiovascular system is to cause tachycardia, but preterminally it may cause bradycardia.

Cyanosis is also a preterminal sign. Hypoxia may also cause peripheral shut down and pallor secondary to sympathetic stimulation. The effect of hypoxia on the brain is to cause initial agitation and irritability in infants, followed by increasing loss of consciousness.

Circulation

Cardiac output is the product of stroke volume and heart rate. The normal heart rate increases with age (Table 19.2). Infants have a small, relatively fixed cardiac stroke volume; thus they must increase rate to respond to increase demand.

Infants have a relatively larger intravascular volume (85 ml/kg) which decreases with age to 60 ml/kg in the teenager. The normal ranges for blood pressure increase with age (Ch. 62). This is due to the fact that systemic vascular resistance increases as the child gets older.

Assessment of circulation

An increase in heart rate is the earliest response to any reduction in intravascular volume. As shock progresses, bradycardia may develop as a preterminal sign. Pulse volume is important to assess both peripherally and centrally. Weak central pulses indicate severe shock. Capillary refill can be a sensitive indicator of vascular status. To assess this, light pressure should be applied to the skin over the sternum for 5 seconds. In the normal individual, capillary return of blood, seen as a slight flush of the pallid area where pressure was applied, will occur in less than 3 seconds. Caution should be used in interpreting this sign in the child who has been exposed to a cold environment.

In the shocked child, hypotension is a late preterminal sign.

Effects of circulatory inadequacy on other organs

Circulatory inadequacy leads to poor tissue perfusion, which in turn leads to metabolic acidosis. Tachypnoea occurs to compensate for this.

Initial sympathetic stimulation may cause agitation, but later poor cerebral perfusion causes increasing drowsiness and coma in the preterminal phase.

Prerenal failure develops with hypovolaemia and hypotension, with reduction of urine output. Normal urine output is greater than 1 ml/kg/h in the child and greater than 2 ml/kg/h in the infant.

Signs of cardiac failure

The signs of cardiac failure should be looked for. Raised jugulovenous pulse is important in the older child but may be difficult to determine in the younger child due to the relatively short, often chubby neck. Listen for a gallop rhythm and lung crepitations. Palpation of the abdomen may reveal an enlarged liver.

Disability

The assessment of neurological function as part of the primary assessment has three main aims:
- to rapidly determine the level of consciousness
- to find localising intracranial lesions
- to determine whether there is raised intracranial pressure.

It must be remembered that respiratory and cardiovascular failure can cause decreased consciousness and must be dealt with first.

Conscious level

Conscious level can be rapidly assessed using the AVPU method:
A Alert
V responds to Voice
P responds to Pain
U Unresponsive

The child who is unresponsive or only responds to pain has a Glasgow coma scale (GCS) score of 8 or less. The GCS has no place in the primary survey, but it is a useful tool for monitoring changes in neurological status after initial stabilisation.

Posture and tone

Hypotonia may be seen in the seriously ill child no matter what the underlying diagnosis. Hypertonia and posturing should be observed, if present, and any asymmetry noted. Decorticate posturing is evidenced by flexed upper limbs and extended lower limbs, whereas in decerebrate posturing both the upper and lower limbs are extended. These are both preterminal signs and must be acted on immediately.

Pupils size and reactivity

Examination of the pupils can give valuable information. It is important to determine whether there is dilatation, non reactivity or inequality. Most importantly, unequal pupils may indicate tentorial herniation or a rapidly expanding lesion on one side of the brain. Small, reactive pupils may indicate a metabolic disorder or medullary lesion.

Respiratory patterns in neurological failure

Raised intracranial pressure can lead to a number of breathing patterns, ranging from hyperventilation to apnoea.

Circulatory changes in neurological failure

Hypertension, bradycardia and hypoventilation form the Cushing triad. These are late signs of raised intracranial pressure and must be acted on immediately. Hypotension is a preterminal event.

Exposure

Infants and small children have a proportionately greater surface area and therefore lose heat more rapidly than older children and adults. Infants are also less able to respond to hypothermia. Early measurement of temperature is therefore important, and appropriate warming during resuscitation should be maintained.

Fever may indicate infection.

It is important to fully expose the child, as valuable clues such as rashes in meningococcal disease or bruises in inflicted injury may be missed.

The child may respond with fear or embarrassment to exposure and therefore it must be undertaken sensitively.

Reassessment

Frequent reassessment should be undertaken, especially if there is any deterioration during the resuscitation. A search for a definitive diagnosis should now be completed.

Now, putting it all together... (Fig. 19.1) overleaf.

Key learning points

- In the collapsed child, a careful and orderly primary assessment and timely resuscitation measures are of more importance than the diagnosis.
- Children differ from adults physiologically and anatomically.
- Conditions affecting respiration are a common pathway to collapse in the child.
- Cyanosis and hypotension are preterminal signs.
- Decerebrate and decorticate posturing are preterminal signs.

Airway — Assess patency
- **Look for**
  Movement of the chest wall
  Intercostal and accessory
  muscle use

- **Listen for**
  Air movement
  Abnormal sounds — stridor

- **Feel for**
  Air movement

Breathing — Assess the adequacy of breathing
- **Effort of breathing**
  Recession
  Respiratory rate
  Inspiration or expiration noises
  Grunting
  Accessory muscle use
  Flare of the alae nasi

- **Effectiveness of breathing**
  Breath sounds
  Chest expansion
  Abdominal excursion

- **Effects of inadequate respiration**
  Heart rate
  Skin colour
  Mental status

Circulation — Assess adequacy of circulation
- **Cardiovascular status**
  Heart rate
  Pulse volume
  Capillary refill
  Blood pressure

- **Effects of circulatory inadequacy
  on other organs**
  Respiratory rate and character
  Skin appearance and temperature
  Mental status
  Urinary output

- **Signs of cardiac failure**
  Raised JVP (not in infancy)
  Gallop rhythm
  Crepitations in lungs
  Enlarged liver

Disability — Assess neurological function
- A rapid measure of level of consciousness should be recorded — AVPU
- Note the child's posture and tone — especially any lateralising features
- Check pupils for size, equality and reactivity
- Note the presence of convulsive movements

Exposure
- Take the child's core temperature
- Look for a rash or injury

Reassessment
- Should be performed regularly, especially if there is deterioration

Fig. 19.1 Now, putting it all together: the primary assessment.

Emergency care of the collapsed child

M. South

The term 'collapsed' is used to describe a child whose neurological state is acutely and abnormally impaired, leading to loss of normal consciousness and muscular tone.

Diagnosis

Collapse may occur because of a primary neurological process; when there is loss or reduction of oxygen supply to the brain; or when metabolic disturbance or toxins affect brain function. Collapse may be the result of many different disease processes, some examples of which are shown in Table 20.1. A more thorough differential diagnosis and approach to assessment of the collapsed child are presented in Chapter 19.

Sometimes the cause of collapse is immediately obvious, as in head injury or drowning, but sometimes it may be a diagnostic problem initially, e.g. sepsis or drug ingestion. In this latter setting, resuscitation will usually have to take priority over obtaining a complete history, examination and investigation. With sufficient personnel available, diagnostic and resuscitative procedures may progress in parallel. One investigation to consider early when the cause of collapse is unknown is a blood glucose estimation.

Clinical example

Terry, a 3 year old boy, was found collapsed in the bathroom while visiting his grandmother's house. He was taken immediately to a local hospital where he was noted to be floppy and poorly responsive to voice or physical stimulation. He had an adequate airway, his breathing was a little shallow and slow, and he was slightly dusky in colour. His limbs were pink, felt warm and he had strong pulses. Terry was placed on his side and an oxygen mask was applied to his face: his colour improved immediately. He was afebrile, with normal blood glucose on bedside testing, and no other physical abnormalities were found.

A careful history showed that he had been very well all day. He had been playing unobserved in his grandmother's bedroom for about an hour before he was found. His grandmother keeps some sedative drugs (nitrazepam) in the bedside cabinet and a telephone call back to the house revealed that the tablet bottle was lying open on the bedroom floor.

Terry continued to receive oxygen and close observation and his clinical condition improved steadily over the next 12 hours. He was discharged home well the following day.

Table 20.1 Some causes of collapse in children	
Category	Diagnosis
Primary neurological process	Meningitis Head injury Encephalitis Seizures
Failure of oxygen supply to brain	Acute asphyxia (e.g. drowning, birth asphyxia) Respiratory causes (e.g. severe asthma, croup) Cardiac causes (e.g. arrythmias, myocarditis) Hypovolaemia (e.g. dehydration, haemorrhage) Sepsis Anaphylaxis
Metabolic disturbance or toxins	Hypoglycaemia Hyponatraemia Drug or other toxic ingestion Envenomation Bacterial toxins

Resuscitation

If you might find yourself responsible for the immediate care of a collapsed child, you should be familiar with at least the procedures used in basic life support. The general principles might be the same as used in the resuscitation of adults but specific techniques are required in children.

The primary aim is to restore an adequate supply of oxygenated blood to the brain — to prevent secondary brain damage. The resuscitation procedures required will vary, depending on the degree of physiological impairment, from simple ones, such as application of an oxygen facemask or administration of a bolus of intravenous fluid; through basic cardiopulmonary resuscitation; to advanced life support measures including endotracheal intubation, mechanical ventilation and the use of vasoactive drugs.

Life support

The environment is important: make sure you are in a safe situation — you will be of no value to the collapsed child if you, the rescuer, become a second victim (e.g. at a road accident scene). Get someone to summon sufficient extra help.

> ### Clinical example
>
> Miah, an 8 year old girl, was a rear seat passenger when her family's car was involved in an accident while travelling at around 60 km/h. She was not wearing a seat belt. On arrival at hospital, she was awake but agitated with multiple superficial abrasions to her face, trunk and limbs. Within 20 minutes her state of consciousness deteriorated, she developed increasing tachycardia and her blood pressure had fallen.
>
> Miah was intubated to protect her airway; during the procedure careful attention was paid to prevent excessive movement of her cervical spine. The doctor had already inserted a large bore cannula into a vein in her antecubital fossa, and through this she was given 40 ml/kg of saline. She was re-examined for possible sites of hidden bleeding, including the abdomen and limbs (especially fractured femur). Her abdomen was noted to be distended and she underwent CT, which showed a large contusion of the liver. CT of her brain, performed at the same time, was normal. Miah was managed with supportive care, including mechanical ventilation and blood transfusion, and was discharged from the ICU 5 days later.

Quickly evaluate the degree of collapse:

- Assess the child's response to verbal or physical arousal (e.g. gentle shaking).
- Assess the circulation: look for pallor, cold limbs, weak or absent pulses, poor capillary refill (press on the fingers and see how quickly the colour returns) and tachycardia (don't rely on the blood pressure: in young children this may be initially maintained even in the presence of significant hypovolaemia).
- Assess oxygenation (is the face or tongue blue?).

In more advanced states of collapse commence cardiopulmonary resuscitation. The term ABC is a useful reminder of not only the manoeuvres required (Airway, Breathing, Circulation) but also the correct sequence in which to apply them.

Airway

If conscious, the child will usually adopt the best posture to maintain his or her own airway: don't force the child to lie down.

An unconscious child should be placed on the side: this improves the size of the airway (gravity pulls the jaw and tongue forward), allows saliva and other secretions to drain from the mouth and reduces the risk of aspiration of gastric contents should they be regurgitated. Moving the child in this way may be harmful if there is a possibility of cervical spine injury (e.g. following road trauma); in this case, work to obtain an optimal airway in the existing position without excessive rotation, flexion or extension of the neck.

Assess the adequacy of the airway by observing the degree of chest movement and by listening and feeling for breath at the mouth (place your ear close to the child's mouth).

Sometimes the airway may be further improved by extending the neck to the neutral, or slightly extended, position, and supporting the jaw in a forward position (Fig. 20.1). This may be done by placing your fingers behind the angle of the mandible and applying gentle forward pressure. If secretions, gastric contents or food might be obstructing the airway suck them out, preferably with a wide bore rigid sucker. If the airway is still not optimal then an oropharyngeal airway device may be tried. It must be of the correct size, and appropriately inserted. If too large, it may increase airway obstruction and induce laryngospasm; it may also stimulate vomiting if the patient is partially conscious. The best size may be approximated by laying the airway beside the face: select a size that reaches from the front teeth to the angle of the mandible.

If it is not possible to secure an adequate airway by these means then endotracheal intubation will be required (see below).

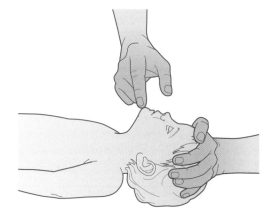

Fig. 20.1 Optimal head and neck position for airway protection in an infant. Do not overextend the neck. This head and neck position may be used with the child on its side or lying on its back.

Breathing

Once you are sure that the airway is patent, assess the adequacy of breathing: look at the rise and fall of the chest and the rate of breathing. If strong breathing movements are present but they appear obstructed (with poor chest expansion and indrawing of the soft tissues) then recheck the airway. If breathing remains inadequate or you are uncertain, commence artificial respiration. Do not delay, as ongoing hypoxaemia and hypercarbia are dangerous to a child whose brain is already compromised by the primary problem.

Artificial respiration may be given to assist existing breathing efforts or as the sole source of respiration. If you are assisting the patient's existing but inadequate breathing efforts, you should attempt to synchronise artificial breaths with any taken by the patient. Additional breaths may also be required.

Respiratory support may take various forms: expired-air breathing, bag and facemask breathing; or endotracheal intubation and mechanical ventilation by machine or bag. The choice will depend on the state of the child, the availability of equipment and your experience. If inexperienced with endotracheal intubation, do not attempt this unless it is not possible to provide adequate respiration by other means (this is unusual in children). Appropriate sizes of endotracheal tube are given in Table 20.2 (see Appendix).

Ideally, any collapsed child should receive high concentrations of inspired oxygen. This may be by simple facemask or through the circuit of the resuscitating bag; there is no indication for using restricted concentrations of oxygen when resuscitating a child.

In children less than 1 year of age, expired air resuscitation should be administered with the rescuer's mouth covering the entire mouth and nose of the infant, in older children, mouth to mouth respiration is used, as for adults.

Facemask and bag resuscitation may be performed with a variety of systems. Those with self-inflating bags are easiest to use. Choose a facemask that provides a good seal around the child's mouth and nose.

Five breaths should be administered initially. Assess their effectiveness by watching the chest move. Ensure the administered breaths are of sufficient volume, but try not to blow excessively hard as this can lead to gastric distension. If there is no adequate chest movement, try re-establishing the airway as described above. After five breaths, move on to assess the circulation, but quickly return to artificial breathing unless adequate spontaneous respiration has commenced.

Circulation

The circulation is inadequate if:
- no central pulses (e.g. carotid or femoral) are palpable
- the heart rate is less than 60 in a collapsed child, or
- the pulses are very weak, with other signs of poor tissue perfusion (pallor, coldness, poor capillary refill).

Cardiac compression is indicated for a child with no pulses or bradycardia in any setting. In a child with very weak pulse, who has intravenous access already established, the first manoeuvre may be a trial of rapid infusion

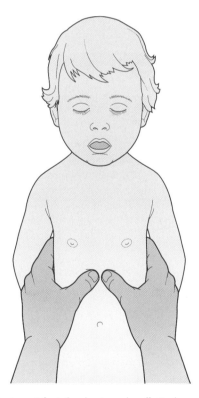

Fig. 20.2 In an infant, the chest may be effectively compressed by encircling the chest with your hands, with the thumbs over the lower sternum. This technique is not very suitable for solo rescuers as it is time consuming to re-establish the position after administering a breath; in this situation compress the chest with two fingers of one hand over the lower sternum.

of a fluid bolus (see below), but in any other setting, or if this fails to rapidly restore the circulation, then cardiac compression is indicated. If in doubt, commence compressions — you will be unlikely to do any harm.

The optimal technique for chest compression varies with age:

- *Infant.* Encircle the chest with the hands, with the thumbs over the lower sternum (Fig. 20.2). This technique is not very suitable for solo rescuers as it is time consuming to re-establish the position after administering a breath; in this situation compress the chest with two fingers of one hand over the lower sternum.
- *Small child.* Use the heel of one hand, centred one fingerbreadth above the xiphisternum.
- *Larger child.* Use the heels of both hands (one atop the other), centred two fingerbreadths above the xiphisternum.

For children of all sizes, the chest should be compressed around 100 times/minute, depressing the anterior chest wall about one third of the anteroposterior diameter.

Any child who requires chest compressions will also require artificial respiratory support; the converse is not always true. Chest compression and artificial respiration should be given at a ratio of approximately 5:1, with resumption of chest compressions towards the end of the child's expiration.

Fluid administration

Hypovolaemia is commonly an important factor in a collapsed child. Rapid infusion of a fluid bolus should be tried in any patient with signs of an inadequate circulation. Again, if in doubt go ahead and give some fluid: you are unlikely to do any harm and you can assess the effects on the patient's circulation. Initial boluses of 10–20 ml/kg are appropriate; these may be repeated as necessary. Normal saline is usually used, but colloid solutions such as 5% albumin may also be used. Avoid hypotonic fluids, such as dextrose solutions with low concentrations of sodium.

Vascular access

A collapsed child will need vascular access for the administration of fluids and drugs.

Cannulation of a peripheral vein will provide adequate initial access. Try to place a large cannula if possible; or more than one cannula, particularly if you suspect the collapse is related to haemorrhage.

Cannulation of a peripheral vein can be very difficult in a collapsed child: do not waste time trying for more than a few minutes. Central venous catheterisation is an option but can be very difficult in this setting, even for experienced operators; it also takes a significant amount

of time. A better alternative is the insertion of an intraosseous needle, whereby a needle is inserted into the bone marrow (which is a vascular space that cannot collapse because of the surrounding bone cortex). This technique is simple, quick and provides access for the administration of fluids and drugs that will reach the central circulation as quickly as if administered into a peripheral vein.

Commercially available intraosseous needles that include a stylet and handle are most commonly used, but a wide bore lumbar puncture needle is a satisfactory alternative. With the stylet in place, insert the needle through the skin, perpendicular to the surface of the bone in all directions. Local anaesthesia is not required unless the patient is conscious. Twist the needle back and forth along its long axis while firmly pushing it into the bone. Do not rock it from side to side. A 'give' is usually felt as the needle tip enters the marrow cavity. Once you feel this, or once the needle has been inserted a centimetre or two into the bone, remove the stylet and aspirate the needle with a small syringe. Aspiration of dark blood-like fluid confirms you are in the correct spot. Commercially available needles usually come with a plastic fixation device. If using a lumbar puncture needle, you can fashion a suitable fixation from plaster of Paris. The aim is for the needle to be well supported, to prevent it being dislodged and to prevent sideways movement and enlargement of the entry hole in the bone. Administration of fluid may require pressure on the infusion bag or the use of a syringe and 3-way tap.

Appropriate sites for intraosseous needle insertion include:

- the distal tibia (the medial aspect where the shaft of the tibia meets the malleolus; Fig. 20.3)
- the proximal tibia, about 1/3 of the way down from the knee to the ankle (on the flat part of the anteromedial aspect of the tibial shaft)
- the anterior iliac crest.

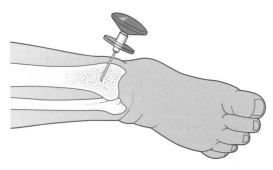

Fig. 20.3 Insertion of a needle into the bone marrow at the distal end of the tibia. The black handle facilitates the twisting motion and application of steady pressure as the needle is inserted. The handle, along with the attached stylet, is removed once the needle is in place.

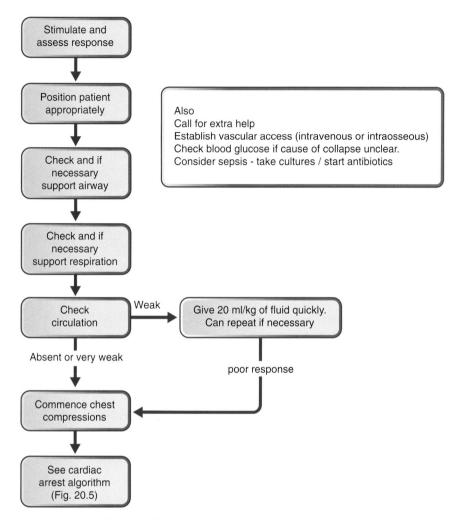

Fig. 20.4 Emergency management of severe collapse.

The tibia is most suitable for children under 5 years of age.

Putting it all together

The general approach to a collapsed child and the management of established paediatric cardiac arrest are summarised in Figures 20.4 and 20.5.

Ongoing resuscitation

In babies and young children, it is important to try to prevent excessive heat loss during resuscitation by the use of clothing, blankets or overhead heaters if available.

If the child has persistently poor circulation despite the presence of sinus rhythm, and after 40–60 ml/kg of intravenous fluid have been given, look for causes of hidden bleeding (especially abdomen, chest and fractured femur); also consider the use of an inotropic infusion such as dobutamine (10 μ/kg/min — put 15 mg/kg of the drug into 50 ml of saline and run at 2 ml/h).

If the child is successfully resuscitated, careful ongoing monitoring will be required. It is a mistake to terminate intubation and mechanical ventilation too soon. Ensuing brain swelling may lead to a secondary deterioration.

It is important to know when to stop if resuscitation efforts are producing no effect. Except in cases of extreme hypothermia, as occur in drowning in near freezing water, persisting cardiac arrest after 20–30 minutes of good resuscitation is an indication of a hopeless prognosis. When hypoxia or hypovolaemia have resulted in cardiac arrest with asystole, particularly in an out of hospital setting, the prognosis for recovery or survival is very poor.

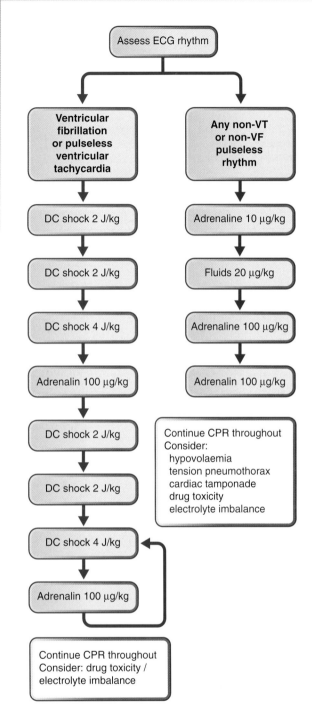

Assess ECG rhythm

Ventricular fibrillation or pulseless ventricular tachycardia

Any non-VT or non-VF pulseless rhythm

DC shock 2 J/kg

Adrenaline 10 µg/kg

DC shock 2 J/kg

Fluids 20 µg/kg

DC shock 4 J/kg

Adrenaline 100 µg/kg

Adrenalin 100 µg/kg

Adrenaline 100 µg/kg

DC shock 2 J/kg

Continue CPR throughout
Consider:
   hypovolaemia
   tension pneumothorax
   cardiac tamponade
   drug toxicity
   electrolyte imbalance

DC shock 2 J/kg

DC shock 4 J/kg

Adrenalin 100 µg/kg

Continue CPR throughout
Consider: drug toxicity /
electrolyte imbalance

Fig. 20.5 *Management of cardiac arrest.*

Key learning points

- Learn the basics of paediatric life support before you need them — you won't have time to consult a text-book in an emergency.
- Learn the technique of intraosseous needle placement — this simple technique can be life saving.
- Never hesitate to give oxygen to a collapsed child.
- Never hesitate to give a trial of an intravenous fluid bolus to a collapsed child.
- Never hesitate to call for extra assistance.

Appendix

Resuscitation guide A

Table 20.2 provides a summary of acceptable physiological parameters for children according to age, along with endotracheal tube sizes, DC shocks, and doses of adrenaline used in resuscitation. This table can be photo-copied (or downloaded and printed from the internet at http://www.rch.unimelb.edu.au/clinicalguide/pages/resus.php. (select 'ID badge size Resuscitation Card'). If folded horizontally at the centre, it can be laminated and punched to attach conveniently to a hospital ID badge, so making it readily available for reference in the clinical setting.

Resuscitation guide B

Another useful aid to resuscitation can be downloaded from the internet at http://www.rch.unimelb.edu.au/clinicalguide/pages/resus.php. (select 'emergency drug and fluid calculator'). It will run as a utility with any recent internet browser (such as Internet Explorer or Netscape). It produces a table of appropriate drug doses, DC shocks, and endotracheal tube sizes according to the age and weight of the patient.

Table 20.2 Resuscitation Card

		Normal values					Resuscitation			
AGE	Wt	Min sys BP	HR	RR	Adren 1st - mls 1:10,000	Adren 2nd - mls 1:1000	ETT	DC 1st joules	DC subseq joules	Fluid Bolus (saline)
Prem	2.5	40	120-170	40-60	0.3	0.3	2.5	5	10	50
Term	3.5	50	100-170	40-60	0.4	0.4	3.5	7	14	70
3m	6	50	100-170	30-50	0.6	0.6	3.5	10	20	120
6m	8	60	100-170	30-50	0.8	0.8	4.0	20	30	160
1y	10	65	100-170	30-40	1.0	1.0	4.0	20	50	260
2y	13	65	100-160	20-30	1.5	1.5	4.5	30	50	260
4y	15	70	80-130	20	1.5	1.5	5.0	30	70	300
6y	20	75	70-115	16	2.0	2.0	5.5	50	70	400
8y	25	80	70-110	16	2.5	2.5	6.0	50	100	500
10y	30	85	60-105	16	3.0	3.0	6.5	70	150	600
12y	40	90	60-100	16	4.0	4.0	7.0	100	150	800
14y	50	90	60-100	16	5.0	5.0	7.5	150	250	1000
17y	70	90	60-100	16	10	10	9.0	150	300	1000

1st dose adren: 10mcg/kg - 0.1ml/kg of 1:10,000
2nd dose adren: 100mcg/kg - 0.1ml/kg of 1:1,000

RECOGNITION OF THE SERIOUSLY ILL CHILD

Features of a seriously ill child are:

AIRWAY and BREATHING - look at trends
- Tachypnoea (see table over)
- Recession, grunting, accessory muscle use
- Low O_2 saturation in air

CIRCULATION - look at trends
- Tachycardia (see table over)
- Increasing systolic-diastolic BP gap
- Low systolic blood pressure (see table over)
- Poor peripheral perfusion (capillary refill time)

CONSCIOUS STATE
- Alteration in conscious state - confusion

FLUIDS IN AND OUT
Consult fluid balance chart re excess losses, gains and trends.

PAEDIATRIC ARREST MANAGEMENT

Call for help

AIRWAY
- Airway opening manoeuvres chin lift, jaw thrust

BREATHING
- Look, listen, feel ?breathing
- Apply 100% O_2 via facial mask or face mask ventilation

CIRCULATION
- Assess pulse
  PULSE Yes Fluids (20mls/kg)
         No   cardiac compressions

- Attach defib-monitor
- IV / IO access

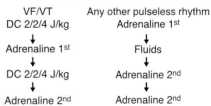

VF/VT	Any other pulseless rhythm
DC 2/2/4 J/kg	Adrenaline 1st
↓	↓
Adrenaline 1st	Fluids
↓	↓
DC 2/2/4 J/kg	Adrenaline 2nd
↓	↓
Adrenaline 2nd	Adrenaline 2nd

Poisoning and envenomation

J. Tibballs

Poisoning and envenomation are two important areas of emergency care that should be familiar to any health practitioner involved with acute care of children and young people.

Poisoning

Poisoning is a common health problem among children. In children's hospitals it is responsible for numerous attendances to casualty and emergency departments: over 3500 children aged 0–4 years are admitted annually to Australian hospitals as a result of poisoning incidents. Worldwide, poisoning is the third most common cause of death among young children. A great deal of effort is expended upon a problem which is largely preventable. A Poisons Information Centre serving a population of 5 million receives approximately 40 000–50 000 telephone inquiries per annum; two thirds concern actual poisoning and, of those, 60–70% concern children aged 4 years and younger.

Epidemiology

The nature of poisoning varies for different age groups in children. Although poisoning in childhood is usually unintentional, the possibility of deliberate poisoning in the younger child as part of child abuse should not be forgotten. Pharmaceutical substances are involved in 70% of poisonings.

Newborns

Poisoning almost always is iatrogenic in this age group. For example, newborns are at risk at delivery, when they may be given ergometrine instead of vitamin K, causing severe hypertension, convulsions and coagulopathy. In intensive care units, the frequent use of potent cardiovascular drugs, chloramphenicol, gentamicin, barbiturates, phenytoin, theophylline, digoxin and opiates predispose the infant to poisoning.

It is not acceptable to perform noxious procedures without analgesia and sedation, and it is commendable that opiates are used in the newborn, but great care should be taken to ensure that overdose does not cause cardiorespiratory failure. Repeated doses or infusions of opiates should be confined to newborns who are mechan-

ically ventilated, and, wherever possible, local or regional anaesthesia should be employed for surgical procedures. Local anaesthetic agents or opiates administered to the mother during labour may poison the newborn.

Care should be exercised with the use of topical antiseptics. Mercurochrome, commonly applied to the umbilical stump, may cause mercury poisoning if used in excess. Hexachlorophane should not be used as a regular bathing solution because it is readily absorbed percutaneously, causing neurotoxicity. If used in excess, iodinated compounds may cause hypothyroidism. Occasionally, mistakes in the preparation of artificial foods may cause serum electrolyte disorders and dehydration.

Age 1–5 years

Poisoning occurs most frequently in this age group. Most instances are said to be accidental, in which the young child discovers a drug or a household cleaning or chemical agent. The majority of serious poisonings occur with prescribed drugs or with over the counter drugs. Parents are often unaware that drugs must be stored safely and they underestimate the capabilities of young children who, at this age, become increasingly mobile and curious. They eat substances that are not palatable to adults, and tablets and capsules which resemble lollies.

The incidence and severity of accidental poisoning from drugs has been reduced markedly by the use of blister packs and bottles with childproof lids. Poisoning in the home often occurs between 10 a.m. and noon and between 6 p.m. and 8 p.m. when the child is active or hungry and when supervision has lapsed because the parent is involved in other household activities.

Clinical example

Simon, a 15 month old toddler, was noted by his mother to be irritable, drooling saliva and have inflamed lips after tasting the residue of the powder in their automatic dishwasher door. On examination, oropharyngeal ulceration was observed. An intravenous cannula was inserted for fluid and nutrition therapy and an endoscopy of the upper gastrointestinal tract was performed. Significant burns to the mid oesophagus were discovered; these healed with stricture formation, necessitating repeated dilatation with bougies.

Age 6–12 years

Poisoning is relatively uncommon in this age group but it may be truly accidental, such as drinking a poison from a bottle which has been labelled wrongly, or when toxic agents have been stored inappropriately. A common example is storage of potentially toxic liquids in soft drink containers in garden sheds. Although uncommon, self-poisoning in this age group may occur as drug abuse or manipulative behaviour.

Age 13–17 years

Emotionally disturbed adolescents and young adults may poison themselves deliberately, usually by ingestion, to manipulate their environment, or they may harbour a genuine suicidal intent. They may seek the thrill of drug abuse by inhalation or injection, sometimes as group behaviour. The peak incidence of poisoning is at 14–16 years of age. Repeated episodes occur more frequently among girls but boys' suicide attempts tend to be more successful.

Management

The immediate aim in the management of poisoning, whether serious or not, is to attend to the effects of the poison on the patient. Later, attention should be given to the circumstances with the aim of preventing a recurrence. There are innumerable poisons. All medicines and many household substances are poisonous if taken in sufficient quantity. Upon presentation, the action to be taken, if any, will be determined by the substance involved, its amount, the interval between ingestion and presentation, and the effect of the poison. The following principles of management may be applied universally.

Support vital functions

It is imperative to maintain and support vital functions if these are depressed. Many poisons are excreted adequately or metabolised by the body if the vital functions are maintained. If the patient is unconscious, the airway, the depth and frequency of breathing and the circulation should be examined for adequacy. Chapter 20 provides a full discussion on the management of deficiencies of the airway, breathing and circulation.

Establish the diagnosis

It is important to establish:
- what poisons are involved
- in what quantity
- when exposure occurred.

Often the diagnosis of poisoning is self-evident, but at times the diagnosis is not obvious. When a poison has been identified, it should never be assumed that other poisons could not be involved. The symptoms and signs of poisoning are diverse but dangerous drugs threaten vital functions. Seriously poisoned patients present commonly with:
- unconsciousness
- cardiorespiratory failure, or
- convulsions.

If any of these are present and the cause is otherwise not known, poisoning should be high on the list of differential diagnoses. A meticulous physical examination and history provides invaluable help in diagnosis and treatment. Laboratory investigations may be necessary to establish a diagnosis, determine the amount of poison in the body and help determine specific treatment for certain poisons.

Clinical example

Amanda, a 3 year old girl, was brought to the emergency department by her parents. Two hours previously she had been perfectly well when they were visiting friends, but since that time had become progressively drowsy and was unconscious on presentation. On examination, her respiration was shallow and her blood pressure was low. No signs of external trauma or infection were obvious. Mechanical ventilation, intravascular volume support and vasopressor therapy were necessary. In spite of the parents' denial of drug ingestion, a high level of amylobarbitone was discovered in her urine and the next day it was revealed that an opened bottle of tablets was found in their friends' house. She recovered completely.

Prevent absorption

Some poisons contaminate the skin, conjunctivae and mucous membranes and other poisons are inhaled as gases. Surface contamination requires copious irrigation with water, while inhalational poisoning may require oxygen therapy and mechanical ventilation. The great majority of poisons are ingested, for which the options for therapy include induced emesis, oral or gastric administration of activated charcoal, gastric lavage and whole bowel irrigation. If the poison has been absorbed already and has reached the vascular compartment, invasive techniques such as:
- plasmapheresis
- plasmafiltration
- haemofiltration
- charcoal haemoperfusion
- haemodialysis
- peritoneal dialysis
- exchange transfusion

may be required.

The treatment of the poisoned patient is determined by the poison, its amount and the seriousness of its effects. These must be weighed against the hazards of removal. Unconscious or drowsy patients or patients who cannot protect their own airway should not undergo induced emesis or gastric lavage or be given activated charcoal or colonic washout solutions. The consequences of aspirating gastric contents during vomiting or regurgitation in a less than fully conscious state far outweigh the dangers of many untreated poisons, as the mortality from severe pneumonitis is approximately 50%. However, it is appropriate to remove a wide variety of ingested poisons with either:

- induced emesis, or
- activated charcoal, or
- whole bowel irrigation, or
- gastric lavage, or
- a combination of these techniques.

Circumstances of presentation and ingestion dictate the choice of technique. To be effective, emesis must be induced within 1 hour of ingestion and is probably most appropriate as a first aid therapy at home.

Activated charcoal is probably the most appropriate therapy in the emergency or casualty department, although whole bowel irrigation may be preferable. Gastric lavage should be reserved for a recent (within 1 hour) serious life threatening ingestion in a conscious patient or for serious poisoning in a less than fully conscious patient who has airway protection. The circumstances for the employment of each technique are summarised in Figure 21.1.

Induced emesis

If induced emesis is indicated, ipecacuanha is used for this purpose. The dose of the syrup according to age is given in Table 21.1. Usually it is administered with a glass of water. The alkaloid content of ipecac irritates the gastric mucosa and stimulates the brainstem chemoreceptor trigger zone. Vomiting in the majority of children is induced within 20–30 minutes. This delay may permit the poison to be absorbed and to produce toxic effects, such as loss of consciousness, which exposes the patient to the risk of aspiration pneumonitis when vomiting does occur. The efficacy of ipecacuanha for removing poison from the stomach is good when administered within 1 hour of ingestion. Complications are infrequent but have been reported as protracted vomiting, oesophageal tears and gastrointestinal haemorrhage. Cardiac toxicity may occur with overdose.

Activated charcoal

Activated charcoal is itself not absorbable but it adsorbs many different poisons in the gastrointestinal tract and thus prevents absorption of poison into the circulation. However, activated charcoal does not adsorb some poisons, including some elemental metals, some pesticides, ferrous sulphate, ethanol, corrosives and petro-

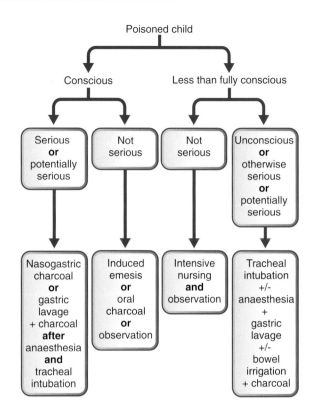

Fig. 21.1 Management of poisoning. Modified from Tibballs J 2000 Poisoning and envenomation. In: Smart J, Nolan T (eds) Royal Children's Hospital Paediatric Handbook. Blackwell Science, Carlton.

chemicals. There are many different preparations of activated charcoal, some with sorbitol as a laxative, but with these excessive diarrhoea and hypernatraemic dehydration may result.

To be effective, activated charcoal should be administered within 1 hour of ingestion by mouth or by a nasogastric tube in a fully conscious patient, or by gastric tube in a less than fully conscious patient after the airway has been secured with an endotracheal tube. The dose of activated charcoal is 10 times the ingested poison by weight or 1–2 g/kg followed by 0.25 g/kg 4–6 hourly. An alternative dosage regimen is 0.25 g/kg hourly for 12–24 hours. Continued or repeated doses of activated charcoal are useful if the poison is in a sustained release preparation or if the charcoal is known to increase the total body

Table 21.1 Dose of ipecacuanha syrup (Australian Pharmaceutical Formulary)	
Age (years)	Liquid extract 6% (ml)
1–2	15
2–3	20
3–4	25
> 4	30

clearance of the poison by interruption of its entero-hepatic circulation or by leaching it from the circulation of the gastrointestinal mucosa. It should not be administered if gastrointestinal ileus is present as this may cause regurgitation. Aspiration of activated charcoal may have a fatal outcome.

Activated charcoal is often administered, probably unnecessarily, with a laxative, notably magnesium sulphate, to prevent constipation. If magnesium sulphate is used, care should be taken to avoid hypermagnesaemia, a potential risk with repeated doses. Activated charcoal does not adsorb ipecacuanha and thus there is nothing to be gained by administering it to the patient whose induced emesis is excessive.

Gastric lavage

This is an invasive procedure and is justified only for significant recent poisoning when other techniques are contraindicated or are unreliable. It may also be indicated when the poison delays gastric emptying or forms concretions in the stomach. To be effective, however, it must be performed well and care taken to prevent complications. It should never be performed in a less than fully conscious patient unless the airway is protected by prior endotracheal intubation. Loss of consciousness due to poisoning may be associated with cardiorespiratory failure. Endotracheal intubation in this situation should be performed only by those experienced in the techniques of rapid intubation and resuscitation.

Gastric lavage should not be performed after the ingestion of a corrosive substance because additional damage to the oesophagus (perforation, mediastinitis) and stomach (perforation) may occur. It is also unwise to perform gastric lavage after ingestion of petrochemicals or hydrocarbons as these substances have very low surface tensions and cause severe pneumonitis, even after minor contamination of the oropharynx, which may occur after the passage of the lavage tube renders the gastro-oesophageal sphincter incompetent. The risk of causing or exacerbating chemical pneumonitis exceeds the benefit of poison removal despite the depression of central nervous system function which may follow. Such patients recover if vital functions are preserved.

Gastric lavage potentially is a traumatic procedure, particularly to the oropharynx, even when indicated. Occasionally the oesophagus and stomach have been perforated. It is psychologically as well as physically traumatic. For physical safety, the child must be restrained: this is best achieved by wrapping the child in a sheet with the arms pinned by the side. The child must be held in a lateral head down position. For gastric lavage to be performed well, safely and atraumatically in a small child, it should be preceded by induction of general anaesthesia with endotracheal intubation.

An indication for gastric lavage would be the recent ingestion of a large amount of paracetamol by a young child. This could be followed by intravenous antidote (*N*-acetylsteine) according to serum levels of paracetamol. In the older, more cooperative child, it would be reasonable to manage this poisoning with oral or nasogastric activated charcoal or whole bowel irrigation with intravenous antidote.

Before commencing gastric lavage, apparatus for oxygen delivery and resuscitation equipment must be functional and ready immediately to hand. Pulse oximetry and ECG monitoring are recommended. A gastric tube, lubricated and of sufficient size (approximated by the child's little finger or appropriate endotracheal tube), is passed by the oral or nasal route. Before instilling lavage fluid, however, the tube must be confirmed to be in the stomach and not in the lungs or oesophagus. This is proven by the aspiration of gastric contents or by performing an X ray. Less reliable evidence of correct positioning is a gurgling sound of air entering the stomach, heard over the anterior abdominal wall on administration of a bolus of air by syringe. Fogging of the proximal end of the tube or coughing suggests that it is in the airways, which can be proven by the wafting of a piece of cotton wool held at the orifice.

Lavage can be performed with tap water, provided that most of it is retrieved to prevent hyponatraemia and convulsions. The water should be warmed to body temperature to prevent hypothermia. The volume instilled should be 50–100 ml and should be removed by aspiration or gravity. This process should be repeated until the return is clear. The first return should be saved for analysis and the total volume instilled and retrieved recorded.

Whole bowel irrigation

This is an effective technique to limit absorption of a poison. It is the preferred technique when the poison has passed beyond the pylorus and therefore cannot be removed by induced emesis or gastric lavage. It is useful also when the substance is a drug or substance not adsorbed by activated charcoal. In the latter category are foreign bodies such as miniature disc batteries. Slow release drug preparations may also be removed with this technique.

The agent used is a mixture of polyethylene glycol and electrolytes that flushes out the contents of the bowel without disturbing the serum volume, osmolality or electrolytes. It is administered via nasogastric tube at a rate of 30 ml/kg/h for 4–8 hours until the rectal effluent is clear. It should not be administered to a less than fully conscious patient or when gastrointestinal ileus is present. Concomitant administration of activated charcoal is counterproductive.

Removal from the circulation

If the poison reaches the circulation, an invasive extracorporeal technique may be necessary to achieve removal. Usual techniques include haemodialysis, plasmapheresis and charcoal haemoperfusion. These techniques are usually reserved for recognised circumstances when there is deterioration of vital functions despite maximal therapy (mechanical ventilation, inotropic/vasopressor therapy and artificial renal therapy) or the lack or failure of an adequate excretory or metabolic pathway (renal, hepatic) to eliminate the poison. For these techniques to be effective, however, the poison must have a relatively small volume of distribution. Peritoneal dialysis is not an efficient technique to remove poisons from the blood. Occasionally, the small size of a patient and the properties of a poison permit its removal by exchange blood transfusion.

Administer an antidote

Only relatively few poisons have antidotes but knowledge and use of these can be life saving. The appropriate dose of each is determined by the amount of poison and its effects. A list of common important antidotes is given in Table 21.2 (see also Further Reading).

Table 21.2   Antidotes to some serious poisons

Poison	Antidotes	Comments
Amphetamines	Esmolol i.v. 500 μg/kg over 1 min, then 25–200 μg/kg/min	Treatment for tachyarrhythmia
	Labetalol i.v. 0.15–0.3 mg/kg or phentolamine i.v. 0.05–0.1 mg/kg every 10 min	Treatment for hypertension
Benzodiazepines	Flumazenil i.v. 3–10 μg/kg, repeat 1 min, then 3–10 μg/kg/h	Specific receptor antagonist. Beware convulsions
Beta blockers	Glucagon i.v. 7 μg/kg, then 2–7 μg/kg/min	Stimulates non catecholamine cAMP, preferred antidote
	Isoprenaline i.v. 0.05–3 μg/kg/min Noradrenaline i.v. 0.05–1 μg/kg/min	Beware β_2 hypotension
Calcium channel blocker	Calcium chloride i.v. 10%, 0.2 ml/kg	
Carbon monoxide	Oxygen 100%	Decreases carboxyhaemoglobin. May need hyperbaric oxygen
Cyanide	Dicobaltedetate i.v. 300 mg over 1 min, then 300 mg at 5 min.	Give 50 mL 50% glucose after each dose
	Sodium nitrite 3% i.v. 0.33 ml/kg over 4 min, then sodium thiosulphate 25% i.v. 1.65 ml/kg (max 50 ml) at 3–5 min	Nitrites form methaemoglobin–cyanide complex. Beware excess methaemoglobin >20%. Thiosulphate forms non toxic thiocyanate from methaemoglobin–cyanide
Digoxin	Magnesium sulphate i.v. 25–50 mg/kg (0.1–0.2 mmol/kg) Digoxin Fab i.v: acute — 10 vials per 25 tablets (0.25 mg each), 10 vials per 5 mg elixir; steady state — vials = serum digoxin (ng/ml) $\times$ BW(kg)/100	
Ergotamine	Sodium nitroprusside infusion 0.5–5.0 μg/kg/min Heparin i.v. 100 units/kg then 10–30 units/kg/h	Treats vasoconstriction. Monitor BP continuously Monitor partial thromboplastin time
Heparin	Protamine 1 mg/100 units heparin	
Iron	Desferrioxamine 15 mg/kg/h 12–24 h if serum iron >90 μmol/l or >63 μmol/l and symptomatic	Give slowly, beware anaphylaxis
Lead	Dimercaprol (BAL) i.m. 75 mg/m^2 4 hourly 6 doses then i.v. CaNa$_2$ edetate (EDTA) 1500 mg/m^2 over 5 days if blood level >3.38 μmol/l. If asymptomatic and blood level 2.65–3.3 μmol/l infuse CaNa$_2$ EDTA 1000 mg/m^2/day 5 days or oral succimer 350 mg/m^2 8 hourly 5 days, then 12 hourly 14 days	

Table 21.2 (Continued)

Poison	Antidotes	Comments
Methaemoglobinaemia	Methylene blue i.v. 1–2 mg/kg over several min	
Methanol, ethylene glycol, glycol ethers	Ethanol i.v. loading dose 10 ml/kg 10% diluted in glucose 5%, then 0.15 ml/kg/h to maintain blood level 0.1% (100 mg/dl)	
Opiates	Naloxone i.v. 0.01–0.1 mg/kg, then 0.01 mg/kg/h as needed	
Organophosphates and carbamates	Atropine i.v. 20–50 µg/kg every 15 min until secretions dry	Blocks muscarinic effects
	Pralidoxime i.v. 25 mg/kg over 15–30 min then 10–20 mg/kg/h for 18 h or more. Not for carbamates	Reactivates cholinesterase
Paracetamol	N-acetylcysteine i.v. 150 mg/kg over 60 min then 10 mg/kg/h for 20–72 h or oral 140 mg/kg then 17 doses of 70 mg/kg 4 hourly (total 1330 mg/kg over 68 h)	Restores glutathione, inhibits metabolites. Give within 18 h according to serum paracetamol
Phenothiazine dystonia	Benztropine i.v or i.m. 0.01–0.03 mg/kg	Blocks dopamine reuptake
Potassium	Calcium chloride 10% i.v. 0.2 ml/kg	Antagonises cardiac effects
	Sodium bicarbonate i.v. 1 mmol/kg	Decreases serum potassium; beware hypocalcaemia
	Glucose i.v. 0.5 g/kg plus insulin i.v. 0.05 units/kg	Decreases serum potassium. Monitor serum glucose
	Salbutamol aerosol 0.25 mg/kg	Decreases serum potassium
	Resonium oral or rectal 0.5–1 g/kg	Absorbs potassium
Tricyclic antidepressants	Sodium bicarbonate i.v. 1 mmol/kg to maintain blood pH>7.45	Reduces cardiotoxicity

Recognition of poisons

There are literally thousands of poisons and no one person can be expected to be familiar with them all. However, it is vital to recognise that any substance which has effects, or side effects, on the central nervous system, cardiovascular system and the respiratory system is a potential serious poison. It is prudent to be familiar with serious poisons that are ingested commonly (Table 21.3) and those that have delayed actions, such as colchicine, paracetamol and paraquat. The content of unfamiliar proprietary preparations should be sought as effects may not be obvious from common usage. For example, the antidiarrhoeal drug Lomotil contains atropine and the opiate diphenoxylate, which may cause respiratory depression. Swallowed disc or 'button batteries' which impact in the gastrointestinal tract may cause ulceration into surrounding structures (trachea, aorta), whether by release of corrosive chemicals or by electrical activity, and may cause mercury poisoning when corroded by gastric acid.

It is important to have access to a Poisons Information Centre by telephone, facsimile machine or electronic mail. These centres maintain a vast store of up to date information and are usually accessible on a 24 hour basis.

Table 21.3   Common lethal/serious poisons and substances

Antihistamines	Hydrochloric acid (spirit of
Aspirin	salts)
Barbiturates	Iron
Carbamazepine	Major tranquillisers
Carbon monoxide	Opiates
Caustic soda	Paracetamol
Chloral hydrate	Theophylline
Digoxin	Tricyclic antidepressants
Disc batteries	Verapamil
Dishwashing powder	Volatile substances

In rural areas/developing countries: paraquat, chloroquine, organophosphate insecticides

While Poison Information Centres provide an invaluable service, the management of the poisoned patient is the responsibility of the treating physician.

Prevention

Too many poisonings are so called 'accidents', particularly among young children. Every opportunity should be taken to educate parents about the dangers of drugs and toxic substances in the home. A warning should be issued whenever a drug is prescribed and counselling given whenever poisoning occurs. It is erroneous to believe that young children cannot open drawers, cupboards and handbags or gain access to bench tops.

All drugs, however common and easily available, should be stored in a locked childproof cabinet. Out of date drugs should be discarded safely. Household cleaning substances, fuels and garden and workshop chemicals should be stored in truly inaccessible places. This applies particularly to automatic dishwasher powders and detergents and to sink and oven cleaners, all of which are highly caustic and corrosive to the gastrointestinal tract. Corrosive poisoning occurs most often when small children have access to dishwashing powder or its residue in the receptacle of an open automatic dishwasher door.

Older children should be taught at home and at school of the dangers of drug abuse, including those of 'street' and pharmaceutical drugs, and that sniffing glue or hydrocarbons imperils their lives. In the case of self-poisoning by adolescents, the provocation is often the result of complex social and psychological disharmony, making remedial action lengthy and difficult (Ch. 18).

All age groups are subject to iatrogenic poisoning at home and in hospital. Most iatrogenic errors result from mistakes in prescription; that is, the dose of a drug and its interval. It is particularly important for doctors to refer always to a recognised prescription manual for children rather than rely upon memory or extrapolation from adult dosages, especially when dealing with infrequently used potent drugs. Prescriptions must be clearly written and if abbreviations are employed, such as 'ug' or 'mcg' for microgram, they must be universally recognised. If in doubt, longhand printing should be used. Care should be taken with a decimal point. Equally, interpretation of a prescription must be with care, and the preparation checked before administration. All too often in hospitals, wrong drugs and wrong doses are given to the wrong patients.

Envenomation

Australia harbours a wide variety of terrestrial and marine creatures. Of these, those that cause the most frequent or serious envenomation are several species of snakes, spiders and jellyfish (Table 21.4). The reader is referred to the Further Reading list for detailed and extensive information.

Snake bite

Australia has over 100 species of snakes, of which a dozen are among the world's most deadly. The average mortality from snake bite in Australia between 1981 and 1999 was 2.6/annum, approximately equal to the mortality from bee sting anaphylaxis. The species that have caused mortality and significant morbidity belong to the genera of:
- Tiger Snakes (*notechis*)
- Brown Snakes (*Pseudonaja*)
- Death Adders (*Acanthophis*)
- Taipan (*Oxyuranus*)
- Black Snakes (*Pseudechis*)
- Copperhead Snakes (*Austrelaps*)
- Rough Scaled Snakes (*Tropidechis*).

Tiger snakes and Brown snakes account for most envenomations. All Australian snakes are elapids, which have relatively small fangs and whose venoms do not cause severe local effects.

The main components of venoms are:
- pre- and postsynaptic neurotoxins, which cause paralysis
- prothrombin activators, which cause disseminated intravascular coagulation and haemorrhage
- anticoagulants, which cause spontaneous haemorrhage
- rhabdomyolysins, which may cause renal failure
- haemolysins.

Different species have different effects but the two most common acute threats to life are neuromuscular paralysis with respiratory failure and coagulopathy causing bleeding with peripheral circulatory failure (shock).

> ### Clinical example
>
> Mario, a 13 year old boy in previous good health but known to have experimented with drugs, collapsed while in the garage of a friend's house. The parents of the friend found him unconscious and summoned an ambulance, whose officers diagnosed ventricular fibrillation. They attempted to resuscitate him with mechanical ventilation and DC shock but were unsuccessful. External cardiac compression was continued, and on arrival at the hospital's emergency department he was still in refractory ventricular fibrillation. Numerous additional attempts at defibrillation using 4 joules/kg of DC shock administered with lignocaine, amiodarone and adrenaline over 45 minutes failed to achieve sinus rhythm. Eventually asystole occurred. Postmortem blood samples revealed high levels of *n*-butane and isobutane, constituents of cigarette lighter fluid which presumably had been inhaled.

Table 21.4   Effects of Australian venomous animals and their treatments

Animal	Main effects	Main treatments
Snakes (many terrestrial and marine species)	Paralysis (rapid) Haemorrhage	Pressure–immobilisation bandage Antivenom with premedication Endotracheal intubation and mechanical ventilation
Funnelweb Spiders	Paralysis (rapid)	Pressure–immobilisation bandage Antivenom Endotracheal intubation and mechanical ventilation
Redback Spider	Pain Paralysis (slow)	Antivenom
Australian Paralysis Tick	Paralysis (slow)	Remove tick Antivenom
Bees, wasps, ants	Anaphylaxis	Adrenaline
Box Jellyfish	Paralysis Hypotension	Pressure–immobilisation bandage after applying vinegar Antivenom Endotracheal intubation and mechanical ventilation
Blue ringed Octopuses	Paralysis (rapid)	Pressure–immobilisation bandage Endotracheal intubation and mechanical ventilation
Stone fish	Pain	Antivenom

Management

Snakes may bite but fail to inject venom on approximately 40–50% of occasions. In young children, particularly, snake bite is suspected even though a snake was not observed. In only 17–20% of such presentations has both a bite and envenomation occurred. Thus one of the difficulties in the management of snake bite is to determine whether envenomation has actually occurred, irrespective of whether or not a bite by a snake was observed.

The syndrome of envenomation is characterised by a rapid onset of paralysis accompanied by coagulopathy over minutes to several hours. However, an early diagnosis may be dependent upon subtle clinical signs and symptoms, abnormal laboratory tests of coagulation and a positive test for venom in the patient's urine or blood. The early reliable symptoms of envenomation are:
- headache
- abdominal pain
- vomiting.

Abnormal laboratory tests of coagulation are also very sensitive and reliable after bite by a species with coagulopathic effects (Death Adders do not cause serious coagulopathy). The onset of weakness of large muscles, including respiratory muscles, is preceded by weakness of the bulbar muscles, so that it is imperative to enquire and seek evidence of dysfunction of the external ocular muscles (double vision, ophthalmoplegia), facial muscles (ptosis) and the muscles of speech and swallowing (dysphonia, dysphagia).

The clinical diagnosis of envenomation may be confirmed with the snake venom detection kit test (CSL Diagnostics, Australia). This is a rapid three step enzyme immunoassay designed for clinical use. It gives a result in approximately 25 minutes and is capable of detecting venom in a concentration of as little as 10 ng/ml. The test can be applied to a swab of the bite site or to the victim's blood or urine. A positive result does not necessarily identify the snake but it stipulates which antivenom to administer, if clinically indicated.

> **Clinical example**
>
> Martina, a $2\frac{1}{2}$ year old child, collapsed with weakness, shallow respiration and weak pulses soon after playing in long grass where tiger snakes had been observed. Mechanical ventilation was necessary. A test of coagulation revealed prolonged prothrombin and activated partial thromboplastin times, a depleted serum fibrinogen level and a low platelet count. Haematuria and melaena were observed. Venom was detected in the child's urine and blood and from scratch and puncture marks on the child's foot. Eight ampoules of tiger snake antivenom and transfusions of platelets, packed cells and fresh frozen plasma were required before her coagulation status returned to normal. Adequate spontaneous respiration was resumed after 48 hours.

The principles of treatment for snake bite are the following:

- to prevent rapid absorption of the venom from the subcutaneous tissue into the circulation by application of a pressure–immobilisation bandage
- to neutralise the venom by the administration of antivenom
- to treat the effects of the venom, namely respiratory failure and bleeding.

The management of suspected and definite envenomation is summarised in Figure 21.2.

Pressure–immobilisation first aid

Snake venoms gain access from the subcutaneous tissue to the circulation via the lymphatics. These channels can be effectively occluded by the application of a firm crepe (or crepe-like) bandage applied over the bite site and whole of the limb (Fig. 21.3), which sustains 95% of all bites. The application of a splint which includes joints on either side of the bite prevents the use of surrounding muscle groups and hence decreases lymph flow. Although the technique is a first aid measure which should be applied at the scene of the snake bite to prevent initial absorption of venom, it is also used in established envenomation in hospital to prevent additional absorption of venom while preparations are being made to administer antivenom.

The bandage can be left in place indefinitely as it should be no tighter than a bandage for a sprained ankle. However, the bandage does not allow substantial inactivation of venom in the tissues and should be removed after the asymptomatic patient reaches a hospital which has a stock of antivenom or after the envenomated patient has been given antivenom. It is dangerous to remove a bandage from an envenomated patient before administration of antivenom because its release allows a substantial additional quantity of venom to gain rapid access to the

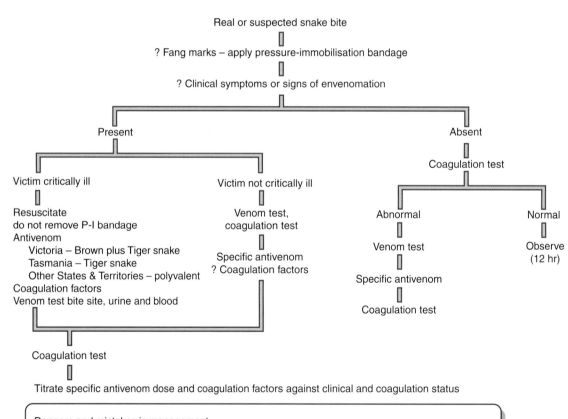

Fig. 21.2 Management of snake bite.

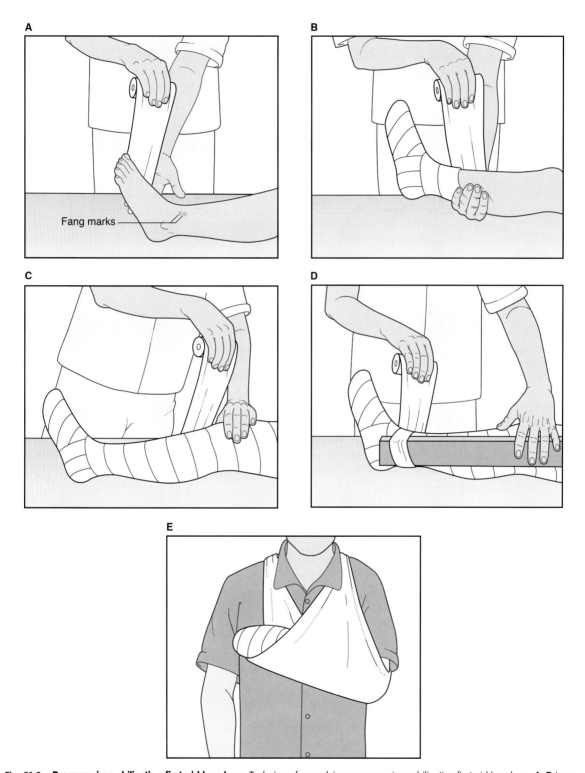

Fang marks (label in panel A)

Fig. 21.3 Pressure–immobilisation first aid bandage. Technique for applying pressure–immobilisation first aid bandage. **A–D** Lower limb; **E** upper limb.

circulation. The splint and bandage should not be removed solely to allow inspection of the bite site of an envenomated patient; instead, the splint should be removed temporarily and a window cut in the bandage to allow a swab of the bite site to be taken for venom testing, then the bandage reinforced and the splint reapplied. Bites are usually visible as scratches or puncture wounds, but not invariably; their presence and appearance or absence does not prove or disprove envenomation and does not allow identification of the snake involved.

Antivenom

Specific monovalent antivenoms (Commonwealth Serum Laboratories Ltd, Melbourne) are manufactured against Tiger, Brown, Taipan, Black, Death Adder and Beaked Sea Snake (*Enhydrina schistosa*) venoms. These are effective against all known snakes in Australia and Papua New Guinea. A mixture of the five terrestrial antivenoms is available as a polyvalent preparation. The antivenoms are highly purified equine immunoglobulins. Crossreactivity between species is limited, so that it is essential to administer the correct antivenom according to the identity of the snake.

If the identity of the snake is not known or uncertain, the type of antivenom to be administered is based on the known geographical snake distribution or according to the result of a venom detection kit test (q.v.). In Tasmania, Australia, where the snakes are (black) Tiger Snakes and Copperheads, the appropriate antivenom is Tiger Snake antivenom. In Victoria, Australia, where the dangerous species are Tiger, Brown, Black and Copperhead Snakes, the appropriate antivenom therapy is Tiger Snake plus Brown Snake antivenom. Everywhere else in Australia additional species exist and the polyvalent preparation should be chosen.

Although essential and life saving, antivenoms are foreign proteins which may cause a life threatening anaphylactoid reaction. However, this may be prevented by premedication with subcutaneous (not intravenous or intramuscular) adrenaline 0.005–0.01mg/kg. Additional protective agents such as a steroid (hydrocortisone) and an antihistamine may be indicated if the patient has a known allergic history. Only one premedication dose of adrenaline is required. The antivenom should be administered intravenously, diluted with a crystalloid solution, over approximately 30 minutes. However, for severe envenomation it may be delivered rapidly. If polyvalent antivenom or multiple doses of monovalent antivenom are required, a course of steroid therapy should be given for several days to prevent serum sickness.

The dose of antivenom is never certain at the beginning of treatment because the amount of venom injected is unknown. Each ampoule of antivenom contains enough to neutralise the average yield from 'milking' — a process whereby venom is collected by inducing a snake to bite a membrane stretched tautly over a vessel. However, the venom injected on biting is highly variable and bites may be multiple. Children are more susceptible than adults because of the larger venom to body mass ratio. The majority of envenomations are treated adequately with 1–3 ampoules but this dose should never be relied upon; many more ampoules are usually required in life threatening envenomations.

Antivenom should not be withheld if indicated, as there is no other satisfactory treatment. Antivenom should be administered either if there are clinical signs or symptoms of envenomation after snake bite, or if in their absence a substantial coagulopathy is present. Occasionally, venom can be detected in the urine but there is no clinical evidence or very mild coagulopathy. In this case antivenom may be withheld, but the patient's clinical and coagulation status should be checked regularly.

Life support

In the severely envenomated patient, endotracheal intubation and mechanical ventilation may be required because of bulbar and respiratory muscle paralysis. If antivenom therapy is delayed, mechanical ventilation may be required for many days.

Coagulopathy may cause massive haemorrhage from mucosal surfaces and subsequent peripheral circulatory failure. Haemorrhage may occur into a vital organ, particularly the brain. It is essential to restore the circulatory volume with blood transfusion and to normalise coagulation with antivenom and coagulation factors (fresh frozen plasma). Antivenom neutralises venom but it does not, per se, restore coagulation. Repeated laboratory tests of coagulation (prothrombin time, activated partial thromboplastin time, serum fibrinogen and fibrin degradation products) or bedside tests of bleeding should be performed repeatedly to determine the need for more antivenom and coagulation factors. The coagulation status is the most sensitive guide to the need for additional antivenom after bite by coagulopathic species.

Spider bite

Several thousand species of spiders exist in Australia. However, only Funnel-web Spiders and Red-back Spiders are known to be potentially lethal or cause significant illness. However, almost all spiders have venom and a few, particularly the White-tailed Spider, may cause severe local injury.

Funnel-web Spider bite

Several species of the genera *Atrax* and *Hadronyche* cause significant illness and are potentially lethal. *A. robustus* (Sydney Funnel-web Spider) is a large aggressive spider which has caused the deaths of more than a dozen people inhabiting an area within an approximate 160 km radius of Sydney, Australia. The male is more dangerous than the female, in contrast to other species, and is inclined to roam after rainfall. In doing so it may enter houses and seek shelter among clothes or bedding and give a painful bite when disturbed.

Bites do not always result in envenomation but envenomation may be rapidly fatal. The early features of the envenomation syndrome include nausea, vomiting, profuse sweating, salivation and abdominal pain. Life threatening features usually are heralded by the appearance of muscle fasciculation at the bite site, which quickly involves distant muscle groups. Hypertension, tachyarrhythmias and vasoconstriction occur. The victim may lapse into coma, develop hypoventilation and have difficulty maintaining an airway free of saliva. Finally, respiratory failure and severe hypotension culminate in hypoxaemia of the brain and heart. The syndrome may develop within several hours but it may be more rapid. Several children have died within 90 minutes of envenomation, and one has died within 15 minutes. The active component in the venom is a polypeptide that stimulates the release of acetylcholine at neuromuscular junctions and catecholamines within the autonomic nervous system.

Treatment consists of the application of a pressure–immobilisation bandage, intravenous administration of antivenom and support of vital functions, which may include artificial airway support and mechanical ventilation. No deaths or serious morbidity have been reported since introduction of the antivenom in the early 1980s.

Red-back Spider bite

This spider is distributed all over Australia and is to be found outdoors in household gardens in suburban and rural areas. Red-back Spider bite is the most common cause for antivenom administration in Australia. The adult female is easily identified. Its body is about 1 cm in size and it has a distinct red or orange dorsal stripe over its abdomen. When disturbed, it gives a pinprick-like bite. The site becomes inflamed and may be surrounded by local swelling. During the following minutes to several hours, severe pain, exacerbated by movement, commences locally and may extend up the limb or radiate elsewhere. The pain may be accompanied by:
- profuse sweating
- headache
- nausea
- vomiting
- abdominal pain
- fever
- hypertension
- paraesthesias
- rashes.

In a small percentage of cases when treatment is delayed, progressive muscle paralysis may occur over many hours and would require mechanical ventilation. Muscle weakness and spasm may persist for months after the bite. Death has not occurred since introduction of an antivenom in the 1950s. If the effects of a bite are minor and confined to the bite site, antivenom may be withheld, but otherwise antivenom should be given intramuscularly, preceded by premedication (see the section on snake bite) to prevent an anaphylactoid reaction. In contrast to a bite from a snake or Funnel-web Spider, a bite from a Red-back Spider is not immediately life threatening. There is no effective first aid but application of a cold pack or ice may relieve the pain.

Jellyfish stings

The most venomous animal in the world is the Box Jellyfish (*Chironex fleckeri*) and related species. It has caused at least 64 deaths in the waters off the north Australian coast. Other unrelated species, notably the 'Irukandji' (*Carukia barnesi*) have caused significant illnesses.

Box Jellyfish

This creature has a cuboid body up to 30 cm in diameter, and numerous tentacles which trail several metres. It is semitransparent and difficult to see by anyone wading or swimming in shallow water. The tentacles are lined with millions of nematocysts which, on contact with skin, discharge a threaded barb which pierces subcutaneous tissue, including small blood vessels. Contact with the tentacles causes severe pain and envenomation which may cause death within several minutes. Death is probably due to both neurotoxic effects causing apnoea and direct cardiotoxicity, although the precise mode of action of the venom is unknown. The skin that sustains the injury may heal with disfiguring scars.

First aid, which must be administered on the beach, consists of dousing the skin with acetic acid (vinegar), which inactivates undischarged nematocysts. Adherent tentacles can then be removed and a pressure–immobilisation bandage applied. Cardiopulmonary resuscitation may be required on the beach. An ovine antivenom is available but prevention is of paramount importance. Water must not be entered when this jellyfish is known to be close inshore. Wet suits, clothing and 'stinger suits' offer protection.

Clinical example

A 12 year old boy sustained a massive jellyfish sting to his legs while wading in water close to the shore. Immediately he experienced excruciating pain but managed to reach the shore, where he became apnoeic. His father gave mouth to mouth breathing. Vinegar was poured over the wounds and typical Box Jellyfish tentacles were removed. Pressure–immobilisation bandages were applied and an ambulance summoned. Shortly before arrival at hospital he became pulseless. Bag–mask ventilation with oxygen, external cardiac compression and intravenous adrenaline were given. Spontaneous circulation was restored and he recommenced spontaneous respiration. In hospital, Box Jellyfish antivenom was infused. Thereafter he made a slow recovery but pulmonary oedema necessitated oxygen therapy and diuretic and inotropic infusion for several days. He recovered fully but the stings healed with disfiguring scars.

PART 5 SELF-ASSESSMENT

Questions

1. **A 13 month old infant is rushed to the emergency department. She is cyanosed with marked respiratory distress.**
   - (A) The most likely diagnosis is severe croup
   - (B) The most likely diagnosis is bronchiolitis
   - (C) She has septicaemia
   - (D) High flow oxygen should be given and assessment of the airway should be undertaken
   - (E) Arterial blood gases should be obtained immediately

2. **A 4 year old boy is brought to the paediatric emergency department by ambulance. His parents are not with him. He is semicomatose, responding only to pain. He is tachypnoeic with a respiratory rate of 50 per minute.**
   - (A) A neurological cause is possible
   - (B) A respiratory cause is possible
   - (C) The airway should be checked first
   - (D) The child may be shocked
   - (E) All of the above

3. **An 8 year old boy is brought to the emergency department. His sister says that he fell several metres from of a tree. He is agitated and confused, with a pulse rate of 150/min.**
   - (A) A CT scan should be obtained immediately
   - (B) The child may have a pneumothorax
   - (C) The child may be shocked
   - (D) The child may have an extradural haematoma
   - (E) High flow oxygen by mask should be given

4. **An 18 month old baby girl is brought to hospital with marked cyanosis and respiratory distress. She is conscious but very agitated.**
   - (A) It is most important to obtain a diagnosis immediately so that this can guide her management
   - (B) An oxygen facemask should be applied immediately
   - (C) She is relying on hypoxic drive to maintain her breathing — no more than 40% oxygen should be given through the facemask
   - (D) Inhaled foreign body is a likely cause
   - (E) Experienced staff should be summoned immediately

5. **A 4 month old baby boy has been non specifically unwell for 2 days. He now presents to hospital drowsy, with cool mottled skin, rapid respirations, a heart rate of 190/minute and he responds poorly to stimulation. His rectal temperature is 36.5°C.**
   - (A) He may be septic
   - (B) He needs an urgent lumbar puncture to diagnose or exclude meningitis
   - (C) He should be given 20 ml/kg of saline intravenously
   - (D) If an intravenous cannula cannot be easily inserted then a central venous line is the best option
   - (E) Intravenous antibiotics should be given, although a diagnosis of serious bacterial infection has not been confirmed

6. **A 9 year old girl was hit by a car as she stepped from behind the school bus. By chance, you arrive in your car on the scene a few minutes later. She is groaning intermittently, talking incoherently, and is holding her left shoulder. Her heart rate is 150/minute and she has a large abrasion visible on her forehead.**
   - (A) You should obtain help from bystanders to move her out of the road and away from the risk of further injury by traffic
   - (B) You should check someone has called an ambulance
   - (C) You should transport her to hospital in your car — it is only 5 minutes drive away
   - (D) You should place her on her side with her neck slightly extended to improve her airway and reduce the risk of aspiration.
   - (E) You should check for any obvious external haemorrhage and apply direct pressure to any bleeding wounds

7. **Mark, a 3 year old boy, was found crying at 7 p.m. with an open half-full 500 ml bottle of kerosene. There was kerosene on the floor and on his clothing. It was not known how much kerosene was in the bottle before 'the accident'. On examination at 8 p.m. the child is alert but crying and coughs occasionally. Would you?**
   - (A) Induce emesis by giving 15 ml of syrup of ipecacuanha orally
   - (B) Give water or milk to dilute the poison
   - (C) Have a chest X ray performed and measure oxygenation
   - (D) Give oral 1 g/kg of activated charcoal
   - (E) Send him home with instructions to return if cyanosis occurs

8. **Annette, a 14 year old girl, ingested 26 slow release theophylline tablets (300 mg each) after an argument with her parents. Three hours later she is brought to the emergency department. On examination she is conscious but agitated and has sinus tachycardia. What would you do first?**

(A) Measure the serum theophylline level

(B) Induce emesis with syrup of ipecacuanha

(C) Perform gastric lavage and administer activated charcoal

(D) Prepare to perform plasmapheresis

(E) Undertake whole bowel irrigation

9. A nurse misinterprets a prescription for an intramuscular injection of morphine sulphate which has been written carelessly by a doctor as premedication for a liver biopsy. The patient, an 18 month old child has impaired liver function and receives 2 mg/kg of the drug (10 times the usual dose for a patient with normal hepatic function) and becomes unconscious. Would you?

(A) Observe the patient closely

(B) Administer naloxone

(C) Ventilate the patient

(D) Administer a CNS stimulant

(E) Check liver function tests

10. A mother telephones for emergency information, stating that her 2 year old son has just swallowed seven of her ferrous sulphate folic acid capsules which were left over from a prescription given to her during pregnancy. Which of the following is correct?

(A) There is no cause for alarm, as iron is a necessary element of diet and is not harmful

(B) A dose of ipecacuanha (15 ml) given now at home would be useful

(C) The mother should arrange transfer to a hospital for evaluation and treatment

(D) Investigations are needed and include measurement of serum iron

(E) An infusion of desferrioxamine will definitely be needed

11. A 15 year old girl claims she consumed 230 mg/kg of paracetamol 12 hours ago in a suicide attempt. Apart from nausea she appears physically well. Should you?

(A) Allow her to return home with her parents but arrange an urgent psychiatric consultation

(B) Determine her serum paracetamol level

(C) Run a urine and blood screen for other drugs

(D) Adminster *N*-acetylcysteine intravenously

(E) Administer activated charcoal

12. You are on cardiac ward duty when a 5 kg patient mistakenly receives a 1 ml intravenous bolus from an infusion of molar potassium chloride instead of the intended flush of normal saline to clear an arterial line. A bradycardia of 25 beats per minute with peaked T waves and hypotension ensues. The first thing you should do is:

(A) Stop the potassium infusion

(B) Give external cardiac compression

(C) Inject calcium chloride

(D) Draw a blood sample for potassium estimation

(E) Arrange an inhalation of salbutamol

13. Greg, a 12 year old boy, is rushed to the emergency department by his parents. He states that he was bitten on the forearm by a brown coloured snake 30 minutes ago. He is vomiting and you can see fang marks. What would you do first?

(A) Do a test of coagulation

(B) Give Brown Snake antivenom

(C) Apply a pressure–immobilisation first aid bandage

(D) Do a venom detection test on a sample of urine

(E) Seek neurotoxic signs

14. Jane, a 4 year old girl who lives in Sydney, Australia, was bitten 45 minutes ago on the arm by an unidentified spider which had been concealed inside her clothing as she was dressing. She is crying, sweating profusely, has muscle fasciculation around the bite site, is mildly hypertensive and is hyperventilating. The spider was not captured. Appropriate actions are:

(A) Give Red-back spider antivenom

(B) Give atropine parenterally

(C) Apply a pressure–immobilisation bandage

(D) Perform endotracheal intubation

(E) Obtain Funnel-web Spider antivenom

Answers and explanations

1. The correct answer is (D). Assessment of the airway is of paramount importance. If it is found to be compromised it must be secured immediately. High flow oxygen should be given to all collapsed children. Severe croup, bronchiolitis and septicaemia may all present with these symptoms. However a primary survey should precede the establishment of definitive diagnosis (A), (B) and (C). Arterial blood gases are not part of the primary survey and initial resuscitation (E).

2. The correct answer is (E). The airway should be checked first. Respiratory, circulatory and neurological causes could all result in the above symptoms. This presentation underlines the importance of a systematic approach to the assessment and initial support of the seriously ill child.

3. The correct answers are (B), (C), (D) and (E). The presenting signs are non specific. Hypoxia from any cause including pneumothorax may cause these signs. Equally, shock with decreased cerebral blood flow could explain the presentation. The child may indeed have an extradural haematoma. It is important to systematically follow the primary assessment to

ensure each possibility is dealt with in a timely manner. CT scan should not be done until this assessment and appropriate resuscitation measures are complete (A).

4. The correct answers are **(B)**, **(D)** and **(E)**. In a collapsed child, resuscitation measures take priority over obtaining a complete diagnosis (A), but with sufficient staff available they may occur concurrently. Cyanosis indicates hypoxaemia and oxygen should be given immediately (B). There is no reason to limit the concentration of oxygen administered to a cyanosed or collapsed child (C), as reliance on hypoxic drive to respiration (as seen in some adults with, for example, chronic obstructive airways disease) is very uncommon in children. Inhaled foreign body (D) is a relatively common cause of sudden onset of cyanosis in a child (aged from around 6 months to 5 years of age especially). It is quite likely this child will need interventions such as endotracheal intubation or instrumental removal of a foreign body: summon extra help (preferably someone experienced in these procedures) quickly (E).

5. The correct answers are **(A)**, **(C)** and **(E)**. The history and presentation are typical for serious bacterial infection (A) in a young baby. Septic babies may present febrile, normothermic or with hypothermia. This baby may indeed have meningitis but a lumbar puncture is contraindicated by his very sick presentation (B). A lumbar puncture at this point could lead to cerebellar coning with brainstem compression. It should be deferred until later and antibiotics should be given immediately to cover the possibility of meningitis. The baby has signs of circulatory insufficiency (cool mottled skin, tachycardia, drowsiness) and administration of a bolus of intravenous fluid is required (C). If an intravenous cannula cannot be easily inserted then insertion of an intraosseous needle is usually the best option because it is a simple and rapid technique for gaining vascular access. Insertion of a central venous line (D) is technically more difficult and time consuming. This child should receive intravenous antibiotics on the presumption he may have serious bacterial infection and while awaiting the results of any cultures taken (E).

6. The correct answers are **(B)** and **(E)**. There is a significant chance that this girl has a spinal injury. She should not be moved (A) and there should be no attempts to move her neck position (D) unless her airway is clearly in danger from her existing posture. Similarly, it would be unsafe to attempt to transfer her to hospital in your car (C). Bystanders should be used to stop or divert the traffic to protect the victim and rescuers from injury. Check someone has called

an ambulance (B): occasionally this is overlooked even when multiple bystanders are present. Any obvious external haemorrhage should be stemmed by the direct application of pressure using a pad of material (E): hypovolaemia will seriously worsen this child's prognosis.

7. The correct answer is **(C)**. Aspiration of petrochemicals causes serious pneumonitis. (C) It is essential to exclude it, as coughing is present. Aspiration must be presumed until proven otherwise. A chest X ray may reveal early involvement, as would some measure of oxygenation such as pulse oximetry or arterial blood gas measurement, although the former would suffice. Clinical examination of the chest of a crying child may be unrewarding at an early stage. (D) Activated charcoal adsorbs kerosene moderately but note that it is not effective for all petrochemicals. A 3 year old would be unlikely to swallow activated charcoal; a nasogastric tube would be necessary and its insertion may cause vomiting. (A) Petrochemicals have very low surface tensions. Vomiting should not be induced with ingested petrochemicals because of the risk of exacerbating or causing pneumonitis. (B) It may be sensible to dilute ingested corrosive substances but not other poisons, the absorption of which may be hastened. (E) Cyanosis is a late sign and unlikely to be detected by unqualified (and sleeping) parents!

8. The correct answer is **(E)**. Whole bowel irrigation, via nasogastric tube, will flush out unabsorbed tablets, particularly slow release tablets, and is a relatively safe procedure. Activated charcoal would be a reasonable alternative to whole bowel irrigation, although the interval between ingestion and presentation would limit its efficacy for direct absorption. However, interruption of the enterohepatic circulation of theophylline would be achieved. Simultaneous administration of whole bowel irrigation and activated charcoal would be counterproductive. (A) The history, if correct, and the clinical signs suggest the serum level will be high but by itself does not dictate treatment, as with theophylline poisoning treatment is directed at the effects of the drug such as loss of consciousness, convulsions, hypotension and hypokalaemia. There are no silent delayed effects. (B) Induction of vomiting is unlikely to be beneficial because the time interval between ingestion and presentation is too long — the drug will have passed beyond the stomach. Spontaneous vomiting may occur. (C) Likewise gastric lavage is unlikely to retrieve any tablets from the stomach at this late stage. (D) Plasmapheresis is invasive and is not indicated at the present stage of management, as the patient's vital functions are not compromised, nor are life threatening toxic effects present. However, it may be required later.

9. The correct answers are **(A)** and **(B)**. (A) The child has one of the life threatening effects of opiate poisoning. Unless nursed in a lateral position, airway obstruction could occur. The other effects of hypotension and hypoventilation may also occur. Close observation is therefore vital. (B) Naloxone is a specific opiate antagonist with an immediate effect. In this child, several doses or an infusion may be required because metabolism of the poison would be slow and the half-life of naloxone is short. (C) Ventilation is not necessary at this moment, based on the information provided, but it may become so and the adequacy of ventilation must be checked immediately. (D) CNS stimulants are not appropriate because a specific antagonist is available. (E) Irrespective of liver function, the present effects of the poison require immediate action.

10. The correct answers are **(B)**, **(C)** and **(D)**. (B) Ipecac, given within 1 hour after ingestion, will be helpful, as it invariably causes vomiting in children and will remove at least some of the poison if given within the hour. It is not usually given in emergency departments, principally because of the delay involved. (C) and (D) A serum level is helpful, along with clinical information about treatment, particularly for chelation therapy. There are two phases of iron poisoning: an initial phase of vomiting and diarrhoea during the first 0.5–2 hours, and a late phase at 6–12 hours of peripheral circulatory collapse and gastrointestinal haemorrhage. (A) Any dose of iron above the therapeutic is potentially harmful. (E) The decision to give desferrioxamine must be related to the serum level and clinical effects. It has a high rate of anaphylaxis and must be done under expert supervision.

11. The correct answers are **(B)** and **(C)**. The serious sequelae of paracetamol poisoning (hepatic failure, and to a lesser extent renal toxicity) only become apparent after several days. Death is due to hepatic coma. (B) The severity of poisoning can be correlated to the serum level of paracetamol at specific times after ingestion. Determination of the serum level will determine if the antidote, *N*-acetylcysteine, should be given. The antidote is effective if given within 24–36 hours after ingestion. It may be given orally or intravenously but the former route precludes the simultaneous administration of activated charcoal, which adsorbs *N*-acetylcysteine. (C) Since this was a suicide attempt, clinical and biochemical evidence of other drug poisoning should be sought. (A) This is a potentially life threatening poisoning and must be treated in hospital immediately. Psychiatric referral should then be obtained to address the problems that led to the poisoning. (D) *N*-acetylcysteine is the antidote for paracetamol poisoning but it may cause an allergic reaction so it should not be given

unless indicated. (E) It is too late to administer activated charcoal to adsorb paracetamol but it may leach some from the gastrointestinal mucosa. Note that *N*-acetylcysteine or activated charcoal may precipitate vomiting in this patient, who already has nausea.

12. The correct answer is **(B)** as the first action but all the others are appropriate. (B) External cardiac compression is necessary to maintain cardiac output while measures are taken to treat hyperkalaemia. Sudden hyperkalaemia is always a possible lethal complication of potassium therapy. Whenever used, measures should be in place to ensure that this accident cannot happen. A bolus of 1 mmol in a 5 kg patient will transiently raise the plasma level by approximately 5 mmol/l, as the plasma volume is approximately 40 ml/kg. (A) Cessation of the potassium infusion is sensible but will not alter the blood level immediately. (C) Injection of calcium chloride (0.2 ml/kg of 10%) will immediately antagonise the cardiac effects and would be the best antidote in this situation because of the simplicity of administration and rapidity of action. (D) This would confirm what otherwise is a clinical diagnosis of potassium toxicity. (E) An inhalation of salbutamol would enhance the intracellular shift of potassium but takes time to prepare and is of relatively slow onset. Other treatments to rapidly decrease blood potassium concentration would be intravenous administration of glucose (0.5 g/kg) with insulin (0.05–0.1 units/kg), or intravenous sodium bicarbonate 1 mmol/kg, or immediate mechanical hyperventilation — an option if the patient is already intubated.

13. The correct answer is **(C)**. Application of a pressure–immobilisation first aid bandage will prevent further absorption of venom from the bite site into the circulation while the appropriate antivenom is selected and preparations are made to administer it, if indicated. Vomiting in this context after observed snake bite is a reliable sign that envenomation has occurred. (A) Although coagulation may be disturbed and hence confirm envenomation, and may require treatment, it does not take precedence. (B) The definitive treatment is antivenom but the type of antivenom needed cannot be decided on the information available. The colour of the snake is not a reliable guide to its identity and hence of appropriate antivenom. If the child was critically ill due to a bite from an unidentified species, Brown Snake antivenom alone would not be sufficient. (D) A venom detection kit (VDK) test of urine, blood or swab from the bite site will indicate the appropriate antivenom to give but not necessarily identify the snake. If the patient's condition is critical and treatment cannot be delayed pending correct identification of the snake or the result of a VDK test, polyvalent antivenom, or mono-

valent antivenom according to geographical location, should be given.

14. The correct answers are **(B)**, **(C)** and **(E)**. Jane has some of the features of Funnel-web Spider envenomation which may advance to become life threatening. (B) Atropine is useful, as some of the effects include excessive secretions such as sweating. Other effects, including salivation, lacrimation and bronchorrhoea, are likely to develop. (C) Pressure–immobilisation will retard further absorption of venom into the circulation and may help inactivate some venom retained at the bite site. (E) Although the signs are not advanced, these are definite signs of envenomation by a Funnel-web Spider, with evidence of acetylcholine release at neuromuscular junctions (fasciculations) and at muscarinic autonomic receptors (sweating) and of catecholamine release (hypertension). In an advanced state of envenomation, the patient has difficulty maintaining the airway free of saliva and bronchorrhoea. The definitive treatment is antivenom, which may obviate the need for airway maintenance, mechanical ventilation and control of hypertension and tachyarrhythmias. (D) Endotracheal intubation is not yet indicated, either to maintain an airway or as a means of giving mechanical ventilation.

PART 2   FURTHER READING

Advanced Life Support Group 2001 Advanced paediatric life support: the practical approach, 3rd edn. BMJ Publishing Group, London

Alperstein G, Vimparni G 1993 Reducing children's body burden of lead: advice for paediatricians. Commonwealth Department of Human Services and Health, Canberra

Barkin R M, Caputo G L, Jaffe D M, Knapp J F, Schafermeyer R W, Seidel J S 1997 Paediatric emergency medicine: concepts and clinical practice, 2nd edn. Mosby-Year Book, St Louis

Bates N, Edwards N, Roper J, Volans G 1997 Paediatric toxicology. Macmillan, London

Burns M 2000 Activated charcoal as the sole intervention for treatment after childhood poisoning. Current Opinion in Pediatrics 12: 166–171

Ellenhorn M J, Schonwald S, Ordog G, Wasserberger J 1997 Ellenhorn's medical toxicology. Williams and Wilkins, Baltimore

Fleisher G R, Ludwig S 2000 Textbook of paediatric emergency medicine, 4th edn. Lippincott, Williams and Wilkins, Philadelphia

Haddad L M, Shannon M W, Winchester J F 1998 Clinical management of poisoning and drug overdose. WB Saunders, Philadelphia

Mackway-Jones K, Molyneux E, Phillips B, Wieteska S (eds) 2000 Advanced paediatric life support, 3rd edn. BMJ Books, London

Quang L S, Woolf A D 2000 Past, present and future role of ipecac syrup. Current Opinion in Paediatrics 12: 153–162

Shannon M 2000 Therapeutics and toxicology. Current Opinion in Paediatrics 12: 151–152

Sutherland S K, Tibballs J 2001 Australian animal toxins. Oxford University Press, Melbourne

Tucker J R 2000 Indications for, techniques of, complications of, and efficacy of gastric lavage in the treatment of the poisoned child. Current Opinion in Pediatrics 12: 163–165

Williamson J A, Fenner P J, Burnett J W, Rifkin J F 1996 Venomous and poisonous marine animals: a medical and biological handbook. University of New South Wales Press, Sydney

Useful links

http://www.ahcpub.com/online.html (The Practical Journal of Paediatric Emergency Medicine — Reports)

http://www.health.gov.au/pubhlth/strateg/injury/index.htm (Australian Department of Health and Aged Care — Injury prevention)

http://www.rch.unimelb.edu.au/clinicalguide/pages/resus.php (Emergency drug doses calculator and resuscitation card)

PART 6

FLUID REPLACEMENT AND THERAPEUTIC AGENTS

The child who needs fluid replacement

D. R. Brewster

Consideration of fluid replacement requires knowledge of body composition, fluid requirements, assessment of dehydration, the various techniques of fluid administration and the composition of the fluids used

Body composition

Body fluids are separated into two compartments, intracellular (ICF) and extracellular (ECF), with the latter subdivided into plasma and interstitial fluid. Total body water (TBW) falls proportionally from about 78% of body weight at birth to 60% in adults (Table 22.1). There is a close linear relationship between TBW in litres and body weight in kilograms (TBW = 0.611 body weight + 0.251). Large changes in body weight over 24 hours or less usually reflect changes in TBW, since growth or subcutaneous tissue wasting result in weight changes over longer periods.

Intracellular water accounts for about 40%, and plasma for about 5%, of body weight. Interstitial fluid is proportionately higher in infants, with an interstitial to plasma volume ratio of 5:1 compared with 3:1 in adults. A 5 kg infant, for example, would have a TBW of 3.5 litres, so a loss of 500 ml as diarrhoea would represent a considerable proportion of his ECF volume. There is also a shift of water from ECF to ICF in the first few days of life when 7% of TBW is lost, so this is a very vulnerable period for dehydration with illness. Body fat contains only 20% water, so obesity implies a relative reduction in expected percentage of body weight as water. Conversely, malnourished infants may have up to 80% of body weight as TBW. The clinical implications are that:
- the severity of dehydration by clinical assessment may be underestimated in obese children

- nutritional wasting is easily confused with dehydration
- fluid loads are poorly tolerated in severe malnutrition.

Water balance depends on an equilibrium between intake and output. The only natural entry points to body fluid compartments are by mouth and the intestinal tract. The four exit routes for ECF are skin, lung, intestine and kidney. Obligatory losses include evaporative losses from skin and lungs, and the urine volume necessary to excrete its solute load. Fluid and energy requirements per kilogram of body weight decrease from infancy to adult life, so on a weight basis infants and children have higher requirements than adults, making them more vulnerable to dehydration.

Extracellular fluid electrolytes are rich in sodium and chloride and are relatively poor in potassium (Fig. 22.1).

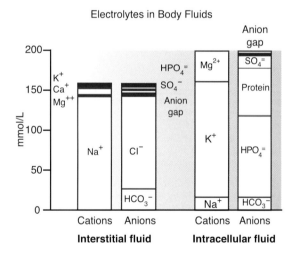

Fig. 22.1 Electrolytes in body fluids.

Table 22.1	Body water distribution				
Age group	Total body water (% of body weight)	Intracellular (% of body weight)	Extracellular (% of body weight)	ECF/ICF ratio	Blood (ml/kg)
Newborn	79	35	44	1.25	100
Infant	60	33	27	0.82	80
Child	62	41	21	0.51	70
Adult	58	39	19	0.49	60

Large increases in plasma lipids due to hyperlipidaemia, nephrotic syndrome or diabetic ketoacidosis may reduce the plasma sodium, but the overall ECF content remains normal. This artefactual hyponatraemia arises from a reduction in the water content of plasma from the increased lipids. But in diabetes mellitus, hyperglycaemia increases ECF osmotic pressure and draws water out of cells, causing a true decrease in the plasma sodium concentration. ICF electrolytes have higher potassium, phosphate, magnesium and protein concentrations. Analysis of the composition of body fluids shows that small intestinal secretions are high in sodium, diarrhoea fluid is high in potassium, gastric juice is high in chloride, and pancreatic secretions are high in bicarbonate (Table 22.2).

The cell membrane is relatively permeable to water, potassium and chloride and is relatively impermeable to sodium, phosphate and protein. The sodium that does enter cells is actively transported out by the energy dependent sodium pump mechanism. There is equilibrium between plasma and interstitial fluid, as well as between hydrostatic and colloid osmotic pressures. Water leaves the arterial end of the capillary and enters the venous end. The result of these processes is a continuous movement of fluid across the capillary wall, and the setting up of a balance between flow in and out of plasma.

The most striking clinical manifestation of a disordered balance of these forces is oedema, which can be caused by:

- increased hydrostatic pressure in the capillaries (venous occlusion, heart failure)
- decreased plasma oncotic pressure (nephrotic syndrome, liver disease, kwashiorkor)
- increased capillary permeability (locally in insect bites, boils).

Oedema may also be lymphatic in origin (lymphoedema in the Turner syndrome, XO).

Table 22.2 Typical composition of body fluids in children (mmol/l)

Source	Na+	K+	Cl-	HCO3-
Blood	140	4	100	25
Normal sweat	22	9	18	0
Bile	150	10	100	20
Gastric	50	15	125	0
Pancreatic	140	10	100	45
Small bowel	140	8	60	70
Diarrhoeal stool	40	50	25	65

These are illustrative mid range values, but there is considerable variation in individual values.

Regulation of extracellular fluids

The plasma osmolality, which is the concentration of solute particles, remains almost constant at 285–295 mosmol/kg H_2O, or approximately 1.86 times the serum sodium if glucose and urea are normal. The osmolality of plasma is controlled through a finely regulated feedback system involving osmoreceptors and volume receptors, the hypothalamus, the posterior pituitary and the collecting duct of the nephron. The intake of water is stimulated by thirst, which is regulated by a centre in the mid hypothalamus, which responds to increases in plasma osmolality of as little as 1–2% or reductions in volume of body fluids. Volume depletion dominates, so that thirst stimulates water intake at the expense of hypotonicity.

Water excretion is regulated by urine volume and concentration through antidiuretic hormone (ADH). The primary action of ADH is to increase the permeability of the renal collecting ducts to water. A rise in osmolality is corrected by increased ADH secretion, resulting in a decreased volume of urine with higher osmolality than plasma. Conversely, a fall in plasma osmolality leads to a decrease in ADH secretion, resulting in excretion of an increased volume of dilute urine. The fluid of plasma volume is contained in arteries (10%), the venous system (55%) and heart, lungs and capillary bed (35%). This is controlled by a rapid feedback loop from baroreceptors and stretch receptors in the heart and large vessels, via the autonomic nervous system, by changes in venous tone, cardiac output and arteriolar resistance. Aldosterone is involved in plasma volume regulation through renal sodium retention via the renin–angiotensin system.

The kidney

The kidney regulates water and electrolytes in the nephron, comprising the proximal tubule, the hypertonic medulla and ascending loop of Henle, the distal tubule and the collecting duct. The precise regulation of fluids and electrolytes in the ECF occurs by two mechanisms:

- reabsorption of the glomerular filtrate into capillaries
- secretion into the lumen and eventual excretion in the urine.

The normal adult kidneys filter 25 000 mmol of sodium, 5000 mmol of bicarbonate, 700 mmol of potassium and 180 litres of water daily, but more than 99% is usually reabsorbed, depending on the body's needs.

Approximately two thirds of the filtered sodium is reabsorbed in the proximal convoluted tubule. Another 25% is reabsorbed in the loop of Henle, which is used to create a concentration gradient for the countercurrent multiplier system, essential for passing concentrated urine. Urine osmolality can vary from a maximal dilution of 100 mosmol/kg to a maximal concentration of 1400 mosmol/kg in adults. The distal tubule only reabsorbs 5% of the filtered sodium, but the electrical gradient generated is used for potassium and hydrogen ion excretion into the distal tubule.

Assessment of dehydration

Clinical history and examination

A full history and examination on admission are important to ensure that the symptom of diarrhoea or vomiting is not part of a disease other than gastroenteritis, such as intestinal obstruction, intussusception, pyloric stenosis, haemolytic–uraemic syndrome, urinary tract infection, etc. The following are some of the important symptoms and signs which may be associated with diarrhoea and dehydration.

History

- Diarrhoea: onset, frequency, volume, consistency, blood, mucus.
- Vomiting: onset, frequency, volume, bilious, projectile.
- Eating and drinking: volumes, frequency, type (e.g. breast milk, oral rehydration solution (ORS), cordials).
- Urine output: volume, frequency, number of wet nappies (often difficult to assess).
- Fever and associated symptoms: cough, shortness of breath, abdominal pain, seizures, rashes, etc.
- Nutritional status: view the child's growth chart or check weight/height (wasting) and height/age (stunting).

Examination

- General condition: drowsy, restless or irritable.
- Vital signs: temperature, pulse (or heart rate), respiratory rate, blood pressure.

- Eyes: sunken, no tears on crying.
- Mouth and tongue: dry mucous membranes.
- Skin: skin turgor reduced or capillary refill time increased.
- Muscle tone: weak, floppy or unable to hold head up.
- Chest: deep acidotic breathing.
- Abdomen: distended or tender, masses.

Weigh the child

If the child has been weighed accurately in the last few days, the percentage weight loss will approximately equal the percentage dehydration. It is highly recommended that the child be reweighed after rehydration (at 24 hours) as a check on whether the admission assessment of percentage dehydration is consistent with the percentage weight change (% weight change = (rehydrated weight – admission weight) ÷ rehydrated weight × 100%). There is often a discrepancy between clinical assessment of dehydration (Table 22.3) and percentage weight change after rapid rehydration. Clinical assessment tends to overestimate the degree of dehydration because in practice the clinical assessor is affected by how sick the child appears clinically, which may be related to sepsis or other associated conditions. On the other hand, percentage weight change will underestimate the severity of dehydration if there is on going osmotic diarrhoea, and may overestimate it with excessive intravenous fluids (for example, puffy eyes). Clinical assessment tends to be more reliable in a setting where severe dehydration is common (e.g. Darwin, Australia), whereas with a lower proportion of cases of severe dehydration (e.g. Melbourne, Australia) percentage weight change is more reliable, but is only known after rehydration unless there is an accurate weight known before the diarrhoea started.

Table 22.3 Signs of dehydration

Degree of dehydration % (deficit)	Mild 3–5% (30–50 ml/kg)	Moderate 6–9% (60–90 ml/kg)	Severe ≥10% (100–150 ml/kg)
General condition	Well, alert	Restless, irritable	Lethargic, drowsy, floppy
Eyes	Normal	Sunken	Sunken
Tears on crying	Present	Absent	Absent
Mouth and tongue	Moist	Dry	Very dry
Thirst	Drinks normally, but may refuse ORS	Thirsty, drinks eagerly	Drinks poorly or not able to drink
Respiratory rate	Normal	Increased	Fast
Pulse	Normal	Fast	Fast, weak
Capillary return	Normal (1 s)	Sluggish (2 s)	Slow (3 s)
Skin pinch	Goes back quickly	Goes back slowly	Goes back very slowly
Hands and feet	Normal	Normal	Cool, blue nail beds

Fluid requirements

Infants and young children are especially susceptible to the consequences of abnormalities of fluid balance, as the usual daily turnover of water is about 25% of TBW, compared with only 6% in adults. Fluid therapy is conventionally divided into:

- maintenance
- deficit
- ongoing losses.

Regardless of the accuracy of fluid calculations, frequent monitoring of children is essential so that appropriate modifications can be made according to clinical assessment, changes in weight, urine output and laboratory tests.

Maintenance fluids

These requirements involve replacement of normal losses from urine, sweat, lungs and faeces. Maintenance fluid and electrolyte requirements are directly related to metabolic rate, which depends on age, body weight, degree of activity and body temperature. The daily maintenance requirement can be simply calculated from the following:

- first 10 kg: 100 ml/kg/day
- 11–20 kg: 1000 ml + 50 ml/kg above 10 kg
- above 20 kg: 1500 ml + 20 ml/kg above 20 kg
- Give oral fluids, ORS or i.v. 4% dextrose + N/5 saline for maintenance requirements.

Conditions affecting normal fluid requirements

- Body temperature: increase for fever, decrease for hypothermia.
- Metabolic rate: increase if high, decrease if low.
- Respiratory rate: increase for fast breathing.
- Humidity: decrease for high humidity.
- Environmental temperature: increase for sweating.

Deficit therapy

The severity of a deficit in body fluids can be gauged from changes in body weight. In children, a weight loss of 3–5% is considered mild, 6–9% moderate, and ≥10% severe dehydration. The speed with which the deficit occurs is important for the body's adjustment.

Dehydration may also be classified as isotonic (serum sodium 130–150 mmol/l), hypotonic or hypertonic. In hypertonic or hypernatraemic dehydration (which is much less common than it used to be) the increase in ECF osmolality results in movement of fluid out of cells, so cells become dehydrated. This has important implications for therapy (see below).

Ongoing losses

It is difficult to quantify the amount of diarrhoea and vomiting, so it is better to review fluid balance, weight changes and clinical assessment frequently and adjust fluid rates accordingly. Run the fluid rate as calculated for rehydration over 4 hours then review: weight, clinical examination including vital signs, ongoing losses, urine output and fluid intake (including breast milk). ***Be prepared to change the rate of administration*** depending on the above findings.

Rehydration

Using the guidelines for assessment of dehydration above, estimate the % dehydration present:

Calculated fluid deficit (ml) =
    % dehydration × weight (kg) × 10
(e.g. 10% dehydration in a 10 kg child = 1000 ml deficit).

Intravenous

If the child is in **shock,** give oxygen and start IV Ringer's lactate 20–40 ml/kg given rapidly, then reassess. If there is no immediate improvement or suggestive clinical features, consider other causes of shock (for example, sepsis, cardiac, metabolic, diabetic ketoacidosis, intussusception, poisoning, etc.). If an intravenous infusion cannot be achieved, use the intraosseous route to the circulation (Ch. 20). Do not use albumin infusions because there is evidence that these are associated with excess mortality in critically ill patients, but this is also the current subject of an Australian multicentre ICU study in adult patients.

For the child who has signs of **severe dehydration,** replace the calculated fluid deficit with intravenous Ringer's lactate (Hartmann's solution) over 4 hours, followed by maintenance requirements with 4% dextrose + N/5 saline. Normal saline rather than Ringer's lactate should be used if there is a lactic acidosis.

For **moderate dehydration**, it may be reasonable to give 20 ml/kg rapidly initially and reassess if you are uncertain of the degree of dehydration but intravenous fluids are appropriate. The response to this therapy should give you the answer in relation to the degree of dehydration, however, a trial of oral rehydration is another option.

Note that rapid rehydration with Ringer's lactate is now the accepted regimen for intravenous rehydration by the World Health Organization (WHO) and the American Academy of Pediatrics, so older regimens of correcting half the deficit over 6 hours and the remainder over 18 hours are outdated (except with hypernatraemic dehydration), as there is no reason to keep children dehydrated that long. Note that rapid intravenous rehydration is ***only***

Table 22.4 Intravenous solutions (mmol/l)

Solution	Sodium	Potassium	Chloride	Lactate	Calcium	Glucose
Ringer's lactate (Hartmann's)	130	5	110	30	2	–
4% glucose & N/5 saline (0.18%)	30	–	30	–	–	222
2.5% glucose & N/2 saline (0.45%)	75	–	75	–	–	139
Normal saline (0.9%)	150	–	150	–	–	–

for Ringer's lactate (or normal saline in older children), **not** for hypotonic fluids such as 4% dextrose with N/5 saline, which could lead to hyponatraemia, seizures and cerebral oedema (Table 22.4).

Nasogastric

For nasogastric rehydration, the maximum safe rate of infusion is 20 ml/kg/h. Nasogastric tubes are unpleasant and carry a risk of pulmonary aspiration, so should be reserved for dehydrated children who cannot drink. Generally, refusal to drink ORS because of the taste means a child is not very dehydrated, as dehydrated children who are alert will not refuse to drink.

Oral

Oral rehydration therapy is usually successful in patients with mild to moderate dehydration. Oral rehydration solution (ORS) is a powder containing a specific balance of electrolytes and glucose, especially formulated for use in children with diarrhoea. It is available as the specific WHO composition but the commercially prepared hypotonic forms are more appropriate for developed countries where there is no cholera. The differences between the two solutions are shown in Table 22.5. ORS is based upon the important principle of glucose facilitated intestinal sodium absorption. Cereal based solutions (for example, rice ORS) are also available but their advantages over glucose solutions in non cholera diarrhoea have not been well documented, and they are not a substitute for early refeeding. Fluids such as soft drinks,

sports beverages and fruit juices are not appropriately constituted to be an effective ORS to treat dehydration.

The main reasons for failure of oral rehydration are:
- persistent vomiting
- high purging rates (stool output)
- electrolyte disturbance (e.g. hypokalaemia)
- excessive drowsiness.

Oral rehydration is a highly effective means of rehydration which is greatly underutilised in developed countries like Australia. Surely the challenge in treating children is to do as little as possible that is unpleasant or painful, provided it is safe management? Teaching hospitals have a tendency to resort too readily to intravenous and nasogastric therapies, allegedly due to 'parental pressure to do something'.

Electrolyte disturbances

Clinically significant electrolyte disturbances occur in about 25% of hospitalised children in whom electrolytes are measured. The risk factors are:
- age ≤6 months
- dry mucous membranes
- vomiting
- delayed capillary refill
- diabetes mellitus
- tachycardia.

Acidosis and hyponatraemia are the most common abnormalities detected, and children with acute gastroenteritis and febrile respiratory infections are most at

Table 22.5 Oral rehydration solutions (mmol/l of made up solution)

Solution	Na$^+$	K$^+$	Cl$^-$	Citrate (base)	Glucose	Osmolality
WHO	90	20	80	10	111	310
Gastrolyte-R	60	20	50	10	111 as rice*	226
Pedialyte	45	20	35	10	126	250
Repalyte	60	20	60	10	90	240

*80% amylopectin, 20% amylose.

Clinical example

How would you manage a 2 year old child weighing 12 kg who is assessed to be 7% dehydrated with serum Na$^+$ 135 mmol/l, K$^+$ 1.8 mmol/l, pH 7.08, bicarbonate 8 mmol/l and base excess –15?

- **Fluids**

I.V. rehydration	Maintenance	Total fluid (24 h)
7% × 10 ml/kg × 12 kg = 840 ml Replace over 4 h 840 ÷ 4 = 210 ml/h as Ringer's lactate	(10 kg × 100) + (2 kg × 50) =1100 ml Over 20 h = 55 ml/h as 4% dextrose + N/5 saline (or ORS, breast milk or formula)	840 + 1100 ml = 1950 ml + ongoing losses

- **Potassium**
1. Rehydration: a. Concentration: 1 g KCl in 1000 ml Ringer's lactate (13.4 + 5) = 18.4 mmol/l (4 h).
                         b. Flow rate: 210 ml/h × 0.0184 mmol/ml K$^+$ ÷ 12 kg = 0.32 mmol K$^+$/kg/h for 4 h.
2. Maintenance: a. Concentration: 2 g KCl in 1000 ml 4% + N/5 saline = 26.8 mmol/l (20 h).
                         b. Flow rate: 55 ml/h × 0.0268 mmol/ml K$^+$ ÷ 12 kg = 0.12 mmol K$^+$/kg/h
(adjust depending on repeat K$^+$ and consider oral therapy).

- **Bicarbonate**
It is not be necessary to add bicarbonate to intravenous rehydration fluid. Ringer's lactate contains base as lactate and ORS as citrate. Bicarbonate has not been shown to be beneficial in diarrhoeal dehydration, and acidosis generally resolves with adequate rehydration alone.

---

risk. In Aboriginal children in northern Australia, on the other hand, two thirds of children have acidosis and/or hypokalaemia on admission for acute gastroenteritis.

Hypokalaemia

Potassium can be lost from the body in diarrhoeal stools, especially with osmotic diarrhoea. It may be lost from the ICF compartment in acidotic children with rotavirus gastroenteritis, for example, and rehydration would lead to hypokalaemia as ECF potassium moves intracellularly. With high aldosterone levels in dehydration, sodium and water retention by the kidney may lead to potassium loss. Hypokalaemia may be manifested as hypotonia, irritability, intestinal ileus with distension, and cardiac arrhythmias with T wave changes. However, it is important to realise that the serum potassium measured by electrolytes may not reflect the actual degree of total body potassium depletion, which is stored intracellularly particularly in muscle and brain tissues. You must ensure that a child with hypokalaemia does not have renal failure (for example, haemolytic uraemic syndrome, acute tubular necrosis, acute glomerulonephritis) before giving potassium. In view of the cardiac effects of changes in plasma potassium levels, ECG monitoring is important in severe hypokalaemia (<2.5 mmol/l) and with intravenous infusions of potassium in concentrations >30 mmol/l.

Management

Intravenous.   Add 1 g (rapid rehydration) or 2 g (maintenance) KCl to 1 litre of Ringer's lactate and run at the rate calculated for rehydration. *Note* Strong KCl ampoules must always be diluted, never infused directly. One gram of KCl = 13.4 mmol K$^+$, so the total concentration of the solutions in mmol/l = 18.4 (for 1 g) or 31.8 (for 2 g), as Ringer's lactate already contains 5 mmol/l K$^+$. You must always calculate ***both*** the K$^+$ infusion rate (mmol/kg/h) and the K$^+$ concentration (mmol/l). Never exceed an infusion rate of 0.4 mmol K$^+$/kg/h (as cardiac arrhythmias may occur) or a K$^+$ concentration of 40 mmol/l (as it is irritating to veins).

Oral.   8–10 mmol K$^+$/kg/day in divided doses 4–6 hourly. Large doses of oral potassium are poorly tolerated, so each individual dose should not exceed about 1.5 mmol/kg/dose.

Hyponatraemia

The common causes of hyponatraemia in young children are hypotonic dehydration and iatrogenic water overload (for example, overestimation of the degree of dehydration, inappropriate use of hypotonic solutions for rehydration and/or too rapid administration of maintenance fluids). Rare causes include salt losing nephropathy, raised intracranial pressure, the sick cell syndrome (such as in kwashiorkor) and the syndrome of inappropriate ADH secretion (SIADH) in meningitis (see below and Chapter 39). Hyponatraemia with dehydration often accompanies acute gastroenteritis and is corrected by the standard rehydration protocols, including treatment of the fluid deficit. The use of hypertonic saline infusions is rarely indicated and should only be done after appropriate consultation.

Management

- Reassess hydration status: is it hyponatraemic dehydration? If the child is >5% dehydrated and the hyponatraemia is due to gastroenteritis, **rehydrate** with Hartmann's solution as above.
- Assess for signs of fluid overload: excessive weight gain, oedema, signs of cardiac failure. If fluid overload is thought to be present, then decreasing the rate of administering fluid or **fluid restriction** is usually all that is necessary. Be cautious about changing the intravenous fluid to normal saline in the mistaken belief that the child is salt depleted or giving diuretics, which could exacerbate the hyponatraemia.
- **Hypertonic saline** solutions may sometimes be necessary with profound hyponatraemia associated with convulsions and cerebral oedema, but usually only in the intensive care setting.

Hypernatraemia

Hypernatraemia (Na$^+$ >150 mmol/l) usually occurs along with moderate or severe dehydration, especially if fluids too high in solutes are used for rehydration. This is now relatively uncommon, but occurred frequently when boiled skim milk and homemade salt–sugar solutions were used to treat diarrhoea, and cows' milk rather than humanised formulas were used for infant feeding. In hypernatraemic dehydration, the degree of dehydration may be underestimated due to the fluid shifts from the intracellular to interstitial compartment, thus expanding the plasma volume.

Hypocalcaemia and hyperglycaemia may accompany hypernatraemia, and the child may have marked irritability and a 'doughy feeling' to the skin. As the main ECF solute, changes in sodium concentration mean changes in body fluid osmolality. It is important to appreciate that rapid changes in cell water content can be devastating, particularly to central nervous system blood vessels, leading to haemorrhage and thrombosis. This is not the case for more gradual changes, so the key to management is to avoid rapid changes in serum sodium.

Management

- Avoid rapid correction of hypernatraemia, as fluid shifts may cause cerebral oedema, seizures and stroke.

Adjust fluids to return the serum sodium to normal slowly (10 mmol/l/24 h). Rapid rehydration, especially with hypotonic maintenance intravenous fluids (4% + N/5 saline), may drop the serum sodium too rapidly.

- Rehydration with oral fluids is often the best policy, correcting the deficit over 24 hours.
- Slow intravenous rehydration and maintenance fluids, replacing losses over 18–24 hours instead of 4–6 hours, is another option when oral rehydration is not feasible.
- Review: the serum sodium and electrolytes and the child's condition need to be monitored closely.

Hypocalcaemia and hypomagnesaemia

Hypocalcaemia and hypomagnesaemia often accompany hypokalaemia. There is complex interplay between these ions and pH changes. Hypomagnesaemia and alkalosis lower the threshold for tetany, whereas hypokalaemia and acidosis raise it. In addition, hypomagnesaemia blunts the parathyroid hormone (PTH) response to hypocalcaemia by blocking the release of PTH, and correction of hypomagnesaemia is often necessary before correction of calcium and potassium levels can occur. Serum calcium is affected by the serum albumin to which it is bound, for which there is usually a laboratory correction as a closer approximation to the ionised calcium level.

Hypocalcaemia may produce clinical features such as tetany (which can manifest as irritability, lethargy, carpopedal spasm, seizures, bronchospasm, laryngospasm), the Chvostek sign (spasm of the facial muscles elicited by tapping the facial nerve in the region of the parotid gland), lengthening of QT interval, arrhythmias and intestinal cramps.

Treatment

For oral correction
- Calcium carbonate; calcium lactate gluconate (e.g. Sandocal 1 g tablets).
- Dose (not per kg): < 4 years — 100 mg 2–5 times daily; 4–12 years — 500 mg b.i.d.

For intravenous correction
- Use calcium gluconate 10% (0.22 mmol Ca^{++}/ml).
- Give stat. dose i.v. 0.5 mmol/kg slowly over 10–20 min or i.m.
- Followed by i.v. infusion of 0.5 mmol/kg over 4–6 h (in fluid calculated for rehydration).
- Note that i.v. calcium cannot be added to bicarbonate (precipitates as chalk); it is irritating to tissues if it extravasates, and it causes bradycardia if infused too rapidly.

Hypomagnesaemia can produce tetany without hypocalcaemia, and should always be thought of in tetany refractory to calcium infusion. Other clinical features are hyperirritability, seizures, increased tone and reflexes, muscle fasciculations, rhabdomyolysis, cardiac arrhythmias and conduction disturbances.

Treatment

For intramuscular or intravenous correction
- 49.3% magnesium sulphate (2 mmol Mg^{++}/ml).
- Dose: 0.2 ml/kg b.d. (give i.v. slowly over 5 min).
- Precautions: high doses of Mg can cause prolongation of PR and QRS intervals and bradyarrythmias, hypotension, neuromuscular blockade and sedation if given too quickly.

For oral treatment
- Use magnesium aspartate tablets (500 mg/1.5 mmol Mg).
- Dose: 3–6 mg/kg/day of elemental magnesium in three divided doses.

Key learning points

- NaCl contains 17 mmol of sodium and chloride per gram
- KCl contains 13 mmol of potassium and chloride per gram, 0.75g/10 ml = 1 mmol/ml K$^+$
- Sodium bicarbonate contains 12 mmol of sodium and bicarbonate per gram, 8.4% = 1 mmol/ml HCO$_3^-$
- Calcium gluconate 10% = 0.22 mmol/ml Ca^{2+}
- Magnesium sulphate 49.3% = 2.465 g/5 ml = 2 mmol/ml Mg^{2+}
- Magnesium chloride 0.48 g/5 ml = 1 mmol/ml Mg^{2+}
- Osmolality of serum = 2 Na$^+$ + glucose + urea, which is normally 270–295 mmol/l
- Anion gap = Na$^+$ + K$^+$ – (HCO$_3^-$ + Cl$^-$), which is normally <12

Acid–base balance

Acidosis commonly complicates severe illness in children but will usually correct itself with treatment of the primary disorder, provided there is normal renal function and bicarbonate production. Acidosis itself only warrants specific treatment if the low pH is interfering with normal cellular function, conventionally considered as a pH below 7.15 (normal range 7.35–7.45). With conditions such as sepsis, injury, poor perfusion and catabolism, excess hydrogen ions (H$^+$) are produced and are buffered by red cells, plasma proteins or bicarbonate. It is important to appreciate that pH and H$^+$ have a logarithmic relationship, such that a fall in the pH to 7.1 means the H$^+$ have doubled from 40 to 80 nmol/l. Bicarbonate reacts with hydrogen ions to produce water and carbon dioxide:

$$H^+ + HCO_3^- \rightleftharpoons H_2O + CO_2$$

Increased production or failure to excrete hydrogen ions results in metabolic acidosis, which can be compensated by increased removal of CO$_2$ by increased breathing to remove H$^+$, or more slowly by buffering via bicarbonate. Acidosis with a high CO$_2$, on the other hand, is respiratory, although often a mixed picture is seen.

Alkalosis is much less common in children, but may occur with severe vomiting and also with hyperventilation due to anxiety. Severe vomiting, such as in pyloric stenosis, may cause alkalosis through both loss of acid and fluid loss (dehydration) with aldosterone secretion, which leads in turn to renal wasting of K$^+$ and H$^+$ with bicarbonate retention and exacerbation of the alkalosis (Table 22.6).

Clinical example

Letisha is a 14 month old Aboriginal girl with acute rotaviral gastroenteritis, assessed to be 10% dehydrated and with the following blood gases on admission:

pH	HCO$_3$ (mmol/l)	PCO$_2$ (mmHg)	BE (mmol/l)
7.16	10	25	–19.6

The pH is below 7.35, indicating acidosis. The negative base excess indicates a metabolic acidosis. The CO$_2$ is below the normal range of 35–45 mmHg, meaning hyperventilation or respiratory alkalosis, which in this case indicates compensation for a metabolic acidosis. Thus, she has a metabolic acidosis that is being partially compensated by a respiratory alkalosis. She was rehydrated with intravenous Ringer's lactate over 4 hours, and her acidosis improved without the need for any sodium bicarbonate.

Table 22.6 Acidosis and alkalosis

Acid–base status	Clinical example	pH	Primary	Compensatory	Clinical feature
Metabolic acidosis	Diabetic ketoacidosis	↓	↓ HCO$_3^-$	↓ PCO$_2$	Kussmaul breathing
Metabolic alkalosis	Pyloric stenosis	↑	↑ HCO$_3^-$	↑ PCO$_2$	Decreased respiration
Respiratory acidosis	Hyaline membrane disease	↓	↑ PCO$_2$	↑ HCO$_3^-$	Drowsiness
Respiratory alkalosis	Hysterical hyperventilation	↑	↓ PCO$_2$	↓ HCO$_3^-$	Tetany

Metabolic acidosis with diarrhoeal disease

Metabolic acidosis often accompanies diarrhoea with dehydration. There are a number of well known causes of acidosis in diarrhoea, such as:
- severe dehydration with decreased tissue perfusion (lactic acidosis)
- bicarbonate loss in stool
- diminished renal function.

Fermentation of dietary sugars from small bowel bacterial overgrowth, leading to absorption of organic acids (for example acetate, butyrate, propionate) may also be a factor in malnourished children.

Measurement of serum chloride and the **anion gap** may be useful in determining the cause of metabolic acidosis:
- Causes of metabolic acidosis with normal anion gap (8–12 mmol/l)
  — gastrointestinal loss of bicarbonate (diarrhoea)
  — renal loss of bicarbonate (renal tubular acidosis).
  Note that the urine anion gap will be negative with gastrointestinal causes of acidosis and positive with renal causes of acidosis (decreased ammonia excretion).
- Causes of metabolic acidosis with increased anion gap (>12 mmol/l):
  — increased organic acid production (e.g. lactic acidosis, diabetic ketoacidosis, organic acidaemias)
  — ingestion of toxic substances (e.g. salicylates, methyl alcohol, ethylene glycol)
  — decreased excretion of acid (e.g. acute renal failure, chronic renal failure).

Metabolic acidosis is often worsened by infection, hypoxia, malnutrition and potassium depletion. A clinical sign of acidosis is tachypnoea with 'air hunger' (deep Kussmaul respirations), but it may be difficult to differentiate from the tachypnoea of heart failure or pneumonia. Acidosis is corrected by fluid replacement, oxygen, provision of calories, and treatment of any infection. Bicarbonate treatment intravenously is rarely indicated in acidosis associated with diarrhoea and has the disadvantage of transiently worsening the hypokalaemia, while the increased sodium load may push the child into cardiac failure, especially if the child is nutritionally wasted. Persisting metabolic acidosis with diarrhoeal disease may indicate the need for further rehydration (that is, the degree of dehydration has been underestimated) or continuing osmotic diarrhoea (for example lactose, sucrose, glucose polymer or monosaccharide intolerance).

Special conditions

Pyloric stenosis

The severe vomiting causes hypochloraemic alkalosis which requires early potassium replacement. Severe intracellular depletion of potassium results in increased exchange of hydrogen ions for sodium in the distal tubule, giving a paradoxically acid urine in the face of systemic alkalosis. Infants with severe vomiting may have a serum chloride concentration <80mmol/l and bicarbonate >50mmol/l. In view of the alkalosis, Ringer's lactate is not an appropriate rehydration fluid in pyloric stenosis, but normal saline with additional potassium can be used to replace the deficit, followed by normal maintenance fluids, and formula or breast milk can be given fairly soon after surgery.

Adrenal insufficiency

With salt losing manifestations, the serum sodium and chloride are low and the potassium is high with increased plasma renin activity. Intravenous administration of 5% glucose in 0.9% saline solution should be given to correct the hypoglycaemia and the sodium loss, along with hydrocortisone.

Burns

For most children with a burn requiring fluid resuscitation, an appropriate starting formula is intravenous Ringer's lactate 4 ml/kg/% burned surface area. Half of this fluid is given in the first 8 hours and the remainder over the next 16 hours, adjusting the rate according to the patient's response. For adequate fluid resuscitation, burn cases may need to gain more than their preburn weight due to intracellular and interstitial oedema. During the second day after the burn, oedema fluid starts to be reabsorbed and urine output should increase. A rough guide to fluid requirements on day two is half of the first day's requirement, but as Ringer's lactate with 5% glucose. There is still controversy about whether colloid should be provided in the early period of burn resuscitation. If 0.5% silver nitrate solution is used as the topical dressing, sodium and potassium losses may be extensive and require supplements. Children with extensive burns are best managed in specialised units.

Bacterial meningitis

There is controversy about fluid management in bacterial meningitis (Ch. 39). There is agreement that rapid or excessive infusion of hypotonic fluids (such as 5% dextrose) is to be avoided, as this may result in hyponatraemic seizures and cerebral oedema. The diagnosis of the syndrome of inappropriate antidiuretic hormone (SIADH) is based upon:
- hyponatraemia (<135 mmol/l),
- plasma osmolality <280 mosmol/kg
- urine osmolality >100 mosmol/kg (i.e. less than maximally dilute with the urinary sodium usually >20 mmol/l).

It also implies the absence of hypovolaemia, oedema, endocrine dysfunction (as in adrenal insufficiency, hypothyroidism), renal failure and drugs impairing water excretion. Hyponatraemia due to SIADH was believed to be a common complication of meningitis, so fluid restriction to two thirds of maintenance requirements was standard practice in order to treat or prevent this syndrome. However, dehydration and circulatory compromise may be features of bacterial meningitis, and do not benefit from fluid restriction. Hyponatraemia in bacterial meningitis may be due to dehydration in which sodium depletion exceeds water depletion with appropriate ADH secretion, which responds to rehydration rather than fluid restriction. The current best practice is *not* to routinely restrict fluids, and to ensure that hyponatraemia is not a feature of dehydration before restricting fluid intake in meningitis.

Acute renal failure

The urine volume is determined by filtration, reabsorption and secretion, so the presence of oliguria should lead to assessment of hydration, sodium excretion and urinary osmolality. Severe oliguria is defined as a urine output <0.5 ml/kg/h. Anuria should raise suspicion of urinary obstruction. The physiological renal response to a decrease in intravascular volume (dehydration, septic shock) is to enhance reabsorption of tubular fluid in the proximal and distal segments of the nephron and to release ADH. This will result in a low urinary sodium (<20 mmol/l) and high osmolarity (>500 mosmol/l). With renal tissue injury, such as in acute glomerulonephritis or haemolytic uraemic syndrome, the urinary sodium is usually >40 mmol/l. Diuretics are indicated in this latter situation, but could exacerbate renal function in the former unless hypovolaemia is treated first.

Intussusception

Intussusception may require careful consideration of fluid needs (see Clinical example below).

Lactose intolerance

The most common carbohydrate intolerance is disaccharide intolerance, which is almost always lactose intolerance. Sucrose or glucose polymer intolerance may accompany lactose intolerance. Occasionally, transient monosaccharide intolerance may also occur, particularly in young infants with *Cryptosporidium* infection, which may necessitate grading of feeds to decrease the carbohydrate intake below the threshold level of intolerance. All carbohydrates in the diet are broken down by digestive processes into monosaccharides, of which glucose is by far the most common. Glucose and galactose are the monosaccharide end products of lactose digestion of milk; glucose and fructose of sucrose breakdown; and glucose of maltose and isomaltose digestion. Starch is the most common carbohydrate in the diet and this is converted to glucose by various steps. All carbohydrates are made up of monosaccharide polymers. Disaccharides contain two monosaccharides, oligosaccharides contain 2–10 monosaccharides, and polysaccharides contain more that 10 monosaccharides. Monosaccharides are absorbed by an active process and the mechanisms are different for glucose and fructose.

Clinical example

A 4 month old girl weighing 5980 g with a presumed urinary tract infection was assessed clinically to be moderately dehydrated at a district hospital. Initial fluid management was calculated for 8.5% dehydration plus ongoing maintenance. She received 510 ml Ringer's lactate solution as rapid replacement over 4 hours, followed by maintenance fluids of 4% glucose and N/5 saline for the next 20 hours. The 8.8% weight gain (577 g) over the first 24 hours confirmed that the initial clinical assessment and fluid replacement were appropriate, although the correct diagnosis was not made.

The following day the child was transferred to a tertiary hospital, where a laparotomy was performed for intussusception. Her ICU postoperative fluid management is summarised below. On day 2 postoperatively, she became oedematous from fluid overload, and received diuretic therapy for the next 48 hours. Intravenous fluids were reduced to maintenance on day 4, with gradual resolution of oedema by day 5.

Postop.	Day 1	Day 2	Day 3	Day 4	Day 5
Total input (ml)	1575	990	905	590	590
Total output	979	501	1081	730	737
Fluid balance	+596	+489	–176	–140	–147

This is an all too common scenario in adult ICUs with inadequate paediatric input: young children are given excessive intravenous fluids postoperatively (240 ml/kg on day 1). Treating this with diuretics may only compound the problem. Regular clinical assessment of the patient, checking the fluid chart and repeat weighing are essential in any patient receiving intravenous fluid therapy. With frequent monitoring and appropriate adjustments to changing requirements, the above errors can be minimised.

The enzymes which allow the breakdown of disaccharides to monosaccharides are present in the brush border of the intestinal mucosa (Ch. 70). Lactase is more superficial and thus more commonly reduced than sucrase or maltase with intestinal mucosal damage. When mucosal damage is more severe the absorption of monosaccharides may also be affected, particularly in non breastfed infants with severe or intractable diarrhoea. Mucosal maltase-glucoamylase and sucrase-isomaltase and glucose cotransporter (SGLT-1) are reduced in villous atrophy. Malnourished children have a reduced mean mucosal lactase specific activity, but have a compensatory increase in sucrase and SGLT-1 levels when controlled for mucosal weight. Malnutrition and small bowel mucosal damage contribute independently to lactose malabsorption.

There is a threshold for lactose intolerance which, when exceeded, may result in profuse osmotic diarrhoea with acidosis and hypokalaemia. Children with tropical enteropathy syndrome (asymptomatic small bowel mucosal damage from poor hygiene living circumstances) have a lower threshold, as lactase is on the tip of the brush border. Recovery of the intestinal mucosa is prompt after rotaviral gastroenteritis, so children with a normal gut before infection will usually tolerate breast milk at least by the third day of infection. However, this threshold is often exceeded in Aboriginal children during early recovery, when their intake of breast milk returns to normal or even increased volumes. The technique for testing for lactose intolerance/intolerance of other sugars is given in Table 22.7.

Table 22.7   Diagnosis of reducing substances in stool (osmotic diarrhoea)

For hot and cold stool testing of reducing substances you need approximately 1 ml of stool fluid. A positive test = >0.5%

Cold test (for monosaccharide or lactose sugars)
1. Mix 1 ml stool with 2 ml water.
2. Take 15 drops from that mixture and place in test tube.
3. Add 1 Clinitest tablet.
4. Wait until tablet stops reacting.
5. Shake and compare with chart.

Hot test (for sucrose, starch sugars or glucose polymers when the cold test is ≤0.5%)
1. Take 10 drops hydrochloric acid 1%.
2. Add 5 drops fluid stool.
3. Mix and bring slowly to boil.
4. Add Clinitest tablet.
5. Wait until tablet stops reacting and compare with chart.

Stool water must be collected directly and tested promptly. If it is scraped from a nappy or tested after 30 minutes, it is likely to give falsely low results.

Clinical example

A 15 month old Aboriginal boy was flown to Royal Darwin Hospital from his Arnhemland community due to diarrhoea, floppiness and fast breathing. He was accompanied by his mother who said that he had had many watery bowel movements over a short period of time. On examination he appeared unwell and was lethargic with sunken eyes. His vital signs were: temperature 37.5°C, heart rate 120/min, respiratory rate 60/min and blood pressure 86/53. Although alert and responsive, he was noted to be floppy, with a dry mouth, absent tears on crying, weak radial pulses, a capillary refill time of over 2 seconds and slow skin pinch recoil. On auscultation his heart sounds were normal and his lung fields were clear. His abdomen was soft and slightly distended with no tenderness, masses or visceromegaly. Bowel sounds were present. Neurological examination was normal except for mild hypotonia.

He was commenced on an intravenous infusion of Ringer's lactate (Hartmann's solution) and blood was taken for full blood count and urea and electrolytes. His weight on admission was 6.1 kg and his height 68 cm. These are all below the 3rd centile and yield a weight for age of 56% of the median (Z-score –4.4), a height for age of 85% (Z-score –4.0) and a weight-for-height of 76% (Z-score –2.6). His head circumference was 43.6 cm which falls well below the 2nd centile for age (Z-score –3.0).

The laboratory findings were as follows (reference ranges are give in parentheses).

Blood count

Haemoglobin (g/l)	**82** (105–135)
MCV (fl)	**53.9** (75–85)
RDW (%)	**24.1** (11.5–14.5)
Platelets (× 10^9/l)	**724** (150–450)
White cells (× 10^9/l)	**15.6** (6.0–11.0)

Blood film report
Marked microcytosis and hypochromia, moderate anisocytosis and poikilocytosis, neutrophil leucocytosis with no toxic changes and moderate eosinophilia.

Electrolytes

Sodium (mmol/l)	138 (132–144)
Potassium (mmol/l)	**2.0** (3.2–4.8)
Chloride (mmol/l)	**111** (98–106)
Total CO_2 (mmol/l)	**6** (18–27)
Anion gap	**23** [(138+2)-(111+6)] (8–12)
Urea (mmol/l)	5.3 (1.4–5.4)
Creatinine (μmol/l)	44 (0–55)

Blood gases

pH	**7.12** (7.35–7.4)
P_{CO_2} (mmHg)	**20.3** (35–45)
Base excess	−18 (−4 to +3)
Blood lactate (mmol/l)	1.6 (0.8–1.8)

He was rehydrated with 600 ml Ringer's lactate with 1 g/l of KCl added (17.4 mmol/l) over 4 hours, followed by maintenance fluids at 30 ml/h with breastfeeding. By 24 hours after admission he had been given 1500 ml of fluids and his condition had much improved. His weight was now 6.7 kg, which implied he had been about 9% dehydrated on admission (6.7 – 6.1 = 0.6 kg; 0.6/6.7 × 100 = 8.96%). His diarrhoea was settling and he was passing dilute urine.

Over the next 24 hours, however, he had six foul watery stools containing large amounts of reducing substances. There was also a decrease in his pH, bicarbonate and magnesium compared with 24 hours previously. This relapse of osmotic diarrhoea was due to breast milk lactose overcoming the lactase threshold in the small intestinal mucosal brush border. He improved on oral lactase drops (β-D-galactosidase) with breastfeeds. The stool microscopy result reported ova of *Strongyloides stercoralis*.

This is a fairly typical case of acute gastroenteritis in an Aboriginal child from northern Australia, whose illness is frequently complicated by osmotic diarrhoea, hypokalaemia, acidosis and iron deficiency. The underlying small bowel damage could be prevented by improving hygiene, reducing overcrowding and prompt treatment of micronutrient deficiencies, which would then make community oral rehydration therapy more effective, without the need for evacuation to hospital.

23 Drugs used in paediatrics

F. Shann

This comprehensive list of drugs used in paediatric practice has been prepared by Dr Frank Shann, Director of Intensive Care, Royal Children's Hospital, Melbourne. It is an extract from Shann F 2001 Drug Doses, 11th edn. Collective Pty Ltd, Parkville, Victoria, Australia. We thank him sincerely for permission to publish it.

The doses of drugs given are indicative, but for some drugs, doses change with new or further knowledge. Therefore further expert advice should be sought, and the user is advised to check the doses carefully. The author, editors and publisher shall not be responsible for any errors in this publication.

It should be noted that paediatric pharmacology is not an exact science and that those caring for children need to be aware of the possible side effects of the drugs they use. With a number of drugs it is both possible and desirable to monitor blood levels. This applies, for example to aminophylline, the aminoglycosides and a number of others. It must also be noted that there are significant differences in tolerance to certain drugs in the neonatal period: where appropriate, neonatal dosages are listed. Only generic names are given and unless otherwise stated dosages are in milligrams per kilogram (Editors).

DRUGS ARE LISTED BY GENERIC NAME

© F. Shann

(*Note* 1/100 = 1% = 10 mg/ml; 1/1000 = 1 mg/ml; 1/10 000 = 0.1 mg/ml;

BE, base excess; FSH, follicle stimulating hormone; INR, international normalised ratio; LH, luteinising hormone; H, hourly; NG, nasogastric tube.)

Acetazolamide 2–7.5 mg/kg/dose (adult 100–350 mg) 8 H oral.

Acetylcholine chloride Adult (NOT/kg): 1% inject 0.5–2 ml into anterior chamber of the eye.

Acetylcysteine Paracetamol poisoning (regardless of delay): 150 mg/kg in 5% dextrose i.v. over 1 h; then 10 mg/kg/h for 20 h (delay <10 h), 32 h (delay 10–16 h), 72 h (delay >16 h) and longer if still encephalopathic. Monitor serum K^+. Give if paracetamol >1000 µmol/l (150 µg/ml) at 4 h, >500 µmol/L 8 h, > 250 µmol/L 12 h. Lung disease: 10% solution 0.1 ml/kg/dose (adult 5 ml) 6–12 H nebulised or intratracheal. Meconium ileus equivalent: 5 ml/dose (NOT/kg) of 20% solution 8 H oral. Cystic fibrosis: 4–8 mg/kg/dose 8 H oral. Eye drops 5% + hypromellose 0.35%: 1–2 drops/eye 6–8 H.

Aciclovir Cutaneous herpes: 5 mg/kg/dose (2–12 weeks), 250 mg/m²/dose (12 weeks–12 years), 5 mg/kg/dose (adult) 8 H i.v. over 1 h. Herpes encephalitis, varicella or Epstein–Barr virus: 500 mg/m²/dose (adult 10 mg/kg) 8 H i.v. over 1 h; neonate 10 mg/kg/dose i.v. over 1 h daily (<30 weeks gestation), 18 H (30–32 weeks), 12 H (1st week of life), 8 H (2–12 weeks).

Genital herpes (NOT/kg): 200 mg/dose oral ×5/day for 10 days, then 200 mg/dose ×2–3/day for 6 months if required. Zoster (NOT/kg): 400 mg/dose (<2 years) or 800 mg/dose (≥2 years) oral ×5/day for 7 days. Cold sores: apply 5% cream ×5/day.

Activated charcoal See charcoal, activated.

Acyclovir See aciclovir.

Adenosine 0.1 mg/kg (adult 3 mg) stat rapid i.v. push, increase by 0.05 mg/kg (adult 3 mg) every 2 min to max 0.35 mg/kg (adult 18 mg).

Adrenaline Croup: 1% (L isomer) or 2.25% (racemic) 0.05 ml/kg/dose diluted to 4 ml by inhalation; or 1/1000 0.5 ml/kg/dose (max 6 ml) by inhalation. Cardiac arrest: 0.1 ml/kg of 1/10 000 i.v. or intracardiac or via endotracheal tube (up to 1 ml/kg/dose if no response). Anaphylaxis: 0.05–0.1 ml/kg/dose of 1/10 000 i.v. s.c.: 0.01 mg/kg (0.01 ml/kg of 1/1000), ×3 doses 20 min apart if required. i.v. infusion 0.05–2 µg/kg/min: for 65 kg adult 5 mg in 50 ml at 2 ml/h is 0.05 µg/kg/min.

Adrenocorticotrophic hormone (ACTH) See corticotrophin.

Agar See paraffin (and phenolphthalein) and agar.

Albendazole Pinworm, threadworm, roundworm, hookworm, whipworm: 20 mg/kg/dose (max 400 mg) oral once (may repeat after 2 weeks). Strongyloides, cutaneous larva migrans, Taenia, *H.nana*, *O.viverrini*, *C.sinesis*: 20 mg/kg/dose (max 400 mg) daily for 3 days, repeated in 3 weeks. 7.5 mg/kg (max 400 mg) 12 H for 8–30 days (neurocysticercosis); 12 H for three 28 day courses 14 days apart (hydatid).

Albumin 20%: 2–5 ml/kg i.v. 4%: 10–20 ml/kg. If no loss from plasma: dose (ml/kg) = 5 × (increase g/l)/ (% albumin).

Alclometasone dipropionate cream or ointment 0.05% Apply 8–12 H.

Aldesleukin (synthetic interleukin-2) See interleukin-2.

Alfacalcidol 0.05 µg/kg (max 1 µg) daily oral or i.v., adjusted according to response.

Alfentanil 10 µg/kg i.v. or i.m. stat, then 5 µg/kg p.r.n. Theatre (ventilated): 30–50 µg/kg i.v. over 5 min, then 15 µg/kg p.r.n or 0.5–1 µg/kg/min. ICU: 50–100 µg/kg i.v. over 10 min, then 0.5–4 µg/kg/min.

Alginic acid (Gaviscon) <1 year: 1–2 g powder with feed 4 H. 1–12 years: liquid 5–10 ml, or granules ½ sachet after meals. >12 years: liquid 10–20 ml, or granules 1 sachet after meals.

Alglucerase Usual initial dose is 60 units/kg every 2 weeks i.v. over 2 h, adjusted according to response; reduce every 3–6 months.

Allopurinol Gout: 2–12 mg/kg/dose (max 600 mg) daily oral. Cancer therapy: 2.5–5 mg/kg/dose (max 200 mg) 6 H.

Alpha1 proteinase inhibitor See alpha1 antitrypsin.

Alpha1 antitrypsin 60 mg/kg once weekly i.v. over 30 min.

Alpha tocopheryl acetate One alpha–tocopheryl (at) equivalent = 1 mg d–at = 1.1 mg d–at acetate = 1.5 mg dl–at acetate = 1.5 units vitamin E. Abetalipoproteinaemia: 100 mg/kg (max 4 g) daily oral. Cystic fibrosis: 45–200 mg (NOT/kg) daily oral. Newborn (high dose, toxicity reported): 10–25 mg/kg daily i.m. or i.v., 10–100 mg/kg daily oral.

Alprenolol 1–4 mg/kg/dose (max 200 mg) 6–12 H oral.

Alprostadil (prostaglandin E1, PGE1) 0.01–0.1 μg/kg/min (10–100 ng/kg/min). To maintain patent ductus arteriosus with 0.01 μg/kg/min (10 ng/kg/min): put 60 μg/kg in 50 ml saline, run at 0.5 ml/h. Pulmonary vasodilation with 0.1 μg/kg/min (100 ng/kg/min) put 500 μg in 83/wt ml saline and run at 1 ml/h (5.0 μg/kg/min nitroglycerine = 2.0 μg/kg/min nitroprusside = 0.1 μg/kg/min PGE1 approximately). Erectile dysfunction (adult NOT/kg): 2.5 μg intracavernous injection, increase in 2.5 μg increments if required to max 60 μg (max of 3 doses/week).

Alteplase (tissue plasminogen activator) 0.2–0.5 mg/kg/h i.v. for 6–12 h (longer if no response); keep fibrinogen >100 mg/dl (give cryoprecipitate 1 bag/5 kg), give heparin 10 units/kg/h i.v., give fresh frozen plasma (FFP) 10 ml/kg i.v. daily in infants. Local i.a. infusion: 0.05 mg/kg/h, give FFP 10 ml/kg i.v. daily.

Aluminium hydroxide 5–50 mg/kg/dose (adult 0.5–1 g) 6–8 H oral. Gel (64 mg/ml) 0.1 ml/kg/dose 6 H oral.

Aluminium hydroxide 40 mg/ml, magnesium hydroxide 40 mg/ml, simethicone 4 mg/ml (Mylanta) 0.2–0.4 ml/kg/dose (adult 10–20 ml) 4–6 H oral. ICU: 0.5 ml/kg/dose 3 H oral if gastric pH <5.

Amantadine hydrochloride 2 mg/kg/dose (adult 100 mg) 12–24 H oral. Flu A prophylaxis (NOT/kg): 100 mg daily (5–9 years), 100 mg 12 H (>9 years).

Amethocaine Gel 4% in methylcellulose (RCH): 0.5 g to skin, apply occlusive dressing, wait 30–60 min, remove gel. Eye drops 0.5%, 1%: 1–2 drops.

Amikacin sulfate Single daily dose i.v. or i.m. Neonate: 15 mg/kg stat, then 7.5 mg/kg (<2.5 kg) or 12 mg/kg (≥2.5 kg) daily. 1 month–10 years: 25 mg/kg stat, then 20 mg/kg daily. >10 years: 20 mg/kg stat, then 15 mg/kg (max 240–360 mg) daily. Trough level <5.0 mg/l.

Amiloride 0.2 mg/kg/dose (max 5 mg) 12 H oral.

Aminocaproic acid 100 mg/kg (adult 5 g) stat, then 30 mg/kg/h (max 1.25 g/h) until bleeding stops (max 18 g/m²/day) oral or i.v. Prophylaxis: 70 mg/kg/dose 6 H.

Aminophylline (100 mg aminophylline = 80 mg theophylline). Load: 10 mg/kg (max 500 mg) i.v. over 1 h. Maintenance: 1st week of life 2.5 mg/kg/dose 12 H; 2nd week of life 3 mg/kg/dose 12 H; 3 weeks–12 months ((0.12 × age in weeks) + 3) mg/kg/dose 8 H; 1–9 years 1.1 mg/kg/h (55 mg/kg in 50 ml at 1 ml/h), or 6 mg/kg/dose i.v. over 1 h 6 H; 10–16 years or adult smoker 0.7 mg/kg/h (<35 kg 35 mg/kg in 50 ml at 1 ml/h; >35 kg 25 mg/ml at 0.028 ml/kg/h), or 4 mg/kg/dose i.v. over 1 h 6 H; adult non smoker 0.5 mg/kg/h (25 mg/ml at 0.02 ml/kg/h), or 3 mg/kg/dose i.v. over 1 h 6 H; elderly 0.3 mg/kg/h (15 mg/kg in 50 ml at 1 ml/h), or 2 mg/kg/dose i.v. over 1 h 6 H. Monitor theophylline level: 60–80 μmol/l (neonate), 60–110 (asthma) (×0.18= μg/ml).

Amiodarone i.v.: 25 μg/kg/min for 4 h, then 5–15 μg/kg/min (max 1.2 g/24 h). Oral: 4 mg/kg/dose (adult 200 mg) 8 H 1 week, 12 H 1 week, then 12–24 H. After starting tabss, taper i.v. infusion over 5 days. Reduce dose of digoxin and warfarin.

Amitriptyline Usually 0.5–1 mg/kg/dose (adult 25–50 mg) 8 H oral. Enuresis: 1–1.5 mg/kg nocte.

Amlodipine 0.05–0.2 mg/kg (adult 2.5–10 mg) daily oral.

Amorolfine Nail lacquer 5%: apply ×1–2/week.

Amoxycillin 10–25 mg/kg/dose (adult 0.25–1 g) 8 H i.v., i.m. or oral. Severe infection: 50 mg/kg/dose (adult 2 g) i.v. 12 H (1st week of life), 6 H (2–4 weeks), 4–6 H or constant infusion (4+ weeks).

Amoxycillin and clavulanic acid Dose as for amoxycillin.

Amphetamine See dexamphetamine.

Amphotericin B 0.5–1.5 mg/kg/day by continuous infusion i.v.; total dose 30–35 mg/kg over 4–8 weeks. Oral (NOT/kg): 100 mg 6 H treatment, 50 mg 6 H prophylaxis. Bladder washout: 25 μg/ml. Cream or ointment 3%: apply 6–12 H.

Amphotericin, liposomal 1 mg/kg daily i.v. over 1 h, increase over 2–4 days to 2–3 mg/kg daily. Total dose typically 20–60 mg/kg over 2–4 weeks.

Ampicillin 10–25 mg/kg/dose (adult 0.25–1 g) 6 H i.v., i.m. or oral. Severe infection: 50 mg/kg/dose (max 2 g) i.v. 12 H (1st week of life), 6 H (2–4 weeks), 3–6 H or constant infusion (4+ weeks).

Ampicillin 1 g + sulbactam 0.5 g. 25–50 mg/kg/dose (adult 1–2 g) of ampicillin 6 H i.m. or i.v. over 30 min.

Amrinone <4 weeks old: 4 mg/kg i.v. over 1 h, then 3–5 μg/kg/min. >4 weeks: 1–3 mg/kg i.v. over 1 h, then 5–15 μg/kg/min.

Amylase See pancreatic enzymes.

Ancestim (human stem cell factor) 20 μg/kg/day s.c.

Aneurine See thiamine.

Antithrombin III Number of IU = (desired − actual level) × wt/2.2.

Antithymocyte (lymphocyte) globulin See immunoglobulin, lymphocyte.

Antivenom to Australian box jellyfish, snakes (black, brown, death adder, sea, taipan, tiger), spiders (funnelweb) and ticks Dose depends on amount of venom injected, not size of patient. Higher doses needed for multiple bites, severe symptoms or delayed administration. Give adrenaline 0.005 mg/kg (0.005 ml/kg of 1 in 1000) s.c. Initial dose antivenom usually 1–2 ampoules diluted 1/10 in Hartmann's solution i.v. over 30 min. Monitor PT, PTT, fibrinogen, platelets. Give repeatedly if symptoms or coagulopathy persist.

Antivenom to black widow spider (USA), redback spider (Australia) 1 ampoule i.m., may repeat in 2 h. Severe envenomation: 2 ampoules diluted 1/10 in Hartmann's solution i.v. over 30 min.

Antivenom, stonefish 1000 units (2 ml) per puncture i.m. Severe envenomation: 1000 units/puncture diluted 1/10 in Hartmann's solution i.v. over 30 min.

Aprotinin (1 kIU = 140 ng = 0.00056 epu, 1 mg = 7143 kIU). 100 000–1 200 000 kIU/m^2 over 1 h, then 100 000–300 000 kIU/m^2/h i.v. ECMO haemorrhage: 10 000 kIU/kg/h i.v.

Arginine hydrochloride Dose (mg) = BE × wt(kg) × 70 (give half this) i.v. over 2 h.

Aspirin 10–15 mg/kg/dose (adult 300–600 mg) 4–6 H oral. Antiplatelet: 2–5 mg/kg daily. Kawasaki: 4 mg/kg daily. Arthritis: 25 mg/kg/dose (max 2 g) 6 H for 3 days, then 15–20 mg/kg/dose 6 H. Salicylate level (arthritis) 0.7–2.0 mmol/l (×13.81 = mg/100ml).

Astemizole 0.2 mg/kg (max 10 mg) daily oral.

Atenolol Oral: 1–2 mg/kg/dose (adult 50–100 mg) 12–24 H. i.v.: 0.05 mg/kg (adult 2.5 mg) every 5 min till response (max 4 doses), then 0.1–0.2 mg/kg/dose (adult 5–10 mg) over 10 min 12–24 H.

Atracurium 0.3–0.6 mg/kg stat, then 5–10 μg/kg/min i.v.

Atropine sulphate 0.02 mg/kg (max 0.6 mg) i.v. or i.m., then 0.01 mg/kg/dose 4–6 H. Organophosphate poisoning: 0.05 mg/kg i.v., then 0.02–0.05 mg/kg/dose every 15–60 min until atropinised (continue 12–24 h). Colic: see phenobarbitone.

Azatadine 0.02–0.04 mg/kg/dose (adult 1–2 mg) 12 H oral.

Azathioprine 25–75 mg/m^2 (approx 1–3 mg/kg) daily.

Azithromycin 15 mg/kg (adult 500 mg) day 1, then 7.5 mg/kg (adult 250 mg) days 2–5 oral.

Azlocillin 50 mg/kg/dose (adult 2 g) 8 H i.v. Severe infection: 100 mg/kg/dose (adult 5 g) 12 H (1st week of life), 8 H or constant infusion (2+ weeks).

Aztreonam 25 mg/kg/dose (adult 1 g) 8 H i.v. Severe infection: 50 mg/kg/dose (adult 2 g) 12 H (1st week of life), 8 H (2–4 weeks), 6 H or constant infusion (4+ weeks).

Baclofen 0.1 mg/kg/dose (adult 5 mg) 8 H oral, increase every 3 days to about 0.4 mg/kg/dose (adult 20 mg) 8 H, max 0.8 mg/kg/dose (adult 35 mg) 8 H.

Intrathecal infusion: 2–20 μg/kg (max 1000 μg) per 24 h.

Beclomethasone dipropionate Rotacap or aerosol (NOT/kg): 100–200 μg (<8 years), 150–500 μg (>8 years) ×2–4/day. Nasal (NOT/kg): aerosol or pump (50 μg/spray): 1 spray 12H (<12 years), 2 spray 12H (>12years).

Benzathine penicillin See penicillin, benzathine.

Benzhexol 0.02 mg/kg/dose (adult 1 mg) 8 H, increase to 0.1–0.3 mg/kg/dose (adult 1.5–5 mg) 8 H oral.

Benzoyl peroxide Liquid, gel 2.5%–10%: apply ×1–3/day.

Benztropine mesylate 0.02 mg/kg (adult 1 mg) stat i.m./i.v., may repeat in 15 min. 0.02–0.06 mg/kg/dose (adult 1–3 mg) 12 24 H oral.

Benzyl benzoate, lotion 25% Scabies: apply from neck down after a hot bath, remove in bath after 24 h; repeat after 5 days. Lice: apply to infected region, wash off after 24 h; repeat after 7 days.

Benzylpenicillin See penicillin G.

Beractant (bovine surfactant, Survanta) 25 mg/ml solution: 4ml/kg intratracheal 4 times in 48 h (each dose in 4 parts: head and body inclined down with head to right, body down head left, body up head right, body up head left).

Betahistine 0.15–0.3 mg/kg/dose (adult 8–16 mg) 8 H oral.

Betamethasone 0.01–0.2 mg/kg daily oral. Betamethasone has no mineralocorticoid action, 1 mg = 25 mg hydrocortisone in glucocorticoid action. Gel 0.05%; cream, lotion or ointment, 0.02%, 0.05%, 0.1%: apply sparingly 12–24 H.

Bethanecol Oral: 0.2–1 mg/kg/dose (adult 10–50 mg) 6–8 H. s.c.: 0.05–0.1 mg/kg/dose (adult 2.5–5 mg) 6–8 H.

Bicarbonate Under 5 kg: dose (mmol) = BE × wt/4 slow i.v. Over 5 kg: dose (mmol) = BE × wt/6 slow i.v. These doses correct half the base deficit.

Biperiden 0.02–0.04 mg/kg/dose (adult 1–2 mg) 8–12 H oral. i.m. or slow i.v.: 0.05–0.1 mg/kg (adult 2.5–5mg), max ×4/day.

Bisacodyl NOT/kg: <12 months 2.5 mg PR, 1–5 years 5 mg PR or 5–10 mg oral, >5 years 10 mg PR or 10–20 mg oral.

Bismuth subcitrate (colloidal) 5 mg/kg/dose (adult 240 mg) 12 H oral 30 min before meal. *H.pylori* (adult, NOT/kg), take 4 doses/day (with meals and at bedtime) oral for 2 week: 107.7 mg/dose, tetracycline 500 mg/dose, and metronidazole 200 mg/dose with meals and 400 mg nocte; see also omeprazole.

Blood 4 ml/kg packed cells raises Hb 1 g%. 1 bag = 300 ml.

Botulinum toxin type A NOT/kg: 1.25–2.5 units/site (max 5 units/site) i.m., max total 200 units in 30 days.

Bromocriptine 0.025 mg/kg/dose (adult 1.25 mg) 8–12 H, increase weekly to 0.05–0.2 mg/kg/dose (adult 2.5–10 mg) 6–12 H oral. Inhibit lactation (NOT/kg): 2.5 mg/dose 12 H for 2 weeks.

Budesonide Metered dose inhaler (NOT/kg): <12 years 50–200 µg 6–12 H, reducing to 100–200 µg 12 H; >12 years 100–600 µg 6–12 H, reducing to 100–400 µg 12 H. Nebuliser (NOT/kg): <12 years 0.5–1 mg 12 H, reducing to 0.25–0.5 mg 12 H; >12 years 1–2 mg 12 H, reducing to 0.5–1 mg 12 H. Croup: 2 mg (NOT/kg) by nebuliser. Nasal spray or aerosol (NOT/kg): 100–200 µg/nostril daily.

Bumetanide 25 µg/kg (adult 1 mg) daily oral, may increase to 8–12 H.

Bupivacaine Max dose: 2–3 mg/kg (0.4–0.6 ml/kg of 0.5%). With adrenaline: max dose: 3–4 mg/kg (0.6–0.8 ml/kg of 0.5%). Epidural: 2 mg/kg (0.4 ml/kg 0.5%) stat intraoperative, then 0.25 mg/kg/h (0.2 ml/kg/h 0.125%) postop. Epidural in ICU: 25 ml 0.5% + 1000 µg (20 ml) fentanyl + saline to 100ml at 2–8 ml/h in adult.

C1 esterase inhibitor 1 unit = activity 1 ml plasma. 10–50 units/kg i.v. over 1 h once (prophylaxis), 12–24 H (treatment).

Caffeine 1–5 mg/kg/dose (adult 50–250 mg) 4–8 H oral, PR. Neonate: 20 mg/kg stat, then 5 mg/kg daily oral or i.v. over 30 min; weekly level 5–30 mg/l midway between doses.

Calciferol (ergocalciferol, D₂). See vitamin D.

Calcitonin Hypercalcaemia: 4 units/kg/dose 12–24 H i.m. or s.c., may increase up to 8 units/kg/dose 6–12 H. Paget: 1.5–3 units/kg (max 160 units) ×3/week i.m. or s.c.

Calcitriol See vitamin D.

Calcium (as carbonate, lactate or phosphate) NOT/kg: <3 years: 100 mg ×2–5/day oral; 4–12 years: 300 mg ×2–3/day; >12 years: 1000 mg ×1–2/day.

Calcium chloride 10% (0.7 mmol/ml Ca) 0.2 ml/kg (max 10 ml) slow i.v. stat. Requirement 2 ml/kg/day. Inotrope: 0.5–2 mmol/kg/day (0.03–0.12 ml/kg/h).

Calcium edetate (EDTA) See sodium calcium edetate.

Calcium folinate NOT/kg: 5–15 mg oral, or 1 mg i.m. or i.v. daily. Rescue starting up to 24 h after methotrexate: 10–15 mg/m²/dose 6 H for 36–48 h i.v. Methotrexate toxicity: 100–1000 mg/m²/dose 6 H i.v. Before a fluorouracil dose of 370 mg/m²: 200 mg/m² i.v. daily ×5, repeat every 3–4 weeks.

Calcium gluconate 10% (0.22 mmol/ml Ca) 0.5 ml/kg (max 20 ml) slow i.v. stat. Requirement 5 ml/kg/day. Inotrope: 0.5–2 mmol/kg/day (0.1–0.4 ml/kg/h).

Calcium polystyrene sulfonate (Calcium Resonium) 0.3–0.6 g/kg/dose (adult 15–30 g) 6 H NG (+ lactulose), PR.

Capreomycin sulphate 20 mg/kg (adult 1 g) i.m. on 2–7 days/week.

Captopril 0.1–1 mg/kg/dose (adult 5–50 mg) 8 H oral.

Carbamazepine 2 mg/kg/dose (adult 100 mg) 8 H oral, may increase over 2 weeks to 5–10 mg/kg/dose (adult 250–500 mg) 8 H. Level 20–50 µmol/l (×0.24 = µg/ml) measured Monday, Wednesday and Friday at RCH.

Carbimazole 0.4 mg/kg/dose (adult 20 mg) 8–12 H oral for 2 week, then 0.1 mg/kg/dose (adult 5 mg) 8–24 H.

Carnitine 20–35 mg/kg/dose (max 1 g) 8 H oral or i.v.

Carob bean gum (Carobel Instant) NOT/kg: 1 scoop (1.8 g) in 100 ml water, give 10–20 ml by spoon; or add ¹/₂ a scoop to every 100–200 ml of milk.

Cefaclor 10–15 mg/kg/dose (adult 250–500 mg) 8 H oral. Slow release tab 375 mg (adult, NOT/kg): 1–2 tab 12 H oral.

Cefadroxil 15–25 mg/kg/dose (adult 0.5–1 g) 12 H oral.

Cefepime 25 mg/kg/dose (adult 1 g) 12 H i.m. or i.v. over 5 min. Severe infection: 50 mg/kg/dose (adult 2 g) i.v. 8–12 H or constant infusion.

Cefixime 5 mg/kg/dose (adult 200 mg) 12–24 H oral.

Cefotaxime 25 mg/kg/dose (adult 1 g) 12 H (<4 weeks), 8 H (4+ weeks) i.v. Severe infection: 50 mg/kg/dose (adult 2–3 g) i.v. 12 H (preterm), 8 H (1st week of life), 6 H (2–4 weeks), 4–6 H or constant infusion (4+ weeks).

Cefotetan 25 mg/kg/dose (adult 1 g) 12 H i.m., i.v. Severe infection: 50 mg/kg/dose (max 2–3 g) 12 H or constant infusion.

Cefoxitin 25–60 mg/kg/dose (adult 1–3 g) 12 H (1st week of life), 8 H (1–4 weeks), 6–8 H (>4 weeks) i.v.

Cefpirome sulfate 25–40 mg/kg/dose (adult 1–2 g) 12 H i.v.

Cefpodoxime 5 mg/kg/dose (adult 100–200 mg) 12 H oral.

Cefprozil 15 mg/kg/dose (adult 500 mg) 12–24 H oral.

Ceftazidime 15–25 mg/kg/dose (adult 0.5–1 g) 8 H i.v. or i.m. Severe infection: 50 mg/kg/dose (max 2 g) 12 H (1st week of life), 8 H (2–4 weeks), 6 H or constant infusion (4+ weeks).

Ceftriaxone 25 mg/kg/dose (adult 1 g) 12–24 H i.v., or i.m. (in 1% lignocaine). Severe infection: 50 mg/kg/dose (max 2 g) daily (1st week of life), 12 H (2+ weeks). Epiglottitis: 100 mg/kg stat, then 50 mg/kg after 24 h. Meningococcus prophylaxis (NOT/kg): child 125 mg, adult 250 mg i.m. in 1% lignocaine once.

Cefuroxime. Oral: 10–15 mg/kg/dose (adult 250–500 mg) 12 H. i.v.: 25 mg/kg/dose (adult 1 g) 8 H. Severe infection: 50 mg/kg/dose (max 2 g) i.v. 12 H (1st week of life), 8 H (2nd week), 6 H or constant infusion (>2 weeks).

Cephalexin 10–25 mg/kg/dose (adult 0.25–1 g) 6–12 H oral.

Cephalothin 15–25 mg/kg/dose (adult 0.5–1 g) 6 H i.v. or i.m. Severe infection: 50 mg/kg/dose (max 2 g) i.v. 4 H or constant infusion. Irrigation fluid: 2 g/l (2 mg/ml).

Cephamandole 15–25 mg/kg/dose (adult 0.5–1 g) 6–8 H i.v. over 10 min or i.m. Severe infection: 40 mg/kg/

dose (adult 2 g) i.v. over 20 min 4–6 H or constant infusion.

Cephazolin 10–15 mg/kg/dose (adult 0.5 g) 6 H i.v. or i.m. Severe infection: 50 mg/kg/dose (adult 2 g) i.v. 4–6 H or constant infusion.

Cephradine Oral: 10–25 mg/kg/dose (adult 0.25–1 g) 6 H. i.m. or i.v.: 25–50 mg/kg/dose (adult 1–2 g) 6 H.

Charcoal, activated Check bowel sounds present: 0.25 g/kg/dose hourly NG. Laxative: sorbitol 1 g/kg (1.4 ml/kg of 70%) once NG, may repeat once.

Chickenpox vaccine See varicella vaccine.

Chloral hydrate Hypnotic: 50 mg/kg (max 2 g) stat (up to 100 mg/kg, max 5 g, in ICU). Sedative: 6 mg/kg/dose 6 H oral.

Chloramphenicol Severe infection: 40 mg/kg (max 2 g) stat, then 25 mg/kg/dose (max 1 g) i.v., i.m. or oral. 1st week of life: daily; 2–4 weeks: 12 H; 5+ weeks: 8 H for 5 days, then 6 H. Ensure serum level 20–30 mg/l peak, <15 mg/l trough.

Chloroquine Oral: 10 mg/kg (max 600 mg) daily ×3 days. i.m.: 4 mg/kg/dose (max 300 mg) 12 H for 3 days. Prophylaxis: 5 mg/kg (adult 300 mg) oral ×1/week. Lupus, rheumatoid arthritis: 12 mg/kg (max 600 mg) daily, reducing to 4–8 mg/kg (max 400 mg) daily oral.

Chlorothiazide 5–20 mg/kg/dose (adult 0.25–1 g) 12–24 H oral, i.v.

Chlorpheniramine 0.1 mg/kg/dose (adult 4 mg) 6–8 H oral.

Chlorpheniramine 1.25 mg + phenylephrine 2.5 mg in 5 ml syrup NOT/kg: 1.25–2.5 ml (0–1 years), 2.5–5 ml (2–5 years), 5–10 ml (6–12 years), 10–15 ml (>12 years) 6–8 H oral.

Chlorpromazine Oral or PR: 0.5–2 mg/kg/dose (max 100 mg) 6–8 H; up to 20 mg/kg/dose 8 H for psychosis. Slow i.v. or i.m.: 0.25–1 mg/kg/dose (usual max 50 mg) 6–8 H.

Chlortetracycline, cream or ointment 3% Apply 8–24 H.

Chlorthalidone 2 mg/kg (max 100 mg) 3 times a week oral.

Cholecalciferol (vitamin D$_3$) 1 unit = 1 unit ergocalciferol. See vitamin D.

Cholera vaccine, parenteral (CSL) Inactivated. 2 doses s.c. 7–28 days apart: 0.1 ml then 0.3 ml (<5 years), 0.3 ml then 0.5 ml (5–9 years), 0.5 ml then 1 ml (>9 years). Boost every 6 months (use 1st dose).

Cholera vaccine, oral (Orochol) Live. >2 years: 1 sachet + 100 ml water. Boost every 6 months.

Cholestyramine 50–150 mg/kg/dose (adult 3–9 g) 6–8 H oral.

Choline salicylate, mouth gel (Bonjela) Apply 3 H p.r.n.

Choline theophyllinate (200 mg = theophylline 127 mg) See theophylline.

Chorionic gonadotrophin Usually 100 IU/kg (max 5000 IU) i.m. ×3/week for 2–8 weeks. After FSH:

10 000 IU (NOT/kg) i.m. once. Men: 7000 IU (NOT/kg) i.m. ×2/week, with 75 IU FSH and 75 IU LH i.m. ×3/week.

Cidofovir 5 mg/kg over 1 h i.v. on day 0, day 7, then every 14 days (given with probenecid).

Cimetidine Oral: 6–8 mg/kg/dose (adult 300–400 mg) 6 H, or 16 mg/kg (adult 800 mg) nocte. i.v.: 10–15 mg/kg/dose (max 200 mg) 12 H (newborn), 6 H (>4 weeks).

Ciprofloxacin 5–10 mg/kg/dose (adult 250–500 mg) 12 H oral, 4–7 mg/kg/dose (adult 200–300 mg) 12 H i.v. Severe infection: 20 mg/kg/dose (max 750 mg) 12 H oral, 10 mg/kg/dose (max 400 mg) 8 H i.v.; higher doses used occasionally. Meningococcus prophylaxis: 15 mg/kg (max 500 mg) once oral. Reduce dose of theophylline.

Ciprofloxacin eye drops 0.3% Corneal ulcer: 2 drops/15 min for 6 h then 2 drops/30 min for 18 h (day 1), 2 drops 1 H (day 2), 2 drops 4 H (day 3–14). Conjunctivitis: 1–2 drops 4 H; if severe 1–2 drops 2 H when awake for 2 days, then 6 H.

Cisapride 0.1–0.3 mg/kg/dose (adult 5–15 mg) (rarely 0.4 mg/kg/dose, max 20 mg) ×3–4/day oral.

Cisatracurium besylate 0.1 mg/kg (child) or 0.15 mg/kg (adult) i.v. stat, then 1–3 µg/kg/min if required. ICU: 0.15 mg/kg stat, then 3 µg/kg/min (0.5–10 µg/kg/min) i.v.

Clarithromycin 7.5–15 mg/kg/dose (adult 250–500 mg) 12 H oral. Slow release tab, adult (NOT/kg): 0.5 g or 1 g daily.

Clavulanic acid with amoxycillin or ticarcillin Dose as for amoxycillin or ticarcillin.

Clindamycin 5–10 mg/kg/dose (adult 150–300 mg) 6 H oral, i.m. or i.v. over 30 min. Severe infection: 10–20 mg/kg/dose (adult 0.5–1 g) 6 H i.v. over 1 h. Acne solution 1%: apply 12 H.

Clobazam 0.1–0.4 mg/kg/dose (adult 10–20 mg) 8–12 H oral.

Clofazimine 2 mg/kg (adult 100 mg) daily oral. Lepra reaction: up to 6 mg/kg (max 300 mg) daily for max 3 months.

Clofibrate 10 mg/kg/dose 8–12 H oral.

Clomipramine 0.5–1 mg/kg/dose (adult 25–50 mg) 8–12 H oral.

Clonazepam 0.02 mg/kg/dose (max 0.5 mg) 12 H oral, slowly increase to 0.05 mg/kg/dose (max 2 mg) 6–12 H oral. Status (may be repeated), NOT/kg: neonate 0.25 mg (if ventilated), child 0.5 mg, adult 1 mg i.v.

Clonidine 3–5 µg/kg slow i.v., 1–6 µg/kg/dose (adult 50–300 µg) 8–12 H oral. Migraine: start with 0.5 µg/kg/dose 12 H oral. Analgesia: 2.5 µg/kg premed oral, 0.3 µg/kg/h i.v., 1–2 µg/kg local block.

Clotrimazole Topical: 1% cream or solution 8–12 H. Vaginal (NOT/kg): 1% cream or 100 mg tab daily for 6 days, or 2% cream or 500 mg tab daily for 3 days.

Coagulation factor, human (Prothrombinex) Factors 2, 9 and 10; 250 units/10 ml. 1 ml/kg slow i.v. daily. Risk of thrombosis in acute liver failure.

Codeine Analgesic: 0.5–1 mg/kg/dose 4 H oral. Antitussive: 0.25–0.5 mg/kg/dose 6 H.

Colfosceril palmitate (synthetic surfactant, Exosurf Neonatal) Solution 13.5 mg/ml. Prophylaxis: 5 ml/kg intratracheal over 5 min immediately after birth, and at 12 h and 24 h if still ventilated. Rescue: 5 ml/kg intratracheal over 5 min, repeat in 12 h if still ventilated.

Colistin sulfomethate sodium (1 mg = 12 500 units = 0.625 mg colistin sulphate) Oral: 30 000–60 000 units/kg/dose (adult 1.5–3 megaunits) 8 H. i.m. or slow i.v.: 40 000 units/kg/dose (adult 2 000 000 units) 8 H, or 3 mg/kg/dose (adult 150 mg) 8 H.

Colonic lavage solution Poisoning: if bowel sounds present, 30 ml/kg/h NG for 4–8 h (until rectal effluent clear).

Coloxyl See dioctyl sodium sulphosuccinate, poloxalkol.

Corticotrophin (ACTH) 1 unit/kg (adult 40 units) i.m. daily.

Cortisone acetate Physiological: 0.2 mg/kg/dose 8 H oral. Cortisone acetate 1 mg = hydrocortisone 1.25 mg in mineralocorticoid and glucocorticoid action.

Cotrimoxazole (trimethoprim 1 mg + sulphamethoxazole 5 mg) TMP 1.5–3 mg/kg/dose (adult 80–160 mg) 12 H i.v. over 1 h or oral. Renal prophylaxis: TMP 2 mg/kg (max 80 mg) daily oral. Pneumocystis: TMP 250 mg/m^2 stat, then 150 mg/m^2 8 H (<11 years) or 12 H (>10 years) i.v. over 1 h; in renal failure dose interval (h) = serum creatinine (mmol/l) × 135 (max 48 h); 1 h postinfusion serum TMP 5–10 μg/ml, SMX 100–200 μg/ml. i.v. infusion: TMP max 1.6 mg/ml in 5% dextrose.

Coumarin Oral: 1–8 mg/kg (adult 50–400 mg) daily. Cream 100 mg/g: apply 8–12 H.

Cromoglycate See sodium cromoglycate.

Crotamiton, cream or lotion 10% Apply ×2–3/day.

Cryoprecipitate Low factor 8: 1 unit/kg increase activity 2% (half-life 12 h); usual dose 5 ml/kg or 1 bag/4 kg 12 H i.v. for 1–2 infusions (muscle, joint), 3–6 infusions (hip, forearm, retroperitoneal, oropharynx), 7–14 infusions (intracranial). Low fibrinogen: usual dose 5 ml/kg or 1 bag/4 kg i.v. A bag is usually 20–30 ml: factor 8 about 5 units/ml and 100 units/bag, fibrinogen about 10 mg/ml and 200 mg/bag.

Cyanocobalamin (vitamin B$_{12}$) 20 μg/kg/dose (adult 1000 μg) i.m. daily for 7 days then weekly (treatment), monthly (prophylaxis). i.v. dangerous in megaloblastic anaemia.

Cyclopentolate hydrochloride, 0.5% or 1% 1 drop/eye, repeat after 5 min. Pilocarpine 1% speeds recovery.

Cyclophosphamide A typical regimen is 600 mg/m^2 i.v. over 30 min daily for 3 days, then 600 mg/m^2 i.v. weekly or 10 mg/kg twice weekly (if leucocytes >3000/mm^3).

Cyclosporin 1–3 μg/kg/min i.v. for 24–48 h, then 5–8 mg/kg/dose 12 H reducing by 1 mg/kg/dose each month to 3–4 mg/kg/dose oral. Juvenile arthritis: 3–5 mg/kg/day. Trough level by Abbott TDx monoclonal specific assay (× 2.5 = non specific assay level) on whole blood (done Tuesday and Friday at RCH): 120–200 ng/ml (marrow), 150–200 ng/ml first 3 months then 100–150 ng/ml (kidney), 100–400 ng/ml (heart, liver).

Cyproheptadine 0.1 mg/kg/dose (adult 4 mg) 8–12 H oral.

Cyproterone acetate 25–50 mg/m^2/dose 8–12 H oral.

Cysteamine 0.05 mg/m^2/dose 6 H oral, increase over 6 weeks to 0.33 mg/m^2/dose (<50 kg) or 0.5 mg/kg/dose (>50 kg) 6 H.

Cytomegalovirus immunoglobulin See immunoglobulin, CMV.

Dalteparin sodium Prophylaxis: 50 units/kg/dose (adult 2500 units) s.c. 1–2 h preop, then daily. Venous thrombosis: 100 units/kg/dose (adult 5000 units) 12 H s.c., or i.v. over 12 h. Haemodialysis: 5–10 units/kg stat, then 4–5 units/kg/h i.v. (acute renal failure, anti-Xa 0.2–0.4 units/ml); 30–40 units/kg stat, then 10–15 units/kg/h (chronic renal failure, anti-Xa 0.5–1 units/ml).

Dantrolene Hyperpyrexia: 1 mg/kg/min until improves (max 10 mg/kg), then 1–2 mg/kg/dose 6 H for 1–3 day i.v. or oral. Spasticity: 0.5–2 mg/kg/dose (adult 25–100 mg) 6 H oral.

Dapsone 1–2 mg/kg (adult 50–100 mg) daily oral. Dermatitis herpetiformis: 1–6 mg/kg (adult 50–300 mg) daily oral. See also pyrimethamine.

Demeclocycline >8 years: 3 mg/kg/dose (adult 150 mg) 6 H, or 6 mg/kg/dose (adult 300 mg) 12 H oral.

Desferrioxamine Antidote: 10–15 mg/kg/h i.v. for 12–24 h (max 6 g/24 h) if Fe > 60–90 μmol/l at 4 h or 8 h; some also give 5–10 g (NOT/kg) once oral. Thalassaemia (NOT/kg): 500 mg per unit blood; and 5–6 nights/week 1–3 g in 5 ml water s.c. over 10 h, 0.5–1.5 g in 10 ml water s.c. over 5 min.

Desipramine 0.5–1 mg/kg/dose (adult 25–50 mg) 8–12 H oral.

Desmopressin (DDAVP) 5–10 μg (0.05–0.1 ml) per dose (NOT/kg) 12–24 H nasal. Low factor VIII: 0.3 μg/kg in 1 ml/kg saline i.v. over 1 H 12–24 H.

Dexamethasone 0.1–0.25 mg/kg/dose 6 H oral or i.v. Bronchopulmonary dysplasia: 0.1 mg/kg/dose 6 H for 3 days, then 8 H 3 days, 12 H 3 days, 24 H 3 days, 48 H 7 days. Severe croup: 0.6 mg/kg (max 12 mg) i.m. stat, then prednisolone 1 mg/kg/dose 8–12 H oral. Eye drops 0.1%: 1–2 drops per eye 3–8 H. Dexamethasone has no mineralocorticoid action, but 1 mg = 25 mg hydrocortisone in glucocorticoid action.

Dexamphetamine 0.2 mg/kg (max 10 mg) daily oral, increase to max 0.6 mg/kg/dose (max 30 mg) 12 H.

Dexchlorpheniramine maleate 0.05 mg/kg/dose (adult 2 mg) 6–8 H oral.

Dextran 1 (Promit) 0.3 ml/kg i.v. 1–2 min before giving dextran 40 or dextran 70.

Dextran 40 10% solution: 10 ml/kg/dose ×1–2 on day 1, then 10ml/kg/day i.v. Half-life about 3 h.

Dextran 70 6% solution: 10ml/kg/dose ×1–2 on day 1, then 10 ml/kg/day i.v. Half-life about 12 h.

Dextrose See glucose.

Diazepam 0.2–0.4 mg/kg (adult 10–20 mg) i.v. or PR. 0.04–0.2 mg/kg/dose (adult 2–10 mg) 8–12 H oral. Do not give by i.v. infusion (binds to PVC).

Diazoxide Hypertension: 1–3 mg/kg (max 150 mg) stat by rapid i.v. injection (severe hypotension may occur) repeat once p.r.n., then 2–5 mg/kg/dose i.v. 6 H. Hyperinsulinism: 30–100 mg/m^2/dose 8 H oral.

Diclofenac 1 mg/kg/dose (adult 50 mg) 8 12 H oral. Eye drops 0.1%: preop 1–5 drops over 3 h, postop 3 drops stat, then 1 drop 4–8 H. Topical gel: apply 2–4 g 6–8 H.

Dicobalt edetate 6 mg/kg (adult 300 mg) i.v. over 1–5 min, repeat ×2 if no response.

Dicyclomine 0.5 mg/kg/dose (max 15 mg) 6 H oral.

Didanosine 50–150 mg/m^2/dose (max 300 mg) 12 H oral.

Diethylcarbamazine Filariasis, onchocerciasis, loiasis: 2 mg/kg/dose 8 H oral for 3–4 weeks. Ascariasis: 6–10 mg/kg/dose 8 H oral 7–10 days. Tropical eosinophilia: 13 mg/kg daily 4–7 days.

Digoxin 15 μg/kg stat and 5 μg/kg after 6 H, then 5 μg/kg/dose (max 200 μg i.v., 250 μg oral) 12 H slow i.v. or oral. Level 0.5–2.5 nmol/l (×0.78=ng/ml).

Digoxin immmune FAB (antibodies) i.v. over 30 min. Dose (to nearest 40 mg) = serum digoxin (nmol/l) × wt (kg) × 0.3, or mg ingested × 55. Give if >0.3 mg/kg ingested, or level >6.4 nmol/l or 5.0 ng/ml.

Dihydrocodeine 0.5–1 mg/kg/dose 4–6 H oral.

Diltiazem 1 mg/kg/dose (adult 60 mg) 8 H, increase to max 3 mg/kg/dose (adult 180 mg) 8 H oral. Slow release (adult, NOT/kg): 120–240 mg daily, or 90–180 mg 8–12 H oral.

Dimenhydrinate 1–1.5 mg/kg/dose (max 50 mg) 4–6 H oral, i.m. or i.v.

Diphenhydramine 1–2 mg/kg/dose (adult 50–100 mg) 6–8 H oral.

Diphenoxylate 2.5 mg and atropine 25 μg tab (Lomotil) Adult (NOT/kg): 1–2 tab 6–8 H oral.

Dipivefrin, eye drops 0.1% 1 drop per eye 12 H.

Dipyridamole 1–2 mg/kg/dose (adult 50–100 mg) 6–8 H oral.

Disodium etidronate 5–20 mg/kg daily oral (no food for 2 h before and after dose) for max 6 months.

Disodium pamidronate 0.3–1.5 mg/kg/dose (adult 15–90 mg) i.v. over 24 h, repeat every 2–3 weeks.

Dobutamine i.v. infusion 1–20 μg/kg/min: for 65 kg adult 250 mg in 50 ml at 2 ml/h is 2.5 μg/kg/min.

Docusate sodium NOT/kg: 100 mg (3–10 years), 120–240 mg (>10 years) daily oral. Enema (5 ml 18% + 155 ml water): 30 ml (newborn), 60 ml (1–12 months), 60–120 ml (>12 months) PR.

Docusate sodium 100 mg + bisacodyl 10 mg, suppository $^1/_2$ suppository (<12 months), 1 suppository (>1 year) when required.

Docusate sodium 50 mg + sennoside 8 mg, tab >12 years: 1–4 tab at night oral.

Dopamine i.v. infusion 1–20 μg/kg/min: for 65 kg adult 200 mg in 50 ml at 2 ml/h is 2 μg/kg/min.

Dopexamine i.v. infusion 0.5–6 μg/kg/min: for 65 kg adult 50 mg in 50 ml at 2 ml/h is 0.5 μg/kg/min.

Dornase alpha (deoxyribonuclease I) NOT/kg: usually 2.5 mg (max 10 mg) inhaled daily (5–21 years), 12–24 H (>21 years).

Dorzolamide 2% eye drops: 1 drop 8 H.

Doxapram 5 mg/kg i.v. over 1 h, then 0.5–1 mg/kg/h for 1 h (max total dose 400 mg).

Doxepin 0.2–2 mg/kg/dose (adult 10–100 mg) 8 H oral.

Doxycycline Over 8 years: 2 mg/kg/dose (adult 100 mg) 12 H for 2 doses, then daily.

Droperidol 0.1–0.4 mg/kg/dose (adult 5–20 mg) 4–8 H oral, 0.1–0.3 mg/kg/dose (adult 5–15 mg) 4–6 H i.m. or slow i.v. Antiemetic: postop 0.02–0.05 mg/kg/dose (adult 1.25 mg) 4–6 H i.m. or slow i.v., chemotherapy 0.02–0.1 (adult 1–5 mg) 1–6 H.

Econazole Topical: 1% cream, powder or lotion 8–12 H. Vaginal: 75 mg cream or 150 mg ovule twice daily.

Ecothiopate eye drops 0.03%, 0.06%, 0.125%, 0.25% Usually 0.125% 1 drop/eye every 1–2 days nocte.

Edrophonium Test dose 20 μg/kg (adult 2 mg), then 1 min later 80 μg/kg (adult 8 mg) i.v. SVT: 0.15 mg/kg (max 2 mg) increase to max 0.75 mg/kg (max 10 mg) i.v., with atropine if required for side effects.

EDTA See sodium calcium edetate.

Eformoterol Caps 12 mg (NOT/kg): 1 cap (child) or 1–2 caps (adult) inhaled 12 H.

Electrolyte solution See glucose electrolyte solution.

EMLA cream See lignocaine + prilocaine.

Enalapril 0.2–1 mg/kg (adult 5–40 mg) daily oral.

Enoxacin 4–8 mg/kg/dose (adult 200–400 mg) 12 H oral.

Enoxaparin (1 mg = 100 units) Prevention of deep vein thrombosis: 0.4–0.8 mg/kg/dose (adult 20–40 mg) 2–12 h preop, then daily s.c. Haemodialysis: 1 mg/kg into arterial line at start 4 h session.

Ephedrine 0.25–1 mg/kg/dose (adult 12.5–60 mg) 4–8 H oral, i.m., s.c. or i.v. Nasal (0.25%–1%): 1 drop each nostril 6–8 H, max 4 days.

Epoetin alfa, beta 20–50 units/kg ×3/week, increase to max 240 units/kg ×1–3/week s.c., i.v. When Hb >10 g%: 20–100 units/kg ×2–3/week.

Epoprostenol (prostacyclin, PGI2) 0.01 μg/kg/min i.v. Pulmonary vasodilation: 0.01 μg/kg/min epoprost = 5 μg/kg/min nitroglycerine = 2 μg/kg/min nitroprusside = 0.1 μg/kg/min PGE1.

Eprosartan mesylate 12 mg/kg (adult 600 mg) daily, increase if required to 6–8 mg/kg/dose (adult 300–400 mg) 12 H oral.

Epsilon aminocaproic acid See aminocaproic acid.

Ergotamine tartrate >10 years (NOT/kg): 2 mg sublingual stat, then 1 mg/h (max 6 mg/episode, 10 mg/week). Suppository (1–2 mg): 1 stat, may repeat once after 1 h.

Erythromycin Oral or slow i.v. (max 5 mg/kg/h): usually 10 mg/kg/dose (adult 250–500 mg) 6 H; severe infection 15–25 mg/kg/dose (adult 0.75–1 g) 6 H. 2% gel: apply 12 H.

Erytropoietin See epoetin.

Esmolol 0.5 mg/kg over 1 min, then 50 μg/kg/min for 4 min; if poor response repeat 0.5 mg/kg and give 50–200 μg/kg/min for up to 48 h.

Ethacrynic acid i.v.: 0.5–1 mg/kg/dose (adult 25–50 mg) 12–24 H. Oral: 1–4 mg/kg/dose (adult 50–200 mg) 12–24 H.

Ethambutol 25 mg/kg once daily for 8 weeks, then 15 mg/kg daily oral. Intermittent: 35 mg/kg ×3/week. i.v.: 80% oral dose.

Ethosuximide 10 mg/kg (adult 500 mg) daily oral, increase by 50% each week to max 40 mg/kg (adult 2 g) daily.

Etomidate 0.3 mg/kg slow i.v.

Factor 8 concentrate (vial 200–250 units), recombinant antihaemophilic factor (rAHF) Joint 20 units/kg, psoas 30 units/kg, cerebral 50 units/kg. 2 × dose (units/kg) = % normal activity, e.g. 35 units/kg gives peak level of 70% normal. See octocog alfa.

Factor 9 i.v. infusion (max 2 units/kg/min): minor haemorrhage 25 units/kg daily, joint 40 units/kg 12–24 H, surgery 50 units/kg stat then 30 units/kg 12–24 H, major surgery 85 units/kg stat then 50 units/kg 12–24 H. Prophylaxis: 25–40 units/kg ×2/week (trough >1 units/dl).

Famciclovir Zoster: 5 mg/kg (max 250 mg) 8 H oral 7 days. Genital herpes: 5 mg/kg/dose (max 250 mg) 8 H oral 5 days, recurrence 2.5 mg/kg/dose (max 125 mg) 12 H 5 days.

Famotidine 0.5–1 mg/kg/dose (adult 20–40 mg) 12–24 H oral. 0.5 mg/kg/dose (max 20 mg) 12 H slow i.v.

Fat emulsion 20% See lipid emulsion.

Felodipine 0.05 mg/kg/dose (adult 2.5 mg), increase to 0.2 mg/kg/dose (adult 10 mg) 12 H oral.

Fenoterol Oral: 0.1 mg/kg/dose 6 H. Respiratory solution 1 mg/ml: 0.5 ml/dose diluted to 2 ml 3–6 H (mild), 1 ml/dose diluted to 2 ml 1–2 H (moderate), undiluted continuous (severe, in ICU). Aerosol (200 μg/puff): 1–2 puffs 4–8 H.

Fentanyl 1–4 μg/kg/dose (adult 200 μg) i.m. or i.v.; infuse 2–4 μg/kg/h (<25 kg: 100 μg/kg in 50 ml at 1–2 ml/h, >25 kg: ampoule 50 μg/ml at 0.04–0.08 ml/kg/h). Ventilated: 5–10 μg/kg stat or 50 μg/kg i.v. over 1 h; infuse 5–10 μg/kg/h (ampoule 50 μg/ml at 0.1–0.2 ml/kg/h). Patch (lasts 72 h) in adult (NOT/kg): 25 μg/h, increase if required by 25 μg/h every 3 days.

Ferrous salts Prophylaxis 2 mg/kg/day elemental iron oral, treatment 6 mg/kg/day elemental iron oral.

Fumarate 1 mg = 0.33 mg iron. Gluconate 1 mg = 0.12 mg iron; so Fergon (60 mg/ml gluconate) prophylaxis 0.3 ml/kg daily, treatment 1 ml/kg daily oral. Sulphate (dried) 1 mg = 0.3 mg iron; so Ferro-Gradumet (350 mg dried sulphate) prophylaxis 7 mg/kg (adult 350 mg) daily, treatment 20 mg/kg (adult 1050 mg) daily oral.

Filgrastim (granulocyte CSF) Idiopathic or cyclic neutropenia: 5 μg/kg daily s.c. or i.v. over 30 min. Congenital neutropenia: 12 μg/kg daily s.c. or i.v. over 1 h. Marrow transplant: 20–30 μg/kg daily i.v. over 4–24 h, reducing if neutrophils >1 × 10^9/l.

Flecainide 2 mg/kg/dose (max 100 mg) 12 H oral, i.v. over 30 min; may increase over 2 weeks to 5 mg/kg/dose (max 200 mg) 12 H.

Flucloxacillin 10 mg/kg/dose (adult 250 mg) 6 H oral, i.m. or i.v. Severe infection: 25–50 mg/kg/dose (adult 1–2 g) i.v. 12 H (1st week of life), 8 H (2–4 weeks), 4–6 H or constant infusion (>4 weeks).

Fluconazole 6 mg/kg (adult 200 mg) stat, then 3 mg/kg (adult 100 mg) daily oral or i.v. Severe infection: 12 mg/kg (adult 400 mg) stat, then 4–12 mg/kg (adult 200–400 mg) daily i.v.

Flucytosine (5-fluorocytosine) 400–1200 mg/m^2/dose (max 2 g) 6 H i.v. over 30 min, or oral. Peak level 50–100 μg/ml, trough 25–50 μg/ml (×7.75 = μmol/l).

Fludrocortisone NOT/kg: 0.05–0.2 mg daily oral. Fludrocortisone 1 mg = hydrocortisone 125 mg in mineralocorticoid activity, 10 mg in glucocorticoid.

Flumazenil 5 μg/kg stat i.v., repeat every 60 s to max total 40 μg/kg (max 2 mg), then 2–10 μg/kg/h i.v.

Flunisolide Asthma (250 μg/puff): 1–2 puffs 12 H. Nasal (25 μg/puff): 1–2 puffs/nostril 8–24 H.

Flunitrazepam Adult (NOT/kg): 0.5–2 mg at night, oral.

Fluorescein, eye drops 1%, 2% 1–2 drops per eye.

9-alpha-fluorohydrocortisone See fludrocortisone.

Fluoxetine 0.5 mg/kg (max 20 mg) daily, increase to max 1 mg/kg/dose (max 40 mg) 12 H oral.

Flupenthixol Oral: 0.05–0.2 mg/kg/dose (adult 3–9 mg) 12 H. Depot i.m.: usually 0.4–0.8 mg/kg (up to 5 mg/kg, max 300 mg) every 2–4 weeks (1 mg flupenthixol deconate = 0.625 mg fluphenazine decanoate = 1.25 mg haloperidol).

Fluphenazine 0.02–0.2 mg/kg/dose (adult 1–10 mg) 8–12 H oral.

Flurazepam Adult (NOT/kg): 15–30 mg at night, oral.

Flurbiprofen 1–2 mg/kg/dose (adult 50–100 mg) 8 H oral or PR. Eye drops 0.03%: 1 drop/eye every 30 min.

Fluticasone Inhaled (NOT/kg): 50–100 μg/dose (child), 100–1000 μg/dose (adult) 12 H. 0.05% solution: 1–4 sprays/nostril daily. 0.05% cream: apply sparingly daily.

Folic acid Treatment: 0.1–0.3 mg/kg (adult 5–15 mg) daily i.v., i.m. or oral. Pregnancy (NOT/kg): 0.5 mg (high risk 4 mg) daily.

Folinic acid See calcium folinate.

Framycetin (Soframycin) Subconjunctival: 500 mg in 1 ml water daily ×3 days. Bladder: 500 mg in 50 ml saline 8 H × 10 days. Eye/ear 0.5%: 2–3 drops 8 H, ointment 8 H.

Framycetin 15 mg/g + gramicidin 0.05 mg/g, cream or ointment (Soframycin topical) Apply 8–12 H.

Framycetin 5 mg + gramicidin 0.05 mg + dexamethasone 0.5 mg/ml eye/ear (Sofradex) 2–3 drops 6–8 H, ointment 8–12 H.

Fresh frozen plasma Contains all clotting factors. 10–20 ml/kg i.v. 1 bag is about 230 ml.

Frusemide Usually 0.5–1 mg/kg/dose (adult 20–40 mg) 6–24 H (daily if preterm) oral, i.m., or i.v. over 20 min (no faster than 0.05 mg/kg/min i.v.). i.v. infusion: 0.1–1 mg/kg/h.

Fusidic acid (1 mg = 0.7 mg sodium fusidate) Suspension (fusidic acid): 15 mg/kg (adult 750 mg) 8 H oral. Tab (sodium fusidate): 10 mg/kg (adult 250–500 mg) 8 H. i.v. over 2–8 h (sodium fusidate): 10 mg/kg (adult 500 mg) 8 H; severe infection 15 mg/kg (adult 750 mg). Peak level 30–200 μmol/l (×0.52 = μg/ml).

Gabapentin 5–15 mg/kg/dose (adult 300–800 mg) 8–12 H oral.

Ganciclovir 2.5–5 mg/kg/dose 8–12 H i.v. over 1 h. Chronic use: 5 mg/kg i.v. over 1 h daily.

Gas gangrene (Clostridia) antitoxin Prophylaxis: 25 000 units i.m. or i.v. Treatment: 75 000–150 000 units i.v. over 1 h, repeat ×1–2 after 8–12 h. Give 100 000 units i.m. as well for severe infection.

Gaviscon See alginic acid.

Gemfibrozil 10 mg/kg/dose (max 600 mg) 12 H oral.

Gentamicin Single daily dose i.v. or i.m. Neonate: 5 mg/kg stat, then 2.5 mg/kg (<2.5 kg) or 4 mg/kg (≥2.5 kg) daily. 1 month–10 years: 8 mg/kg stat, then 6 mg/kg daily. >10 years: 7 mg/kg stat, then 5 mg/kg daily (max 240–360 mg) daily. Trough level <1.0 mg/l.

Glucagon 1 units = 1 mg. 0.04 mg/kg (adult 1–2 mg) i.v. or i.m. stat, then 10–50 μg/kg/h (0.5 mg/kg in 50 ml at 1–5 ml/h) i.v. Beta-blocker overdose: 50–150 μg/kg i.v. stat, then 0.3–2 μg/kg/min.

Glucose. Hypoglycaemia: 1 ml/kg 50% dextrose i.v., then increase infusion rate. Hyperkalaemia: 0.1 u/kg insulin + 2 ml/kg 50% dextrose i.v. Neonates: 6 g/kg/day (about 4 mg/kg/min) day 1, increase to 12 g/kg/day (up to 18 g/kg/day with hypoglycaemia). Infusion rate (ml/h) = (4.17 × wt × g/kg/day)/% dextrose = (6 × wt × mg/kg/min)/% dextrose. Dose (g/kg/day) = (ml/h × % dextrose)/(4.17 × wt). Dose (mg/kg/min) = (ml/h × % dextrose)/(6.0 × wt). mg/kg/min = g/kg/day/1.44.

Glucose electrolyte solution Not dehydrated: 1 heaped teaspoon sucrose in a large cup of water (4% sucrose = 2% glucose); do NOT add salt. Dehydrated: 1 sachet of Gastrolyte in 200 ml water; give frequent small sips, or infuse through a nasogastric tube.

Glyceryl trinitrate Adult (NOT/kg): sublingual tab 0.3–0.9 mg/dose (lasts 30–60 min); sublingual aerosol 0.4–0.8 mg/dose; slow release buccal tab 1–10 mg 8–12 H; transdermal 0.5–5 cm of 2% ointment, or 5–15 mg patch 8–12 H. i.v. infusion 1–10 μg/kg/min: adult 50 mg in 50 ml at 0.8 ml/h is 0.2 μg/kg/min; use polyethylene lined syringe and tubing (not PVC). Pulmonary vasodilation: 5 μg/kg/min nitroglycerine = 2 μg/kg/min nitroprusside = 0.1 μg/kg/min PGE1.

Glycopyrrolate See glycopyrronium bromide.

Glycopyrronium To reduce secretions or treat bradycardia: 4–8 μg/kg/dose (adult 200–400 μg) 6–8 H i.v. or i.m. With 0.05 mg/kg neostigmine: 10–15 μg/kg i.v. Anticholinergic: 0.02–0.04 mg/kg/dose (max 2 mg) 8 H oral.

Goserelin Adult (NOT/kg): 3.6 mg s.c. every 28 days; implant 10.8 mg s.c. every 12 weeks.

Griseofulvin 10–20 mg/kg (adult 0.5–1 g) daily oral.

Griseofulvin (ultramicrosize) 5.5 mg/kg (adult 330 mg) daily oral.

Growth hormone See somatropin.

Guaiphenasin 4–8 mg/kg/dose (adult 200–400 mg) 4 H oral doses.

Halofantrine 10 mg/kg/dose (max 500 mg) 6 H for 3 doses oral, repeat after 1 week if non immune.

Haloperidol 0.01 mg/kg (max 0.5 mg) daily, increase up to 0.1 mg/kg/dose 12 H i.v. or oral; up to 2 mg/kg/dose (max 100 mg) 12 H used rarely. Acutely disturbed: 0.1–0.2 mg/kg (adult 5–10 mg) i.m. Long acting decanoate ester: 1–6 mg/kg i.m. every 4weeks.

Heparin 1 mg = 100 units. Low dose: 75 units/kg i.v. stat, then 10–15 units/kg/h i.v. (500 units/kg in 50 ml at 1 ml/h = 10 units/kg/h). Full dose: 200 units/kg stat, then 15–30 units/kg/h.

Heparin calcium Low dose: 75 units/kg/dose s.c. 12 H.

Heparin, low molecular weight See certoparin, dalteparin, danaparoid, enoxaparin, nadroparin.

Histrelin Usually 10 μg/kg daily s.c.

Homatropine, eye drops 2% 1–2 drops 4 H.

Hyaluronidase Hypodermoclysis: add 1–1.5 units/ml fluid. Local anaesthesia: add 50 units/ml solution.

Hydralazine 0.1–0.2 mg/kg (adult 5–10 mg) stat i.v. or i.m., then 4–6 μg/kg/min (adult 200–300 μg/min) i.v. Oral: 0.4 mg/kg/dose (adult 20 mg) 12 H, slow increase to 1 mg/kg/dose (usual max 50 mg).

Hydrochloric acid Use solution of 150 mmol/l, give i.v. by central line only. Dose (ml) = BE × wt × 2.2 (give half this). Maximum rate = 1.33 ml/kg/h.

Hydrochlorothiazide 1 mg/kg/dose (adult 50 mg) 12–24 H oral.

Hydrocortisone Cream or ointment 0.5%, 1%: apply 8–24 H. Eye drops 0.5%, 1%: 1–2 drops/eye 2–4 H.

Hydrocortisone acetate Cream or ointment 0.5%: apply 6–12 H. Rectal foam 10%: 125 mg/dose (Colifoam). Usually 125 mg 12–24 H for 2–3 weeks, then 48 H.

Hydroxocobalamin (vitamin B$_{12}$) 20 μg/kg/dose (adult 1000 μg) i.m. daily for 7 days then weekly (treatment), every 2–3 months (prophylaxis). i.v. dangerous in megaloblastic anaemia.

Hydroxyapatite 20–40 mg/kg/dose (adult 1–2 g) 8 H oral.

Hydroxychloroquine Malaria: 10 mg/kg (max 600 mg) daily for 3 days; prophylaxis 5 mg/kg (max 300 mg) once a week oral. Juvenile arthritis: 5–6 mg/kg (max 400 mg) daily oral.

Hydroxyzine 0.5–2 mg/kg/dose (adult 25–100 mg) 6–8 H oral.

Hyoscine 0.01 mg/kg/dose (max 0.6 mg) 6 H, i.m. or i.v.

Hyoscine hydrobromide NOT/kg: 0.25 tab (2–7 years), 0.5 tab (7–12 years), 1–2 tab (>12 years) 6–24 H oral.

Hyoscine butylbromide 0.5 mg/kg/dose (max 40 mg) 6–8 H i.v., i.m. or oral.

Hyoscine transdermal 1.5 mg >10years: 1 patch every 72 h.

Hyperimmune bovine colostrum, antirotavirus 5 g sachet + 20 ml warm water + 10 ml milk: 1/3 (10 ml) 8 H until 3 days after infection risk.

Ibuprofen 2.5–10 mg/kg/dose (adult 150–600 mg) 6–8 H oral.

Ichthammol 1–10% cream, ointment. Apply 6–8 H.

Imipenem/cilastatin 15 mg/kg/dose (adult 500 mg) 6 H i.v. over 30 min. Severe infection: 25 mg/kg/dose i.v. over 1 h (adult 1 g) 12 H (1st week of life), 8 H (2–4 weeks), 6–8 H or constant infusion (4+ weeks).

Imipramine hydrochloride 0.5–1.5 mg/kg/dose (adult 25–75 mg) 8 H oral. Enuresis: 5–6 years 25 mg, 7–10 years 50 mg, >10 years 50–75 mg nocte.

Immunoglobulin See also antivenoms.

Immunoglobulin, CMV 100–200 mg/kg i.v. over 2 h. Transplantation: daily for first 3 days, weekly ×6, monthly ×6.

Immunoglobulin, diphtheria 250 units i.m. once.

Immunoglobulin, hepatitis B 400 units i.m. within 5 days of needlestick, repeat in 30 days; 100 units i.m. within 24 h birth to baby of hepatitis B carrier.

Immunoglobulin, lymphocyte (antithymocyte immunoglobulin, equine; Atgam) 10 mg/kg daily for 3–5 days i.v. over 4 h in saline.

Immunoglobulin, normal, human Hypogammaglobulinaemia: 10–15 ml/kg of 6% solution (600–900 mg/kg) i.v. over 5–8 h, then 5–7.5 ml/kg (300–450 mg/kg) over 3–4 h monthly; or 0.6 ml/kg of 16% solution (100 mg/kg) every 2–4 weeks i.m. Kawasaki, Guillain–Barré, ITP, myasthenia gravis, Still disease: 35 ml/kg of 6% solution (2 g/kg) i.v. over 16 h stat, then if required 15 ml/kg (900 mg/kg) i.v. over 8 h each month. Prevention hepatitis A: 0.1 ml/kg (16 mg/kg) i.m. Prevention measles: 0.2 ml/kg (32 mg/kg) i.m. (repeat next day if immunocompromised).

Immunoglobulin, rabies (Hyperab, Imogam) 20 IU (0.133 ml)/kg i.m. once (¹/₂ infiltrated around wound), with rabies vaccine.

Immunoglobulin, Rh 1 ml (625 IU, 125 μg) i.m. within 72 h of exposure. Large transfusion: 0.16 ml (100 IU, 20 μg) per ml Rh positive red cells (maternal serum should be anti-D positive 24–48 h after injection).

Immunoglobulin, respiratory syncytial virus 750 mg/kg every month i.v. (50 mg/ml: 1.5 ml/kg/h for 15 min, 3 ml/kg/h for 15 min, then 6 ml/kg/h).

Immunoglobulin, tetanus (TIG) i.m. preparation: 250–500 IU (1–2 ampoules). i.v. preparation: 4000 IU (100 ml) at 0.04 ml/kg/min for 30 min, then 0.075 ml/kg/min.

Immunoglobulin, zoster Prevention of chickenpox in immunocompromised, 0.4–1.2 ml/kg (max 6 ml) i.m.

Indomethacin 0.5–1 mg/kg/dose (adult 25–50 mg) 8 H (max 6 H) oral or PR. Patent ductus arteriosus: 0.1 mg/kg (<1 kg) or 0.2 mg/kg (≥1 kg) day 1, then 0.1 mg/kg daily days 2–7 oral, or i.v. in saline over 1 h.

Insulin Regular insulin: 0.05–0.2 units/kg p.r.n., or 0.1 units/kg/h; later 1 units/10 g dextrose i.v. For hyperkalaemia: 0.1 units/kg insulin and 2 ml/kg 50% dextrose i.v. In TPN: 5–25 units/250 g dextrose. s.c.: insulin lispro onset 10–15 min, peak 1 h, duration 2–5 h; regular insulin onset 30–60 min, peak 4 h, duration 6–8 h; isophane (NPH) insulin onset 2–4 h, peak 4–12 h, duration 18–24 h; zinc (Lente) insulin onset 2–3 h, peak 7–15 h, duration 24 h; crystalline zinc (Ultralente) insulin onset 4–6 h, peak 10–30 h, duration 24–36 h; protamine zinc insulin onset 4–8 h, peak 15–20 h, duration 24–36 h.

Interferon alfa-2a, recombinant 1 700 000 units/m^2 (max 3 000 000 units) s.c. or i.m. daily for 16–24 weeks, then ×3/week.

Interferon alfa-2b, recombinant Leukaemia: 2 000 000 units/m^2 s.c. ×3/week. Condylomata: 1 000 000 units into each lesion (max 5) ×3/week for 5 weeks. Hepatitis B: 200 000 units/kg (adult 10 000 000 units) ×3/week s.c., i.m. for 4 months. Hepatitis C: 60 000 units/kg (adult 3 000 000 units) ×3/week s.c. or i.m. for 24 weeks.

Interferon alfa-n3 Adult: 250 000 units injected into base of wart (max 10 doses per session) ×2/week for max 8 weeks.

Interferon beta-1a Adult (multiple sclerosis): 30 μg i.m. once a week.

Interferon beta-1b Adult (multiple sclerosis): 0.25 mg (8 million IU) s.c. alternate days.

Interferon gamma-1b 1.5 μg/kg/dose (body area ≥0.5 m^2) or 50 μg/m^2 (area >0.5 m^2) ×3/week s.c.

Interleukin-2 Malignancy: constant i.v. infusion less toxic than bolus injection: 3 000 000–5 000 000 units/m^2/day for 5 days, repeat ×1–2 if tolerated (5 days between courses).

Ipecacuanha syrup (total alkaloids 1.4 mg/ml) 1–2 ml/kg (adult 30 ml) stat oral, NG.

Ipratropium Respiratory solution (250 μg/ml): 0.25–1 ml diluted to 4 ml 4–6 H. Aerosol 20 μg/puff: 2–4 puffs 6–8 H.

Iron See ferrous gluconate, ferrous sulphate.

Iron dextran, iron polymaltose Fe 50 mg/ml: dose (ml) = 0.05 × wt in kg × (15 – Hb in g%) i.m. (often in divided doses). i.v. infusion possible (but dangerous).

Isoniazid 10 mg/kg (max 300 mg) daily oral, i.m. or i.v. TB meningitis: 15–20 mg/kg (max 500 mg) daily.

Isoprenaline Aerosol 80–400 μg/puff: 1–3 puffs 4–8 H. i.v. infusion <33 kg: 0.3 mg/kg in 50 ml at 1 ml/h = 0.1 μg/kg/min; >33 kg: 0.1 μg/kg/min using 1/5000 (0.2 mg/ml) solution = 0.03 × wt ml/h; for 65 kg adult 4 mg in 50 ml at 2 ml/h is 0.05 μg/kg/min.

Isotretinoin Adult: 0.5–1 mg/kg daily oral for 2–4 weeks, reducing if possible to 0.1–0.2 mg/kg daily for 15–20 weeks. Gel 0.05%: apply sparingly at night.

Itraconazole 2–4 mg/kg/dose (adult 100–200 mg) 12–24 H oral after food.

Ivermectin 0.15–0.2 mg/kg (max 12 mg) oral every 6–12 months.

Josamycin 10–15 mg/kg/dose (adult 500–750 mg) 8–12 H oral.

Kanamycin Single daily dose i.v. or i.m. Neonate: 15 mg/kg stat, then 7.5 mg/kg (<2.5 kg) or 12 mg/kg (≥2.5 kg) daily. 1 months–10 years: 22.5 mg/kg daily. >10 years: 18 mg/kg (max 240–360 mg) daily. Trough level <5.0 mg/l.

Ketamine 1–2 mg/kg i.v., 5–10 mg/kg i.m. Infusion: anaesthesia 10–20 μg/kg/min, analgesia 4 μg/kg/min.

Ketoconazole Oral: 5 mg/kg/dose (adult 200 mg) 12–24 H. Cream 2%: apply 12–24 H. Shampoo 2%: wash hair, apply liquid for 5 min, wash off.

Ketorolac Oral: 0.2 mg/kg/dose (max 10 mg) 4–6 H (max 0.8 mg/kg/day or 40 mg/day). i.m.: 0.6 mg/kg (max 30 mg) stat, then 0.2–0.4 mg/kg/dose (max 20 mg) 4–6 H for 5 days, then 0.2 mg/kg/dose (max 10 mg) 6 H.

Ketotifen Child >2 years (NOT/kg): 1 mg/dose 12 H oral with food. Adult (NOT/kg): 1–2 mg/dose 12 H oral with food.

Labetalol 1–2 mg/kg/dose (adult 50–100 mg) 12 H oral, may increase weekly to max 10 mg/kg/dose (max 600 mg) 6 H.

Lactulose 3.3 g/5 ml. Laxative: 0.5 ml/kg/dose 12–24 H oral. Hepatic coma: 1 ml/kg/dose hourly until bowel cleared, then 6–8 H.

Lamivudine 4 mg/kg/dose (adult 150 mg) 12 H oral.

Lamotrigine 0.5 mg/kg (adult 25 mg) oral daily for 2 weeks, then 1 mg/kg (adult 50 mg) daily 2 weeks, then 1–4 mg/kg/dose (adult 50–200 mg) 12 H (double dose if taking carbamazepine, phenobarbitone, phenytoin or primidone; halve dose if taking valproate).

Lenograstim (rHuG-CSF, Granocyte) 150 μg/m² daily s.c. or i.v. over 30 min. Keep WCC 5000–10 000/mm³.

Levamisole Anthelmintic: 3 mg/kg (adult 150 mg) oral once (ascaris), repeat in 1 week (hookworm). Adeno-carcinoma colon (with 5-fluorouracil 450 mg/m² i.v.

weekly): 1 mg/kg (adult 50 mg) 8 H oral for 3 days every 2 weeks.

Levorphanol 0.03–0.1 mg/kg/dose 12–24 H oral or s.c.

Levothyroxine sodium See thyroxine.

Lignocaine i.v. 1 mg/kg (0.1ml/kg of 1%) over 2 min, then 15–50 μg/kg/min: for 65 kg adult 1 g in 50 ml at 5 ml/h is 25 μg/kg/min. Nerve block: without adrenaline max 4 mg/kg (0.4 ml/kg of 1%), with adrenaline 7 mg/kg (0.7 ml/kg of 1%). Topical spray: max 3–4 mg/kg (xylocaine 10% spray pack: about 10 mg/puff). Topical gel 2%, solution 2% and 4%, ointment 5%, dental ointment 10%: apply p.r.n.

Lincomycin 10 mg/kg/dose (max 600 mg) 8 H oral, i.m. or i.v. over 1 h. Severe infection: up to 20 mg/kg/dose (max 1.2 g) i.v. over 2 h 6 H.

Lindane, cream or lotion 1% Scabies: apply from neck down, wash off after 8–12 h. Lice: rub into hair for 4 min, then wash off; repeat after 24 h (max ×2/week).

Liothyronine (T$_3$) Oral: 0.2 μg/kg/dose (adult 10 μg) 8 H, may increase to 0.4 μg/kg/dose (adult 20 μg) 8 H. i.v.: 0.1–0.4 μg/kg/dose (adult 5–20 μg) 8–12 H.

Liotrix Liothyronine (T$_3$) plus thyroxine (T$_4$) mixture.

Lipase, lipolytic enzymes See pancreatic enzymes.

Lipid emulsion 20% 1–3 g/kg/day i.v. (ml/h = g/kg/day × wt × 0.21).

Lisinopril 0.1 mg/kg (adult 5 mg) daily oral, may increase over 4–6 weeks to 0.2–0.4 mg/kg (adult 10–20 mg) daily.

Lithium (salts) 5–20 mg/kg/dose 12–24 H to maintain trough serum level 0.8–1.6 mmol/l (>2 mmol/l toxic).

Lofepramide Adult (NOT/kg): 70 mg morning, 70–140 mg night oral.

Loperamide 0.05–0.1 mg/kg/dose (max 2 mg) 8–12 H oral.

Loratadine 0.2 mg/kg (adult 10 mg) daily oral.

Lorazepam i.v.: 0.05–0.2 mg/kg i.v. over 2 min, then 0.01–0.1 mg/kg/h. Chronic: 0.02–0.06 mg/kg/dose (adult 1–3 mg) 8–24 H oral.

Lymphocyte immune globulin. See immunoglobulin, lymphocyte immune.

Lypressin (lysine-8-vasopressin) 1 spray (2.5 IU) into 1 nostril 4–8 H, may increase to 1 spray both nostrils 4–8 H.

Lysuride Migraine: 0.5 μg/kg/dose (adult 25 μg) 8 H oral. Parkinson, adults (NOT/kg): 0.2 mg daily, increase by 0.2 mg daily each week to max 1.6 mg/dose 8 H oral.

Magnesium chloride 0.48 g/5 ml (1 mmol/ml Mg). 0.4 mmol (0.4 ml)/kg/dose 12 H slow i.v. Myocardial infarction (NOT/kg): 5 mmol/h i.v. for 6 h, then 1 mmol/h for 24–48 h.

Magnesium hydroxide Antacid: 10–40 mg/kg/dose (max 2 g) 6 H oral. Laxative: 50–100 mg/kg (max 5 g) oral.

Magnesium sulphate Deficiency: 50% mag sulph (2 mmol/ml) 0.2 ml/kg/dose (max 10 ml) 12 H i.m., slow i.v. Asthma: 25–40 mg/kg (max 1.2 g) i.v. over 30 min once. Digoxin tachyarrhythmia: 50% mag sulph 0.1 ml/kg (max 5 ml) i.v. over 10 min, then infuse 0.4 ml/kg (max 20 ml) over 6 h, then 0.8 ml/kg (max 40 ml) over 18 h (keep serum Mg 1.5–2.0 mmol/l). Laxative: 0.5 g/kg/dose (max 15 g) as 10% solution 8 H for 2 days oral. Myocardial infarction (NOT/kg): 5 mmol/h i.v. for 6 h, then 1 mmol/h for 24–48 h. Pulmonary hypertension of newborn: aim for 3–4 mmol/l.

Malathion See maldison.

Maldison, liquid 0.5% 20 ml to hair, wash off after 12 h.

Mannitol 0.25–0.5 g/kg/dose i.v. (2–4 ml/kg of 12.5%, 1.25–2.5 ml/kg of 20%, 1–2 ml/kg of 25%) 2 H p.r.n, provided serum osmolality <320–330 mmol/l.

Mebendazole NOT/kg: 100 mg/dose 12 H ×3 days. Enterobiasis (NOT/kg): 100 mg once, may repeat after 2–4 weeks.

Meclozine 0.5–1 mg/kg/dose (adult 25–50 mg) 12–24 H oral.

Medroxyprogesterone Adult (NOT/kg): 5 mg daily for 5–10 days per month oral; malignancy 0.5 g daily i.m. or oral for 4 weeks, then 1 g weekly.

Medrysone, eye drops 1% 1 drop/eye 6–12 H.

Mefenamic acid 10 mg/kg/dose (adult 500 mg) 8 H oral.

Mefloquine 15 mg/kg (adult 750 mg) stat, then 10 mg/kg (adult 500 mg) after 6–8 h. Prophylaxis: 5 mg/kg (adult 250 mg) once a week.

Melatonin Usually 0.1 mg/kg (adult 5 mg) at night oral.

Meprobamate 5–10 mg/kg/dose (max 800 mg) 8–12 H oral.

Meropenem 10–20 mg/kg/dose (adult 0.5–1 g) 8 H i.v. over 5–30 min. Severe infection: 20–40 mg/kg/dose (adult 1–2 g) 8 H or constant infusion.

Mesalazine 10–15 mg/kg/dose (adult 500–800 mg) 8 H oral. Suppository: 5–10 mg/kg (max 500 mg) 8 H. Enema: 20 mg/kg (max 1 g) nocte.

Metaraminol i.v.: 0.01 mg/kg stat (repeat p.r.n.), then 0.1–1 µg/kg/min and titrate dose against BP. s.c.: 0.1 mg/kg.

Methotrexate Leukaemia: typically 3.3 mg/m² i.v. daily for 4–6 weeks; then 2.5 mg/kg i.v. every 2 weeks, or 30 mg/m² oral or i.m. ×2/week; higher doses with folinic acid rescue. Intrathecal: 12 mg/m² weekly for 2 weeks, then monthly. Juvenile arthritis: 10–15 mg/m² weekly oral, i.v. or i.m. Adult psoriasis: 0.2–0.5 mg/kg weekly oral, i.v. or i.m. until response, then reduce.

Metylcellulose Constipation: 30–60 mg/kg/dose (adult 1.5–3 g) with at least 300 ml fluid 12 H oral.

Methyldopa 3 mg/kg/dose (adult 150 mg) 8 H oral, may increase to max 15 mg/kg/dose (adult 750 mg).

Methylene blue 1–4 mg/kg/dose i.v. Septic shock: 0.5 mg/kg over 15 min i.v., then 0.1–0.25 mg/kg/h.

Methylprednisolone Asthma: 0.5–1 mg/kg/dose 6 H oral, i.v. or i.m. day 1, 12 H day 2, then 1 mg/kg daily,

reducing to minimum effective dose. Severe croup: 4 mg/kg i.v. stat, then 1 mg/kg/dose 8 H. Severe sepsis before antibiotics (or within 4 h of 1st dose): 30 mg/kg i.v. once. Spinal cord injury (within 8 h): 30 mg/kg stat, then 5 mg/kg/h 2 days. Lotion 0.25%: apply sparingly 12–24 H. Methylprednisolone 1 mg = hydrocortisone 5 mg in glucocorticoid activity, 0.5 mg in mineralocorticoid.

Methysergide 0.02 mg/kg/dose (adult 1 mg) 12 H oral, increase if required to max 0.04 mg/kg/dose (adult 2 mg) 8 H for 3–6 months.

Metirosine 5–20 mg/kg/dose (adult 0.25–1 g) 6 H oral.

Metoclopramide 0.12 mg/kg/dose (adult 10–15 mg) 6 H i.v., i.m. or oral. 0.2–0.4 mg/kg/dose (adult 10–20 mg) 8 H PR.

Metoprolol i.v.: 0.1 mg/kg (adult 5 mg) over 5 min, repeat every 5 min to max 3 doses, then 1–5 µg/kg/min. Oral: 1–2 mg/kg/dose (adult 50–100 mg) 6–12 H.

Metronidazole 15 mg/kg stat, then 7.5 mg/kg/dose (max 800 mg) 12 H in neonate (1st maintenance dose 48 h after load in preterm, 24 h in term baby), 8 H (4+ weeks) i.v., PR or oral. Topical gel 0.5%: apply daily. Level 60–300 µmol/ml (×0.17 µg/ml).

Mexiletine i.v. infusion: 2–5 mg/kg (max 250 mg) over 15 min, then 5–20 µg/kg/min (max 250 mg/h). Oral: 8 mg/kg (max 400 mg) stat, then 4–8 mg/kg/dose (max 400 mg) 8 H starting 2 h after loading dose.

Miconazole 7.5–15 mg/kg/dose (adult 0.6–1.2 g) 8 H i.v. over 1 h. Topical: 2% cream, powder, lotion, tincture or gel 12–24 H. Vaginal: 2% cream or 100 mg ovule daily.

Midazolam Sedation: usually 0.1–0.2 mg/kg i.v. or i.m.; up to 0.5 mg/kg used safely in children. Anaesthesia: 0.5 mg/kg, then 2 µg/kg/min (3 mg/kg in 50 ml at 2 ml/h) i.v.

Milrinone 50 µg/kg i.v. over 10 min, then 0.375–0.75 µg/kg/min (max 1.13 mg/kg/day).

Minocycline Over 8 years: 4 mg/kg (max 200 mg) stat, then 2 mg/kg/dose (max 100 mg) 12 H oral or i.v. over 1 h.

Minoxidil 0.1 mg/kg (max 5 mg) daily increase to max 0.5 mg/kg/dose (max 25 mg) 12–24 H oral. Male baldness: 2% solution 1 ml 12 H to dry scalp.

Misoprostol (PGE1 analogue) 5 µg/kg/dose (max 200 µg) 4–6 H oral.

Mivacurium 150 µg/kg stat, then 100 µg/kg/dose i.v. Infusion: 5–15 µg/kg/min.

Moclobemide 2–3 mg/kg/dose (adult 100–150 mg) 6–12 H oral.

Molgramostim 5–10 µg/kg daily s.c. or i.v. over 6 h.

Montelukast NOT/kg: 5 mg (6–14 years) 10 mg (>14 years) daily at bedtime, oral.

Morphine Half-life 2–4 h. i.m.: neonate 0.1 mg/kg, child 0.2 mg/kg, adult 10–20 mg. i.v. (ventilated): 0.1–0.2 mg/kg/dose (adult 5–10 mg). Infusion of 1 mg/kg in 50 ml 5% dextrose: ventilated neonate 0.5–1.5 ml/h

(10–30 µg/kg/h), child or adult 1–3 ml/h (20–60 µg/kg/h). Patient controlled: 20 µg/kg boluses (1 ml of 1 mg/kg in 50 ml) with 5 min lockout time + (in child) 5 µg/kg/h. Oral: double parenteral dose; slow release, start with 0.6 mg/kg/dose 12 H and increase every 48 h if required.

Mupirocin, ointment 2% Apply 8–12 H.

Muromonab-CD3 (Orthoclone OKT3) 0.1 mg/kg (adult 5 mg) daily for 10–14 days i.v. over 1 min.

Mycophenolate mofetil 600 mg/m^2/dose 12 H oral.

Nadroparin Venous thrombosis: 90 anti-XaU/kg 12 H s.c. Prophylaxis: general surgery 2850 anti-XaU (adult, NOT/kg) daily s.c.; orthopaedics 40 anti-XaU/kg 24 H (start 12 h presurgery) s.c., then 55 anti-XaU/kg daily. Haemodialysis: 65 anti-XaU/kg into arterial line at start of 4 h session.

Nafarelin Adult (NOT/kg): 200 µg spray to 1 nostril 12 H.

Nafcillin Oral: 15–30 mg/kg/dose 6 H. Severe infection (slow i.v., i.m.): 40 mg/kg/dose (max 2 g) 12 H (1st week of life), 8 H (2nd week), 6 H or constant infusion (>2 weeks).

Nalidixic acid 15 mg/kg/dose (adult 1 g) 6 H oral, reducing to 7.5 mg/kg/dose (adult 500 mg) 6 H after 2 weeks.

Naloxone Opiate intoxication (including newborn): 0.1 mg/kg (max 2 mg) stat i.v., i.m., s.c. or intratracheal, then 0.01 mg/kg/h i.v. Postop sedation: 0.002 mg/kg/dose repeat every 2 min, then 0.01 mg/kg/h (0.2 µg/kg/min) i.v.

Naltrexone 0.5 mg/kg (adult 25 mg) stat, then 1 mg/kg (adult 50 mg) daily oral.

Nandrolone decanoate Anaemia: 1–4 mg/kg (adult 50–200 mg) weekly deep i.m. Osteoporsis: adult (NOT/kg) 50 mg deep i.m. every 3 weeks.

Naphazoline 0.025–0.1%: 1–2 drops each nostril or eye 3 H.

Naproxen 5–10 mg/kg/dose (adult 250–500 mg) 12–24 H oral.

Naratriptan 0.05 mg/kg (adult 2.5 mg), repeated once after 4 h if required.

Nedocromil Inhalation: 4 mg/dose (NOT/kg) 6–12 H. Eye drops 2%: 1 drop/eye 6–24 H.

Neomycin 12.5–25 mg/kg/dose (adult 0.5–1 g) 6 H oral. Bladder washout: 40–2000 mg/l.

Neostigmine Oral: 0.3–0.6 mg/kg/dose 3–4 H (max 400 mg/day). i.v., i.m.: 0.01–0.05 mg/kg/dose 3–4 H (max 20 mg/day). Reverse relaxants: 0.05–0.07 mg/kg/dose i.v.; suggested dilution: neostigmine (2.5 mg/ml) 0.5 ml + atropine (0.6 mg/ml) 0.5 ml + saline 0.5 ml, give 0.1 ml/kg i.v.

Netilmicin Single daily dose i.v. or i.m. Neonate: 5 mg/kg stat, then 2.5 mg/kg (<2.5 kg) or 4 mg/kg (≥2.5 kg) daily. 1 month–10 years: 7.5 mg/kg daily. >10 years: 6 mg/kg (max 240–360 mg) daily. Trough level <1.0 mg/l.

Nicardipine 0.4–0.8 mg/kg/dose (adult 20–40 mg) 8 H oral.

Niclosamide 40 mg/kg (max 2 g) oral.

Nicotinic acid Hypercholesterolaemia and hypertriglyceridaemia: 5 mg/kg/dose (adult 200 mg) 8 H, gradually increase to 20–30 mg/kg/dose (adult 1–2 g) 8 H oral.

Nifedipine Caps 0.25–0.5 mg/kg (adult 10–20 mg) 6–8 H, tabs 0.5–1 mg/kg/dose (adult 20–40 mg) 12 H oral or sublingual.

Nimodipine 10–15 µg/kg/h (max 1 mg/h) i.v. for 2 h, then 10–45 µg/kg/h.

Nitrazepam NOT/kg: 1.25–5 mg/dose 12 H oral. Hypnotic: 2–5 mg.

Nitric oxide 5–40 p.p.m. (up to 80 p.p.m. used occasionally). 0.1 l/min of 1000 p.p.m. added to 10 l/min gas gives 10 p.p.m. [NO] = cylinder [NO] × (1 − (patient FiO$_2$/supply FiO$_2$)). [NO] = cylinder [NO] × NO flow/total flow.

Nitrofurantoin 1.5 mg/kg/dose (adult 100 mg) 6 H oral. Prophylaxis: 1–2.5 mg/kg at night.

Nitroglycerine See glyceryl trinitrate.

Nitroprusside See sodium nitroprusside.

Noradrenaline i.v. infusion: 0.05–0.5 µg/kg/min.

Norethisterone Contraception: 350 µg daily, starting 1st day of menstruation. Menorrhagia: 10 mg 3 H until bleeding stops, then 5 mg 6 H for 1 week, then 5 mg 8 H for 2 weeks.

Norfloxacin 10 mg/kg/dose (adult 400 mg) 12 H oral.

Normacol granules 6 months–5 years $^1/_2$ teaspoon 12 H, 6–10 years 1 teaspoon 12 H, over 10 years 1 teaspoon 8 H.

Nortriptyline 0.5–1.5 mg/kg/dose (adult 25–75 mg) 8 H oral.

Nystatin 500 000 units (1 tab) 6–8 H NG or oral. Neonates: 100 000 units (1 ml) 8 H, prophylaxis 50 000 units (0.5 ml) 12 H. Topical: 100 000 units/g gel, cream or ointment 12 H. Vaginal: 100 000 units 12–24 H.

Octocog alfa (recombinant factor 8) See factor 8.

Octreotide 1 µg/kg/dose 12–24 H s.c., may increase to 4 µg/kg/dose (max 250 µg) 8 H. i.v.: 1 µg/kg stat, then 1–5 µg/kg/h.

Oestradiol Transdermal patch 1.5 mg (releases 50 µg/day): apply twice a week.

Oestradiol 2 mg or 4 mg (×12 tab), oestradiol 1 mg (×6 tab), oestradiol 2 mg or 4 mg + norethisterone 1 mg (×10 tab). 1 tab daily, starting 5th day of menstruation. Vaginal tab 25 µg: 1 tab daily for 2 weeks, then 1 tab ×2/week. See also norethisterone + oestradiol.

Oestriol Vaginal: 0.5 mg daily, reducing to ×2/week. Patches (Menorest) 37.5 (3.28 mg), 50 (4.33 mg), 75 (6.57 mg), 100 (8.66 mg): apply 1 patch ×2/week (adjust dose monthly), with medroxyprogesterone acetate (if uterus intact) 10 mg daily oral for 10 days each month.

Oestrogen See ethinyloestradiol.

Ofloxacin 5 mg/kg/dose (adult 200 mg) 8–12 H, or 10 mg/kg/dose (adult 400 mg) 12 H oral or i.v. over 1 h.

OKT3 See muromonab-CD3.

Olanzapine Adult (NOT/kg): 5–10 mg daily oral, increase gradually up to 20 mg daily if required.

Omeprazole Usually 1.0 mg/kg (adult 20–40 mg) 12–24 H oral. Zollinger–Ellison syndrome: 0.4–1 mg/kg (adult 20–60 mg) 12–24 H oral. i.v.: 2 mg/kg (max 80 mg) stat, then 1 mg/kg (max 40 mg) 8–12 H. *H.pylori*: 0.8 mg/kg/dose (adult 40 mg) daily with metronidazole 8 mg/kg/dose (adult 400 mg) 8 H + amoxycillin 10 mg/kg/dose (adult 500 mg) 8 H oral for 2 weeks.

Ondansetron i.v.: 0.1–0.2 mg/kg (usual max 8 mg) over 15 min, then 0.25–0.5 µg/kg/min. Oral: 0.1–0.2 mg/kg/dose (usual max 8 mg) 8–12 H.

Oral rehydration solution (ORS) See glucose electrolyte solution.

Orciprenaline Oral: 0.25–0.5 mg/kg/dose (adult 20 mg) 6 H. Respiratory solution (2%): 0.5 ml/dose diluted to 4 ml 3–6 H (mild), 1 ml/dose dilute to 4 ml (moderate), undiluted continuously (severe, in ICU). Aerosol 750 µg/dose: 2 puffs 4–6 H.

Orlistat 3 mg/kg/dose (adult 120 mg) with each main meal containing fat (max 3 doses/day).

Ornipressin (POR 8) i.v.: 0.1 unit/kg/h (max 6 units/h) for max 4 h, then 0.03 unit/kg/h (max 1.5 units/h). s.c.: 5 units in 30 ml saline, max total dose 0.1 unit/kg.

Orphenadrine 1–2 mg/kg/dose (adult 50–100 mg) 8 H oral.

Oxacillin Oral: 15–30 mg/kg/dose 6 H. Severe infection (i.v., i.m.): 40 mg/kg/dose (max 2 g) 12 H (1st week of life), 8 H (2nd week), 6 H or constant infusion (>2 week).

Oxandrolone 0.05–0.1 mg/kg/dose (adult 2.5–5 mg) 6–12 H oral.

Oxaprozin Usually 20 mg/kg (max 1200 mg), range 10–26 mg/kg (max 1800 mg), daily oral.

Oxazepam 0.2–0.5 mg/kg/dose (adult 10–30 mg) 6–8 H oral.

Oxcarbazepine Initially 4–5 mg/kg/dose (adult 300 mg) 12 H oral; increase weekly by max 5 mg/kg/dose (adult 300 mg) to usually 15 mg/kg/dose (adult 750 mg), max 23 mg/kg/dose (adult 1200 mg).

Oxerutin 10 mg/kg/dose (adult 500 mg) 12 H oral.

Oxitropium Inhalation: 200 µg/dose (NOT/kg) 8–12 H.

Oxpentifylline Slow release tab: 8 mg/kg/dose (adult 400 mg) 8–12 H oral.

Oxprenolol 0.5–2 mg/kg/dose (adult 30–120 mg) 8–12 H oral.

Oxybuprocaine 4 mg/ml (0.4%): 1–2 drops/eye 8–12 H. Deep anaesthesia: 2 drops/eye every 90 s ×3 doses.

Oxymetazoline, nasal 0.25 mg/ml (<6 years), 0.5 mg/ml (>6 years): 2–3 drops or sprays in each nostril 8–12 H.

Oxytetracycline >8 years (NOT/kg): 250–500 mg/dose 6 H oral, or 250–500 mg/dose 6–12 H slow i.v.

Oxytocin Labour (NOT/kg): 1–4 munits/min i.v., may increase to 20 munits/min max. Lactation: 1 spray (4 IU) into each nostril 5 min before infant feeds.

Packed cells 4 ml/kg raises Hb 1 g%. 1 bag is about 300 ml.

Paclitaxel 100–250 mg/m^2 i.v. over 24 h each 3 weeks, total of 3–6 doses.

Palivizumab 15 mg/kg i.m. once a month.

Pamidronate See disodium pamidronate.

Pancreatic enzymes With meals (NOT/kg): 1–3 Cotazyme-S Forte cap, 1–5 Pancrease cap oral.

Pancuronium ICU: 0.1–0.15 mg/kg i.v. p.r.n. Theatre: 0.1 mg/kg i.v., then 0.02 mg/kg p.r.n. Infusion: 0.25–0.75 µg/kg/min.

Pantoprazole 1.0 mg/kg (max 40 mg) 12–24 H oral. Zollinger–Ellison syndrome: adjust dose to achieve acid <10 mmol/l.

Papaveretum (Omnopon) 0.2 mg/kg/dose i.v., 0.4 mg/kg/dose i.m. (half-life 2–4 h). ICU: 0.3 mg/kg/dose i.v., 0.6 mg/kg/dose i.m.

Papaveretum (20 mg/ml) and hyoscine (0.4 mg/ml) 0.4 mg/kg (P) + 0.008 mg/kg (H) = 0.02 ml/kg/dose i.m.

Papaverine Adult (NOT/kg): 150–300 mg 12 H oral, 12–40 mg ×1–2/week intracavernosal. i.a. lines: 0.12 mg/ml.

Paracetamol Oral: 20 mg/kg stat, then 15 mg/kg/dose 4 H (max 4 g/day). Rectal: 40 mg/kg stat, then 30 mg/kg/dose 6 H (max 5 g/day). Overdose: see acetylcysteine.

Paraffin Liquid: 1 ml/kg (max 45 ml) daily oral. Liquid 50% + white soft 50%, ointment: apply 6–12 H.

Paraffin 65% + agar NOT/kg: 6 months–2 years 5 ml, 3–5 years 5–10 ml, >5 years 10 ml 8–24 H oral.

Paraffin, phenolphthalein and agar (Agarol) NOT/kg: 6 months–2 years 2.5 ml, 3–5 years 2.5–5 ml, >5 years 5 ml 8–24 H oral.

Paraldeyde i.m.: 0.2 ml/kg (adult 10 ml) stat, then 0.1 ml/kg/dose 4–6 H. i.v.: 0.2 ml/kg (adult 10 ml) over 15 min, then 0.02 ml/kg/h (max 1.5 ml/h). Rectal or NG: 0.3 ml/kg/dose diluted 1:10.

Parathyroid hormone See teriparatide.

Paroxetine 0.4–1 mg/kg (adult 20–50 mg) daily oral.

Penbutolol 0.4–1.5 mg/kg (adult 20–80 mg) daily oral.

Penicillamine 5–10 mg/kg/dose (adult 250–500 mg) 6 H oral.

Penicillin, benzathine 1 mg = 1250 units. Usually 20 mg/kg (max 900 mg) i.m. once. Venereal disease: 40 mg/kg (max 1.8 g) i.m. once. Streptococcal prophylaxis: 20 mg/kg (max 900 mg) i.m. 3–4 weekly, or 10 mg/kg i.m. 2 weekly.

Penicillin, benzathine 900 mg + procaine 300 mg in 2 ml. 0–2 years $^1/_2$ vial, 3 years or more 1 vial i.m. once.

Penicillin, benzyl (penicillin G, crystalline) 1 mg = 1667 units. 30 mg/kg/dose 6 H. Severe infection:

60 mg/kg/dose (max 3 g) i.v. 12 H (1st week of life), 6 H (2–4 weeks), 4 H or constant infusion (>4 weeks).

Penicillin, procaine 1 mg = 1000 units. 25–50 mg/kg (max 1.2–2.4 g) 12–24 H i.m. Single dose: 100 mg/kg (max 4.8 g).

Penicillin V See phenoxymethylpenicillin.

Pentagastrin 6 μg/kg s.c., or 0.6 μg/kg/h i.v.

Pentamidine isethionate 3–4 mg/kg (1.7–2.3 mg/kg base) i.v. over 2 h or i.m. daily for 10–14 days (1 mg base = 1.5 mg mesylate = 1.74 mg isethionate).

Pentastarch 10% solution: 10–40 mg/kg i.v.

Pentazocine Oral: 0.5–2.0 mg/kg/dose (adult 25–100 mg) 3–4 H. s.c., i.m. or slow i.v.: 0.5–1 mg/kg/dose (adult 30–60 mg) 3–4 H. PR: 1 mg/kg/dose (adult 50 mg) 6–12 H.

Pentobarbital See pentobarbitone.

Pentobarbitone 0.5–1 mg/kg/dose (adult 30–60 mg) 6–8 H oral, i.m., slow i.v. Hypnotic: 2–4 mg/kg (adult 100–200 mg).

Pericyazine 0.15–2 mg/kg/dose (adult 7.5–100 mg) 12 H oral.

Perindopril 0.05–0.15 mg/kg (adult 2–8 mg) daily oral.

Permethrin. Cream rinse 1% (head lice): wash hair, apply cream for 10 min, wash off; may repeat in 2 weeks. Cream 5% (scabies): apply to whole body except face, wash off after 12–24 h.

Perphenazine 0.1–0.3 mg/kg/dose (adult 5–20 mg) 8–12 H oral.

Pethidine 0.5–1 mg/kg/dose (adult 25–50 mg) i.v., 0.5–2 mg/kg/dose (adult 25–100 mg) i.m. (Half-life 2–4 h). Infusion: 5 mg/kg in 50 ml at 1–3 ml/h (100–300 μg/kg/h).

Phenazone 5.4% + benzocaine 1.4% otic (Auralgin) 3 drops 6–8 H.

Phenelzine 0.3–2 mg/kg/dose (adult 15–90 mg) 8 H oral.

Phenindamine 0.5–1 mg/kg/dose (adult 25–50 mg) 8–12 H oral.

Peniramine 0.5–1 mg/kg/dose (adult 25–50 mg) 6 H oral.

Phenobarbitone Loading dose in emergency: 20–30 mg/kg i.m. or i.v. over 30 min stat. Ventilated: repeat doses of 10–15 mg/kg up to 100 mg/kg in 24 h (beware hypotension). Usual maintenance: 5 mg/kg (max 300 mg) daily i.v., i.m. or oral. Infant colic: 1 mg/kg/dose 4–8 H oral. Level 80–120 μmol/l (×0.23 = μg/ml) done Monday, Wednesday, Friday at RCH.

Phenoxybenzamine 0.2–1 mg/kg (adult 10–50 mg) 12–24 H oral. Cardiac surgery: 1 mg/kg i.v. over 1 h stat, then 0.5 mg/kg/dose 6–12 H i.v. over 1 h or oral.

Phenoxymethylpenicillin (penicillin V) 7.5–15 mg/kg/dose (adult 250–500 mg) 6 H oral. Prophylaxis: 12.5 mg/kg/dose (adult 250 mg) 12 H oral.

Phentolamine 0.1 mg/kg stat, then 5–50 μg/kg/min i.v.

Phenylephrine i.v.: 2–10 μg/kg stat (adult 500 μg), then 1–5 μg/kg/min: for 65 kg adult 25 mg in 50 ml at 8 ml/h is 1 μg/kg/min. s.c. or i.m.: 0.1–0.2 mg/kg (max 10 mg). Oral: 0.2 mg/kg/dose (max 10 mg) 6–8 H. Eye drops (0.12%, 10%): 1–2 drops/eye 6–8 H. Nose drops (0.25%, 0.5%): 1–3 drops/sprays per nostril 6–8 H.

Phenytoin Loading dose in emergency: 15–20 mg/kg (max 1.5 g) i.v. over 1 h. Maintenance, oral or i.v.: 2 mg/kg/dose 12 H (preterm); 4 mg/kg/dose 12 H (1st week of life), 8 H (2nd week), 6 H (3 weeks–12 month), 8 H (1–2 years), 8–12 H (3–12 years); 2 mg/kg/dose (usual max 100 mg) 6–12 H >12 years. Level 40–80 μmol/l (×0.25 = μg/ml), done Monday, Wednesday and Friday at RCH.

Pholcodine 0.1–0.2 mg/kg/dose (adult 5–10 mg) 6–12 H oral.

Phosphate, potassium (1 mmol/ml) 0.1–1 mmol/kg/day (max 20 mmol/day) i.v. infusion.

Phosphate, sodium (500 mg tab) 0.5–1 g (NOT/kg) 8 H oral.

Physostigmine 0.02 mg/kg (max 1 mg) i.v. every 5 min till response (max 0.1 mg/kg), then 0.5–2.0 μg/kg/min.

Phytomenadione 0.3 mg/kg (max 10 mg), i.m. or i.v. over 1 h. Prophylaxis in neonates (NOT/kg): 1 mg i.m. at birth; or 1 mg oral or 0.1 mg i.m. at birth, at 4–7 days, and 3–4 weeks (give half dose if weight <1500 g).

Pilocarpine 0.1 mg/kg/dose (adult 5 mg) 4–8 H oral. Eye drops 0.5%, 1%, 2%, 3%, 4%: 1–2 drops 6–12 H.

Pimozide 0.04–0.4 mg/kg (adult 2–20 mg) daily oral.

Pindolol 0.3 mg/kg/dose (adult 15 mg) 8–24 H oral.

Pipecuronium 20–85 μg/kg i.v. stat, then 5–25 μg/kg p.r.n.

Piperacillin 50 mg/kg/dose (adult 2–3 g) i.v. 6–8 H (1st week of life), 6–8 H (2+ weeks). Severe infection: 100 mg/kg/dose (adult 4 g) 4–6 H or constant infusion.

Piperacillin + tazobactam (1 g/125 mg) Dose as for piperacillin.

Pirbuterol Oral: 0.2–0.3 mg/kg/dose (adult 10–15 mg) 6–8 H. Inhalation (NOT/kg): 0.2–0.4 mg/dose 4–6 H.

Piroxicam 0.2–0.4 mg/kg (adult 10–20 mg) daily oral. Gel 5 mg/g: apply 1 g (3 cm) 6–8 H for up to 2 weeks.

Pizotifen NOT/kg: 1–3 mg daily oral, usually 0.5 mg morning, 1 mg night.

Platelets 10ml/kg i.v. stat, then daily if necessary. 1 unit is about 60 ml.

Podophyllotoxin, paint 0.5%. Apply 12 H for 3 days, then none for 4 days; 4 weeks course.

Podophyllum, solution or ointment 15%–25%. Apply to wart ×2/day.

Poloxamer 10% solution 8 H oral: <6 months 10 drops/dose, 6–18 months 15 drops/dose, 18 months–3 years 25 drops/dose.

Polyethylene glycol See colonic lavage solution.

Polymyxin B See bacitracin + neomycin + polymyxin.

Poractant alfa (porcine surfactant, Curosurf) Intratracheal: 200 mg/kg stat, then up to 4 doses of 100 mg/kg 12 H if required.

POR 8 See ornipressin.

Potassium Max i.v. 0.4 mmol/kg/h. Max oral 1 mmol/kg/dose (<5 years), 0.5 mmol/kg/dose (>5 years). Need 2–4 mmol/kg/day. 1 g KCl = 13.3 mmol K, 7.5% KCl = 1 mmol/ml.

Pralidoxime 25–50 mg/kg (adult 1–2 g) over 30 min, then up to 10 mg/kg/h (max 12 g/day).

Pravastatin 0.2–0.4 mg/kg (adult 10–20 mg) at bedtime oral.

Praziquantel 20 mg/kg/dose 4 H for 3 doses oral.

Prazosin 0.005 mg/kg (max 0.25 mg) test dose, then 0.025–0.1 mg/kg/dose (adult 1–5 mg) 6 H oral.

Prednisolone Asthma: 0.5–1 mg/kg/dose 6 H for 24 h, 12 H for the next 24 h, then 1 mg/kg daily. Severe croup: 4 mg/kg stat, then 1 mg/kg/dose 8–12 H oral. Prednisolone 1 mg = hydrocortisone 0.8 mg in mineralocorticoid action, 4 mg in glucocorticoid. See also methylprednisolone.

Prilocaine Max dose 6 mg/kg (0.6 ml/kg of 1%). With adrenaline max dose 9 mg/kg (0.9 ml/kg of 1%).

Primaquine Usually 0.3 mg/kg (max 15 mg) daily for 14–21 days oral. Gameteocyte: 0.7 mg/kg (max 45 mg) once.

Primidone 5–15 mg/kg/dose (adult 250–750 mg) 12 H oral.

Probenicid 25 mg/kg (adult 1 g) stat, then 10 mg/kg/dose (adult 500 mg) 6 H oral.

Procainamide i.v.: 0.4 mg/kg/min (adult 20 mg/min) for max 25 min, then 20–80 µg/kg/min. Oral: 2–8 mg/kg/dose 4 H.

Procaine Max dose 20 mg/kg (1 ml/kg of 2%).

Prochlorperazine (1 mg base = approximately 1.5 mg edisylate, maleate or mesylate) Only use if >10 kg. i.m. or slow i.v.: 0.1–0.2 mg/kg (adult 12.5 mg salt) 6–8 H. Oral or PR: 0.1–0.4 mg/kg/dose (max 25 mg salt) 6–8 H, slow increase to max 0.6 mg/kg/dose (max 35 mg) 6 H in psychosis. Buccal: 0.05–0.1 mg/kg (max 6 mg salt) 12–24 H.

Progesterone Adult (NOT/kg). Premenstrual syndrome: 200–400 mg/dose PV or PR 12–24 H (last $^1/_2$ cycle). dysfunctional uterine haemorrhage: 5–10 mg/day i.m. for 5–10 days before menses. Prevention of abortion: 25–100 mg i.m. every 2–4 days.

Proguanil 3.5 mg/kg (adult 200 mg) daily oral after food.

Promethazine 0.2–0.5 mg/kg/dose (adult 10–25 mg) 6–8 H i.v., i.m. or oral. Sedative, hypnotic: 0.5–1.5 mg/kg/dose (adult 25–100 mg).

Propafenone Oral: 3–5 mg/kg/dose (adult 150–300 mg) 8 H. i.v.: 1–2 mg/kg over 15 min, then 10–20 µg/kg/min.

Propantheline bromide 0.3–0.6 mg/kg/dose (adult 15–30 mg) 6 H oral.

Propofol 1–3 mg/kg stat, then 4–12 mg/kg/h i.v. Beware acidosis and myocardial depression.

Propranolol i.v.: 0.02 mg/kg (adult 1 mg) test dose then 0.1 mg/kg (adult 5 mg) over 10 min (repeat ×1–3 p.r.n.), then 0.1–0.3 mg/kg/dose (adult 5–15 mg) 3 H.

Oral: 0.2–0.5 mg/kg/dose (adult 10–25 mg) 6–12 H, slow increase to max 1.5 mg/kg/dose (max 80 mg) 6–12 H if required.

Prostacyclin See epoprostenol.

Prostaglandin See alprostadil (PGE1), carboprost (15-Me-PGF2-alpha), dinoprost (PGF2-alpha), dinoprostone (PGE2), epoprostenol (PGI2, prostacyclin), gemeprost (PGE1 analogue), and misoprostol (PGE1 analogue).

Protamine i.v. 1 mg/100 units heparin (or 1 mg per 25 ml pump blood) i.v. stat; subsequent doses of protamine 1 mg/kg (max 50 mg). Heparin 1 mg = 100 units (half-life 1–2 h).

Prothrombinex See coagulation factor, human.

Protirelin NOT/kg: 200 µg i.v. stat.

Protriptyline 0.1–0.4 mg/kg/dose (adult 5–20 mg) 6–8 H oral.

Proxymetacaine, eye drops 0.5% 1–2 drops stat, then 1 drop every 10 min.

Pseudoephedrine 1 mg/kg/dose (adult 60 mg) 6 H oral.

Pumactant (ALEC) Preterm babies (NOT/kg): disconnect endotracheal tube, rapidly inject 100 mg in 1 ml saline via catheter at lower end of endotracheal tube, flush with 2 ml air; repeat after 1 h and 24 h. Prophylaxis if unintubated: 100 mg into pharynx.

Pyrantel embonate 10 mg/kg (adult 500 mg) once oral. Necator: 20 mg/kg (adult 1 g) daily ×2 doses. Enterobius: 10 mg/kg (adult 500 mg) each 2 weeks ×3 doses.

Pyrazinamide 20–35 mg/kg/dose (max 3 g) daily oral.

Pyridostigmine 1–3 mg/kg/dose (usual max 200 mg) 4–12 H oral. 180 mg slow release tab (Timespan), adult (NOT/kg): 1–3 tab 12–24 H. 1 mg i.v., i.m. or s.c. = 30 mg oral.

Pyridoxine With isoniazid (NOT/kg): 5–10 mg daily i.v. or oral. Fitting: 10–15 mg/kg daily i.v. or oral. Sideroblastic anaemia: 2–8 mg/kg (max 400 mg) daily i.v. or oral.

Pyrimethamine 12.5 mg and dapsone 100 mg (Maloprim) 1–4 years quarter tab weekly, 5–10 years half tab, >10 years 1 tab.

Pyrimethamine 25 mg and sulphadoxine 500 mg (Fansidar) <4 years half tab once, 4–8 years 1 tab, 9–14 years 2 tab, >14 years 3 tab. Prophylaxis: <4 years quarter tab weekly, 4–8 years half tab, 9–14 years three-quarter tab, >14 years 1 tab.

Quinapril 0.2–0.8 mg/kg (adult 10–40 mg) daily oral.

Quinidine, base 10 mg/kg stat, then 5 mg/kg/dose (max 333 mg) 4–6 H oral. i.v.: 6.3 mg/kg (10 mg/kg of gluconate) over 2 h, then 0.0125 mg/kg/min. i.m.: 15 mg/kg stat, then 7.5 mg/kg/dose (max 400 mg) 8 H. Note: 1 mg base = 1.2 mg sulphate = 1.3 mg bisulphate = 1.6 mg gluconate.

Quinine, base Oral: 8.3 mg/kg/dose (max 500 mg) 8 H for 7–10 days. Parenteral: 16.7 mg/kg (20 mg/kg of dihydrochloride) i.v. over 4 h or i.m., then 8.3 mg/

kg/dose 8 H i.v. over 2 h or i.m. for 2–3 days, then 8.3 mg/kg/dose 8 H oral for 5 days. Note: 1 mg base = 1.7 mg bisulphate = 1.2 mg dihydrochloride = 1.2 mg ethyl carbonate = 1.3 mg hydrobromide = 1.2 mg hydrochloride = 1.2 mg sulphate.

Quinupristin + dalfopristin (Synercid i.v.) 7.5 mg/kg/dose 8 H i.v. over 1 h.

Raloxifene 1 mg/kg (adult 60 mg) daily oral.

Ramipril 0.05 mg/kg (adult 2.5 mg) oral daily, may increase over 4–6 weeks to 0.1–0.2 mg/kg (adult 5–10 mg) daily.

Ranitidine i.v.: 1 mg/kg/dose slowly 6–8 H, or 2 µg/kg/min. Oral: 2 mg/kg/dose (max 150 mg) 12 H, or 4 mg/kg (max 300 mg) at night.

Ranitidine bismuth citrate 8 mg/kg/dose (adult 400 mg) 12 H oral; to eradicate *H.pylori*, add an antibiotic.

Remifentanil 1 µg/kg i.v. over 30 s, then 0.05–0.2 µg/kg/min. Ventilated: 1 µg/kg, then 0.5–4 µg/kg/min.

Repaglinide Adult (NOT/kg) before main meals, oral: initially 0.5 mg, increase every 1–2 weeks to 4 mg (max 16 mg/day).

Reproterol Aerosol 0.5 mg/puff: 1–2 puffs 3–8 H.

Reserpine 0.005–0.01 mg/kg/dose (adult 0.25–0.5 mg) 12–24 H oral.

Resonium See sodium polystyrene sulphonate.

Reteplase Adult (NOT/kg) for myocardial infarction: give heparin 5000 units i.v. + aspirin 250–350 mg oral; then reteplase 10 units i.v. over 2 min with a second dose 30 min later; then heparin 1000 units/h for 24–72 h and aspirin 75–150 mg/day until discharge.

Retinol A See vitamin A.

Ribavirin Inhalation (Viratek nebuliser): 20 mg/ml at 25 ml/h (190 µg/l of gas) for 12–18 h/day for 3–7 days. Oral: 5–15 mg/kg/dose 8–12 H.

Riboflavine NOT/kg: 5–10 mg daily oral. Organic acidosis (NOT/kg): 50–200 mg daily oral, i.m. or i.v.

Rifabutin 3–12 mg/kg (adult 150–600 mg) daily oral.

Rifampicin 10–15 mg/kg (max 600 mg) daily oral fasting, or i.v. over 3 h (monitor AST). Prophylaxis — *N. meningitidis*: 10 mg/kg daily (neonate), 10 mg/kg (max 600 mg) 12 H for 2 days; *H.influenzae*: 10 mg/kg daily (neonate), 20 mg/kg (max 600 mg) daily for 4 days.

Rimantadine 2.5 mg/kg/dose (max 100 mg) 12 H oral.

Risedronate Osteoporosis: 0.1 mg/kg (adult 5 mg) daily oral. Paget: 0.5 mg/kg (adult 30 mg) daily oral.

Risperidone 0.02 mg/kg/dose (adult 1 mg) 12 H, increase to 0.02–0.15 mg/kg/dose (usually 2–4 mg, max 8 mg) 12 H oral.

Rivastigmine Adult (NOT/kg): initially 1.5 mg 12 H, increase every 2 weeks to max 6 mg 12 H oral.

Rocuronium 0.45–1.2 mg/kg i.v. stat, then 0.1–0.2 mg/kg.

Rofecoxib 0.25–0.5 mg/kg/dose (adult 12.5–25 mg) daily oral.

Ropivacaine 4–5 mg/kg (adult max 200–250 mg). Postop infusion 0.25–0.4 mg/kg/h (adult 12–20 mg/h).

Rotavirus See hyperimmune bovine colostrum, rotavirus.

Roxithromycin 2.5–4 mg/kg/dose (adult 150 mg) 12 H oral before meals.

Salbutamol 0.1–0.15 mg/kg/dose (adult 2–4 mg) 6 H oral. Inhalation — mild: respiratory solution (5 mg/ml, 0.5%) 0.5 ml/dose diluted to 4 ml, or nebule 2.5 mg/2.5 ml 3–6 H; moderate: 0.5% solution 1 ml/dose diluted to 4 ml, or nebule 5 mg/2.5 ml 1–2 H; severe (in ICU): 0.5% solution undiluted continuous. Aerosol 100 µg/puff: 1–2 puff 4–6 H. Rotahaler: 200–400 µg 6–8 H. i.m. or s.c.: 10–20 µg/kg/dose (adult 500 µg) 3–6 H. i.v.: child 5–10 µg/kg/min for 1 h, then 1–2 µg/kg/min (1 µg/kg/min using 1 mg/ml solution = 0.06 × wt ml/h); adult 5 mg in 50 ml at 4 ml/h is 0.1 µg/kg/min.

Salcatonin Hypercalcaemia: 5 units/kg/dose 12–24 H i.m., s.c. or i.v. over 6–12 h. Paget: adult 50–100 units daily. Cancer bone pain: 4 units/kg/dose (adult 200 units) up to ×4/day.

Salicylic acid Cradle cap: 6% solution (Egocappol) 12 H 3–5 days. Plantar warts: 15% solution ×1–2/day, 40% medicated disc 24–48 H.

Salicylsalicylic acid See salsalate.

Salmeterol Aerosol, diskhaler (NOT/kg): 50–100 µg 12 H.

Salsalate 10–20 mg/kg/dose (adult 0.5–1 g) 6 H oral.

Saquinavir 12 mg/kg/dose (adult 600 mg) 8 H oral.

Sargramostim (GM-CSF, Leucomax) 3–5 µg/kg daily s.c., or i.v. over 6 h. Keep WCC 5000–10 000/mm^3.

Scopolamine See hyoscine.

Secretin (1 cu = 4 chr units) 1–2 cu/kg slow i.v.

Sennoside Tab 7.5 mg daily (NOT/kg): 6 months–2 years $^1/_2$–1 tab, 3–10 years 1–2 tab, >10 years 2–4 tab. Granules 22.5 mg/teasp, 12–24 H (NOT/kg): <6 months $^1/_4$–$^1/_2$ teasp, 6 months–2 years $^1/_2$–1 teasp, 3–10 years 1–2 teasp.

Sermorelin (GHRH) 1 µg/kg fasting in morning i.v.

Sertraline 1–2 mg/kg (adult 50–100 mg) daily oral; may give 3–4 mg/kg (adult 150–200 mg) daily for up to 8 weeks.

Sildenafil Adult sexual dysfunction: 25–100 mg (NOT/kg) oral 1 h before sexual activity (max once/day). Pulmonary hypertension: 0.3–2 mg/kg 3–6 H oral.

Silver nitrate, stick Apply daily to affected area only.

Silver sulfadiazine 1% + chlorhexidine 0.2%, cream Apply in 3–5 mm layer.

Simethicone See aluminium hydroxide compound.

Simvastatin Initially 0.2 mg/kg (adult 10 mg) daily, may increase every 4 weeks to max 1 mg/kg (adult 40 mg) daily oral.

Sodium Deficit: to increase serum Na by 2 mmol/l/h (maximum safe rate), infusion rate (ml/h) = 8 × wt(kg)/(% saline infused); number of hours of infusion = (140 – serum Na)/2. 4 ml/kg of X% saline raises serum

Na by X mmol/l. Need 2–6 mmol/kg/day. NaCl MW = 58.45, 1 g NaCl = 17.1 mmol Na, NaCl 20% = 3.4 mmol/ml.

Sodium alginate See alginic acid.

Sodium aurothiomalate 0.25 mg/kg weekly i.m., increase to 1 mg/kg (max 50 mg) weekly for 10 weeks, then every 2–6 weeks. i.m., then every 1–4 weeks.

Sodium benzoate Neonate: 250 mg/kg over 2 h stat, then 10–20 mg/kg/h i.v.

Sodium bicarbonate See bicarbonate.

Sodium calcium edetate (EDTA) 30–40 mg/kg/dose 12 H i.m. or i.v. over 1 h for 5 days.

Sodium chloride See sodium.

Sodium citrotartrate 40–80 mg/kg/dose (adult 2–4 g) in 50 ml water 8–12 H oral.

Sodium clodronate 6 mg/kg (adult 300 mg) i.v. over 2 h daily for 7 days, then 15–30 mg/kg/dose (adult 0.8–1.6 g) 12 H oral.

Sodium cromoglycate Inhalation (Intal): 1 cap (20 mg) 6–8 H, 2 ml solution (20 mg) 6–8 H, aerosol 1–10 mg 6–8 H. Eye drops (2%): 1–2 drops per eye 4–6 H. Oral: 5–10 mg/kg/dose (max 200 mg) 6 H oral. Nasal (Rynacrom): insufflator 5 mg in each nostril 6 H, spray 1 puff in each nostril 6 H.

Sodium fluoride NOT/kg: <2 years 0.55 mg oral daily, 2–4 years 1.1 mg, >4 years 2.2 mg. Osteoporosis, Paget, bone secondaries in adult: 20–40 mg/dose (NOT/kg) 8–12 H.

Sodium fusidate See fusidic acid.

Sodium nitrite 3% solution: 0.2 ml/kg (max 10 ml) i.v. over 5 min.

Sodium nitroprusside i.v. infusion 0.5–10 μg/kg/min: for 65 kg adult 50 mg in 50 ml at 2 ml/h is 0.5 μg/kg/min. If used for >24 h, max rate 4 μg/kg/min. Max total 70 mg/kg with normal renal function (or sodium thiocyanate <1725 μmol/l, ×0.058 = mg/l). Pulmonary vasodilation: 5 μg/kg/min nitroglycerine = 2 μg/kg/min nitroprusside = 0.1 μg/kg/min PGE1 approx.

Sodium picosulpate 0.1–0.3 mg/kg (adult 5–15 ml) at night oral.

Sodium polystyrene sulphonate (Resonium) 0.3–0.6 g/kg/dose (adult 15–30 g) 6 H NG (give lactulose) or PR.

Sodium thiosulphate 1 ml/kg (adult 50 ml) 25% solution i.v. over 10 min.

Sodium valproate 5–15 mg/kg/dose (max 1 g) 8–12 H oral. Level 0.3–0.7 mmol/l (×144 = μg/ml).

Somatostatin See octreotide.

Somatropin Usually 2–3 IU/m^2 on 5–7 days a week s.c., or 4–6 iuIU/m^2 on 3 days a weeks i.m.

Sorbitol 70% 0.2–0.5 ml/kg/dose (adult 20–30 ml) 8–24 H oral. With activated charcoal: 1g/kg (1.4 ml/kg) NG, ×1–2.

Sorbolene cream; pure, with 10% glycerin, or with 5% or 10% olive oil or peanut oil. Skin moisturiser, apply p.r.n.

Sotalol i.v.: 0.5–2 mg/kg/dose (adult 25–100 mg) over 10 min 6 H. Oral: 1–4 mg/kg/dose (adult 50–200 mg) 8 H.

Spectinomycin 40–80 mg/kg (adult 2–4 g) i.m. once.

Spironolactone Oral (NOT/kg): 0–10 kg 6.25 mg/dose 12 H, 11–20 kg 12.5 mg/dose 12 H, 21–40 kg 25 mg/dose 12 H, over 40 kg 25 mg/dose 8 H. i.v.: see potassium canrenoate.

Stanozolol 0.05–0.2 mg/kg oral (adult 2.5–10 mg) daily at first, then every 2–3 days.

Stavudine (d4T) 20 mg/m^2/dose 12 H oral.

Streptokinase (SK) Short term (myocardial infarction): 30 000 units/kg (max 1 500 000 units) i.v. over 60 min, repeat if occlusion recurs <5 days. Long term (DVT, pulmonary embolism, arterial thrombosis): 5000 units/kg (max 250 000 units) i.v. over 30 min, then 2000 units/kg/h (max 100 000 units/h); stop heparin and aspirin, if PTT <×2 normal at 4 h give extra 10 000 units/kg (max 500 000 units) i.v. over 30 min, stop SK if PTT >×5 normal then give 1000 units/kg/h. Local infusion: 50 units/kg/h (continue heparin 10–15 units/kg/h). Blocked i.v. cannula: 5000 units/kg in 2 ml in cannula for 2 h then remove, may repeat ×2.

Streptomycin 20–30 mg/kg (max 1 g) i.m. daily.

Sucralfate 1 g tab NOT/kg: 0–2 years $^1/_4$ tab 6 H, 3–12 years $^1/_2$ tab 6 H, >12 years 1 tab 6 H oral.

Sufentanil 2–50 μg/kg slow i.v.; may then infuse so that total dose is 1 μg/kg/h of expected surgical time.

Sulbactam See ampicillin + sulbactam.

Sulfadiazine 50 mg/kg/dose (max 2 g) 6 H slow i.v.

Sulindac 4 mg/kg/dose (adult 200 mg) 12 H oral.

Sulphamethoxazole See cotrimoxazole.

Sulphasalazine Active colitis: 12.5 mg/kg/dose (max 1 g) 4–6 H oral; remission 7.5 mg/kg/dose (max 0.5 g) 6–8 H, suppository (NOT/kg) adult 0.5–1 g 12 H. Juvenile arthritis 15 mg/kg/dose 8–12 H (max 2 g/day) oral.

Sulphinpyrazone 2–3 mg/kg/dose (max 200 mg) 6–12 H oral.

Sulpiride 4 mg/kg/dose (adult 200 mg) 12 H, slow increase to 4–24 mg/kg/dose (adult 0.2–1.2 g) 12 H oral.

Sulthiame 1 mg/kg/dose (adult 50 mg) 8–12 H oral, may increase to 5 mg/kg/dose (adult 200 mg) 8 H.

Sumatriptan Oral: 1–2 mg/kg (adult 50–100 mg) stat, may repeat twice. s.c.: 0.12 mg/kg (max 6 mg) stat, may repeat once after 1 h.

Surfactant See beractant (Survanta), colfosceril palmitate (Exosurf), poractant alfa (Curosurf), pumactant (ALEC).

Suxamethonium. i.v.: neonate 3 mg/kg/dose, child 2 mg/kg/dose, adult 1 mg/kg/dose. i.m.: double i.v. dose.

Tacrine (THA) 0.5–2 mg/kg/dose (adult 30–120 mg) 3 H i.v.

Tacrolimus i.v. infusion: 2 mg/m^2/day. Oral: 3 mg/m^2/dose 12 H. Maintain trough plasma level 0.4–1.2 ng/ml, whole blood level 10–20 ng/ml.

Tazobactam + piperacillin (125 mg/1 g) See piperacillin.

Teicoplanin 250 mg/m^2 i.v. over 30 min stat, then 125 mg/m^2 i.v. or i.m. daily. Severe infection: 250 mg/m^2 12 H ×3 doses, then 250 mg/m^2 i.v. or i.m. daily.

Telmisartan 1 mg/kg (adult 40 mg) daily, increase if required to 2 mg/kg (adult 80 mg) daily oral.

Temazepam Adult (NOT/kg): 10–30 mg at night, oral.

Tenoxicam 0.2–0.4 mg/kg (adult 10–20 mg) daily oral.

Terazosin 0.02 mg/kg test, then 0.04–0.4 mg/kg (adult 2–20 mg) daily oral.

Terbinafine 5 mg/kg (adult 250 mg) daily oral. 1% cream, gel: apply 12–24 H to clean dry skin.

Terbutaline Oral: 0.05–0.1 mg/kg/dose (adult 2.5–5 mg) 6 H. s.c.: 5–10 μg/kg/dose (adult 0.25–0.5 mg). i.v.: child 3–6 μg/kg/min for 1 h, then 0.4–1 μg/kg/min; adult 0.25 mg stat over 10 min, then 1–10 μg/kg/h. Inhalation — mild: respiratory solution (1%, 10 mg/ml) 0.25 ml/dose diluted to 4 ml 3–6 H; moderate: 0.5 ml of 1% diluted to 4 ml, or respule 5 mg/2 ml 1–2 H; severe (in ICU): undiluted continuous. Aerosol 250 μg/puff: 1–2 puffs 4–6 H.

Terfenadine 1 mg/dose (adult 60 mg) 12 H oral.

Terlipressin 0.04 mg/kg/dose (adult 2 mg) i.v., then 0.02–0.04 mg/kg/dose (adult 1–2 mg) 4–6 H for max 72 h.

Testolactone 5–10 mg/kg/dose (max 250 mg) 6 H oral.

Testosterone Esters: 100–500 mg (NOT/kg) i.m. every 2–4 weeks. Implant: 8 mg/kg (to nearest 100 mg). Undecanoate: 40–120 mg (NOT/kg) daily oral. Testosterone level: <16 years 5–10 nmol/l, >16 years 10–30 nmol/l.

Tetrabenazin 0.5–2 mg/kg/dose (adult 25–100 mg) 12 H oral.

Tetracosactrin zinc injection (Synacthen Depot) 600 μg/m^2 (max 1mg) i.m. every 1–7 days.

Tetracycline Over 8 years (NOT/kg): 250–500 mg/dose 6 H oral.

Tetrahydrobiopterin Defective synthesis: 20 mg/kg daily oral. Defective regeneration: 5 mg/kg/dose 6 H oral. Loading test: 20 mg/kg oral, 2 mg/kg i.v.

Thalidomide 4 mg/kg/dose (adult 200 mg) 12 H oral, reducing over 2–4 weeks to 0.5–1 mg/kg/dose (adult 25–50 mg) 12 H.

THAM See trometamol.

Theophylline (80 mg theophylline = 100 mg aminophylline) Loading dose: 8 mg/kg (max 500 mg) oral. Maintenance: 1st week of life 2 mg/kg/dose 12 H; 2nd week of life 3 mg/kg/dose 12 H; 3 weeks–12 months (0.1 × age in weeks) + 3 mg/kg/dose 8 H; 1–9 years 4 mg/kg/dose 4–6 H, or 10 mg/kg/dose slow release 12 H; 10–16 years or adult smoker 3 mg/kg/dose 4–6 H, or 7 mg/kg/dose 12 H slow release; adult non smoker 3 mg/kg/dose 6–8 H; elderly 2 mg/kg/dose 6–8 H. Monitor serum level: neonate 60–80 μmol/l, asthma 60–110 (×0.18 = μg/ml).

Thiabendazole 25 mg/kg/dose (max 1.5 g) 12 H oral for 3 days.

Thiamine Beriberi: 1–2 mg/kg i.v., i.m. or oral daily.

Thiopentone 2–5 mg/kg slowly stat (beware hypotension), then 1–5 mg/kg/h i.v. Level 150–200 umol/l (×0.24 = μg/ml).

Thioridazine 0.5–3 mg/kg/dose (adult 25–150 mg) 6–8 H oral or i.m.

Threonine 15–30 mg/kg/dose (adult 0.75–1.5 g) 8 H oral.

Thrombin gluc 10 000 units thrombin in 9 ml mixed with 1 ml 10% calcium chloride in syringe 1, 10 ml cryoprecipitate in syringe 2: inject into bleeding sites together.

Thrombin topical 100–2000 units/ml onto bleeding surface.

Thyroxine Infants: 8–12 μg/kg/day oral. Adult (NOT/kg): 100–200 μg daily.

Tiagabine Usually 0.1 mg/kg/dose (adult 5 mg) 12 H, increase weekly to 0.1–0.5 mg/kg/dose (adult 5–15 mg) 8 H oral.

Tiaprofenic acid 2–4 mg/kg/dose (adult 100–200 mg) 8 H oral.

Ticarcillin 50 mg/kg/dose (adult 3 g) i.v. 6–8 H (1st week of life), 4–6 H or constant infusion (2+ weeks). Cystic fibrosis: 100 mg/kg (max 6 g) 8 H.

Ticarcillin and clavulanic acid Dose as for ticarcillin.

Ticlopidine 5 mg/kg/dose (adult 250 mg) 12 H oral.

Tilactase 200 units/drop: 5–15 drops/l added to milk 24 h before use. 3300 units/tab: 1–3 tabs with meals oral.

Timolol 0.1 mg/kg/dose (adult 5 mg) 8–12 H, increase to max 0.3 mg/kg/dose (adult 15 mg) 8 H. Eye drops (0.25%, 0.5%): 1 drop/eye 12–24 H.

Tinidazole Giardia: 50 mg/kg (max 2 g) stat, repeat after 48 h. Amoebic dysentery: 50 mg/kg (max 2 g) daily for 3 days.

Tinzaparin (1 mg = 75 anti-Xa IU) 50 units/kg s.c. 2 h before surgery, then daily for 7–10 days.

Tiopronin 3–10 mg/kg/dose (adult 150–500 mg) 6–8 H oral.

Tirilazad 1.5 mg/kg/dose 6 H i.v. over 30 min.

Tirofiban 0.4 μg/kg/min for 30 min, then 0.1 μg/kg/min for 2–5 days; also give heparin to APTT ×2 normal.

Tissue plasminogen activator See alteplase.

Tobramycin Single daily dose i.v. or i.m. Neonate: 5 mg/kg stat, then 2.5 mg/kg (<2.5 kg) or 4 mg/kg (≥2.5 kg) daily. 1 month–10 years: 7.5 mg/kg daily. >10 years: 6 mg/kg (max 240–360 mg) daily. Trough level <1.0 mg/l.

Tocainide 5–10 mg/kg/dose (max 400–800 mg) 8–12 H i.v. over 30 min or oral.

Tocopherol See alpha-tocopheryl acetate, and vitamin E.

Tolazamide 2–5 mg/kg/dose (adult 100–250 mg) 6–24 H oral.

Tolmetin 5–10 mg/kg/dose (adult 400–600 mg) 8 H oral.

Tolnaftate, cream, ointment, powder, solution 1% Apply 8–12 H.

Topiramate 1 mg/kg/dose (adult 50 mg) 12–24 H oral, increase gradually to 4–10 mg/kg/dose (adult 100–500 mg) 12 H.

Topotecan 1.5 mg/m^2 daily ×5 i.v. over 30 min, repeat every 3 weeks for at least 4 courses.

Torasemide 0.1–1 mg/kg (adult 5–50 mg) daily oral or i.v. Rarely up to 4 mg/kg (adult 200 mg) daily in renal failure.

Tramadol 1–2 mg/kg/dose (adult 50–100 mg) 4–6 H (max 400 mg/day) oral.

Tramazoline Nasal: 82 μg/dose each nostril ×3–6/day.

Tramazoline 20 μg + dexamethasone 20 μg per dose, nasal. Aerosol: 1 puff in each nostril 4–8 H.

Trandolapril 0.01–0.1 mg/kg (adult 0.5–4 mg) daily oral.

Tranexamic acid Oral: 15–25 mg/kg/dose (adult 1–1.5 g) 8 H. i.v.: 10–15 mg/kg/dose (adult 0.5–1 g) 8 H.

Trastuzumab 4 mg/kg i.v. over 90 min loading dose, then 2 mg/kg i.v. over 30 min weekly.

Trazodone 1–4 mg/kg/dose (adult 50–200 mg) 8 H oral.

Tretinoin 22.5 mg/m^2 12 H oral. Cream or lotion 0.05%, gel 0.01%: apply daily for 3–4 months, then ×1–3/week.

Triacetyloleandomycin 6–12 mg/kg/dose (adult 250–500 mg) 6 H oral.

Triamcinolone Joint, tendon (NOT/kg): 2.5–15 mg stat. i.m.: 0.05–0.2 mg/kg every 1–7 days. Cream or ointment 0.02%, 0.05%: apply sparingly 6–8 H. Triamcinolone has no mineralocorticoid action, 1 mg = 5 mg hydrocortisone in glucocorticoid action.

Triamcinolone 0.1% + neomycin 0.25% + gramicidin 0.025% + nystatin 100 000 units/g. Kenacomb ointment: apply 8–12 H. Kenacomb otic ointment, drops: apply 8–12 H (2–3 drops).

Triamterene 2 mg/kg/dose (adult 100 mg) 8–24 H oral.

Triclosan, emulsion 2% 2 ml to wet skin for 20 s, rinse and repeat.

Trientine 10 mg/kg/dose (adult 500 mg) 6–12 H oral.

Trifluoperazine 0.02–0.2 mg/kg/dose (adult 1–10 mg, occasionally 20 mg) 12 H oral.

Triiodothyronine (T$_3$) See liothyronine.

Trilostane 0.5–4 mg/kg/dose (adult 30–240 mg) 6 H oral.

Trimeprazine 0.05–0.5 mg/kg/dose (adult 2.5–25 mg) 6 H oral. Sedation: 0.5–1 mg/kg i.m., 2–4 mg/kg oral.

Trimethobenzamide 5 mg/kg/dose (adult 250 mg) 6–8 H oral, i.m. or PR.

Trimethoprim 3–4 mg/kg/dose (usual max 150 mg) 12 H, or 6–8 mg/kg (usual max 300 mg) daily oral or i.v. Urine prophylaxis: 1–2 mg/kg (adult 150 mg) at night oral.

Trimethoprim–sulphamethoxazole See cotrimoxazole.

Trimipramine 1–2 mg/kg/dose (adult 50–100 mg) 8–24 H oral.

Tripelennamine 1.25 mg/kg/dose (adult 75 mg) 6 H oral.

Tripotassium dicitratobismuthate See bismuth sub-citrate (colloidal).

Triprolidine 2.5 mg + pseudoephedrine 60 mg (Actifed) 10 ml elixir = 1 tab. NOT/kg: 2.5 ml (<2 years), 2.5–5 ml (2–5 years), 0.5 tab (6–12 years), 1 tab (>12 years) 6–8 H oral.

Trisodium edetate 40–70 mg/kg (max 3 g) i.v. over 6 h daily for 5 days; max 3 courses each 2 days apart.

Trometamol (THAM) ml of 0.3 molar (18 g/500 ml) solution = wt × BE (give $^1/_2$ this) i.v. over 30–60 min.

Tropicamide, eye drops 0.5%, 1% 1–2 drops/eye, repeat after 5 min.

Tropisetron 0.1 mg/kg (adult 5 mg) slow i.v. just before chemotherapy, then oral 1 h before breakfast for 5 days.

Tulobuterol 0.04 mg/kg/dose (adult 2 mg) 8–12 H oral.

Urokinase 4000 units/kg i.v. over 10 min, then 4000 units/kg/h for 12 h (start heparin 3–4 h later). Blocked cannula: instil 5000–25 000 units (NOT/kg) in 2–3 ml saline for 2–4 h. Empyema: 2 ml/kg of 1500 units/ml in saline, position head up/down and right side up/down 30 min each, then drain.

Ursodeoxycholic acid 4–8 mg/kg/dose (adult 200–400 mg) 12 H oral.

Valaciclovir 20 mg/kg/dose (adult 1 g) 8 H oral.

Valproic acid, valproate See sodium valproate.

Vancomycin 15 mg/kg/dose (max 750 mg) i.v. over 2 h: daily (preterm), 12 H (1st week of life), 8 H (2+ weeks). Oral: 10 mg/kg/dose (adult 500 mg) 6 H. Intraventricular (NOT/kg): 10 mg/dose 48 H. Peak 25–40 mg/l, trough <10 mg/l; done Monday–Friday RCH.

Vasopressin Aqueous: put 2–5 units in 1 litre fluid, and replace urine output + 10% i.v.; or 2–10 units i.m. or s.c. 8 H. Brain death: 0.0003 units/kg/min (1 units/kg in 50 ml at 1 ml/h) + adrenaline 0.1–0.2 μg/kg/min. Oily: 2.5–5 units (NOT/kg) i.m. every 2–4 days. Gastrointestinal haemorrhage (aqueous solution): 0.4 units/min i.v. in adult; 0.1 units/min local i.a. in adult. See desmopressin and lypressin.

Vecuronium ICU: 0.1 mg/kg p.r.n. Theatre: 0.1 mg/kg stat, then 1–10 μg/kg/min i.v.

Venlafaxine 0.5 mg/kg/dose (adult 25 mg) 8 H oral, increase to max 2.5 mg/kg/dose (adult 125 mg) 8 H if required.

Verapamil i.v.: 0.1–0.2 mg/kg (adult 5–10 mg) over 10 min, then 5 μg/kg/min. Oral: 1–3 mg/kg/dose (adult 80–120 mg) 8–12 H.

Versenate See sodium calcium edetate.

Vidarabine Eye ointment: ×5/day until epithelialised, then 12 H 7 days. i.v. infusion: 10 mg/kg/day 5–10 days (varicella/zoster), 15 mg/kg/day 10 days (herpes encephalitis).

Vigabatrin Initially 40 mg/kg (adult 2 g) daily oral, may increase to 80–100 mg/kg (max 4 g) daily (given in 1–2 doses).

Viloxazine 2–5 mg/kg (adult 100–250 mg) morning, and 2–3 mg/kg (adult 100–150 mg) noon oral. Elderly: 100 mg daily.

Vitamin A High risk (NOT/kg): 100 000 IU (<8 kg), 200 000 IU (>8 kg) oral or i.m. every 4–6 months. Severe measles: 400 000 IU (NOT/kg) once. >10 000 IU daily may be teratogenic.

Vitamin A, B, C, D compound (Pentavite, infant) <3 years (NOT/kg): 0.15 ml daily, increase by 0.15 ml/day to 0.45 ml/day.

Vitamin A, B, C, D compound (Pentavite, child) <3 years (NOT/kg): 2.5 ml daily. >3 years (NOT/kg): 5 ml daily.

Vitamin B group Ampoule: i.v. over 30 min. Tab: 1–2/day.

Vitamin B$_1$ See thiamine.

Vitamin B$_{12}$ See hydroxocobalamin.

Vitamin C See ascorbic acid.

Vitamin D Nutritional rickets: ergocalciferol (D$_2$) 10–250 µg (400–10 000 units) daily (NOT/kg) for 30 days oral, calcifediol (25-OH D$_3$) 1–2 µg/kg daily oral. Renal rickets or hypoparathyroidism: calcitriol (1,25-OH D$_3$) start 0.01 µg/kg daily; dihydrotachysterol (1-OH D$_2$) 20 µg/kg/day; ergocalciferol (D$_2$): 50 000– 300 000 units/day (NOT/kg).

Vitamin E (Copherol E) Preterm babies (NOT/kg): 40 units (2 drops) daily oral. 1 unit = 1 mg. See also alpha-tocopheryl.

Vitamin K$_1$ See phytomenadione.

Vitamins, parenteral MVI–12 (for adult): 5 ml in 1 litre i.v. fluid. MVI Paediatric, added to i.v. fluid: 65% of a vial (<3 kg), 1 vial (3 kg to 11 years).

Warfarin Usually 0.2 mg/kg (adult 10 mg) stat, 0.2 mg/kg (adult 10 mg) next day providing INR <1.3, then 0.05–0.2 mg/kg (adult 2–10 mg) daily oral. INR usually 2–2.5 for prophylaxis, 2–3 for treatment. Beware drug interactions.

Whole blood 6 ml/kg raises Hb 1g%. 1 bag = 400 ml approximately.

Xamoterol 4 mg/kg/dose (adult 200 mg) 12–24 H oral.

Xipamide 0.5–1.5 mg/kg (adult 20–80 mg) daily oral.

Xylometazoline <6 years: 0.05% 1 drop or spray 8–12 H. 6–12 years: 0.05% 2–3 drops or sprays 8–12 H. >12 years: 0.1% 2–3 drops or sprays 6–12 H.

Yohimbine 0.05–0.1 mg/kg/dose (adult 2.7–5.4 mg) 8 H oral.

Zalcitabine 0.005–0.015 mg/kg/dose (adult 0.25–0.75 mg) 8 H oral.

Zidovudine (AZT) Child: 90–180 mg/m^2/dose (max 150 mg/dose) 6 H oral, 8 H i.v. Adult (NOT/kg): usually 200 mg/dose 8 H oral, or 150 mg/dose 8 H i.v.

Zinc sulphate Adult (NOT/kg): 50–220 mg 8–24 H oral. Acrodermatitis enteropathica (child): (NOT/kg) 25 mg 12 H oral.

Zolmitriptan 0.05–0.1 mg/kg (adult 2.5–5 mg) oral, repeated 2 H if required; max 0.3 mg/kg (adult 15 mg) in 24 h.

Zolpidem 0.1–0.4 mg/kg/dose (adult 5–20 mg) nocte oral.

Zopiclone 0.1–0.3 mg/kg (adult 5–15 mg) at bedtime oral.

Zuclopenthixol 0.4–3.0 mg/kg (adult 20–150 mg) daily oral.

Drugs and breastfeeding

Breastfeeding is the best method of feeding human infants; however, some drugs may harm the baby if they are taken by a woman who is breastfeeding. Table 23.1 provides a guide to some of the drugs that may cause problems.

Table 23.1 Use of drugs by women who are breastfeeding

Drug type	Usually contraindicated	Use rarely, with caution	Usually safe
Analgesics	Meperidine, oxycodone		Flurbiprofen, ibuprofen, ketorolac, mefenamic acid, morphine, paracetamol
Antibiotics	Cloramphenicol, tetracycline		
Anticoagulants	Phenindione		Heparin, warfarin
Anticonvulsants		Ethosuximide, phenobarbitone, primidone	Carbamazepine, phenytoin, sodium valproate
Antidepressants		Doxepin, thioxetine, lithium	Sertraline, tricyclics
Antimigraine	Ergotamine, ergometrine		Sumatriptan
Antineoplastic	All: stop breastfeeding		

Table 23.1 (Continued)

Drug type	Usually contraindicated	Use rarely, with caution	Usually safe
Cardiovascular		Acebutolol, amiodarone, atenolol, nadolol, sotalol	Labetalol, propranolol
Endocrine drugs	Bromocriptine, oestrogens		
Immunodepressants		Azathioprine, cyclosporin	
Iodides, iodine	Iodides, iodine		
Radioactive substances	Withhold breastfeeding		
Recreational drugs	Drugs of abuse (e.g. amphetamines, cocaine, heroin, LSD, marijuana, mescaline, phencycladine), smoking		Alcohol (one drink at least 2 h before breast feed), buprenorphine (safer than methadone), caffeine (up to 2 coffees or colas per day)
Sedatives	Long term: alprazolam, diazepam		

PART 6   SELF-ASSESSMENT

Questions

1. **Which of the following would be an adequate rehydration treatment for a 10 kg child who is assessed to be 7.5% dehydrated with normal electrolytes?**
   (A) 200 ml/h of oral rehydration solution for 4 hours
   (B) Double maintenance fluid intravenously for 18 hours
   (C) 750 ml of Ringer's lactate over 4 hours
   (D) 45 ml/h of 4% dextrose in 0.18% saline
   (E) 5 ml of Ringer's lactate intravenously over 4 hours

2. **A normal anion gap acidosis occurs in which of the following conditions?**
   (A) Diabetic ketoacidosis
   (B) Renal tubular acidosis
   (C) Salicylate poisoning
   (D) Acute gastroenteritis
   (E) Septic shock

3. **Oral rehydration is the treatment of choice for all children with acute gastroenteritis, with the following exceptions:**
   (A) High fever
   (B) Ileus and coma
   (C) Vomiting
   (D) Sunken fontanelle
   (E) Shock

4. **Regarding clinical assessment of dehydration, which of the following is/are true?**
   (A) The degree of dehydration may be underestimated in obesity
   (B) Sunken eyes are a sign of moderate to severe dehydration
   (C) There are no clinical signs of mild dehydration
   (D) A high urine specific gravity is a reliable indicator of dehydration
   (E) The degree of dehydration may appear exaggerated by wasting

5. **Hypokalaemia in acute gastroenteritis may be associated with which of the following features?**
   (A) Rhabdomyolysis
   (B) Hypotonia
   (C) Prolonged QT interval
   (D) Strongyloidiasis
   (E) Ileus

Answers and explanations

1. The correct answers are **(A)** and **(C)**. Rapid rehydration over 4–6 hours is now recommended standard treatment for significant dehydration in hospital. For rapid rehydration, this child requires either approximately 750 ml i.v. or 200 ml/h of oral rehydration (provided the child is able to drink) over 4 hours. Rapid rehydration with maintenance fluid (4%

dextrose in 0.18% saline) is dangerous because it can cause hyponatraemia and seizures.

2. The correct answers are **(B)** and **(D)**. Renal tubular acidosis and acute gastroenteritis (usually) produce a normal anion gap acidosis due to the loss of bicarbonate by the kidney and gut, respectively, whereas ketones, salicylates or lactate are unmeasured ions, so increase the anion gap when they cause acidosis.

3. The correct answers are **(B)** and **(E)**. Ileus, coma (with the risk of aspiration) and shock are contraindications to oral rehydration therapy. Fever, and signs of 5% dehydration are not necessarily reasons not to commence oral rehydration, at least in the first instance.

4. The correct answers are **(A)**, **(B)**, **(C)** and **(E)**. Clinical signs of dehydration appear later with

obesity than in normally nourished children. Marasmus or severe wasting with no dehydration may be mistaken for dehydration due to abnormal skin turgor. A concentrated urine with high specific gravity merely reflects a renal response to decreased fluid intake and does not necessarily imply dehydration. The clinical signs of dehydration such as sunken eyes and skin turgor changes do not appear until the degree of dehydration is moderate.

5. The correct answers are **(A)**, **(B)**, **(C)**, **(D)** and **(E)**. Hypotonia, ileus and ECG changes are classic features of hypokalaemia. Rhabdomyolysis and inability to concentrate the urine have been described with hypokalaemia. *Strongyloides stercoralis* and *Cryptosporidium parvum* are parasitic causes of diarrhoea that are more likely to cause hypokalaemia than other viral or bacterial causes.

PART 6   FURTHER READING

Alderson P, Schierhout G, Roberts I, Bunn F 2000 Colloids versus crystalloids for fluid resuscitation in critically ill patients. Cochrane Database of Systematic Reviews (2): CD000567

Andriske L 1997 Drugs and breast feeding. Royal Women's Hospital, Melbourne

Anonymous 1996 Practice parameter: the management of acute gastroenteritis in young children. American Academy of Pediatrics, Provisional Committee on Quality Improvement, Subcommittee on Acute Gastroenteritis. Pediatrics 97: 424–435

Blaser M J, Smith P D, Ravdin J I, Greenberg H B, Guerrant R L 1995 Infections of the gastrointestinal tract. Raven Press, New York, 635–649

Duggan C, Refat M, Hashem M, Wolff M, Fayad I, Santosham M 1996 How valid are clinical signs of dehydration in infants? Journal of Pediatric Gastroenterology and Nutrition 22: 56–61

Fontaine O, Gore S M, Pierce N F 2000 Rice-based oral rehydration solution for treating diarrhoea. Cochrane Database of Systematic Reviews (2): CD001264

Gorelick M H, Shaw K N, Murphy K O 1997 Validity and reliability of clinical signs in the diagnosis of dehydration in children. Pediatrics 99(5): E6

Howard C R, Lawrence R A 1999 Drugs and breast feeding. Clinics in Perinatology 26: 447–478

Ito S 2000 Drug therapy for breast-feeding women. New England Journal of Medicine 343: 118–126

Mackenzie A, Barnes G, Shann F 1989 Clinical signs of dehydration in children. Lancet ii: 605–607

Murphy M S 1998 Guidelines for managing acute gastroenteritis based on a systematic review of published research. Archives of Disease in Childhood 79: 279–284

Narchi H 1998 Serum bicarbonate and dehydration severity in gastroenteritis. Archives of Disease in Childhood 8: 70–71

Reid S R, Bonadio W A 1996 Outpatient rapid intravenous rehydration to correct dehydration and resolve vomiting in children with acute gastroenteritis. Annals of Emergency Medicine 28: 318–323

Rothrock S G, Green S M, McArthur C L, DelDuca K 1997 Detection of electrolyte abnormalities in children presenting to the emergency department: a multicenter, prospective analysis. Detection of Electrolyte Abnormalities in Children Observational National Study (DEACONS) Investigators. Academic Emergency Medicine 4: 1025–1031

Valentiner-Branth P, Steinsland H, Gjessing H K et al 1999 Community-based randomized controlled trial of reduced osmolarity oral rehydration solution in acute childhood diarrhea. Pediatric Infectious Disease Journal 18: 789–795

Useful links

Useful links

http://www.breastfeedingbasics.org/cgi-bin/deliver.cgi/content/Drugs/index.html (Module on breastfeeding)

http://www.drreddy.com/gastro.html (Gastroenteritis symptoms and treatment)

http://www.emedicine.com/emerg/topic275.htm (Hyponatraemia)

http://emedicine.com/emerg/topic312.htm (Metabolic acidosis)

http://www.intox.org/pagesource/treatment/english/hypokalaemia.htm (Hypokalaemia)

http://www.niddk.nih.gov/health/digest/pubs/lactose/lactose.htm (Lactose intolerance)

http://www.nutramed.com/nutrition/minerals.htm (Minerals in nutrition)

http://www.oucom.ohiou.edu/CVPhysiology//BP016.htm (Cardiovascular physiology)

http://www.rehydrate.org/ (Rehydration project: focus on diarrhoea, dehydration and rehydration)

http://www.virtual-anaesthesia-textbook.com/vat/acidbase.html (water, electrolytes, renal and acid–base)

http://www.who.int/chd/publications/cdd/meded/1med.htm (Child and adolescent health and development)

PART 7

PRINCIPLES OF IMAGING IN CHILDHOOD

24 Diagnostic imaging in infancy and childhood

R. Teele

Paediatric radiology became a subspecialty of Radiology and of Paediatrics because of two men: John Caffey, paediatrician, and Edward B.D. Neuhauser, radiologist. A quirk of fate resulted in this 'infant' subspecialty, born in the1940s, being affiliated with Radiology rather than with Paediatrics — and the fact that ionising radiation as a means of imaging was the province of Radiology. Paediatric radiology has developed dramatically in the interim. Now, the tools of the radiologist include plain radiography, fluoroscopy (screening), intravenous, intracavitary and gastrointestinal contrast media, angiography, nuclear medicine, ultrasonography, computerised tomography and magnetic resonance imaging.

There are many differences between imaging the child and imaging the adult. Most importantly, the diseases are different. Congenital disease as well as acquired disease must be considered in the differential list. Usually a child has a single diagnosis to explain symptoms. History taking and clinical examination is not easy for infants and children and thus information from imaging is crucial in certain situations. Radiation protection is important both for the child and for the society as a whole. The child's physical and psychological welfare during diagnostic imaging must also be considered.

Imagine yourself as a 4 month old infant, starving hungry, being held down on a cold hard table by strangers. A rubber nipple is being pushed into your mouth and it is full of strawberry flavoured chalk fluid that you are supposed to swallow while a machine makes horrible noises over your head. Now imagine yourself as a 2 year old, (on the same hard cold table) being held down and catheterised. Soon, your bladder feels like it will burst and you have to micturate all over the table (in the presence of your mother who has just started to toilet train you!).

The upper gastrointestinal series and micturating cystourethrogram are touted as both anatomical and physiological studies but, if you reread the paragraph above, you can understand why they may be lacking in their representation of normal human physiology. Paediatric radiologists play an important intermediary role between Paediatrics and Radiology, both in the conduct and the interpretation of an examination. They are the clinician's friend and the patient's advocate.

Imaging has to be problem oriented. The most important information on a requisition form, apart from the child's name and age, is the question to be answered. The next most important items are the legible name and contact number of the person asking the question. In this age of computerisation, the telephone remains an invaluable instrument of technology because it allows one person to talk to another person. As a paediatric radiologist, it is imperative to do the least possible in the way of investigation to achieve the most information possible about that child's condition.

In concluding this introductory section, it is important to recognise that there is little evidence based information to support many of the recommendations that are in print regarding appropriate algorithms for paediatric imaging. There are few clinical situations and ethical guidelines that allow the performance of several studies on a child simply to compare their utility. Clinical information is frequently imperfect; 'comparable' studies are rarely comparable (for example, consider the problems in defining infection of the urinary tract). Furthermore, local traditions, biased by the practitioners of the area, available facilities and economic conditions, usually prevail over expert opinions and recommendations in textbooks. If you have any question about a patient, ask a radiologist with paediatric experience for help. With these caveats, and encouragement to you, the reader, to challenge algorithms when they seem less than sensible, the following sections outline appropriate imaging considerations for particular situations, and are arranged anatomically, for easy reference.

Neurology

Newborn

- Portable ultrasonography when screening for germinal matrix/intraventricular and intraparenchymal haemorrhage in the premature infant.
- CT for suspected extra-axial collections.
- MRI for:
  - suspected non haemorrhagic parenchymal disease
  - neuronal migrational disorders.

Acute trauma, all ages

- CT scanning when neurological signs/symptoms present.
- MRI when CT scanning is negative in an infant/child with abnormal neurological signs.

Notes

Radiographs of the skull are poorly predictive of intracranial pathology. Their only use is in the situation of suspected inflicted injury (non accidental injury) where multiple fractures or fractures of different ages are helpful in establishing the diagnosis.

Seizures

- CT scanning:
  — without intravenous contrast media, and
  — with intravenous contrast media or MRI.

Notes

A single febrile seizure does not warrant imaging.

Altered neurological state

- CT scanning
  — without intravenous contrast media, and
  — with intravenous contrast media or MRI.

Cardiology (see Chs 51 and 52)

Suspected congenital heart disease (for example, abnormal prenatal ultrasonogram, cyanosis, murmur, unexplained oxygen requirement)
- PA and lateral chest film to include upper abdomen.
- Cardiology referral/echocardiography.
- CT or MRI for anatomical detail of vascular rings as necessary.

Central/cardiac pain

- PA and lateral chest film to include upper abdomen.
- Cardiology referral/echocardiography.

Notes

Plain films of the chest can be remarkably uninformative in some infants with complex congenital heart disease; echocardiography is the gold standard. There can be clues to the presence of congenital heart disease on plain films. Check the six Ss: cardiac **s**ize, cardiac **s**hape, **s**ide of aortic arch, **s**tatus of pulmonary vasculature, abdominal **s**itus, and **s**keletal anomaly. Barium swallow is a very useful ancillary study for characterising a suspected vascular ring if CT or MRI is unavailable. In most centres, echocardiography is the province of the cardiologist. Transoesophageal echocardiography gives excellent detail of the heart and great vessels but the child needs sedation for the procedure. Most echocardiographic examinations are time consuming; some centres use sedation for transthoracic scanning.

Pulmonary/airway

Cough and fever

- PA and lateral chest film.

Pleuritic chest pain

- PA and lateral chest film.

Suspected sepsis in an infant

- PA and lateral chest film.

First episode of wheezing

- PA and lateral chest film.
- Fluoroscopy/screening if foreign body is suspected.

Unexplained stridor

- PA and lateral chest film.
- Lateral film of the neck.
- Fluoroscopy/screening/barium swallow.

Trauma to the chest

- AP supine chest film.
- CT with intravenous contrast if mediastinal injury suspected.
- Angiography for rare situation of traumatic dissection.

Notes

There is great debate as to whether a previously well child, who has clinical symptoms and signs of pneumonia, requires radiography at all. Likewise, there is argument as to whether the workup of sepsis in an infant, and the first episode of wheezing (without history of aspiration of foreign body) requires imaging. Remember that normal radiographs and fluoroscopy do not rule out the presence of an endobronchial foreign body. There has to be enough obstruction of an airway to provide radiographic evidence of its presence. Bronchoscopy should follow if there is a good history of aspiration, even if films are normal.

There is no good prospective study that compares the utility of the PA only radiograph with PA and lateral views of the chest. There is plenty of anecdotal evidence that supports the acquisition of both views. In many cases, lower lobe pneumonia is difficult to diagnose from the PA view alone. The cardiac size is easier to judge when the shape of the chest is defined by two views. When both films are normal, the radiologist can state with certainty that the chest is normal to radiographic examination. It is just as important to document normalcy in some situations as to find an abnormality.

There is general consensus that follow up radiography for an uncomplicated pneumonia is unnecessary. Follow up films are reserved for children who have persisting symptoms of chest disease or who have had unusual radiographs on presentation.

Stridulous breathing implies narrowing of the trachea. A vascular ring, endotracheal haemangioma, tracheitis or epiglottitis are all possible causes. No child or infant with respiratory compromise should be sent for imaging without adequate safeguards for provision of an airway.

Gastroenterology

Non bilious vomiting (Ch. 68)

- Ultrasonography when pyloric stenosis is suspected but a pyloric mass is not palpable.
- Upper gastrointestinal series with barium.

Bilious vomiting

- Upper gastrointestinal series with barium.

Diarrhoea

- Upper gastrointestinal series with follow through examination of small bowel when the cause is not obvious from clinical and laboratory data, cultures, small bowel biopsy, or when idiopathic inflammatory bowel disease is suspected.

Failure to thrive

- Upper gastrointestinal series with follow through examination of small bowel when all other investigations and therapeutic interventions are unhelpful.

Constipation

- Plain radiograph of the abdomen only if a rectal examination is unrevealing.
- Plain radiograph then contrast enema for the neonate who fails to pass meconium.

Gastrointestinal bleeding

- Technetium-99m pertechnetate scintiscan when a Meckel diverticulum is suspected.
- Upper gastrointestinal series with follow through examination of small bowel and antegrade evaluation of colon and/or air contrast barium enema when all other investigations are unhelpful (for example, upper gastrointestinal endoscopy and colonoscopy).

Notes

The availability of consultants trained in paediatric gastroenterology and their skill in endoscopy affects the role of Radiology in gastrointestinal diseases. If there is no one available to perform colonoscopy, there is reliance on air contrast barium enema for evaluation of the colon.

Normal infants vomit, spill, regurgitate and posset. If an infant younger than 6 months is 'a happy chucker', imaging is unnecessary. Pulmonary symptomatology, failure to thrive, feeding difficulty and gastrointestinal blood loss are reasons to pursue imaging with upper gastrointestinal series.

Problems in the neonatal period, such as failure to pass meconium, bilious vomiting and distention, tend to be congenital in origin and the appropriate sequence of imaging requires close cooperation between Paediatric surgery and Radiology. One cannot rely on ultrasonography to confirm or exclude malrotation; a contrast study of the upper gastrointestinal tract is the gold standard. Where there are appropriate ultrasonic facilities and practitioners, pyloric stenosis should be diagnosed with ultrasonography if the pyloric tumour is impalpable.

Hepatobiliary (see Chs 26 and 28)

Neonatal jaundice (Ch. 33)

- Ultrasonography to establish anatomy.
- MRC or radionuclide study with technetium-99m IDA derivative when biliary atresia is a consideration.

Right upper abdominal pain

- Plain radiograph, and sometimes with the addition of ultrasonography.

Notes

Right lower lobe pneumonia may present as severe right upper abdominal pain; therefore, always look at the bases of the lungs on abdominal radiographs. Gallstones in childhood are more likely to be pigment stones than cholesterol stones and may contain enough calcium to be visible on radiography.

Juvenile/adolescent jaundice

- Ultrasonography of liver, biliary tract, pancreas and spleen.
- CT or MRI, depending on the results of ultrasonography.

Abnormal hepatic function

- Ultrasonography when the clinical situation is atypical for hepatitis.
- Ultrasound guided biopsy if the diagnosis is uncertain.

Nephrology/urology

Urinary infection

- Ultrasonography of the urinary tract in neonates, at the time of infection, to rule out an obvious surgical problem, such as obstruction.
- Ultrasonography and MCU in infants and children who have had a documented urinary tract infection.
- IVU or technetium-99m DTPA or Mag 3 scans, with furosemide, for evaluation of the child with possible obstruction at the pelviureteric junction or ureterovesical junction.
- Technetium-99m DMSA or Mag 3 scans during the acute illness can support the diagnosis of pyelonephritis, and/or after infection has cleared can document renal scars.
- RNC for follow up of known reflux.

Notes

The type of imaging, the timing of investigation and the age of the child requiring radiological evaluation are some of the most contentious issues in Paediatrics today (Ch. 61). The American Academy of Pediatrics has issued guidelines regarding diagnostic imaging in young children (aged 2 months to 2 years) but has not addressed the issue of whether children to the age of 5 years should have MCU as part of their evaluation. Many hospitals follow protocols that require MCU for the first documented urinary infection in those 5 years and younger. There are data to suggest that reflux is just one of many factors that result in symptomatic, culture positive urinary infection.

Radionuclide cystogram is a method of documenting reflux with far less radiation than standard MCU. The availability of this study is often limited to tertiary centres. Ultrasonographic MCU requires catheterisation, the instillation of ultrasonographic contrast medium, a cooperative patient and technical expertise; it is not currently available as a routine study.

Renal failure

- Ultrasonography of urinary tract.
- Ultrasound guided biopsy of kidney if necessary for diagnosis.

Note

Ultrasonography, which does not rely on renal function for images, can usually aid in triage of the patient by determining a surgical or medical cause for renal failure.

Hypertension

- Ultrasonography of urinary tract and adrenal glands.

- Abdominal CT if an endocrine tumour is suspected from laboratory data (for example, phaeochromocytoma).
- Nuclear medicine for quantitative, divided renal vascular flow and function.
- Angiography in the rare situation of renal vascular disease.

Haematuria unrelated to trauma

- Ultrasonography of urinary tract.
- MCU or retrograde urethrography if a distal site of bleeding is suspected and cystoscopy is unavailable.
- CT if a renal tumour is suspected.

Notes

See below for renal/abdominal trauma.

Musculoskeletal

Trauma

- Two orthogonal views of the bone or joint that has been injured. Oblique/special views as needed of areas such as scaphoid, radial head, shoulder.
- CT for special cases such as intra-articular fractures of ankle, pelvic fracture.

Fever/pain/swelling in the musculoskeletal system (see Chs 38 and 44)

- Two orthogonal views of the symptomatic bone or joint.
- Nuclear medicine technetium-99m diphosphonate bone scan.
- MRI for difficult diagnoses, tumour, occult infection.
- Ultrasonography for specific questions: localisation of collection of fluid, joint effusion.

Metabolic disease

- AP plain radiograph of wrist and/or knee.

Notes

Because metabolic disease such as rickets is more obvious in areas of rapid bone growth, the wrists and knees are more revealing of abnormality than other sites. Other views (hands, clavicles) may show changes of secondary hyperparathyroidism in those with renal failure.

Possible syndrome with potential skeletal involvement

- Plain radiographs of chest, spine, pelvis, skull, leg and arm to include hand for determination of bone age.

Developmental dysplasia of the hip (DDH)
(Ch. 25)

- Ultrasonography at 4–6 weeks of age if DDH suspected but not obvious on physical examination, or if risk factors (female, breech, positive family history) present;
  or
- Plain radiograph at 4–6 months of age if DDH suspected but not obvious on physical examination.

Notes

This is another area of contention. Ultrasonography of the infant's hips requires training and practice. Early radiography of neonates is unhelpful because so much of the anatomy is cartilaginous. Radiographs at 4–6 months are more informative and still allow intervention if necessary. In some areas of Europe, ultrasonography is used to screen all newborns. Such studies have a high false positive rate of diagnosis of DDH. Repeated physical examination is the cornerstone of diagnosis. Infants may not have an obvious problem until after the neonatal period; hence the change in name from CDH (congenital dysplasia of the hip) to DDH. The availability of experienced paediatric orthopaedic surgeons has an effect on the local imaging protocols.

Abdomen (see Chs 26 and 28)

Abdominal mass

- Plain radiograph of abdomen except for adolescent female with pelvic mass.
- Ultrasonography.
- CT if necessary.
- MRI for neurogenic tumour, soft tissue tumour or bony involvement by tumour, choledochal cyst or an unusual mass.

Notes

Plain radiography provides a road map; it also provides information regarding the bases of the lungs, presence of calcification, effects of the mass on contiguous organs and/or gastrointestinal tract. Most abdominal masses in childhood are related to the retroperitoneum and, in particular, the kidney, such as obstructive hydronephrosis or multicystic dysplastic kidney. A mass that is gastrointestinal in origin, for example intussusception, requires a different approach to that of a mass that is hepatobiliary such as a choledochal cyst. The plain film and ultrasonography, together, provide a triage for further imaging. Remember to consider pregnancy in an adolescent female who has a pelvic mass! If a malignant tumour is

diagnosed, the affected child may be enrolled in treatment protocols that have very specific requirements in terms of imaging at staging and follow up.

Abdominal pain (Ch. 68)

- Supine and upright or decubitus plain radiography for acute abdominal pain.
- No imaging, or ultrasonography only, for non specific, periumbilical abdominal pain.

Notes

A patient who has periumbilical abdominal pain unassociated with any of the objective measures of weight loss, fever, abnormal urinalysis or culture, gastrointestinal blood loss, abnormal FBC, elevated ESR, and who has a normal physical examination, does not require imaging. Ultrasonography is often used as a means of reassuring parents, child and clinician that there is no anatomical abnormality of the liver, spleen, pancreas and kidneys. Limiting radiographs to patients who have had prior abdominal surgery, suspected ingestion of foreign body, abnormal bowel sounds, abdominal distention or peritoneal signs identifies virtually all patients with significant disease.

Abdominal trauma

- Supine radiograph, with decubitus if possible, and lateral view of lumbar spine if there has been hyperflexion of the spine, such as with a lapbelt injury.
- CT with intravenous contrast.

Notes

Many trauma protocols for evaluating the severely injured child have been based on the approach to adults, who have different mechanisms and types of abdominal injury. Peritoneal lavage is not a helpful diagnostic test in paediatric trauma. Major organ injury can occur without there being free intra-abdominal fluid. Ultrasonography is not as sensitive a method as CT but in some remote areas may be the only tool available to search for free fluid, intraparenchymal laceration/haematoma, and renal perfusion.

A child should be stabilised before moving to CT. Cervical spine and head injury should be considered. Oral contrast medium is not usually used for the following reasons: risk of aspiration; time needed to allow contrast to pass through intestinal tract; and relative ileus in the situation of severe injury. However, some centres use positive contrast and some instil water through the nasogastric tube to outline the duodenum.

Inflicted injury (non accidental injury) (Ch. 12)

- CT or MRI of brain to assess extra-axial spaces, parenchymal injury.
- Complete skeletal survey (infants) with high detail images to search for evidence of fracture.
- Nuclear medicine technetium-99m diphosphonate bone scan in unusual cases.
- CT of abdomen, with intravenous contrast, if evidence of abdominal trauma.

Notes

Often a follow up skeletal survey or limited survey may be very revealing. Periosteal reaction takes about 7–10 days to appear. The acute fracture may be occult.

Abbreviations

The following abbreviations are in common use in imaging:

AP Anteroposterior
PA Posteroanterior

These terms relate to the course of the X ray beam through the body. Anteroposterior, supine, chest radiographs are much easier to accomplish in infants who cannot sit without support. Magnification of the heart is not as significant an issue as it is in adults.

CR computerised radiography

Radiographs, films, or images are the result of X rays passing through part of the body. 100 years ago, the images were on glass plates — hence the use of the term 'plate' by some radiologists and clinicians. You may also read of 'roentgenogram' — another relatively old fashioned term highlighting Roentgen's contribution. With computerised radiology now routine, the image is likely to be digital, and viewed on a computer screen.

CT computerised tomography
IVU intravenous urography, synonymous with the old term of intravenous pyelogram (IVP)
MCU micturating cystourethrography
MRC magnetic resonance cholangiography
MRI magnetic resonance imaging
NM nuclear medicine
RNC radionuclide cystography
US ultrasound or ultrasonography

PART 7   SELF-ASSESSMENT

Questions

1. **Cranial ultrasonography of the neonate is a sensitive and specific diagnostic study for diagnosing:**
   (A) Germinal matrix haemorrhage
   (B) Degree of ventricular dilatation (assessment)
   (C) Suspected subdural haematoma
   (D) Hypoxic–ischaemic encephalopathy
   (E) Agenesis of the corpus callosum

2. **Which of the following should you request before obtaining radiographs in a child who has abdominal pain and a normal physical examination?**
   (A) Urinalysis
   (B) Full blood count
   (C) Sedimentation rate or C reactive protein
   (D) Serum amylase
   (E) Sigmoidoscopy

3. **The initial imaging for a neonate who presents with bilious vomiting may be:**
   (A) Plain abdominal radiographs then upper gastrointestinal series with barium
   (B) Plain abdominal radiographs then contrast enema

   (C) Plain abdominal radiographs then magnetic resonance cholangiography
   (D) Ultrasonography then plain radiographs

4. **Intussusception can be diagnosed on:**
   (A) Plain abdominal radiographs
   (B) Ultrasonography of the abdomen
   (C) CT of the abdomen
   (D) Technetium-99m labelled red blood cell study
   (E) Air enema

5. **What is reasonable imaging for a child who has sustained witnessed, significant trauma to the head and who has neurological signs?**
   (A) Plain radiographs of the skull
   (B) MRI of the brain
   (C) CT of the brain
   (D) Electroencephalography of the brain
   (E) Chest, abdomen and lateral neck radiographs

Answers and explanations

1. The correct answers are **(A)**, **(B)** and **(E)**. (A) Germinal matrix and intraventricular haemorrhage are usually easy to diagnose on ultrasonographic exami-

nation through the anterior fontanelle of the neonate. (B) Ventricular size is likewise easy to assess. (C) The extra-axial spaces are not easily visualised by ultrasonography; CT or MRI is far superior. (D) The parenchymal changes from hypoxic–ischaemic encephalopathy are much more obvious on CT or MRI, although the use of good equipment in ultrasonography can allow diagnosis of parenchymal abnormality in some cases. (E) Agenesis of the corpus callosum, as well as other major structural anomalies, can be readily diagnosed with ultrasonography. Subtle abnormalites of grey matter, such as focal migrational abnormality, will only be apparent with MRI.

2. The correct answers are **(A)**, **(B)**, **(C)** and **(D)**. The overuse of abdominal radiography and ultrasonography in the setting of abdominal pain and normal physical examination could be prevented by the judicious selection of these studies. Imaging should follow only when there is some objective measure of abnormality. This is not to suggest that children do not have abdominal pain; rather, that they do not need imaging. (E) Children who have abdominal pain do not need screening sigmoidoscopy; they do need evaluation of their stool for occult blood.

3. The correct answers are **(A)** and **(B)**. The diagnosis that must always be considered in the setting of bilious vomiting is malrotation with midgut volvulus. The upper gastrointestinal series with barium is the diagnostic gold standard in imaging. Bilious vomiting may occur with any level of obstruction distal to the duodenum. Therefore, a neonate with bilious vomiting, failure to pass meconium, dilated small bowel and no colonic gas on plain films may proceed to contrast enema in a search for a colonic obstruction such as atresia or Hirschsprung disease. Enemas are not performed to diagnose malrotation. Magnetic resonance cholangiography (C) is performed when there is concern regarding biliary atresia. Ultrasonography (D) is not the appropriate first study for a neonate with bilious vomiting. Plain films should always be obtained first. Ultrasonography, although diagnostic of malrotation and midgut volvulus in some cases, is not specific or sensitive enough to replace upper gastrointestinal series.

4. Actually, **intussusception can be diagnosed with all of these methods** but the usual protocol involves supine and decubitus plain radiographs, ultrasonography if the diagnosis is in doubt, and air enema for treatment of the intussusception if it is considered to be idiopathic, i.e. without obvious leadpoint and in a patient younger than 5 years of age. Occasionally CT of the abdomen may reveal an occult intussusception, and a labelled red blood cell study would show leakage of radionuclide into the lumen at the site of the intussusception if there is active bleeding of the mucosa. Neither of these methods is recommended for routine diagnosis!

5. The correct answers are **(C)** and **(E)**. Plain radiographs are poorly predictive of significant intracranial injury, may give false reassurance if negative, and take time and further manipulation of the child. CT is the most appropriate initial imaging in this situation, with the objective being delineation of injury that requires immediate surgical intervention. Significant trauma to the chest, abdomen and cervical spine can be screened for with portable, plain radiographs in the emergency department. Findings may modify further imaging; for example, inclusion of cervical spine views or chest and/or abdominal CT. MRI (B) may be useful in the recovery phase to better demonstrate subtle parenchymal damage/axonal sheer injury. It is not usually a tool for the evaluation of acute injury. Electroencephalography (D) is not appropriate in the acute setting.

PART 7 FURTHER READING

Benya E C, Lim-Dunham J E, Landrum O, Statter M 2000 Abdominal sonography in examination of children with blunt abdominal trauma. American Journal of Roentgenology 174: 1613–1616

Carty H 1997 Non-accidental injury: a review of the radiology. European Radiology 7: 1365–1376

Goske M J, Mitchell C, Reslan W A 1999 Imaging of patients with Wilms' tumor. Seminars in Urologic Oncology 17: 11–20

Jaw T S, Kuo Y T, Liu G C, Chen S H, Wang C K 1999 MR cholangiography in the evaluation of neonatal cholestasis. Radiology 212: 249–256

Kirks D R 1998 Practical pediatric imaging: diagnostic radiology of infants and children, 3rd edn. Little, Brown, Boston

Kramer M S, Roberts-Brauer R, Williams R L 1992 Bias and 'overcall' in interpreting chest radiographs in young febrile children. Pediatrics 90: 11–13

Lauu L 2001 Imaging guidelines, 4th edn. The Royal Australian and New Zealand College of Radiologists

Ment L R, Schneider K C, Ainley M A, Allan W C 2000 Adaptive mechanisms of developing brain. The neuroradiologic assessment of the preterm infant. Clinics in Perinatology 27: 303–233

Rockney R M, McQuade W H, Days A L 1995 The plain abdominal roentgenogram in the management of encopresis. Archives of Pediatric and Adolescent Medicine 149: 623–627

Rothrock S G, Green S M, Hummel C B 1992 Plain abdominal radiography in the detection of major disease in children: a prospective analysis. Annals of Emergency Medicine 21: 1423–1429

Shahdadpuri J, Frank R, Gauthier B G, Siegel D N, Trachtman H 2000 Yield of renal arteriography in the evaluation of pediatric hypertension. Pediatric Nephrology 14: 816–819

Taylor J A, Del Beccaro M, Done S, Winters W 1995 Establishing clinically relevant standards for tachypnea in febrile children younger than 2 years. Archives of Pediatric and Adolescent Medicine 149: 283–287

Wren C, Richmond S, Donaldson L 1999 Presentation of congenital heart disease in infancy: implications for routine examination. Archives of Disease in Childhood. Fetal and Neonatal Edition 80: F49–53

Useful links

http://www.acr.org/departments/stand_accred/standards/dl_list.html (Radiology guidelines from the American College of Radiology)

http://www.aap.org/policy/paramtoc.html (Practice Guidelines from the American Academy of Pediatrics)

http://www.pediatricradiology.com (Catalogue of pediatric radiology web sites)

http://www.pedrad.org/html/education.shtml (Education page of the Society for Pediatric Radiology)

PART 8

COMMON ORTHOPAEDIC PROBLEMS

Common paediatric orthopaedic problems

P. Cundy

Skeletal variations during growth

Adult posture should not be used as a criterion for the proper posture in infancy and childhood. During development in childhood a number of different limb shapes (or postures) may be noted and these can cause parental anxiety. These transitory postures can be due to:

- **Intrauterine posture**, sometimes described as 'packaging'.
- **Developmental variants** — that is, not present at birth, but may appear during growth and then disappear spontaneously. These include the common conditions of bow legs, knock knees, flat feet and in toeing. These conditions seldom require active treatment but parents do need informed reassurance, which must be based on accurate knowledge of the natural history of the variations of posture of infants and children.

Intrauterine posture

The position of the child before birth normally is one of flexion. The spine is flexed so that it forms a long curve with a concavity forward, the arms and legs are flexed, and the feet may assume a variety of postures. In the newborn the intrauterine posture can be readily reconstructed by 'folding' the baby into his or her most comfortable position and this may indicate any postural abnormality present.

Posture of the spine

After birth, 'stretching out' occurs. There are two primary curves in the spine, both convex backwards: one is in the dorsal region and the other at the sacrum. On the assumption of the erect posture two secondary curves appear, both convex forward: one is in the cervical region and one in the lumbar region (which appears after the child stands).

Sometimes children display an increase in the normal thoracic and lumbar curves; this may merely reflect ligamentous laxity, poor muscle tone, fatigue and/or a listless mood. These curves do not tend to become fixed and generally no action is called for.

When the newborn infant is viewed from behind, the spine generally is quite straight. However, some babies have a persistent scoliosis in the form of a long curve which extends from the base of the neck to the sacrum. This is generally a 'packaging' defect and, like other packaging defects, will correct itself spontaneously. It is merely necessary to note the curvature and to confirm, at subsequent examinations, that this spontaneous correction is taking place. Very rarely there may be a progressive scoliosis in infancy and generally the curve is over a short length of the spine.

Posture of the feet

Two common foot postures are seen in newborns:

- *Talipes calcaneovalgus*. Many babies are born with the foot turned upwards at the ankle so that the toes lie close to the front of the shin: this is known as talipes calcaneovalgus. This posture can be corrected passively so that the foot can be brought down to a plantigrade position or even into equinus. The condition has a strong tendency to correct itself spontaneously over a period of 2–3 months.
- *Postural talipes equinovarus*. Some babies are born with one or both feet in a position of plantar flexion at the ankles, and inversion of the remainder of the foot, so that the sole of the foot faces the opposite foot. This is postural talipes equinovarus and may be distinguished from true talipes equinovarus by the fact that the former condition is easily correctable, either actively by the baby's movement, or passively by the attendant. The foot can be readily held in normal alignment to the leg or even in a position of calaneovalgus, whereas in true congenital talipes equinovarus (club foot) the deformity is rigid. All mobile foot postures correct themselves spontaneously, whereas fixed deformities require treatment.
- *Out toeing (external rotatory contracture of the hip).* This condition is rare. Between the ages of 6 and 10 months some infants have a tendency to lie or stand with one foot directed outward from the midline. The condition usually is unilateral and is seen most commonly in the left leg. Closer inspection reveals that not only is the foot turned out but also the knee on that side lies in an externally rotated position. When the child is examined lying, one finds that the hip on the affected side has an excessive range of external rotation and a limited range of internal rotation. This was the posture assumed by this leg while the child was in utero.

Children who have this condition will tend to walk with an out toe gait at first. The condition invariably corrects itself by the age of 2 years. Some parents are keen to treat the problem and they can be taught to stretch the legs inwards at each nappy change.

Developmental variants

Many developmental variants are seen in early and later childhood and often cause concern for parents.

Bow legs

Bow legs (Fig. 25.1) are common up to 2 years of age: the parents will often be concerned that the legs are bowed and the feet turn in. The condition is not caused by bulky nappies, because the bowing is in the tibiae. It is a normal developmental process and seldom requires treatment

Knock knees

A high proportion of the population between the ages of 2 and 7 years have knock knees (Fig. 25.2). This condition has a very strong tendency to correct itself by the age of 7 years and as a rule the only management necessary is parental reassurance that improvement will occur.

There is a rare form of knock knees which presents in obese children over the age of 12 years and which does require treatment.

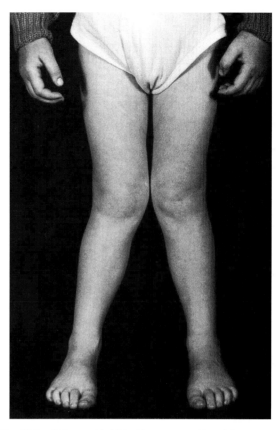

Fig. 25.2 A 5 year old child with pronounced knock knees.

Rolling in of ankles

Parents will frequently mention this, especially after it has been noticed by a concerned grandparent or shoefitter. The rolling of the hindfoot into valgus is due to physiological joint laxity and requires no treatment. The clinician can show the parents how the hindfoot straightens when the child stands up on high tiptoes. This is the **tiptoe test**, which also demonstrates development of the medial longitudinal arch (Fig. 25.3).

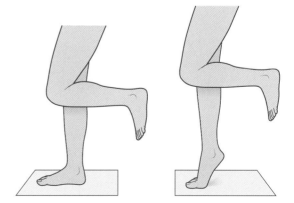

Fig. 25.3 If the arch appears when standing on tiptoe then the feet are flexible. The flat arch is of no significance and requires no treatment apart from explanation.

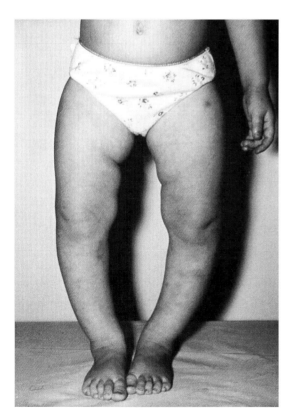

Fig. 25.1 Bow legs in a toddler: a normal phenomenon.

Flat feet

Flat feet in children are a frequent cause for parental concern. Usually this concern is unwarranted and the child's foot is normal for age (Fig. 25.4). Often parents notice that their child's foot appears flat. Sometimes the attendant fitter at the shoe shop may comment on the shape of the child's foot. Children usually have low arches because they are loose jointed and flexible. The arch flattens when they are standing. However, the arch can be better seen when the feet are hanging free or the child stands on tiptoes.

When a child first learns to walk, the stance is usually wide to assist balance, and the feet roll. As the child grows and ankle muscles strengthen, the foot gradually develops its mature shape with some medial arch. Flat feet are common in preschoolers and are present in less than 10% of teenagers. The final shape of the foot may also be influenced genetically, in that one or both parents may have low arches.

When children start walking they do so on feet that appear flat, partly because there is true flatness of the medial longitudinal arch and partly because the arch is filled in by a fat pad. Between the ages of 2 and 8 years, mothers are often concerned because a 'second ankle bone' appears on the medial aspect of the foot. They are referring to prominence of the navicular bone, which is present in most children who have flat feet. Unless the prominence of this bone is causing symptoms, it can be ignored. Children with flat feet generally have some valgus deformity of the heel: when viewed from behind the heels do not point straight up and down, but tend to slope outwards and downwards. This seldom persists into adult life.

During the first 7 or 8 years of life the majority of children develop a medial longitudinal arch but approximately 15% do not. Clearly the results of any form of treatment for flat feet are going to be excellent, as some 85% will get better whether or not they are treated. Sometimes treatment with shoe inserts (orthotics) or other forms of arch supports/shoe modifications are recommended by therapists. These may satisfy concerned parents but do little, if anything, to correct the 'flat foot' and certainly do not make an arch where one is not present. Most of the time orthotics such as these are not necessary for children.

Other treatments, such as splints, massage or special shoes, may be offered but there is little evidence that these interventions alter the foot for the better.

Shoes. The only essential is that children's shoes should be roomy enough. Shoes themselves are not necessary to promote normal foot growth and development; they are only worn for protection and need not be worn until activities demand this protection. Boots are no better than shoes, although in toddlers boots may be more satisfactory in that they are less likely to fall off or be taken off.

It is not harmful to use 'hand down' shoes from older children in the family provided they are roomy enough. There is no evidence that sandals, thongs or sneakers have any harmful influence on the feet. While wedging of the soles and heels has long been employed for in toeing and out toeing, such footwear modifications have no influence either on the gait itself or on the natural history. Thomas heels are of little or no value in the management of flat feet. If the child has excessive wear on the inner side of the sole of the shoes, advise parents to look for shoes which have a stiffer heel area. Some children with flexible flat feet are rather hard on their shoes and this can be dealt with by selecting shoes of stronger construction. This is usually much less expensive than elaborate and unnecessary orthotics.

Accessory navicular bone

The child with a prominent accessory navicular may have some temporary discomfort which may be relieved by wearing arch supports for a period of a year or two. Frequently the ossicle either unites with the main navicular bone or just becomes asymptomatic. Excision of the accessory navicular bone is required only rarely.

Curly middle toe

Sometimes the third toe curls inwards under the second toe so that the second toe tends to lie above the level of the first and third toes. Parents generally notice the abnormal posture of the second toe, but it is the third toe which is the cause of the problem. This can be safely ignored until the child is at least 2 years old. Occasionally a flexor tenotomy is required and provides excellent correction.

In toe gait (pigeon toeing)

In toeing in childhood is common. It may appear worse when the child is running or tired. It does not cause

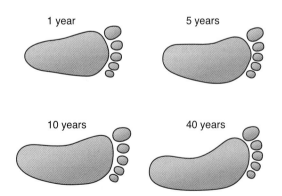

Fig. 25.4 Flexible flat feet are normal in infants and children. The arch develops whether the child wears shoes or goes barefoot.

arthritis or back problems later in life. It can be due to one or more of the following:

- inset hips
- internal torsion of the tibia
- metatarsus adductus.

Inset hips (persistent femoral neck anteversion) have internal rotation in excess of the range of external rotation. It is more common in girls and the feet seem to fly out sideways when running. The pathology lies in the top of the femur where there is a normal twist of 30° at birth, which unwinds gradually by the age of 7 years. In severe cases, when there is a major cosmetic problem unresolved by about 10 years, derotation femoral osteotomy can be performed but this is rarely required.

Children with inset hips commonly sit between their feet with their hips in full internal rotation, the knees flexed and the legs splayed outwards (the 'W' position) (Fig 25.5). This is the only way they can sit comfortably as they cannot externally rotate their hips sufficiently to sit in a crosslegged fashion. There is no evidence that this sitting posture should be discouraged in children and it is worthwhile remembering that it is almost unknown for an adult to present with a complaint of in toeing.

Internal tibial torsion (a twist in of the shin bone) is usually due to intrauterine pressure and can persist up to the age of 3 years and then spontaneously corrects.

Metatarsus adductus (Fig. 25.6) is a condition in which the feet are banana shaped, with the convexity of the banana outwards and the toes directed towards each other. This may be due to intrauterine pressure; however, if it persists it is called metatarsus adductus. It is passively correctable and slowly rights itself, especially after walking commences. Very rarely manipulation and plaster immobilisation is necessary.

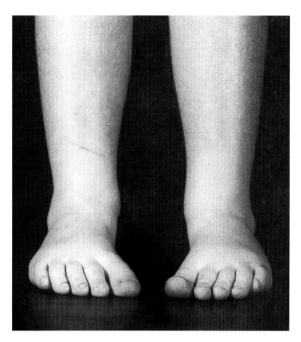

Fig. 25.6 A 3 year old child with metatarsus adductus.

Congenital abnormalities

Developmental dysplasia of the hip

This condition was previously called congenital dislocation of the hip (CDH); however, developmental dysplasia of the hip (DDH) is now the preferred term as it implies that some of these hip problems develop after birth. DDH is the most common musculoskeletal abnormality in neonates. The incidence of this condition in Australia and North America is 7 per 1000 live births. In some regions of Europe it is more common. These figures would be much increased if every child who had a 'clicky' hip at birth were diagnosed as having a congenitally dislocated hip. Many of these hips click for a few days only and they are almost always normal.

Clinical classification

DDH can be classified clinically as follows:

- stable
- subluxatable
- dislocatable
- dislocated, reducible
- dislocated, irreducible
- teratologic.

Main risk factors

Some of the important risk factors for DDH (with the degree of increased risk) are:

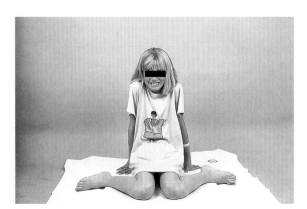

Fig. 25.5 'W' sitting is easy for the child with inset hips.

- breech presentation (10 times)
- female baby (4 times)
- oligohydramnios (4 times)
- big baby > 4 kg (2 times)
- firstborn baby (2 times)
- family history.

When diagnosed and treated from birth, it is possible to produce a normal hip joint after a few months treatment in an abduction splint. However, if the diagnosis is not made until after the child begins to walk, the treatment is long and tedious and often ends with an imperfect joint.

Diagnosis in the newborn

The Barlow and Ortolani tests are used for diagnosis (Fig. 25.7). Every baby should be examined for hip dislocation during the first day of life and again at discharge from the maternity ward, and at ages 6 weeks, 3 months, 6 months and 1 year. The baby is stripped and examined on a large firm bench. If the baby is crying, a bottle or pacifier is offered, as the baby must be relaxed or the examination will not be useful. With the legs extended, any asymmetry of the legs or adductor creases is noted. The examiner then holds the leg to be examined (using the opposite hand to the side of the hip to be examined). With the knee flexed, the thumb is placed over the lesser trochanter and the middle finger over the greater trochanter. The pelvis is steadied by the other hand and the flexed thigh is abducted and adducted and any clunk or jerk is noted.

It is very important to note that frequently a fine click can be felt in the hip joint without any laxity or abnormal movement. Sometimes the click comes from the knee joint. This is very common and is of no significance. Also, it is common in the first 2 or 3 days of life for the hip to be felt to subluxate smoothly without any clunk. This is especially felt in premature and shocked babies and requires repeated examination; frequently the hip becomes normal without treatment.

Radiography has no place in the diagnosis of developmental dysplasia of the hip in the neonatal period (Ch. 24). Ultrasound examination of the hips gives the clinician useful information as to the relationship of the femoral head to the acetabulum and the existence of any acetabular dysplasia during the first 6 months of life. Ultrasound has a **high false positive rate** in babies under 6 weeks of age and scans should only be performed under 6 weeks to either check whether a hip is 'in joint' or not. Over the age of 4 months the degree of ossification of the upper femur and acetabulum enables X rays to be of value.

If the dislocatable or dislocated hip is held in a flexed and abducted position for 8 to 12 weeks, it will usually develop normally. The Pavlik harness or Denis Browne splint is used to maintain this position. Subluxatable hips can be observed with a later ultrasound after 6 weeks or radiograph at 4 months. The use of double nappies is not recommended.

All abnormal or treated hips require follow up until normal hip morphology is ascertained.

Teratologic hip. If there is considerable restriction of abduction in flexion and the 'clunk' sign cannot be elicited, it usually means that the hips are dislocated and irreducible, a condition referred to as teratological dislocation because the hip has been manufactured in the dislocated position. These hips require operative reduction at a later date.

Diagnosis in the older infant

Palpable dislocation and reduction becomes more difficult to elicit after 6 weeks of age. As this physical sign disappears, new signs appear because the head of the femur is never in the acetabulum; there is now limited abduction of the flexed hip. This sign is not diagnostic, but an X ray is indicated when there is asymmetry in the range of the abduction of the hips, or when the range of abduction of both hips is inappropriate for the age of the child. In the first year of life the range of abduction in flexion is usually 60–90°; this arc normally lessens with age.

The physical signs of late presenting dislocation include:
- higher greater trochanter
- wide perineum
- asymmetric gluteal buttock crease
- short leg
- abnormal gait.

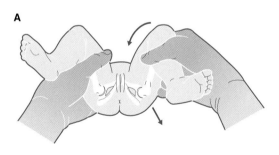

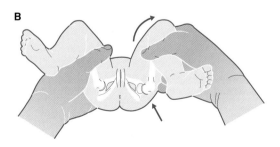

Fig. 25.7 **A** The Barlow test is positive if the hip can be manually dislocated. **B** The Ortolani test is positive if the hip is lying in a dislocated position and is manually reducible.

If dislocation is not diagnosed or presents after walking age, usually an open reduction operation is required.

Congenital talipes equinovarus (congenital club foot)

Congenital talipes equinovarus is the commonest congenital abnormality of the foot, occurring in about 1 per 1000 live births. The male:female ratio 2:1. The condition is bilateral in 40% of cases, and there is a 2% chance of a subsequent child being affected if there is a positive family history.

The deformity is a combination of:
- equinus of the hindfoot
- varus of the hindfoot
- adductus of the midfoot
- cavus of the medial arch.

The degree of each deformity is variable, but all are rigid and are incapable of being corrected manually. This is distinct from the 'postural clubfoot', which is due to intrauterine pressure and is fully passively correctable and resolves without treatment, as described above.

Club feet should be treated from the first day of life. Treatment involves serial plaster casting for 6–12 weeks and usually surgical intervention is required at 3–6 months of age, with a posterior or posteromedial release.

Scoliosis

Scoliosis (lateral curvature of the spine) is most commonly seen in its adolescent idiopathic form (Fig. 25.8). However, there are other forms of scoliosis. The common ones are:
- *Congenital*: vertebral anomalies are responsible for the curvature. Usually the deformity is minor and may be present at birth or develop during growth. In only 5% is the deformity progressive.

- *Neuromuscular*: such as Duchenne muscular dystrophy, cerebral palsy or spina bifida.
- *Idiopathic*: this is usually seen as adolescent idiopathic scoliosis.

Idiopathic scoliosis can be seen in younger children as either:
- *Infantile idiopathic scoliosis*: most commonly seen in males and may be seen in association with congenital dislocation of the hip and other congenital anomalies. The natural history is for the curve to resolve in a high proportion of cases
- *Juvenile idiopathic scoliosis*: a curve in children between the age of 3 years and the onset of puberty; it is uncommon.

Adolescent idiopathic scoliosis

Ninety per cent of cases occur in girls and the scoliosis progresses during the rapid growth spurt years.

For diagnosis, the child must remove all clothing above the waist and stand with the back facing the examiner (Fig. 25.9). In all but very minor curves the deformity will be readily apparent. Signs to look for are:
- uneven shoulders
- waist (flank) line asymmetry
- a unilateral rib prominence when the child bends forward (Fig. 25.10).

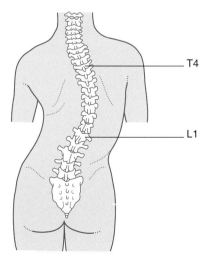

Fig. 25.8 Adolescent idiopathic scoliosis; the curve is usually convex to the right side.

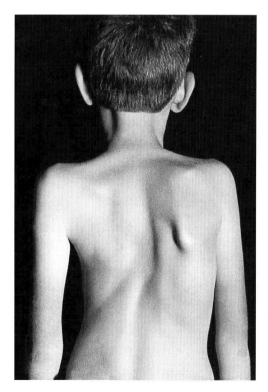

Fig. 25.9 Adolescent scoliosis in a male; 90% occur in females.

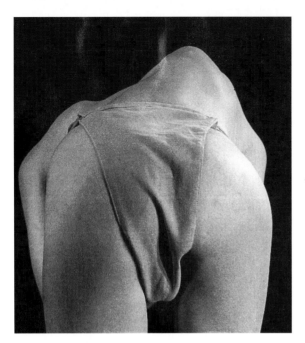

Fig. 25.10 On flexion, a rib hump becomes readily visible.

When the child is bent forwards the curve may disappear completely, in which case it can be labelled 'postural' and treatment is not required. Should a rib hump become visible (due to rotation of the vertebrae and consequent rib deformity) (Fig. 25.10) the curve is labelled 'structural'.

There are three main treatment options:
- observation for curves less than 20°
- bracing for curves 20–40°
- surgery for curves greater than 40°.

These are broad guidelines only. Larger curves may not be treated if proven to be non progressive in a skeletally mature patient. Several studies have investigated the role of exercises in improving the curve or preventing progression, but there is no evidence that exercises alone are able to achieve this.

Congenital muscular torticollis

Torticollis usually presents in the first few months of life when the tilt of the head and limited lateral flexion is noted. Sometimes it can remain undetected for 1–2 years. The head is held with a lateral flexion toward the shoulder and with rotation of the face towards the opposite side. The face on that side is smaller and the eye is lower on the side of the tight sternomastoid. Most patients will have presented in the first few months of life with a sternomastoid tumour; that is, a palpable lump in the middle of the sternomastoid muscle.

The cause of this condition is unknown. Treatment in the first 6 months of life with a stretching programme supervised by a physiotherapist is usually effective,

with full resolution. If the condition does not resolve then surgical correction at 2–4 years of age is required. At operation, the muscle is divided transversely and the corrected position maintained by the use of a collar.

Alexander the Great (354 BC) is reported to have had this condition, with statues showing a persistent head tilt!

Osteochondroses (osteochondritis)

These conditions involve the epiphysis. The pathology consists of localised areas of ischaemic bone necrosis and sometimes oedema of adjacent soft tissues. The tendency is for healing to occur, but this is dependent on a number of factors, which include age, the site of the lesion, its blood supply and perhaps the method of treatment. Any bone having a cartilaginous area at the site of either the primary or secondary centre of ossification may be affected. The aetiology is uncertain.

Scheuermann's condition

The epiphyseal plates of the vertebral bodies are involved. Usually it is seen in the thoracic vertebrae, but occasionally in the lumbar spine. Occurrences are almost always in the adolescent. Usually children present in early adolescence because of an increase in the normal thoracic kyphosis, so that the child appears round shouldered. Many do not progress much and merely require observation, whereas others progress rapidly and require management in a brace.

The condition it is frequently 'overdiagnosed' in radiology reports and causes anxiety in families, especially when the radiological changes are described as Scheuermann's '*disease*'. The term '*condition*' is preferred.

Slipped capital femoral epiphysis

This is primarily a disorder of the adolescent between the ages of 10 and 15 years. Approximately 40% of cases are bilateral. Its aetiology is unknown but recent reports suggests that hormonal factors may be of importance. Most cases present with pain and limp; pain is often referred to the knee and it is important to consider a hip radiograph when children present with distal thigh pain.

Types of slip

- Acute: the child feels the hip 'collapse' and is unable to walk. This is uncommon and needs urgent treatment.
- Acute on chronic: the child has months of discomfort and then a worsening over a few weeks with a pronounced limp.
- Chronic: many months of thigh ache and a mild limp.

Examination reveals limited internal rotation of the hip compared with the other side and some joint irritability. The diagnosis is confirmed radiologically, especially with a frog lateral view.

All cases of slipped capital femoral epiphysis require surgery with screw fixation across the physis to prevent further slip.

Chondromalacia patellae

This condition has a number of other names, including:
- anterior knee pain
- lateral pressure syndrome
- maltracking of the patella.

It is particularly common over the age of 10 years. It is characterised by pain in the knee after activities which involve flexing the knee and quadriceps contraction. The child complains of aching around the patella during or especially after exercise. Stairs precipitate discomfort, particularly walking down stairs. It is more common in adolescent females, in both those who enjoy sport and those who wish to avoid physical education lessons at school.

Clinically there is little to find, although occasionally there is some patellofemoral crepitus and rarely an effusion in the knee. Ensure that the hips are normal and that the symptoms do not relate to a slipped hip. The diagnosis is based upon obtaining the relevant history.

Treatment involves education of the child and concerned parents (explain that the 'back of the knee cap is soft' and will toughen up with time), some limitation of flexed knee/jumping activities, quadriceps stretches, elastic knee support and tincture of time. Frequently children tolerate their symptoms and continue with their sport. The natural history suggests spontaneous resolution of symptoms over 1–2 years.

Osgood–Schlatter's condition

This is an apophysitis of the tibial tubercle and presents with pain and swelling. Children notice the pain and then an adult sees the swelling and can be concerned about a sinister cause such as malignancy. The common age of presentation is 10–14 years and the natural history is resolution over a 12–18 month period. Warn the parents that a lump will remain permanently but it will be smaller than when first seen. Normal activities within the limits of the child's comfort are allowed. The tibial tubercle does not detach or pull off. Radiographs are not necessary for diagnosis. Simple measures such as quadriceps stretches and massage with a linament can provide some symptomatic relief. Rarely a small loose ossicle remains and can be excised after the child reaches 15 years.

Sever condition

This is an apophysitis of the os calcis (heel) bone where the tendo achilles attaches. It is seen in children aged between 10 and 12 years. It resolves over 12 months and is best treated by reassurance, calf stretches and sometimes a simple rubber heel raise. Sport is allowed within the child's level of comfort.

Injuries in infancy and childhood

Children are susceptible to injury because of their carefree play habits, and skeletal injuries are common. For practical purposes sprains do not occur in children: **'children break bones and adults tear ligaments'**. Post-traumatic pain, swelling and loss of function are nearly always the result of a fracture or growth plate separation; therefore X rays are obligatory. Dislocations are rare in childhood. The type of injury which may produce dislocation of an adult joint usually gives rise to a fracture or growth plate separation in a child.

Fractures are the commonest type of skeletal injury in childhood; these generally unite in less than half the time the equivalent injury would take to heal in an adult, and non union is almost unknown. Childhood fractures may unite in a position of deformity, with the deformity correcting itself spontaneously over the ensuing 6–12 months, especially if the fracture is near the ends of the bone where there is most growth. Some shortening of bones also can be expected to correct spontaneously following childhood fractures.

Child abuse is an important cause of childhood injury; it is important because, if unrecognised, further abuse is likely to occur and might even be fatal. The subject of child abuse is discussed in Chapter 12. When assessing a child after trauma, ensure that you check the whole child, using the principles of EMST (emergency management of severe trauma), and look for hidden injuries (Ch. 19).

Clavicle fractures

These are the most common fractures seen in children. The fracture is usually midshaft and is of greenstick type. Complete fractures with overlap of the ends are seen in older children and unite well. It is important to warn the parents at the beginning that they must expect to see a large lump develop: this is healing callus, which will remodel over 6–12 months without any cosmetic or functional deficit.

Treatment is with a triangular sling inside the clothes to suport the elbow, regular analgesia and rest. The clavicle will start to join within a week and the sling can usually be discarded by 3 weeks.

Forearm fractures

Children's bones can break in several ways, namely:
- *bend*
- *buckle*
- *greenstick*
- *complete with/without displacement and overlap.*

Most forearm fractures are of the buckle or greenstick variety and if there is minimal tilt or deformity they can be treated in an above elbow cast for 5 weeks. It is important to do a check radiograph after 7–10 days to ensure that the fracture has not tilted more. If it has tilted to an unacceptable position, the fracture can still undergo a closed reduction before firm union occurs.

Fractures with visible deformity or significant tilt/displacement require closed reduction and a similar time of cast immobilisation.

Ensure that you complete and document a neurovascular examination of the limb initially. Provide the parents with written instructions for neurovasular observations at home and provide them with emergency contact details if excessive swelling or symptoms develop. Look for the five *P*s:
- excessive *Pain*
- *Paraesthesia* (compresssion of the sensory nerves)
- *Paleness* of the fingers
- *Plum* coloured (venous congestion)
- *Pulseless.*

Approximately 30% of children's fractures involve the growth plate (physis). If the physis suffers permanent damage, the bone can end up:
- short (all physeal growth stops), or
- angulated (one side of the physis stops growing).

The Salter–Harris classification is used for growth plate fractures (Fig. 25.11). Type I is often seen in the distal fibula as the childhood equivalent of the adult ankle sprain. Type II is the commonest variety and frequent in the distal radius. Types III and IV have a much higher risk of growth disturbance and usually require accurate reduction and fixation to minimise the risk to growth arrest.

Supracondylar fracture of the humerus

This fracture is often seen in children of 4–10 years after a fall from a height, such as from monkey bars, or when running. The mechanism is usually hyperextension of the elbow joint with the olecranon acting as a fulcrum lever to cause the fracture.

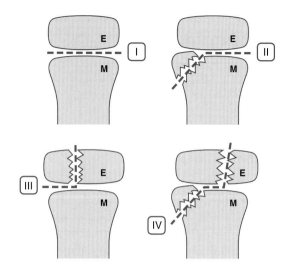

Fig. 25.11 Salter–Harris fracture: type I, the fracture passes directly through the physis; type II, a corner of the metaphysis (M) is broken off; type III, the fracture passes through the physis and the epiphysis (E); type IV, the fracture passes through the epiphysis and the metaphysis, causing a high risk of growth arrest.

Neuropraxia of the radial, median, ulna nerve is common. Occasionally displaced fractures cause damage to the brachial artery. Again, neurovascular assessment is mandatory. Minimally tilted fractures can be treated in a collar and cuff under the clothes for the first 2 weeks, then outside the clothes for a further 2 weeks. Warn the parents to expect elbow stiffness, especially loss of elbow extension for several months.

Displaced fractures require accurate reduction to avoid later deformity. Often the fracture will be held with K wires, which are removed at 4 weeks.

Toddler fracture of the tibia

This distal shaft fracture may not be visible on initial radiographs and often perplexes clinicians faced with a toddler who refuses to walk for days after a seemingly minor trauma. The fracture can be diagnosed clinically by twisting the good leg first and then noting the cry or facial expression when twisting the affected side. Warn the parents what you are going to do first!

Treat the fracture in an above knee cast and allow weight bearing as the child dictates. Most will walk after 1 week in the cast and the cast can be removed at 3 weeks. Warn the parents to expect a limp for 1–2 months: the limp will resolve spontaneously.

PART 8   SELF-ASSESSMENT

Questions

1. **List the three common causes of in toe gait in children.**

2. **Write brief notes on flat feet in children, with an emphasis on your explanation to the parents.**

3. **Successful treatment of fractures in childhood depends upon many factors: list as many as you can.**

4. **Name two tests for developmental dysplasia of the hip in newborns and briefly describe them.**

5. **When would you do an ultrasound for hip dysplasia and when would you ask for a radiograph?**

Answers and explanations

1. Inset hips (persistent femoral neck anteversion); tibia in torsion (twist in of shin bones); metatarsus adductus (hook or banana foot).

2. You should include mention of flexibility of children; normal to have flat feet in children; arch develops with age; 10% of teenagers have flat feet; flexible flat feet do not cause long term disability; orthotics are not necessary and do not alter the natural history.

3. Check for other injuries; neurovascular examination of the limb; adequate analgesia; appropriate radiographs; plaster cast and instructions; check X rays at 7–10 days.

4. Barlow test: tests to see if the hip can be manually dislocated by pushing posteriorly with the hip flexed 90° and slightly adducted. It is essential that the child is relaxed and not crying or upset. Ortolani test: a 'jerk of re-entry' when the dislocated hip is manually reduced by upward pressure and abduction of the hip. Sometimes a clunk can be palpated. Again the child must be relaxed. The answer could also mention signs of uneven buttock creases, short leg, or higher greater trochanter for the older child.

5. Ultrasound has a high false positive rate in children less than 6 weeks of age and can lead to unnecessary treatment. An ultrasound can be performed before 6 weeks of age to check that a hip joint is enlocated (i.e. 'in joint'). Ultrasound has its main role in children aged 6 weeks to 6 months, as it demonstrates both the bony outline and the cartilaginous components of the hip joint. Over 4 months of age a radiograph can be of value and plain films remain the gold standard of hip investigation. At 4 months there is usually sufficient ossification of the femoral head and acetabulum to enable adequate interpretation.

PART 8   FURTHER READING

Chan A 1997 Perinatal risk factors for developmental dysplasia of the hip. Archives of Disease in Childhood 76: 94–100

Editorial 1990 Flat feet in children. BMJ 301: 942–943

Morrissey R T, Weinstein S L 2001 Lovell and Winter's Pediatric orthopaedics, 5th edn. Lippincott, Williams and Wilkins, Philadelphia

Price CT 1985 Lower extremity rotational problems in children. Normal values to guide management. Journal of Bone and Joint Surgery 67A: 823–824

Staheli L T et al 1987 The longitudinal arch. Journal of Bone and Joint Surgery, 69A: 426–428

Wenger D et al 1989 Corrective shoes and inserts as treatment for flexible flat foot in infants and children. Journal of Bone and Joint Surgery 71A: 800–810

Useful links

http://www.aaos.org (Website of the American Academy of Orthopaedic Surgeons with adult and paediatric information and links)

http://www.posna.org (Website of the Pediatric Orthopaedic Society of North America. Contains useful links and parent information)

PART 9

COMMON PAEDIATRIC SURGICAL PROBLEMS

26 Common surgical conditions in children

S. W. Beasley

The penis and foreskin

The glans of the uncircumcised penis is protected by a layer of loose skin called the foreskin or prepuce. The amount of foreskin present varies between boys. At birth, and for many years afterwards, it is normal for part or all of the undersurface of the foreskin to be adherent to the glans penis. This adherence slowly separates during childhood. Forcible retraction of the foreskin before it is ready can damage the glans and may cause secondary phimosis. Therefore, the foreskin should not be retracted forcibly unless a circumcision is being performed. Spontaneous separation of these adhesions is normally complete by puberty.

Smegma

Smegma accumulates beneath the adherent foreskin. It appears as asymmetrical accumulations of yellow tinged material in the coronal groove beneath the foreskin (Fig. 26.1). There may be sufficient smegma to produce a noticeable swelling that may be misdiagnosed as a dermoid cyst or tumour. It is often misinterpreted as being mid shaft because a small child's coronal groove may be a long way from the tip of the foreskin. Smegma is normal, and is released spontaneously as the foreskin separates from the glans penis. When it is released, it may be associated with some redness and irritation of the foreskin for a day or so: this, too, is a normal process.

Balanitis

Infection can develop beneath the foreskin, and, if severe, pus may appear from the end of the foreskin. Balanitis is often associated with phimosis. Infection may cause considerable redness and swelling of the penile shaft, necessitating treatment with either topical or oral antibiotics.

Phimosis

In phimosis the opening at the tip of the foreskin has narrowed down to such a degree that the foreskin cannot be retracted (Fig. 26.2). The external urethral meatus is not visible. Phimosis must be distinguished from the normal adherence of the foreskin to the glans. In most boys, phimosis can be treated by application of steroid ointment

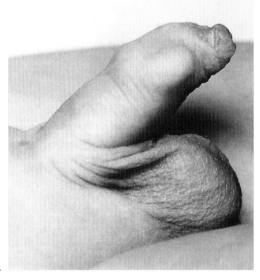
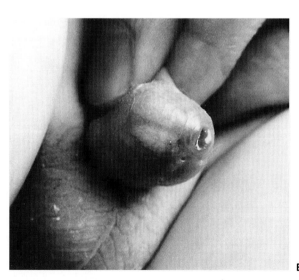

Fig. 26.1 **A** The normal foreskin with accumulation of smegma beneath it. The swellings caused by the smegma are in the region of the coronal groove. **B** On retraction, smegma appears as accumulations of material beneath a foreskin that has not yet separated from the glans.

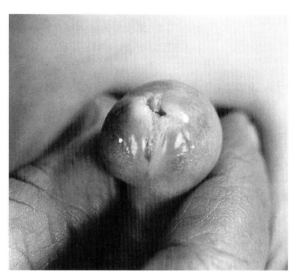

Fig. 26.2 In phimosis, the foreskin is narrowed and cannot be retracted.

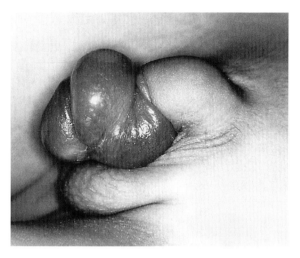

Fig. 26.3 Paraphimosis: the foreskin has become stuck behind the coronal groove.

(for example, half strength betamethasone valerate oint-ment) to the tight shiny part of the foreskin. This usually obviates the need for circumcision. However, marked previous inflammation, infection, skin splitting and bal-anitis xerotica obliterans can lead to marked scarring of the foreskin and phimosis, and in many of these children the only reasonable treatment is circumcision. Sometimes the severity of phimosis is such that there is ballooning of the foreskin on micturition, and on rare occasions it may even cause urinary retention with a dis-tended bladder.

> ### Clinical example
>
> James was a 7 year old boy who presented following two episodes of balanitis. He also complained of discomfort on micturition. Examination revealed a tight foreskin that could not be retracted; the urethral meatus could not be seen. After 1 month of topical application of betamethasone ointment to the tight part of the foreskin he was able to fully retract it. Circumcision was not necessary.

Paraphimosis

Paraphimosis occurs when a mildly phimotic foreskin has been retracted over the glans and has become stuck behind the coronal groove, causing oedema of itself and the glans penis (Fig. 26.3). It is a painful and progressive process. Treatment involves gentle manipulation of the foreskin forwards, which may require a general anaesthetic. Circumcision is not performed at this time, but a few chil-dren may need it subsequently if the phimosis does not respond to topical application of steroid ointment.

Hypospadias

It is important to recognise hypospadias when it is present. The foreskin looks square and hangs off the penis, and the shaft is bent ventrally. The two main problems in hypospadias are:

- the location of the urethra (which can be found on the ventral side of the shaft of the penis, proximal to its correct position)
- chordee (ventral angulation of the shaft and glans) (Fig. 26.4).

Correction of chordee is required to allow later success-ful sexual function. Surgery is usually performed as a single stage procedure at 9–12 months of age, often as day surgery.

Circumcision is absolutely contraindicated in hypo-spadias because the skin of the prepuce is used during repair of the hypospadias. Severe hypospadias may be indicative of an intersex abnormality. For example, when there is penoscrotal hypospadias and a bifid scrotum, the scrotum should be examined carefully for testes, because some of these children may be females with congenital adrenal hyperplasia; the labioscrotal folds are labia rather than scrota, and the presumed urethral opening may in fact be the entrance to the vagina (Ch. 65).

Circumcision

The indications for circumcision remain controversial. In many countries, circumcision has been abandoned in the neonatal period because of its relatively high complica-tion rate. Apart from the risk of septicaemia and menin-gitis when performed in the immunologically immature neonate, there are a number of problems that may occur during circumcision at any age. These include removal of too much or too little foreskin, postoperative bleeding

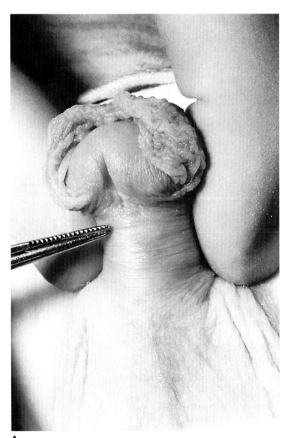

A

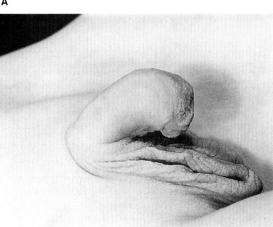

B

Fig. 26.4 In hypospadias the ventral shaft of the penis is angulated and shortened (chordee), the urethral meatus is ventrally placed and the foreskin is deficient on the underside. **A** Ventral aspect; **B** appearance from above.

and infection. Haemorrhage postoperatively occasionally requires surgical reintervention. The most troublesome and common complication of circumcision is abrasion and ulceration of the sensitive glans penis, particularly near the urethral meatus. As the meatal ulceration heals it may produce meatal stenosis and require a meatotomy to re-establish an adequate urinary stream.

Epispadias

In epispadias, the urethra opens on to the dorsal aspect of the base of the penis, and is part of a spectrum of lower abdominal wall defects in which ectopia vesicae (bladder exstrophy) and cloacal exstrophy are the most severe forms. Boys with epispadias are often incontinent of urine because the sphincter of the bladder neck is also deficient.

The inguinoscrotal region

Inguinal hernia

After the testis has descended into the scrotum during the 7th month of pregnancy, the canal down which it migrates, the processus vaginalis, should obliterate. Failure of obliteration of the processus vaginalis may produce an inguinal hernia, hydrocele or an encysted hydrocele of the cord.

A widely patent proximal processus vaginalis allows bowel (and in girls, the ovary as well) to enter the inguinal canal, producing a reducible lump in the groin, called an indirect inguinal hernia (Fig. 26.5). This occurs in about 2% of live male births, but is less frequent in girls. The greatest incidence is in the first year of life.

The usual presentation is that of an intermittent swelling overlying the external inguinal ring, that has been noticed by a parent. At times it may appear to cause discomfort. It is most likely to be present during an episode of crying or straining, and in infants may be seen during nappy changes. Inguinal hernias should be repaired as soon as practicable.

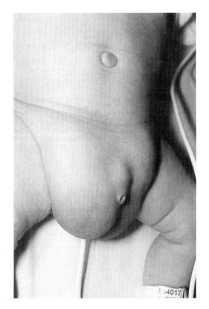

Fig. 26.5 Large bilateral inguinal herniae.

Strangulation of inguinal herniae is common, particularly during the first 6 months of life. Strangulation can be recognised when the groin swelling becomes irreducible. If left untreated a strangulated hernia may damage the incarcerated bowel and, occasionally, by compressing the testicular vessels may lead to testicular atrophy. For this reason, an immediate attempt should be made to reduce the hernia manually. This is done by:

- first disimpacting the hernia at the external inguinal ring, and then
- reducing it along the line of the inguinal canal.

Fortunately, most hernias that become stuck can be reduced manually; the hernia can then be repaired as an elective procedure within a few days.

Hydrocele

A hydrocele presents as a painless cystic swelling around the testis in the scrotum (Fig. 26.6). It contains peritoneal fluid that has tracked down a narrow but patent processus vaginalis. It transilluminates brilliantly. When the hydrocele is lax, the testis can be felt within it. The upper limit of the hydrocele can be demonstrated distal to the external inguinal ring, distinguishing it from an inguinal hernia, where the swelling extends through the external inguinal ring. There is no impulse on crying or straining.

Hydroceles are common in the first few months of life, do not cause symptoms, and usually disappear sponta-neously. Surgery is only indicated if the hydrocele persists beyond 2 years of age.

Undescended testis

Undescended testis (or cryptorchidism) is a term used to describe the testis that does not reside spontaneously in the scrotum. Undescended testes occur in about 2% of boys, being more common in premature infants. Spontaneous descent of the testis is unlikely beyond 3 months post term. Cryptorchidism is important to detect because it will result in reduced fertility if left untreated. It is suspected that the higher temperature to which an undescended testis is subject impairs spermatogenesis.

The diagnosis is made by examining the inguinoscrotal region. Normally the testis should be found within the scrotal sac. In cryptorchidism the scrotum looks empty (Fig. 26.7). The testis is 'milked' down the line of the inguinal canal towards the scrotum and is pulled gently towards the scrotum. If the testis cannot be brought into the scrotum or will not remain there spontaneously it is considered undescended.

Clinically, it may be difficult to distinguish a retractile testis from an undescended testis. In most normal boys the testis resides in the bottom of the scrotum, but the cremasteric reflex, which is prominent during mid childhood, may cause it to move upwards, sometimes completely out of the scrotum. A retractile testis found outside the scrotum initially can be brought down into the

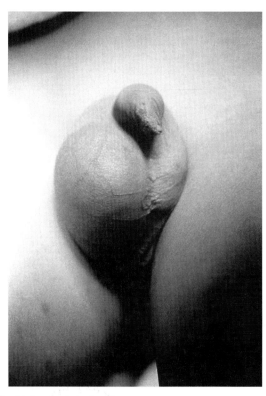

Fig. 26.6   A right hydrocele.

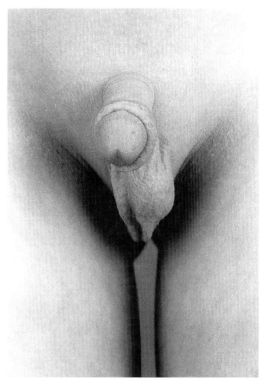

Fig. 26.7   Undescended right testis.

Table 26.1 Comparison of undescended and retractile testes		
Feature	Undescended testis	Retractile testis
Can be brought fully to bottom of scrotum	No	Yes
Remains in scrotum spontaneously for a period before retracting	No	Yes
Resides spontaneously in scrotum at times	No	Yes
Normal size	Normal or small	Normal

Table 26.2 Causes of an acutely painful scrotum		
Condition	Comment	Frequency
Torsion of testicular appendix	Peak age 11 years Unilateral tenderness	>75%
Torsion of testis	Peaks in neonatal and adolescent age groups Surgical emergency	20%
Epididymo-orchitis	Usually in infancy Association with urinary tract abnormalities	Rare
Idiopathic scrotal oedema	Usually in young child Bilateral oedema Testes not tender	Rare

normal position and should stay there spontaneously, at least until a cremasteric reflex is stimulated (Table 26.1). An undescended testis will not stay in the scrotum spontaneously and usually cannot even be coerced beyond the neck of the scrotum. It is often smaller than a normal testis on the other side.

Undescended testes should be brought down into the scrotum surgically between 9 and 12 months of age. Unfortunately, in many boys the diagnosis is not made until the child is older. The later the testis is brought down, the more likely it is that there will be damage to spermatogenesis. Orchidopexy is performed as a day case procedure. In general, the results are excellent when the procedure is performed by a specialist paediatric surgeon.

The acutely painful scrotum

There are a number of conditions that cause an acutely painful or enlarged scrotum (Fig. 26.8), of which torsion of a testicular appendage is the most common, and torsion of the testis itself the most important (Table 26.2). In both conditions the boy complains of severe pain in the scrotum. In the early stages of torsion of a testicular appendage, a blue-black 'pea sized' swelling which is extremely tender to touch may be seen through the skin of the scrotum near the upper pole of the testis. Palpation of the testis itself causes no discomfort. Later, a reactive hydrocele develops, the tenderness becomes more generalised and the clinical features may make it difficult to distinguish from torsion of the testis. Where torsion of the testis has occurred, both the testis and the epididymis are exquisitely tender (unless necrosis has already occurred) and the testis may be lying high within the scrotum. In older boys the pain radiates to the ipsilateral iliac fossa and may be associated with nausea and vomiting.

Treatment

Urgent surgical exploration of the scrotum is required to untwist the testis and epididymis and to suture both testes to prevent subsequent torsion. A completely necrotic testis should be removed. A torted and infarcted testicular appendix should be removed. In this situation the testis should be checked to make sure that it has not twisted, but otherwise it requires no other treatment. Epididymo-orchitis is unusual in children: it is most often seen during the first year of life, where it may signify an underlying structural abnormality of the urinary tract. For this reason, a renal ultrasound and micturating cystourethrogram should be arranged. Examination of the urine may show leucocytes and bacteria. Mumps orchitis is extremely rare prior to puberty. Infiltration of the testis is occasionally seen in leukaemia or with a primary testicular neoplasm.

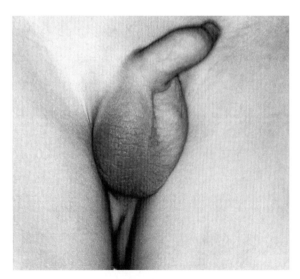

Fig. 26.8 An acutely painful scrotum in a child is most likely to be caused by torsion of an appendix testis or torsion of the testis.

Abnormalities of the umbilicus

(Table 26.3)

The umbilical cord desiccates and separates several days after birth, allowing the umbilical ring to close. Sometimes the stump of the cord may become infected, the umbilical ring may not close, or there may be remnants of the embryonic channels which pass through the umbilicus.

Umbilical hernia

Failure of the umbilical ring to close after birth produces an umbilical hernia (Fig. 26.9). Umbilical hernias are common in neonates, but most close spontaneously in the first year of life. The skin overlying the umbilical hernia never ruptures and strangulation of the contents is virtually unknown. The swelling will become tense when the infant cries or strains. Umbilical hernias are probably symptomless. No treatment is required during the first few years of life. If the hernia is still present after the age of 3 years it can be repaired as a day surgical procedure.

Discharge from the umbilicus

Discharge from the umbilicus may be pus, mucus, urine or faeces. An umbilical granuloma is a common lesion which first becomes evident after separation of the umbilical cord. There is a small accumulation of granu-

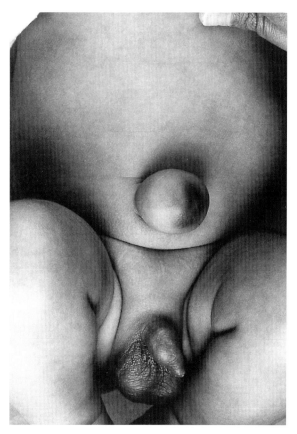

Fig. 26.9 Umbilical hernia.

Table 26.3   Abnormalities of the umbilicus

Abnormality	Comment
1. Exomphalos	See Chapter 36
2. Gastroschisis	See Chapter 36
3. Umbilical hernia	Common, most resolve Asymptomatic Skin covered
4. Umbilical sepsis ('omphalitis')	Neonatal, serious condition
5. Umbilical granuloma	Common, treat with silver nitrate Often pedunculated
6. Ectopic bowel mucosa	Treat with silver nitrate
7. Patent vitellointestinal duct	Sinus opening at umbilicus Communication with ileum Discharges faecal fluid and gas
8. Patent urachus	Communication with bladder Discharges urine

lation tissue in the umbilicus, accompanied by a sero-purulent discharge. If it has a definite stalk it can be ligated without anaesthesia, but most often it is treated by topical application of silver nitrate. Ectopic bowel mucosa has a similar appearance but has a smooth red glistening surface and discharges mucus. It is treated in the same way. Persistence of part or all of the vitello-intestinal (omphalomesenteric) duct produces one of a number of abnormalities which usually present in early infancy, but which may not be evident for some years. Complete patency of the tract allows ileal fluid and air to discharge from the umbilicus. Persistence of one part produces a sinus or cyst, which may become infected to form an abscess and may discharge pus. A vitello-intestinal band attaching the ileum to the deep surface of the umbilicus may cause intestinal obstruction. A Meckel diverticulum represents persistence of the ileal part of the duct. Vitellointestinal duct remnants are excised.

Urinary discharge from the umbilicus suggests a persistent communication with the bladder in the form of a patent urachus. Sometimes it may produce a cystic mass or abscess in the midline just below the umbilicus. Urachal remnants should be excised.

The anus and perineum

A variety of unrelated conditions affect the anus and perineum in children.

Anal fissure

These are usually seen in infants and toddlers when passage of a hard stool splits the anal mucosa, causing sharp pain and a few drops of bright blood. The condition is of little consequence and the fissure usually heals within days. Examination of the anal margin shows a split in the epithelium anteriorly or posteriorly in the midline. An anal fissure may occur in an older child, in which situation it tends to be secondary to constipation. The child gets severe pain on defecation, and becomes reluctant to defecate, further worsening the constipation. Treatment is directed at overcoming the underlying constipation. A stool softener and lubricant, for example, paraffin oil, maybe helpful. A chronic indolent, often non painful, fissure away from the midline may indicate inflammatory bowel disease, such as Crohn's disease.

Perianal abscesses

These are most likely to occur in the first year of life from infection of an anal gland. The abscess points superficially, a centimetre or two from the anal canal. The abscess should be drained and the fistula between the abscess and the anal canal laid open to reduce the likelihood of recurrence.

Rectal prolapse

Rectal prolapse tends to occur in the second and third years of life in otherwise normal children. The rectum prolapses during defecation and returns spontaneously afterwards. In some, manual reduction is required. The prolapsed mucosa may become congested and bleed but causes little discomfort. Clinically, it needs to be distinguished from prolapse of a benign rectal polyp (a benign hamartomatous lesion seen in children) and the apex of an intussusception (the child would have other symptoms of intussusception). The passage of time, and treatment of any underlying constipation, is all that is required in the majority of toddlers. Occasionally, a sclerosant is injected into the submucosal plane of the rectum for persistent cases.

In a few patients there is an underlying organic cause for the rectal prolapse. Usually the reason is obvious, as in paralysis of anal sphincters in spina bifida and sacral agenesis, undernourished hypotonic infants, bladder exstrophy, cloacal exstrophy, following surgery for imperforate anus, or malabsorption.

Labial adhesions

This common condition is often detected on routine examination in infant girls. The epithelium of the labia minora has fused, and sometimes may cause discomfort on micturition. Labial adhesions are not present at birth. Gentle lateral traction on the labia may assist their separation. They have a tendency to recur after separation.

The neck

Lesions of the neck fall into two broad groups: developmental anomalies and acquired lesions. The exact location of the lesion will usually provide a clue as to its nature.

Midline neck swellings (Table 26.4)

The most common midline neck swelling in children is a thyroglossal cyst. Typically, there is a swelling overlying and attached to the hyoid bone which moves on swallowing and tongue protrusion. It may become infected to form an abscess with overlying erythema. The thyroglossal cyst and the entire thyroglossal tract is best excised before it becomes infected. Excision must include the middle third of the hyoid bone (Sistrunk operation); otherwise, recurrence is common. Ectopic thyroid tissue is a less common cause of a midline neck swelling. Clinically, it may be difficult to distinguish from a thyroglossal cyst. If suspected preoperatively, a thyroid isotope scan will clarify the distribution of all functioning thyroid tissue.

Table 26.4	Midline neck swellings
1. Thyroglossal cyst	Most common (80% of midline neck swellings) Moves with tongue protusion and swallowing Attached to hyoid bone
2. Ectopic thyroid	May be only thyroid tissue present Do thyroid isotope scan
3. Submental lymph node/abscess	Check inside mouth for primary infection Other cervical lymph nodes may be enlarged
4. Dermoid cyst	Small, mobile, non tender Yellow tinge through skin In subcutaneous layer
5. Goitre	Lower neck
6. Cystic hygroma	Hamartoma Usually evident from birth May be extensive

Congenital dermoid cysts can occur along any line of fusion, including the neck where they are situated in the midline. A midline cervical dermoid is occasionally mistaken for a thyroglossal cyst. It contains sebaceous material surrounded by squamous epithelium. The most common congenital dermoid cyst is the external angular dermoid which is found at the orbital margin. Dermoid cysts enlarge slowly and it is appropriate for them to be removed.

Cystic hygromas are congenital hamartomas of the lymphatic system. They vary greatly in size and may involve the front of the neck or extend to one or both sides asymmetrically. Some complex cystic hygromas may contain cavernous haemangiomatous elements and may extend upwards into the floor of the mouth, or downwards into the thoracic cavity. They may enlarge rapidly from viral or bacterial infection, or from haemorrhage. Depending on their extent and location, the airway may be compromised, leading to life threatening respiratory obstruction. Surgery involves excision or debulking of the lesion.

Lateral neck swellings

Most lateral neck swellings are acquired, being due to infection of one or more of the cervical lymph nodes. Persistently enlarged cervical lymph nodes are normal in children with frequent upper respiratory infections: they represent a normal response to infection (that is, reactive hyperplasia), and require no treatment. Lymph nodes may enlarge rapidly and become tender during active infection, but usually settle with rest, analgesia and antibiotics as required. In children aged 6 months to 3 years lateral cervical lymphadenitis may progress to abscess formation: the lymph nodes enlarge over 4 or 5 days and become fluctuant, although deeper nodes may not exhibit fluctuation. The overlying skin becomes red. Treatment involves incision and drainage of the abscess under general anaesthesia.

MAIS lymphadenitis

Cervical lymphadenitis due to atypical mycobacterial infection is common in preschool children. The MAIS (*Mycobacterium avium, intracellulare, scrofulaceum*) infection produces chronic cervical lymphadenitis and collar stud abscesses (so called MAC or *Mycobacterium avium* complex), and usually affects the jugulodigastric, submandibular or preauricular lymph nodes. The involved lymph node increases in size over several weeks before erupting into the subcutaneous tissue as a collar stud 'cold' abscess. Eventually, if untreated, it may cause purple discoloration of the overlying skin and will ulcerate through the skin to produce a chronic discharging sinus. MAIS mycobacterial infections respond poorly to antibiotics. Treatment involves surgical removal of the collar stud abscess and excision of the underlying infected lymph nodes.

Lymph node tumours

Primary tumours involving the lymph nodes occur in older children. Both Hodgkin and non Hodgkin lymphomas may involve cervical lymph nodes. Rarely, other tumours may metastasise to the cervical lymph nodes, for example, neuroblastomas and nasopharyngeal tumours.

Branchial remnants

Branchial remnants arise from the branchial arch system. A variety of abnormalities occur, including branchial cysts, branchial sinuses, branchial fistulae and persistent cartilaginous remnants. Branchial fistulae are present from birth but because the opening is so tiny, they may not be noticed for some years. A drop of mucus or saliva may be observed leaking from the external orifice near the anterior border of the sternomastoid muscle in the lower neck. Branchial cysts present later in childhood with a mass beneath the anterior border of the sternomastoid near its upper third. They may become infected and should be removed. Sinuses or fistulae usually arise from the second branchial cleft, although sometimes the first and third clefts are responsible.

Torticollis

Torticollis, or wry neck, has many causes in childhood (Table 26.5). A sternomastoid tumour presents in the third week of life when the parents notice a hard lump in the neck or that the head cannot be turned to one side. The head is flexed slightly to the side of the shortened sternomastoid muscle, and is turned to the contralateral side. There may be a history of breech delivery or forceps delivery. There is a hard painless swelling, usually 2–3 cm long, in the shortened sternomastoid

Table 26.5	Causes of torticollis	
1. Sternomastoid tumour		Not present at birth Present at 3 weeks of age Tight shortened sternomastoid muscle Most resolve without treatment
2. Postural torticollis		Present at birth Disappears in months From intrauterine position
3. Cervical hemivertebrae		
4. Imbalance of ocular muscles (strabismus)		
5. Lateral cervical lymphadenitis		
6. Tumours		
7. Atlanto-occipital subluxation		

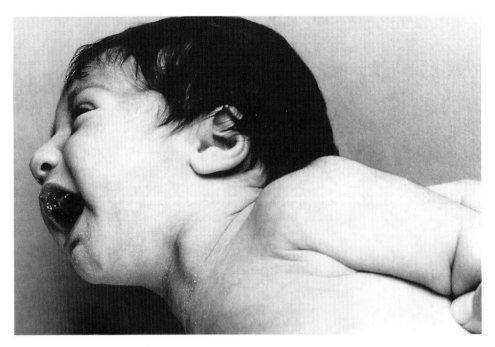

Fig. 26.10   Sternomastoid tumour in torticollis.

muscle (Fig. 26.10). Sometimes the whole muscle may be involved. Rotation of the head to the side of the tumour is limited. Hemihypoplasia of the face may develop in subsequent months. The 'tumour' disappears within 9–12 months in the vast majority of affected infants. Where fibrosis persists and causes permanent shortening of the muscle with persistent torticollis, the sternomastoid muscle should be divided. Occasionally, older children present with torticollis due to a short, tight and fibrous sternomastoid muscle; the ipsilateral shoulder is elevated, there may be compensatory scoliosis, and the child has difficulty rotating the head towards the affected side. These children require surgical division of the muscle.

PART 6   SELF-ASSESSMENT

Questions

1. **Which of the following are true in relation to the penis and foreskin?**
   (A) It is wise to retract the foreskin in the early days of life to prevent the accumulation of smegma and subsequent balanitis
   (B) In phimosis, the opening of the urethra is not visible and the condition is an absolute indication for circumcision
   (C) Paraphimosis is a painful and progressive lesion which may require treatment under general anaesthetic
   (D) In hypospadias, the opening of the urethra is located on the ventral surface of the shaft of the penis and proximal to its correct position
   (E) Severe hypospadias may be an indication for karyotyping

2. **Which of the following are correct in relation to inguinoscrotal abnormalities?**
   (A) An indirect inguinal hernia is the result of failure of closure of the processus vaginalis
   (B) Indirect inguinal hernias occur in approximately 2% of boys; an ovary may be palpable in association with an indirect inguinal hernia in girls

(**C**) There is no urgency to correct a non strangulated indirect inguinal hernia in infancy as complications are uncommon

(**D**) Most hydroceles in infants and young children resolve spontaneously by the age of approximately 2 years

(**E**) Failure to recognise and surgically correct an undescended testis may result in reduced fertility

3. **In swellings of the neck in infancy and childhood:**
   (**A**) A thyroglossal cyst is situated in the midline and moves upwards with swallowing and protrusion of the tongue
   (**B**) Thyroglossal cysts are cured by simple excision of the cyst
   (**C**) In children between the ages of approximately 6 months and 3 years, acute cervical adenitis may suppurate and require surgical incision and drainage
   (**D**) MAIS lymphadenitis is readily treated and cured with antituberculous therapy
   (**E**) A cystic hygroma may enlarge rapidly and may compromise respiration

4. **Which of the following are true?**
   (**A**) Most umbilical hernias close spontaneously by the end of the first year of life
   (**B**) An umbilical granuloma or ectopic bowel mucosa may be accompanied by a seropurulent discharge or by a mucous discharge
   (**C**) Prolapse of the rectum is most commonly due to constipation and responds to treatment of the constipation
   (**D**) Labial adhesions are due to fusion of the labia minora and require surgical incision
   (**E**) Persistence of the vitellointestinal (omphalomesenteric) duct may result in a discharge of ileal fluid and air from the umbilicus

Answers and explanations

1. The correct answers are (**C**), (**D**) and (**E**). Retraction of the foreskin is contraindicated in infancy and early childhood, as usually it will retract spontaneously by about the age of 4 years. Forcible retraction before spontaneous separation will result in the formation of adhesions, paraphimosis and infection (A). The application of a steroid cream will usually relieve the phimosis and obviate the need for circumcision (B). The treatment of paraphimosis is gentle manipulation of the foreskin forwards. This may require anaesthesia in some instances (C). The urethral opening in hypospadias is on the ventral aspect of the penis, proximal to its correct position; additionally, chordee

(ventral angulation of the shaft of the penis) may be present (D). Severe hypospadias may be indicative of an intersex abnormality, and karotyping is sometimes indicated (E).

2. The correct answers are (**A**), (**B**), (**D**) and (**E**). A widely patent proximal processus vaginalis allows bowel (and ovary in girls) to enter the inguinal canal to form an indirect inguinal hernia (A, B). Surgical repair of a non strangulated inguinal hernia should occur as soon as possible after diagnosis because of the risk of strangulation, which is particularly common in the first 6 months of life (C). Most hydroceles which are present in the first few months of life will disappear spontaneously (D). Undescended testes should be brought down into the scrotum surgically between 9 and 12 months of age (E).

3. The correct answers are (**A**), (**C**) and (**E**). The swelling of a thyroglossal cyst typically overlies and is attached to the hyoid bone: it moves on swallowing and protrusion of the tongue (A). Excision must include the cyst, the entire thyroglossal tract and the middle third of the hyoid bone; otherwise recurrence is common (B). Cervical lymphadenitis may progress to fluctuant abscess formation in children aged 6 months to 3 years: surgical incision and drainage will be necessary under general anaesthetic (C). MAIS infection of the cervical lymph nodes is common in preschool children and does not respond well to antituberculous drugs: surgical excision of the infected nodes is necessary (D). Cystic hygromas may enlarge rapidly from viral or bacterial infection or from haemorrhage, leading to respiratory embarrassment: excision is necessary (E).

4. The correct answers are (**A**), (**B**), (**C**) and (**E**). Umbilical hernias are common in neonates most close spontaneously in the first year of life (A). If the umbilical discharge contains mucus, the lesion is likely to have ectopic bowel mucosa (B). Prolapse of the rectum is usually associated with constipation, with prolapse during defecation (C); however, it may also be due to an underlying organic cause. Labial adhesions may be separated by gentle lateral pressure and/or the application of an oestrogen cream (D). Persistence of the vitellointestinal duct may result in a variety of symptoms. If the patency is complete, there may be discharge of ileal fluid and air from the umbilicus (E). If infection is superimposed, there may be pus, and intestinal obstruction may occur if a band connects the ileum to the umbilicus. If urine discharges from the umbilicus, there is a connection to the bladder in the form of a patent urachus.

PART 9 FURTHER READING

Ashcroft K W, Holder T M 1993 Paediatric surgery, 2nd edn. W B Saunders, Philadelphia

Beasley S W, Hutson J M, Myers N A 1993 Pediatric diagnosis: an illustrated guide to disorders of clinical significance. Chapman and Hall, London

Hilton S V W, Edwards D K 1994 Practical pediatric radiology, 2nd edn. W B Saunders, Philadelphia

Hutson J M, Beasley S W 1988 The surgical examination of children: an illustrated guide. Heinemann, Oxford

Hutson J M, Beasley S W, Woodward A A 1999 Jones' clinical paediatric surgery, 5th edn. Blackwell Scientific, Carlton, Australia

Nakayama D K 1992 Pediatric surgery: a color atlas. Gower, New York

Spitz L, Coran A G 1995 Pediatric surgery, 5th edn. Chapman and Hall, London

INHERITED AND METABOLIC PROBLEMS

Birth defects, prenatal diagnosis and teratogens

J. Liebelt, N. J. Hotham

Birth defects

A birth defect is any abnormality, structural or functional, identified at any age, which began before birth, or the cause of which was present before birth. Examples of structural birth defects include spina bifida, congenital heart malformations and cleft lip. Phenylketonuria, Duchenne muscular dystrophy and Huntington disease are examples of functional birth defects.

With continued advances in obstetric and paediatric medicine, birth defects have become the most important cause of perinatal and postneonatal mortality in developed countries.

Birth defects:

- are the leading cause of perinatal death (20–25% of deaths)
- are now the leading cause of postneonatal deaths (25–30%), as deaths due to sudden infant death syndrome continue to decline
- are responsible for a major proportion of the morbidity and disability experienced by children and young adults
- are the cause for 20–30% of the admissions to a tertiary paediatric hospital
- have an immense impact on the emotional and physical wellbeing of the children and their families
- have a significant financial cost for the community.

Types of structural birth defects

Structural birth defects may be classified on the basis of the mechanism by which they arise:

- *Malformations* arise during the initial formation of the embryo and fetus as a result of genetic and/or environmental factors during organogenesis (2–8 weeks postconception). Malformations may include failure of formation, incomplete formation or abnormal configuration. Examples include spina bifida, cleft palate, hypospadias.
- *Disruptions* result from a destructive process which alters structures after formation. Examples include early amnion rupture causing amputation defects of digits or an abdominal wall defect.
- *Deformations* result from moulding of a part by mechanical forces, usually acting over a prolonged period. Examples include talipes, congenital hip dislocations and plagiocephaly associated with oligohydramnios.

Causes of birth defects

Birth defects can be caused by a wide variety of mechanisms. These range from genetic abnormalities, both monogenic and polygenic, through presumably accidental events within the developing embryo, such as vascular accidents, to environmental factors, including teratogens generated by the mother, such as maternal phenylketonuria and maternal diabetes, and those originating outside the fetomaternal unit, for instance medications, infectious agents and high dose X irradiation. Table 27.1 provides a framework for thinking about causes of birth defects. Most have a multifactorial basis, reflecting interaction between genes, environment and chance events within the developing embryo and fetus.

Genes and birth defects

Early human development from fertilised ovum to fetus involves numerous processes controlled by genes, expressed sequentially in a defined cascade. The processes and developmental phases include such things as definition of polarity, cell division, formation of the germ layers, segmentation of the embryo, cell migration, organ formation, cell differentiation, interactions between cells, tissues and organs and programmed cell death.

There has been a recent rapid increase in knowledge of the genes that determine or predispose to birth defects. This has resulted from technological advances in molecular genetics, in phenotype delineation, gene mapping and gene discovery in humans and other species, and an understanding of the cascade of sequential gene expression during embryonic development in other species.

Examples of these genes include the homeotic (HOX) and paired box (PAX) gene families. HOX genes are involved in the formation of structures developing from specific segments of the embryo and PAX genes have an important role in eye development. Birth defects caused by mutations in selected developmental genes are shown in Table 27.2

Table 27.1 Causes of birth defects

Mechanism	Example	Cause
Whole chromosome missing or duplicated	Down syndrome Turner syndrome	Trisomy 21 Monosomy X
Part of chromosome deleted or duplicated	Cri du chat syndrome Cat eye syndrome	Deletion 5p Duplication 22q
Submicroscopic deletion or duplication of chromosome material	Williams syndrome Velocardiofacial syndrome Charcot–Marie–Tooth disease 1A	Deletion 7q Deletion 22q Duplication 17p
Mutation in single gene	Smith–Lemli–Opitz syndrome Holt–Oram syndrome Apert, Crouzon and Pfeiffer syndrome	7-Dehydrocholesterol reductase TBX5 Fibroblast growth factor receptor 2
Consequence of normal imprinting	Prader–Willi syndrome	Maternal uniparental disomy or paternal deletion for 15q12
Imprinting errors	Beckwith–Wiedemann syndrome Angelman syndrome	Multiple mechanisms resulting in overexpression of IGF2 Mutations in UBE3A gene
Multifactorial/polygenic: one or more genes and environmental factors	Isolated heart malformations, neural tube defects and facial clefts	Complex interactions between genes and environmental factors not yet defined
Non genetic vascular and other 'accidents during development'	Poland anomaly Oculoauriculovertebral dysplasia	Subclavian artery ischaemia Stapedial artery ischaemia
Uterine environment	Talipes. hip dysplasia Plagiocephaly	Oligohydramnios Twins, bicornuate uterus
Maternal environment	Mental retardation Caudal regression	Maternal phenylketonuria Maternal diabetes mellitus
Wider environment	Fetal rubella syndrome Fetal alcohol syndrome Microcephaly Limb deficiency	Rubella infection in pregnancy Maternal alcohol ingestion High dose X irradiation Thalidomide

Frequency of birth defects

Major birth defects

Major birth defects:
- are those with medical and social consequences
- are present with the highest prevalence among miscarriages, intermediate in stillbirths and lowest among liveborn infants
- are recognised at birth in 2–3% of liveborn infants.

The birth prevalences of the more common birth defects are shown in Table 27.3. They represent the frequency with which the defect occurred during development (its incidence), less the spontaneous loss of affected fetuses during pregnancy. An almost equal number of additional major abnormalities, particularly heart defects and urinary tract abnormalities, will be recognised by 5 years of age during clinical examinations or because of symptoms.

Minor birth defects

Minor birth defects:
- are relatively frequent but pose no significant health or social burden
- are recognized in approximately 15% of newborns
- are important to recognise, as their presence prompts a search for coexistent, more important abnormalities.

Infants free of minor defects have a low incidence of major malformations, approximately 1%. Those with one, two or three minor defects have risks of 3%, 10% and 20%, respectively.

Multiple birth defects

Various terms have been used to classify multiple birth defects in the hope that the terminology will convey information about aetiology, pathogenesis and the relationship between the birth defects. However, no system of naming

Table 27.2   Some developmental genes that, when mutant, cause birth defects in humans

Gene	Disorder	Features
CBP	Rubinstein–Taybi syndrome	Mental retardation, broad thumbs/toes, facial features
DAX1	X linked adrenal hypoplasia	Adrenal insufficiency
ENDR3B	Hirschsprung disease	Megacolon
FGFR2	Apert, Crouzon, Pfeiffer syndrome	Craniosynostosis, faciostenosis, +/– brachysyndactyly
FGFR3	Achondroplasia	Short limbed dwarfism, macrocephaly
GL13	Grieg cephalopolysyndactyly	Polysyndactyly, frontal bossing
HOXD13	Dominant polysyndactyly	Polysyndactyly
L1 CAM	X linked hydrocephalus	Aqueduct stenosis, mental retardation, adducted thumbs
MITF	Waardenburg syndrome type 2	Deafness, pigmentary disturbance
MSX2	Craniosynostosis (Boston type)	Craniosynostosis, short metatarsals
Myosin 7A	Usher syndrome type 1B	Congenital deafness, prepubertal retinitis pigmentosa
PAX2	Coloboma	Coloboma, urinary tract abnormalities
PAX3	Waardenburg syndrome type 1	Deafness, pigmentary disturbance, dystopia canthorum
PAX6	Aniridia	Aniridia
SHH	Holoprosencephaly	Holoprosencephaly
SOX9	Campomelic dysplasia	Short limbed dwarfism, bowed bones, abnormal brain development, sex reversal, cleft palate
TBX5	Holt–Oram syndrome	Variable upper limb defects, heart malformations

Table 27.3   Prevalence of some common birth defects. (Source: South Australian Birth Defects Register 1986–1998)

Defect	Rate
Malformations of heart and great vessels	11.9
Developmental hip dysplasia	7.0
Hypospadias	3.4
Talipes equinovarus	2.2
Hypertrophic pyloric stenosis	1.9
Down syndrome	1.6
Cleft lip with or without cleft palate	1.1
Spina bifida	1.0
Anencephaly	0.8
Renal agenesis and dysgenesis	0.6
Tracheo-oesophageal fistula, oesophageal atresia and stenosis	0.5
Abdominal wall defects: exomphalos and gastroschisis	0.6

*Rate per 1000 births including terminations of pregnancy, stillbirths and livebirths.

meets all these criteria or is able to meet all the situations encountered in clinical practice. Some commonly used terms are *syndrome, association, sequence* and *field defect*: these are defined in Chapter 29. *Phenotype* is a useful general term that makes no assumptions about aeti-ology or pathogenesis but registers the fact that multiple birth defects are present and are related in some way. *Complex* and *spectrum* are alternative terms that have been used in this context.

Diagnosis of birth defects

Hundreds of patterns of multiple birth defects have been defined and the diagnosis for a child with multiple birth defects is often not obvious.

The primary reasons for pursuing a diagnosis are that this allows:

- discussion with the parents regarding the prognosis for their child
- parents to develop an understanding of how the birth defect arose
- counselling of the parents regarding recurrence risk and possibilities for prenatal diagnosis in future pregnancies.

Thorough investigation, including autopsy if the child dies, may lead to a diagnosis, and referral to a clinical geneticist should be considered. Diagnosis is aided by computerised syndrome identification systems such as POSSUM and the London Dysmorphology Database. In spite of the large number of known syndromes, clinicians continue to encounter children with birth defects that cannot be diagnosed.

Birth defect/congenital malformation registers

Birth defects registers were established in many countries following the 'thalidomide tragedy' in which hundreds of children were born with a range of anomalies following maternal use of thalidomide in pregnancy as an antiemetic.

Registers serve a number of purposes, including:
- provision of early warning of new environmental teratogens
- provision of precise prevalence figures for individual birth defects and syndromes
- monitoring of geographic and temporal trends in birth defects
- comparison of birth defect prevalence in different populations
- assessment of the impact of population based prevention strategies and prenatal diagnosis
- research into the epidemiology of birth defects.

Prevention of birth defects

Despite considerable research efforts there are very few preventive strategies that effectively reduce the incidence of birth defects. Some effective population based examples include:
- Oral folic acid supplementation at least 1 month prior to and in the early months of pregnancy can reduce the incidence of neural tube defects by up to 70%.
- Education and legislation to reduce potential exposure to teratogens:
  — public health policy on rubella immunisation
  — restrictions on prescribing of known teratogens such as thalidomide and retinoids
  — education about avoidance of foods in pregnancy which may predispose to maternal infection with known teratogenic agents, e.g. toxoplasmosis and uncooked meat.
- Genetic counselling and the development of alternative reproductive options, including donor gametes and embryos to allow avoidance of the risk of conception of a child with a birth defect related to a specific genetic condition.
- Neonatal screening to detect children with those types of birth defect which do not cause permanent damage before birth, with a view to early treatment and improved prognosis. Neonatal screening for phenylketonuria, hypothyroidism and cystic fibrosis, and clinical examination for hip dislocation are examples of highly successful screening programmes.

At present, the primary approach to the prevention of the birth of children affected by birth defects is prenatal diagnosis.

Prenatal diagnosis

Prenatal diagnosis refers to testing performed in pregnancy aimed at the detection of birth defects in the fetus. Depending on the type of birth defect identified, the gestation of the pregnancy and the perceptions of the parents, prenatal detection of a birth defect may allow:
- termination of an affected fetus
- potential treatment in utero or postnatally to improve prognosis related to the defect
- preparation for the birth of a child with a specific medical condition.

The number of prenatal tests available and the range of birth defects that may be detected is expanding rapidly. Many chromosome abnormalities, structural anomalies, enzymatic and single gene defects are already potentially detectable prenatally. Advances in knowledge regarding the aetiology of birth defects and technical aspects of testing will expand this range further. Despite these advances, the majority of birth defects remain undetected until after birth.

In our society, it is an individual decision whether or not to utilise prenatal testing in a pregnancy. The provision of antenatal care must therefore ensure that parents are able to make informed decisions about testing and are supported throughout the testing process.

Types of prenatal tests

Prenatal tests fall into two main categories.

1. screening tests
2. diagnostic tests.

Screening tests

Prenatal screening tests:
- are aimed at *all* pregnant women
- assess whether an individual pregnancy is at increased or low risk of a particular birth defect
- generally pose no risk to maternal or fetal wellbeing
- are followed by an offer of a diagnostic test if an increased risk is identified
- are aimed primarily at the detection of structural anomalies and chromosomal abnormalities, in particular Down syndrome.

Screening tests in pregnancy are evolving rapidly, with the aim being earlier, more accurate and more accessible tests.

Screening tests available

Currently, screening tests are either performed on a serum sample from the mother, or utilising ultrasound.

Maternal serum screening (MSS)

- MSS is primarily aimed at the detection of Down syndrome and, in some programmes trisomy 18.
- MSS involves measuring the levels of a number of different analytes produced by the fetus in a blood sample from the mother.
- The analytes have been selected on the basis that large population studies have shown that the levels of the analytes in maternal serum differ significantly between pregnancies in which the fetus does or does not have Down syndrome.
- MSS is most commonly offered in the second trimester (around 15–18 weeks) using various combinations of three or four analytes. These may include, estriol (oestriol), alphafetoprotein (AFP), inhibin, and the alpha and beta subunits of human chorionic gonadotrophin (hCG).
- A computer based algorithm, which takes into account the mother's age related risk, the gestation of the pregnancy and the analyte levels, is used to calculate a risk figure for Down syndrome in that pregnancy.
- If the risk figure is greater than a predetermined 'cutoff' risk, the risk is considered to be increased and a diagnostic test is offered to clarify the situation.
- Most programmes are designed so that 5% of women having the test will receive an increased risk result. The majority of these women will go on to have healthy babies.
- If all of these women chose to have a diagnostic test, the screening programme would be expected to detect about 60–70% of cases of Down syndrome.
- If AFP is one of the analytes used in second trimester MSS, then the test can also be used to screen for open neural tube defects, as AFP will be elevated if neural tissue is exposed to the amniotic fluid. If it is elevated, then the diagnostic test is a tertiary level ultrasound to examine the fetal spine.
- First trimester maternal serum screening programmes are being developed using inhibin and pregnancy associated protein A (PAPP-A) as analytes.

Ultrasound

Ultrasound utilises sonar waves to allow real time, two dimensional visualisation of the fetus in utero. The fetus can be examined in different views and fetal movements can be studied. Improved technology and training allow excellent views to be obtained to allow detection of many specific structural anomalies. Most antenatal care programmes now offer an ultrasound between 18–20 weeks gestation to screen for fetal anomalies.

Ultrasound is usually considered a screening rather than a diagnostic test as:

- some structural anomalies may not be readily detected, e.g. cleft palate
- interpretation of a possible anomaly and its impact on fetal development may be limited
- detection rate of anomalies is dependent on the skill of the operator, equipment and fetal views obtained.

Potential advances which may enhance the value of fetal imaging as a screening test in pregnancy include 3D ultrasound and alternative imaging techniques such as fetal MRI.

Nuchal translucency screening

- Over the last decade, a new form of ultrasound based screening for Down syndrome in the first trimester has been developed, based on the MSS model.
- All fetuses have a collection of fluid in the nuchal region that can be visualised as a translucent area and measured by ultrasound at the end of the first trimester (11–13 weeks gestation).
- Large population studies have shown that on average this nuchal translucency measurement is increased in pregnancies in which the fetus has Down syndrome.
- As with MSS, a computer algorithm which takes into account the mother's age related risk, the gestation, and the thickness of the nuchal translucency measurement is used to calculate a risk for that individual pregnancy.
- If the risk is above a predetermined 'cutoff risk' a diagnostic test is offered.
- The detection rate of a nuchal translucency screening programme is dependent on the skill of the operator; however, detection rates of up to 70–80% of cases of Down syndrome have been reported.
- Other chromosome abnormalities, in particular Turner syndrome (45,XO) and triploidy also are often associated with an increased nuchal translucency measurement.
- An increased nuchal translucency measurement in the presence of normal chromosomes may be an indicator of other types of fetal anomaly, such as cardiac malformations or skeletal dysplasias. Detailed ultrasound follow up is recommended.

Combined screening

In order to increase the detection rates of screening tests, combinations of the different tests are being explored. The most promising at present is the combination of a nuchal translucency measurement with the measurement of two first trimester maternal serum analytes to give a combined first trimester risk. Early data suggest this may allow increased detection rates for Down syndrome of up to 90% for a 5% false positive rate. The best combination of screening tests is yet to be firmly established and a number of large multicentre trials are in progress to address this issue.

Diagnostic tests

Prenatal diagnostic tests:

- are aimed at pregnant women identified to be at increased risk of having a baby with a particular birth defect (see below)
- allow accurate clarification of whether an individual fetus is affected or not
- usually pose a small risk of fetal loss; this risk relates to the need to sample fetal tissue for testing
- are primarily aimed at the detection of chromosomal abnormalities, enzymatic and single gene defects.

New diagnostic tests continue to be developed, with the principal aim of increasing both the safety of the tests and range of conditions that may be tested for.

Indications for diagnostic prenatal tests

Although all women are at risk of conceiving a baby with a birth defect, there are a number of risk factors that increase the risk of an individual woman above the background population risk. In general, diagnostic prenatal tests are offered to women whose risk of conceiving a baby with a specific birth defect is considered to be above an arbitrary level. This 'cutoff' level takes into account the risk of fetal loss related to the test and economic issues relating to the number of women who would be offered testing.

Some of the reasons why a woman may be offered a prenatal diagnostic test include:

- advanced maternal age (see below)
- increased risk identified by a screening test, for example, maternal serum screening
- previous child with a birth defect for which a prenatal test is available and an increased risk of recurrence is recognised, e.g. chromosome abnormality, neural tube defect, single gene disorder such as cystic fibrosis
- a parent or couple known to carry a genetic mutation for which testing is available and which poses a risk of abnormality in offspring, e.g. chromosome translocation or single gene defects
- other factors known to increase the risk of birth defects, e.g. exposure to teratogens such as maternal infection

Advanced maternal age

As maternal age increases, there is an increased risk of conception of a fetus with some specific chromosomal anomalies, primarily trisomies (an additional copy of a single chromosome). Most fetuses conceived with a trisomy miscarry, however trisomy 21, 13 and 18 are potentially viable chromosomal anomalies leading to the potential birth of baby with specific constellations of birth defects (Ch. 29). Maternal age is not associated with an increased risk of other birth defects.

Table 27.4 Age specific risks for a liveborn child with Down syndrome (After Gardner & Sutherland, 1996)

Maternal age (years) at expected time of delivery	Risk (1 in)
20	1540
25	1350
30	890
34	445
35	335
36	300
37	220
38	165
39	125
40	90
42	50
44	30
46	17

The risk of any chromosome abnormality is approximately double these risks.

Trisomy 21 (Down syndrome) is the most common chromosome abnormality seen at livebirth in our population. Many screening and diagnostic prenatal tests are therefore aimed at detection of this condition. Population data exist on which to counsel women regarding their 'age related' risk in order that they may make informed decisions about prenatal testing (Table 27.4).

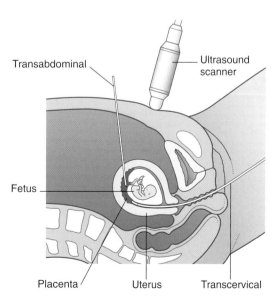

Fig. 27.1 Schematic representation of CVS showing transabdominal and transcervical routes. Illustration courtesy of Ultrasound Department, Royal Women's Hospital, Melbourne.

Diagnostic tests available

Most diagnostic tests involve sampling of fetally derived tissue which can be directly analysed for abnormalities. The most common test performed is chromosomal analysis. However, tissue may also be utilised as a source of DNA for molecular genetic tests, for metabolic tests or more rarely to look for evidence of fetal infection or histological confirmation of abnormality of a specific tissue; for example, the skin for the diagnosis of epidermolysis bullosa.

Amniocentesis and chorionic villus sampling (CVS) are the two principal diagnostic tests used; however, fetal blood samples, skin, liver or kidney biopsies may be required in very specific, rare circumstances. Amniocentesis, CVS and fetal blood sampling are performed as outpatient procedures under ultrasound guidance (Fig. 27.1). Each of these tests has advantages and disadvantages in certain situations (Table 27.5)

Imaging techniques

In some circumstances, ultrasound or other forms of fetal imaging such as MRI, or even plain X rays, are considered diagnostic and may be the only tool available for diagnosis of genetic conditions that do not have a chromosomal, enzymatic or known molecular basis. Examples include neural tube defects, skeletal dysplasias and congenital heart defects. Imaging techniques, however, are dependent on gaining adequate views and appropriate interpretation of the views and are limited by the gestation at which some defects may be identifiable; for example, hydrocephalus may not become apparent in a fetus until the third trimester.

Future options

Hope for a 'non invasive' diagnostic test has rested on the concept of isolation of fetal cells found within the mater-

Table 27.5	Prenatal diagnostic tests		
	Chorionic villus sampling (CVS)	Amniocentesis	Fetal blood sampling or fetal biopsies
Tissue sampled	Chorionic villi derived from the same initial fertilised ovum as the fetus	Amniotic fluid containing fetal cells	Fetal blood, liver skin or skin
Indications for test	1. Increased risk of fetal chromosomal anomaly 2. Increased risk of specific genetic conditions for which a molecular or enzymatic test exists.	1. As for CVS 2. Increased risk of fetal infection 3. Other less common indications, AFP measurements to assist in diagnosis of neural tube defects	1. Increased risk of fetal chromosome anomaly when rapid results are required 2. Diagnosis of fetal haemoglobinopathy 3. Diagnosis of fetal conditions by tissue histology (e.g. some skin disorders)
Gestation at which test is performed	Can be performed safely after 10 weeks gestation; most often done at 11–13 weeks gestation	Can be performed safely after 15 weeks gestation; most often done between 16–18 weeks gestation	Can be performed after 18 weeks gestation
Risks	0.5–1% rate of miscarriage related to the test	0.5% rate of miscarriage related to the test	1–5% rate of miscarriage related to the test, depending on the indication for the test
Other issues	1% risk of a discrepant result between fetal and placental tissue (confined placental mosaicism), requiring amniocentesis to clarify	1% risk of failure of the amniocytes to culture, requiring a repeat test	Potentially difficult access
Timing of results	Rapid chromosome analysis by FISH 24–48 hours. * Final chromosome, DNA or enzyme test results 7–21 days	As for CVS	Dependent on test performed

*FISH (fluorescent in situ hybridisation) involves the use of labelled DNA probes designed to bind to specific regions of individual chromosomes. This allows the number of a specific chromosome in an interphase cell to be ascertained within 24–48 hours.

nal circulation during pregnancy. This would allow collection of fetal tissue for the purpose of testing without risk to fetal wellbeing. Current techniques do not yet allow this option to be used in a clinical setting; however, research continues.

Prenatal diagnosis for specific genetic conditions

Rapid progress in knowledge of the underlying molecular genetic aetiology of specific conditions allows an increasing number of genetic conditions to be diagnosed prenatally by utilising specific DNA based technology. In order that this can occur for any individual couple known to have an increased risk of conceiving a child with such a disorder, a number of conditions must be satisfied:

- accurate diagnosis of the condition in the affected family member
- confirmation of the aetiology of the condition by identification of a mutation in the causative gene or an enzymatic defect that can be tested for accurately in fetal tissue (a process that may take many months and may not be possible in some cases)
- appropriate pretest (preferably prepregnancy) counselling regarding the process of testing and implications and options relating to the potential results of testing
- appropriate support throughout the process.

Prenatal diagnosis in these circumstances is best provided by an experienced multidisciplinary team consisting of an obstetrician, clinical geneticist, genetic counsellor and experienced laboratory staff. CVS is usually the preferred method for DNA based and enzymatic prenatal tests, as it often allows direct testing rather than a need for culturing of tissue prior to testing. Examples of conditions that DNA based prenatal diagnosis may be available for include: Duchenne and Becker muscular dystrophy, fragile X syndrome, cystic fibrosis, haemoglobinopathies and metabolic defects such as maple syrup urine disease.

In some families, although the specific mutation causing the condition in the family has not been identified, linkage studies using polymorphic DNA markers close to or within the gene may be possible. This requires further testing of family members and has a margin of error related to the possibility of genetic recombination. For X linked conditions in which the gene has not yet been identified or a mutation cannot be identified, identification of the gender of the fetus by chromosome analysis and termination of males (50% of whom would be unaffected) may be the only available option.

Preimplantation genetic diagnosis

Prenatal diagnosis in an already established pregnancy may not be an option for some couples for ethical and

---

Clinical example

Jennifer is aged 39 years and is 8 weeks pregnant with her third child. Jennifer's second child Amy was diagnosed with cystic fibrosis on the basis of a positive sweat test, which was performed because of failure to thrive in the first year of life. DNA testing confirmed she is homozygous for the ΔF508 mutation in the cystic fibrosis gene and that both Jennifer and her husband Peter are carriers of this mutation. Having received genetic counselling, Jennifer and Peter are aware that there is a 1 in 4 chance that any child that they conceive as a couple will be affected by cystic fibrosis. They are also aware of the 1 in 125 risk of having a baby with Down syndrome, based on Jennifer's age. They wish to know if their current pregnancy is affected by either of these conditions. Following counselling regarding the process of prenatal testing, they elect to undergo a CVS at 11 weeks of pregnancy. The molecular genetics laboratory extracts DNA from a portion of the CVS sample and tests specifically for the ΔF508 mutation in the cystic fibrosis gene. This takes several days and the results indicate that the fetus has not inherited a copy of the ΔF508 mutation from either Jennifer or Peter and therefore is not expected to be affected by cystic fibrosis. The cytogenetics laboratory concurrently cultures the remainder of the CVS sample and performs a chromosome analysis. These results, which are available in about 8 days, identify a normal male chromosome complement. Jennifer and Peter are relieved and feel they are now able to look forward to the birth of their third baby with no more anxiety than other couples.

---

moral reasons. Following advances during the last decade in both reproductive and molecular genetic technology, the technique of preimplantation genetic diagnosis (PGD) has become a potential alternative option.

The principle of this technique is the genetic analysis of an embryo produced by in vitro fertilisation (IVF) technology, in order to select those embryos free of a specific genetic condition for transfer to the women's uterus to establish a pregnancy.

A single cell can be removed for genetic analysis on day 3 postconception from an embryo cultured in vitro. Genetic analysis may consist of specific mutation detection or a limited analysis of chromosomes. The limited amount of material and the limited time frame available for analysis have provided the impetus for the development of specialised techniques to prevent misdiagnosis. Hundreds of babies have now been born worldwide following PGD in a number of highly specialised centres. Continual improvements in genetic techniques and pregnancy rates following IVF will mean that PGD will become a viable alternative to the well established methods of CVS and amniocentesis.

Teratogens

A teratogen is an environmental agent that can cause abnormalities of form or function in an exposed embryo or fetus. It is estimated that between 1 and 3% of birth defects may be related to teratogenic exposure.

A teratogen may cause its effect by a number of different pathophysiological mechansims, including:

- cell death
- alteration of cell division and tissue growth, including cell migration
- interference with cellular differentiation.

Examples of the different ways in which teratogens may have their effects are seen with alcohol and sodium valproate, which are believed to cause dysmorphic facial features with underdevelopment of the mid face and philtrum due to cell death in these areas, whereas syndactyly can result from failure of programmed death of cells between the digits.

Factors modifying the effects of a teratogen

In theory, to produce a malformation a teratogen must be present in a sufficient amount, at the appropriate time, in a genetically susceptible individual, where other conditions do not prevent the effects occurring. In other words, there are a number of factors that can modify the effects of a teratogen, including:

- timing of exposure
- dose to the fetus
- genetic susceptibility
- access of the drug to the fetus
- interaction between teratogens.

Timing of exposure

The effect of an environmental agent may differ depending on the gestational age at which exposure occurs:

- Exposure very early in embryogenesis, prior to organogenesis (<2 weeks after conception), is likely to cause embryonic death rather than malformations. This is seen as an 'all or nothing' effect.
- During organogenesis (2–8 weeks after conception) malformations can occur if the exposure is not lethal.
- Each organ develops during a specific time period and will be susceptible to the malforming effects of teratogens only during that critical period.
- During fetal development (after organogenesis) functional effects, such as mental retardation, are most likely, although malformations can still occur, for example in slowly forming organs such as the brain and kidney.

An example of this effect is seen with thalidomide, which affects limb development only at the time when limb buds are developing between 27 and 41 days, and causes ear abnormalities between 21 and 27 days. Another example is the effect of tetracycline, which only causes tooth discoloration with fetal exposure after about 16 weeks. Angiotensin converting enzyme (ACE) inhibitors in the third trimester can affect fetal kidneys and cause anuria.

Dose

The harmful effects of teratogens are dose dependent. Similarly, fetal alcohol syndrome can occur when a mother drinks 4–8 standard measures of alcohol per day but not if she drinks only one. There is no observed effect of X rays at doses routinely used in diagnostic radiology, while doses associated with nuclear explosions cause microcephaly, mental retardation and growth failure.

Genetic susceptibility

There are marked differences in genetic susceptibility to environmental agents, both between species and between individuals of one species. It is likely that the susceptibility to the harmful effects of many teratogens depends on the genetically determined efficiency of both the mother's and fetus's detoxifying metabolic pathways. Thalidomide again forms an example of this, in that it is not teratogenic in a large number of species but is teratogenic in some rabbits and some primates, including humans. Phenytoin metabolism by a fetus with low epoxide hydrolase activity may put the fetus at risk of fetal phenytoin syndrome.

Access

In order to have an effect, a teratogen must gain access to the fetus. Some potentially harmful agents are not teratogens because their size, means of transport or binding properties prevent or restrict them from crossing the placenta. Clinically this is seen with heparin, and pancuronium.

Interaction between teratogens

The ingestion of multiple medications can have additive effects. An example is that the risk of fetal effects is greater if a mother with epilepsy is taking multiple anticonvulsants (polypharmacy) rather than a single one.

Some important teratogens

Selected teratogens that cause common clinical issues are discussed below; a more extensive list is provided in Table 27.6.

Table 27.6	Environmental agents that can adversely affect human development

Infectious agents
Viruses: rubella, cytomegalovirus, varicella-zoster, Venezuelan equine encephalitis, herpes simplex, [parvovirus B19]
Bacteria: syphilis, [listeria]
Parasites: toxoplasmosis

Physical agents
Ionising radiation, carbon monoxide, (heat)

Drugs and chemicals
Environmental chemicals: organic mercury compounds, (polychlorinated biphenyls, i.e. 'PCBs')
Non prescription drugs: ethanol, cocaine, (amphetamine), [tobacco smoking, marijuana smoking]
Prescription drugs

Anticancer drugs:	aminopterin, busulphan, chlorambucil, cyclophosphamide, plicamycin, methotrexate, cytarabine, (dacarbazine, fluorouracil, procarbazine)
Anticonvulsants:	phenytoin, sodium valproate, carbamazepine, trimethadione, (primidone, phenobarbitone)
Hormones:	diethylstilboestrol, male sex hormones, strongly androgenic progestogens
Antibacterials:	tetracyclines, streptomycin, (gentamicin, quinolones)
Antivirals:	ribavirin, (ganciclovir. zalcitabine)
Anthelmintics:	(albendazole)
Antimalarials:	(chloroquine when used to treat malaria but not when used for prophylaxis)
Retinoids:	systemic isotretinoin, etretinate, acitretin, (vitamin A, topical tretinoin and isotretinoin)
Immunomodifiers:	(methotrexate), [interferon beta-1b]
Miscellaneous	thalidomide, misoprostol, penicillamine, warfarin, phenindione, lithium, intra-amniotic methylene blue, (diazepam, antithyroid drugs), [angiotensin converting enzyme inhibitors, angiotensin II receptor antagonists]

Maternal disorders
Insulin dependent diabetes mellitus, maternal phenylketonuria

No brackets, teratogen; (   ), possible teratogen; [   ] not known to be teratogenic but may cause other effects including embryonic/fetal death and/or growth retardation.
The above list should be considered illustrative only and may change in the light of new knowledge.

Rubella virus

- Infection of the fetus by the rubella virus in the first trimester can cause devastating birth defects, including mental retardation, short stature, deafness, blindness and congenital heart defects.
- The risk is greatly reduced if the mother has been immunised prior to pregnancy.
- Many countries have implemented preventive public health programmes to immunise either adolescent girls or all children.
- Affected children can be born to previously immunised mothers, due to initial failure of seroconversion or waning immunity with age; therefore immune status of women planning pregnancy should be reviewed.

Alcohol

- The harmful effects of ethanol on the developing human are well documented.
- Teratogenic effects of alcohol are dose related, ranging from clinically unapparent effects to the fetal alcohol syndrome of prenatal and postnatal growth failure, microcephaly, intellectual disability, a characteristic facial appearance, cleft palate, microphthalmia and heart defects.
- Heavy drinking throughout pregnancy is associated with a 10% risk of fetal alcohol syndrome and a 30% risk of observable fetal alcohol effects.
- No minimum safe dose has been defined and some evidence suggests that effects may be seen after as little as two standard measures of alcohol daily or periodic heavier drinking in early pregnancy, e.g. five or more drinks on each occasion.
- Consumption of a significant amount of alcohol prior to diagnosis of pregnancy is a frequent clinical scenario. It is difficult to estimate the risk of harm to the baby because of lack of good data, although in most cases it appears to be small.
- Women should be advised to avoid alcohol during pregnancy.

Antiepileptic medication

- Women with epilepsy receiving treatment with anticonvulsant medication have a two- to threefold risk of giving birth to a child with a birth defect.

- No anticonvulsant has been shown to be safe in pregnancy and specific teratogenic effects have been defined for phenytoin, sodium valproate, carbamazepine and trimethadione, particularly for neural tube defects.
- The risk to the fetus increases if multiple anticonvulsants are needed to prevent seizures.
- It is likely that individual susceptibility exists, based on the activity of genetically determined detoxifying metabolic pathways for disposal of the drug and/or its metabolites.
- Epileptic women must accept some additional risk of birth defects in their infants, but the risk can be minimised if epileptic control can be achieved with a single drug at the lowest possible dose.
- Periconceptional folic acid supplementation at a dose of 5 mg daily should be recommended for women on anticonvulsant medication because of the increased risk of neural tube defects in offspring.

Vitamin A analogues: isotretinoin, etretinate and acitretin

- These highly potent analogues of vitamin A are extremely teratogenic.
- Their systemic use in early pregnancy is associated with a high (25–30%) risk of birth defects, including serious abnormalities of brain development, with microcephaly, hydrocephalus, cortical blindness and intellectual disability, cranial nerve palsies, dysmorphic facial features, microtia, cleft palate, heart defects, thymic hypoplasia and genitourinary abnormalities.
- There is no 'safe' period in early pregnancy from the teratogenic effects of these drugs.
- The teratogenic dose has not been determined.
- Many countries have restricted the right to prescribe these drugs to particular groups of doctors and recommend that women should have a pregnancy test before commencing treatment and should use effective contraception for 1 month before treatment begins, throughout treatment and for a period after treatment stops.
- Isotretinoin is used to treat severe cystic acne. Although it has a short elimination half-life, it is recommended that pregnancy should be avoided for at least 1 month after the last dose.
- Etretinate is used to treat psoriasis and other disorders of keratinisation. Etretinate is readily taken up into adipose tissue, is slowly released from it, and has a long elimination half-life of 120 days. Acitretin has a relatively short half-life but is converted to etretinate during therapy. It is therefore recommended that pregnancy be avoided for 2 years following use of these drugs.

Warfarin

- Warfarin is used in the treatment of thromboembolic disease and for individuals with artificial heart valves.
- Warfarin crosses the placenta, is teratogenic and may cause haemorrhage in the fetus.
- The teratogenic effects appear to result from inhibition of vitamin K and/or arylsulphatase E activity during skeletal development.
- The fetal warfarin syndrome comprises nasal hypoplasia, short fingers with hypoplastic nails, low birth weight, stippling of epiphyses on X ray and intellectual disability.
- Recent estimates indicate that the risk of fetal warfarin syndrome in the babies of women who require warfarin throughout pregnancy is low, around 5%.
- The period of greatest embryonic susceptibility is between 6 and 9 weeks after conception, although it is recommended that the drug should be avoided throughout the first trimester, if possible.
- It has been suggested that warfarin exposure limited to the second and third trimesters can cause brain and eye damage, presumably as a result of haemorrhage, but, if so, the risk also appears low.
- Heparin is not a teratogen. It is used in the treatment of thromboembolic disease but does not cross the placenta.
- Use of heparin instead of warfarin may be appropriate when the indication is venous thrombosis but not when it is used for artificial heart valves. Low dose heparin carries a significant risk of valve thrombosis, and high dose heparin in the outpatient setting carries a risk of serious maternal and retroplacental haemorrhage.

Ionising radiation

- Very high doses of X rays can affect the developing fetus, resulting in growth failure, microcephaly, intellectual disability and ocular defects.
- The sensitive period for these effects appears to be between 2 and 4–5 weeks after conception.
- The doses delivered to the appropriately shielded uterus by modern X ray equipment in the course of standard diagnostic radiology are well below the level which is teratogenic.
- Women who are inadvertently exposed to diagnostic X rays in early pregnancy can usually be reassured, although they may find it hard to understand that, while public health policy strongly recommends avoidance of diagnostic X rays in pregnancy, the absolute risk to the baby of an exposed woman is negligible.
- If an undiagnosed pregnancy is irradiated during radiotherapy, the dose must be calculated and the risk assessed.
- Ionising radiation is not only potentially teratogenic but also potentially mutagenic and carcinogenic. It is likely that even low dose irradiation of the fetus, as

with the child and adult, does have mutagenic and carcinogenic potential but the absolute size of the risk increase is very small.

- In general, if there is a good clinical reason for performing diagnostic radiology in pregnancy, it can be done knowing that the risks to the fetus are very low.

Diethylstilboestrol (DES)

- This drug (diethylstilboestrol USP, stilboestrol BP), widely used in the 1950s and 1960s in the belief that it prevented miscarriage, is both a teratogen and a prenatal carcinogen.
- Exposure, especially before 10 weeks gestation, can cause vaginal adenosis in girls and these areas of epithelium have an increased risk of progressing to vaginal adenocarcinoma years later.
- This knowledge highlights that there can be a delay of many years before the effects of fetal exposure to environmental agents become apparent, and absence of birth defects in the earliest years of life is not sufficient evidence to declare a drug safe in pregnancy.
- Exposed girls also appear to have an increased risk of cervical abnormalities and uterine malformations.
- Exposed boys appear to have an increased risk of testicular abnormalities, infertility and, possibly, testicular malignancy.

Paternal exposures

To date there has been no convincing evidence that preconception paternal exposures to environmental chemicals are teratogenic, although paternal drugs may affect fertility. For paternal exposure to be teratogenic, it would have to involve mutagenesis of paternal DNA. A mutagenic agent could affect any part of the genome, resulting in the spread of risk of mutation across a very large number of individual genes. While new dominant and X linked mutations could potentially occur, one would not expect a consistent pattern of birth defects in the children of exposed men. At present, any teratogenic risk from paternal exposures should be considered negligible, although it is admitted that it would be very hard to see an effect against the significant background prevalence of birth defects in humans. It is theoretically possible that environmentally induced mutations could contribute to the known paternal age related risk of new dominant mutations, such as for achondroplasia.

Teratogen advisory services

Appropriate public concern about the possible effects of exposure to environmental agents in pregnancy, as a result of the thalidomide experience and a more general uneasiness about environmental agents and health, has resulted in the establishment of services to provide information to health professionals and women with concerns. Teratogen advisory services have access to online databases such as TERIS, containing the most recent distillation of information about individual agents, have experience in assessing the significance of an exposure and counselling skills, and can usually be contacted by phone when the need arises.

28 Modern genetics

G. Suthers

Most of the chapters of this book describe abnormalities of function in children, that is, the ways that such abnormalities present in clinical practice, how to identify the underlying dysfunction, and how to correct or ameliorate the problem. These abnormalities of function may reflect a problem that is intrinsic to the child or be primarily due to external factors. More usually the abnormality of function reflects a combination of both intrinsic and extrinsic factors.

The cells of the human body need a source of information to direct those activities that are primarily intrinsic in nature, such as prenatal development. A source of information will also be essential for consistently regulating the body's responses to external factors. Both types of information must be passed from parent to child (during reproduction) and from cell to cell (during development) so that the next generation will benefit from the information that allowed the parents (or cells) to reproduce successfully.

The study of this information is called genetics. There has been an explosion in the amount of information available about human genetics in the last decade. Most medical practitioners are unable to keep abreast of all the advances in genetic knowledge pertinent to their field. A clinical geneticist, a medical specialist with an expert knowledge of this information, can assist a patient or medical colleague to obtain the genetic information that is relevant to the situation; however, genetic information underlies the development and responses of every individual and an understanding of human genetics is essential for every medical practitioner.

The pervasive and complex nature of human genetics cannot be encompassed in a single chapter. This chapter will provide a brief overview of genetics as it pertains to paediatrics, but the reader is cautioned that there is much that is both important and fascinating that cannot be covered in the space available. It is also important to realise that the genetic information available today may be outdated within a matter of months. It is strongly recommended that the reader utilise other resources, such as those listed in the Further Reading list at the end of this chapter.

The nature of genetic information is reviewed briefly in the next section of this chapter. Although many technical terms are used in this section, most will be familiar from courses in genetics or biochemistry. Readers will need to be familiar with these terms to ensure that their genetic education keeps pace with the advances in genetic knowledge in the years ahead.

The focus of the remainder of the chapter is genetic errors, or mutations:
- What causes mutations?
- What types of mutations cause disease?
- When do mutations occur?
- How are mutations inherited?

The nature of genetic information

Genetic information is encoded in DNA, a double strand of simple molecules

Genetic information is encoded in the structure of a chemical within the nucleus of each cell. The chemical is deoxyribonucleic acid (**DNA**). A DNA molecule consists of a long string made up of four simple molecules, **adenosine** (A), **thymidine** (T), **cytosine** (C) and **guanidine** (G); these molecules are collectively termed **nucleotides**. The sequence of nucleotides provides a basic but robust code to record all the information needed by the cell. The genetic instructions required to run a human cell are encoded by approximately three billion (3×10^9) nucleotides. The entire DNA sequence is called the human **genome**.

This long sequence of nucleotides must be copied correctly and passed on to the next cell prior to cell division to ensure that the next cell benefits from the survival of its predecessor. The process of accurately copying this many nucleotides is somewhat simplified by the duplex structure of DNA. Each of the nucleotides has chemical affinity for one of the other nucleotides. Adenosine consistently pairs with thymidine, and cytosine pairs with guanidine. As a result the entire string of three billion nucleotides has an adjacent and complementary strand of paired nucleotides. DNA is, in fact, a double stranded string in which one strand encodes the information and the second represents the complementary sequence (Fig. 28.1). The two strands are parallel and the attraction between the nucleotide pairs of A-T and C-G can be represented as rungs on a very long ladder. The entire ladder is twisted along its length and the end result is a 'double helix' of DNA.

The benefit of this structure is most readily evident during the copying (or **replication**) of DNA. If the

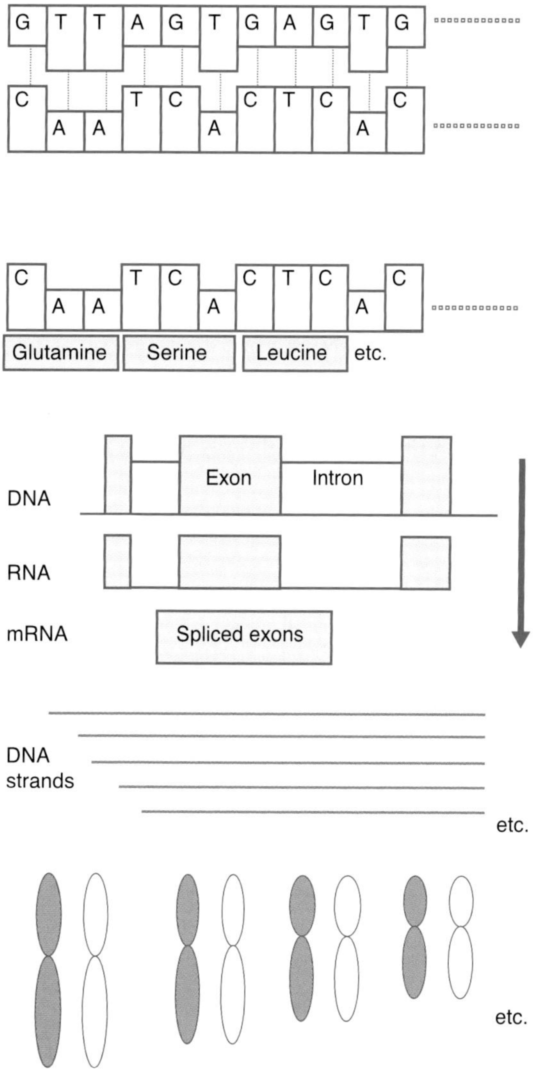

The double-stranded structure of DNA is represented as a series of squares and rectangles representing the four nucleotides. The molecular forces between A-T and C-G (shown as dashed lines) provide a template for accurate copying of the DNA strand.
This long thin strand is twisted lengthwise to form a double helix.

A triplet of nucleotides (or codon) represents the genetic code for a single aminoacid. A sequence of three codons is shown (with the corresponding aminoacids indicated below). A typical gene has a few hundred codons encoding a protein of the same number of aminoacids.

A gene consists of regions of codons (called exons; shown as grey boxes) separated by regions of non coding DNA called introns (white boxes). An exon may consist of 100 or so codons. A gene is transcribed into RNA and the introns are spliced out to form messenger RNA (mRNA). The spliced mRNA then directs the formulation of the specified protein.

The DNA required to encode all the genes in the human genome is present as 23 fragments of varying length. The total length of these fragments is approximately one metre.

Each DNA fragment is coiled into a short bundle called a chromosome. The chromosomes are numbered in decreasing order of size (except for the X and Y chromosomes). With the exception of sperm and ova, all cells have two copies of each chromosome. One chromosome of each size is inherited from each parent (as shown by the different shading). Each cell has a total of 23 pairs of chromosome (46 in all).

Fig. 28.1 The packaging of DNA.

strands of DNA are separated, each nucleotide in each strand will attract a complementary nucleotide that is free floating in the nucleus. With assistance from a variety of enzymes, each strand of the original DNA molecule will act as a template for the production of its own complementary strand, and two double stranded DNA molecules will be formed from the original double helix.

A gene is a single item of genetic information encoded in the DNA sequence

A unit of genetic information is called a **gene**. A gene usually encodes a particular **protein**, or it may provide a regulatory function within the nucleus. Each gene consists of a sequence of between several hundred and many thousands of nucleotides. There are specific DNA sequences which define the beginning and end of a gene. It has been estimated that there are 30 000–50 000 genes encoded by the three billion paired nucleotides of human DNA.

By international convention each human gene is known by a sequence of capital letters and numbers. The choice of characters is idiosyncratic and often reflects the history of the research that led to the isolation of the gene. Typical gene symbols include HBA, F8C, FRAXA and COL2A1. The convention is mentioned here because this nomenclature frequently appears in laboratory reports.

Most genes consist of essential sequences of nucleotides (**exons**) which alternate with dispensable sequences that are not essential for the gene's function (**introns**) (Fig. 28.1). Exons are usually a few hundred nucleotides long, while introns may be many thousands of nucleotides in length.

To access the information encoded in a gene, the enzyme **RNA polymerase** generates a short lived transcript of the gene made from the chemical ribo-nucleic acid (**RNA**). RNA is similar in structure to single stranded DNA but has the great advantage that it is degraded rapidly within the cell. If a cell is to react quickly to its environment it must be able to regulate the level of RNA (and hence the synthesis of specific proteins) with speed and precision.

The RNA will initially contain both exons and introns. The introns are carefully **spliced** out of the message by a family of molecules within the nucleus, and the completed RNA strand (called messenger RNA or **mRNA**) is moved to the cytoplasm to direct the synthesis of the protein encoded by the gene.

An amino acid is encoded by a triplet of DNA nucleotides

Proteins are made of many amino acids joined end to end in a long chain. This chain of amino acids then folds to form a specific three dimensional shape that is the essential feature of each protein. Each amino acid of the protein is encoded in DNA as a triplet of nucleotides (or **codon**). For example, the codon ATG encodes the amino acid methionine and the codon CGC encodes the amino acid arginine. During protein synthesis each successive codon of the mRNA directs the addition of the appropriate new amino acid to the growing sequence of amino acids. There are also specific **stop codons** (such as TAG) that indicate the end of a gene.

There is no gap or boundary between adjacent codons. For example, the DNA sequence ...AATCGCTATGGC... could be interpreted as ...-AAT-CGC-TAT-GGC-..., or ..A-ATC-GCT-ATG-GC., or .AA-TCG-CTA-TGG-C.., and each codon sequence would encode a different sequence of amino acids. In practice, the sequence of codons in a DNA sequence (or **reading frame**) is simply determined by the point from which the first codon is 'read', and this starting position is dictated by the specific sequence that identifies the start of a gene.

A gene is regulated by DNA sequences that lie adjacent to the gene

The amount of protein synthesised from a gene is regulated by molecules that interact with DNA sequences lying to one side or other of the gene. Regulatory regions may also be chemically altered by the addition of methyl groups ($-CH_3$) to nucleotides of the sequence. These methyl groups interfere with the binding of regulatory molecules and the net effect is inactivation of the gene. The methyl groups may also be removed and so provide a means for varying gene activity. A gene may be inactivated by this process of **methylation** in normal cells in a specific tissue or at certain times during development.

Certain genes are selectively inactivated by methylation when transmitted by sperm, and selectively activated when transmitted by an ovum; other genes demonstrate the reciprocal pattern of activation. This is a normal process that persists for the life of the individual and results in there being just one active copy of the gene in the cell. This selective inactivation of genes by methylation according to the parental gender is called **imprinting**.

Chromosomes are tightly coiled lengths of DNA

A DNA double helix of three billion nucleotides is approximately one nanometre (10^{-9} metre) wide and 1 metre long. This represents an enormous length of DNA within the tiny volume of a cell's nucleus (which is approximately 10^{-5} metres in diameter). The metre of DNA is packaged into 23 fragments that are of varying length. During cell division each of these fragments is tightly coiled into a short bundle (or **chromosome**) which is visible down the light microscope. The division of the genetic code into these fragments is very consistent between individuals. As a result a gene that is located at a specific point on a chromosome will be found at the same location on the equivalent chromosome in any other individual.

Evolutionary processes have dictated that virtually all human cells have two copies of the entire genetic code, with one copy being inherited from each parent. Thus the nucleus of each cell contains two copies of the metre long DNA sequence, and this DNA is packaged into a total of 46 chromosomes.

The only cells that have less DNA are sperm and ova. These cells contain just a single copy of the genetic code, that is, 1 metre of DNA packaged as 23 chromosomes. The fertilisation of an ovum by a sperm cell restores the amount of DNA to the usual 2 metres (46 chromosomes).

Within the cell each chromosome can usually be paired with an equivalent chromosome inherited from the other parent, that is, there are 23 pairs of chromosomes in the nucleus. The chromosome pairs are ranked according to length, and 22 of the pairs are identified by their relative size (that is, each copy of chromosome 1 is slightly longer than each copy of chromosome 2, which is longer than chromosome 3, etc.). These 22 pairs of chromosomes are collectively called **autosomes**.

Men and women have different types of sex chromosomes

Two of the chromosomes are referred to as **sex chromosomes** and they are the important exception to this concept of pairs of chromosomes within the cell. In women the sex chromosomes consist of two equivalent chromosomes that are relatively long (similar in size to chromosome 6); for historical reasons these two chromosomes are referred to as **X chromosomes**. In men the sex chromosomes consist of one X chromosome and a very small **Y chromosome**. The Y chromosome is the smallest of all the human chromosomes. It encodes a few genetic instructions which trigger a cascade of other processes which result in the developing embryo becoming male.

All human embryos inherit an X chromosome from their mothers; the inheritance of an X or Y chromosome from the father determines whether the embryo will develop as a female (XX) or as a male (XY). Gender is one of the few elements of human variation that is visible at the chromosomal level; almost all of the genetic variation in the population occurs at the level of individual genes and cannot be identified by examining the chromosomes.

Women compensate for the presence of two X chromosomes by inactivating one X chromosome

The difference in the number of X chromosomes between men and women represents a profound difference in the amount of genetic information in the cell. A woman has two copies of the thousands of genes located on the X chromosome, but the fact that men survive as well as they do indicates that a single copy is sufficient. Although this genetic information is duplicated in half the human race, it is made functionally equivalent in both sexes by an intriguing process in women. At the time of conception both X chromosomes in a female conceptus are active, but at a very early stage (after just a few cell divisions) one of the X chromosomes is rendered inactive in each cell by extensive methylation. The choice of X chromosome is usually random but the same X chromosome remains inactive in all the cells derived from that ancestral cell. This process was first described by Mary Lyon and is called **lyonisation**.

Each mitochondrion contains its own DNA strand

Mitochondria are small organelles within the cell which are the major energy source for all cellular functions. A cell typically has a few hundred mitochondria. Within each mitochondrion there is a complex array of proteins. As one might expect, many of the genes that encode these proteins are located on chromosomes within the nucleus of the cell. But each mitochondrion also has its own DNA strand that encodes some of the proteins located within mitochondria. The **mitochondrial DNA** is a double stranded loop that is 16 000 nucleotides long and is joined end to end in a circle. Each mitochondrion has 10 or so copies of this DNA loop.

Mitochondria (and their DNA) are copied independently of the process of copying DNA within the cell's nucleus. The number of mitochondria within a cell can vary without the need for cell division. When a cell does divide into two, approximately half of the mitochondria present are distributed to each new cell.

The mitochondria in all the cells of a person are maternally inherited, that is, all the mitochondria are derived from the original ovum. A sperm has mitochondria which provide energy to the cilium that propels it, but these mitochondria do not enter the ovum at fertilisation. The exclusive maternal inheritance of the mitochondrial DNA is in marked contrast to the inheritance of the DNA in the cell's nucleus, which is inherited from both parents.

Detailed information about human genes is accumulating very rapidly

In recent years there has been a dramatic increase in the rate at which new genes have been identified. The major factor accounting for this progress has been the injection of many millions of dollars into human genome research and infrastructure by numerous public and private sources. This large scale project has been called the **Human Genome Project**. The aim of the project was the definition of the DNA sequence of the entire human genome. This short term goal was achieved during the year 2000, but evaluation of the significance of this sequence will take many years.

The Human Genome Project encompasses many issues, including the ethical use of this new genetic knowledge, the development of new computational methods for analysing the sequences of billions of nucleotides, and the development of new genetic therapies. There are many technical and general resources dealing with the Human Genome Project available on the internet. The ramifications of the Human Genome Project are also discussed with increasing frequency in the medical literature and the general media.

What causes mutations?

DNA replication consists of accurately copying the six billion nucleotides which are spread along the 2 metres of DNA within the few microns of space within the nucleus of a cell. The resulting 4 metres of DNA must be carefully separated into two equivalent portions and normal cellular functions must be maintained all the while. The process of copying DNA and dividing into two equivalent cells is called **mitosis**.

The penalty for failing to copy DNA accurately is the generation of new genetic errors (or **mutations**) that are transmitted to all of the cell's progeny. The enzyme **DNA polymerase** is very good at copying DNA accurately. It has an error rate of approximately one wrong nucleotide pair per million processed. This is impressive, but it would amount to thousands of new mutations at every cell division. There is an additional proofreading mechanism which compares the original with the copied strand and corrects any mismatched nucleotides on the new strand. This mechanism reduces the overall mutation rate to approximately one wrong nucleotide per billion processed. As a consequence, the division of any cell results in approximately six new mutations in DNA sequence.

The accumulation of these new mutations is relentless. Each person consists of billions of cells, each of which was derived from the original fertilised egg. Every mutation that was generated during any cell division will be present in the descendants of that cell. By the time we reach adulthood, every cell in the body has accumulated hundreds of new mutations that were not present at the moment of conception.

Despite the frequency of mutations, most of them have no adverse effect on the information encoded in the DNA. Approximately 95% of the DNA in the nucleus does not have any genes. This vast amount of geneless DNA is referred to as **non coding DNA**. The role of this DNA is not known; some portions are presumably involved in the activation or regulation of specific genes and in maintaining chromosome structure. Mutations in non coding DNA have little effect. They are usually referred to as **polymorphisms** (meaning 'many forms') because they do not reduce an individual's ability to survive.

Polymorphisms are very common. On average the sequences of non coding DNA in two individuals differ by one nucleotide pair in every 300. These polymorphisms have played a central role in identifying and analysing genes because they can act as landmarks along the DNA within a cell.

Mutations in genes are much less common than polymorphisms. Genes account for only 5% or so of all of the DNA within a cell's nucleus. Mutations which occur in this small component of the DNA may interfere with the function of a gene, compromise the cell's function, and cause a disorder. Subtle variation in certain DNA sequences (and hence in the functions of certain genes) is also the basis for much of the variation in human structure that makes us individually different.

The versions of a specific gene that are present in the population are referred to as **alleles**. This term includes mutated versions of the gene that cause disease and benign variants in gene sequence that are found in the normal population. Some genes have only one allele. The role of such a gene is so critically dependent on the specific DNA sequence that any change results in the death of the cell and loss of the mutant gene. Other genes demonstrate many alleles. For example, the MC1R gene has a role in the regulation of melanocytes. It has nine alleles which are present in the normal Caucasian population; some of these alleles are found in healthy people with red hair or fair skin, while others are usually noted in healthy dark haired people.

What types of mutations cause disease?

It is convenient to divide mutations into groups according to the scale of the mutation (a portion of DNA sequence versus entire chromosomes) and the type of mutation (affecting primarily the structure or the function of the genetic information). This distinction is a little artificial, but it provides a basis for classifying various mutations (as summarised in Table 28.1).

Structural mutations of genes

The simplest mutation is the loss (or **deletion**) of all or part of a gene's DNA sequence. A deletion could involve as little as one or two nucleotides. A deletion could alter the sequence of codons (or reading frame) of the gene, which would result in disruption of the information encoded by the gene.

A deletion of three nucleotides could involve the loss of a single codon and the consequent absence of a single amino acid from the mature protein. The impact of such a mutation would depend on the role of the specific amino acid. For example, the most common mutation in the genetic disorder cystic fibrosis is the loss of the three nucleotides that encode the 508th amino acid, phenylalanine. The absence of this one amino acid renders the protein inactive.

Another type of mutation is **duplication** of the DNA sequence. A small duplication of one or two nucleotides will disrupt the reading frame of the gene and, as with a small deletion, will render the gene inactive. Larger duplications may also disrupt the reading frame.

Very large deletions or duplications may encompass one or more genes. The presence of one or three active copies of a gene (instead of the normal two copies) may be sufficient to cause a disorder.

A change in the DNA sequence may not alter the overall length of the sequence but may introduce a new stop codon. For example, an alteration in just one nucleotide would change the codon TAC (which encodes the amino acid tyrosine) to TAG (which is one of the stop codons). The presence of a premature stop codon results in a shortened (or **truncated**) protein. This type of mutation is called a **nonsense** mutation.

A small change in DNA sequence also may alter the amino acid encoded by the codon. For example, achondroplasia is a relatively common familial bone dysplasia that causes short stature; the underlying mutation is a change in DNA sequence from GGG to AGG. The effect of this mutation is that the 380th amino acid in the protein is arginine rather than glycine. The total length of the protein is normal but the altered amino acid sequence at

Table 28.1 Types of mutations that occur during DNA replication

Scale and type of error	Mutation	Description	Examples of diseases due to these mutations *
Structural errors of genes	Deletion	Loss of all or part of a gene, resulting in little or no protein product	Duchenne muscular dystrophy
	Duplication	Duplication of all (or part) of a gene resulting in excess (or deficiency) of the protein product	Charcot–Marie–Tooth disease
	Nonsense/ truncation	Mutation involving one or more nucleotides which prevents the cell generating a complete RNA strand	Hurler syndrome
	Missense	Mutation involving one codon that causes a critical alteration in the protein sequence	Cystic fibrosis
	Splicing error	Mutation involving the nucleotides which identify the junction between exons and introns resulting in generation of an abnormal RNA strand	Crouzon syndrome
Functional errors of genes	Regulatory mutation	Mutation in the regulatory region of a gene causing inappropriate activation or silencing of gene	Thalassaemia
	Abnormal imprint	Reversal of the normal silencing or activation of specific genes in the maternal or paternal germline	Beckwith–Wiedemann syndrome
	Unstable triplet repeat	Increase in the number of copies of a repeated triplet of nucleotides causing impairment of function of gene or protein	Fragile X syndrome
Structural errors of chromosomes	Monosomy (deletion)	Loss of whole (or part) of a chromosome	Turner syndrome
	Trisomy (duplication)	Excess of the whole (or part) of a chromosome	Down syndrome
	Triploidy	Presence of an extra copy of each chromosome	Miscarriage
Functional errors of chromosomes	Uniparental disomy	Both copies of all or part of a chromosome inherited from just one parent	Prader–Willi syndrome

*Note that different patients with the same genetic disorder may have different types of mutations in the same gene.

this point causes a major change in bone formation. This type of mutation is called a **missense** mutation.

The mutations described above occur primarily in exons, which are those portions of a gene that contain essential information. The exons of a gene are separated by non essential DNA sequences called introns. When an RNA transcript is first synthesised from a gene it includes sequences from both introns and exons. The introns are then spliced out of the RNA before protein synthesis is begun. A **splicing mutation** is an abnormality in the DNA sequence of an intron that indicates its boundary with an adjacent exon. A splicing mutation will cause the splicing process to fail, with the result that an intron may be left inappropriately in the mRNA or an exon may be spliced out inappropriately. In either case the end result is the synthesis of an abnormal protein.

Functional mutations of genes

The activity of a gene is controlled by proteins that bind to regulatory regions of DNA close to the gene. A muta-

tion in a regulatory sequence may interfere with the binding of regulatory molecules and so may interfere with the normal control of gene activity. For example, deletion of a regulatory region of the DMD gene causes muscle weakness and wasting. This **regulatory mutation** lies thousands of nucleotides away from the nearest exon of the DMD gene and the DNA sequence of all the exons and introns of the gene is normal.

Imprinting involves the selective methylation (and hence inactivation) of a regulatory region according to the gender of the parent. A failure of the imprinting process will cause problems. For example, the maternal copy of the IGF2 gene is normally imprinted, leaving the paternal copy as the only active copy in the cell. Failure to imprint the maternal IGF2 gene results in there being two active copies of the gene, producing excess growth in the developing baby (Beckwith–Wiedemann syndrome). The specific cause of abnormal methylation and **imprinting mutations** is not known.

Triplet repeat mutations are a special class of mutation that have features of both structural and functional mutations, as well as having unique characteristics of their own. Throughout the genome there are many nucleotide triplets that are present as many adjacent copies. Most of these triplet repeats occur in non coding DNA and are of no consequence. However, some triplets occur within genes (in exons or introns) or within nearby regulatory regions. A number of genes contain the DNA sequence CAG-CAG-CAG repeated many times within an exon. The codon CAG encodes the amino acid glutamine and the proteins synthesised from these genes contain regions of polyglutamine. Other genes have the sequence CCG repeated many times in the regulatory region of the gene.

The number of triplet repeats varies widely (approximately 5–40 copies) in the normal population. An abnormal expansion outside this range in the number of the triplet repeats in an exon will result in an increased length of polyglutamine in the protein and usually interferes with protein function. An increase in the number of repeats in a regulatory region may inactivate the gene. Larger degrees of expansion tend to be associated with more severe disruption of normal function of the gene or protein.

One of the most striking features of these expanded triplet repeat mutations is that they tend to increase in size during cell division. The increase may occur during ovum or sperm formation and so may be transmitted from parent to child, or it may occur during normal cell division during development and growth (mitosis). The effect of this increase in size over time is that a genetic disorder due to a triplet repeat mutation often becomes progressively more severe when passed from parent to child, or during the life of the individual.

Structural mutations of chromosomes

With the exception of the sex chromosomes, chromosomes are normally present in the nucleus in pairs. The presence of two copies of a chromosome in a normal cell is called **disomy**. A deletion involving all or part of one chromosome is equivalent to the loss of hundreds or thousands of genes and is called **monosomy**. Conversely, the duplication of part or all of a chromosome results in the cell having three copies of many genes (**trisomy**). The commonest cause of moderate intellectual disability in children is the Down syndrome; this condition is due to the presence of an extra copy of chromosome 21 (trisomy 21).

Monosomy and trisomy interfere with a multitude of cellular functions. The majority of developing embryos that have monosomy or trisomy will have such severe abnormalities in development that the pregnancy will miscarry. The surviving children with monosomy or trisomy always have major developmental problems but they represent the relatively mild end of the spectrum. Approximately 1 in every 200 babies is born with a chromosome abnormality, and structural chromosome abnormalities are a major cause of morbidity and mortality in childhood.

It is important to note that these concerns do not apply to abnormalities in the number of sex chromosomes within the cell. The observation that normal men and women have different numbers of X and Y chromosomes highlights the fact that alterations in the number of sex chromosomes are of less significance than monosomy or trisomy involving autosomes. The Y chromosome is very small and boys with an extra Y chromosome usually demonstrate normal growth and development. The X chromosome is much larger. Children with abnormalities in the number of X chromosomes may have abnormalities of pubertal development and growth but their intellectual development is frequently normal.

An extreme form of trisomy frequently occurs in early pregnancy. The cells of a developing embryo may contain an extra copy of each chromosome, that is, 23 chromosome triplets, or 69 chromosomes in all. This condition is called **triploidy**. It is compatible with survival during the first (and even second) trimester of pregnancy but inevitably results in a miscarriage.

Functional mutations of chromosomes

Occasionally a child will be found to have inherited two copies of a particular chromosome from one parent and none from the other, rather than having one copy from each parent. This is called **uniparental disomy**. If none of the genes on the chromosome involved are imprinted there will be two active copies of each of the genes on that chromosome; this is the same as would be found in the normal situation and the child is healthy. But if one or more genes on the chromosome are imprinted, the child could have zero or two copies of the active gene instead of the normal single copy. This will result in serious problems. For example, the Prader–Willi syndrome is a cause of intellectual disability and obesity in children. It is due to an abnormality involving a gene on chromosome 15. In normal children the maternal copy of the Prader–Willi gene is imprinted; only the paternal copy is active. Some children with this condition have inherited two copies of chromosome 15 from their mothers. The total number of chromosomes and genes is normal but they have no active (paternal) copy of this essential gene.

When do mutations occur?

Conception is the time when the genetic code is most vulnerable

The significance of any mutation depends on when it occurs during development. The moment of conception could be regarded as the time when the genetic code is at its most vulnerable. Any mutation present at that time will be replicated in all the cells of the body. The significance of each mutation will be tested again and again in billions of cells in various stages of growth and differentiation.

Many of the mutations present at conception are new mutations that occurred during the formation of the individual ovum or sperm (or **germ cell**). The process of DNA replication during germ cell formation (or **meiosis**) is even more challenging than that confronting a cell undergoing normal cell division. A germ cell contains one copy of the pairs of chromosomes present in other cells in the body. To create such a cell the germ cell's precursor first duplicates the initial 23 chromosome pairs and then parcels the resulting 92 chromosomes into four equivalent sets of 23 each.

The error rate during meiosis is higher than during mitosis. Approximately 10% of sperm and over 20% of ova have new chromosome errors and many more are presumed to have errors in the DNA sequence. The frequency of new mutations in germ cells accounts for much of the high failure rate of human conception. It is estimated that three quarters of all human conceptions fail to survive longer than the first 6 weeks of a pregnancy; the majority of these miscarriages occur before a woman is aware that she is pregnant. Furthermore, many birth defects are due to new mutations that had occurred during the formation of the egg or sperm from which the baby developed.

If a mutation is present at conception the gonads of the developing baby will also consist of cells with this mutation. This mutation can then be passed on to the child's progeny. In this way a **sporadic mutation** that occurred during the formation of a germ cell in one generation can be transmitted to the next generation and become a **familial mutation**.

Mutations occurring during embryogenesis are limited to specific lineages of cells

Embryogenesis encompasses the first 12 weeks of a pregnancy. It is the period when the organs of the body are formed. A new mutation that occurs during embryogenesis may affect the structure, function or even survival of tissues in that cell lineage; the other cells of the body which lack this mutation will function normally. A mixture within the body of normal cells and cells with a defined mutation is called **somatic mosaicism**; the term 'somatic' refers to the cells of the body other than germ cells. The clinical hallmark of somatic mosaicism is a focal birth defect or (in the skin) a birthmark.

If a mosaic mutation is not present in the gonads it will not be transmitted to the next generation and hence will not be familial. However, if a new mutation occurs in a cell which contributes to the formation of an ovary or testis the mature gonad will contain a mixture of germ

cell precursors which either have or lack the mutation; this situation is called **gonadal mosaicism**. This can result in a healthy person having a number of children with the same 'new' mutation in a certain gene. For example, the condition osteogenesis imperfecta type II is a severe bone dysplasia that is fatal in the newborn period. Each affected baby has a new mutation that occurred in one of the germ cells from which the baby developed. Although each affected baby has a new mutation, the parents are at a 5% risk of having a second affected child. These familial cases are due to one parent having a mixture of mutant and normal germ cells in their testes or ovaries; this is known as gonadal mosaicism. The mutant germ cells had derived from a single mutant precursor cell in the parent.

It is important to recognise that the focal effects of a mosaic mutation can be mimicked by a non mosaic phenomenon. As noted earlier in this chapter, all women inactivate one X chromosome in each cell of the body (lyonisation). In normal individuals there is little to distinguish cells which have inactivated different X chromosomes. However, a mutation on one X chromosome can result in patchy birth defects. If a girl is conceived with a mutation in an essential gene located on one X chromosome, the mutation will interfere with the development of cells in which the mutant X chromosome is left active; cells which *in*activate the mutant X chromosome will function normally. This patchwork of functionally normal and abnormal cells is not due to a mutation which has occurred during embryogenesis but reflects the patchy inactivation of an abnormal gene that is present in every cell of the girl's body. The cells in the girl's ovaries will also have the mutation and the mutation may be transmitted to her children.

Mutations occurring after embryogenesis cause many of the features of ageing

After embryogenesis is completed, the impact of new mutations becomes less apparent. A new mutation cannot wind the developmental clock back and cause a malformation in a previously normal organ or tissue. However, new mutations continue to be generated, and these are transmitted to all the progeny of a cell. These mutations accumulate within a cell's genetic code and eventually interfere with cellular function. If the cellular dysfunction results in cell death, the loss of an individual cell will probably go unnoticed. If a cell accumulates mutations in a number of growth limiting genes, the consequence will be failure to regulate cell division, that is, cancer.

The progressive accumulation of mutations in the nuclear DNA is compounded by a similar process occurring in mitochondrial genes. The rate at which mutations accumulate in mitochondrial DNA is 10–20 times faster than the rate in nuclear genes. This is due to the relatively high exposure of mitochondrial DNA to oxygen radicals (a byproduct of ATP synthesis) and the lack of protective proteins and effective DNA repair mechanisms in mitochondria. The mitochondrial mutation rate is increased even further by hypoxia, which may be a consequence of coronary or cerebral vascular disease. Mitochondrial DNA is replicated independently of nuclear DNA and, as a result, mitochondrial mutations accumulate in cells (such as neurones) that are not actively dividing.

We are usually unaware of our accumulating mutation load but at some point the mutations must inevitably cause problems. The mitochondrial mutations may be so widespread that energy production in many cells is compromised and causes problems such as cardiac failure or dementia, or accumulated mutations in nuclear genes may cause a cell to become malignant.

How are mutations inherited?

The previous section of this chapter has highlighted the fact that an individual's genetic code is not static but is accumulating mutations constantly from the moment of conception. Mutations that are present only in cells outside the gonads are not familial. These mutations may account for the development of clinical problems in an individual, but they will not result in a familial disorder. On the other hand, mutations that are present in the cells of the gonads may be transmitted to a fertilised egg in the next generation. A mutation that is present at conception will subsequently be present in the ovaries or testes of the developing child. If these children then survive to have children of their own, the mutation may be transmitted again to the next generation.

An autosomal recessive disorder is due to mutations in both copies of a gene

With the exception of sperm and ova, the cells of the body have two copies of the genes present on the autosomes (that is, on chromosomes other than the sex chromosomes). If a mutation interferes with the function of one copy of a gene, the presence of the other normal copy of the gene may be sufficient to prevent the development of a medical problem. This type of mutation could be inherited by many family members who remain healthy and are unaware that they are carrying the mutation. It is called an **autosomal recessive** mutation. We all have at least 2–3 different genes with recessive mutations affecting just one copy. A person who has a recessive mutation in a particular gene is called a **carrier** of that mutation.

It is much more serious if a person has recessive mutations in both copies of a particular gene. This situation could arise if both parents are carriers of mutations in the gene and the child has inherited the mutant gene from each parent (Fig. 28.2). In the absence of a normal copy of the gene the child will develop an autosomal recessive

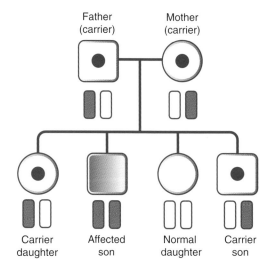

Fig. 28.2   An example of a pedigree demonstrating autosomal recessive inheritance. Both parents are carriers of mutations in a particular gene and hence have one normal and one abnormal copy of the gene (indicated as white and grey rectangles, respectively). There is a 50% (1/2) chance that a child will inherit the mutant gene from one parent, and a 50% (1/2) chance that the mutant gene will be inherited from the other parent. The chance that the child will inherit the mutant genes from **both** parents and develop the disorder in question is 25% (1/2 × 1/2 = 1/4). By similar reasoning, the chance of this couple having a child with no mutations (i.e. two normal genes) is also 25%; the risk of the child being a carrier is 25% + 25% = 50%. The symbols used for males, females, carriers and affected people are those in common use.

disorder related to the absence of the specific protein encoded by that gene. Autosomal recessive disorders affect both boys and girls.

The hallmark of autosomal recessive inheritance is the presence of affected siblings with other members of the extended family being unaffected. Some of the unaffected family members will, of course, be carriers, but if their partner is not a carrier of the same disorder they will not have affected children and their carrier status will not be suspected.

Thousands of autosomal recessive disorders have been identified. The frequency of an autosomal recessive disorder will be determined by the frequency of carriers in the population. The carrier frequencies for many autosomal recessive conditions vary in different ethnic groups and may be quite high. For example, the carrier frequency for mutations causing cystic fibrosis (among Caucasians) and β-thalassaemia (in some Mediterranean populations) is approximately 5–10%. As a consequence, these disorders are relatively common in those populations. However the carrier frequency of most autosomal recessive disorders is approximately 1%, and the chance of both parents being carriers for the same disorder is very small. Consanguinity represents an important exception; a couple who are biologically related are more likely to be carriers of the same disorder than a couple picked at random from the general population, and parental consanguinity increases the chance of their children having an autosomal recessive disorder.

An autosomal dominant disorder is due to a mutation in one copy of a gene

For certain autosomal genes and mutations, the presence of one abnormal gene may be sufficient to cause a clinical disorder. In this situation most of the family members who have the mutated gene will be affected. This type of mutation is called an **autosomal dominant** mutation. Dominant mutations are less common than recessive mutations. Autosomal dominant disorders affect both boys and girls.

In contrast to an autosomal recessive disorder, an autosomal dominant disorder may be passed down successive generations (Fig. 28.3). In some large families with an autosomal dominant disorder it may be apparent that an individual has the mutation, yet is unaffected. The reasons why some individuals remain healthy despite having a dominant mutation are not usually known.

An autosomal dominant disorder may be due to a new mutation that occurred for the first time in the egg or sperm from which the affected person developed. For this reason a child may have a dominant disorder yet may be the only affected person in the family. In this situation, the recurrence risk of the disorder in the siblings of the affected child would be very low, but the recurrence risk among the offspring of the affected child would be 50%. A new dominant mutation may cause such a severe disorder that the affected child does not survive to reproduce. Many abnormalities of chromosome structure fall into this category. These disorders are never familial because the severity of the dominant mutation precludes the possibility of reproduction.

It is often not clear why some genes or mutations cause a recessive rather than a dominant disorder. Some genes produce an abundance of the particular protein from each copy of the gene, and the presence of one normal gene is more than sufficient to meet the cell's needs. Mutations in these genes will cause a recessive disorder. For other genes it may be essential that both are active for sufficient protein to be produced. A mutation in just one gene may cause such a reduction in protein production that cell function is compromised. A mutation in this type of gene would result in a dominant disorder. A dominant disorder may also be due to abnormal interactions between different proteins. Certain proteins bind together in the normal cell to form a complex of proteins that has a particular function. A mutant gene may produce a protein of abnormal structure that interferes with the function of the protein complex even though the other proteins in the complex are normal.

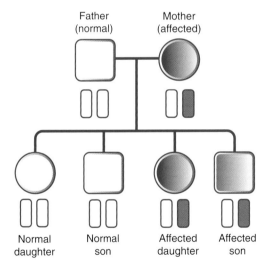

Father (normal) Mother (affected)

Normal daughter   Normal son   Affected daughter   Affected son

Fig. 28.3   An example of a pedigree demonstrating autosomal dominant inheritance. One parent has a mutation in a particular gene and hence has one normal and one abnormal copy of the gene (indicated as white and grey rectangles, respectively). A child will inherit a normal gene from the unaffected parent. The child could inherit a normal gene from the affected parent (as shown for the first and second children; 50% (1/2) chance for each child) or the abnormal gene from the affected parent (third and fourth children; 50% (1/2) chance for each child). The symbols used for males, females and affected people are those in common use.

An X linked recessive disorder is due to a recessive mutation on the X chromosome

Mutations on the X chromosome demonstrate an important and common mode of inheritance. If a girl has a recessive mutation on one X chromosome the presence of the normal gene on the other X chromosome usually prevents the development of a severe genetic disorder. The girl would be a carrier of the mutation. On the other hand, a boy has just one X chromosome and a mutation on the X chromosome will result in a genetic disorder. A disorder due to a recessive mutation on the X chromosome is referred to as an **X linked recessive** disorder. A family with an X linked disorder will have affected males and carrier females (Fig. 28.4).

If there is only one boy in the family with an X linked recessive disorder, his mother may be a carrier and the absence of affected male relatives may be due to chance. In this situation the recurrence risk among the boy's brothers would be 50% (1/2). On the other hand, the absence of affected male relatives could indicate that the boy has a new mutation which occurred for the first time during the formation of the egg from which he developed. In this situation the recurrence risk among his brothers would be very low. The distinction between these two possibilities is usually of great concern to the parents and represents a major task for the clinical geneticist.

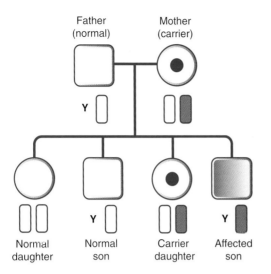

Father
(normal)

Mother
(carrier)

Y

Normal
daughter

Normal
son

Y

Carrier
daughter

Affected
son

Y

Fig. 28.4 An example of a pedigree demonstrating X linked recessive inheritance. The mother is a carrier of a mutant gene on the X chromosome. She has one normal and one abnormal copy of the gene (indicated as white and grey rectangles, respectively). Her husband has a single normal X chromosome (white rectangle) and a normal Y chromosome (as shown). A child could inherit the normal gene from the mother (as shown for the first two children; 50% (1/2) chance for each child) or inherit the abnormal gene from the mother (as shown for the third and fourth children; 50% (1/2) chance for each child). Each child could inherit the father's normal X chromosome (and be female, as shown for the first and third children; 50% (1/2) chance for each child) or his Y chromosome (and be male, as shown for the second and fourth children; 50% (1/2) chance for each child). Overall there is a 25% (1/2 × 1/2 = 1/4) chance of each of the following outcomes: normal daughter, normal son, carrier daughter and affected son.

It is important to note that some female carriers of an X linked recessive disorder may be mildly affected. This is in contrast to the situation with carriers of an autosomal recessive disorder. A woman inactivates one X chromosome in every cell (lyonisation). The normal and mutant X chromosomes within a cell are usually equally likely to be inactivated. On average 50% of the cells will have inactivated the normal X chromosome. The other cells will have inactivated the mutant X chromosome and the woman is unlikely to demonstrate any features of the X linked recessive disorder. But some women tend to inactivate their normal X chromosome, and the mutant X chromosome may be left activated in the majority of cells. In this situation a woman may demonstrate mild features of an X linked recessive disorder.

A polygenic disorder is due the interaction of a number of different genes

Many common genetic disorders cannot be attributed to a mutation in a single gene but are due to the interaction of a number of genes. Examples of such **polygenic**

disorders include common congenital malformations, such as cleft lip, and disorders of later life, such as asthma, diabetes and schizophrenia. These conditions result from the interaction of a number of genes, each of which has some mutation or polymorphism that increases the risk of the condition. Any one of these mutations or polymorphisms cannot cause the disorder on its own.

Even if a fetus has inherited a number of mutations that place it at increased risk of a birth defect, non genetic factors, such as maternal nutrition or chance, may ultimately determine whether the malformation occurs. A disorder due to the interaction of multiple genes and non genetic factors is called a **multifactorial** disorder. An example is spina bifida.

Polygenic and multifactorial disorders typically affect between 0.1% and 1% of the population. The recurrence risk among close relatives is usually 10–20 times higher (that is, 1–2%). Few of the genes responsible for polygenic disorders have been identified, and this remains a major objective in genetic research.

Disorders due to mutations in mitochondrial DNA exhibit maternal inheritance

Mitochondria are essential for providing chemical energy to the cell. Some mitochondrial proteins are encoded by genes within the nucleus, while the remainder are encoded by a small loop of DNA within the mitochondrion itself. Mutations in either the nuclear or mitochondrial genes will result in impairment of normal energy production by the mitochondrion. An abnormality of mitochondrial function due to a mutation in a nuclear gene demonstrates autosomal recessive or X linked inheritance (Figs 28.2 and 28.4). A mutation in a nuclear gene will affect all of the mitochondria and all the affected children in a family will have similar problems.

A mitochondrial abnormality due a mutation in a mitochondrial gene will be maternally inherited, that is, the abnormal mitochondria will always have been inherited from the child's mother (Fig. 28.5). A child with such a mutation may have a mixture of normal and mutant mitochondria in each cell. The impact of the mutation on cell function will depend on what proportion of mitochondria are affected. A small number of mutant mitochondria may have little impact on cell function in a woman and she may be asymptomatic. The distribution of mitochondria to new cells during cell division is random and it is possible that an ovum could have a relatively high proportion of mutant mitochondria. During subsequent development the many cells of the fetus could inherit varying proportions of mutant mitochondria. Those tissues that have a high proportion of mutant mitochondria will not function correctly, while other tissues with comparatively low proportions of mutant mitochondria may function normally. For this reason disorders due to mutations in mitochondrial genes demonstrate marked

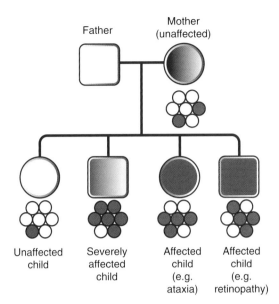

Father

Mother
(unaffected)

Unaffected
child

Severely
affected
child

Affected
child
(e.g.
ataxia)

Affected
child
(e.g.
retinopathy)

Fig. 28.5 An example of a pedigree demonstrating mitochondrial inheritance. The cells of the mother have a mixture of normal and mutant mitochondria (shown as a mixture of white and grey circles, respectively); the majority of the mitochondria are normal and the woman is unaffected. Her husband has normal mitochondria; these are not transmitted to his children and are not shown. A child could inherit predominantly normal mitochondria from the mother and be unaffected (first child); a child could inherit predominantly abnormal mitochondria and be severely affected (second child); or the child could inherit an intermediate proportion of mutant mitochondria and the manifestations of the disease would depend on the proportion of mutant mitochondria in various tissues (third and fourth children). The probabilities of each of these outcomes cannot be predicted.

variability in both severity and the type of tissue involved within the one family. Disorders due to mitochondrial mutations affect both boys and girls.

The practical application of genetics

The application of the genetic principles outlined in this chapter will primarily be found in the other chapters of this book. The pattern of inheritance of a child's disorder is clearly a major issue in counselling parents about their child's condition. An understanding of the different types of mutation will become essential for interpreting laboratory reports. The ability to define the molecular basis of a disorder may also make prenatal diagnosis in the next pregnancy an option for the parents.

The ability to define specific mutations may also raise ethical issues. Should there be widespread screening for carriers of common autosomal recessive disorders? Should children be tested to determine carrier status at a

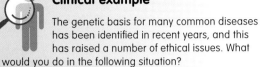

Clinical example

The genetic basis for many common diseases has been identified in recent years, and this has raised a number of ethical issues. What would you do in the following situation?

Preamble
Cystic fibrosis is a common autosomal recessive disorder that affects approximately 1:2000 Caucasian children. It causes recurrent lung infections and malabsorption of food. Children with cystic fibrosis die during infancy unless they are treated. With intensive (and expensive) therapy at home and in hospital the median life span of these children has increased to 30–40 years. With improvements in therapy, this outlook will probably improve in the future.

Approximately 1:20 healthy Caucasian adults are carriers of a mutation that can cause cystic fibrosis. Over 600 different mutations have been identified. One mutation (deletion of codon 508 that encodes phenylalanine) accounts for 80% of all mutations; the other mutations are all much less common. A simple and cheap test for the common mutation is available.

Proposal
It has been proposed that all people in Caucasian communities could be screened for the presence of this mutation. The aim would be to identify couples who are both carriers and hence would be at 25% risk of having an affected child. The couple could opt for prenatal diagnosis (and termination of affected fetuses) or consider other reproductive options.

Arguments in favour
● Cystic fibrosis is expensive in financial, social and emotional terms. Any cost effective means for reducing the frequency of the disorder should be considered.
● Couples who are carriers are not obliged to consider prenatal diagnosis and termination of affected fetuses; other reproductive options are available, such as insemination with donor semen.

Arguments against
● Screening implies prenatal diagnosis and termination of pregnancy. Termination of pregnancy is not acceptable because conventional therapies have been very successful in improving the survival and quality of life of people with cystic fibrosis.
● Screening for cystic fibrosis carriers is incomplete. Genetic testing cannot identify all mutations and 20% of the carriers will be missed. If one person is identified as a carrier and the partner is not, there remains a 1% chance that the partner has a rare mutation and is a carrier.
● Genetic testing will result in attention being inappropriately focused on a single gene. Those who are identified as carriers may be subject to discrimination or may consider themselves to be unhealthy. The survival and value of an individual involves far more than one gene.

Similar arguments could be made for (and against) screening for carriers of other autosomal recessive disorders. Do you think that such screening programmes should be established? You may wish to explore this issue further at the following web site: www.exploratorium.edn/genepool/ETHEX.html

young age so that they can grow up mindful of this knowledge, or should genetic testing be deferred until a child can give informed consent to have the DNA test performed?

The parents of a child who has a genetic disorder due either to a new mutation or to inherited mutations are usually stunned. They may be angry or confused, blaming themselves for causing the problem, or they may search for some environmental agent to blame. It can be very difficult for them, indeed for anyone, to accept the genetic basis of the disorder. It is often helpful to highlight the universality of mutations. We are all conceived with mutations inherited from both of our parents, and we all create new mutations throughout development and postnatal life. The processes that caused the mutations responsible for the child's condition are the same processes which ultimately cause our own demise.

The dysmorphic child

E. Thompson

Dysmorphic, which literally means 'abnormal form', refers to an unusual appearance, usually of the face. A dysmorphic child may have an underlying diagnosis that could have implications for the health not only of the child but also of other family members if the condition is inherited. The child may present as a neonate with one or more birth defects, such as a missing hand, or with developmental delay or intellectual disability, an organ defect such as congenital heart disease, failure to thrive or obesity, short or tall stature, a behavioural disturbance or a metabolic problem.

Birth defects can be classified as deformations, disruptions, dyplasias or malformations (Ch. 27). It is important to distinguish between abnormalities and minor variants which are common in the general population. These can, however, appear in syndromes. For example, a unilateral single transverse palmar crease is seen in 4% of normal people but is more common in Down syndrome. Some physical traits, such as an unusual shaped nose, are a harmless family variant but, again, could be part of an undiagnosed syndrome in the family.

Making an overall diagnosis relies on recognising a pattern of problems. The types of pattern include:

- *Syndrome*. This is from the Greek 'running together' and refers to a cluster of physical and other features occurring in a consistent pattern, with an implied common specific cause which may be unknown. The word syndrome is often used loosely to describe any of the other diagnostic patterns described below.
- *Association*. This is a group of physical features that tends to occur together but the link is not consistent enough to allow the term syndrome to be used. An example is the VATER association (see below)
- *Sequence*. This refers to a group of abnormalities caused by a cascade of events beginning with one malformation. An example is the Potter sequence which can result from any cause of severe oligohydramnios, such as renal agenesis. For example: renal agenesis → no fetal urine → severe oligohydramnios → lung hypoplasia and intrauterine constraint → limb deformities, such as talipes and a compressed facial appearance.
- *Developmental field defect*. This refers to a group of malformations caused by a harmful influence in a particular region of the embryo. Abnormalities of blood flow are thought to underlie many of these. An example is hemifacial microsomia with unilateral facial hypoplasia and ear anomalies relating to an abnormality in development of first and second branchial arch structures.

Why is it important to recognise an underlying diagnosis? Some important reasons are:
- avoiding unnecessary investigations
- providing information about prognosis for doctors and family
- recognising complications that need to be looked for prospectively
- determining the pattern of inheritance and recurrence risk
- enabling support from other families. Individual syndromes are rare and parents become the experts in day to day management of the child and can share this with other families.

Are there any pitfalls in making a diagnosis? Some areas for consideration are:
- The diagnosis must be correct. Often the diagnosis is based on clinical assessment alone with no confirmatory tests. Diagnosis must not be not undertaken lightly as it can be difficult to remove or alter a diagnosis once it has been made, with harmful consequences for the child and family.
- Parents do not wish their child to be labelled, especially if the child is young and they do not yet perceive any problems themselves.
- Doctors may attribute all new problems to the syndrome.

How to assess the dysmorphic child

Instant recognition

A 'waiting room diagnosis' based on the facial 'gestalt' might be made if the doctor has seen a person with the particular syndrome before, just as most people are able to recognise if a person in the street has Down syndrome. Often, however, the diagnosis is not apparent initially, and the following approach is recommended.

History

A detailed medical history is important. Special points to note include:

- Antenatal history:
  — Teratogens, such as drugs, viruses, maternal diabetes, maternal hyperthermia (Ch. 27)
  — Fetal movements. A neuromuscular disorder may cause reduced fetal movements resulting in arthrogryposis (multiple fixed deformities of joints).
  — Prenatal screening and diagnostic tests.
- Perinatal history, weight, length and head circumference and Apgar scores at birth.
- Growth and development, behaviour, sleep patterns.
- Family history; draw a family tree noting the following:
  — Miscarriages, stillbirths and deaths of siblings.
  — Information about other family members with the same features.

Examination

Observe before undressing or disturbing the child. On the other hand, the examination is not complete until the child has been fully undressed. Especially note:

- Behaviour and alertness.
- Body size and proportions, relative head size, asymmetry, chest shape and spinal curvature.
- Height, weight, head circumference, arm span, upper and lower body segments.
- Always plot measurements on standard normal charts. Charts are available for many different body parts, e.g. hand measurements, foot and ear length. Special charts are available for certain disorders, such as Down syndrome, and various bone dysplasias, such as achondroplasia.
- Facial features:
  — Shape of the head and face
  — Spacing of the eyes (hyper- or hypotelorism, i.e. wide or closely spaced); slant of the palpebral fissures (up or down)
  — Shape and size of the nose and mouth
  — Structure and position of the ears.
- Proportions of the limbs, muscle bulk and tone, joint contractures and mobility.
- Structure of hands and feet (shape, length, number of digits, dermal ridges, nails).
- Skin pigmentary or vascular markings.
- External genitalia.
- Any birth defects (for example, cleft palate)?
- Auscultate the chest for any cardiac nurmurs.
- Palpate the abdomen for organomegaly.

A *photograph* (with parental consent) is useful for:
- comparing later on to see how the face has changed
- consulting colleagues.

Examining the family of a child with unusual facial features:

- Parents and siblings should be examined to see if this is a family characteristic.
- Photographs of them at a younger age and of other family members may be helpful.
- In the event of a syndrome being diagnosed, the family should also be examined for its specific features.

Putting it all together

- *Check textbooks of syndromes* (see Further Reading list) by trying to match the most important dysmorphic features and comparing the photographs with those of the patient.
- *Consultation:*
  — **Paediatricians** will recognise the more common syndromes, for example Down syndrome
  — **Clinical geneticists** have experience in identifying many more syndromes. Some have a special interest and expertise in syndrome diagnosis (**dysmorphologists**)
  — It's not easy! A skilled dysmorphologist makes a syndrome diagnosis in a dysmorphic child in only 20% of cases referred from an experienced paediatrician.
  — If an overall diagnosis is not made, the recognised problems must still be managed.
- *Review* in a few years may allow a diagnosis to be made, as the features of many syndromes evolve with time and new information or laboratory techniques may be available for specific diagnoses.
- *Computerised databases*
  — Several thousand syndromes are published, and many are individually rare.
  — Computerised databases combine pictures and descriptions of syndromes.
  — Searches are made using a few key dysmorphic features and a number of possible diagnoses are suggested which can be compared with the patient.
  — Occasionally, a match will be achieved!
  — Success is more likely if relatively rare features are used for the search. For example, a common feature such as hypertelorism (wide spaced eyes) would give a long list of suggested syndromes, whereas imperforate anus would give a more manageable list to consider.
  — Training and experience are needed to use these databases effectively.

Examples of these databases are:
- POSSUM (Pictures Of Standard Syndromes and Undiagnosed Malformations) developed by the Genetic Health Services, Victoria, Australia
- The London Dysmorphology Database
- REAMS (a Radiological Electronic Atlas of Malformation Syndromes and Skeletal Dysplasias).

Investigation

Chromosome analysis:

- A routine chromosome study (karyotype) on blood lymphocytes should be done on all children with an intellectual disability, especially when dysmorphic features and birth defects are present.
- Submicroscopic deletions or duplications of a gene or cluster of genes underlie some syndromes. These may be detected by FISH (fluorescence in situ hybridisation). Examples of these are Williams syndrome with an elastin gene deletion.
- Subtelomeric rearrangements detectable by FISH occur in about 7% of children with an unexplained intellectual disability, often with dysmorphic features. The subtelomeres are just next to the ends of the chromosomes and are prone to structural rearrangement.
- Parental chromosomes may need to be examined if a structural alteration is found, in order to clarify the abnormality and to facilitate genetic counselling in the family.

Other investigations such as metabolic studies or radiology should be done as clinically indicated.

The following are some of the more common dysmorphic syndromes seen in childhood.

Common chromosomal disorders

Children with chromosome disorders, particularly of the autosomes (chromosomes 1–22), tend to be small, dysmorphic and have an intellectual impairment.

Numerical chromosome disorders

Trisomy 21 (Down syndrome) (Fig 29.1, p. 290)

- Commonest chromosome disorder in liveborn babies and commonest genetic cause of intellectual disability.
- Birth incidence is about 1 in 1200 live births; the overall incidence rises after maternal age of 35 years.
- Maternal serum screening and ultrasound can be offered to all pregnant women to identify those at high risk, who may then opt for prenatal diagnosis by amniocentesis.
- Features include:
  - Flat midface, flat occiput, upward slanting eyes with medial epicanthic folds, Brushfield spots in the iris, palpebrae 'purse' on laughing or crying, small down turned mouth and protruding tongue, small ears, excess nuchal skin in the neonate.
  - Short fingers, clinodactyly of the fifth fingers (short middle phalanges lead to incurving), single palmar creases, widened gap between 1st and 2nd toes.
  - Birth defects may be present; for example, congenital heart disease in 40–50%, duodenal atresia, anal atresia and many others.
  - Intellectual disability of varying degree, mean IQ < 50, up to about 70 and declines with age; all have neuropathological changes of Alzheimer disease by 35–40 years with clinical onset in early 50s; is an important cause of death in adults.
  - Slightly reduced life span (around 60 years if no organ defects).
- Follow up is necessary for children with Down syndrome to monitor for:
  - Cataracts, strabismus (30–40%), leukaemia, hypothyroidism, obesity, infections, constipation, obstructive sleep apnoea, dental problems and atlantoaxial instability, but only a minority develop neurological complications from this.
  - Behaviour: often happy, affectionate, friendly but anxiety and depression often occur with age.
- Cause:
  - 95% have trisomy for chromosome 21 with a low recurrence risk.
  - The rest have either a Robertsonian translocation (a chromosome 21 attached to another similar chromosome, usually chromosome 14), or
  - Mosaicism (some cells with trisomy 21 and some with a normal karyotype).
  - Half of the translocation cases are inherited from a parent, so parental chromosomes should be checked *only* if there is a translocation. An inherited translocation is associated with an increased risk of recurrence.

Trisomy 18 (Edwards syndrome)

- Birth incidence is about 1 in 8000 live births.
- Many have prenatal ultrasound abnormalities and are then detected at amniocentesis.
- Low birth weight, prominent occiput, dysplastic low set ears, micrognathia (small chin), short palpebral fissures, small mouth.
- Characteristic clenched hand posture (5th and 2nd fingers overlap 4th and 3rd); prominent heels.
- Malformations are common; for example, heart, brain, exomphalos, kidney.
- Behaviour: poor feeding and neurological development, about one third die in the first month, less than 10% live beyond 1 year.
- Most have trisomy for chromosome 18, which is associated with advanced maternal age; a few have translocations.
- Recurrence risk for trisomy or non inherited translocation is low and prenatal diagnosis is available.

Trisomy 13 (Patau syndrome)

- Birth incidence is about 1 in 30 000 live births.
- Many have prenatal ultrasound abnormalities and are then detected at amniocentesis.

- Low birth weight, microcephaly with sloping forehead, scalp defects, cleft lip and palate, broad flat nose, polydactyly (extra digits).
- Birth defects such as holoprosencephaly and heart defects are common.
- Very poor neurological status and 50% of babies die within the first month.
- Most have trisomy 13 associated with advanced maternal age; some have translocations.
- Recurrence risk for trisomy is low and prenatal diagnosis is available.

Turner syndrome

- One of the commonest chromosome defects at conception but the majority miscarry, usually at an early stage of pregnancy.
- Birth incidence is around 1 in 3000 liveborn girls.
- Lymphoedema of hands and feet and redundant nuchal skin are common in neonates.
- May present in childhood with short stature, or in adolescence with failure of puberty.
- Variable features, which include: webbed neck, increased carrying angle of elbows, broad chest, pigmented naevi, narrow deep set hyperconvex nails, coarctation of the aorta, idiopathic hypertension, renal anomalies.
- Intelligence normal but specific learning problems are common.
- Most are infertile because the ovaries are dysplastic.
- Pregnancy has been achieved by in vitro fertilisation using donor eggs.
- The mean untreated adult height is around 140 cm. Refer early for assessment regarding growth hormone treatment.
- Cause: 60% have 45,X, others have a structural defect in which one X chromosome is missing all or part of the p (short) arm, or there is mosaicism 46,XX/45,X.
- Not associated with advanced maternal age, recurrence risk not increased.

Klinefelter syndrome

- Birth incidence is about 1 in 700 liveborn males.
- Many present as adolescents with delayed puberty, or as adults with infertility.
- May present in childhood with developmental delay, especially of speech or with learning disabilities, often involving reading and mathematics.
- Overall, IQ is reduced compared to siblings but can be normal.
- Features: tall stature, long limbs, small testes, undescended testes, gynaecomastia and female fat distribution with age, infertility, behaviour problems.
- Treatment with testosterone at puberty will bring about a more normal virilisation.

- Cause: 47, XXY karyotype.
- Recurrence risk is low.

Triple X syndrome

- Birth incidence is about 1 in 1500 liveborn females.
- Features: tall stature, few dysmorphic features.
- Intellect: can be normal, but overall the IQ is lower than that of siblings. Learning difficulties, delayed speech and motor milestones, poor coordination and behaviour problems are common.
- Pubertal development and fertility are generally normal.
- Cause: 46,XXX karyotype.
- Recurrence risk low to sibs and offspring.

Structural chromosome disorders

Fragile X syndrome (Fig. 29.1b, p. 290)

- This is the commonest familial form of intellectual impairment affecting 1 in 4000 males and 1 in 10 000 females.
- Features:
  — intellectual disability of varying degree, usually more severe in males than females.
  — mild dysmorphism with macrocephaly, high forehead, long face, large jaw, big ears, post-pubertal macro-orchidism (large testes).
  — soft skin, joint laxity.
  — shy personality, autistic features.
- Cause:
  — A mutation called an 'unstable triplet repeat' in the FMR1 gene on the X chromosome.
  — A normal FMR1 gene contains a sequence with 5–55 copies of a CCG triplet.
  — A *premutation* contains 55–230 CCG repeats. Male and female carriers of this are clinically normal (note that normal male carriers are unusual in X linked disorders).
  — A *full mutation* contains more than 230 CCG repeats. All males and about 60% of females with a full mutation show clinical features of the syndrome. The full mutation in males and some females is associated with the appearance of a 'fragile site' on light micoscopy when cells are cultured in folate deficient medium.
  — When the CCG repeat is passed from a carrier mother to a child (but not from a carrier father), it is unstable and tends to enlarge.
  — Intellectual impairment increases with CCG repeat number.
  — Female carriers pass the abnormal gene to 50% of their children but only males with the full mutation and 60% of females with the full mutation will be affected with the syndrome.

— Male premutation carriers pass the premutation unchanged to their daughters and both are clinically normal.

- DNA testing can identify carriers of the pre- and full mutation.
- Female premutation carriers are at risk of premature menopause.
- Prenatal diagnosis on chorionic villus sampling or amniocentesis is available but is complicated by the uncertainty of clinical outcome in a female fetus carrying a full mutation.
- The above is called fragile XA syndrome. There is also a much less common fragile XE syndrome which is similar clinically and at the DNA level but involves a CCG repeat in the FMR2 gene on the X chromosome.

Velocardiofacial syndrome (also called VCFS, Shprintzen, 22q deletion, DiGeorge, Cayler and Sedlacková syndromes) (Fig 29.1c, p. 290)

- Estimated birth incidence may be as high as 1 in 2000.
- Very variable syndrome with > 180 clinical features described!
- Suspect the diagnosis if a child has the following two features:
  — Cleft palate. VCFS is found in 8% of children with cleft palate and 5% with cleft lip and palate.
  — Conotruncal congenital heart defects (aortic arch defects, ventricular septal defect, pulmonary atresia/stenosis, tetralogy of Fallot and truncus arteriosus). VCFS is found in about 5% of children with a congenital heart defect.
- Facial appearance variable but often there is a prominent nasal bridge, narrow nostrils, bulbous nasal tip.
- Older children often have developmental delay and learning disabilities, social immaturity, anxiety and phobias.
- Up to 20% of adults have psychiatric illness.
- Cause:
  — Deletion of 22q11, visible in only 15%, detectable by FISH in the others.
  — Up to 5% who clinically appear to have the syndrome have no detectable deletion.
  — Parents should be tested, as features can be mild and risk to each child of a carrier is 50%.
- Prenatal diagnosis is available.

Other common disorders

VATER association

- An acronym for **V**ertebral anomalies, **A**nal malformations, **T**racheo-**E**sophageal fistula with (o) esophageal atresia (American spelling), **R**adial and **R**enal anomalies.

- **C**ardiac and non-radial **L**imb abnormalities are common and the association is sometimes enlarged to **VACTERL**.
- No particular facial appearance is associated and mental development usually is normal.
- Cause unknown.
- Recurrence risk is low.

Noonan syndrome

- Can present in utero with fetal nuchal oedema.
- Birth incidence 1 in 1000 to 1 in 2500 live births.
- Main features:
  — Short stature. Some have growth hormone deficiency.
  — Short neck with webbing or redundancy of skin.
  — Cardiac defect, especially pulmonary stenosis, atrial septal defect, ventricular septal defect, patent ductus arteriosus, hypertrophic cardiomyopathy.
  — Characteristic chest deformity with pectus carinatum superiorly and pectus excavatum inferiorly.
  — Broad chest with widespaced nipples.
  — Characteristic facial appearance which changes with age:
  > hypertelorism, broad forehead, ptosis, down slanting eyes in infancy, epicanthic folds, posteriorly rotated ears
  > similar facial appearance to Turner syndrome but affects both sexes and chromosomes are normal.
- Developmental delay is common and mild intellectual disability occurs in about 1/3 of cases.
- Look for:
  — Hearing loss (1/3 of cases).
  — A bleeding diathesis (1/3 of cases).
  — Visual problems (in most children with the syndrome).
- Many are sporadic but is transmitted to offspring as an autosomal dominant.
- Mutations in a gene called PTPN11 on chromosome 12q24.1 have been identified in about 50% of 22 Noonan syndrome patients (other loci may be involved).
- Prenatal diagnosis is not routinely available.

Marfan syndrome

- Incidence 1–2 in 10 000 individuals.
- Connective tissue disorder caused by mutations in the fibrillin gene (at chromosome 15q21.1).
- Diagnosis is clinical and is based on established criteria (the Ghent criteria, 1996).
- Features include:
  — Musculoskeletal:
  > tall stature, long limbs with significantly increased arm span and reduced upper to lower body segment ratio

long fingers (arachnodactyly)

joint laxity and flat feet

chest deformity and kyphoscoliosis

long narrow face with deep set eyes, a high narrow palate and dental crowding.

— Cardiovascular:

mitral valve prolapse

dilatation of the ascending aorta in 50% of children, which requires drug therapy to prevent or delay development of aortic dissection and rupture.

— Eye:

ectopia lentis (dislocation of the lens, often upward)

myopia

retinal detachment.

- Other problems such as spontaneous pneumothorax, striae (stretch marks of the skin) and herniae can occur.
- Mental develpment is normal.
- Autosomal dominant, 25% of cases are new mutations (that is, parents are normal).
- Prenatal diagnosis is possible in some families in which the fibrillin mutation has been identified.

Achondroplasia

- Commonest and most widely recognised skeletal dysplasia affecting about 1 in 26 000–28 000 newborns.
- Main features:
  - Short stature. Mean adult height is 130 cm in males and 125 cm in females.
  - Short limbs, most marked in the upper segments of the limbs (rhizomelic Shortening).
  - Short fingers with 'trident' hand shape.

— Relatively large head, depressed nasal bridge.

— Small chest.

- The radiological features are also characteristic and allow a firm diagnosis to be made soon after birth.
- Length can be within the normal range at birth. Occasionally the diagnosis is unrecognised for a few months.
- Regular follow up is required throughout childhood to monitor for complications such as:
  - Hydrocephalus.
  - Constriction of the cervicomedullary junction, mainly in the first 2 years.
  - Upper airway obstruction, especially during sleep, due to small upper airway size.
  - Middle ear dysfunction and hearing loss.
  - Kyphosis.
  - Lumbosacral spinal stenosis causing symptoms in older children and adults.
  - Hypermobile joints, knee instability.
  - Varus deformity (bow legs).
  - Dental crowding.
  - Adverse psychosocial impact of the disorder on the child and family.
- Treatment:
  - Growth hormone transiently increases growth velocity but it is not known if final adult height is increased.
  - Limb lengthening by cutting and stretching the long bones with an external distractor is controversial. Many families believe it is better to modify the environment rather than the child.
- Autosomal dominant inheritance is usual but most cases result from a new mutation in the FGRF3 (fibroblast growth factor receptor 3) gene.

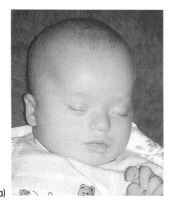 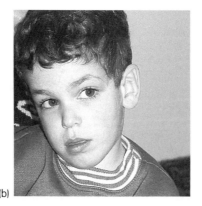 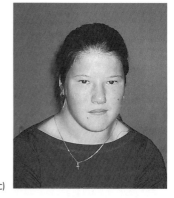

(a) (b) (c)

Fig 29.1 (a) Down syndrome. Note round face, small mouth, upward-slanting palpebral fissures. (b) Fragile X syndrome. Note long face, macrocephaly, big ears. (c) Velocardiofacial syndrome. Note long mid-face, prominent nose with a squared-off nasal tip and notched alae nasi.

Genetic counselling 30

M. B. Delatycki

Genetic counselling is what happens when an individual, a couple or a family asks questions of a health professional about a medical condition or disease that is, or may be, genetic in origin. Genetic counselling is not always provided by genetic specialists (clinical geneticists or genetic counsellors). It is appropriate for paediatricians and disease oriented specialists to counsel in their own area of expertise. It may be difficult, however, for the doctor who looks after a child with a genetic condition to challenge a family to look at their feelings in the genetic counselling context. Even when another practitioner provides genetic counselling to the immediate family, the genetic specialists will often be involved in counselling the broader family.

The provider of counselling for any particular condition or situation tends to evolve with time. As new technology arises it is often the genetic specialist who will counsel the family, but with time this often falls to the disease oriented specialist and general practitioner. An example is counselling for advanced maternal age and tests to diagnose Down syndrome prenatally. In the 1980s medical geneticists and some specialised obstetricians largely undertook this. It is now done by obstetricians and general practitioners in most instances.

Genetic specialists

Clinical geneticists are medical practitioners who undertake specialist training in this discipline. Their primary training is usually in paediatrics or adult internal medicine but can be in other areas, such as obstetrics and gynaecology.

Genetic counselling is a relatively young paramedical profession in Australasia. Genetic counsellors come from a range of different backgrounds, such as science, nursing and teaching. They undertake a basic training programme in both genetics and counselling, followed by on the job training.

Areas that are covered by genetic specialist practice include:
- dysmorphology
- prenatal counselling and testing
- neurogenetics
- cancer genetics
- bone dysplasias
- metabolic diseases.

As can be seen, it covers a wide age range of patients — pre conception to post mortem! Traditionally a paediatric specialty, the genetic specialist is increasingly involved in diagnosis and counselling for adult onset disease as more and more genes are discovered for these conditions.

Indications for formal genetic counselling

Anybody who suspects that there might be an increased risk of a genetic condition or producing a child with a genetic condition or birth defect may wish to receive formal genetic counselling. This includes:
- individuals who themselves have a genetic disorder (e.g. myotonic dystrophy)
- couples who have had a stillbirth
- couples who have had a child with a birth defect
- couples who have had a child with mental retardation
- family history of any of the above
- family history of known genetic disorders, such as Huntington disease, muscular dystrophy
- multiple miscarriages
- exposure to radiation or drugs during pregnancy
- advanced maternal age
- consanguinity
- chromosome translocations
- cancers.

For appropriate genetic counselling, the following are essential:
- diagnostic precision
- knowledge of risk
- knowledge of burden
- knowledge of reproductive options
- knowledge of scientific advances
- counselling skills.

Process of genetic counselling

The genetic specialist needs to allow each family at least 1 hour in quiet surroundings. Medical records and doctors' reports are best obtained before undertaking counselling as this will make the consultation more efficient.

Detailed histories or records of probands (the affected individual through whom a family with a genetic disorder is ascertained) need to be obtained. A pedigree is drawn with a minimum of three generations. This should include information about stillbirths, deaths and health problems. Probands and other members of the family are examined carefully and investigated as necessary. Only then can counselling be undertaken properly.

A genetic specialist will not tell the family what they should do, but will help them reach an informed and reasoned decision based on their own sets of values. Thus, when a family asks 'Should we have another child?', instead of a direct answer the geneticist might ask 'How would you feel about having another child with cystic fibrosis?' In this way families are encouraged to explore their own feelings. For many families it is possible to be counselled in a single visit, but some families need to return for further discussions.

It is excellent practice to write to all families seen for counselling, restating the advice given to them at the time. This letter should be written in simple clear language and outline the discussion that has taken place. A copy of this letter is sent to the family doctor and other specialists so that everybody involved has the same information. This document then serves as a valuable family record, can be shown to other professionals, and overcomes the problem of selective recall.

A postmortem examination may be necessary to establish a precise diagnosis. This can be of particular importance in a child with malformations or retardation when a diagnosis is not possible, and in adults with neurological disorders. Postmortems need to be planned in advance so that specific tissues can be obtained for biochemical study, electron microscopy or histochemistry. When death can be anticipated, it is best to raise the issue of a postmortem before death occurs. In practice it works better than asking permission immediately after the death, when families are bound up in their own grief. When permission for a postmortem has been granted, it is of the greatest importance that the parents return to fully discuss the autopsy findings.

Collection of samples for DNA

With advances in DNA technology it has become essential to store samples of DNA from family members with the condition in question who are likely to die, as well as relatives such as grandparents. This enables subsequent family members to benefit from advancing knowledge. Such samples can also be obtained at the time of postmortem if not collected earlier. Appropriate samples to allow DNA to be stored include blood and fibroblasts from a small skin biopsy.

Diagnostic precision

A critical element in genetic counselling is establishing the correct diagnosis. When considering the need for investigations, a precise diagnosis may not influence treatment, but appropriate genetic counselling may be of extreme importance to the patient and his or her family. An example is muscular dystrophy. There are many different forms of muscular dystrophy. The principles of management are similar for these; for example, appropriate splints, physiotherapy and occupational therapy. The risk for other family members, however, varies considerably between these disorders because muscular dystrophies may be autosomal dominant, autosomal recessive, X linked recessive or mitochondrial. To counsel a family appropriately, the exact diagnosis must be known.

Clinical example

Andrew died from Hunter syndrome at 10 years of age in 1975. Hunter syndrome is a rare X linked recessive neurodegenerative disorder. In 1999 his sister Jane came for advice about her risk of having a son with Hunter syndrome. Fibroblasts were stored from Andrew. A gene mutation was found in DNA extracted from the fibroblasts, even though the gene was cloned 15 years after his death. Jane was shown not to carry the mutation. She could therefore be reassured that she is at low risk to have a son with Hunter syndrome.

Diagnostic precision may require the help of specialists who are expert in differentiating various neuromuscular diseases, retinal dystrophies and other complex problems. Dysmorphic and retarded children often require investigation before counselling can be given. An underlying chromosomal or metabolic basis should always be excluded and specific dysmorphic syndromes identified where possible (Ch. 27, 29 and 31).

Clinical example

Anne and her partner Bob are planning to start a family. They see you because Anne's sister has a son with muscular dystrophy. They have been told that it is an X linked condition and that there is a significant risk that they could have a son with the same condition. After gaining permission from Anne's sister, you find that the child's muscle biopsy revealed the diagnosis of limb girdle muscular dystrophy 2B, an autosomal recessive condition. You are able to reassure Anne and Bob that the risk for their own children is low.

Genetic counselling without a diagnosis

Of children presenting with intellectual disability or dysmorphic features, approximately one half will not have a precise diagnosis. There is a large body of empirical data that can be used for counselling in this group. The only caveat is that appropriate examination and investigation should be done by an experienced clinician to exclude known disorders. While an inability to label a child with a specific diagnosis is disappointing and frustrating to both parents and doctors, it should not disadvantage the child, as management can be based on periodic assessment and planning.

The evolution of knowledge and new techniques make it necessary to look again at old problems. Thus patient review is of the greatest importance. For example, when the fragile X chromosome became recognised as a major cause of intellectual disability, many families required further study utilising new chromosome techniques. This required further repetition using DNA studies when the triplet repeat abnormality was recognised as the cause. Also, new approaches, using DNA, for diagnosis and identification of carriers will require recall and further study of affected families. In addition, the clinical features making up a syndrome may become more apparent with increasing age and thus allow for better diagnostic precision.

Counselling for risk

Following diagnostic evaluation, an estimate of risk can be made. Risk is a numerical estimate of the likelihood of a particular disorder occurring in a current or future pregnancy.

Risk in specific situations

Mendelian disorders

These are conditions which are autosomal dominant, autosomal recessive or X linked. Some 6500 mendelian disorders have been described in humans. They are comprehensively catalogued in Online Mendelian Inheritance in Man (OMIM). Where the disorder follows mendelian inheritance, risk calculation is based on the mode of inheritance and other factors, such as carrier testing. DNA testing has improved the precision of counselling in some cases.

Polygenic or multifactorial inheritance

There are many common disorders in which there is a genetic component and where the inheritance pattern cannot be explained simply in terms of mendelian inheritance or chromosomal rearrangement. It appears that these disorders are due to the cumulative action of a number of genes together with environmental influences. This is called polygenic or multifactorial inheritance and numerically is the commonest pattern of inheritance

Clinical example

Lara's brother James recently had a child, Craig, with cystic fibrosis. Lara and her partner Ivan are planning a family and come to you to seek advice about their risk of having a child with this condition. Based on a community carrier rate of 1:25, you inform Lara and Ivan that their risk is 1:200. Mutation testing of the CFTR gene reveals that Craig is homozygous for the ΔF508 mutation, the commonest mutation that leads to cystic fibrosis. Lara is tested and is shown to carry this mutation. Ivan is then tested and is shown to carry another cystic fibrosis mutation, G551D. This means that they have a 1:4 risk of having a child with cystic fibrosis and that it is possible for them to have prenatal testing by DNA analysis for this condition.

responsible for the family tendency or predisposition to various disorders. The recurrence risk of multifactorial disorders after a single affected child or with a single affected parent depends on the condition and can often be estimated from empirical data. The following are examples of conditions that generally follow multifactorial inheritance:

- congenital cardiac anomalies
- neural tube defects, such as spina bifida and anencephaly
- club foot
- cleft lip and cleft palate
- congenital dislocation of the hip
- pyloric stenosis.

Clinical example

Sonya and her partner Joe had a child with anencephaly, a neural tube defect. This is an invariably fatal condition where the skull and brain do not fully form. They seek counselling about the risk of recurrence and what can be done to avoid this and detect it if it does recur. They are informed that the risk of a neural tube defect (anencephaly, spina bifida, encephalocele) in her next pregnancy is about 1:25. This risk can be reduced by Sonya taking folate 5 mg daily for 3 months prior to conception and the first 3 months of pregnancy. Sonya and Joe are told that detailed expert ultrasound at about 11 and 18 weeks gestation are the best tests to detect a neural tube defect.

Unknown diagnosis

The commonest example here is where one child in a family has a syndrome with dysmorphic features and intellectual disability. Despite expert evaluation and investigation, no diagnosis is made. Again here empiric data are used, with the recurrence risk usually being in the order of 1:20 (5%).

Interpretation of risk

Many families do not have a good grasp of probability and careful discussion is needed to give meaning to any risk estimate. While it might be clear to the doctor what is meant by a one in four risk, many people believe that if they have had one abnormal child they can have another three before they need worry again. It is important to emphasize to families that chance has no memory. Simple illustrations and a concrete example such as tossing two coins are often helpful. Describing the risk in more than way can also be helpful for some people. Thus some may understand a 25% recurrence risk better than one in four.

It can be helpful to put risk into the perspective of how their risk compares with that of other families. In Australia there is approximately a 1 in 30 risk that any child will be born with a major defect. This is the risk that any family either accepts or ignores and is a useful point of comparison. While genetic counselling does not aim to tell a person what to do, it is important for a counsellor to see that parents understand the meaning of any numbers used.

From the nuclear to the extended family

Where a disorder is identified in a family that puts other family members at significant risk of either a problem themselves or of having a child with a problem, the extended family needs to be offered the opportunity to discuss this and have testing. An example of this is the case of Lara and Ivan, above, where their risk of having a child with cystic fibrosis only came to light because a child was born into the family with this condition. This form of testing is called cascade testing. Examples of conditions where the extended family may be at risk are a chromosome translocation, a dominant disorder such as Marfan syndrome, common recessive disorders such as cystic fibrosis and haemochromatosis, or sex linked disorders such as Duchenne muscular dystrophy. Where members of the extended family need to be informed that there is a risk to them or their offspring of having a genetic disorder, a letter for the genetic specialist can be very helpful in conveying this sensitive information.

Predictive testing

Predictive or presymptomatic testing is defined as a test on an asymptomatic person that allows that individual to know whether or not he or she will go on to develop the condition in question. The test may be genetic (e.g. the identification of the causative gene mutation in Huntington disease) but may not be (e.g. nerve conduction studies in an asymptomatic person at risk of Charcot–Marie–Tooth disease).

Predictive testing is mainly available for neurodegenerative diseases (for example, Huntington disease, autosomal dominant spinocerebellar ataxia) and some cancers (familial breast/ovarian cancer, familial bowel cancer). It is conducted in the setting of a counselling protocol to give those undertaking the testing the opportunity to understand what a gene positive or negative result would mean for them. Where no preventative treatment is available (for example, Huntington disease), the majority of those at risk choose not to be tested. Predictive testing for

---

Clinical example

Frank had symptoms of lethargy, joint pain and abdominal pain. Extensive medical evaluation eventually revealed that the underlying cause for this was iron overload due to hereditary haemochromatosis. He was shown to be homozygous for the common C282Y mutation in his HFE gene. Frank has a brother Graham. Graham is found to be C282Y homozygous and iron studies show a moderately raised ferritin and transferrin saturation. He has had no symptoms referable to haemochromatosis. He has regular venesections to return his iron indices to normal. By doing this Graham will avoid the risk of developing symptomatic haemochromatosis.

Clinical example

Sue and David are 12 year old twins and are at 50% risk of having familial polyposis coli (FAP). FAP results in a sufferer having 100s or 1000s of bowel polyps which, if untreated, invariably leads to malignant change in one or more polyps. Sue and David's mother, uncle and grandfather, as well as many other relatives, have suffered from FAP. The causative mutation in the APC gene in Sue and David's family has been found. Because polyposis and malignant change may occur in the teens, it is recommended that surveillance by sigmoidoscopy begin in the early teens. Sue and David undergo predictive testing. It is found that Sue does not have the familial mutation but David does. David therefore is recommended to have yearly colonoscopies but Sue does not need to do so. Prior to the availability of molecular diagnosis, Sue would have had yearly sigmoidoscopies until she reached her 30s before a confident diagnosis that she did not have FAP could be made.

conditions where no preventative treatment is available is not generally undertaken on minors.

The burden

The burden of an actual or possible genetic diagnosis is of great importance in genetic counselling. This can be considered in two contexts: in prenatal diagnosis and a diagnosis in a child. Where a diagnosis is made pre-natally, the couple need to be fully informed about the problems a child with that condition may face. This is to allow an informed decision about pregnancy termina-tion but also allows couples who choose not to terminate the pregnancy to prepare for that child's birth. Where there is a strong family history of a condition, the couple may be well aware of the burden. An example is a woman who has grown up with a brother with Duchenne muscular dystrophy who has prenatal testing that reveals that the male she is carrying has this condition. More difficult is where a diagnosis is made that was not specifically being looked for. An example is the diagno-sis of Klinefelter syndrome (47,XXY) on a prenatal chromosome test done to look for Down syndrome. Here much time is often required to help the couple under-stand what that diagnosis will mean for their child and the rest of the family.

Similar issues exist where a child is diagnosed with a particular condition. For example, parents of a baby recently diagnosed as having cystic fibrosis or mental retardation may have little idea of what lies ahead for the child and themselves. It is necessary to give parents an understanding of what is going to be involved in the care of a child with that particular disorder, including the life expectancy, the quality of life, treatment and variability which exists for that disorder. Just as importantly, it is vital that, in situations where the prognosis cannot be pre-dicted, this uncertainty is conveyed to the parents. For instance, with tuberous sclerosis, a child may present with hypsarrhythmia and profound retardation, or may be normal.

Alternatives for families at risk

Where a couple have a child, or they know they at risk of having a child, with a genetic condition, there are a number of reproductive options available to them. These include:
- childless lifestyle
- acceptance of risk
- adoption
- intrauterine diagnosis
- donor sperm
- donor ova
- donor embryo
- preimplantation genetic diagnosis.

Childless life style

A family may choose not to have children where there is a risk of a genetic condition or where a child has been born with a genetic condition.

Acceptance of risk

For some couples the risk of the disorder may be accept-able compared to the burden of other alternatives. This may relate to the perceived severity of the disorder. Thus prenatal diagnosis is requested much more often when the disorder is lethal in childhood (e.g. Duchenne muscular dystrophy) than when it frequently leads to many years of health before its onset (e.g. Huntington disease) or where its severity is unpredictable and is often relatively mild (e.g. neurofibromatosis type I). There are religious and cultural factors that may contribute to this decision.

Adoption

The number of young babies available for adoption is very limited because of the increase in single parent fam-ilies and in termination of pregnancies. Thus adoption is rarely a practical alternative in Australia.

Intrauterine diagnosis

Intrauterine diagnosis provides an option for many couples. This can be offered to families who feel that ter-mination of pregnancy is an acceptable approach. The range of disorders that can be recognised by intrauterine diagnosis is constantly increasing (Ch. 27).

Donor sperm

Artificial insemination by donor (AID) is of limited appeal. Many couples and ethnic groups find it unac-ceptable. This, however, should never be assumed and couples should be informed about this option to find whether or not it is acceptable to them. AID can provide an alternative when the father has an autosomal dominant disorder, carries a chromosome translocation or produces a child with an autosomal recessive disorder.

Donor ova

In vitro fertilisation (IVF) using donor ova can be offered when a woman carries a sex linked disorder, has an autosomal dominant disorder, carries a chromosome translocation, has a mitochondrial DNA mutation or produces a child with an autosomal recessive disorder. Parents may find this more acceptable as the mother still experiences the pregnancy.

Donor embryo

Donor embryos are usually donated by couples who have utilised IVF and have stored embryos but do not require them as they have completed their family. Some couples prefer this to donor sperm or ovum, as they feel uncomfortable about one partner being genetically related to their offspring but the other partner not being related.

Preimplantation genetic diagnosis

This state of the art technology is not currently available in all Australian states. In preimplantation genetic diagnosis, cells from an embryo produced by IVF are tested for the disorder in question. This may be through DNA analysis or chromosome examination by fluorescence in situ hybridisation (FISH). Only those embryos where the disorder is excluded are returned to the uterus. The advantage of preimplantation genetic diagnosis is that termination of pregnancy is not required. The disadvantages are that it is expensive, labour intensive and for each cycle of IVF there is well below 50% completed pregnancy rate.

Emotional impact of genetic counselling

Patients often feel very vulnerable when referred for genetic counselling. This may be because of the recent arrival of a child with a birth defect, a stillbirth or a neonatal death. People might be concerned about details of their family history and worry that they might be blamed for any abnormality.

In counselling, the emotional impact of a birth defect, and the risk of producing a child with a birth defect, are carefully explored. People need an opportunity to vent their fears and anxieties. Discussions of emotional issues are of equal importance to discussions of risk, burden and alternatives. Families who have recently lost a child may need understanding and reassurance about the process of mourning and may need to allow time before they are ready for a further pregnancy.

Acknowledgements

The author wishes sincerely to thank Dr John Rogers for teaching him about the practice of genetic counselling. Dr Rogers was the author of this chapter in the first four editions of *Practical Paediatrics* and the current chapter draws much from that work.

Inborn errors of metabolism 31

J. McGill

Metabolic disorders, particularly those presenting acutely, remain seriously underdiagnosed. This is because the presentation is often precipitated by or mimics infection and so the possibility of an inborn error of metabolism is overlooked. Diagnostic clues such as:

- ketosis
- hypoglycaemia
- metabolic acidosis

are often misinterpreted as being due to the precipitating infection. The possibility of a metabolic disorder needs to be considered so that specific diagnostic tests such as urine organic acids, plasma amino acids and ammonium estimation are undertaken. Rapid diagnosis is needed and appropriate therapy should be instituted to avoid death or permanent neurological damage.

Although individually uncommon, collectively metabolic disorders are frequent. The main forms of presentation are acutely in the neonatal period and associated with intercurrent illness in childhood, the storage disorders, organ dysfunction and the mitochondrial disorders.

Acute metabolic decompensation

Neonatal

In the neonatal period, metabolic disorders can be grouped into those that become symptomatic because of the accumulation of a toxin (Fig. 31.1) or an energy deficiency. The toxin accumulation group are usually well until 2–5 days of age, as the placenta has usually cleared the toxin in utero. Poor feeding and lethargy are frequent early symptoms, followed by decreased conscious state and abnormalities of tone and movement.

The energy deficient group can present at any time from birth, with seizures, acidosis, hypertrophic cardiomyopathy, hypotonia and malformations being common features.

The history can be helpful and questions should be asked regarding consanguinity, history of previous neonatal deaths or stillbirths and dietary exposures such as galactose (breast or cow's milk) or fructose (honey on a dummy). Most of the disorders are due to an enzyme deficiency and have an autosomal recessive inheritance.

A very useful approach to diagnosis in the newborn period utilises the measurement of glucose, ketones, lactate, ammonium and acidosis.

Older children

Acute metabolic presentations in children are often precipitated by a viral illness associated with loss of appetite or vomiting. This causes catabolism and the gluconeogenic, fat and protein metabolic pathways are stressed. Ingestion of large amounts of protein or deliberate fasting (for example, prior to surgery) can also precipitate an acute decompensation in some disorders.

For all age groups the presentation can be as decreased conscious state, hypoglycaemia, metabolic acidosis or seizures.

Decreased conscious state

A decreased conscious state may be the result of:
- a metabolic encephalopathy
- hypoglycaemia
- hyperammonaemia
- amino acidopathies, for example maple syrup urine disease.

Diagnosis of the last condition is based on plasma and urine amino acids which show elevated concentrations of the branched chain amino acids: valine, leucine and isoleucine.

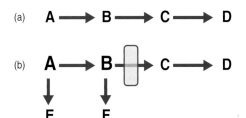

Fig. 31.1 This schematically shows a metabolic pathway in which A is converted to D by two chemical reactions (**a**). If there is a block in the pathway due to an enzyme deficiency (**b**) then there is an accumulation of the compounds proximal to the block and a deficiency of the products distal to the block. Alternate pathways may become activated (E, F). Symptoms may be due to the toxicity of accumulating compounds (A,B,E,F), a deficiency of compounds distal to the block (C,D) or both.

Hyperammonaemia

This often causes a respiratory alkalosis. The absence of ketosis can be important in distinguishing these disorders from the secondary hyperammonaemia of patients with an organic acidosis. Causes and associated findings may be:

- normal anion gap
  — high amino acids
  — urea cycle disorders: citrullinaemia, argininaemia, argininosuccinic aciduria
- low/normal amino acids
  — urea cycle disorders: ornithine transcarbamylase (OTC) deficiency, carbamyl phosphate synthetase (CPS) deficiency
  — lysinuric protein intolerance
  — transient hyperammonaemia of the newborn (premature babies with respiratory distress)
- increased anion gap
  — liver disease/failure
  — organic acidaemia.

The presence of raised urinary orotic acid concentrations distinguishes OTC from CPS deficiency. Ornithine transcarbamylase deficiency is an X linked disorder so an extended family pedigree on the maternal side may provide useful information. Females heterozygous for the gene may be symptomatic.

Children with milder or partial deficiencies of urea cycle enzymes, including some females heterozygous for OTC deficiency, present later in life, usually after a high protein intake or with catabolism with an intercurrent illness. Abdominal pain and vomiting are early symptoms.

> ### Clinical example
>
> Baby Thomas presented at 3 days of age as he was difficult to arouse and had fed poorly the day before. He was afebrile and investigations for sepsis were negative. Blood gas measurements revealed a respiratory alkalosis and his alert paediatrician ordered a plasma ammonium, which was 530 mmol/l (NR < 60). Plasma amino acid measurement showed a low citrulline but was otherwise normal. Urine orotic acid was normal. He was treated with peritoneal dialysis, sodium benzoate, sodium phenylbutyrate (alternative pathways to excrete nitrogen) and arginine and his ammonium level returned to normal in 48 hours. He has been well on the above medications and a low protein diet. A liver biopsy was performed and carbamyl phosphate synthetase (CPS) deficiency was confirmed.

Hypoglycaemia

The causes of hypoglycaemia can be grouped according to the presence or absence of ketones, hepatomegaly and lactic acidosis, and the rapidity of onset after the last feed.

Tests to be performed at the time of hypoglycaemia (that is, before it is corrected)

- Glucose
- Insulin
- C-peptide
- Growth hormone
- Cortisol
- ACTH
- Free fatty acids
- b-hydroxybutyrate
- Acylcarnitine profile
- Lactate
- Plasma amino acids
- Organic acids (the first urine passed after the episode)

Causes

- Hypoketotic hypoglycaemia
  — fatty acid oxidation disorder producing a block to ketone production, as in medium chain acyl CoA dehydrogenase (MCAD) deficiency
  — hyperinsulinism due to inhibition of fat mobilisation (persistent hyperinsulinaemic hypoglycaemia of infancy, Beckwith–Wiedemann syndrome, small for gestational age infants, infants of diabetic mothers, hyperammonaemic hyperinsulinism or insulinoma)
  — occasionally panhypopituitarism in which there is a lack of cortisol and growth hormone, resulting in a functional excess of insulin
  — growth hormone deficiency
- Hypoketotic hypoglycaemia and hyperammonaemia
  — glutamate dehydrogenase upregulation (hyperammonaemic hyperinsulinism)
- Ketotic hypoglycaemia
  — organic acidurias
  — recurrent functional ketotic hypoglycaemia, usually in the mornings and not a problem after 6–8 years of age
  — adrenal insufficiency
  — panhypopituitarism
- Hepatomegaly with liver dysfunction
  — galactosaemia
  — tyrosinaemia type 1
  — neonatal haemochromatosis
  — alpha 1 antitrypsin deficiency
  — respiratory chain disorders
  — hereditary fructose intolerance
- Hepatomegaly without liver dysfunction
  — glycogen storage diseases types I and III
- Transient hepatomegaly
  — fatty acid oxidation disorders
  — gluconeogenic disorders, e.g. fructose-1,6-bisphosphatase deficiency
- Onset within 2–6 hours postprandial

— hyperinsulinism
— glycogen storage diseases
- + Lactic acidosis
  — glycogen storage disease type 1
  — gluconeogenic disorders.

Some babies with hypopituitarism present with hypoglycaemia and obstructive jaundice.

Children with disorders of hyperinsulinism usually require a higher glucose intake to control the hypoglycaemia than do children with disorders of fatty acid oxidation.

Metabolic acidosis (excluding lactic acidosis)

These infants and children are severely ill, but the presentation is often similar to severe infection, which is the usual initial diagnosis. The associated tachypnoea can be mistaken for respiratory disease. The metabolic acidosis has a high anion gap. Associated laboratory abnormalities can include neutropenia, thrombocytopenia, hypoglycaemia or hyperglycaemia, hypocalcaemia and moderate hyperammonaemia. The diagnosis is reached by assessment of urine organic acids or the blood acylcarnitine profile. It is essential that the first urine passed is analysed, as the diagnostic metabolites can clear quickly once intravenous glucose is given. Common disorders in this group are methylmalonic, propionic and isovaleric acidaemias.

Clinical example

Baby Mohammed became unwell at 4 days of age. He was vomiting, lethargic and tachypnoeic. A blood gas revealed a mixed acidosis. Infection was suspected and feeds were ceased. Intravenous antibiotics were started and intravenous 10% dextrose, $^1/_4$ normal saline fluids were given. He improved during the next 36 hours and feeds were restarted. Two days later the symptoms recurred and the possibility of a metabolic disorder was considered. Questioning of his parents revealed that they were first cousins. Urine organic acids meaurement showed methylmalonic acidaemia and he was not vitamin B_{12} responsive. He is now growing and developing normally at 4 years of age but averages five admissions per year with decompensations with infections.

Lactic acidosis

These patients have an energy deficiency. The main symptoms are due to the high anion gap acidosis. In neonates, ketosis is an important clue and the presence of ketosis increases the likelihood of a metabolic disease as it is rarely present with hypoxia. Some patients have associated dysmorphic features and malformations. Causes and features of lactic acidosis may be:

- high lactate to pyruvate ratio
  — respiratory chain defects
  — pyruvate carboxylase deficiency type B (+ hyperammonaemia and citrullinaemia)
- normal lactate to pyruvate ratio
  — pyruvate dehydrogenase deficiency
  — pyruvate carboxylase deficiency type A
  — glycogen storage disease type 1
  — fructose-1,6-bisphosphatase deficiency
- abnormal organic acids
  — organic acidaemias, for example methylmalonic acidaemia
  — fatty acid oxidation disorders.

Clinical example

Brendan is a 2 year old boy who was being reviewed regularly for failure to thrive and developmental delay. The whole family developed gastroenteritis. While his parents and sibling recovered quickly, he remained unwell and became drowsy. He was rushed to the local hospital where tests showed a high anion gap acidosis and hypoglycaemia. Assessment of urine organic acids showed lactate and ketones present, but no other abnormalities. His plasma lactate concentration was 12mmol/l (NR 1.0–2.0) on blood collected at presentation and a second test showed a normal lactate: pyruvate ratio. His lactate fluctuated inversely to the glucose input. He remained intolerant of food and hepatomegaly developed but resolved again when his nutrition improved. A liver biopsy showed that he had fructose-1, 6-bisphosphatase deficiency. Overnight studies showed that he developed a lactic acidosis and low glucose and this may have contributed to his growth and development problems. He requires overnight cornstarch to maintain his sugar and lactate.

Seizures

Seizures in this group of energy deficient disorders may be present from birth. The most common disorders in this group are non ketotic hyperglycinaemia (diagnosed by an elevated CSF: plasma glycine ratio); sulphite oxidase deficiency (diagnosed by urine metabolic screen); and peroxisomal disorders (diagnosed by plasma very long chain fatty acids and phytanic acid). This last group are usually dysmorphic and hypotonic. It is important to identify pyridoxine dependent seizures, and the diagnosis is confirmed by improvement of the EEG during injection of pyridoxine.

Treatment

The basis of treatment is to reverse the catabolism and this is usually achieved by intravenous 10–20% dextrose with maintenance salts. Sometimes it is necessary to remove the toxins by dialysis or haemoperfusion. Many of the enzymes have vitamin cofactors, and in a small proportion giving pharmacological doses of the vitamin can overcome the defect, for example vitamin B_{12} for methylmalonic acidaemia and biotin for multiple carboxylase deficiency. A secondary carnitine deficiency may develop in many of these disorders and correction of that is essential.

In the long term the disorders of protein metabolism require a low protein diet supplemented by amino acid formulas lacking the amino acid(s) that accumulates proximal to the block and boosted in those deficient distal to the block.

Non acute metabolic decompensation

Splenomegaly with or without hepatomegaly

The majority of the disorders with this type of presentation are due to lysosomal storage diseases. In these children, the lack of one of the enzymes involved in the lysosomes results in the accumulation of the structural substrate in a variety of tissues. Other presenting features include developmental regression, coarsening of the facial features and clouding of the cornea. Radiological examination often reveals changes in the spine (dysostosis multiplex) and long bones. Not all types have CNS involvement. Storage bodies may be seen in white blood cells on a blood film. Disorders in this group include the mucopolysaccharidoses (such as Hurler and Sanfilippo syndromes), Gaucher and Niemann–Pick diseases. Diagnosis is made by urine screens for mucopolysaccharides and oligosaccharides and lysosomal enzyme analysis.

A new form of therapy is available for this group of disorders. Enzyme replacement therapy (ERT) is already commercially available for Gaucher type 1, which does not have involvement of the brain. The enzyme is produced by recombinant DNA technology and is then modified so that it is delivered to the target tissues. Trials of ERT are currently underway for Pompe disease, Hurler syndrome, Hunter syndrome and Fabry disease.

Bone marrow transplantation has been an effective treatment for several lysosomal disorders, with the outcome depending on the neurological status at the time of transplant.

Multisystem disease

Mitochondrial respiratory chain disorders

These are increasingly being recognised as a cause of progressive neurological disease, and multisystem disease. The range of symptoms is vast and mitochondrial disorders can present at any age, with any combination of symptoms and with any pattern of inheritance. Tissues which depend on mitochondrial ATP production, such as brain, skeletal muscle and heart, are more susceptible to disorders of the mitochondrial respiratory chain. Common presentations in childhood include seizures, developmental delay and regression, strokes, lactic acidosis, myopathy, cardiomyopathy, liver failure, renal disorders, ophthalmoplegias, retinitis pigmentosa and deafness. There is a mitochondrial mutation that predisposes to aminoglycoside toxicity, and many of the patients who developed liver failure after sodium valproate therapy had a mitochondrial disease.

The diagnosis should be suspected in any child with a combination of symptoms, particularly if they appear unrelated, for example CNS and liver disease or renal tubular acidosis and a neurodegenerative disease.

Mitochondria have their own DNA, inherited from the mother via the ovum (maternal inheritance). Some mitochondrial diseases are inherited as mutations in the mitochondrial DNA, such as MELAS (mitochondrial encephalopathy, lactic acidosis and stroke-like episodes), MERRF (myoclonic epilepsy, ragged red fibres), NARP (neurogenic muscle weakness, ataxia and retinitis pigmentosa) and Leigh disease. Others, such as complex IV deficiency, are inherited from nuclear genes.

The diagnosis of mitochondrial diseases is difficult. The screening tests include elevated lactate in the blood or CSF and histological changes on muscle biopsy, including ragged red fibres. Only a small proportion of children have one of the common mutations of mitochondrial DNA and these may only be present in some tissues, such as muscle. The next stage of investigation is to assay the enzyme complexes of the respiratory chain in muscle, liver or skin. Because the disorder involves enzyme complexes, the results are often suggestive rather than diagnostic of a respiratory chain disorder. It is important to realise that there is no test that can exclude a disorder of the mitochondrial respiratory chain.

Clinical example

Christina, a 12 year old girl, presented with severe migraines. She had a history of migraines about once every few months but her mother had noted that they had become more frequent during the previous 6 months. She was otherwise a well and active girl. Routine biochemistry showed a low bicarbonate and high anion gap. A plasma lactate was ordered and was 6.0 mmol/l (NR 1.0–2.0). Mitochondrial DNA analysis showed that she had the common mutation for MELAS. She continued to have severe migraines and 14 months later presented with a left hemiplegia. She progressed to coma within a few days and died a week later.

Congenital disorders of glycosylation (CDG)

This group of disorders is being increasingly recognised and delineated. Glycoproteins are those proteins that require the attachment of specific sugars for their function. These proteins have important functions, for example as receptors and transporters. Clinical presentations include multiorgan failure, neuropathies, strabismus, dysmorphic features, coagulation disorders, cardiomyopathy, ataxia, psychomotor retardation, gastrointestinal bleeding and hormonal disorders.

The most useful diagnostic test is to look for abnormalities in transferrin isoforms.

Table 31.1 lists other non acute presentations for metabolic disorders.

Newborn screening

Newborn screening is performed from a blood sample collected onto a blotting paper at 2–5 days of age. Tests are performed to identify disorders that are difficult to recognise clinically and for which early treatment is beneficial. The first and most successful disorder so diagnosed is phenylketonuria (PKU). Prior to newborn screening, children with PKU were not diagnosed until they presented in childhood with intellectual impairment. With treatment from the neonatal period, intelligence is normal.

All States in Australia screen for PKU, cystic fibrosis and hypothyroidism, and most screen for galactosaemia. A new form of screening based on tandem mass spectroscopy has started in several States and this allows the diagnosis of organic acidaemias (such as methylmalonic acidaemia), amino acidopathies (such as maple syrup urine disease) and disorders of fatty acid oxidation (such as MCAD) in addition to the above disorders. Trials have started in detecting lysosomal storage disorders by newborn screening, and screening techniques for identifying other disorders, such as the peroxisomal group of disorders, are also being investigated.

Phenylketonuria (PKU)

Phenylketonuria is usually diagnosed by newborn screening. Untreated, it causes mental retardation, eczema and behavioural problems. It occurs in 1 in 15 000 newborns and is an autosomal recessive disorder. It is due to a deficiency of the enzyme phenylalanine hydroxylase (Fig. 31.2). About 1% of cases are due to a deficiency of the cofactor, tetrahydrobiopterin (BH_4). These are more severe as BH_4 is a cofactor for two other enzymes in the neurotransmitter pathway.

Treatment is by a very restrictive low protein diet, which is essentially a vegan diet with some further restrictions and the need to weigh and measure all protein-containing food. This is supplemented by special amino acid formulae which lack phenylalanine and are boosted in tyrosine (examples of such formulae are XP Analog, XP Maxamaid, XP Maxamum, Phenex 1 and 2, and PKU gel).

Perimortem protocol

If the possibility of a metabolic disorder is considered in an infant or child who is dying and cannot be treated, it is important that arrangements are made to collect appropriate samples either before or as soon as possible after death (within 1–2 hours but the sooner the better). This needs to be discussed with the parents before death and the parents must be allowed some time with their child after death before the procedure is undertaken.

Table 31.1 Non acute presentations for metabolic disorders

Sign	Common metabolic causes
Cataract	Galactosaemia, galactokinase deficiency, peroxisomal disorders
Cardiomyopathy	Respiratory chain disorders, CDG, carnitine deficiency
Strokes	Homocystinuria, CDG, MELAS
Retinal haemorrhages	Glutaric aciduria type 1
Retinitis pigmentosa	Peroxisomal disorders, NARP, CDG
Abnormal hair	Menke syndrome, argininosuccinic aciduria
Dislocated lenses	Homocystinuria, sulphite oxidase deficiency
Endocrine abnormalities	Respiratory chain defects, CDG
Renal cysts	Glutaric aciduria II, CDG, peroxisomal disorders

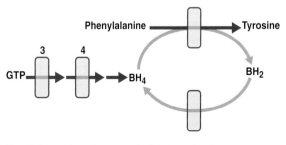

Fig. 31.2 In phenylketonuria the block can be due to a deficiency of phenylalanine hydroxylase, a defect in the biosynthesis of the cofactor, tetrahydrobiopterin, or a defect in recycling the tetrahydrobiopterin. Symptoms are due to the accumulation of phenylalanine and the deficiency of tyrosine.

Samples of blood (plasma and serum), CSF and urine should be collected and frozen. Vitreous fluid may be used if there is no urine available. Muscle, liver and, if indicated, heart tissue should be collected. This is best achieved by a right upper quadrant incision taking liver, rectus muscle and cardiac muscle. The tissue samples should be no greater than 1 ml and should be wrapped in alfoil, labelled and put onto dry ice until storage at −70°C. A small sample of each tissue should be collected into glyceraldehyde for electron microscopy.

PART 10   SELF-ASSESSMENT

Questions

1. **Mrs A is 8 weeks pregnant at the age of 36 years. She is considering prenatal testing. Which of the following statements are correct?**
   - (A) Mrs A's risk of having a baby with spina bifida is significantly increased above that of a woman aged 25 years
   - (B) A chorionic villus sample has a higher rate of detection for Down syndrome than a nuchal translucency scan
   - (C) An amniocentesis will exclude the possibility that Mrs A's baby could have a genetic disorder
   - (D) Mrs A is eligible for preimplantation genetic diagnosis in this pregnancy
   - (E) Mrs A will only be offered prenatal diagnosis if she agrees to terminate a pregnancy in which the fetus is shown to have a significant birth defect

2. **Which of the following statements relating to birth defects are correct?**
   - (A) The term 'birth defect' only applies to medical conditions which are evident at the time of birth
   - (B) Birth defects play a role in up to a quarter of perinatal deaths
   - (C) The majority of birth defects are readily preventable by public health measures
   - (D) Most birth defects have a multifactorial basis
   - (E) Minor birth defects are a marker for the presence of major birth defects

3. **Mrs B has discovered that she is unexpectedly 9 weeks pregnant. She is concerned, as she has been taking several medications. Mrs B has epilepsy and is well controlled on valproate 500 mg b.d. In addition, she has been taking doxycycline 50 mg orally daily and using 0.5% retinoic acid cream topically to help control her acne. Which of the following statements are correct?**
   - (A) Mrs B should be told to cease all medications immediately
   - (B) Mrs B should be told that provided she ceases the doxycycline now, her baby is not at risk of staining of the teeth related to the use of doxycycline in this pregnancy
   - (C) Mrs B should be counselled to consider termination of the pregnancy due to the very high risk of damage to the fetus related to the use of retinoic acid in the first trimester
   - (D) All women taking anticonvulsant medication should be advised to also take 5 mg of folic acid daily, if there is any chance they may conceive
   - (E) Mrs B cannot contact the local teratogen advisory service for further information directly, as she is not a medical practitioner

4. **A girl has been found to have inherited retinitis pigmentosa, a form of degeneration of the retina. She is the only person with visual symptoms in the family. The family history is unremarkable, but her parents are first cousins. Various mutations in different genes can cause retinitis pigmentosa. The pattern of inheritance may be autosomal dominant, autosomal recessive, X linked recessive, or reflect mitochondrial inheritance. What modes of inheritance should be considered in this case?**
   - (A) Autosomal dominant
   - (B) Autosomal recessive
   - (C) X linked recessive
   - (D) Mitochondrial
   - (E) All of the above

5. **Haemophilia is an X linked recessive disorder of clotting. A number of males in an extended family**

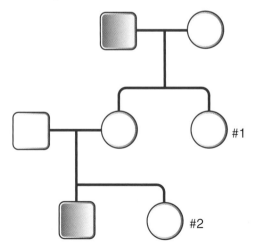

Fig. SA10

have this condition. Two women in the family (indicated on previous page) want to know their risk of being carriers.

For each woman, what is the carrier risk?

(A) 100%

(B) 50%

(C) 25%

(D) 1%

(E) 0%

6. **A father and two of his children have the same autosomal dominant condition. DNA studies of part of a certain gene have shown that each affected person has one gene with the sequence ACACCAGGA (which encodes the amino acids threonine–proline–glycine) and one gene with the sequence TCACCAGGA (which encodes the amino acids serine–proline–glycine). Other family members (who are all healthy) have only the first sequence described above. There is insufficient information presented here to differentiate between a polymorphism and a mutation. What approaches would you consider to determine if the difference in DNA sequence is likely to be responsible for the autosomal disorder?**

7. **Baby Sarah has the facial features of Down syndrome and a VSD. Which of the following are correct:**

(A) There is no need to test her chromosomes as it is inappropriate to take blood from a baby just for academic interest

(B) Her chromosomes have been tested and confirm trisomy 21, so parental bloods need not be checked

(C) If her chromosome test showed the translocation form of Down syndrome involving chromosomes 21 and 14, this automatically means that there is a significantly increased risk of Down syndrome for the parents' next pregnancy.

(D) If the diagnosis of Down syndrome is confirmed, Sarah's mother must be 35 years old or more

(E) If the diagnosis of Down syndrome is confirmed, Sarah should be followed up and have an annual blood test to monitor thyroid function

8. **Which of the following are correct in relation to syndrome diagnosis:**

(A) Is now mainly done by computers

(B) Is just esoteric 'stamp collecting' by the doctor and provides no benefit to the child

(C) A child and her father have the same unusual facial appearance, but the child has a significant intellectual disability and the father is mentally normal. They could have the same syndrome

(D) There is no need to go through the usual medical model of history and examination when trying to make a syndrome diagnosis, as the diagnosis will be apparent as soon as the doctor sees the child

(E) Parents often want a diagnostic label for their child once they have perceived a problem, as it is easier for them to explain the problem to friends and relatives

9. **Which of the following are true of chromosome disorders?**

(A) All chromosome disorders cause an intellectual disability

(B) A woman could have triple X syndrome and not know it

(C) A male with Klinefelter syndrome is at risk of having a daughter with triple X syndrome

(D) If a woman has a child with Turner syndrome, there is quite a high risk that this could happen again in her next pregnancy

(E) Fragile X is the commonest inherited form of intellectual disability

10. **A child whose father has Marfan syndrome is unusually tall. Which of the following are correct?**

(A) There is a 50% chance that she does have Marfan syndrome

(B) It is very likely that a simple blood test to look at the fibrillin gene will resolve whether or not she has Marfan syndrome

(C) If she has the necessary skeletal criteria, referral for an echocardiogram and cardiology opinion as well as to an ophthalmologist is recommended

(D) It is generally recommended that individuals with Marfan syndrome do not play body contact sports or lift heavy weights

(E) None of the child's grandparents has Marfan syndrome, so the diagnosis must be incorrect

11. **A newborn baby has achondroplasia and the parents are not affected. Which of the following are correct?**

(A) The chance that their next baby will have achondroplasia is 50%

(B) When telling parents that their newborn baby has achondroplasia, it is best to speak with both parents at once

(C) It is preferable to try to tell the parents everything about the condition in the first meeting, as they will go and look it up on the internet anyway

(D) The child is now 3 years old and attends for her regular follow up appointment. Father mentions that she snores a lot. Is this something that needs further investigation?

(E) At the 6 year check up, you notice that the child is now on the 90th centile on the 'weight versus height' chart for achondroplasia, having been on the 50th centile last year. You decide to just

303

reassure the parents that this is fine. After all, the child needs her comfort foods, as she has discovered that she cannot do all the things that other children are doing

12. **Which of the following is true of genetic counselling?**
    (A) Genetic counselling is always done by clinical geneticists or genetic counsellors
    (B) The testing of extended family members where a family member is diagnosed with a genetic disease is called cascade testing
    (C) Having a confirmed diagnosis is essential when counselling about risk
    (D) Predictive testing is not always by molecular genetic tests
    (E) Risk for polygenic disorders requires the use of empiric data

13. **Regarding reproductive options for a couple who have a child, or who know they are at risk of having a child with a genetic condition, which of the following is correct?**
    (A) The severity of the genetic disorder plays an important role in what couples decide
    (B) Some couples choose not to have further children or to remain childless
    (C) Adoption is commonly utilised in this setting
    (D) Donor ovum will overcome recessive, X linked, dominant and mitochondrial conditions
    (E) Preimplantation genetic diagnosis means that no couple need face the option of intrauterine diagnosis and termination of pregnancy

14. **Lisa is a 4 day old baby who was admitted because she was needing to be woken for feeds. When feeding, she is difficult to feed initially, then seems to become more alert half way through and after the feed. Testing shows that she becomes hypoglycaemic about 3–4 hours after a feed. A urine sample collected immediately after an episode of hypoglycaemia shows that no ketones are present. Which of the following are true?**
    (A) The absence of ketones suggests the possibility of a disorder of fatty acid oxidation
    (B) Glycogen storage diseases should be considered in the differential diagnosis because of the rapidity of onset
    (C) Hyperinsulinism is a likely diagnosis
    (D) The rapidity of onset favours a diagnosis of hyperinsulinism more than a disorder of fatty acid oxidation
    (E) The absence of ketones in the urine is not significant because babies of this age can't make ketones

15. **Justine is a 6 year old girl who has learning problems. She presents on the third day of a febrile** illness with a history of uncontrollable behaviour during the morning. She is now asleep and is difficult to rouse. She was adopted at 2 months of age. Compared to other family members, she tends to tolerate viral infections poorly, being ill for longer and becoming drowsy. She has needed hospital admission on 4 occasions and has responded to intravenous fluids. Physical examination findings are consistent with an upper respiratory tract viral illness. Laboratory tests show a normal blood glucose and pH. Plasma amino acid measurements show a high glutamine concentration and a citrulline concentration at the lower end of the normal range. Which of the following are true?
    (A) The plasma ammonium concentration should be measured on the basis of the history
    (B) As she is a girl, ornithine transcarbamylase deficiency (OTC), which is X-linked, is excluded
    (C) If the plasma ammonium concentration is elevated, the most useful additional test would be assessment of urine orotic acid
    (D) Assuming this is a metabolic disorder, appropriate treatment will restore her academic abilities to normal
    (E) Blood collected for an ammonium estimation should be collected on ice and then measured quickly or the plasma frozen.

16. **Jacob, an 18 month old boy, presents with a febrile illness associated with weakness on his right side. With two previous febrile illnesses he developed weakness, once on the left and the other time on the right. He has recently learned how to pull to a standing position, but is not saying any words, suggesting developmental delay. His parents are non-consanguineous and an older brother and sister are normal. Physical examination reveals strabismus and inverted nipples but is otherwise normal. Glucose, lactate, ammonium, acid–base studies and electrolytes are all normal. Which of the following are true?**
    (A) Mitochondrial respiratory chain disorders often present with symptoms during intercurrent illnesses, so MELAS syndrome is a possible diagnosis even though the lactate is normal
    (B) Urinary homocystine should be measured
    (C) An MRI scan of the brain looking for cerebellar hypoplasia is a useful diagnostic investigation
    (D) Measurement of transferrin isoforms is indicated to assist with diagnosis of a congenital disorder of glycosylation
    (E) The physical findings of inverted nipples and strabismus support the diagnosis of a congenital disorder of glycosylation

Answers and explanations

1. The correct answer is **(B)**. Although the risk of conceiving a baby with specific birth defects related to chromosomal trisomies increases with increasing maternal age, the risk of conceiving a baby with spina bifida does not (A). A chorionic villus sample is a diagnostic test for Down syndrome, as it allows direct analysis of fetal chromosomes. It therefore has a higher detection rate for Down syndrome than a nuchal translucency, scan which is a screening test that has a detection rate for Down syndrome of around 70–80% (B). It is a common misconception that if a baby has 'normal' chromosomes this means that he or she will be free from any 'genetic disorder'. Most birth defects are not the result of chromosomal abnormalities, and most genetic conditions are not related to a visible chromosomal abnormality (C). Preimplantation genetic diagnosis implies genetic analysis of embryos prior to transfer to the womb during IVF. As Mrs A has an already established pregnancy, this is not an option for her in this pregnancy (D). Although prenatal diagnosis is primarily aimed at detection of birth defects to allow the option of termination of pregnancy of an affected fetus, some women choose to have prenatal testing in order to be prepared for the possibility of the birth of a child with a birth defect and to allow optimal treatment to be provided (E).

2. The correct answers are **(B)**, **(D)** and **(E)**. To be defined as a birth defect, an abnormality must either be present at birth or the cause must be present at birth (A). Many conditions, particularly those caused by genetic mutations, do not become evident until well after birth, unless specific tests are performed. Examples are Duchenne muscular dystrophy and Huntington disease. Birth defects are the cause of 20–25% of perinatal deaths (B). Despite a number of effective population based preventive programmes (e.g. folate supplementation and rubella immunisation) and extensive research, the majority of birth defects remain non preventable by population public health measures (C). Most birth defects are the result of interaction between genes, environment and chance events occurring within the developing embryo or fetus, rather than a single event; i.e. they are multifactorial (D). The presence of a minor birth defect in an infant should prompt investigation to exclude major birth defects, as there is an association between the two (E).

3. The correct answers are **(B)** and **(D)**. Although it is appropriate to recommend cessation of any non essential medication in this situation, e.g. acne medication, It may be inappropriate to cease an anticonvulsant medication (A). This may predispose Mrs B to uncontrolled seizures which may be damaging to both her own and the baby's wellbeing. In general, if a woman has epilepsy and her seizures are well controlled on monotherapy, this treatment should be sustained throughout pregnancy with a discussion with the woman regarding the potential teratogenic issues (A). Doxycycline is known to cause fetal teeth discoloration only if there is fetal exposure after 18 weeks gestation (B). Although oral use of retinoic acid in the first trimester is associated with a high risk of fetal defects, topical use has not been proven to have the same association, as the dose reaching the fetus is minimal (C). Anticonvulsant medications increase the risk of conceiving a baby with a neural tube defect (D). Taking 5 mg folic acid supplementation at least 1 month prior to conception and through the first trimester has been shown to reduce the risk of neural tube defects. Therefore, any woman taking anticonvulsants should be advised to take folic acid supplements in case she conceives unexpectedly. Teratogen advisory services are set up to provide information to the public and health professionals. In general, most of the calls they take are from concerned members of the public, like Mrs B (E).

4. The correct answer is **(E)**. The girl could have a new dominant mutation that occurred during the formation of the ovum or sperm from which she developed. It is also possible that one of her parents has the mutation responsible for retinitis pigmentosa but has not developed symptoms. She could also have an autosomal recessive disorder. The fact that her parents are cousins makes this the most likely mode of inheritance, but other modes cannot be excluded. Some women with X linked recessive mutations causing retinitis pigmentosa do develop symptoms. This is due to inactivation of the normal X chromosome in the majority of their cells. In this case an X linked recessive mutation could be a new mutation or be inherited from the girl's mother. A mutation in mitochondrial DNA would be inherited from the mother. She may have a predominance of normal mitochondria and so be unaffected.

5. The correct answers are **(A)** for woman #1, and **(B)** for woman #2. Woman #1 is the daughter of an affected man. She has inherited one of her mother's X chromosomes and must have inherited her father's only X chromosome. This has the mutation and so she must be a carrier. Woman #2 has a brother who is affected. Her mother is a carrier and there is a 50% chance that woman #2 will have inherited her mutant X chromosome.

6. This is a recurring problem in genetic research. Variation in DNA sequences between people are very common, and sometimes it is difficult to know if a variation is pathogenic or not. There are a number of possible approaches to this question: (1) Determine whether all the affected members of the family have the same variation (as noted in this family). (2) Examine this portion of the same gene from many healthy members of the population. If one variant sequence is not found in the normal population this would clearly be in favour of it being pathogenic. (3) Examine this portion of the gene in other mammalian species. If the aminoacid sequence is the same in many species, this would suggest that variations in the sequence are pathogenic. (4) Synthesise the two proteins encoded by these DNA sequences and examine their function in vitro. If one protein exhibits a reduction in function, the underlying variation in DNA sequence is pathogenic.

7. The correct answers are **(B)** and **(E)**. The diagnosis must be confirmed as this is a serious condition with important consequences for the child and her family (A). In addition, parental chromosomes will need to be checked if there is a translocation, as half of the translocations are inherited. (B) is true. Parental chromosomes will be normal when the child has trisomy 21. The only exception to this is if a parent is a mosaic, that is, with some normal and some trisomy 21 cells, but usually this will be suspected clinically. This is a very rare situation. (C) is false. Parental chromosomes need to be checked, and a translocation will be found in half of the cases; there is then an increased risk of recurrence in future pregnancies, which varies according to the type of translocation and sex of the parent. (D) is false. Women of any age can have a child with Down syndrome, but the incidence rises with maternal age. (E) is correct.

8. The correct answers are **(C)** and **(E)**. Computerised databases are only a helpful adjunct to clinical diagnosis of syndromes (A). There are several advantages in making a diagnosis (B). Parents usually want to know the reason for their child's problem, the prognosis and recurrence risk, and can meet other families and receive enormous support through them. Many syndromes have variable features, even within a family (C). Immediate recognition of syndromes does occur but is uncommon (D). The usual medical model of detailed history and examination must be followed. Parents often say they find it easier to explain to others what is wrong with their child if there is a diagnosis (E). Care agencies also often respond more favourably to a known diagnosis in terms of offering support. Parents are not so keen on a diagnostic label if they themselves do not perceive or accept that their child has a problem.

9. The correct answers are **(B)** and **(E)**. Abnormalities of the sex chromosomes can be associated with normal intellect, particularly Turner syndrome and also triple X and Klinefelter syndromes (A). Disorders of the autosomes are virtually always associated with a degree of intellectual disability. (B) is correct. The clinical features of triple X syndrome are often very mild. Males with Klinefelter syndrome are almost always infertile (C). If they could have a child, there might be a theoretical chance of them having a daughter with triple X. There is no increased risk of recurrence after having a baby with Turner syndrome (D). (E) is correct. There is sometimes confusion between the terms 'inherited' and 'genetic'. Down syndrome is the commonest genetic cause of intellectual disability but is rarely inherited, whereas fragile X syndrome is genetic and is always inherited.

10. The correct answers are **(A)**, **(C)** and **(D)**. Marfan syndrome is autosomal dominantly inherited, so there is a 1 in 2 or 50% chance that each child of an affected person has inherited the gene and will show signs of the disorder (A). At the present time, the diagnosis is made on the basis of clinical assessment in most cases (B). In a minority of families, the mutation in the fibrillin gene has been identified and so a blood test would allow the diagnosis to be made in family members at risk. (C) is correct and the recommended assessments are appropriate. (D) is correct: these type of activities increase the risk of dilatation of the aorta. The father could have a new mutation in the gene, as do 25% of cases (E).

11. **(B)** and **(D)** are correct. It is most likely that the child has a new mutation in the FGFR3 gene, with no increased risk of recurrence to sibs (A). There is, however, a small theoretical risk of recurrence due to parental gonadal mosaicism, that is, one parent carries the mutation in the ovary or testis and so is clinically normal. Many parents who are unaffected opt for prenatal diagnosis in the next pregnancy on the basis of this small risk. (B) is correct. It is always best when breaking serious news to parents about their child to see the them together if possible, in privacy and with ample time allowed. In general, because there is a lot of information to tell parents about achondroplasia, they would not be able to absorb it all in one session (C). In addition, parents often say that once they hear that their child has a serious problem, they find it hard to take much in during that session. They need to know the outline of the problem, that long term follow up will be required and to have their questions answered honestly. However, parents vary enormously in their reaction to this kind of news, so the doctor must be flexible, and realise that some people cope by amassing information. It is true that many parents will then look on

the internet and may need assistance interpreting the information they find. They also need to realise that not all information on the internet is correct. Another appointment to discuss the diagnosis should be scheduled soon after the initial one. Further investigation is needed if she is snoring (D). Snoring indicates upper airway obstruction which could be associated with significant lowering of oxygen levels. Referral for ear, nose and throat assessment is required, and a sleep study to assess the degree of obstruction and its effect on P_{O_2} levels may be needed. Being overweight in achondroplasia puts unnecessary strain on the spine, hips, knees and ankles, which will be associated with pain and restricted mobility, especially in adult life. Dietary assessment and advice is required (E). Non weight bearing sports such as swimming are helpful to reduce weight gain and improve muscle strength.

12. **(A)** Incorrect. Genetic counselling is not always provided by genetic specialists (clinical geneticists or genetic counsellors). It is appropriate for paediatricians and disease oriented specialists to counsel in their own area of expertise. **(B)** Correct. (C) Incorrect-It is often possible to give general advice even when a specific diagnosis is not made. Here empiric data is used. **(D)** Correct. The test may be genetic (e.g. the identification of the causative gene mutation in Huntington disease) but may not be (e.g. nerve conduction studies in an asymptomatic person at risk of Charcot–Marie–Tooth disease). **(E)** Correct.

13. **(A)** Correct. Prenatal diagnosis is requested much more often when the disorder is lethal in childhood (e.g. Duchenne muscular dystrophy) than when it often leads to many years of health before its onset (e.g. huntington disease) or where its severity is unpredictable and is often relatively mild (e.g. neurofibromatosis type I). **(B)** Correct. (C) Incorrect. Availability of children for adoption is very limited in Australia due to increased acceptance of social pregnancy termination and single parenthood. **(D)** Correct. (E) Incorrect. Preimplantation genetic diagnosis is only available for limited conditions, and even then only in some Australian states. This may change as the technology improves.

14. The correct answers are **(A)**, **(B)**, **(C)** and **(D)**. Hypoketotic hypoglycaemia is most common with hyperinsulinism or a disorder of fatty acid oxidation (A),(C). The latter tend to present after prolonged periods of fasting, especially when associated with a viral illness, but may occur in the neonatal period. The onset after only 3–4 hours is characteristic of both hyperinsulinism and glycogen storage disorders (B,D), but the latter are usually ketotic. Infants are not efficient at making ketones but can (E) and their presence is a useful marker for some metabolic disorders.

15. The correct answers are **(A) (C)**, and **(E)**. This is a typical pattern for mild disorders of the urea cycle. Although OTC is X-linked, females can be symptomatic (due to random X-chromosome activation — Lyonisation) (B). An elevation of plasma glutamine is a useful marker for hyperammonaemia (A). With OTC deficiency and carbamylphosphate (CPS) deficiency, plasma amino acids are relatively normal with the only clues being mild elevation of ornithine and a low citrulline concentration. Urine orotic acid is increased in OTC deficiency but is normal in CPS deficiency (C). A respiratory alkalosis occurs with severe hyperammonaemia but the pH may be normal with lesser elevations. Once brain damage has occurred, it cannot be reversed but treatment should prevent further damage (D). The ammonia concentration increases in blood left standing at room temperature so collection on ice and rapid processing is recommended (E).

16. The correct answers are **(A), (C), (D), (E)**. Metabolic strokes can occur with homocystinuria, mitochondrial encephalopathies including MELAS, and congenital disorders of glycosylation (A), (B). Lactate is a useful screening test for disorders of the mitochondrial respiratory chain but may be normal (A) as may be the DNA test for MELAS. Urinary homocystine is not reliable so a plasma homocystine or homocysteine should be measured on an appropriately handled specimen (B). Inverted nipples, strabismus and cerebellar hypoplasia all occur with increased frequency in congenital disorders of glycosylation (C), (E). The best screening test for these disorders is transferrin isoforms (D).

PART 10 FURTHER READING

Aase J M 1990 Diagnostic dysmorphology. Plenum, New York, London

Anonymous 2000 Molecular genetic testing in pediatric practice: a subject review. Committee on Genetics. Pediatrics 106: 1494–1497

Bankier A, Rose C 2001 POSSUM. Version 5.5. Murdoch Children's Research Institute, Australia

Bennett M J, Rinaldo P, Strauss A W 2000 Inborn errors of mitochondrial fatty acid oxidation. Critical Reviews in Clinical Laboratory Sciences 37: 1–44

Briggs G G, Freeman R K, Yaffe S J 1998 Drugs in pregnancy and lactation. 5th edn. Williams and Wilkins, Baltimore

Broadstock M, Michie S, Marteau T 2000 Psychological consequences of predictive genetic testing: a systematic review. European Journal of Human Genetics 8(10): 731–738

Buyse M L 1990 Birth defects encyclopedia. Blackwell Scientific, Cambridge, MA

Cassidy S B, Allanson J E 2001 Management of genetic syndromes. Wiley-Liss, New York

Clarke A 1994 Genetic counselling: practice and principles. Routledge, London

Eng C M, Guffon N, Wilcox W R et al Safety and efficacy of recombinant human a-galactosidase: a replacement therapy in Fabry's disease. New England Journal of Medicine 345: 9–16

Fernandes J, Saudubray J M, Van den Berghe G 2000 Inborn metabolic diseases — diagnosis and treatment, 3rd edn. Springer

Gardner R J M, Sutherland G R 1996 Chromosome abnormalities and genetic counselling, 2nd edn. Oxford University Press, Oxford

Gorlin R J, Cohen M M, Levin L S 1990 Syndromes of the head and neck, 3rd edn. Oxford University Press, New York

Gottlieb B, Beitel L K, Trifiro M A 2001 Somatic mosaicism and variable expressivity. Trends in Genetics 17: 79–82

Gould S J, Valle D 2000 Peroxisome biogenesis disorders: genetics and cell biology. Trends in Genetics 16: 340–345

Hall J G, Froster-Iskenius U G, Allanson J E 1989 Handbook of normal physical measurements. Oxford University Press, Oxford

Hall C, Washbrook J 2001 A radiological electronic atlas of malformation syndromes and skeletal dysplasias (REAMS). Oxford University Press, Oxford

Hanahan D, Weinberg R A 2000 The hallmarks of cancer. Cell 100: 57–70

Harper P 1998 Practical genetic counselling. Butterworth-Heinemann, Oxford

Jaeken J, Carchon H 2000 What's new in congenital disorders of glycosylation? European Journal of Paediatric Neurology l4: 163–167

Jones K L 1997 Smith's recognizable patterns of human malformation, 5th edn. WB Saunders, Philadelphia

Kalousek D K, Vekemans M 2000 Confined placental mosaicism and genomic imprinting. Baillières Clinical Obstetrics and Gynaecology 14: 723–730

Koren G et al 1998 Drugs in pregnancy. New England Journal of Medicine 338: 1128–1137

Korson M S 2000 Advances in newborn screening for metabolic disorders: what the pediatrician needs to know. Pediatric Annals 29: 294–301

Lachmann R H, Platt F M 2001 Substrate reduction therapy for glycosphingolipid storage disorders. Expert Opinion on Investigational Drugs 10: 455–466

Leonard J V, Schapira A H 2000 Mitochondrial respiratory chain disorders I: mitochondrial DNA defects. Lancet 355: 299–304

Leonard J V, Schapira A H 2000 Mitochondrial respiratory chain disorders II: neurodegenerative disorders and nuclear gene defects. Lancet 355: 389–394

Marteau T, Richards M 1996 The troubled helix. Cambridge University Press, Cambridge

Milunsky A (ed.) 1998 Genetic disorders and the fetus: diagnosis, prevention and treatment, 4th edn. John Hopkins University Press, Baltimore

Moser H W 2000 Molecular genetics of peroxisomal disorders. Frontiers in Bioscience 5D: 298–306

Newberger D 2000 Down syndrome: prenatal risk assessment and diagnosis. American Family Physician 62: 825–832

Richards R I, Sutherland G R 1997 Dynamic mutation: possible mechanisms and significance in human disease. Trends in Biochemical Sciences 22: 432–436

Robertson S C, Tynan J A, Donoghue D J 2000 RTK mutations and human syndromes: when good receptors turn bad. Trends in Genetics 16: 265–271

Saudubray J M, Ogier H, Bonnefont J P et al 1989 Clinical approach to inherited metabolic diseases in the neonatal period: a 20-year survey. Journal of Inherited Metabolic Disease 12(suppl 1): 25–41

Schardein J L 2000 Chemically induced birth defects, 3rd edn. Marcel Dekker, New York

Scriver C R, Beaudet A L, Sly W S, Valle D 2000 The metabolic and molecular bases of inherited disease, 8th edn. McGraw-Hill, New York

Strachan T, Read A P 1999 Human molecular genetics, 2nd edn. Bios, Oxford

Suthers G 1996 Mutations, malformations and mortality. Journal of Paediatrics and Child Health 32: 10–15

Trent R J A 1997 Molecular medicine, 2nd edn. Churchill Livingstone, Edinburgh

Wallace D C 1999 Mitochondrial diseases in man and mouse. Science 283: 1482–1488

Weaver D 1999 Catalog of prenatally diagnosed conditions, 3rd edn. John Hopkins University Press, Baltimore

Williamson R 1993 Universal community carrier screening for cystic fibrosis? Nature Genetics 3: 195–201

Winchester B, Vellodi A, Young E 2000 The molecular basis of lysosomal storage diseases and their treatment. Biochemical Society Transactions 28: 150–154

Winter R M, Baraitser M 2000 The London dysmorphology database: a computerised database for the diagnosis of rare syndromes. Oxford University Press, Oxford

Useful links

http://www.birthdefects.org/ (The Association for Birth Defects Research for Children)

http://www.cpdx.com/ (Centre for Prenatal Diagnosis)

http://www.growthcharts.com/charts/ds/charts.html (Growth charts for Down syndrome: height and weight (metric and imperial))

http://www.health.gov.au/tga/docs/html/medpreg.htm (Australian Drug Evaluation Committee — prescribing medicines in pregnancy — categorisation of risk of drug use in pregnancy)

http://www.lda.org.au (Lysosomal Diseases Australia)

http://www.ncbi.nlm.nih.gov/entrez/query.fcgi?db=OMIM (Catalogue of genetic disorders)

http://www3.ncbi.nlm.nih.gov/Omim/ (Online Mendelian Inheritance in Man (OMIM))

http://www.ndss.org (US National Down Syndrome Society)

http://www.ornl.gov/TechResources/Human_Genome/home.html (Human Genome Project)

http://www.otispregnancy.org/fact_sheet.htm (Organisation of Teratology Information Services fact sheets)

http://www.pbs.org/gene/ (Ethics and the application of genetic knowledge)

http://www.possum.net.au (OMIM (Online Mendelian Inheritance in Man))

http://www.umdf.org (United Mitochondrial Diseases Foundation)

PART 11

NEONATAL PROBLEMS

The normal newborn

N. Campbell

Most babies are born at term gestation (37–42 weeks), following normal pregnancy and labour, and are healthy. Having a baby is for most people one of life's most joyous and enriching experiences. Health professionals should keep these matters in mind and be as unobtrusive as possible with medical interventions, remembering we are, in a way, privileged to share in this special experience.

Medical care of such babies consists of:
- ensuring normal adaptation to extrauterine life
- assessing intrauterine growth and development
- checking for birth defects
- supporting and advising the parents in their new role.

Birth: a transition

Birth triggers a series of transitional processes which adapt the fetus to life outside the womb. Only the most important are outlined here.

Respiration

Before birth, exchange of oxygen and carbon dioxide are performed by the placenta. The fetal lung has no respiratory function, although the fetus makes small intermittent breathing movements. The birth process stimulates continuous regular breathing, the lungs are expanded rapidly with air resulting in oxygen and carbon dioxide exchange, and the respiratory functions of the placenta cease. The onset of effective breathing may be delayed if the baby has been depressed by asphyxia or maternal analgesics, especially opiates, during labour.

Circulation

The fetus has in effect a single circulation, both ventricles pumping to the fetal systemic circulation and placenta, with minimal circulation through the lungs. This changes quickly after birth into two separate circulations, the right (pulmonary) and the left (systemic), and the placental circulation ceases. Before birth there is a high resistance to blood flow through the unexpanded lungs, so blood returning to the right side of the heart bypasses the lungs through the foramen ovale and the ductus arteriosus. Breathing expands the lungs, resulting in a rapid fall in pulmonary vascular resistance and a rise in pulmonary blood flow. The foramen ovale and ductus arteriosus close and thus separate

pulmonary and systemic circulations are established. Most of this transition occurs with the first few breaths. Occasionally it is delayed, usually because pulmonary vascular resistance fails to fall despite adequate breathing. This delay is called persistent fetal circulation. The baby remains cyanosed (blue) despite apparently adequate breathing. Life threatening hypoxia can result (Ch. 34).

Metabolism

Many metabolic transitions must occur in the minutes and hours after birth. For example, the fetus does not have to generate metabolic heat energy to keep warm, the temperature being maintained by the maternal environment. From birth, diverse and complex adaptations must be brought into play to produce suffficient heat energy to maintain the core temperature. These adaptations progress over many days, but even though they occur, babies can become cold easily and careful attention to maintenance of temperature is important.

Nutrition

Fetal nutrition is supplied by the placenta. The fetal gastrointestinal tract has little function. From birth, placental nutrition ceases and gastrointestinal motility and secretory and digestive functions are 'switched on' over days so that the gut can take over nutrition. Breast milk production increases progressively during the days after birth, complementing the progressive development of gut motility and digestive capacity. There are factors in breast milk which trigger or promote gastrointestinal adaptation.

Bilirubin clearance

Before birth unconjugated bilirubin is excreted by the placenta. Conjugation of bilirubin by the fetal liver is suppressed, as it cannot be excreted by the placenta. From birth hepatic conjugation of bilirubin is 'switched on' allowing bilirubin to be excreted in bile. This transition takes days, so that transient accumulation of bilirubin — jaundice — is common in babies (Ch. 33).

Glucose homeostasis

Fetal blood glucose levels are maintained by the placenta. The complex hormonal and metabolic mechanisms responsible for blood glucose homeostasis in adults are inactive. From birth these complex mechanisms are 'switched on' over several days. Babies have lower, less stable blood glucose levels than older age groups. Failure or delay in these adaptations can lead to serious hypoglycaemia (Ch. 33).

By definition, normal babies undergo normal physiological adaptations after birth. Conversely there are 'diseases' babies may suffer which are simply failures or delays in normal adaptation, for example, persistence of the fetal circulation. Additionally, many diseases of babies cause delays in adaptation; for example, intrapartum asphyxia may delay the onset of breathing, glucose homeostasis and gut motility.

Care after birth

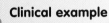

Clinical example

Baby Nguyen, born by spontaneous vaginal delivery after a normal pregnancy and labour, breathed within 20 seconds and rapidly became pink. Nurse Jones passed a suction catheter to the back of his mouth and applied suction, as she had been taught to do in her midwifery training. Baby Nguyen immediately made choking noises, turned blue, and stopped breathing for more than 20 seconds. His mother and father cried out, thinking he was dying. Nurse Jones's supervisor put the baby in his mother's arms, spoke quietly and reassuringly and he resumed breathing and cried.

Normal babies establish effective breathing and normal colour within 1 or 2 minutes. They require no immediate medical intervention. As long as it is obvious that a baby is breathing well, becoming pink, is roughly the expected size (not unexpectedly premature or very small from intrauterine growth retardation), and free of gross malformations requiring immediate care (for example, a myelomeningocele), he or she should be passed quickly to the parents. A common practice is to place the baby on the mother's lower abdomen or in her arms, lightly covered in previously warmed wraps.

Catheter suction of mucus or liquor from the nose and mouth used to be performed routinely in all babies at birth. It is now known that it provides no benefit to normal babies and sometimes causes harm. It is distressing and should not be done.

Occasionally babies establish normal breathing and colour quickly, but then develop respiratory distress, hypoventilation, or even apnoea. If unrecognised, such babies can become hypoxic and seriously ill. To avoid this they should be observed for 5–10 seconds every 10 minutes or so during the first hour. Many families choose

to experience labour and delivery in semi-darkness. Attendants can use small bright clinical torches with good batteries to make observations after birth, taking care not to shine them directly in the baby's or parents' eyes.

Babies lose large amounts of heat through evaporation of amniotic fluid from the skin and wet wraps. After the first 10 minutes or so from birth, attendants should assist parents in wiping the baby dry and replacing wet wraps with prewarmed dry wraps.

Apgar scores

Some babies are born unexpectedly asphyxiated. Because hypoxia and acidosis in labour depress brain and cardiac function, asphyxiated babies fail to establish effective breathing and circulation after birth. Analgesics or anaesthetics given to mother in labour, and rare developmental abnormalities, also can depress brain function at birth.

The Apgar score is used to evaluate:
- brain function at birth
- circulatory status at birth
- the effectiveness of respiratory and circulatory adaptations thereafter
- which babies need active assistance (resuscitation).

Five indicators of status at birth and adaptation are each assigned a score between 0 and 2. This scoring is performed at 1 minute and 5 minutes of age. The indicators are as follows:
- *Heart rate.* The heart rate is counted over 15–30 seconds by auscultation. An undetectable heart beat scores 0; less than 100 beats/minute scores 1; and greater than 100 scores 2.
- *Respiratory effort.* Breathing movements are counted over 15–30 seconds and their quality assessed. No respiratory efforts, or only occasional gasps score 0; irregular or inefficient efforts score 1; and regular effective breathing, including crying, scores 2.
- *Reflex irritability.* A tactile stimulus is applied, such as inserting a suction catheter into the nose, and the reflex response observed: facial grimacing or withdrawal away from the stimulus. No response scores 0; a weak or incomplete grimace scores 1; and a complete grimace or withdrawal scores 2.
- *Muscle tone and movements.* A floppy baby with no tone and no limb movements scores 0; babies with partial flexion or weak movements of the limbs score 1; and babies with well flexed limbs and active movements score 2.
- *Colour.* Fetuses are blue. When breathing is effective and the fetal circulation undergoes its usual transition rapidly they become pink. Babies who remain centrally cyanosed, with blue lips and oral mucosa, score 0; they are often also very pale due to poor cardiac output and

circulation. Babies who become centrally pink, but whose body or limbs remain blue (peripheral cyanosis) score 1; and babies pink all over score 2.

Apgar scores, at 1 minute, of:
- 8–10 indicate a baby in good condition adapting well and not in need of assistance.
- 4–7 indicate a baby who may have suffered mild to moderate asphyxia. Such a baby warrants continuous observation and may need assistance if not improving.
- 0–3 indicate a baby with moderate to severe asphyxia or other serious illness, and urgent active resuscitation is needed.

The Apgar score at 5 minutes reassures that adaptation is successful in well babies. It is a guide to how well resuscitative measures are succeeding in very sick babies. In the sickest babies requiring prolonged resuscitation the Apgar score is repeated at 5 minute intervals (10, 15 and 20 minutes) until recovery.

Although it has been used for decades, the Apgar score does not correlate very well with asphyxia and outcome. Some babies with low scores at 1 minute quickly improve without assistance; some babies with reasonable 1 minute scores subsequently turn out to have serious asphyxia. Nor does it predict long term outcome very well. Most babies with Apgar scores of 0–3, even at 5 minutes, survive without brain damage and permanent handicaps.

Many hospitals and governments require that Apgar scores be recorded for every baby born, for legal and statistical reasons. However, properly performed Apgar scores require close observation of a near naked baby for at least 30 seconds, with auscultation of the heart and tests of tone and reflex irritability. They are thus intrusive and potentially distressing for baby and family. For these reasons most experienced doctors and midwives perform prospective Apgar scores only on very sick babies. For all other babies Apgars are often assigned retrospectively by inference. For example, in the well baby, obviously breathing and perhaps crying, turning quickly pink and wrapped up in its mother's arms by 1 minute, an Apgar score of 9–10 can be assigned by inference. Five seconds of visual inspection of the baby's face, hand and upper chest at 5 minutes can allow an Apgar score of 9–10 at that time also by inference.

Tests of reflex irritability should never be performed on babies who are clearly in good condition; performed on conscious babies they are distressing and serve no purpose. In such babies a score of 2 can always be inferred.

Resuscitation

The birth of an asphyxiated fetus usually can be predicted. There are risk factors or warning signs in pregnancy or labour. When these occur, advance preparations can be made. These include:

- transferring the mother to a specialised unit for delivery
- having a paediatrician skilled in resuscitation present for the delivery
- ensuring necessary equipment is available and functioning.

However, in about 30% of babies born with serious asphyxia, the condition is unexpected. It is therefore important that all facilities delivering babies have all the equipment necessary for resuscitation available in good working order, and personnel skilled in its use.

The principles of resuscitation of babies failing to breathe and adapt at birth are the same as for 'collapse' in older age groups ('ABC'; Chs 19, 20) but babies also need special measures to maintain temperature. The immediate aim is to ensure, as quickly as possible, adequate perfusion of the brain and heart with oxygenated, glucose-containing blood, at the same time reducing respiratory and metabolic acidosis.

Babies can become cold quickly when they are exposed at normal room temperatures for the 10–30 minutes required for resuscitation. Mortality and morbidity rise when babies become cold. A radiant heater or other effective heat source is essential. The room should be warm, with doors and windows closed to prevent draughts. The baby should be dried and kept at least partially covered with prewarmed wraps.

The airway (nose, mouth, and pharynx) should be cleared by suction of meconium, blood or infected liquor if present.

Breathing should be assisted artificially, to establish oxygenation and ventilation as quickly as possible. This can be achieved by a bag and facemask designed specifically for babies if the baby is already making some respiratory effort. Endotracheal intubation is essential in babies making no effort or if bag and mask ventilation are not effective rapidly.

External cardiac massage may be needed if the heart rate and circulation do not improve with effective artificial ventilation (Ch.20). An intravenous catheter can be inserted easily into the umbilical vein for drugs and infusions. This should be done only *after* effective ventilation is established and maintained. Most asphyxiated babies are hypovolaemic. Normal saline or 5% albumin can be given to improve circulating blood volume. Hypoglycaemia is common; intravenous 10% dextrose can be given. Metabolic acidosis can be corrected with intravenous sodium bicarbonate. Occasionally babies are depressed by maternal opiates; naloxone can be given to reverse this effect.

Although babies requiring active resuscitation at birth may appear relatively well by 30–60 minutes of age, they must be admitted to a special care unit or intensive care unit for close observation, as they may develop apnoea, respiratory distress, hypoglycaemia or convulsions.

Examination of the newborn

This is best performed in three episodes, each with different purposes.

The initial examination

The initial examination has already been described. It is performed in the first minutes of life, and at regular intervals for the first hour or so thereafter. Its purpose is to ensure that the baby is roughly the expected size and gestation, is free of gross malformations requiring immediate attention, and is adapting successfully. Every effort should be made to be as unobtrusive as possible.

The subsequent examinations: general points

Two further examinations, much more thorough, are performed, one within the first 4–8 hours, the other around the time of discharge.

The following description of the newborn examination is meant to provide a technique of examination, and is a starting point rather than an exhaustive description. Examination of babies, like many things in medicine, is learnt by practice over time. It is different from that of older age groups, both in method and information sought. Many babies are distressed by the handling required: for example, undressing, opening the eyes and mouth, palpating the abdomen, and examining the hips. Auscultation of the chest, feeling the pulses, assessing tone and reflexes, and examining the hips are not possible in a crying struggling infant.

Distress can be avoided by:
- examining in a warm, quiet environment;
- beginning at the completion of a breastfeed;
- returning the baby to the mother to settle if he or she becomes distressed,
- performing first those parts of the examination that are least likely to disturb, leaving the potentially upsetting parts till the end.

If the baby has been dressed, it is best that he or she be undressed well before the examination, and either breastfed or cuddled in warm wraps until the examination. Although it is disruptive of busy schedules, it as well to abandon the examination if the baby becomes markedly upset, and resume at another time.

One or both parents should be present. It is educational, reassuring, and of great interest to most parents to have parts of the examination discussed and questions answered as it proceeds. It also can be rewarding to both parents and examiner (and is good manners) if the examiner makes admiring comments about the baby, and congratulates the parents on their achievement.

The first 'thorough' examination

At the first thorough examination:
- the progress of adaptation is reassessed
- gestational age is confirmed
- a careful search for birth defects is made
- neurological status is assessed
- the baby is weighed and measured
- if the baby is at the breast, rooting and sucking reflexes can be observed, as well as colour.

The rooting reflex consists of the baby turning the head vigorously towards the nipple (or finger) stroking the cheek and attempting to grasp the stimulus with the mouth. The baby's colour should be pink, although hands and feet may normally be blue (peripheral cyanosis). Jaundice in the first 24 hours is always pathological and requires investigation (Ch. 33).

After unwrapping, posture (slightly curled up with limbs flexed) and spontaneous movements (equal on both sides) can be observed, together with respiratory rate and quality. The heart and lungs should then be auscultated. The respiratory rate changes from 60–80 breaths per minute in the first 15–20 minutes of life, to 40–60 breaths per minute after 30 minutes. Although breathing is often irregular (changing rate rapidly), difficult and laboured breathing suggests lung disease or upper airway obstruction. The heart rate reduces from 150–180 beats per minute in the first 15–20 minutes to 90–120 beats per minute at rest, and to up to 180 beats per minute when crying. The brachial and femoral pulses should be felt at this stage.

Close examination by inspection and palpation from head to toes can then be performed.

Head and neck

The head circumference is measured and compared to the appropriate percentile charts. The scalp is often swollen by oedema over the presenting part, the caput succedaneum. This is normal, painless and resolves quickly. A cephalhaematoma is a large fluctuant swelling covering the entire surface of a single skull bone (usually the parietal bone), due to bleeding under the periosteum. It is alarming to parents but is benign, painless, does not imply undue birth trauma and resolves over weeks. The fontanelles and sutures should all be felt. Any birthmarks should be pointed out to parents. Flat capillary naevi, known as 'naevus flammeus', are very common on the eyelids, in the midline of the upper lip and forehead, and at the nape of the neck (here called a 'stork bite'). They are benign and fade with time.

A good view of the eyes can often be obtained when the baby opens them spontaneously. Subconjunctival haemorrhages are common and do not imply birth trauma. Note should be taken that the eyes are equal in size, that the corneas are not opaque, and are also of normal size, around 11 mm in diameter.

The mouth and palate should be examined, looking for clefts of the palate or alveolar margin. Mucous retention cysts of the gums are common and are benign. Oral inspection can often be done whenever the baby spontaneously opens the mouth: if the examiner has to open the mouth it is best done towards the end of the examination as it may be distressing.

The face as a whole, including the ears, should be evaluated for its symmetry and the presence of any dysmorphic features, which may indicate the presence of a congenital syndrome (Ch. 29).

Chest, abdomen and genitalia

The chest and abdomen should then be inspected, noting birthmarks, the nipples and breast tissue, and the umbilicus. The breasts are often prominent with 10–15 mm of breast tissue palpable under the nipple. Milky fluid ('witches milk') can sometimes be seen coming from the nipple. Occasionally the defect of the abdominal muscle wall at the umbilicus is wider than usual, presenting as an umbilical hernia.

The abdomen should be palpated. In a relaxed baby, 1–2 cm of liver edge can be felt under the right costal margin, extending across the midline. Occasionally the tip of the spleen can be felt; more than this may be abnormal. With experience, and a relaxed baby, the lower poles of both kidneys can be felt in each upper quadrant. Although it is higher than in older age groups, the bladder should not be palpable, except briefly when the baby is about to pass urine.

The genitalia should be examined carefully. In boys, the urethral opening should be identified, and both testes sought gently. There are wide variations in the shape, size and pigmentation of the male genitalia, learnt by practice. In girls, the labia minora and clitoris are often partly exposed, visible between the labia majora. The anus should be assessed for patency, tone and position. An anus very close to the genitalia (anterior) may indicate stenosis or underlaying genitourinary malformations. Digital examination (PR) is not part of routine examination. It is distressing and should only be done by an experienced person if there is a specific question to be answered.

Other examinations

Turning the baby prone, the spine should be examined from neck to anus. Grey-purple birthmarks, often extensive, occur in the lumbosacral region. These are known as 'Mongolian blue spots'. They are commoner in non Caucasian babies. Hairy tufts or patches over the sacral area may indicate spina bifida occulta (Ch. 59) There is often a dimple or pit in the mid line at the base of the sacrum: the 'sacral dimple' or 'pit'. As long as the bottom of the dimple is clearly visible and intact it is normal. If the floor of the dimple cannot be seen, there may be an abnormal sinus track in communication with the spinal canal. The hands, arms, legs and feet should be inspected and digits counted with the baby again supine. The pattern of the palmar creases should be noted: they are abnormal in some congenital syndromes. The limbs should be gently put through a wide range of passive movements evaluating joint mobility, muscle tone and strength.

During the course of these examinations observations of the baby's neurological state can be made incidentally, including the level of consciousness or awareness; the quality and symmetry of spontaneous limb movements; tone and strength, and rooting and sucking reflexes. The baby will often grasp the examiner's fingers or stethoscope, exhibiting the grasp reflex, which is the automatic grasping of objects touching the baby's palm. The walking reflex consists of walking movements of the legs stimulated by the soles of the feet touching a surface when the baby is held vertical. It is not necessary to elicit this reflex if the baby otherwise appears normal, but it is often of great interest to parents.

The Moro reflex is a primitive reflex of academic interest. Eliciting it is distressing to the babies. It should not be performed in infants who appear otherwise neurologically normal. It can be of value in babies and infants who for other reasons are suspected of having serious neurological abnormalities.

Finally the hips should be examined to ensure enlocation (Ch. 25); the mouth and eyes can be opened by the examiner if the baby has not already done so spontaneously, and the length and weight can be measured.

The 'discharge' examination

The second thorough examination is best performed around 7 days of age. Its purposes are:
- to evaluate feeding and weight progress
- to ensure jaundice has resolved
- to recheck for minor birth defects and major malformations not apparent on the first day
- to discuss the baby's progress with the parents.

Major social and economic changes in the organisation of normal baby care have made this second examination problematic. Mothers and babies used to stay in hospital for 7–10 days. To contain costs, and for social reasons, length of stay is becoming shorter. The average in many places is now 3 days, and many families leave after stays as short as 4, 24 or 48 hours.

Health workers have been concerned that early discharge for the purpose of reducing costs will lead to harm; for example, failure of breastfeeding, severe jaundice, or major malformations or serious infections going unrecognised until the affected baby has become very ill. So far the evidence for this is inconclusive. There are published reports of babies requiring readmission for the above reasons, but far fewer than was feared. It remains to be seen whether early discharge will turn out to be a net benefit or not. In the meantime a careful examination and evaluation of the normal baby as either an inpatient or outpatient at around 1 week of age should be the aim.

For this examination a history should be taken, enquiring into the baby's general behaviour, feeding, bladder and bowel function, weight progress and any parental concerns.

The same techniques of physical examination as described previously should be used. A few minutes of feeding should be observed to ensure that the mother's technique is correct and that the baby is sucking and swallowing normally.

Neurological assessment can be more refined:

- Does the baby 'attend', that is, suddenly become still, and possibly turn towards her when the mother speaks to him?
- Does he 'fix' with his eyes on his mother's face, and follow the face when it moves?
- Visual fixing and following are tested as follows: the baby is held so that his face is 15–20 cm from the examiner's face and in the *en face* position; that is, the baby's and examiner's faces have the same orientation. A relaxed alert baby will fix the eyes on the examiner's face and follow movements sideways. Though not conclusive, attending, fixing and following are a reassurance that a baby is normal.

The complete physical examination is repeated. Jaundice should have resolved by 7 days of age.

Some major malformations may not be apparent at birth, but may start to become apparent after the first week. For example, in some cases of congenital hydrocephalus, the fontanelles, sutures and head circumference are normal at birth, but signs of rising intracranial pressure slowly appear during the following days and weeks. There may be no signs at birth of major heart malformations, such as ventricular septal defect or coarction of the aorta, but signs emerge thereafter, such as murmurs, hepatomegaly, tachypnoea and abnormal pulses.

Examining babies should be a pleasant experience for the examiner, the parents and the baby. Patience is essential: if battles arise, the baby always wins!

Other first week care

Vitamin K

All babies are given vitamin K (phytomenadione) soon after birth to prevent haemorrhagic disease of the newborn. It is usually given as an intramuscular injection within minutes of birth. Alternatively, it can be given orally but this is less effective and has to be repeated at around 4 days and again at 4 weeks of age.

Some parents are concerned about vitamin K administration because of past reports that it increased the risk of childhood cancers. These reports have been proven wrong and parents can be reassured. The issue should be discussed and decided in the antenatal period well before birth.

Immunisations

Babies born to mothers who are hepatitis BSAg positive are given hepatitis B vaccine and hepatitis B immune globulin)(HBIG) at birth. All babies should receive hepatitis B vaccine (HBV) at birth (Ch. 8).

Biochemical screening

All babies have blood tests at around 4 days of age to screen for rare biochemical diseases. The diseases screened for vary between States in Australia, but usually include phenylketonuria, hypothyroidism and cystic fibrosis (Ch. 31).

Protection from infection

All normal babies are born microbiologically sterile. The skin, mouth and pharynx, gastrointestinal tract and respiratory tract become colonised with environmental bacterial flora, including the flora of people who handle the babies, in the first 72 hours. Babies have reduced immunity and a correspondingly high risk of infection from colonising organisms. Various measures are taken to minimise these risks. Breastfeeding is the most important mechanism. It provides antibodies and other factors which protect against a range of infections. It also reduces the numbers of people handling the baby for feeding and thus the range of organisms to which the baby is exposed. Careful handwashing by all health workers handling babies also is very important.

'Rooming in' rather than 'nursery nursing' also reduces infection. Rooming in means that from birth the mother and baby stay together in the same room, with mother being the main person handling her baby. In contrast, nursery nursing means many babies are nursed together in a common nursery, away from their mothers, in contact with other babies, and handled by many people, for example three shifts of nurses each day.

There are various procedures for skin and umbilical care which are aimed at reducing infection, but their efficacy is much less clear than the measures described above. For example, from time to time various antiseptics have been used to bathe babies to reduce or control skin colonisation. In the past, nursery epidemics of *Staphylococcus aureus* have been managed this way, but if rooming in and handwashing are practised, it is doubtful that antiseptic soaps or lotions are efficacious.

The umbilical stump is a potential site of entry for infections. In the past, various regimens, including anointing the stump every 4 hours with antiseptic or alcohol, have been used to try to minimise bacterial colonisation. As with skin washing, it is doubtful whether such practices are useful or necessary.

Other normal baby matters

Weight

Normal babies lose up to 5% of their birth weight in the first 3–5 days, and regain birth weight by 7–10 days.

Micturition

Normal babies often pass urine soon after birth, then infrequently for the next 24 hours. As feeding is established urine is passed more often, usually every 3–4 hours.

Bowel actions

Twenty per cent of babies pass meconium before delivery or during the first 4 hours afterwards; 96% pass meconium by 24 hours; and 99.9% by 48 hours. Failure to pass meconium by 48 hours is almost always abnormal, and may indicate Hirschsprung disease, meconium plug syndrome or meconium ileus.

Jaundice

Around 40% of normal babies develop transient physiological jaundice. By definition it is never present in the first 24 hours, peaks during day 3, and is rapidly resolving by day 5. Variations from this pattern may indicate a pathological cause.

Vomiting

Small volume (<5 ml) occasional vomits are common, as all babies have some degree of gastro-oesophageal reflux in the first week of life. 'Possets' are tiny 1–2 ml vomits. Larger, more frequent vomits may be a normal variation, but also may be the first signs of illness, for example a bacterial infection. Vomits containing bile (which is green, not yellow) are almost always abnormal, strongly suggesting bowel obstruction, and should always be investigated even if other indicators of bowel obstruction (distension and constipation) are absent.

Temperature

Normal babies maintain their core temperature in the same range as older age groups if they are dressed adequately and wrapped. Elevated or low temperatures must be taken seriously as they can be early indicators that a baby is ill, especially with serious infections. Skin temperature measurements can be unreliable in babies; a high or low skin temperature should be checked by measuring rectal temperature.

Waking, sleeping, crying

Normal babies are usually awake and active for 30 minutes or so after birth. Thereafter patterns of sleep, wakefulness and crying are extremely variable. On average, babies sleep for at least 18 hours per 24 hours in the first week. They may cry for an average of 4 hours or more per 24 hours. Babies appear to have complex visual experiences: they can distinguish the human face from other objects, and show other distinguishing behaviours to a range of visual stimuli. They can hear and distinguish their mother's voice from other sounds. They have a sense of smell and can distinguish their mother's smell from others. They distinguish between several tastes. They move in characteristic ways to different rhythms of speech, and they mimic adult facial movements, including tongue protrusion.

We attribute many human experiences, emotions and moods to babies, and rightly so, but no one really knows what it is like to be a baby. Health workers should strive to make this episode in life as rewarding as possible for babies and their parents. The rewards for health workers who achieve these goals are also great.

Low birth weight, prematurity and jaundice in infancy

J. Harding

Principles of care

Care of the sick newborn is usually thought of as complex and requiring specialised training and equipment. However, remembering the basic principles will allow you to provide emergency care for the sick newborn, regardless of diagnosis, until such specialised help is available:

- *Keep the baby pink.* Initial resuscitation should follow the usual ABC guidelines (Chs 19, 20). After that, many babies will maintain breathing with supplemental oxygen until more sophisticated respiratory support is available. The right amount of oxygen is the least amount that is needed to keep the baby pink.
- *Keep the baby warm.* Cooling increases the baby's oxygen and glucose requirements and is associated with increased mortality. Dry the baby promptly after birth and put a hat on the baby to reduce heat loss while you are assessing other problems. Use a radiant heater, electric blanket or incubator if available.
- *Keep the baby fed.* Sick babies are at risk of hypoglycaemia, which can cause brain damage. If milk feeds are not possible, give intravenous dextrose 60 ml/kg/day (2.5 ml/kg/h).
- *Consider infection.* Almost any signs and symptoms of illness in the newborn can be caused by infection, and untreated septicaemia can cause death within hours. If specialised care is likely to be delayed by more than an hour or two, take blood cultures if possible and give intravenous or intramuscular antibiotics.

Definitions

Babies are commonly classified into groups associated with different disease patterns and different outcomes (Fig. 33.1). These include:

- **Gestation**
  Term: ≥ 37 completed weeks gestation
  Preterm: <37 completed weeks gestation
  Post-term: >42 completed weeks gestation

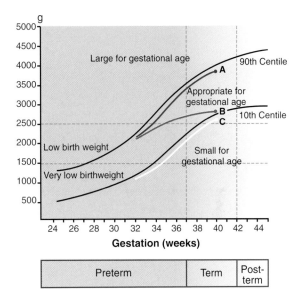

Fig. 33.1   Common definitions of size at birth, illustrating the difference between intrauterine growth restriction (IUGR) and small for gestational age (SGA). Baby A is an appropriately grown term baby. Baby B is also born appropriate size for gestational age (AGA), but has suffered reduced intrauterine growth compared to baby A and thus has intrauterine growth restriction (IUGR). Baby C has had normal intrauterine growth, but is born small for gestational age (SGA).

- **Birth weight**
  Low birth weight (LBW):   <2500 g
  Very low birth weight (VLBW):   <1500 g
  Extremely low birth weight (ELBW):   <1000 g
- **Weight for gestational age**
  Appropriate for gestation (AGA): birth weight between 10th and 90th centiles for gestation
  Small for gestational age (SGA): birth weight <10th centile for gestation
  Large for gestational age (LGA): birth weight >90th centile for gestation.

The premature infant

Causes of premature birth

Major risk factors for preterm birth are well recognised (Table 33.1), although approximately half of preterm births occur in the absence of recognised risk factors. There is an increased risk of recurrence in mothers with a previous history of preterm labour. Mortality is inversely related to gestational age and birth weight (Fig. 33.2).

> ### Clinical example (part A)
>
> George is a 900 g (extremely low birth weight) baby born to a 16 year old mother who received no prenatal care. His mother was admitted after the membranes ruptured and she began to have contractions. She did not remember the date of her last menstrual period and had not had any antenatal ultrasound scans. She smoked a pack of cigarettes per day during the pregnancy. At delivery, George had poor respiratory effort and marked retractions so he was intubated in the delivery room and was brought to the neonatal intensive care unit. He required moderate ventilator settings and 50% oxygen. Chest X ray showed a diffuse ground glass appearance with air bronchograms consistent with respiratory distress syndrome. A dose of surfactant was given through the endotracheal tube. Gestational age was estimated at approximately 27 weeks based on the Ballard examination, which assesses physical and neuromuscular development. Based on this estimated gestation, the infant's weight, length and head circumference were all at the 25th centile, and were appropriate for his gestational age.

Table 33.1 Risk factors for preterm birth

Maternal	Placenta and membranes
Extremes of maternal age	Placenta previa
High gravidity	Abruptio placentae
Low prepregnant weight	Premature rupture of
Acute abdomen	membranes
Pyelonephritis	Chorioamnionitis
Uterine anomalies	
Cervical incompetence	**Social**
Pre-eclampsia/ eclampsia	Low socioeconomic status
Prior termination of	Smoking
pregnancy	Alcohol abuse
History of infertility	Illicit drug abuse
Genital infection	Fatigue and psychological
	stress
Fetal	
Multiple gestation	**Idiopathic**
Fetal anomalies	Previous preterm delivery
Polyhydramnios	
Fetal demise	
First trimester threatened	
abortion	

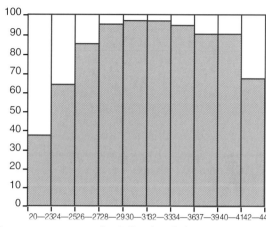

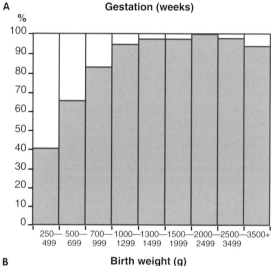

Died ☐   Survived ▨

Fig. 33.2 Survival of preterm infants according to **A** gestational age and **B** birth weight. From Donoghue and Cust, 1999, with permission.

Short term complications of prematurity

The incidence and severity of all complications of prematurity are inversely related to gestation and birth weight (Fig. 33.3, Table 33.2).

Respiratory

Respiratory distress syndrome (RDS). This disorder is also called hyaline membrane disease or surfactant deficiency syndrome. Immaturity of the respiratory system with surfactant deficiency results in respiratory distress. This is managed with oxygen, nasal continuous positive airway pressure (NCPAP), or, when more severe, surfactant administration and mechanical ventilation. Corticosteroids given to the mother before preterm birth can reduce the incidence and severity of RDS.

Periodic breathing, apnoea of prematurity. Premature infants commonly experience periodic breathing due to immaturity of the respiratory centres of the brain. Cessation of breathing persisting for >20 seconds is termed apnoea. This often results in bradycardia and desaturation, so premature infants require cardiorespiratory and pulse oximetry monitoring. Apnoea of prematurity occurs in almost all extremely preterm infants, and usually improves around 34–36 weeks postmenstrual age. Pharmacological treatment includes methylxanthines such as caffeine or theophylline, which improve diaphragmatic contraction and stimulate the respiratory centres. NCPAP is also helpful, partly by reducing any obstructive component to the apnoea and reducing the work of breathing. If apnoea is severe the infant may have to be ventilated mechanically. Apnoea can also be caused by many

Table 33.2 Complications of preterm birth

	Common	Rare except in VLBW
Early		
Respiratory	Respiratory distress syndrome Apnoea	
Cardiac		Patent ductus arteriosus
Neurological		Periventricular haemorrhage Periventricular leucomalacia
Hepatic	Hypoglycaemia Hyperbilirubinaemia	Hyperglycaemia
Renal	Hyponatraemia	Hyperkalaemia Metabolic acidosis
Gastrointestinal	Feeding problems	Necrotising enterocolitis
Other	Anaemia Infection Poor thermo- regulation	
Late	Delayed growth	Retinopathy of prematurity Chronic lung disease Neurodevelopmental delay

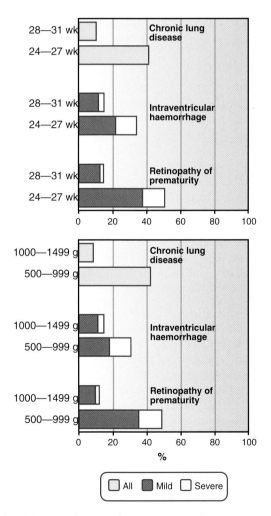

Fig. 33.3 Complications of prematurity according to **A** gestational age and **B** birth weight. From Donoghue and Cust, 1999, with permission.

other complications of prematurity, such as infection, neurological problems, anaemia, hypoxia, patent ductus arteriosus and upper airway obstruction, so these need to be considered in infants experiencing apnoea.

Cardiac

Patent ductus arteriosus (PDA). Before birth the ductus arteriosus diverts blood from the right ventricle away from the lungs to the aorta. After birth it normally closes functionally within a few days. In preterm babies, closure may be delayed, leading to left to right shunting of blood from the aorta through the ductus to the lungs. This results in pulmonary congestion, worsening lung disease, and decreased blood flow to the gastrointestinal tract and brain. These changes have been implicated in the pathogenesis of necrotising enterocolitis and intraventricular haemorrhage. Clinical signs of a PDA include a continuous heart murmur, hyperdynamic precordium, bounding pulses and widened pulse pressure. Diagnosis is made by echocardiogram. Treatment is by giving antiprostaglandins (indomethacin or ibuprofen). If these are unsuccessful, surgical ligation may be necessary.

Neurological

Periventricular or intraventricular haemorrhage (IVH). This is due to bleeding from the immature rich capillary bed of the germinal matrix lining the ventricles. Risk factors include asphyxia and changes in cerebral blood flow due to hypotension or rapid intravenous fluid infusion. Intraventricular haemorrhage often occurs within the first 48 hours of life. It is diagnosed by cranial ultrasound, and is graded by severity from grade I IVH (germinal matrix haemorrhage) to grade IV (intra-parenchymal haemorrhage). Although lower grades of IVH have a good prognosis, grades III and IV IVH are often associated with hydrocephalus and neurological abnormalities such as cerebral palsy.

> ### Clinical example (part B)
>
> George improved significantly after the administration of surfactant. He was extubated and was placed on nasal continuous positive airway pressure (NCPAP) by age 36 hours. Caffeine was given before extubation in anticipation of apnoea of prematurity. Small feedings of expressed breast milk were started on day 3. Electrolytes were monitored closely because of the potential for large insensible water losses.
>
> On day 4, George began to deteriorate with increasing apnoeas and respiratory distress. A continuous murmur was noted along the left sternal border. The pulses were bounding and the precordium was very active. An echocardiogram confirmed the presence of a large patent ductus arteriosus and a course of indomethacin was commenced.
>
> George did well during the next week. At 2 weeks of age, he again developed worsening apnoea with feed intolerance and temperature instability. A full blood count revealed anaemia and an increase in immature white cells. Blood cultures, a lumbar puncture, chest X ray and bladder tap were performed. George was treated with a blood transfusion and antibiotics, with gradual improvement during the next 2 days.

Periventricular leucomalacia (PVL). This is an uncommon problem, characterised by necrosis of the periventricular white matter surrounding the lateral ventricles. It is caused by ischaemic damage to that region of the brain. PVL is diagnosed on head ultrasound, commonly at 4–6 weeks of age. It commonly results in cerebral palsy.

Hepatic

- *Hypoglycaemia* is common due to decreased glycogen stores and increased glucose requirements in premature infants.

- *Hyperglycaemia* can also occur in VLBW infants because of high glucose infusion rates, reduced insulin secretion and impaired insulin sensitivity.
- *Hyperbilirubinaemia* occurs due to hepatic immaturity coupled with a shorter half-life of red blood cells. Premature infants require treatment at lower bilirubin levels than term infants because their low albumin levels and immaturity of the blood-brain barrier place them at greater risk of bilirubin encephalopathy.

Renal

Immaturity of the kidneys is associated with poor ability to concentrate or dilute the urine. This leads to:
- dehydration
- hyper- and hyponatraemia
- hyperkalaemia
- metabolic acidosis due to inability to conserve bicarbonate.

Skin immaturity leading to high insensible water losses may also aggravate these problems.

Gastrointestinal

Necrotising enterocolitis (NEC). This is an uncommon inflammatory process in the bowel wall that can lead to bowel necrosis. Alterations in gut blood flow, hypotension, hypoxia, infection and feeding practices have all been implicated but their exact contribution remains unclear. Presentation of NEC can be non specific, including apnoea, bradycardia and temperature instability, then more focal abdominal signs such as distension, tenderness, feed intolerance, bloody stools and bilious gastric aspirates. Occasionally there may be rapid progression to sepsis, shock and death. Classic X ray findings are air in the bowel wall (pneumatosis intestinalis) and perforation of the gut. Treatment is by withholding of feeds, antibiotics and, if necessary, surgery.

Feeding problems: Preterm babies have weak and uncoordinated suck and swallow reflexes, delayed gastric emptying and immature gut motility. Feed intolerance and gastro-oesophageal reflux are common. Parenteral nutrition is usually required initially in extremely preterm infants, with gradually increasing volumes of milk given by tube. Once full milk feeds are established, supplemental vitamins, minerals, protein and calories may also be required to allow adequate growth. Sucking feeds are usually established at 34–36 weeks postmenstrual age.

Haematological

Anaemia. Anaemia of prematurity is almost universal, due to low iron stores and red cell mass at birth, rapid growth, reduced erythropoiesis and decreased survival of red blood cells, aggravated by multiple blood sampling. Treatment is supportive with transfusion in the early period, iron supplementation and sometimes erythropoietin.

Immunological

Infection. Preterm babies have increased susceptibility to infection due to impaired cell mediated immunity and reduced concentrations of complement and immunoglobulins, together with invasive procedures and monitoring. Signs of sepsis are extremely non specific, including lethargy, temperature instability, apnoea, tachypnoea, feed intolerance and jaundice. Investigation usually requires a full blood count, blood culture, chest X ray, bladder tap urine and lumbar puncture. Because deterioration can be rapid, early treatment with antibiotics is essential pending culture results.

Thermoregulation

This is a significant problem in the premature infant due to a relatively large body surface area, thin skin and subcutaneous tissues and lack of keratinised epidermal barrier.

Clinical example (part C)

George did well throughout the remainder of his hospitalisation. He began to suck some feeds by 34 weeks corrected age, and by 37 weeks he was fully breastfed. His eyes were examined for retinopathy of prematurity (ROP) at 6 weeks of age and were found to be immature but with no evidence of ROP. He would be followed every 2–3 weeks until his retinae were fully mature. His head ultrasound scans were normal at 5 and 28 days of age. He continued to have occasional episodes of desaturation until 36 weeks corrected age and required oxygen 100 ml/min by nasal cannula to maintain adequate oxygenation. An audiology referral was arranged prior to discharge. He was discharged at 38 weeks postmenstrual age with an appointment to be seen in the high risk follow up clinic 6 weeks later. He also was followed by home health nurses while on oxygen.

Late onset complications of prematurity

Retinopathy of prematurity (ROP)

This results from disruption of the normal process of vascularisation of the retina, with new vessel formation and fibrous scarring. Although ROP can result from excessive oxygen exposure, most cases occur in extremely preterm babies with multiple other problems even when oxygen monitoring has been meticulous. Severity is classified based on the location and extent of ROP, from grade 1 (mild changes, resolves spontaneously) to grade 4

(retinal detachment). Most mild ROP regresses spontaneously; however, regular eye examinations are required to detect progressive ROP requiring laser therapy to reduce the chances of myopia and blindness.

Chronic lung disease (CLD)

This is usually defined as the need for supplemental oxygen at 36 weeks postmenstrual age. It results from a combination of lung immaturity, oxygen toxicity, barotrauma, volutrauma, inflammatory and free radical mediated lung injury. Babies with CLD may require supplemental oxygen for months or even years, and are at increased risk of respiratory infections in the first year and adverse developmental outcome.

Growth

Because preterm babies often do not grow for 2–3 weeks after birth, most are still below birth centiles at discharge; however, steady catch up growth is usual during the first 2 years of life. Permanent growth failure is more likely in preterm infants who were also small for gestational age.

Neurodevelopmental impairments

Severe impairments (cerebral palsy, mental retardation, blindness, deafness) occur in 10–15% of VLBW babies. More subtle delays in language, attention deficits and social/behavioural difficulties are common. Regular developmental assessment is recommended for all VLBW infants.

Small for gestational age

Clinical example (part A)

Rachel was born at 36 weeks gestation to a 30 year old mother in her first pregnancy. Labour was induced because of poor growth and maternal pregnancy induced hypertension. Delivery was by emergency caesarean section for fetal distress. Rachel was vigorous at birth with a birth weight of 1800 g, which was less than the 3rd centile. Her length was 45 cm, on the 10th centile, and her head circumference was 33 cm, at the 50th centile. Apart from her small size, no abnormalities were detected on initial examination. In particular, there were no dysmorphic features or signs of congenital infection. She was initially nursed in an incubator because of poor temperature maintenance in a cot. Blood glucose concentrations were monitored because of her small size. Despite early milk feeds, Rachel required intravenous glucose infusion for the first 24 hours to maintain adequate blood glucose concentrations. She also became jaundiced and required phototherapy from days 3 to 6 after birth.

Terminology

Clinically, smallness for gestational age (SGA) is usually defined as birthweight below 10th centile for gestation. The distinction between SGA babies and those with intrauterine growth restriction (IUGR) would be useful but is difficult to make clinically (Fig. 33.1). SGA is measured by birth weight because this is easy and accurate, but babies with IUGR suffer a variety of complications even if birthweight is in the normal range. Similarly, some SGA babies are small normal babies. An example is the small infant of a small mother in some ethnic groups. Clinical assessment of gestation such as the Ballard assessment tends to underestimate gestational age in SGA babies because of delayed physical maturation due to reduced subcutaneous fat and cartilage formation.

Causes of SGA

It is useful to think of the causes and complications of SGA in two main groups (Table 33.3):

- Intrinsic fetal problems: altered fetal potential for growth, such as chromosomal anomalies, intrauterine infection and congenital anomalies. Complications and outcome in this group depend on the underlying cause.
- Extrinsic problems in fetal supply: the baby is undernourished in utero due to factors limiting nutrient supply at one or more places along the fetal supply line. Complications and outcome can be thought of as those of intrauterine starvation (Table 33.4).

Table 33.3 Causes of being small for gestational age

Intrinsic: altered growth potential
Chromosomal
Congenital anomalies
Dysmorphic syndromes
Congenital infections

Extrinsic: reduced fetal nutrient supply
Reduced substrates in maternal blood (e.g. severe maternal undernutrition, eating disorders, chronic illness)
Reduced uterine blood flow (e.g. hypertension, renovascular disease, vigorous exercise)
Reduced placental transfer of substrates to the fetus (e.g. placental infarcts, abruption)
Factors acting at all these points (e.g. drugs, smoking, alcohol)

However, in a large proportion (perhaps 30%) of cases no cause is identified.

Clinical example (part B)

Clinically Rachel did well. She fed vigorously, lost little weight after birth and by 12 days she was weaned from the incubator to the cot. Her weight at that time was 1900 g. She was discharged home at 2 weeks of age. On follow up at 2 years of age all her measurements were at the 10th percentile and she had normal developmental milestones.

Table 33.4 Pathophysiology of intrauterine growth restriction

Fetal nutrient limitation	Consequences for the fetus	Possible clinical consequences for the newborn	Long term consequences
Reduced supply of glucose	Reduced body fat Reduced glycogen stores	Hypothermia Hypoglycaemia	Increased mortality Neurological damage
Reduced supply of oxygen	Stillbirth	Meconium aspiration	
	Asphyxia Increased haematopoiesis	Hypoxic ischaemic encephalopathy Coagulopathy Polycythaemia Jaundice	Neurological damage
	Redistributed cardiac output Cardiac failure	Relatively big head (head sparing) Pulmonary haemorrhage	
Reduced supply of amino acids	Impaired immune function Delayed bone maturation Reduced muscle mass	Infection Hypocalcaemia Insulin resistance	Poor growth

Prognosis

- *General.* Prognosis depends on the cause of growth restriction. For the intrinsic group, outcome is that of the underlying problem. For the extrinsic group, outcome depends on severity and time of onset of the growth restriction. In general, the earlier the onset in gestation and the more severe the growth restriction, the greater the likelihood of permanent growth and developmental problems.
- *Growth.* Most SGA babies catch up in the first 6 months after birth. However, babies born short tend to remain short, and being an SGA baby is the cause of short stature in approximately 20% of adults who are short.
- *Neurodevelopment.* If growth restriction is of late onset and head size is preserved, outcome may be good. However, many of the complications of growth restriction impair developmental outcome, and on average performance is reduced (Table 33.4).
- *Adult disease.* Babies born small are at increased risk of a number of chronic diseases in adulthood, particularly coronary heart disease, stroke, hypertension and non insulin dependent diabetes. This is thought to be because fetal adaptations to undernutrition in utero result in both small size at birth and permanent resetting of homeostatic mechanisms (programming), which lead to later disease (the fetal origins of adult disease or Barker hypothesis).

Jaundice

Jaundice is the visible yellow coloration of the skin due to elevated bilirubin levels. It is extremely common in neonates, affecting approximately 50% of all newborns. In most infants jaundice is physiological; however, it should always be taken seriously, as it is a common sign of illness in the newborn, and at high levels bilirubin can cause permanent brain damage (kernicterus).

Bilirubin synthesis

Bilirubin is derived primarily from haemoglobin, and to a lesser degree from myoglobin and the cytochromes. These haem proteins are oxidised in the reticuloendothelial system to form biliverdin and then *unconjugated bilirubin.* Because unconjugated bilirubin is not water soluble, most of it circulates bound to albumin. Circulating bilirubin is taken up by the liver, is bound to the intracellular proteins Y (ligandin) and Z and is then conjugated in the endoplasmic reticulum by the enzyme glucuronyl transferase to form bilirubin mono- and diglucuronides. *Conjugated bilirubin* is excreted via the biliary tree into the gastrointestinal tract and then into the faeces. However, some of the conjugated bilirubin is converted back to unconjugated bilirubin and is reabsorbed by the intestine into the circulation by a process known as *enterohepatic circulation.*

Evaluation of jaundice

Jaundice usually becomes visible at serum bilirubin levels of 85–120 µmol/l; however, the depth of jaundice is an extremely unreliable guide to the bilirubin level. Unconjugated hyperbilirubinaemia is the most common type of hyperbilirubinaemia and can be physiological or pathological. Conjugated hyperbilirubinaemia is defined as a serum conjugated bilirubin > 35 µmol/l and *always* requires urgent evaluation. Conjugated hyperbilirubinaemia is discussed in more detail in Chapter 72.

The extent of evaluation required in a jaundiced infant depends on the wellness or otherwise of the infant and the pattern of jaundice (Fig. 33.4). As a minimum, all jaundiced babies should have a history taken, and physical examination and measurement of the serum bilirubin level should be performed.

History

- Family history: previous sibling, other family members with jaundice
- Maternal history: history of splenectomy, haemolytic anemia, gallstones, blood type
- Pregnancy history: gestational diabetes, illnesses
- Delivery history: type of delivery (forceps, vacuum extraction), medications, length of rupture of membranes, delay in cord clamping (suggests polycythaemia), Apgar score (evidence of asphyxia)
- Newborn history: feeding history (dehydration, starvation) including volume and type of feeding, stool pattern (delayed passage suggests Hirschsprung disease), vomiting (intestinal obstruction, pyloric stenosis).

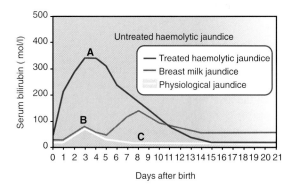

Fig. 33.4 Trends in serum bilirubin levels in common types of jaundice: **A** Early onset haemolytic jaundice (Dotted line indicates possible pattern if untreated); **B** Prolonged breast milk jaundice; **C** Physiological jaundice.

Physical examination

- Measurements: small for gestational age (poly-cythaemia) or infant of a diabetic mother
- Colour: plethora due to polycythaemia, pallor due to anaemia
- Wellness: activity, tone, cry
- Presence of bruising, petechiae, cephalhaematoma
- Umbilical cord: infection or umbilical hernia suggesting hypothyroidism
- Hepatosplenomegaly suggesting haemolysis or intrauterine infection
- Neurological examination: evidence of bilirubin encephalopathy.

Laboratory evaluation

Early jaundice (< 24 hours age)
- Always pathological.
- Evaluate for haemolysis and sepsis:
  — full blood count
  — maternal and infant blood type
  — Coombs test
  — assess risk for hereditary haemolytic diseases
  — consider cultures for infection.

Jaundice at > 24 hours age
- Is it physiological? (Normal history and examination, normal pattern of jaundice.)
  — Monitor, no further investigations.
- Not definitely physiological?
  — Assess for haemolysis and sepsis as above.
  — Assess for gastrointestinal obstruction.
  — Urinalysis for reducing substances (galactosaemia).

Persistent or late jaundice (>1 week in term baby, >2 weeks in preterm baby)
- Confirm bilirubin is unconjugated (conjugated requires immediate investigation).
- Breast milk jaundice?
- Thyroid function tests.
- Liver function tests.

Physiological jaundice

Physiological jaundice begins after 24 hours of age, peaks on approximately day 3, and resolves around the end of the first week (Fig. 33.4). It is unconjugated and caused by a number of factors, including increased bilirubin load and impaired excretion (Table 33.5). The infant is healthy with a relatively slow rise in serum bilirubin ($< 85\ \mu$mol/day), which does not generally exceed $250\ \mu$mol/l. Other factors, such as race and breastfeeding, can cause exaggeration of physiological jaundice. In the premature infant the bilirubin peaks towards the end of the first week and resolves in the second week.

Table 33.5   Causes of physiological jaundice

Increased bilirubin load
Increased red blood cell volume
Decreased red blood cell survival
Increased enterohepatic circulation

Defective hepatic uptake
Low levels of protein Y, protein Z
Relative hepatic uptake deficiency

Defective bilirubin conjugation
Decreased synthesis and activity of glucuronyl transferase

Defective bilirubin excretion
Higher concentration of β-glucuronidase in intestinal mucosa increasing bilirubin breakdown
More alkaline pH in proximal small intestine causing breakdown of conjugated bilirubin
Lack of intestinal flora

Physiological jaundice is a diagnosis of exclusion. In a well infant whose jaundice is following the predicted course, no further investigation or treatment is required; however, any signs of illness in the baby or alterations in the pattern of jaundice require immediate investigation.

Breast milk jaundice

Breast milk jaundice is a prolonged unconjugated hyperbilirubinaemia common in breastfed babies. The jaundice peaks in the second week but resolves only very slowly and may last up to 3 months (Fig. 33.4). The infant is healthy and thriving. Breast milk jaundice is thought to be due to a factor in breast milk that causes increased enteric absorption of bilirubin.

Diagnosis is based on the pattern of jaundice and wellness of the infant. As for any prolonged jaundice, conjugated hyperbilirubinaemia must be excluded. The diagnosis can be confirmed by improvement of the jaundice on temporary interruption of breastfeeding, but this is rarely required.

Pathological unconjugated jaundice

Haemolysis

The onset of jaundice before 24 hours of life is always pathological, and usually caused by haemolysis (Table 33.6). Haemolytic jaundice is most commonly immune mediated due to blood group incompatibilities, such as ABO and rhesus incompatibility. If investigations for immune mediated haemolysis are negative then further investigations are necessary to determine whether haemolysis is due to other causes such as glucose-6-phosphate dehydrogenase deficiency (G6PD), an X linked disorder seen in Mediterranean and Asian ethnic

Table 33.6 Causes of haemolytic jaundice

Immune mediated
ABO incompatibility
Rhesus disease
Minor blood group incompatibilities
Drug induced
Maternal autoimmune haemolysis

Acquired, non immune
Congenital intrauterine infection
Bacterial sepsis

Hereditary
Membrane defects: hereditary spherocytosis, elliptocytosis,
   and others
Enzyme abnormalities: G6PD deficiency, pyruvate kinase
   deficiency

Haemoglobinopathies

Clinical example

David is a term male infant born to a 33 year old G2P1 blood group O+ serology negative mother by normal vaginal delivery. Jaundice was noted at 18 hours of life, with an unconjugated bilirubin of 220 μmol/l.

A full blood count showed a normal haemoglobin. The peripheral smear showed occasional spherocytes and some fragmented red blood cells, and the reticuloctye count was significantly elevated. The baby was found to be blood type A+ with a positive direct Coombs test. A diagnosis of ABO incompatibility jaundice was made. Phototherapy was started and serum bilirubin was monitored. The bilirubin rose to near exchange transfusion levels on day 2 before stabilising. On day 7 a full blood count showed a slightly low haemoglobin due to haemolysis. Phototherapy was stopped on day 14. Blood counts were monitored after discharge to look for worsening anaemia.

groups, or hereditary spherocytosis, an autosomal dominant disorder affecting the cell membrane.

Non haemolytic jaundice

Unconjugated hyperbilirubinaemia can be caused by increased production or decreased clearance of bilirubin, or sometimes by a combination of these factors (Table 33.7).

Table 33.7 Other causes of unconjugated hyperbilirubinaemia

Increased haem load
Hemorrhage
   Haematoma (especially cephalohaematoma), pulmonary
      haemorrhage, cerebral haemorrhage, occult, birth
      trauma
Polycythaemia
Swallowed blood

Increased enterohepatic circulation
Bowel obstruction or ileus
Pyloric stenosis

Impaired hepatic uptake and conjugation
Inborn errors of bilirubin metabolism
   Non haemolytic inherited disorders: type I, type II, Gilbert
      disease
   Metabolic disease: galactosaemia, tyrosinosis,
      hypermethionaemia
Endocrine
   Hypothyroidism, hypopituitarism, drugs
Inhibitors
   Lucey–Driscoll syndrome, breast milk

Mixed
Asphyxia
Prematurity
Sepsis
Infants of diabetic mothers

Complications of jaundice

Unconjugated bilirubin is water insoluble and is toxic to cells, especially the brain. *Kernicterus* is a term used to describe the yellow staining of the brain and the associated neuronal death seen on histologoical examination of the brain. The cerebellum, basal ganglia and cranial nerve nuclei tend to be the most severely affected regions. *Bilirubin encephalopathy* refers to the clinical manifestations of bilirubin injury to the central nervous system. These can include reversible or irreversible abnormalities of muscle tone, lethargy, seizures, opisthotonus (arching of back), cerebral palsy and high frequency hearing loss. The risk of brain damage can be increased by:

- High unconjugated serum bilirubin concentration.
- Reduced binding of bilirubin to albumin. This can be caused by a number of conditions, including prematurity with low serum albumin concentrations, acidosis, displacement of bilirubin by fatty acids such as intralipids, and by certain drugs.
- Impairment of the blood–brain barrier, due to prematurity, asphyxia, meningitis.

Treatment of jaundice

The aim of treatment is to prevent bilirubin encephalopathy by reducing bilirubin levels.

General. Ensure adequate calorie and fluid intake and adequate stool production to reduce enterohepatic circulation. Treat with antibiotics if sepsis is suspected.

Phototherapy, which consists of nursing the baby under blue light at wavelengths of 450–460 nm. This transforms bilirubin near the skin into a water soluble

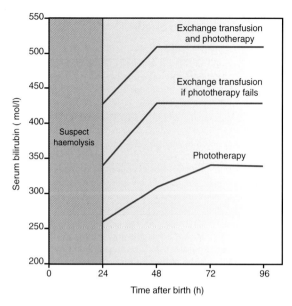

Fig. 33.5 Example of a nomogram for treatment of jaundice in healthy term infants.

form through photoisomerisation. Bilirubin can then be excreted in the bile and urine. This is a safe, simple treatment, designed to avoid exchange transfusion.

Exchange transfusion. This involves replacing the baby's blood with donor blood in order to rapidly decrease the bilirubin levels. The procedure is now rarely undertaken and has a small risk of morbidity and mortality.

The levels at which phototherapy and exchange transfusion are performed are usually determined using standard hospital nomograms. An example is illustrated in Figure 33.5. The threshold for treatment is lower if the infant is premature, asphyxiated, ill or haemolysing.

Intravenous immunoglobulin is a new therapy that may be helpful in the treatment of immune mediated haemolytic disease, probably by blocking the Fc receptors on the red blood cells and thereby inhibiting haemolysis.

Breathing problems arising in the newborn period

34

D. Tudehope

The establishment and maintenance of respiratory function is one of the most important features of the perinatal period. It is at this time that transition from dependence on placental function occurs.

The fetus

The placenta is a fetal organ with two major functions: transport and metabolism. Its transport role of gaseous exchange of oxygen and carbon dioxide, maintenance of acid–base status, diffusion of nutrients and excretion of waste products is essential for fetal homeostasis.

The fetal circulation consists of two umbilical arteries and an umbilical vein. Pulmonary blood flow is kept to a minimum by high pulmonary vascular resistance and three right to left shunts:
- Ductus venosus shunts blood away from the liver.
- Foramen ovale shunts blood from right to left atrium.
- Ductus arteriosus shunts blood from pulmonary artery to aorta.

Cardiopulmonary adaptations for extrauterine life

- Expulsion of fetal lung fluid and inflation of lungs with air.
- Decrease in pulmonary vascular resistance and increase in pulmonary blood flow.
- Closure of fetal shunts.
- Extrauterine breathing, increases in pulmonary compliance and lung volumes.

Maladaptation at birth

Conditions that interfere with normal oxygenation and lung expansion after birth may delay the physiological drop in pulmonary vascular resistance. This results in persistence of the fetal circulation, leading to severe hypoxia and acidosis.

Other clinical sequelae of maladaptation at birth are:
- perinatal asphyxia
- excessive placental transfusion — hypervolaemia, polycythaemia, hyperviscosity
- transient tachypnoea of the newborn
- meconium aspiration syndrome
- respiratory distress syndrome.

Respiratory disorders in the newborn

Respiratory problems are perhaps the commonest of all disorders in the newborn period and present clinically in three different ways:
- respiratory distress
- upper airways obstruction
- apnoea and bradycardia.

Respiratory distress

Respiratory distress is the generic term used to describe the following clinical signs persisting for more than 4 hours:
- tachypnoea — respiratory rate in excess of 60 per minute
- chest retraction or recession — intercostal, subcostal, sternal or substernal
- cyanosis in room air — central
- flaring of ala nasae — use of accessory respiratory muscles
- expiratory grunt — particularly in preterm infants.

Diagnosis is made by a careful perinatal history, physical examination and appropriate investigation. Investigations include:
- chest X rays — anteroposterior and sometimes lateral films
- bacteriology — deep cultures: blood, urine, CSF, gastric aspirate
- virological studies — nasopharyngeal aspirate, blood
- haematocrit and full blood count — ancillary evidence for sepsis
- chest transillumination with cold light source — diagnosis of pneumothorax
- passage of nasogastric catheters — diagnosis of choanal atresia, oesophageal atresia
- hyperoxia or nitrogen washout test — to distinguish cyanotic heart disease from respiratory disorders.

Transient tachypnoea of the newborn (TTN)

- Benign disorder in 1–2% of newborn infants.
- Onset of tachypnoea, cyanosis and grunt in first 1–3 hours.

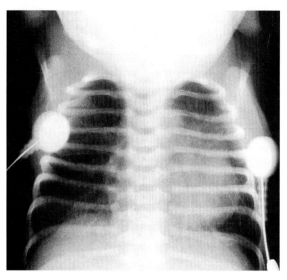

Fig. 34.1 Chest X ray of transient tachypnoea of the newborn showing cardiomegaly, perihilar cuffing, fluid in the horizontal fissure and coarse streaking in the lungs.

- Usually responds to 30–40% oxygen and settles in 24–48 hours but may persist for 3–5 days.
- Term or near term infant, caesarean section, breech delivery, male sex, birth asphyxia, heavy maternal analgesia.
- Chest X ray reveals coarse streaking, fluid in fissures giving 'wet lung' appearance (Fig. 34.1).

Respiratory distress syndrome (RDS)

Clinical example

Baby Chyle was born by caesarean section to a 17 year old single primigravida, who had no antenatal care, and who spontaneously ruptured her membranes at 29 weeks gestation. His mother was given one dose of betamethasone, in an attempt to accelerate fetal lung maturity, but despite an infusion of tocolytics, she delivered 4 hours later. At birth he weighed 1250g and had Apgar scores of 3 and 6 at 1 and 5 minutes of age. He received nasopharyngeal CPAP from birth and was transferred to the intensive care nursery in 50% oxygen. Chest X ray revealed hypoinflated lungs with a granuloreticular pattern and air bronchograms consistent with RDS. After taking bacteriological cultures he was commenced on amoxycillin and gentamicin. After inserting an umbilical catheter an arterial blood gas revealed pH 7.18, Pco_2 55 mmHg, Po_2 40 mmHg, and BE −7 while on CPAP of 6 cmH_2O and 70% O_2. He was intubated and mechanically ventilated with positive pressure ventilation. Following intratracheal administration of exogenous surfactant at 4 and 10 hours of age his condition improved. He had a diuresis at 48 hours and was able to be extubated at 72 hours. He remained oxygen dependent for a further 21 days.

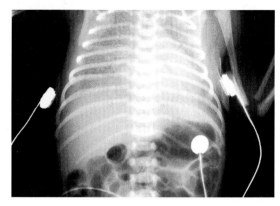

Fig. 34.2 Chest X ray of respiratory distress syndrome with hypoaeration, air bronchograms and diffuse granuloreticular pattern — almost a 'white out'.

RDS, also known as hyaline membrane disease, is a specific entity in preterm infants; it is caused by a lack of surfactant (a surface tension lowering agent) in the alveoli. It has a characteristic clinical picture and chest X ray shows hypoaeration, a diffuse granuloreticular pattern, air bronchograms and, in its most severe form, a diffuse 'white out' (Fig. 34.2).

Clinical features

- Diagnosed at birth or first 4 hours
- Signs of respiratory distress
  — tachypnoea, cyanosis
  — nasal flaring, expiratory grunt
  — harsh, diminished breath sounds
- Oedema
- Apnoea
- Course of RDS
  — classically increases for 24–72 hours then diuresis and recovery 48–96 hours
  — if severe and requiring mechanical ventilation, slow recovery over weeks to months.

Epidemiology

- Common condition occurring in 1% of all newborn infants.
- Incidence relates to degree of prematurity (Table 34.1).
- Predisposing factors: maternal diabetes mellitus, antepartum haemorrhage, second twin, hypoxia/acidosis at birth, male gender, caesarean section not in labour, positive family history.
- RDS, including extreme prematurity, and its complications contribute 37% to all causes of neonatal death.

Pathophysiology

Surfactant is a phospholipid secreted by the type II alveolar cells of the fetal lung from about 28–32 weeks

Table 34.1 Incidence and survivial rates for respiratory distress syndrome in the intensive care nursery, Mater Mothers' Hospital, Brisbane, Australia 1996–2000

Birth weight (g)	Incidence of RDS (%)	Survival rate with RDS (%)	Gestational age (weeks)	Incidence of RDS (%)	Survival rate with RDS (%)
500–999	81	69	23–27	81	66
1000–1499	52	95	28–30	64	94
1500–1999	26	97	31–33	27	99
2000–2499	11	95	34–36	11	97
≥ 2500	Not available	99	≥ 37	Not available	96

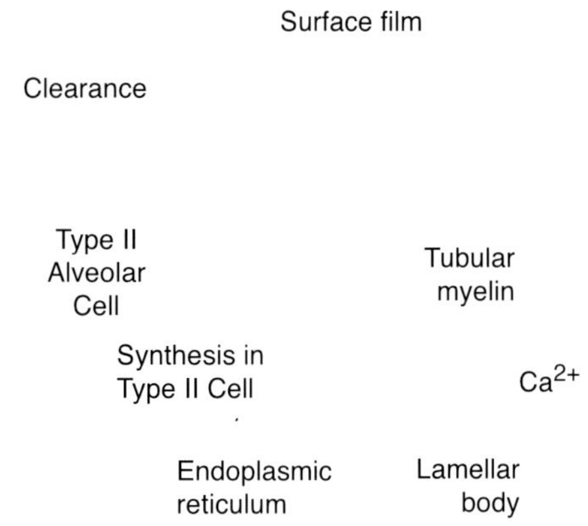

Surface film

Clearance

Type II
Alveolar
Cell

Tubular
myelin

Synthesis in
Type II Cell

Ca²⁺ Ca^{2+}

Endoplasmic
reticulum

Lamellar
body

Fig. 34.3 Life cycle of surface active material.

gestation. The major phospholipid is lecithin but other phospholipids and surfactant proteins A, B and C must be present for full activity (Fig. 34.3).

The action of surfactant can be understood by the LaPlace equation:

$$P = \frac{2\Upsilon}{r}$$

where P = pressure, Υ = surface tension, r = radius. The equation explains why, in the presence of high surface tension, large alveoli tend to get larger and small ones remain collapsed.

When the lungs of an infant who has survived for several hours are examined at autopsy, hyaline membranes are demonstrated lining respiratory bronchioles and alveolar ducts.

Prognosis

Acute, subacute and chronic complications are summarized in Table 34.2. The prognosis for RDS relates to severity and gestational age but has improved since the availability of exogenous surfactant.

Neurosensory disabilities may be divided into major handicaps (spasticity, posthaemorrhagic hydrocephalus,

Table 34.2 Complications of RDS

Acute	Subacute	Chronic
Cardiopulmonary		
Perinatal asphyxia	→ Encephalopathy	→ Neurosensory disability
Pulmonary air leak	Consolidation/collapse	Bronchopulmonary dysplasia
Patent ductus arteriosus	Lung oedema	SIDS
Pulmonary hypertension	Opportunistic infection	Subglottic stenosis
Pulmonary haemorrhage		Chronic obstructive pulmonary disease
Cerebral		
Cerebroventricular haemorrhage	→ Ventricular dilatation	→ Hydrocephalus
Periventricular leucomalacia	→ Cysts	→ Porencephaly
		Cerebral atrophy
Gastrointestinal tract		
Necrotising enterocolitis	→ Bowel obstruction	→ Malabsorption

blindness, deafness, mental retardation) and minor handicaps (hyperactivity attention deficit disorder, incoordination, speech and language delay).

Pneumonia

Presentation

- Early or late onset respiratory distress.
- Pulmonary component of severe, early onset septicaemic illness.
- Often non specific with lethargy, apnoea, bradycardia, temperature instability and intolerance to feeds.
- May be early onset (perinatal acquisition) or late onset (nosocomial).

Perinatal acquisition or congenital pneumonia

- Usually presents as pulmonary component of severe early onset septicaemic illness, or
- Isolated primary neonatal pneumonia.

Predisposing factors

- Prolonged rupture of membranes → group B β haemolytic streptococcus, Gram negative bacilli.
- Colonization → ascending infection → chorio-amnionitis → fetal and neonatal infection.
- Transplacental infection → group B β haemolytic streptococcus, *Listeria monocytogenes*.
- Maternal bacteraemia.

Late onset

Late onset nosocomial infection occurs in ventilated infants who exhibit ventilatory deterioration, worsening chest X ray, mucous plugging and increased secretions. Diagnosis is by isolation of pathogenic organisms cultured from endotracheal tube or nasopharyngeal aspirate and toxic full blood count.

Diagnosis

- Diminished air entry, increased crepitations, consolidation and effusions.
- Chest X ray essential for diagnosis but appearance often non specific. Lobar pneumonia rarely occurs, sometimes widespread diffuse or patchy coarse changes (Fig. 34.4).

Organisms

- Bacteria
  - Gram negative bacilli (*Escherichia coli, Klebsiella* spp, *Pseudomonas* spp)

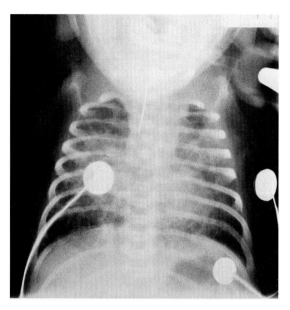

Fig. 34.4   Chest X ray of group B streptococcus pneumonia.

  - Group B β haemolytic streptococcus
  - *Staphylococcus aureus*
  - *Listeria monocytogenes*
- Non bacterial pathogens
  - *Chlamydia trachomatis, Ureaplasma urealyticum. Candida albicans, Pneumocystis carinii*
  - Viral pneumonitis is rare but may occur with cytomegalovirus, coxsackie, respiratory syncytial virus and rubella.

Pulmonary air leaks

Pulmonary air leaks are more common in the neonatal period than at any other time of life. There are several types:
- pneumothorax: air in the pleural cavity
- pneumomediastinum: air in the mediastinum
- pneumopericardium: air in the pericardial sac
- pulmonary interstitial emphysema (PIE): air in the interstitial lung spaces
- pneumoperitoneum: air in the peritoneal cavity
- air embolus: air dissecting into pulmonary veins and disseminating through the bloodstream.

The pathophysiology of these conditions is similar, in that the alveoli become hyperinflated and rupture. Air escapes into the lung interstitium (PIE) or tracks along the perivascular spaces and ruptures into the mediastinum (pneumomediastinum), through the visceral pleura (pneumothorax), or rarely into the pericardium (pneumopericardium) (Fig. 34.5).

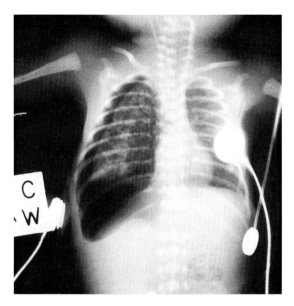

Fig. 34.5 Chest X ray showing right tension pneumothorax with underlying pulmonary intersititial emphysema.

Predisposing factors

- Spontaneous pneumothorax in 1% of vaginal and 1.5% of caesarean section deliveries. Usually asymptomatic.
- Active resuscitation at birth.
- Other lung disorders — RDS, hyperinflated lungs, hypoplastic lungs, meconium aspiration syndrome, transient tachypnoea of the newborn.

Treatment of RDS with exogenous surfactant decreases the likelihood of a pulmonary air leak.

Presentation

- Respiratory distress.
- Sudden deterioration with mediastinal shift, asymmetrical chest expansion, cardiorespiratory collapse.
- Prominent sternum suggests pneumomediastinum.

Diagnosis

- Aided by chest transillumination with powerful cold light source.
- Confirm by chest X ray.
- In an emergency, 'needle' aspiration and then drainage with an intercostal catheter.

In term infants reabsorption may be facilitated by breathing 100% oxygen for 12–24 hours.

Meconium aspiration syndrome (MAS)

- Meconium staining of liquor occurs in 10–15% of births, especially breech, post-term and fetal distress.

- Staining may be mild, moderate or severe (with oligohydramnios).
- Aspiration into the lungs occurs within a few breaths of birth.
- Once spontaneous respirations occur, meconium migrates into distal airways.
- Clinical and pathological features interact.

Chest X ray reveals hyperinflated lungs with widespread, coarse pulmonary infiltrate and collapse (Fig. 34.6).

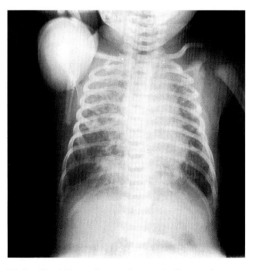

Fig. 34.6 Chest X ray of meconium aspiration syndrome. Hyperinflated lungs with widespread coarse pulmonary infiltration.

Management

Morbidity and mortality from MAS can be prevented or minimised by optimal perinatal management (Fig. 34.7). Treatment for established MAS is as for respiratory distress, with emphasis on humidification of inspired gases, postural drainage and airway suction, and antibiotics.

Pulmonary hypoplasia

Normal fetal lung development requires adequate amniotic fluid volume and fetal breathing movements.

Although unilateral lung hypoplasia may be an isolated developmental anomaly, bilateral hypoplasia is secondary to other factors, such as:

- Oligohydramnios, e.g. prolonged membrane rupture, severe renal disease. The baby may exhibit additional features of Potter syndrome, with facial dysmorphism, joint contractures and amnion nodosum of the placenta.
- Decreased intrathoracic space, e.g. diaphragmatic hernia, hydrops fetalis, cystic adenomatoid malformation of the lung.
- Chest wall deformities, e.g. skeletal dysplasia.

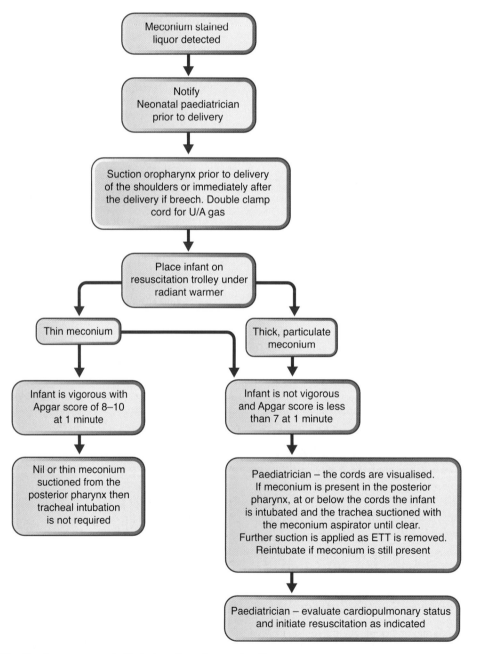

Fig. 34.7 Algorithm for management of baby born through meconium liquor.

Clinical features

- Progressive respiratory failure from birth, with marked hypoxia, hypercarbia and metabolic acidosis.
- Pneumothorax is common.
- Death, ventilator dependence or bronchopulmonary dysplasia may result.

Pulmonary haemorrhage

- Usual presentation is haemorrhagic pulmonary oedema coming up the endotracheal tube, compromising ventilation and resulting in cardiovascular collapse.
- Complicates severe perinatal asphyxia, coagulation disturbances, severe intrauterine growth restriction, hypothermia or congenital heart disease and occasionally following exogenous surfactant therapy for RDS.
- Additional treatment is required for shock, metabolic acidosis, coagulation disturbance, pulmonary oedema (frusemide/morphine), and positive end expiratory pressure to splint lungs.

Pulmonary collapse

- Pulmonary collapse or atelectasis may be segmental or lobar, most commonly of the right upper lobe after extubation from ventilation (Fig. 34.8)
- It occurs after aspiration of meconium, blood or milk and is common following muscle paralysis for surgery and when an endotracheal tube is inadvertently pushed down into right main stem bronchus.
- Thick pulmonary secretions → mucous plugs → migratory pulmonary collapse.
- Prevention is by adequate humidification, postural drainage, chest physiotherapy and exogenous surfactant therapy.

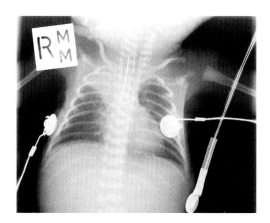

Fig. 34.8 Chest X ray right upper lobe collapse. Endotrachael tube located too far down trachea with associated right upper lobe collapse.

Congenital diaphragmatic hernia (Ch. 36)

> **Clinical example**
>
> Mrs T's fetus was diagnosed as having a left diaphragmatic hernia on her routine ultrasound scan at 17 weeks gestation. Serial ultrasound examinations revealed progressive polyhydramnios, with a gastric shadow in the left chest and mediastinal displacement. Lucas was born at 36 weeks gestation after spontaneous rupture of membranes. He was in good condition at birth, with an Apgar score of 7 at 1 minute, and an umbilical cord pH of 7.3, but there was rapid deterioration with cyanosis and bradycardia. A tube was passed and his stomach aspirated, then he was intubated and ventilated. He was paralysed with a muscle relaxant, and narcotic and alkali solutions were infused.
>
> Intratracheal exogenous surfactant was given but inhaled nitric oxide did not improve oxygenation. Intravascular volume replacement and a dopamine infusion improved BP and oxygenation. Corrective surgery was delayed until he was more stable on day 6. After a stormy postoperative period he was finally extubated on day 16 but required continuous low flow intranasal oxygen for 3 months and marked delay in achieving full oral feeding.

Abdominal contents herniate through a muscular defect in the diaphragm into the chest. The incidence is 1 in 3800 births, with 60% isolated and 40% associated with other anomalies or chromosomal defects.

Clinical presentation

- Most cases diagnosed by routine obstetric ultrasound at 17–19 weeks gestation or following investigation for polyhydramnios.
- Typically rapidly progressive respiratory failure after birth.
- Less acute cases present in the nursery with respiratory distress, dextracardia or scaphoid abdomen.

Diagnosis

Diagnosis is confirmed by demonstration of bowel loops in the thorax on chest X ray (Fig. 34.9)

Management

Management involves gastric decompression, cardio-respiratory support and avoidance of hypoxia. Surgical repair is typically delayed 3–7 days to enable maximum stabilisation. Overall only 40–60% of children with an isolated lesion survive. All infants with other anomalies die.

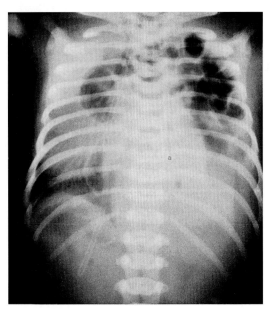

Fig. 34.9 Chest X ray of left diaphragmatic hernia with mediastinal shift to the right and gas pattern within the thorax.

Prognosis

Prognosis depends on age at presentation, degree of pulmonary hypoplasia, presence of polyhydramnios and development of persistent pulmonary hypertension.

Oesophageal atresia and tracheo-oesophageal fistula

With this congenital anomaly, there is usually complete interruption of the lumen of the oesophagus, resulting in a blind upper pouch. This generally is associated with a tracheo-oesophageal fistula. The various types are shown in Figure 34.10.

Maternal hydramnios occurs in 60% of cases and is largely responsible for the high frequency of premature births.

The outlook for oesophageal atresia is good, but complications and sequelae from surgery are frequent.

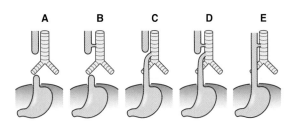

Fig. 34.10 Anatomical types of oesophageal atresia; 85% of all cases are type C.

These include a brassy cough associated with coexistent tracheomalacia, oesophageal stricture, breakdown of anastomosis, recurrence of the tracheo-oesophageal fistula and gastro-oesophageal reflux. Preterm birth worsens prognosis.

Congenital lobar emphysema

- Rare anomaly due to cartilaginous deficiency in lobar bronchus (upper lobe > right middle lobe).
- Insidious onset of respiratory distress over 2–3 weeks.
- Hyperinflated lobe causes surrounding pulmonary collapse and mediastinal displacement.
- Surgical lobectomy is usually curative.

Acquired lobar emphysema may be secondary to an extrinsic or intrinsic bronchial obstruction.

Cystic adenomatoid malformation

Often diagnosed on antenatal ultrasound. Polyhydramnios, hydrops fetalis, prematurity or still birth may result. There are three types:
- type 1 (70%) — single or multiple large cysts in one lobe
- type 2 (18%) — multiple medium sized cysts
- type 3 (10%) — large cysts containing smaller cysts.

Differential diagnosis is from lobar emphysema, sequestration of lung and pulmonary lymphangiectasia. Surgical resection is usually curative.

Other lung diseases

Other disorders presenting in the newborn include sequestration of lung, pulmonary lymphangiectasia, lung cysts (especially bronchogenic), pleural/chylous effusions and eventration of the diaphragm.

Treatment of the neonate with respiratory distress

The supportive care of the infant with respiratory distress is similar regardless of aetiology.

Observation and monitoring

- Observation for colour, chest recession, expiratory grunt, flaring of ala nasae.
- Continuous monitoring — heart rate, respiratory rate, skin temperature, blood pressure.
- Fluid balance chart.
- Thermoregulation in servocontrol incubator (open or closed).
- Maintain mean BP > 30 mmHg using volume expanders and inotropic support.

Oxygen

- Monitor percentage delivered continuously with analyser.
- Monitor oxygenation continuously with pulse oximetry and transcutaneous P_{O_2} + P_{CO_2} monitor.
- Warm to 36–37°C and humidify to 90–100%.
- Delivery into head box (if >30%) or servocontrol incubator.
- Indwelling arterial catheter enables blood sampling and continuous BP monitoring.

Fluids

- Avoid oral feeding, gavage feed if mild respiratory distress.
- Intravenous fluids and electrolytes (added after 24 hours) for moderate/severe distress.
- Total parental nutrition after 72 hours of no feeding.

Acid–base balance

- Normal range of blood gases (Table 34.3).
- Metabolic acidosis — volume replacement, inotropic support, $NaHCO_3$.
- Respiratory acidosis — pH < 7.20 and P_{CO_2} > 60 mmHg → provide assisted ventilation.

Assisted ventilation

In more severe cases, respiratory support may be necessary but further management is influenced by the weight of the infant.

Infants < 1500 g. Although continuous positive airway pressure (CPAP) may be administered shortly after birth, most will require mechanical ventilation. The indications for mechanical ventilation are:

- if inspired O_2 exceeds 60% to maintain P_{aO_2} > 60 mmHg
- apnoea
- rising P_{CO_2} which exceeds 60 mmHg, particularly if pH is <7.25.

Infants >1500g. CPAP is indicated if the inspired O_2 exceeds 60% to maintain P_{O_2}>60 mmHg. Mechanical ventilation is recommended in the following circumstances:
- P_{O_2}>60 mmHg while receiving CPAP
- inspired O_2 exceeds 80% to maintain
- apnoea
- rising P_{CO_2} which exceeds 65 mmHg, with pH (<7.25).

Techniques for mechanical ventilation vary between neonatal units and include intermittent mandatory ventilation, patient triggered ventilation, high frequency ventilation and high frequency oscillation. Large infants often struggle or 'fight' the ventilator and benefit from analgesia and sedation or paralysis with a non depolarising muscle relaxant.

Surfactant replacement

Exogenous surfactant (natural, synthetic, partially synthetic) administered via endotracheal tube, both in prophylactic (infants < 30 weeks) and rescue modes, has resulted in a 40% reduction in mortality from RDS. Pulmonary air leaks have been dramatically reduced but not so bronchopulmonary dysplasia or patent ductus arteriosus. Exogenous surfactant may benefit selected infants with meconium aspiration, congenital pneumonia and congenital diaphragmatic hernia.

Management and prevention of infection

- Bacteriological investigation, which includes cultures of blood, tracheal and gastric aspirate, is essential before commencing antibiotics.
- A penicillin (penicillin G or amoxycillin) and an aminoglycoside (gentamicin or tobramycin) are used when infection is suspected.
- Prevention of infection involves meticulous hand washing for all procedures, the use of gloves for tracheal toilets and routine bacteriological surveillance and swabbing of all infants in intensive care nurseries.
- Active chest physiotherapy may be required for pneumonia, collapsed segments of lungs, and aspiration syndromes.
- All infants with respiratory distress require correct positioning with frequent changes to facilitate ventilation and lung drainage.

Specific treatment

- Tension pneumothorax: drainage with intercostal catheter.
- Pleural/chylous effusion: thoracentesis or indwelling pleural drain.
- Symptomatic polycythaemia (venous Hct.>66%): dilutional exchange transfusion.

Table 34.3 Normal ranges for arterial blood gases in term and preterm infants

Parameter	Term	Preterm
P_{O_2} (mmHg)	60–90	50–80
P_{CO_2} (mmHg)	35–42	35–45
pH	7.35–7.42	7.30–7.40
Base excess (mmol/l)	–2 to 0	–0.4 to 0
Bicarbonate (mmol/l)	22–26	18–24

- Diaphragmatic hernia, oesophageal atresia, lobar emphysema, choanal atresia, lung cysts, and sometimes Pierre Robin sequence require surgery.

Chronic neonatal lung disease

Two definitions are in common usage:
- preterm infant with parencyhmal lung disease requiring increased inspired O_2 > 28 days from birth
- preterm infant requiring increased or inspired O_2 beyond 36 weeks postmenstrual age.

Bronchopulmonary dysplasia (BPD)

The classification of chronic neonatal lung disease is given in Table 34.4; the most common type is characteristically associated with the healing phase of severe RDS in extreme prematurity but it may complicate meconium aspiration, diaphragmatic hernia, apnoea or congenital pneumonia.

Clinical features

Wide spectrum of severity, from prolongation in plateau phase of wean from mechanical ventilation to failure to wean 24–28 week infant from O_2, to progressive respiratory failure and death.

Complications

- Pulmonary — collapse, pneumonia, gastro-oesophageal reflux, aspiration
- Apnoea — central, obstructive
- Systemic hypertension
- Bronchospasm — wheezing
- Progressive pulmonary hypertension
- Cor pulmonale
- Postnatal growth failure
- Sudden, unexpected death in infancy.

Pathogenesis

It is a multifactorial disease relating to the severity of RDS and degree of prematurity. Other factors in its causation are positive pressure ventilation, high inspired O_2 tensions and pulmonary complications such as air leaks, oedema, mucous plugging, recurrent aspiration and infection.

Chest X ray

Radiological appearances of BPD are staged as 1–4. Stage 4 has an irregular honeycomb appearance with overinflated lung fields, extensive fibrosis and lung cysts (Fig. 34.11) Most infants with BPD have less severe changes consisting of a fine, homogeneous pattern of abnormality with some dense streaks.

Management

The stratagem of modern mechanical ventilation is to obtain acceptable blood gases with the minimum of barotrauma and volutrauma to preterm lungs. Exogenous surfactant for RDS reduces pulmonary air leaks and duration of assisted ventilation but has only a modest reduction in BPD. Low dose dexamethasone for ventilated infants accelerates time to extubation. Diuretics may reduce interstitial lung fluid and inhaled bronchodilators decrease airway reactivity. For established BPD the mainstay of therapy is prolonged supplemental O_2 to maintain high O_2 saturations, adequate nutrition, physiotherapy and parental support.

Table 34.4   Classification of chronic neonatal lung disease
Bronchopulmonary dysplasia (BPD)
Wilson–Mikity syndrome
Chronic pulmonary insufficiency of prematurity (CPIP)

Recurrent aspiration
    Pharyngeal incoordination
    Gastro-oesophageal reflux
    Tracheo-oesophageal fistula

Interstitial pneumonitis
    Cytomegalovirus
    Candida albicans
    Chlamydia trachomatis
    Pneumocystis carinii

Chronic pulmonary oedema due to a left to right shunt
Rickets of prematurity

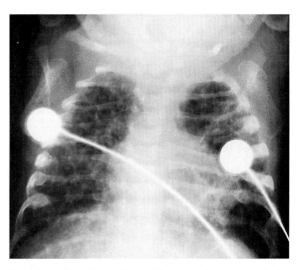

Fig. 34.11   Chest X ray of stage 4 bronchopulmonary dysplasia showing gross hyperinflation, large cysts and bullae and fractured ribs.

Prognosis

Death from BPD is now rare, and occurs in infants with multiple complications of extreme prematurity or following respiratory syncytial virus infection. The healing stage is associated with continued lung growth and may take 2–3 years. Survivors are prone to recurrent wheezing episodes associated with viral infection in the first 2 years of life. The incidence of oxygen dependence at 36 weeks for infants of birth weight 500–749 g, 750–999 g and 1000–1499 g was 71.2%, 44.5% and 12.6%, respectively, in Australian and New Zealand intensive care nurseries in 1999.

Wilson–Mikity syndrome (or pulmonary dysmaturity)

This syndrome used to be common in preterm infants of <32 weeks gestation but is now rarely diagnosed. It occurred in the absence of RDS and had an insidious onset in second and third weeks of life.

Upper airway obstruction

Frequently, upper airway obstruction presents in the delivery room or nursery due to foreign material in the airway. This can be readily relieved by suction to the airway. Upper airway obstruction not relieved by suction is unusual and may be mild, occurring only at times of stress or during feeds, or may be life threatening, presenting acutely in the delivery room.

Clinical features

The cardinal signs of upper airway obstruction are:
- stridor (inspiratory if obstruction is extrathoracic or expiratory if obstruction is intrathoracic)
- suprasternal retraction
- a croupy cough
- a hoarse cry.

With severe increasing upper airway obstruction, the infant may develop cyanosis followed by a secondary apnoea and bradycardia.

Aetiology

The causes of upper airway obstruction may be classified according to the site of obstruction.

Intraluminal obstruction from foreign material, such as mucus, blood, meconium or milk, may be relieved by suction. Vocal cord paralysis is a rare complication of traumatic birth.

Intramural obstruction in the larynx is due to subglottic stenosis, laryngeal oedema, a laryngeal web, diaphragm, papilloma or haemangioma. Transient stridor is a frequent consequence of neonatal resuscitation in the delivery room. The most common cause of persistent upper airway obstruction is subglottic oedema/stenosis following prolonged intubation of the trachea.

Extramural obstruction may occur with a goitre, vascular ring or cystic hygroma. Nasal obstruction may be due to choanal atresia or nasal congestion.

Infants with Pierre Robin sequence (micrognathia, cleft palate and glossoptosis) are prone to severe upper airway obstruction, especially when asleep, and require careful nursing in the prone position or insertion of a long nasopharyngeal tube. Stridor due to an infantile larynx (laryngomalacia) usually improves after 6 months of age but requires careful medical supervision, particularly during intercurrent respiratory tract infection.

Apnoea and bradycardia

Apnoea is defined as a cessation of breathing lasting for 20 seconds or more. Apnoea lasting for less than 20 seconds is also significant if accompanied by colour change, bradycardia of less than 100 beats per minute or hypotonia.

Physiology

The control of breathing in the neonate is complicated and poorly understood. The regulation of breathing in premature infants is unstable and shows a variety of patterns. These may be regular, irregular or periodic, in which cycles of hyperventilation alternate with periods of hypoventilation, with eventual apnoea lasting between 3 and 10 seconds. With advancing gestation to term, the proportion of time the infant is breathing regularly increases and phases of irregular, periodic and apnoeic periods decline. Further maturation occurs in the months after birth. Infants revert to shorter periods of regular respiration and longer periods of less stable forms of breathing during rapid eye movement (REM) sleep.

Infants, particularly preterm, have less well developed chemoreceptor responses to hypoxia and hypercapnia. A low Po_2 initially stimulates respiratory effort for only a short time before irregular respiration and apnoea occur, which induce further hypoxia. Hypercapnia may also fail to stimulate respiration, particularly in the presence of hypoxia.

Aetiology

All babies who suffer from apnoea must be fully investigated. In the term infant the aetiology is usually identified, whereas in the preterm infant it is unusual to find a cause. Recurrent apnoea of prematurity is presumed to be due to immaturity of the respiratory centre in the brainstem and immaturity of the chemoreceptor response to hypoxia and acidosis. Apnoea is common in more immature babies, occurring in 25% of infants <2500 g and in over 80% of infants <1000 g birth weight.

Central apnoea is due to factors affecting the respiratory centre in the brainstem or higher centres in the cerebral cortex. Causes include:

- prematurity
- hypoxia/acidosis
- drugs (for example, maternal narcotics, tromethamine (THAM), prostacyclin, magnesium sulphate)
- metabolic (for example, hypoglycaemia, hypocalcaemia, hypomagnesaemia, hypermagnesaemia)
- sepsis — generalised or a specific infection
- intracranial haemorrhage
- polycythaemia with hyperviscosity
- necrotising enterocolitis
- patent ductus arteriosus
- convulsions
- brain maldevelopment
- temperature instability (for example, incubator temperature too high, hypothermia, too rapid warming or cooling).

Obstructive apnoea

Babies are obligatory nose breathers and if their nares are obstructed, especially while sleeping, they are prone to severe apnoea. Obstructive apnoea occurs with some congenital malformations, such as choanal atresia and the Pierre Robin sequence. Preterm infants with small upper airways may have apnoea when lying in the supine position, especially during active (REM) sleep. Babies who have milk, mucus or meconium lodged in the airways are likely to have episodes of obstructive apnoea.

Mixed apnoea

This is difficult to diagnose clinically. It resembles central apnoea, initially, with the cessation of respiration, but then the baby makes intermittent respiratory efforts without achieving gas exchange.

Reflex apnoea

Reflex or vagally mediated apnoea may be due to suction of the phyarynx or stomach or from passage of a nasogastric tube, physiotherapy or even in response to defecation. Apnoea associated with gastro-oesophageal reflux may be reflex and/or obstructive.

Investigation of apnoea

Initially the infant must be examined carefully to exclude respiratory or remote disease. Investigations will depend to a large extent on the suspected cause but at times may be extensive.

Apnoea monitoring

A variety of monitors are available but none will detect obstructive apnoea until the baby stops fighting for breath. The use of an ECG monitor together with an apnoea monitor is recommended in order to recognise bradycardia occurring with an obstructed airway.

Treatment of apnoea and bradycardia

Prevention and early detection

Infants at risk should have continuous heart rate and respiratory monitoring with appropriate set alarms. Low birth weight infants must be carefully handled, and attention paid to feeding techniques, with avoidance of stomach distension and rapid feeding. Temperature must be maintained in the thermal neutral range. Nursing the infant in the prone position and careful suctioning of the airway will minimise obstruction to the airway.

Treatment of the underlying cause

This will depend on the findings on examination and of relevant investigations.

Management of the acute apnoeic episode

- *Stimulation of the infant.* This may be all that is required. Suction of the upper airways is indicated when obstruction is the likely cause.
- *Manual ventilation with a facemask and bag.* Intubation and intermittent positive pressure ventilation will be necessary when the baby fails to respond to bag and mask ventilation or when severe apnoeic attacks occur frequently.

Treatment of recurrent apnoea

Recurrent apnoea usually occurs in preterm babies and may be very difficult to manage; however, before undertaking sophisticated therapy the potential hazards of therapy need to be carefully balanced against the brain damaging effects of the apnoeic episodes.

Pharmacological treatment
- Methyl xanthines
  — Aminophylline
  — Theophylline

— Caffeine. The neonate methylates theophylline to caffeine and caffeine may be used to treat apnoea.

- Doxapram. This has recently been shown to be effective in infants in whom recurrent apneoa cannot be controlled by methyl xanthines. Severe jitteriness is a well recognised side effect.

Dosages of these drugs are given in Chapter 23.

Continuous positive airway pressure (CPAP)

CPAP may be effective in treating or preventing apnoea. The use of nasal prongs to administer CPAP may produce additional effects by local stimulation.

Stimulation

Tactile stimulation, which has been shown to be effective in reducing the number of apnoeic episodes, cannot be used as a routine; however, a variety of rocking mattresses have been devised for use as a means of stimulation and appear to reduce the number of apnoeic episodes in some infants.

Prognosis

This will depend on the underlying cause of the apnoea. Although modern management has decreased the incidence and severity of apnoea, in very low birth weight infants, the long term outlook has not yet been fully evaluated.

Recurrent apnoea of prematurity usually resolves by 37 weeks postmenstrual age but in some instances it may persist beyond the expected date of delivery and no cause can be found. In some cases, discharge home on methyl xanthine drugs is recommended and home apnoea monitors may be of some benefit.

Home apnoea monitors

The parents of a preterm infant may request a monitor for use at home There is no evidence that home monitoring reduces the risk of a life threatening event occurring out of hospital, nor does it prevent death; babies have died despite being monitored. One consensus view for indications for home monitoring includes the following:

- One or more apparently life threatening events associated with apnoea and requiring vigorous resuscitation.
- Symptomatic preterm infants.
- Siblings of two or more victims of sudden infant death syndrome (SIDS). The consensus view is that monitoring of subsequent infants after a single case of SIDS could not be justified.
- Infants with hypoventilation conditions.

Most paediatricians believe that the use of monitors at home for less rigorous indications than those listed above is justified if it is felt that it will reduce parental anxiety. It is essential that, before parents are given an apnoea monitor they are shown how to apply basic resuscitation skills to the infant in case the baby is found apnoeic or collapsed at home. Most important of all is the education of parents in the strategies to reduce the risk of SIDS.

35 Congenital and perinatal infections

L. Gilbert

General considerations

Defence mechanisms that protect the fetus and newborn from infection include:

- the placenta — separates maternal and fetal circulations
- chorioamniotic membranes and cervical mucus — prevent upward spread of vaginal organisms
- antimicrobial activity of amniotic fluid — from about 20 weeks' gestation
- maternal IgG — crosses the placenta in the third trimester to reach adult levels by term
- fetal specific immune responses — from early second trimester
- breast milk — contains secretory IgA, lymphocytes, macrophages and other antimicrobial substances.

Routes of fetal infection include:

1. Before birth
   a. haematogenous — across the placenta
   b. ascent from the maternal genital tract — across intact membranes, or after the membrane rupture
2. During delivery
   a. from maternal genital secretions
   b. from maternal blood
3. After birth
   a. from breast milk
   b. by conventional (horizontal) routes from mother or other contacts.

Some pathogens can infect the fetus or neonate by more than one route (Fig. 35.1).

The outcome of intrauterine infection depends when, during gestation, it occurs. Only a minority of exposed infants are infected and, of these, a minority will be damaged. Many infections which can damage the fetus are mild or asymptomatic in the mother and diagnosis may depend on routine antenatal screening. Whether this is appropriate depends on the frequency and severity of fetal or neonatal disease and the availability of a suitable screening test and effective intervention. The clinical features of some important congenital and perinatal infections are described in Table 35.1.

Rubella

In 1941, the Australian ophthalmologist, Norman Gregg, first described a syndrome of cataracts, deafness and congenital heart disease in infants of women who had had rubella during pregnancy. Rubella virus causes cellular growth retardation, endothelial damage and vascular insufficiency in affected tissues, decreased organ weight and overall fetal growth retardation. If it occurs during crucial stages of organogenesis, structural abnormalities, for example of the heart, can occur.

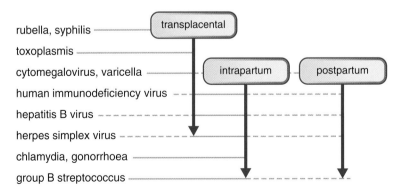

dashed lines indicate less common routes of transmission

Fig 35.1 Some vertically transmissible infections and their routes of transmission.

Table 35.1 Some common clinical manifestations of symptomatic congenital infection

Spontaneous abortion or stillbirth
Growth retardation
Hepatosplenomegaly, hepatitis, jaundice, hepatic calcification
Haematological abnormalities, especially thrombocytopenia
Microcephaly, intracerebral calcification
Pneumonitis, osteitis
Skin rash
Chorioretinitis*
Long term sequelae*: deafness, neurological defects

*May develop or be detected months or years later in an infant who is apparently normal at birth.

Clinical features

The risk of fetal infection and damage is greatest during the first 8 weeks of pregnancy and damage is rare after 16 weeks. Specific serious effects of intrauterine rubella (in addition to those listed in Table 35.1 include:

- cardiac abnormalities: pulmonary artery hypoplasia, patent ductus arteriosus
- eye abnormalities: cataract, retinopathy; microphthalmia
- diabetes mellitus — developing later.

Infected infants can excrete virus for many months; those who are apparently normal at birth can later develop deafness, other neurological abnormalities or diabetes. Follow up is important to allow appropriate management.

Diagnosis

Congenital rubella is confirmed by:

- isolation of rubella virus from saliva, tears, urine, cerebrospinal fluid (CSF) or tissue during the first 3 months of life
- demonstration of specific IgM antibody or persistence of IgG antibody beyond 6 months of age.

Prevention

Congenital rubella is preventable by immunisation. A combination of universal infant immunisation, supplemented by a booster dose at school entry, provides a high enough level of immunity to prevent sustained transmission. Remaining susceptible individuals are at risk from occasional imported cases. Routine antenatal screening and postpartum immunisation of susceptible women provides additional protection.

If rubella infection or contact is suspected during pregnancy, investigation to detect or exclude infection (specific IgM or IgG seroconversion) should be done even in women with known past immunity, as reinfection occasionally occurs. Therapeutic abortion is usually recommended after proven infection during the first trimester.

Syphilis

Clinical example

Cathy was an 19 year old single woman who, 2 years before, had delivered a stillborn infant at 36 weeks gestation, for which no cause was found; an autopsy was not performed. She presented at term, in her second pregnancy, having had no antenatal care, and delivered a baby boy who had hepatosplenomegaly. Investigations included tests for intrauterine infection. Serological tests for syphilis were positive in both Cathy and her baby: rapid plasma reagin test (RPR) reactive (titre 1:8); *Treponema pallidum* particle agglutination test (TPPA) reactive. Both Cathy and her baby were treated with a full course of parenteral penicillin. Examination of the baby's cerebrospinal fluid showed no evidence of neurosyphilis.

Cathy had a history of occasional intravenous drug use but no past history or clinical signs of syphilis; the diagnosis was therefore latent syphilis. Her HIV antibody and hepatitis B surface antigen tests were negative, but she had a positive hepatitis C antibody test. The baby recovered without serious sequelae and at 12 months of age his hepatitis C antibody test was negative and RPR was non reactive.

Congenital syphilis may present in a variety of ways. It is important to screen for maternal syphilis following stillbirth or if an unusual lesion or condition consistent with syphilis is present in the newborn infant. Routine antenatal screening for syphilis is cost effective and still recommended, although the prevalence in Australia is low. Adequate treatment of an infected mother during pregnancy will prevent fetal damage.

Syphilis is a sexually transmitted infection caused by *Treponema pallidum*. Congenital syphilis is preventable by routine antenatal screening for, and treatment of, asymptomatic maternal syphilis. *T. pallidum* can be transmitted to the fetus at any stage of pregnancy, especially during early (primary or secondary) syphilis. If infection is detected and treated early, irreversible fetal damage can be prevented. Later treatment of the mother may cure the fetal infection but cannot reverse tissue damage.

Diagnosis

Maternal syphilis is often asymptomatic and recognised only because of a positive routine antenatal serological test. If the mother has been appropriately treated, the infant is usually not infected. If not, and the infant is normal at birth, congenital syphilis is suggested by antibody titres significantly higher than the mother's or the presence of specific IgM.

Clinical features

The fetal outcome of untreated maternal syphilis depends on the stage of the disease:

- primary or secondary: premature delivery or perinatal death ~50%; congenital syphilis ~ 50% (few normal infants)
- early latent syphilis (or indeterminate): at least 50% normal, 20–40% congenital syphilis; increased risk of perinatal death and preterm birth.

Specific clinical features typical of symptomatic congenital syphilis (in addition to those listed in Table 35.1) include:

- an abnormally bulky placenta — histological examination should be done
- hydrops fetalis due to severe anaemia and/or severe liver disease
- lymphadenopathy
- osteochondritis with typical radiological changes; arthropathy or pseudoparalysis
- persistent nasal discharge
- vesiculobullous rash involving palms and soles, followed by desquamation
- condylomata lata — fleshy lesions in moist areas of skin.

The diagnosis is made by serological tests. The mother's serum should be tested or retested, even if antenatal screening was negative; infection can occur late in pregnancy. Cerebrospinal fluid (CSF) should be examined — neurosyphilis is suggested by CSF pleocytosis, raised protein level and positive CSF serology, but not excluded by normal CSF.

Treatment

Congenital syphilis is treated with parenteral penicillin. Serological and clinical follow-up is needed to confirm successful treatment and exclude neurological or ophthalmological abnormality or deafness.

Cytomegalovirus (CMV) infection

CMV is a member of the herpes group of viruses. Primary CMV infection is usually asymptomatic or causes a non specific illness with fever, atypical lymphocytosis and mild hepatitis. The virus remains in a latent state with periodic asymptomatic reactivation and excretion in urine, saliva or genital secretions. Note that:

- Primary maternal infection or reactivation can result in fetal CMV infection.
- Only the primary infection commonly causes fetal damage.
- The best evidence of primary maternal infection is seroconversion but this may not be demonstrable if investigation is delayed.

Clinical example

Jacqueline was 32 year's old when her second child, Ben, was born at 38 weeks gestation. Her pregnancy was uneventful, except that clinical and ultrasound examination shortly before delivery had shown that the fetus was mildly growth retarded. On examination at birth, the baby weighed 2400 g. His head circumference was smaller than expected for his weight and hepatosplenomegaly was noted. There was a moderate thrombocytopenia. Intrauterine infection was suspected. Serological tests on sera from mother and infant were performed to determine the cause.

The results were:

		Maternal	Infant
Rubella	IgG	Positive	Positive
	IgM	Negative	Negative
CMV	IgG	Positive	Positive
	IgM	Negative	Positive
Toxoplasma	IgG	Negative	Negative
	IgM	Not done	Not done
VDRL		Non reactive	Non reactive

Serum from Jacqueline's first antenatal visit had been stored and was retested for rubella and CMV antibody. The rubella result was the same but CMV IgG and IgM were detected in this earlier sample, suggesting maternal infection early in pregnancy. Her husband Nick was seronegative and she had had no other sexual contact. The couple's first child, Eliza, aged 2 years, had been attending day care for approximately 6 months before the beginning of Jacqueline's second pregnancy. Subsequently, CMV was isolated from Ben's urine and throat swabs which were collected within 5 days of delivery.

The possibility of treating Ben with ganciclovir was discussed with Jacqueline and Nick. This would have involved intravenous therapy in hospital for 6 weeks and the likelihood of an improved outcome was uncertain. They decided to take him home, but he was followed up to detect deafness as early as possible. He was moderately deaf but was fitted with a hearing aid during the first year of life and his speech developed well. He had mild developmental delay.

CMV spreads readily between toddlers in close contact with each other. Adults most commonly acquire infection either from a sexual partner or by close contact with an infected child. Jacqueline probably acquired her infection, early in pregnancy, from Eliza.

- Specific IgM may indicate recent infection but is unreliable: it may be detectable for months; can rise after reactivation, and false positive results are not uncommon.

Epidemiology of maternal and congenital (CMV) infection in Australia (and other developed countries)

Primary infection

- 40–60% of young women are seronegative (susceptible).

- ~1% of them seroconvert during pregnancy.
- 40% of fetuses of women with primary infection are infected.
- Infection is transplacental; severe fetal damage is more likely early in gestation.
- ~10% of infants infected during primary maternal infection are abnormal at birth and usually have significant long term handicap.
- 10–15% of infected but initially asymptomatic infants later develop deafness or intellectual handicap.
- Overall incidence of congenital infection due to primary maternal infection is 1/1000.

Reactivation

- 20–30% of seropositive women reactivate latent infection during pregnancy.
- 2–5% of their infants are infected in utero but significant CMV disease is rare; mild sequelae (unilateral deafness) occur infrequently (<10%).
- Overall incidence of congenital infection is 1–2% — usually benign.
- ~10% of the infants of seropositive women are benignly infected during or after delivery by contact with maternal genital secretions or breast milk.

In developing countries and lower socioeconomic groups, primary infection occurs at a younger age and fewer adult women are susceptible.

Clinical features

The clinical features of severe intrauterine CMV infection include:
- Intrauterine growth retardation.
- Hepatosplenomegaly, hepatitis.
- Anaemia, thrombocytopenia.
- Pneumonitis.
- Microcephaly, encephalitis, cerebral calcification and chorioretinitis.
- Deafness, which is the commonest long term consequence.
- Cerebral palsy, intellectual handicap, epilepsy and visual impairment, which can occur.

Diagnosis

If primary maternal infection is suspected or cannot be excluded, fetal infection can be diagnosed by amniotic fluid culture and/or polymerase chain reaction (PCR) at about 18 weeks gestation. Depending on when maternal infection occurred, the risk of fetal damage may justify termination of pregnancy. Antiviral drugs active against CMV are too toxic for use during pregnancy but have been used with limited success in congenitally infected infants. Early diagnosis is important to ensure optimal management of the infant.

Congenital CMV infection is diagnosed by a positive culture of urine or saliva collected in the first 2 weeks of life; after that it is difficult to distinguish congenital from perinatal infection. Testing for CMV IgM in the infant's serum is less sensitive and specific.

There is no CMV vaccine. Normal hygiene, especially handwashing after changing nappies, can reduce the risk of transmission of CMV to seronegative carers of infected infants.

Toxoplasmosis

The protozoan *Toxoplasma gondii* infects many types of animal, including humans (and meat-producing animals). Sexual reproduction of the organism occurs only in the small intestine of members of the cat family. Oocysts shed in cat faeces are distributed widely in soil. Human infection occurs by ingestion of soil contaminated with mature oocysts or undercooked or raw meat containing tissue cysts.

Toxoplasmosis is usually asymptomatic or causes a mild illness with lymphadenopathy and fever. Infection during pregnancy involves the placenta and fetus in about 50% of cases overall. The risk of fetal infection increases but that of fetal damage decreases with advancing gestation. There is geographic variation in the incidence of congenital infection; in Australia it is estimated to be less than 1:1000 births.

Clinical features

- Most congenitally infected infants are asymptomatic at birth.
- Many later develop signs and sometimes symptoms of chorioretinitis (up to 80% ophthalmoscopic evidence, with some visual impairment in about half).
- ~10% develop neurological sequelae and/or hearing deficit.
- Signs of severe symptomatic congenital toxoplasmosis include:
  — anaemia, hepatosplenomegaly, jaundice
  — lymphadenopathy, chorioretinitis
  — central nervous system damage (intracranial calcification, hydrocephalus and microcephaly)
  — neurological and/or visual impairment, in most survivors.

Diagnosis and treatment

Toxoplasmosis during pregnancy is diagnosed, ideally, by showing seroconversion. More commonly it is suspected because specific IgM is detected in serum by antenatal screening. IgM can remain detectable for many months and, in the absence of symptoms, further testing is needed. If recent infection is confirmed or not excluded, treatment of the mother with spiramycin can reduce the risk of fetal infection. Appropriate management depends on diagnosis of intrauterine infection by amniotic fluid PCR at about 18 weeks gestation. Although rare, fetal infection during the first trimester is associated with a high risk of damage and termination of pregnancy is often recommended. Infection during the second or third trimester is more common but less likely to cause damage. The outcome is probably improved by treatment of the mother with a combination of pyrimethamine and a sulphonamide.

Specific IgM in the infant's serum or persistence of IgG beyond the first few months of life are evidence of congenital toxoplasmosis. *T. gondii* may be detected in tissue by histological examination or PCR, or in CSF by PCR. Treatment of a congenitally infected infant with spiramycin and/or pyrimethamine plus a sulphonamide can reduce progressive damage after birth.

Herpes simplex virus (HSV) infection

Perinatal HSV infection is acquired from the maternal genital tract during delivery (usually HSV-2), maternal viraemia during primary infection (HSV-1 or -2), or contact after birth with cold sores, infected saliva or hands (usually HSV-1). Often the source is unknown. Primary maternal HSV infection can cause fever, systemic symptoms and severe mucocutaneous lesions, but is often asymptomatic (and diagnosed by seroconversion). Transplacental infection is rare but spontaneous abortion or preterm labour can occur. Vertical transmission:
- is seen in up to 40% of cases when primary maternal HSV infection occurs around the time of delivery:
  - treating the mother with aciclovir and delivery by caesarean section will reduce the risk, if maternal infection is recognised.
- during vaginal delivery in the presence of recurrent genital herpes is less than 5%:
  - the amount of virus present is relatively small and the infant is protected by maternal antibody.

Clinical features

Neonatal herpes occurs in about 1:5000–1:10 000 infants. It may start with skin or mucocutaneous lesions but often disseminates; disseminated infection can occur without obvious skin lesions. Symptoms are similar to those of sepsis: fever, disseminated intravascular coagulation, shock and/or hepatitis, pneumonia, encephalitis. If untreated, the mortality is about 80%, with a high incidence of sequelae in survivors.

Neonatal herpes encephalitis can be due to either HSV-1 or -2. The mortality from untreated encephalitis is about 50%, with a high incidence of severe neurological sequelae in survivors. HSV-2 causes more severe disease, which is more likely to recur and cause permanent sequelae than HSV-1 disease. Infants with apparently localised mucocutaneous HSV infection may have neurological sequelae from unrecognised encephalitis.

Diagnosis and treatment

Neonatal HSV infection is diagnosed by isolation or detection of HSV by immunofluorescence or PCR in skin lesions, blood, CSF, saliva, urine or tissue biopsy. Early treatment with aciclovir reduces the mortality and morbidity and should be given for proven neonatal HSV infection, whatever its severity, or, after collection of appropriate specimens, if there is reasonable suspicion of HSV infection.

Varicella

Fewer than 5% of women of child bearing age are susceptible to varicella but exposure during pregnancy is common. Fetal outcomes following maternal infection early in pregnancy include:
- uncomplicated self-limiting infection (~10%)
- herpes zoster (shingles) in the first year of life (2–3%)
- fetal varicella syndrome (2–3% of cases), manifestations of which include:
  - growth retardation
  - skin scarring over a dermatomal distribution
  - ipsilateral limb or other skeletal hypoplasia
  - encephalopathy and abnormalities of various organs.

If maternal varicella occurs within 5 days of labour or in the immediate postpartum period, infection of the infant, at 5–10 days of age, may be complicated by pneumonia, hepatitis or encephalitis and a high mortality. When maternal infection occurs more than 5 days before delivery, infection in the infant is usually mild. Infants exposed to varicella after the first few days of life also usually have mild disease, although this is variable and depends on, among other factors, the mother's immune status.

Prophylaxis and treatment

Zoster immune globulin (ZIG) can prevent or modify varicella if given within 4 days (preferably 48 hours) of exposure to:
- pregnant women with no past history of varicella who are seronegative or whose immune status is unknown

- newborn infants of women who develop varicella within 5 days before or 48 hours after delivery.

Severe varicella in mother or infant should be treated with aciclovir.

Varicella vaccine has recently become available. Immunisation of susceptible women of child bearing age will protect the fetus from the risk of congenital varicella.

Chlamydial and gonococcal infection

Neisseria gonorrhoeae and *Chlamydia trachomatis* are sexually transmitted organisms that cause cervicitis in women and can be vertically transmitted during delivery. Gonorrhoea is more likely to be symptomatic and is easier to diagnose than chlamydial infection. In most Western countries, the incidence of both has fallen, but chlamydial infection, in particular, remains an important cause of pregnancy complications and secondary infertility.

Chlamydial infection

In Western countries, chlamydial infection in women is relatively uncommon (<5%), with wide variation in different geographic and socioeconomic groups. The incidence is relatively high in young, single women with multiple sexual partners, in socially disadvantaged groups and in developing countries. Most infants of infected women are normal at delivery but about 60% of those exposed are infected and, of these, about half develop symptoms.

Clinical features

- Conjunctivitis and/or pneumonia, in 15–30% of infants exposed.
- Conjunctivitis:
  — Incubation period: a few days to about 2 weeks.
  — Symptoms are often persistent, but are eventually self-limited.
- Pneumonia:
  — Incubation period: 2–6 weeks.
  — Subacute onset and an insidious course; history of conjunctivitis ~50%.
  — Paroxysmal coughing, vomiting and weight loss; often misdiagnosed as pertussis.
  — Systemic symptoms are minimal and fever absent.
  — Prolonged but eventually self-limited course, if untreated.
- Diagnosis: culture, immunofluorescence or nucleic acid test (e.g. PCR) of conjunctival scrapings or nasopharyngeal aspirate.

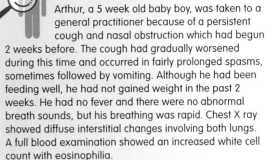

Clinical example

Arthur, a 5 week old baby boy, was taken to a general practitioner because of a persistent cough and nasal obstruction which had begun 2 weeks before. The cough had gradually worsened during this time and occurred in fairly prolonged spasms, sometimes followed by vomiting. Although he had been feeding well, he had not gained weight in the past 2 weeks. He had no fever and there were no abnormal breath sounds, but his breathing was rapid. Chest X ray showed diffuse interstitial changes involving both lungs. A full blood examination showed an increased white cell count with eosinophilia.

Arthur's mother, Sally, was an 18 year old single woman who had had an uneventful pregnancy apart from some frequency and dysuria at 36 weeks gestation which had been treated with trimethoprim. She had a normal vaginal delivery, induced at term because of mild hypertension. Arthur was well apart from 'sticky eyes' in the first week of life, which responded to saline eye toilets.

Laboratory investigations included examination of a nasopharyngeal aspirate (NPA) for respiratory pathogens, and cervical Gram stain and culture from the mother. Neither respiratory viruses nor *Bordetella pertussis* were detected in the NPA but *Chlamydia trachomatis* was detected by immunofluorescence. The Gram stain of the mother's cervical swabs showed an increased number of pus cells but few bacteria. There was a scanty growth of normal flora only, but immunofluorescence for *C. trachomatis* was positive. *Neisseria gonorrhoeae* was not isolated.

The mother's boyfriend, Barry, was contacted and gave a history of having been treated for urethritis 3 months previously. The couple had not seen each other since then. Sally (who was breastfeeding) and Arthur were treated with erythromycin (1 and 3 week courses, respectively). Arthur's symptoms resolved slowly.

There were several missed opportunities for prevention of Arthur's illness. Barry had been asked to contact his sexual partner(s), but there was no follow up to ensure that he had done so. Frequency and dysuria during pregnancy can be due to urethritis. Women in high risk groups for sexually transmissible infection (young, single) should be investigated for genital as well as urinary tract infection before being treated. Babies with sticky eyes should be investigated for chlamydial infection.

Treatment

Infection in an infant is a marker of maternal infection; if untreated, it can cause postpartum salpingitis with a risk of secondary infertility. Thus, it is important for both mother and infant that a specific diagnosis be made, even if mild conjunctivitis is the only symptom. The mother and her sexual partner(s) should be treated. Treatment of chlamydial pneumonia should reduce the duration of illness. Treatment of:

- Conjunctivitis: oral erythromycin for 2 weeks. Topical therapy with tetracycline or erythromycin eye drops does not eradicate *C. trachomatis* from the nasopharynx or prevent pneumonia.

- Pneumonia: oral erythromycin for 3 weeks.

Gonococcal infection

Gonorrhoea during pregnancy is comparatively rare — less than 1 per 1000 — in most Western communities. About 50% of infants of infected mothers develop conjunctivitis after an incubation period of 3–7 days. Usually, it is mild but, in a small minority, it is sight-threatening, with copious purulent exudate and corneal ulceration. Rarely, neonatal gonococcal infection causes meningitis or septic arthritis.

Diagnosis: Gram stain of a conjunctival smear; plus culture for confirmation and antibiotic susceptibility testing.

Treatment: third generation cephalosporin intravenously for 7 days (change to intravenous penicillin if the isolate is susceptible); frequent eye irrigation with sterile saline or chloramphenicol eye drops.

Hepatitis B virus (HBV) infection

Women who are chronic carriers of HBV (that is, have persistently detectable hepatitis B surface antigen (HBsAg) in serum) or who have acute hepatitis B late in pregnancy often transmit the virus to their infants. The risk and the outcome depend on the amount of live virus in maternal serum. A relatively high level of infectivity is indicated by the presence in serum of the hepatitis B e antigen (HBeAg) or DNA polymerase, both of which are associated with active viral replication.

About 95% of infants of HBeAg positive carriers are infected during delivery and will become chronic carriers; they are at risk from chronic liver disease, cirrhosis and hepatocellular carcinoma in early adult life or even childhood. Children who are HBsAg carriers are a potential source of horizontal transmission of HBV to other young children.

The risk of becoming carriers is much lower (approximately 5%) for infants of HBsAg carriers with antibody to HBeAg (indicating lower infectivity) but they can develop acute HBV infection, which is occasionally life threatening.

Prevention

Routine antenatal screening and immunisation of infants of HBsAg carriers can prevent neonatal HBV infection. The infant should be given hepatitis B immune globulin (HBIG) as soon as possible after birth (no later than 48 hours) and a course of hepatitis B vaccine starting in the first week, with second and third doses at 4–6 weeks and 6 months of age, respectively.

This prevents HBV infection in more than 95% of infants at risk.

Parvovirus infection

Human parvovirus B19 is the cause of erythema infectiosum or fifth disease (Ch. 37). At least 50% of women reach child bearing age without developing immunity and may become infected during pregnancy. Seroconversion occurs at the rate of about 50% after household contact, 20–30% after occupational exposure to infected children (e.g. in primary school teachers) and 10–15% overall. Infection in pregnancy is associated with:

- 10% excess pregnancy loss when infection occurs in the first half of pregnancy
- ~3% risk of hydrops fetalis, due to severe fetal anaemia, when infection occurs between 9 and 20 weeks gestation
- hydrops, which is diagnosed by ultrasound examination and may result in:
  — spontaneous resolution (one third of cases)
  — fetal death (usually without intrauterine transfusion; occasionally despite it)
  — resolution after intrauterine transfusion (most cases in which it is attempted)
- no increase in the incidence or any specific type of congenital abnormalities associated with maternal parvovirus infection.

Human immunodeficiency virus (HIV) infection

Women infected with HIV (the cause of the acquired immune deficiency syndrome (AIDS)) can transmit virus to their infants in utero, at delivery or after birth through breast milk. It is a serious problem in populations with a high or increasing incidence of HIV infection in heterosexuals; for example, among intravenous drug users and in countries where HIV infection occurs equally in both sexes. The risk of transmission is 25–30% and mainly depends on the degree of maternal viraemia. It can be reduced significantly by antiretroviral therapy of the mother during pregnancy and delivery, and/or of the infant immediately after birth. The diagnosis, clinical manifestations and management of HIV infection and AIDS in children are discussed in Chapter 41.

Neonatal sepsis

Aetiology

The bacterial pathogens that classically cause neonatal sepsis are:

- *Streptococcus agalactiae* (group B streptococcus, GBS) — the commonest
- *Escherichia coli* serotype K1.
- *Listeria monocytogenes* — uncommon but often occurring in clusters.

Numerous other bacteria, including other Gram negative bacilli, other streptococci, anaerobes, *Staphylococcus aureus* and genital mycoplasmas, can be involved.

Premature neonates are more susceptible to infection than term infants and premature delivery can be caused by intrauterine infection; however, sepsis can occur, albeit rarely, in apparently normal fullterm infants.

Source

The mother is the usual source of infection occurring in the first week of life, but infants remain susceptible to neonatal pathogens for several weeks. Infection can occur in utero — across the placenta or from the maternal genital tract — or exposure may occur during delivery. After birth, potential pathogens can be acquired from other adults or indirectly from other infants within the nursery or from the environment. Nosocomial infection is more likely in premature neonates who need prolonged intensive care.

Clinical features

Intrauterine infection can cause premature labour or fetal distress with or without maternal fever. The clinical manifestations of perinatal sepsis are non specific:
- respiratory distress, tachypnoea, apnoea
- temperature instability, irritability
- feeding difficulty, vomiting, diarrhoea and jaundice
- haematological changes:
  — neutrophilia or neutropenia
  — increased proportion of immature neutrophils
  — thrombocytopenia and coagulopathy.

Focal disease such as pneumonia, meningitis or urinary tract, bone, soft tissue or middle ear infections may complicate disseminated sepsis or occur alone, often with only non specific systemic symptoms.

Diagnosis

Investigations for suspected neonatal sepsis should include:
- Full blood examination and acute phase reactants such as C reactive protein.
- Culture of blood, CSF (if indicated) or urine collected by suprapubic bladder aspiration.
- CSF examination (if indicated): typical findings in bacterial meningitis are pleocytosis, with a predominance of polymorphonuclear leucocytes, a raised protein and decreased glucose level; in viral meningoencephalitis the cell counts are lower, mononuclear cells usually (not always) predominate and glucose levels are normal.
- Gram stain and culture of gastric contents or meconium immediately after delivery, and tracheal aspirate at the time of intubation: may suggest the causative pathogen if there is no growth from other specimens.
- Antigen tests for common pathogens (GBS and *E. coli* K1) in CSF or urine: rapid presumptive diagnosis in selected cases.

Specific pathogens

Group B streptococcus (GBS)

- Commonest cause of neonatal sepsis.
- Carried in vaginal flora of 25% of healthy women.
- <1% of the infants of carriers are infected; overall incidence 1–2/1000.
- Main risk factor for perinatal infection is lack of maternal (and hence fetal) serotype specific IgG antibody against GBS; tests for GBS antibody are not generally available.
- ~50% of infections begin in utero; associated with preterm labour, prolonged rupture of membranes and chorioamnionitis.
- 10–15% mortality.
- Incidence can be reduced (but not eliminated) by intrapartum antibiotic prophylaxis for women at risk; none of various strategies for identifying these women is particularly specific. They include routine antenatal screening for vaginal GBS carriage and/or identification of clinical risk factors during labour.
- All strategies involve administration of penicillin to a substantial proportion of healthy women, with associated risk of adverse effects, including emergence of antibiotic resistance.

Gram negative bacteria

- *E. coli* is the second most common cause of neonatal meningitis — most often serotype K1 — mainly in premature infants.
- *Proteus*, *Klebsiella* and *Salmonella* spp. are implicated uncommonly.
- Gram negative meningitis is associated with a significant risk of long term neurological sequelae.

L. monocytogenes

- Listeriosis is usually acquired from contaminated food such as dairy products and processed meats.
- Pregnant women, neonates, the elderly and the immunocompromised are most at risk.
- Maternal infection is often asymptomatic or mild.
- Spontaneous abortion, stillbirth or premature delivery and neonatal sepsis or meningitis can occur.

Treatment

Antibiotic therapy is started as soon as the diagnosis of neonatal sepsis is suspected and appropriate specimens have been collected for culture. The choice depends on the site of infection and the most likely pathogen:

- For sepsis (in the first week of life) without suspected meningitis:
  - penicillin and gentamicin (gentamicin is included even if the pathogen is susceptible to penicillin, because of its synergistic activity);
  - continue for 7–14 days.

- For suspected meningitis:
  - penicillin (active against *L. monocytogenes* and GBS) plus a cephalosporin such as cefotaxime (which is active against GBS, *E. coli* and most other Gram negative bacilli but not *L. monocytogenes*)
  - continue for 2–4 weeks
  - relapse occurs in about 5% of cases, even after apparently adequate therapy.
- Other treatment modalities used include pooled human gammaglobulin and irradiated leucocyte transfusion.

Acute neonatal surgical conditions

S. W. Beasley

The majority of the conditions discussed in this chapter will present initially to the paediatrician, general practitioner or obstetrician as emergencies. Delay in diagnosis may seriously compromise recovery and will almost certainly increase morbidity. Disorders that are obvious at birth but do not require urgent surgical referral have not been included in this chapter. For information on these, the reader is referred to paediatric surgical texts.

Oesophageal atresia

Any newborn infant who appears to salivate excessively at birth (drooling) should be suspected of having oesophageal atresia. This is a congenital abnormality where the mid portion of the oesophagus is missing. In most there is an abnormal communication between the lower oesophagus and the trachea, called a distal tracheo-oesophageal fistula (Ch. 34, Fig. 34.10).

The diagnosis is confirmed by passing a large firm catheter, for example a 10 French gauge orogastric tube, through the mouth and finding that it cannot be passed more than about 10 cm from the gums. The child must not be fed; otherwise, aspiration of feeds into the lungs is likely to occur. A plain X ray of the torso will show gas in the bowel, confirming the presence of a distal tracheo-oesophageal fistula. About 50% of these infants have other congenital abnormalities, most of which form part of the VATER association (vertebral, cardiac, renal, anorectal and radial abnormalities) (Ch. 29). Major chromosomal abnormalities are seen in 5%, of which trisomy 18 and trisomy 21 are the most frequent. Many are premature and a history of maternal polyhydramnios is common.

Initial management involves regular suctioning of the upper oesophageal pouch to prevent aspiration until the tracheo-oesophageal fistula has been divided. The oesophageal ends are anastomosed at the time of thoracotomy to close the fistula.

Duodenal obstruction

Bile stained vomiting starts soon after birth. The obstruction may be:

- intrinsic, as in duodenal atresia, or
- extrinsic, when it is the result of malrotation with volvulus.

In duodenal atresia there may be other abnormalities such as Down syndrome and imperforate anus (Ch. 29). In the absence of birth asphyxia these infants are usually alert and feed well, but they vomit bile stained material almost immediately. There may be epigastric distension. The diagnosis of duodenal atresia is made on plain X ray of the abdomen, which reveals a characteristic 'double bubble' due to gas in the stomach and proximal duodenum (Fig. 36.1). Little or no gas will be visible distal to the obstruction. Duodenoduodenostomy is performed after resuscitation and correction of any fluid and electrolyte disturbance.

Bile stained vomiting may also be an indication of malrotation in which volvulus has supervened. The midgut twists around the superior mesenteric vessels, which have a narrow attachment to the abdominal wall, the so called 'universal mesentery'. This is a true surgical emergency as the blood supply to the midgut may be cut off as the midgut twists around this axis.

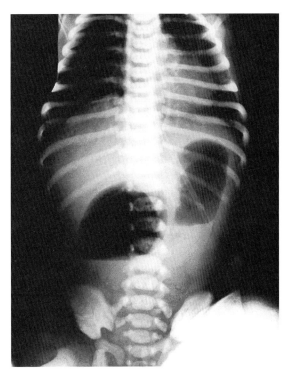

Fig. 36.1 X ray of the abdomen in a neonate demonstrating the 'double bubble' sign. Note the absence of gas in the bowel distal to the second bubble. This child had duodenal atresia.

The diagnosis can be confirmed with an urgent barium meal. If signs of peritonitis with abdominal distension and guarding are already present, the infant should be taken immediately to theatre.

Distal bowel obstruction

In more distal bowel obstructions, vomiting remains a major feature, but tends to occur later and is associated with abdominal distension. The more distal the obstruction, the later the vomiting and the more pronounced the distension (Fig. 36.2). The vomitus may become faeculent. An erect film of the abdomen will show distended loops of bowel and fluid levels (Fig. 36.3). The number of loops is dependent on the level of obstruction. The radiological appearances of ileal atresia, meconium ileus and Hirschsprung disease may be similar, and a contrast study, rectal biopsy or laparotomy may be required to make the definitive diagnosis.

Hirschsprung disease

Hirschsprung disease (congenital megacolon) is the most common cause of neonatal bowel obstruction. There is an absence of ganglion cells for a variable distance proximal to the anus. Peristalsis is abnormal in the aganglionic segment and results in severe constipation and an incomplete lower intestinal obstruction. The bowel proximal to the aganglionic segment becomes dilated and hypertrophied. The diagnosis is confirmed on rectal suction biopsy. Most of these infants present at 3 or 4 days of age with increasing abdominal distension, and delay in the passage of meconium. Surgical correction involves:

- excision of the aganglionic segment, and
- anastomosing ganglionated bowel to the anus.

It is often performed as a single stage procedure at diagnosis, but in certain circumstances requires staging.

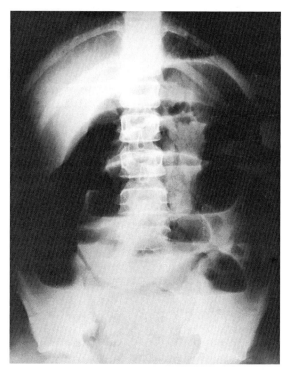

Fig. 36.2 Erect plain X ray of the abdomen, showing marked dilatation of multiple loops of bowel and several fluid levels. The most likely diagnoses include Hirschsprung disease, meconium ileus and ileal atresia.

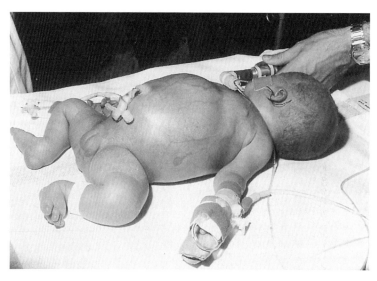

Fig. 36.3 Distal bowel obstruction in a neonate. Gross abdominal distension is evident, and was associated with vomiting of faeculent material.

Thomas was born normally after an uneventful pregnancy and labour. Meconium was first passed at 36 hours. At the age of 4 days he was noted to be feeding poorly and his abdomen was becoming increasingly distended but no mass was palpable. He vomited twice. On rectal examination a 'squirt' of meconium was passed. A plain upright film of the abdomen revealed several fluid levels suggestive of intestinal obstruction. A provisional diagnosis of Hirschsprung disease was made. This was confirmed on suction rectal biopsy which demonstrated the absence of ganglion cells in the submucosa. At laparotomy the transition zone was determined by frozen section. A primary pull through procedure was performed under the same anaesthetic.

Meconium ileus

Meconium ileus occurs in infants with cystic fibrosis. In this condition meconium becomes excessively thick and tenacious, causing obstruction, and the distal ileum is jammed with hard pellets of inspissated meconium. The colon is empty and no meconium is passed after birth. The infant has a distended abdomen and commences vomiting shortly after birth. A contrast enema will demonstrate a microcolon.

Sometimes the impacted pellets can be dislodged with a gastrograffin enema, but usually surgery is required. A temporary ileostomy allows the bowel to be irrigated. The diagnosis of cystic fibrosis is confirmed subsequently.

Small bowel atresias

Atresias of the jejunum are often multiple (Fig. 36.4). There is gross distension of the proximal jejunum, followed by multiple short segments of jejunum, and normal bowel distally. Ileal atresia tends to be an isolated lesion. Colonic atresia is extremely rare.

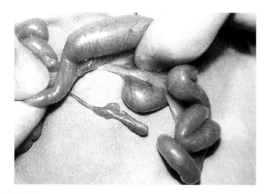

Fig. 36.4 Intraoperative photograph showing multiple areas of jejunal atresia in a neonate who presented with vomiting after the first two feeds after birth.

Neonatal necrotising enterocolitis

Neonatal necrotising enterocolitis is an acquired condition that predominantly afflicts premature infants who have undergone severe perinatal stress (Ch. 33). The infant becomes lethargic and unwell, usually between 2 days and 2 weeks after birth. There is bile stained vomiting and the abdomen becomes distended. Loose stools are passed, which may contain blood. As the disease progresses, signs of peritonitis develop: there is redness and oedema of the abdominal wall and increasing abdominal tenderness. Both small and large bowel may be involved. Plain X rays of the abdomen show:
- dilated loops of bowel.
- intramural gas (pneumatosis intestinalis). Gas may outline the portal venous system, and if full thickness perforation has occurred, free gas within the peritoneal cavity will be evident.

Initial management involves cessation of all oral feeds, decompression of the gastrointestinal tract by nasogastric aspiration, fluid resuscitation and antibiotics. Where there is continued clinical deterioration despite appropriate resuscitation, or there is evidence of full thickness bowel necrosis (for example, free gas on X ray), surgery is indicated. Necrotic bowel is excised and a defunctioning stoma may be required. Mal-absorption, short gut syndrome and colonic strictures may complicate the condition.

Anorectal anomalies

There is a spectrum of abnormalities that affect the anorectum, loosely called 'imperforate anus' (Fig. 36.5). They fall into two main groups: high lesions, where the rectum stops at or above the pelvic levator ani musculature (Fig. 36.5A), and low lesions where it continues beyond this point. Low lesions usually have a fistulous communication with the skin as an anocutaneous fistula (Fig. 36.5B). High lesions tend to be more complicated and are more likely to be associated with other congenital abnormalities. In the male with a high lesion there is either no opening at all, or the rectum communicates with the urinary tract via a rectourethral or rectovesical fistula (Fig. 36.5C). In the female the rectum usually communicates with the vestibule or vagina as a rectovestibular or rectovaginal fistula, respectively (Fig. 36.5D). In addition, a rare but even more severe group of abnormalities may occur in the female: in these cloacal malformations there is only one opening for the rectum, vagina and urinary tract.

In general, low lesions are treated by cutback anoplasty on the day of birth. High lesions require an anorectoplasty — a considerably more complicated procedure, performed either at birth or as a staged procedure later.

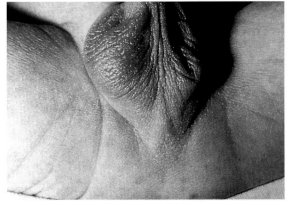

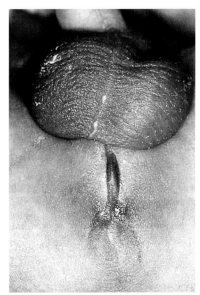

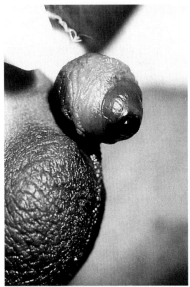

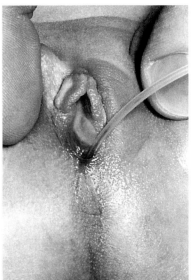

Fig. 36.5 Anorectal anomalies presenting as imperforate anus in the neonatal period. **A** A high imperforate anus, the lesion being above the levator ani musculature. **B** Imperforate anus due to a low lesion. Meconium is visible behind the distended skin of the median raphe. **C** Passage of meconium from the urethra. This has occurred in a neonate with a high imperforate anus and an associated rectourethral fistula. **D** Anorectal anomaly in a newborn girl. The catheter has been passed into the rectum.

Abdominal wall defects

The two main major abdominal wall defects are:
- exomphalos
- gastroschisis.

Frequently, both diagnoses are made on antenatal ultrasonography, although this does not influence the mode of delivery.

Exomphalos

This is a large defect at the umbilicus with herniation of bowel and liver into a sac which is covered by fused amniotic membrane and peritoneum (Fig. 36.6). The sac is translucent at birth but quickly becomes opaque as it desiccates. Coexisting abnormalities are common, and usually involve the heart and kidneys. Beckwith–Wiedemann syndrome may also be present and should be

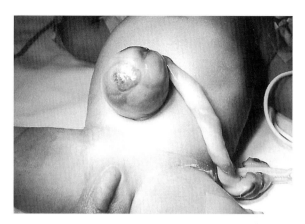

Fig. 36.6 Exomphalos, showing the site of the defect at the umbilicus. In some affected neonates the lesion is much larger and may contain most of the bowel and liver.

recognised as it is associated with severe hypoglycaemia that requires immediate correction at birth.

The early management of exomphalos involves placing the baby in a warm humidicrib incubator and wrapping the entire torso, including the exposed viscera, in clear plastic wrap to prevent evaporative heat loss. A nasogastric tube keeps the stomach empty, aiding subsequent closure of the defect. The defect can usually be repaired at birth, but the largest defects, particularly those which contain liver, may require a staged procedure.

Gastroschisis

In gastroschisis there is a small defect immediately to the right of the umbilicus through which bowel (and sometimes the gonads) herniate (Fig. 36.7). The eviscerated small and large bowel is thickened and densely matted

with exudate as a result of amniotic peritonitis before birth. These infants have a significant risk of hypothermia and exposed bowel should be wrapped in a plastic sheet to avoid evaporative heat loss. Surgery is directed at returning the bowel to the peritoneal cavity and repairing the defect. Where the peritoneal cavity is too small to accept the bowel it may be necessary to create a temporary prosthetic silo. After surgical repair the bowel may take many weeks to function normally. Coexisting abnormalities are normally confined to the gastrointestinal tract.

Diaphragmatic hernia

In the most common type of congenital diaphragmatic hernia (Bochdalek hernia) there is a defect of the left posterolateral part of the diaphragm which allows the contents of the abdomen to herniate into the left thoracic cavity. This limits the space available for the lungs to develop in utero. The resulting pulmonary hypoplasia creates severe respiratory distress within minutes of birth, and in many infants is not compatible with long term survival. The more severe the lung hypoplasia, the earlier the infant becomes symptomatic, and the poorer the prognosis. Diagnosis of the condition may be made antenatally on routine ultrasonography.

The diagnosis is confirmed by a plain chest X ray, which shows loops of bowel in the left chest (Ch. 34, Fig. 34.9). The heart is displaced to the contralateral side and there is little room available for the lungs. Right sided diaphragmatic hernias account for only 15% of such lesions. Early treatment involves aggressive cardiorespiratory support and decompression of the bowel. When the child is stable, operative repair of the diaphragm is undertaken.

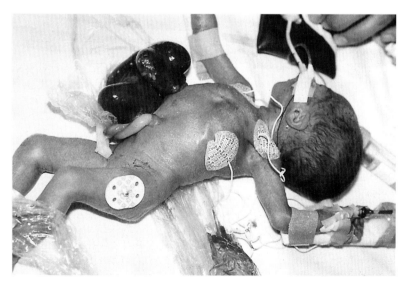

Fig. 36.7 Gastroschisis, with herniation of abdominal contents through an abdominal wall defect lateral to the umbilicus.

Sacrococcygeal teratoma

This is a rare tumour that is usually evident at birth; the baby is born with a large mass protruding from the lower back and arising from the tip of the coccyx or sacrum. In other infants it may expand predominantly into the pelvis. It may be extremely large and cause obstetric difficulties. A few become malignant. Malignant change is more likely if surgery is delayed, or where the tumour is uniformly solid and devoid of cysts. They are removed at birth.

PART 11   SELF-ASSESSMENT

Questions

1. **For the newborn infant:**
   - (A) The initial examination should be performed without the parents present in case an unsuspected abnormality is found
   - (B) A caput succedaneum suggests bleeding under the periostium of one of the skull bones.
   - (C) All newborn infants should be given intramuscular vitamin K
   - (D) The most important means of providing protection from infection is breastfeeding
   - (E) Normal infants lose up to 5% of their body weight during the first 3–5 days of life and usually regain their birth weight by 7–10 days of life

2. **The following are signs of significant prematurity:**
   - (A) Absence of palmar skin creases
   - (B) An empty scrotum in males with no scrotal rugae visible
   - (C) Flat pinnae of the ears, with the ears remaining folded when the pinna is rolled forwards
   - (D) Absence of palpable breast tissue
   - (E) Clitoris and labia minora visible only with difficulty in the female

3. **Which of the following are true?**
   - (A) A low Apgar score at 5 minutes of age accurately predicts brain damage from birth asphyxia
   - (B) Normal babies are able to breast feed immediately after birth
   - (C) Capillary naevi on the nape of the neck indicate underlying spina bifida occulta
   - (D) Although babies' hearts beat much faster than adults, the resting heart rate can be as low as 80 beats per minute

4. **You have been asked to see a 12 hour old term European baby girl who looks jaundiced. What should you do next?**
   - (A) Order a serum bilirubin
   - (B) Observe the jaundice clinically and obtain a serum bilirubin if getting worse
   - (C) Order a blood type on mother and infant and a Coombs test on the cord blood
   - (D) Order a G6PD screen
   - (E) Plot the serum bilirubin on a standard curve for healthy term newborns in order to decide whether phototherapy is necessary

5. **Which of the following is/are true about premature babies?**
   - (A) There is no increased chance of preterm labour in mothers with a history of previous preterm labour
   - (B) The incidence and severity of respiratory distress syndrome (RDS) is reduced when steroids are given to the mother before birth
   - (C) Chronic lung disease is one of the long term complications of prematurity. These infants sometimes go home on supplemental oxygen
   - (D) Hypoglycaemia is an uncommon problem in the premature baby
   - (E) The Ballard test is the most accurate assessment of gestational age

6. **You are asked to evaluate a newborn whose weight is at the 3rd centile, length at the 3rd centile, and head circumference at the 50th centile. Which of the following is/are likely to be true about this infant?**
   - (A) If there is no other abnormality on history or examination, the most likely cause is congenital infection
   - (B) This infant is likely to become hypoglycaemic
   - (C) This infant may remain short in adult life
   - (D) This infant is likely to be anaemic
   - (E) This infant is likely to be at risk of hypothermia

7. **Baby Andrew was born at 35 weeks gestation after 22 hours of membrane rupture and through meconium stained liquor. He presented with respiratory distress at 1 hour of age.**
   - (A) Meconium aspiration syndrome could be eliminated because he was suctioned as head crowned and again after delivery
   - (B) Broad spectrum antibiotics are indicated until culture results are available
   - (C) Transient tachypnoea of newborn (wet lung disease) is most likely diagnosis

(D) Intrapartum penicillin for the mother was indicated

(E) Intratracheal administration of surfactant would have a dramatic benefit

8. **Lucy was born at 42 weeks gestation by emergency caesarean section because of fetal bradycardia, thick meconium stained liquor and a fetal scalp blood lactate of 5.5 mmol/l. At birth she was apnoeic, cyanosed and had a heart rate of 50/min. Meconium was suctioned from the oropharynx. You would:**

(A) Provide cutaneous stimulation and then bag and mask ventilation

(B) Intubate the trachea and provide suction with the aid of a meconium aspirator

(C) Provide tracheoalveolar lavage with normal saline

(D) Give positive pressure ventilation if the heart rate was persistently 50/min

(E) Give corticosteroids after admission to the intensive care nursery

9. **True or false? The congenital rubella syndrome:**

(A) Can be prevented by immunisation of pregnant women

(B) Can be eliminated by routine immunisation of teenaged girls

(C) Is most likely to occur if maternal infection occurs between 9 and 16 weeks gestation

(D) Results in virus induced growth retardation

(E) Can occur after asymptomatic maternal infection

10. **True or false? Congenital syphilis:**

(A) Does not occur if the mother is infected in the first trimester

(B) Can be prevented by early treatment of maternal syphilis

(C) Is most likely to occur if the mother has had undiagnosed syphilis for 2 years or more

(D) Can first cause clinical manifestations a year or more after birth

(E) Can be confirmed by a positive VDRL in the first week of life

11. **True or false? Cytomegalovirus (CMV) infection:**

(A) Causes damage only from reactivation of maternal infection

(B) Can be diagnosed by culture of the infant's urine in the first week of life

(C) Can be excluded by a negative CMV specific IgM in the first week of life

(D) Can be cured by treatment with intravenous ganciclovir

(E) Symptomatic infection can occur in successive pregnancies

12. **True or false? Neonatal chlamydial pneumonia:**

(A) Is often preceded by conjunctivitis

(B) Is often misdiagnosed as early whooping cough

(C) Can be prevented by treatment of maternal infection during pregnancy

(D) Usually occurs in the first week of life

(E) Indicates that the mother is infected and should be treated after appropriate investigations

Answers and explanations

1. The correct answers are **(C)**, **(D)** and **(E)**. It is important that parents are present when their newborn baby is examined for the first time so that they can see that their baby is normal, can ask questions, and can learn about their baby (A). If abnormalities are found, there can be immediate and open discussion and management approaches can be communicated immediately. A caput succedaneum is an area of soft tissue oedema relating to pressure over the presenting part (usually the occipital area of the skull) during labour and delivery; (B) the above description is of a subperiosteal haematoma. Previous concerns that intramuscular administration of vitamin K may be associated with the later development of cancers have been proven to be unfounded. Oral vitamin K is less effective in preventing haemorrhagic disease of the newborn and needs repeated doses. Therefore intramuscular vitamin K administration is recommended for all newborn babies at the time of delivery (C). Breastfeeding is the most important protective mechanism against infection in the newborn. Careful hand washing and rooming in with the mother in the maternity facility are also important (D). It is normal for the newborn to lose some weight in the first few days of life as oral feeding becomes established (E). If the weight loss is greater than 10%, serious consideration should be given to an underlying abnormality.

2. The correct answers are **(A)**, **(B)**, **(C)** and **(D)**. Plantar skin creases appear with increasing maturity in utero and are seen readily by 33–34 weeks gestation (A). The testes are palpable in the upper scrotum by 36 weeks gestation and scrotal rugae are evident at 36 weeks (B). Thin cartilage imparting some resistance to folding of the pinnae is present in the ears by 35–36 weeks gestation, with only scant cartilage being present from 32 to 35 weeks (C). Breast tissue becomes palpable at about 35–36 weeks (D). In marked prematurity, the labia minora and clitoris are readily visible, and become obscured by the labia majora with increasing gestation (E).

3. **(A)** False. The 5 minute Apgar correlates poorly with established brain damage. More than 90% of babies with a 5 minute Apgar score of 0–3 grow up neurologically normal. **(B)** True. Babies are able to seek

355

out and attach to the nipple (rooting reflex) and suck well from birth. (C) False. Capillary naevi at the nape of the neck (stork bites) are benign. Hairy tufts over the sacral area may indicate an underlying spina bifida occulta. **(D)** True.

4. The correct answers are **(A)** and **(C)**. Early jaundice (before 24 h) must always be evaluated and is likely to be due to haemolysis. A serum bilirubin should be obtained (A). The most likely cause of haemolytic jaundice in this newborn is blood group incompatibility. Therefore it is important to know both mother and infant's blood type (C). Both ABO and rhesus incompatibility are immune mediated. Group A or B babies born to group O mothers are most likely to have ABO incompatibility because of the presence of anti-A and anti-B antibodies. Similarly, Rhesus disease is seen in Rh+ babies born to Rh− mothers. The Coombs test looks for antibodies either on the red blood cells or in the serum (C). Glucose-6-phosphate dehydrogenase deficiency would be unlikely in this infant, as it is an X linked disorder that primarily affects males and occurs in Asian and Mediterranean ethnic groups (D). Because haemolytic disease is suspected, the threshold for treatment is lower than that for healthy term infants, who should not require phototherapy at < 24 hours (E).

5. The correct answers are **(B)** and **(C)**. The incidence of preterm labour is increased in mothers who have had previous preterm labour (A). Hypoglycaemia is very common in preterm infants due to their decreased glycogen stores and increased glucose needs (D). The Ballard test assesses neuromuscular and physical maturity based on a scoring system. It is not as accurate as the first day of the last menstrual period or an early antenatal ultrasound in estimating gestational age, and gestational age can be underestimated in small for gestational age babies (E).

6. The correct answers are **(B)**, **(C)** and **(E)**. Smallness at birth can be a presenting feature of congenital infection, but commonly other features are also present and asymptomatic infection is a rare cause of SGA (A). Most babies in whom a cause for SGA is identified have relevant features on history and examination. In the absence of any of these a cause for SGA is rarely identified. Hypoglycaemia and hypothermia are common problems in SGA infants due to decreased glycogen and fat stores, and relatively increased surface area (B, E). These infants may be polycythaemic rather than anaemic (D) due to

reduced oxygen supply in utero leading to increased haematopoiesis. Babies born short are at increased risk of remaining small throughout life (C).

7. The correct answers are **(B)**, **(C)** and **(D)**. Although the most likely diagnosis is transient tachypnoea of the newborn (C), congenital pneumonia could not be excluded and antibiotics are indicated (B). Because membranes were ruptured 22 hours, prophylactic, intrapartum penicillin is indicated (D). Meconium aspiration syndrome could not be excluded on history (A). Although RDS is a differential diagnosis, intratracheal instillation of surfactant is not indicated without further evidence (E).

8. The correct answers are **(B)** and **(D)**. The primary treatment for probable meconium aspiration for a depressed infant born through thick meconium and who has meconium visualised in the oropharynx is endotracheal intubation for suction of the trachea with the aid of a meconium aspirator (B). If the baby is persistently bradycardic a decision must be made to cease tracheal suction and give positive pressure ventilation (D). Cutaneous stimulation and bag and mask ventilation is inappropriate (A). Instillation of normal saline into the airway to lubricate meconium to facilitate suctioning is contraindicated because it washes out surfactant (C). There is no evidence that postnatal steroids are beneficial (E).

9. (A) False. It may be too late. (B) False. Vaccine is not totally reliable and antibodies may fall over 10 or more years. (C) False. It is most likely to occur in the early weeks of pregnancy — the period of organogenesis. **(D)** True. **(E)** True.

10. (A) False. Congenital syphilis does occur if the mother is infected in the first trimester. **(B)** True. Early treatment of maternal syphilis with penicillin will prevent congenital syphilis. (C) False. It is more likely, to occur if the mother has early syphilis. **(D)** True. Congenital syphilis can be asymptomatic for many months. (E) False. In the first week of life a positive VDRL may be the result of cured maternal syphilis.

11. (A) False. CMV causes fetal damage only from primary maternal infection. **(B)** True. (C) False. only 60–70% of congenitally infected infants have CMV specific IgM antibodies. (D) False. CMV does not respond to treatment with ganciclovir. (E) False. Infection may occur in subsequent pregnancies but it is asymptomatic.

12. (A) False. **(B)** True. **(C)** True. (D) False. **(E)** True.

PART 11   FURTHER READING

Bancalari E 2000 Epidemiology and risk factors for the 'new' bronchopulmonary dysplasia. Pediatrics in Review Neonatal Reviews 1:e2–e5

Breton J R 1998 Early perinatal hospital discharge. Clinics in Perinatology 25:2

Cashore W J 2000 Bilirubin and jaundice in the micropremie. Clinics in Perinatology 27: 171–179

Chatelain P 2000 Children born with intra-uterine growth retardation (IUGR) or small for gestational age (SGA): long term growth and metabolic consequences. Endocrine Regulations 34: 33–36

Donoghue D, Cust A 1999 Report of the Australian and New Zealand Neonatal Network. AIHW National Perinatal Statistics Unit, Sydney

Dunn D, Wallon M, Peyron F, Petersen E, Peckham C, Gilbert R 1999 Mother-to-child transmission of toxoplasmosis: risk estimates for clinical counselling. Lancet 353: 1899–1900

Gartner L 1994 Neonatal jaundice. Pediatrics in Review 15: 422–428

Godfrey K M, Barker D J 2000 Fetal nutrition and adult disease. American Journal of Clinical Nutrition 71(5 Supplement): 1344S–1352S

Hager W D, Schuchat A, Gibbs R et al 2000 Prevention of perinatal group B streptococcal infection: current controversies. Obstetrics and Gynecology 96: 14–15

Hammerman C, Kaplan M 2000 Recent developments in the management of neonatal hyperbilirubinemia. Pediatrics in Review Neonatal Reviews 1: e19–e24

Lazzarotto T, Varani S, Guerra B, Nicolosi A, Lanari M, Landini M P 2000 Prenatal indicators of congenital cytomegalovirus infection. Journal of Pediatrics 137: 4–6

Levene M I, Tudehope D I, Thearle M J 2000 Essentials of Neonatal Medicine, 3rd edn. Blackwell Science, Oxford

Lorenz J M 2000 Survival of the extremely preterm infant in North America in the 1990s. Clinics in Perinatology 27: 255–262

Miller E, Fairley C K, Cohen B J et al 1998 Immediate and long term outcome of human parvovirus B19 infection in pregnancy. British Journal of Obstetrics and Gynaecology 105: 174–178

Msall M E, Tremont M R 2000 Functional outcomes in self-care, mobility, communication, and learning in extremely low-birth weight infants. Clinics in Perinatology 27: 381–401

O'Shea M T, Dammann O 2000 Antecedents of cerebral palsy in very low-birth weight infants. Clinics in Perinatology 27: 285–302

Rennie J M, Roberton D M 1999 Textbook of neonatology, 3rd edn. Churchill Livingstone, Edinburgh

Sheffield J S, Wendel G D 1999 Syphilis in pregnancy. Clinical Obstetrics and Gynecology 42: 97–106

Sommerfelt K, Andersson H W, Sonnander K et al 2000 Cognitive development of term small for gestational age children at five years of age. Archives of Disease in Childhood 83: 25–30

Strauss R S, Dietz W 1998 Growth and development of term children born with low birth weight: effects of genetic and environmental factors. Journal of Pediatrics 133: 67–72

Wallon M, Liou C, Garner P, Peyron F 1999 Congenital toxoplasmosis: systematic review of evidence of efficacy of treatment in pregnancy. BMJ 318: 1511–1514

Useful links

http://www.aap.org/sections/sperintl.htm (American Academy of Pediatrics, Section on Perinatal Pediatrics)

http://www.cochrane.org (Cochrane Database of Systematic Reviews, The Cochrane Library. Issue 1, 2001. Update Software, Oxford)

http://www2.hawaii.edu/medicine/pediatrics/neoxray/neoxray.html (Radiology cases in neonatology)

http://www.med.jhu.edu/peds/neonatology.poi.html (Harriet Lane www links)

http://neonatol.peds.washington.edu (NICU — WEB)

http://www.neonatology.org (Neonatology on the web)

http://www.nichd.nih.gov/cochraneneonatal (Cochrane Neonatal Group)

http://www.vh.org/ (Virtual hospital)

PART 12

INFECTIONS IN CHILDHOOD

Infectious diseases of childhood

D. Isaacs

Infectious diseases of childhood are still a significant cause of illness in children, especially in the first years of life. Although immunisation has resulted in a very marked reduction in many of the childhood infections that in previous times caused significant morbidity and mortality (Ch. 8), some of these infections are still seen, and others have yet to have effective vaccines developed. This chapter describes the features of some of these infections.

Measles (rubeola, morbilli)

Measles (Figs 37.1, 37.2) is one of the most important of the childhood exanthems, due to its high infectivity and virulence. At the end of the twentieth century it still caused a million childhood deaths a year worldwide. It is a paramyxovirus, one of the RNA viruses.

The rash of measles is mediated by T cells: infected subjects with defective T cells (cellular immunity) get little or no rash, but classically develop a giant cell pneumonia. Measles infection also causes significant

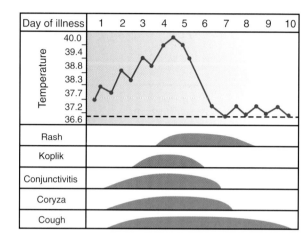

Fig. 37.2 The development of measles.

suppression of host T cell immunity, resulting in anergy to tuberculin (negative Mantoux) and increased susceptibility to diarrhoeal and respiratory illness.

Epidemiology

- From 1978 to 1992 in Australia over 10 children a year died from measles, due to acute encephalitis or pneumonia.
- As immunisation levels improved, the number of deaths has fallen to 1–2 per year since 1992.
- In developing countries, the high mortality is mainly due to pneumonia, often with bacterial (staphylococcal or pneumococcal) superinfection.
- Children in developing countries who recover from measles have increased mortality for a year afterwards due to the resultant suppression of cellular immunity.
- Measles is highly contagious, and over 98% of adults in unimmunised communities are seropositive.

Complications

See Table 37.1.

Differential diagnosis

- In roseola infantum (see below), the rash can be identical to measles, but appears as the fever subsides, and the child looks well.

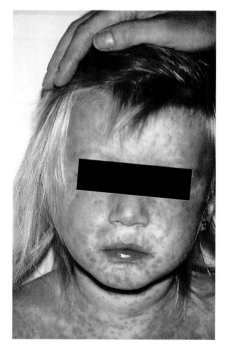

Fig. 37.1 Measles: blotchy, raised rash.

Clinical example

Harriet, 3 years old, was in preschool with a friend who, 2 weeks earlier (1) had a cough and fever (2) and later came out in a measles rash. Neither had been immunised (3). Harriet developed a high fever, runny nose and cough (4) and was irritable. Her eyes became red and weepy (5) and her ears were sore (6). After 3 days (2) her doctor found bilateral otitis media (6) and white spots on a red background on her buccal mucosa (7). Next day she remained miserable and hot, and developed a rash behind her ears, which spread over the next 2 days to her face, trunk and limbs, and was pink to red and blotchy (8). In some areas the rash joined up and was raised. She had scattered rhonchi bilaterally (4). She remained febrile and unwell for 3 days, then the rash faded, leaving a brown discoloration of the skin with desquamation of the fingers and toes (9).

The following are features typical of measles infection. Incubation period 10–14 days (1). Infectious during the prodromal period, which lasts 3–5 days (2). Immunisation over 95% protective (3). Bronchitis (4), exudative conjunctivitis (5) and otitis media (6) almost invariable features. Enanthem called Koplik spots (7). Rash is classically descending, blotchy to confluent, maculopapular (8), with desquamation, often more marked in children from developing countries (9).

Table 37.1 Major complications of measles in industrialised countries

	Incidence	Clinical features	Outcome
Neurological			
Acute encephalitis	1 in 1000 to 1 in 5000	Onset usually day 4–7 after rash, i.e. postinfective	10–15% die, 15–40% brain damage
Subacute			
Sclerosing panence-phalitis (SSPE)	1 in 25 000	Intellectual deterioration, myoclonic jerks	Invariably fatal
Respiratory			
Pneumonia	1 in 25	Viral pneumonitis or secondary bacterial infection	Occasional deaths
Otitis media	1 in 40	During prodrome	Transient hearing loss

- Other viruses causing morbilliform (measles-like) rash on occasions: enteroviruses, Epstein–Barr virus (EBV), influenza, parinfluenza.
- Antibiotics, especially amoxycillin or ampicillin, may cause a rash.
- Kawasaki disease.
- Scarlet fever.

Laboratory diagnosis

- Serology: measles-specific IgM or four fold or greater rise in IgG titre.
- Antigen detection: immunofluorescent antibody stain on nasopharyngeal secretions.

Treatment

- Mainly symptomatic in industrialised countries.
- Vitamin A therapy recommended for severe cases and malnourished children.
- Antibiotics for bacterial complications, particularly pneumonia.

Prevention

- Measles is a **vaccine preventable disease.**
- There are effective live, attenuated vaccines.
- There is only one serotype of measles.
- Humans are the only host.
- It should be possible to eradicate measles from the world by immunisation.

In developing countries, routine vitamin A supplementation reduces the mortality of measles. In Australia measles-mumps-rubella (MMR) vaccine is given at 1 year of age and a second dose at 4–5 years of age. (Note that maternal antibody is generally protective before 1 year, and interferes with immunogenicity if vaccine is given earlier.)

Measles vaccine is contraindicated for immuno-suppressed children. If exposed to measles, they should be given normal human immunoglobulin, as 'passive' protection.

Rubella (German measles)

The main importance of rubella virus is its teratogenic effect on the fetus, causing congenital rubella syndrome.

Epidemiology

- Respiratory droplet spread.
- Causes spring and summer epidemics in unimmunised communities.
- Mainly affects children aged 5–10 years, but also non-immune pregnant women.
- Less infectious than measles: 15–20% of adults in unimmunised populations (including South East Asia) are non immune.
- Most rubella infections are subclinical.

Clinical features (Figs 37.3, 37.4)

- Incubation period 14–21 days.

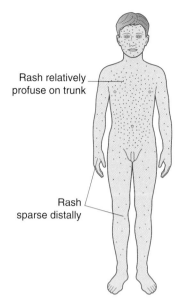

Fig. 37.3 The distribution of rash in rubella.

Rash relatively profuse on trunk

Rash sparse distally

Day of illness	1	2	3	4	5	6	7	8	9	10
Temperature 40.0 39.4 38.8 38.3 37.7 37.2 36.6										
Rash										
Lymph nodes										
Malaise										
Conjunctivitis										
Coryza										

Fig. 37.4 The development of rubella.

- Rash much fainter and less florid than measles.
- Rash often starts on face in young children, spreads to neck, trunk and extremities.
- Lymphadenopathy, particularly suboccipital, post-auricular and cervical, usual.
- In adolescents and adults, often get more constitutional symptoms: conjunctivitis, arthralgia or arthritis, malaise, fever.
- Encephalitis, purpura are rare complications.
- Congenital rubella syndrome results from first trimester rubella infection (Ch. 35).

Diagnosis

A non immune pregnant woman exposed to possible rubella should have acute serum for rubella-specific IgM and IgG and a convalescent titre 2–4 weeks later, looking for a rising IgG titre. These are usually measured by ELISA.

Differential diagnosis

Many other viruses cause rubelliform rashes. Clinical diagnosis of rubella is notoriously unreliable. Rubella is very rare in infancy: other viruses, e.g. enteroviruses, HHV-6 are much more likely to cause infantile rashes.

Prevention

Live attenuated rubella vaccine is usually given universally as MMR in industrialised countries. Congenital rubella syndrome is rare in industrialised countries like Australia, but common in developing countries.

Roseola infantum (exanthem subitum)

- Caused by infection with human herpesvirus 6 (HHV-6) and occasionally HHV-7.
- Affects infants aged 6–18 months.

Clinical example

Mark, a 9 month old baby who was previously well, developed a runny nose, fever and irritability (1) and went off his feeds. After 2 days, he had a generalised, tonic–clonic seizure (2) which stopped after 2 minutes. He was admitted to hospital, where he was found to have a fever of 40°C, cervical lymphadenopathy (3) but no rash or enanthem (4). A lumbar puncture was normal. After 24 hours observation in hospital his fever subsided, but he developed a maculopapular rash, thought at first to be measles (5). He was well and was discharged home. Serology was positive for IgM to HHV-6.

The following are features typical of roseola infantum. (1), (3) Usual presenting features, lasting 2–3 days. Febrile convulsion (2) is a recognised complication. No enanthem (4). Child well and fever falls as rash appears (5), in contrast to measles.

Erythema infectiosum (slapped cheek disease, fifth disease)

- Caused by human parvovirus B19 (parvo = small).
- Spread by respiratory route.
- Causes epidemics in school aged children, which mimic rubella outbreaks.
- Initial presentation is with fever, cervical lymphadenopathy and facial rash resembling sunburnt cheeks (viraemic phase).

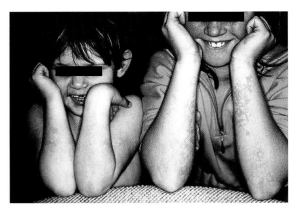

Fig. 37.5 Fifth disease: slapped cheeks and lacy rash (with kind permission of Dr Maureen Rogers).

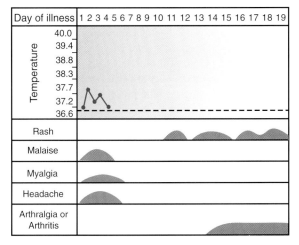

Fig. 37.6 The development of erythema infectiosum (fifth disease).

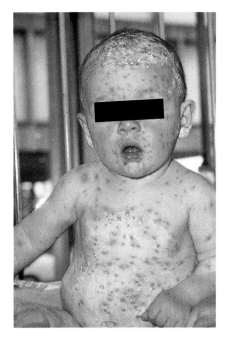

Fig. 37.7 Chickenpox: vesicles and pustules on trunk and scalp.

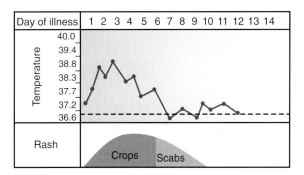

Fig. 37.8 The development of chickenpox.

- Subsequently develop lacy, reticular rash on limbs and trunk, sometimes with arthralgia or arthritis (immune complex mediated) (Figs 37.5, 37.6).
- The virus infects red cell precursors in the bone marrow, causing no effect in normals (Hb drops by 1 g/dL) but severe anaemia in those with shortened red cell survival.
- In sickle cell disease and other hereditary anaemias, infection causes aplastic crises due to red cell aplasia.
- Infection during the 2nd or 3rd trimester of pregnancy can cause fetal hydrops due to fetal anaemia.

Varicella (chickenpox)

Chickenpox (Figs 37.7, 37.8) is a highly infectious disease causing a bullous (pox-like) rash. The DNA virus responsible, varicella-zoster virus (VZV), is a herpes-virus and, as such, has the ability to remain dormant, in the dorsal root ganglia of nerves, and reactivate as herpes zoster (shingles).

Epidemiology

- Occurs worldwide, although spreads less readily in tropical countries.
- Highly infectious, spread by respiratory route, due to infectious particles from burst vesicles and from respiratory tract.
- Peak age incidence is 2–8 years.

Complications

- Bacterial superinfection of skin.
- Pneumonia/pneumonitis

363

Charles, aged 6, had been in contact with a schoolfriend who was off school 2 weeks ago with chickenpox (1). Charles had a sore throat and fever of 38°C but no spots (2). Next day, a few small red spots like mosquito stings appeared on his trunk and limbs and on his scalp under the hair (3). These became raised (4), then developed into small fluid-filled blisters surrounded by a small area of erythema (5). They were intensely itchy, and when scratched readily became superinfected and left a scar (6). These spots crusted over within hours but fresh crops of vesicles kept appearing on his face, trunk and limbs (7). He had difficulty swallowing (8) and his eyes were red and sore (9). He was miserable but not unwell and was troubled by the intense pruritus. After a week, the last spot had crusted (10) and the scabs disappeared over the next 2 weeks.

The following are features typical of varicella. (1) Incubation period 10–21 days. Short 1–2 day prodrome (2) during which infectious (not infectious during the incubation period). Spots under hairline (3) characteristic and distinguish from insect bites. Start as macules (3), then progress to papules (4), vesicles or pustules (5). If scratched they may become infected, the commonest complication, and leave a scar or pockmark (6). They come in crops (7), and can infect the pharynx, palate (8) and conjunctivae of the lids (9). The child is infectious until the last spot crusts (10).

— Varicella pneumonitis occurs in immunocompromised children, but also in pregnant women and normal adults.
— Bacterial pneumonia (pneumococcal or staphylococcal) can rarely complicate varicella pneumonitis.
- Encephalitis
— Incidence about 1 in 1000 cases.
— Most common form is pure cerebellar ataxia, with complete recovery over days to weeks.
— Severe form is acute disseminated encephalomyelitis (ADEM), a postinfectious demyelinating illness, with high morbidity and mortality.
- Haemorrhagic chickenpox — severe illness in subjects with profound defect in cellular immunity, indicating importance of T cells in recovery from VZV infection.
- Congenital varicella syndrome — affects 2% of babies whose mothers develop 2nd trimester chickenpox.

Diagnosis

Usually clinical. Can grow virus from blister fluid in tissue culture or detect antigen by immunofluorescence or serology (IgG, IgM) available.

Prevention

- Live attenuated VZV vaccines are now available and are highly protective.

- Varicella zoster immune globulin (ZIG or VZIG) is an immunoglobulin preparation with a high titre of anti-VZV IgG antibodies. It is used for passive prophylaxis of immunocompromised patients (e.g. oncology patients, neonates) exposed to VZV.

Treatment

The antiviral drug acyclovir inhibits viral thymidine kinase, and can be used to treat children with severe varicella.

Zoster (herpes zoster, shingles)

VZV can remain dormant in the dorsal root ganglia of sensory nerves after primary infection, and reactivate many years later as zoster. Zoster follows a dermatome distribution, and was indeed the means by which the distribution of the sensory nerves was mapped. Vesicles form a band and do not usually cross the midline. They can occur on the trunk and limbs or follow cranial nerves. The Ramsay Hunt syndrome presents with vesicles on the pinna of one ear and facial nerve palsy due to zoster of the geniculate ganglion.

- Zoster infection in a previously well child is almost always benign and not suggestive of underlying malignancy.
- About 10% of children whose mothers developed chickenpox during pregnancy will develop zoster in early childhood: if a young child gets zoster, ask about chickenpox in pregnancy.
- Immunocompromised children are at increased risk of zoster.
- Neuralgia, before, during and after zoster, is very uncommon in children, in contrast to adults.
- Most childhood zoster does not need specific treatment, but aciclovir is indicated for ophthalmic zoster (to prevent eye damage) or if the child is immunocompromised (to prevent life threatening disseminated infection).

Mumps (epidemic parotitis)

- Infectious disease of childhood, 90% before adolescence.
- Preventable by immunisation with live attenuated virus (usually given as MMR vaccine).
- Causes swelling, pain and tenderness of the parotid glands.
- Can rarely be unilateral, but unilateral neck swelling more suggestive of alternative diagnoses (e.g. lymphadenopathy, autoimmune parotitis).
- Other salivary glands, sublingual and submandibular, may be involved.

- Complications include viral meningitis (symptomatic in 10% of children with mumps, asymptomatic in over 50%), encephalitis, orchitis, oophoritis, pancreatitis, thyroiditis, deafness, and rarely ophthalmitis, arthritis, myocarditis and nephritis.

Scarlet fever and scarlatina

(Figs 37.9, 37.10)

Scarlet fever is a toxin mediated disease caused by exotoxins elaborated by Group A streptococcus (*Streptococcus pyogenes*) and coded by plasmids. These toxins act as 'superantigens', causing widespread T cell activation because they can bind to the edge of the T cell receptor and bypass its usual highly specific recognition of antigens. Analogous superantigen mediated diseases include toxic shock syndrome and Kawasaki disease.

Scarlatina is a mild form of scarlet fever, often affecting preschool age children, whereas scarlet fever is commonest at age 5–10 years. In both, the primary site of group A streptococcal infection is the throat, causing exudative tonsillitis and/or pharyngitis.

In preantibiotic days, scarlet fever, and the related erysipelas, was a quarantinable disease, highly contagious and with a high mortality. Although scarlet fever became less common after the 1940s, it has re-emerged, perhaps due to the re-emergence of strains with virulent exotoxins.

> ### Clinical example
>
> Anna, 7 years old, presented with fever and sore throat for 2 days, followed by a rash. Her tonsils were red and covered in spots of white exudate (1). Her tongue had prominent red papillae (2). Her face looked red, but was white around the mouth, like a clown (3). The rash was red, patchy and rough to the touch (4), and covered her whole body. In the axillae and groins there were lines of petechiae (5). Her cervical lymph nodes were enlarged and tender (6). She was treated with penicillin and rapidly improved. Two weeks later she had extensive peeling of her hands and feet (7).
>
> The following are features typical of scarlet fever. Exudative tonsillitis (1); strawberry tongue (2); circumoral pallor (3); sandpaper rash (4); Pastia lines (5); tender cervical lymphadenitis (6); peripheral desquamation (7).

Diagnosis

Positive throat swab or positive serology: high or rising titre to streptolysin O (ASOT) or deoxyribonuclease B (anti-DNAase B).

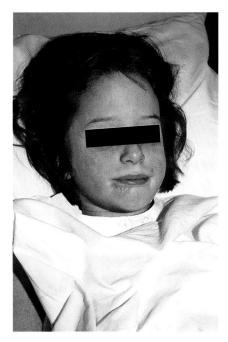

Fig. 37.9 Scarlet fever: generalised erythema with circumoral pallor.

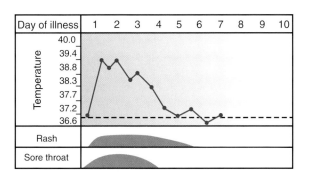

Fig. 37.10 The development of scarlet fever.

Glandular fever (infectious mononucleosis)

Classical glandular fever is caused by Epstein–Barr virus (EBV) and is associated with atypical mononuclear cells in the blood, giving the name infectious mononucleosis. A similar syndrome can be produced by infection with cytomegalovirus (CMV) and *Toxoplasma gondii* (toxoplasmosis).

Adolescence is a common time of presentation, with transmission from infected saliva by the oral route ('kissing disease'). However, EBV can also present in infancy and early childhood with an 'anginose' form, mainly affecting the tonsils.

Clinical example

Beth, 6 years old, presented with fever, sore throat and malaise. She was treated with amoxycillin for exudative tonsillitis (1). Two days later, she developed a florid rash (2). When reviewed, she had marked tonsillar enlargement and large matted nodes in the neck, which were moderately tender (3). She had petechiae on the soft palate (4). Her eyelids were puffy (5) and her spleen was palpable 2 cm below the costal margin (6). Pulse oximetry, performed overnight to exclude significant upper airways obstruction, was normal, so dexamethasone (7) was withheld and she was sent home.

'Purulent' exudative tonsillitis (1) may be due to group A streptococcus or EBV at this age. Ampicillin or amoxycillin cause a dramatic rash in EBV infection (2). Tender lymphadenitis occurs in both (3), but palatal petechiae (4), puffy eyelids (5) and splenomegaly (6) are typical features of EBV infection. There is no specific treatment, but steroids are sometimes used to reduce upper airway obstruction (7).

Diagnosis

Serological: specific IgM or rising IgG titre to EBV. The Paul-Bunnell test and monospot test detect non specific antibodies produced due to the polyclonal B cell proliferation caused by EBV. They have low sensitivity in children. The blood film is often strongly suggestive, showing many atypical mononuclear cells.

Herpes simplex virus (HSV)

- HSV is a DNA herpesvirus, with two serotypes, HSV-1 and HSV-2.
- HSV-1 is primarily oropharyngeal.
- HSV-2 is primarily genital.
- Neonates can catch HSV around delivery, usually (about 90%) HSV-2.
- The commonest childhood HSV infection is gingivostomatitis, due to primary HSV-1 infection: it causes nasty ulceration of the gums (gingivae), buccal mucosa (stoma = mouth) and pharynx.
- HSV infection can disseminate in the skin of children with eczema (eczema herpeticum, Kaposi varicelliform eruption) if not treated promptly with aciclovir.
- Neonatal HSV infection may be localised to skin, eye (conjunctivitis) and/or mouth, may cause isolated encephalitis or isolated pneumonitis or, if not treated with aciclovir, will usually disseminate to cause hepatitis, DIC, encephalitis and death.
- Herpes encephalitis can occur at any age, may be primary or secondary, due to HSV-1 or HSV-2, and has a poor prognosis, even if treated with aciclovir.

- As a herpesvirus, local recurrences of HSV are common, often at the mucocutaneous junction of the lip ('cold sores') but can be on the finger ('whitlow') or on the skin anywhere.

Diagnosis

Rapid diagnosis by immunofluorescence of blister fluid or polymerase chain reaction (PCR) of blister fluid or CSF is preferred to culture or serology (IgM).

Enteroviruses

- The enteroviruses, as the name suggests, are gut viruses, transmitted mainly faecal-orally, although respiratory spread probably occurs.
- They are picornaviruses (pico = small, RNA).
- They can affect the central nervous syndrome, causing a variety of syndromes.
- The major groups of enteroviruses are:
  — Coxsackieviruses (Coxsackie is a town in New York State where an outbreak occurred).
  — Echoviruses *e*nteric *c*ytopathic *h*uman *o*rphan).
  — Polioviruses types 1–3.
  — Enterovirus 71 (EV 71).
- Fever: common cause of isolated fever in infancy.
- Rashes:
  — Hand, food and mouth disease: blistering rash on palms, soles and palate caused by Coxsackie virus A16 and other enteroviruses, including enterovirus 71.
  — Various non specific rashes: macular, maculopapular, papulourticarial, vesicular, morbilliform, rubelliform, etc.
- Enanthem: herpangina (= ulcerative pharyngitis) due to Coxsackie virus A.
- Neurological:
  — Paralytic: poliomyelitis due to infection of anterior horn cells by poliovirus, but similar syndrome can be caused by other enteroviruses.
  — Monoplegia: EV 71, other enteroviruses.
  — Aseptic meningitis, meningoencephalitis: coxsackieviruses, echoviruses, EV 71.
- Cardiac: myocarditis — mainly Coxsackie virus B.
- Liver: hepatitis — mainly echoviruses.
- Eyes: epidemic conjunctivitis — EV 71
- Muscles: Bornholm disease (epidemic pleurodynia) due to Coxsackie virus B).
- Spread: Swimming and wading pools, direct contact, mainly in summer and autumn.
- Treatment: the antiviral drug, pleconaril, has activity against enteroviruses.

Adenoviruses

- Multiple serotypes.
- In infancy, adenoviruses are an important cause of exudative tonsillitis with high fever (at this age, group A streptococcal infection is rare).
- Can cause epidemics of conjunctivitis, often with red throat (pharyngoconjunctival fever).
- Rarely they can cause disseminated infection with pneumonia, hepatitis and encephalitis, particularly adenovirus 7 and 21, which is often fatal.
- Enteric adenoviruses can cause gastroenteritis.

Diagnosis

Culture or immunofluorescence.

Infections of bones and joints

H. K. Graham

There are some conditions in clinical medicine where the outcome can vary from cure to lifelong disability, depending on early diagnosis and adequate treatment. The diagnosis and initial management of bone and joint infection in children is an example. The early presentation of bone and joint infection may be confusing to the most experienced clinician and diagnostic delay is common. Later the picture is often obvious and the diagnosis may be made with ease. In the interval between the earliest signs and the diagnosis being obvious, the important opportunity for early intervention may have been lost.

There are few diagnoses which can be more puzzling to a clinician in the first 24 hours than bone and joint infection. The illustrations in this chapter have been chosen to demonstrate the gross pathological features of

Clinical example

Jennifer, aged 6 months, was admitted to hospital with a diagnosis of 'pyrexia of unknown origin'. She was investigated extensively. Eventually she was treated with oral antibiotics for a 'possible urinary tract infection'. Septic arthritis of the right hip and proximal femoral osteomyelitis was diagnosed 3 weeks after the onset of fever. She progressed to develop septic dislocation of the right hip, avascular necrosis of the femoral capital epiphysis, and growth arrest. She required more than 20 hospital admissions for orthopaedic operations throughout childhood. At the age of 15 years, she is a disturbed teenager with a painful hip, short leg and severe limp. She has twice been admitted to psychiatric institutions after drug overdoses.

Clinical example

Michael, aged 15 months, was noted by his parents to be reluctant to weight bear on his right leg and he had a low grade fever. He was seen by his general practitioner and referred immediately to the emergency department, from where he was admitted as 'possible osteomyelitis' of the right distal femur because of mild metaphyseal tenderness and refusal to weight bear. Osteomyelitis was confirmed by positive blood culture (*S. aureus*) and a positive bone scan. Plain X rays were normal throughout.

He was managed with intravenous flucloxacillin for 7 days, followed by oral flucloxacillin for 3 weeks. He was followed for 6 months and had no long term sequelae.

late presenting osteomyelitis with modern imaging. Such cases should be rare. Given early diagnosis and effective early treatment, the ideal scenario would be a positive bone scan with no changes seen on serial plain X rays, apart from minor soft tissue swelling (Fig. 38.1).

Pathogenesis

The pathogenesis of bone and joint infection is not fully understood but useful insights have been gained from research using animal models. These studies indicate that normal bone is resistant to infection but that trauma or the

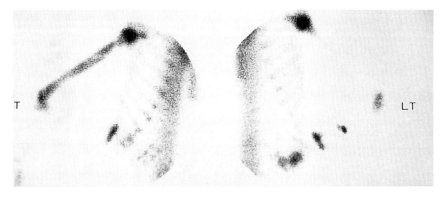

Fig. 38.1 Bone scan of the right humerus in a 4 year old girl with florid signs of acute osteomyelitis. Note the hot area of markedly increased isotope uptake in the proximal metaphysis. (see also Fig. 38.2).

presence of foreign bodies increases susceptibility. Acute haematogenous osteomyelitis results from bacteraemia; however, although bacteraemia is a daily event in childhood, few episodes result in clinical infection. *Staphylococcus aureus* is the most common agent causing osteomyelitis.

The acute inflammatory response to infection results in the release of oxygen radicals and proteolytic enzymes (proteases, peptidases, collagenases) from phagocytes which have ingested bacteria. These enzymes destroy the various components of connective tissue, firstly the glycosaminoglycans of articular cartilage matrix and later the collagen itself. The sequelae of infection depend on the susceptibility of these proteins to destruction and the ability of the intrinsic repair mechanisms. Bone may heal with little or no scarring, but both growth cartilage and articular cartilage have limited repair mechanisms.

The typical metaphyseal focus of bone infection results in an acute inflammatory mass in the medullary canal which decompresses through the haversian canals in the cortex, elevating the periostium. As the pressure under the periostium rises, the blood supply to the cortex and medulla is compromised, resulting in further bone necrosis and the presence of bony sequestra. New bone is formed by attempts at repair resulting in formation of an involucrum. Subperiosteal pus may discharge spontaneously through an enlarged opening in the cortical bone (cloaca) and form a discharging sinus. The distinguising feature of chronic osteomyelitis is necrotic bone.

Bacteria may reach synovial joints from adjacent metaphyseal infection, especially in sites where the metaphysis is in part intraarticular, including:
- femur–hip
- humerus–shoulder
- radial head–elbow
- fibula–ankle joint.

Direct blood borne spread and inoculation from penetrating injury are other mechanisms. Synovial joints have a poor ability to clear bacterial infection, and the connective tissues are sensitive to damage from collagenase and other lysozymal enzymes. A florid synovitis is seen with the production of increased amounts of joint fluid, leading to an effusion which becomes more viscous and organised with time as fibrin levels increase. Neglected joint infection may result in destruction of articular cartilage and growth cartilage, softening of the joint capsule, dislocation, avascular necrosis of intra-articular epiphyses and joint destruction.

Clinical syndromes

It is useful to consider bone and joint infection under the following headings:
- possible bone and joint infection
- probable bone and joint infection
- proven bone and joint infection.

Possible bone and joint infection

This is the largest and least well defined category. It is defined as a history suggestive of infection in the absence of corroboration by major physical signs or investigations. In the lower limb this usually means pain and limping, or refusal to weight bear. In the upper limb the history is of pain and loss of function. In infants this may present as 'pseudoparalysis'; in older children there may be a reduction in activity or an inability to use the limb properly. There often is a history of minor trauma or recent infection of the respiratory tract or skin.

Possible bone and joint infection therefore overlaps clinically with the presentation of trauma and tumours. Children who are injured may not give a history of injury if the injury is not observed (toddler's fracture of the tibia), is inflicted deliberately or is repetitive and not considered significant (stress fracture).

Probable bone and joint infection

This is when a suggestive history is accompanied by supporting physical findings such as fever, metaphyseal tenderness, restricted joint range of motion and swelling. Supporting investigations include a raised C reactive protein (CRP), erythrocyte sedimentation rate (ESR), white cell count (WCC), and positive radiology such as ultrasound for hip effusions or bone scan for osteomyelitis.

It should be noted that it is expected that plain X rays will be normal in the acute phase of bone and joint infection, or will at most show signs of soft tissue swelling.

Proven bone infection

This is when a typical history and physical examination is confirmed by culture of an organism from blood, aspirated fluid or tissue sample, the drainage of pus or unequivocal serial changes on X ray.

Implications of the approach outlined above

This clinical approach has management implications.
- Children who have 'possible' bone and joint infection require careful re-examination over a period of time, preferably by the same examiner, to exclude the presence of evolving infection and to observe resolution of the presenting symptoms or the establishment of an alternative diagnosis.
- Children with 'probable' bone and joint infection need to be admitted to hospital urgently for investigation and treatment.

During investigation and treatment either the 'probable' infection will become 'proven', the condition will resolve or an alternative diagnosis will become apparent.

- All children with 'proven' infection must be managed rigorously, preferably according to established medical and surgical protocols adjusted by the medical team in the light of changing patterns of microorganism identification and sensitivity or resistance to antibiotics.

Osteomyelitis

Acute haematogenous osteomyelitis (AHO) is the most common and the most important clinical presentation. Children usually present with:

- a short febrile illness
- bone pain, and
- limping or loss of upper limb function.

The key physical sign is metaphyseal tenderness, a sign which is often undervalued or ignored. Signs of acute inflammation, such as swelling or redness, are evidence of abscess formation and therefore are late signs.

Neonates and infants may present with an acute septicaemic illness without an obvious bony focus. The bone infection may be multifocal in these very ill children. Alternatively, neonates may present non specifically with irritability and poor feeding. The differences in presentation may reflect altered pathogenicity of the organism or differences in the immune response by the host.

Subacute osteomyelitis is characterised by a focal rather than systemic response to infection, with signs of bone destruction on X rays at presentation. The differential diagnoses here are subacute osteomyelitis (Brodie's abcess), bone tumour and stress fracture. Chronic osteomyelitis usually is the result of delayed diagnosis and/or inadequate treatment of AHO. The features are of chronic bone pain, swelling and intermittently discharging sinuses. The X rays will show evidence of bone destruction, bone healing and often a sequestrum or involucrum.

Laboratory investigations

The correct sequence is:

1. clinical diagnosis
2. baseline radiology
3. blood tests
4. appropriate sample collection before treatment.

However, the procurement of specimens and radiological investigations must under no circumstances delay treatment.

Blood is collected for culture at presentation and during spikes of fever. Samples are sent for CRP, ESR and a full blood examination. The most useful acute phase reactant is CRP both in diagnosis and management. The CRP rises with the onset of the illness before the ESR, and starts to fall with the administration of effective treatment, in parallel with clinical improvement. The ESR may remain elevated for weeks after effective therapy for AHO.

The blood count usually shows a leucocytosis with a left shift and sometimes a thrombocytosis or anaemia in severe or neglected cases.

Between 40 and 50% of blood cultures will be positive in the presence of osteomyelitis. Aspiration of the affected metaphysis may increase the percentage of positive cultures but is hard to justify because of the pain and invasiveness of the procedure. If there is failure to respond to antibiotic therapy, surgery may be indicated. This provides an opportunity to obtain further specimens for culture, from pus or bone biopsies.

Radiology

Plain films

Standard X rays of the area are obtained as a baseline for comparison with later changes and to exclude other diagnoses, principally trauma. It is expected that they will be normal initially in the majority of cases of AHO. Some may show subtle signs of soft tissue swelling.

Ultrasound

Ultrasonography is a sensitive method of detecting soft tissue swelling and subperiosteal abscesses in children who are not responding to therapy, especially if the need for surgical drainage is contemplated.

Bone scans

The three phase technetium-99m bone scan is very sensitive and is reasonably specific in the early diagnosis of AHO. There can be false negatives early in the clinical course, especially in neonates. In AHO of the pelvis or spine and in multifocal infections, the value of bone scans is unquestioned.

Magnetic resonance imaging (MRI)

MRI also is very sensitive in the acute phase, but is limited by cost and availability. Marrow oedema is the earliest sign, seen as a decrease in signal intensity on T1 and increased signal on T2 weighted scans (Fig. 38.2). Soft tissue swelling effusions, cartilage injury and oedema are very well demonstrated using MRI, but cortical bone changes are appreciated more easily on computed tomography.

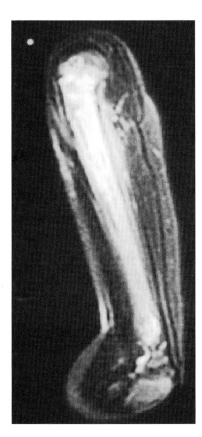

Fig. 38.2 An MRI scan of the patient in Figure 38.1 was done because of failure to improve clinically. The bright area seen in this T2 weighted scan is an intramedullary abscess in the proximal metaphysis.

Computed tomography (CT)

In subacute and chronic osteomyelitis, CT is useful to stage the disease by documenting the degree of bony destruction, growth plate involvement and the presence of sequestra.

Management

The management of AHO primarily is medical, with surgery reserved for late presenting cases or failure to respond to initial medical treatment. Given that the most frequently cultured organism at all ages is *S. aureus,* the most useful antibiotic is flucloxacillin. Group A and B beta haemolytic streptococci usually but not invariably are sensitive to benzylpenicillin, which is used routinely unless sensitivities indicate otherwise. With increasing uptake of Hib vaccine, *Haemophilus influenzae* infections are rapidly decreasing. When *H. influenzae* is isolated, a third generation cephalosporin is appropriate.

Intravenous antibiotics are required in uncomplicated early cases for between 2 and 4 days, followed by 3 weeks of oral therapy. After 3 weeks there may be no changes seen on plain X rays or there may be minor areas of bone destruction which usually heal uneventfully.

In later presenting cases with more advanced bone changes, intravenous antibiotics are required for between 5 and 10 days; immobilisation is helpful, using a plaster backslab or splint, and the duration of oral therapy should be 6 weeks.

Failure to improve quickly with intravenous antibiotics usually implies the presence of a subperiosteal or intramedullary abscess. In this event, surgery to drain the abscess by incision of the periosteum or drilling the medulla is essential to effect a cure and to reduce the risk of further bone destruction and chronicity.

Chronic osteomyelitis (Figs 38.3 and 38.4) is managed surgically, with antibiotics playing a supporting role. Areas of chronic infection must be debrided radically to remove avascular and necrotic material which cannot be sterilised by antibiotics. Cavities must be filled with healthy tissue and covered with healthy skin. Combined approaches by plastic and orthopaedic surgeons to introduce new tissue may have a major role. This may include bone grafts, muscle flaps and skin grafts or flaps.

Osteomyelitis: other syndromes

Osteomyelitis of the calcaneum

This is an important clinical problem, seen most frequently in the emergency room of children's hospitals. The history usually is typical: an adventurous child stands on a nail and sustains a minor puncture wound to the sole of the foot. During the initial visit to the emergency room the wound is inspected, tetanus prophylaxis is given and a broad spectrum antibiotic may be given. Usually the puncture wound heals but 5–10 days later an acute infection develops with a bone and soft tissue abscess. In more than 90% of cases the offending organism is a *Pseudomonas* species. The nail puncture inoculates the wound with several organisms including Pseudomonas. The oral broad spectrum antibiotics deal with all but the Pseudomonas, which results in a Pseudomonas osteomyelitis. The characteristic odour of children's sports footwear is in part due to colonisation with Pseudomonas.

The management involves antibiotics with anti-Pseudomonas activity. Drainage of the bone and soft tissue abscess is often required.

Meningococcal septicaemia

This is a devastating illness which, when survived, can result in long term orthopaedic complications. In the early stages, necrosis of skin and soft tissues leads to 'purpura fulminans' and the need for amputation and skin grafting. Later, many epiphyseal centres will show growth arrest, leading to angular deformities and limb shortening.

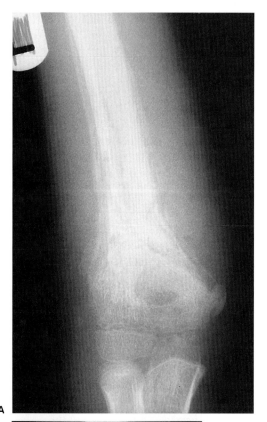

A

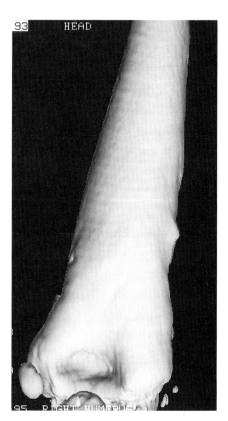

Fig. 38.4 CT scan with three dimensional reconstruction from the patient of Figure 38.3 at a later stage. There is now exuberant involucrum encasing the entire distal humeral shaft and metaphysis. Fortunately this was adequate to maintain the integrity of the humerus following surgical sequestrectomy.

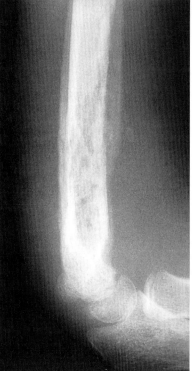

Fig. 38.3 **A** Anteroposterior (AP), and **B** lateral, right distal humerus in a 7 year old child with a delayed diagnosis of osteomyelitis. On both the AP and lateral views there is patchy osteolysis of the humerus because of local bone destruction. Pus has escaped under pressure from the medullary canal and has stripped the periosteum circumferentially. Exuberant new bone (involucrum) is seen encasing the humeral shaft. Eventually, most of the diaphysis became a 'sequestrum' and had to be excised to gain control of the infection. The organism involved was *Staphylococcus aureus* (see also Fig. 38.4).

B

Sickle cell osteomyelitis

Children with sickle cell disease are subject to attacks of acute bone pain (Ch. 53). The two principal causes are a 'sickle cell crisis' leading to infarction of bone, or acute osteomyelitis. The organism involved is almost invariably a Salmonella species.

Inflammation of a lumbar disc in children ('discitis')

This probably is secondary to a localised staphylococcal osteomyelitis, centred on the disc but also involving the adjacent vertebral bodies. However, there is uncertainty about the pathogenesis because the site is difficult to aspirate or biopsy. Note that:

- Toddlers usually present with a deterioration in gait or have difficulties standing (Fig. 38.5).
- Older children complain of back pain or stiffness.

Diagnosis often is delayed, but eventually the plain X rays will be diagnostic, by which time the MRI will be alarming. Organisms are recovered infrequently from blood culture or from aspiration of the disc space.

Treatment with intravenous flucloxacillin results in such rapid improvement in the majority of children that the staphylococcal aetiology is plausible.

Pelvic osteomyelitis

This also can result in puzzling clinical syndromes because the pain may be referred to the abdomen, buttock or leg. Diagnosis often is delayed when alternative diagnoses such as appendicitis or a lumbar disc protrusion are being considered. More than 80% are due to staphylococcal infections. The bone scan is diagnostic and rapid recovery is the rule following administration of intravenous flucloxacillin.

Septic arthritis

The presentation, investigation and management of acute haematogenous osteomyelitis and acute suppurative septic arthritis overlap to a considerable degree, especially in younger children. In neonates and infants the two con-

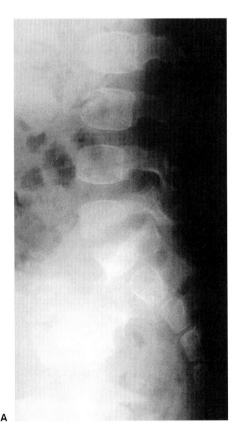
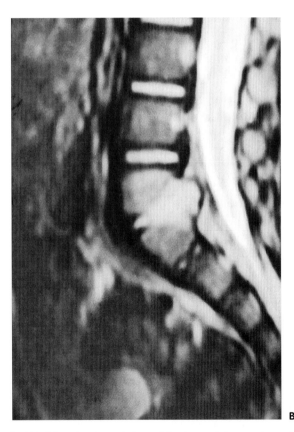

A   B

Fig. 38.5 **A** Lateral lumbosacral spine X ray in a 15 month old toddler who showed signs of developmental regression and gait disturbance. There is narrowing of the L5–S1 disc space with regular bony destruction on either side of the disc. **B** The T2 weighted MRI scan shows a large inflammatory mass centred on the disc space, involving the bodies of the vertebrae and protruding into the spinal canal and causing pressure on the lumbosacral nerve roots. Diagnosis: acute 'discitis' with vertebral osteomyelitis.

ditions coexist so frequently that the preferred term is 'osteoarticular infection'. In older children, infection of bone and joint are distinguished more easily and management should be tailored accordingly.

Infections of the shoulder and hip are more difficult to detect clinically because there is no visible joint swelling in the early stages, and diagnosis and treatment may be delayed with serious consequences. Effusions are detected readily in the knee, elbow, wrist and ankle where the diagnosis is easier and can usually be made at an earlier stage.

Acute septic arthritis occurs most frequently in a child with a bacteraemia or septicaemia as part of a systemic illness. Less frequently there is a history of a penetrating injury from a nail, wood splinter or needle, including iatrogenic causes. The synovial joint environment has a limited ability to deal with suppuration and responds non specifically by the increased production of synovial fluid, leading to an effusion and acute inflammation of the synovium.

The clinical signs include:
- fever
- swelling
- warmth
- tenderness
- restricted range of joint motion.

Pain tends to be more rapidly progressive than in osteomyelitis and is worse at rest. The range of motion is often much more restricted in septic arthritis than in osteomyelitis.

The CRP, ESR and WCC are elevated, as in acute osteomyelitis. Plain X rays are either normal or show soft tissue swelling. Ultrasound examination of the hip is a very sensitive method of detecting small effusions, but gives no guide as to the cause.

Differential diagnosis

'Irritable hip' or transient synovitis is a much more common condition than septic arthritis and may follow minor injury or viral illness. Management is by exclusion of septic arthritis (and other conditions), followed by rest and observation until resolution occurs. In the early stages of septic arthritis, there is no definitive way of distinguishing an irritable hip from septic arthritis on clinical grounds alone. Children with septic arthritis usually are more ill with a higher fever and more severe joint signs. When doubt exists, the only acceptable policy is to admit the child to hospital for observation and to aspirate the hip joint.

Acute arthritis with a negative culture may be the result of a pyogenic infection, but other syndromes should be considered. These should include juvenile arthritis, arthritis associated with inflammatory bowel disease, psoriasis and ankylosing spondylitis. Reactive arthritis may result from a number of triggers, including enteric infections such as *Salmonella*, *Shigella* and *Campylobacter* species. Acute arthritis also is a major feature of rheumatic fever, Kawasaki disease and Henoch–Schönlein purpura (Ch. 44).

The differential diagnosis of subacute or chronic arthritis is a partially treated acute septic arthritis, tuberculosis or foreign body arthritis. Tuberculous arthritis is suggested by a history of contact with the disease and is confirmed by a Mantoux test, chest X ray, and/or culture of acid fast bacilli from joint fluid or synovial biopsy.

Management

The organisms responsible for acute suppurative septic arthritis in childhood are similar to those which cause AHO, but there are notable differences. In all joints and at all ages, *S. aureus* is the most common organism identified and the antibiotic policy is similar in both conditions. *H. influenzae* is recovered more commonly from the shoulder, especially in children with chest infections. In neonates the spectrum of organisms is wide, sensitivities vary and antibiotic policy should be decided by ongoing audit of all microbiological data. Cover for Gram negative organisms with gentamicin or a third generation cephalosporin is frequently required. It is emphasised that a complete history and physical examination are required to exclude other causes of an acute (non bacterial) arthritis. Appropriate investigations should be undertaken:
- Blood for CRP, ESR, blood film and blood culture.
- Ultrasound examination of the hip to confirm or exclude the presence of joint fluid.
- Plain X rays are taken as a baseline, but are expected to be normal or show soft tissue swelling only.

All joints which are suspected of harbouring an acute pyogenic infection must be aspirated under sterile conditions urgently. Ideally this should be in an operating room with the child under general anaesthesia so that arthroscopic washout or arthrotomy can be performed without delay. Septic joints cannot be managed adequately by repeated aspiration. Aspiration is a diagnostic procedure; arthroscopic washout or arthrotomy are the definitive therapeutic procedures. Aspiration alone is justified only as a temporising measure when the diagnosis is in doubt or there is an unavoidable delay in proceeding to arthrotomy.

Joint fluid is sent for Gram stain and culture. The Gram stain results can be a helpful guide to antibiotic choice pending more definitive information from bacterial culture and sensitivity testing.

When a specific organism is cultured, the appropriate antibiotic is administered intravenously for between

3 and 5 days, followed by 3 weeks of oral therapy. Splintage of an infected joint provides welcome pain relief in the early stages, but motion should be encouraged once the acute signs have settled. An infected hip may require abduction bracing to prevent or treat septic dislocation in the younger child.

If frank pus or turbid fluid is recovered but the Gram stain and cultures are negative, it is often wise to presume there is an *S. aureus* infection and to treat as above.

Prognosis

Early diagnosis and prompt, effective treatment of acute suppurative arthritis should result in a rapid cure and a normal joint. Delayed diagnosis and late and inadequate treatment, especially failure to drain the joint, may result in loss of articular cartilage and degenerative arthritis. Damage to physeal cartilage results in growth arrest with limb shortening or angular deformity.

Meningitis and encephalitis

K. Grimwood

Meningitis and encephalitis are potential life threatening disorders that demand prompt recognition and management.

Bacterial meningitis

Bacterial meningitis is a medical emergency requiring rapid diagnosis and treatment. Equal attention must be paid to specific antimicrobial and supportive therapy, including the immediate treatment of:
- seizures
- cerebral oedema
- circulatory collapse.

Epidemiology

The annual incidence of bacterial meningitis is 30–50 cases per 100 000 children aged 0–5 years. Rates are highest in infants and indigenous populations and during late winter and spring. The events that cause meningitis are incompletely understood, but are likely to include a combination of microbial, host and environmental factors:
- microbe
  — polysaccharide capsule
- host
  — young age
  — recent respiratory infection
  — ? genetic susceptibility
  — impaired immunity
  — neuroanatomical defects
- environment
  — household crowding
  — poverty
  — tobacco smoke exposure
  — season
  — daycare attendance
  — sharing food, drink, pacifiers.

Aetiology

The most common pathogens in each age group are:
- infants and children
  — *Streptococcus pneumoniae*
  — *Neisseria meningitidis*
  — *Haemophilus influenzae* type b (Hib) — rare in areas with routine immunisation

- children older than 5 years
  — *Streptococcus pneumoniae*
  — *Neisseria meningitidis*.

Pathogenesis

As outlined in Figure 39.1, the development of bacterial meningitis follows (1) the colonisation of the nasopharynx by encapsulated bacteria, (2) invasion of the host with infection of the meninges, (3) bacterial multiplication and induction of inflammation within the subarachnoid space, and (4) neuronal injury.

Clinical presentations

Infants and toddlers

Symptoms and signs of serious infection within this age group are often non specific:
- fever, irritability, vomiting
- drowsiness
- neck stiffness or a bulging fontanelle.

Both neck stiffness and a bulging fontanelle may be absent, especially during infancy and early in the illness.

Children over the age of 3 years

The signs of meningeal irritation are more obvious:
- fever, severe headache, vomiting, photophobia
- neck stiffness
- delirium or deteriorating consciousness follow rapidly.

Infants and children with meningococcal meningitis may have a petechial or purpuric rash over the trunk and limbs (Fig. 39.2).

Diagnosis

Immediate tests should include:
- lumbar puncture for microscopy, culture and biochemistry
- blood culture
- suprapubic aspirate or catheter urine specimen (if less than 6 months old)
- full blood count
- serum electrolytes, glucose and creatinine
- needle aspirate of any focal areas of infection.

Microbial factors		Host and environmental factors
Adhesions, proteases	Bacterial colonisation and local invasion	Viral infection, crowding, tobacco smoke exposure
Polysaccharide capsule	Bacteraemia and meningeal invasion	Absence of complement and/or specific anticapsular antibodies
Bacterial cell wall products	Multiplication within the subarachnoid space and induction of inflammation	Inflammatory cytokines and chemotaxins
Bacterial cell wall products polysaccharide capsule	Meningeal inflammation, altered microvascular endothelium and cerebral vasculitis	Neutrophil infiltration, inflammatory cascade
	Neuronal injury	Ischaemia, cerebral oedema, oxygen radicals, NO, cytokines, excitory amino acids

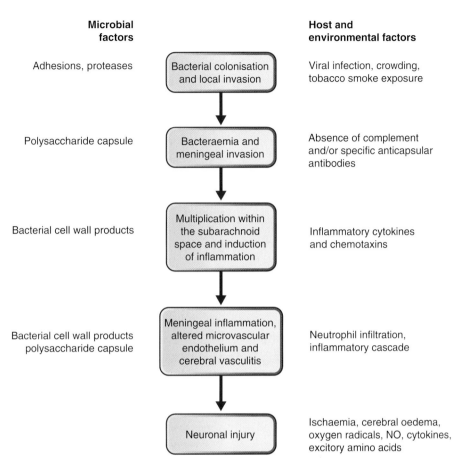

Fig. 39.1 The pathophysiological cascade of meningitis.

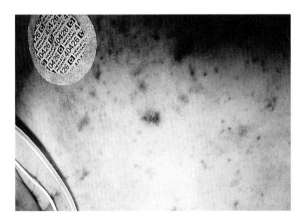

Fig. 39.2 The purpuric rash of meningococcal disease.

Lumbar puncture establishes the diagnosis and aids identification of the causative organism and its antibiotic sensitivities. It is postponed when there are signs of cerebral herniation, circulatory compromise or disseminated intravascular coagulation (DIC). A lumbar puncture is delayed for patients with any of the following:

• absent or non purposeful responses to pain

• focal neurological signs
• abnormal pupil size or reaction
• decerebrate or decorticate posturing

> ### Clinical example
>
> Jordan, a 7 month old infant presented following a brief right sided focal seizure. He had been 'off colour' for 24 hours with a clear nasal discharge and had been feeding poorly. His past medical history was unremarkable. Growth and development were both normal. He had received his primary immunisations and there was no family history of seizures. His temperature was 39.3°C; he was pale with cool extremities; and he was very irritable when handled. Neck stiffness, bulging fontanelle and rash were absent, but a mild weakness of the right arm was present.
>
> A lumbar puncture revealed turbid CSF. Numerous Gram positive diplococci were seen in the CSF, and a penicillin susceptible strain of *S. pneumoniae* was isolated. Less than 1% of children with febrile seizures have meningitis. Infants and those with complex febrile seizures are at greatest risk. It is important that all children are carefully evaluated for signs of meningitis following a febrile seizure.

- irregular breathing
- papilloedema.

In these situations, blood cultures are collected and antibiotics started immediately. Such patients require intensive care management and the necessary measures to reduce intracranial pressure (Ch. 20).

The typical CSF changes in bacterial meningitis are outlined in Table 39.1. Organisms are often seen on Gram stain of the CSF and a presumptive diagnosis may be made. Rapid diagnostic tests are also available to detect specific bacterial antigens or DNA in the CSF. The major value of these tests is in partly treated meningitis, when cultures may be negative.

Occasionally the CSF examination is difficult to interpret, especially when antibiotics have been given before lumbar puncture. The decision to treat a child for bacterial meningitis is a clinical one and antibiotics are continued until the CSF is found to be sterile on culture. Parameningeal foci, such as brain abscess and tuberculous meningitis can have a similar CSF profile to partially treated bacterial meningitis and should be considered. However, if they are not ill, it is reasonable to observe some children closely in hospital without specific therapy until the pattern of illness becomes apparent.

Cerebral imaging by either CT or MRI is not recommended unless conditions that may mimic meningitis, such as intracranial mass lesions, are suspected and a lumbar puncture is contraindicated.

Antibiotic treatment

Antibiotics are selected that are effective against commonly encountered causative bacteria. The emergence of penicillin and cephalosporin non susceptible strains of *S. pneumoniae* means that vancomycin is often added to a third generation cephalosporin for the initial empiric treatment of bacterial meningitis. Subsequent therapy is adjusted according to culture and sensitivity results. Dosage and duration of antibiotic treatment are outlined in Table 39.2.

Supportive treatment

Clinical observations

Regular recording of the pulse, respiratory rate, blood pressure, temperature and conscious state is required. The head circumference in infants with meningitis should be measured daily as part of the neurological assessment.

Fluid therapy

Intravenous fluids are administered initially to restore circulating blood volume, to correct glucose or electrolyte disturbance and to minimise the risk of aspiration.

As meningitis is frequently accompanied by increased secretion of antidiuretic hormone (see below), once any

---

Table 39.1   Cerebrospinal fluid: normal values and typical changes in some pathological conditions

	Total WCC (× 10⁶/ml)ᵃ	Predominant cell type	Glucose (mmol/l)	Protein (g/l)
Normal	<5	Lymphocytes	2.5	<0.4
Normal neonate	<20	Lymphocytes	Normal	Mildly elevated
Bacterial meningitis	1000s	Polymorphs	Reduced or undetectable	Moderately elevated
Partially treated bacterial meningitisᵇ	100–1000s	Polymorphs	Reduced or undetectable	Moderately elevated
Tuberculous meningitis	50–100s	Polymorphs/mononuclear cells	Reduced or undetectable	Moderately to markedly elevated
Viral meningitis	<10–100s	Lymphocytesᶜ	Usually normal	Normal to <1 g/l
Encephalitis	<10–100s	Lymphocytes	Usually normal	Mildly to moderately elevated
Brain abscess and other mass lesionsᵈ	Normal to mild increase	Variable polymorphs	Normal	Normal to mildly elevated

ᵃWCC = white cell count. A traumatic tap is the commonest cause of blood stained CSF; for every 1000 × 10⁶/l of red blood cells add 2 × 10⁶/l of white blood cells and 0.01 g/l of protein to normal values.
ᵇPartially treated meningitis is seen when children in the early phase of illness are thought to have other infections, for example an upper respiratory infection, and receive oral antibiotics before the diagnosis of meningitis is made.
ᶜNeutrophil predominance may be present in enterovirus meningitis.
ᵈLumbar puncture is not done if a mass lesion is suspected. CSF changes depend on the site of the lesion, for example if near the cerebral surface pleocytosis occurs.

Table 39.2 Antibiotic therapy for bacterial meningitis

Pathogen	Antibiotic	Dose (mg/kg)	Duration (days)
Streptococcus pneumoniae			
Penicillin susceptible	Penicillin G	30 i.v. 4 h	7–10
Penicillin non susceptible	Cefotaxime*	50 i.v. 6 h	7–10
Penicillin + third generation non susceptible	Vancomycin + cefotaxime*	15 i.v. 6 h 75 i.v. 6 h	10–14
Neisseria meningitidis	Penicillin G	30 i.v. 4 h	5–7
Haemophilus influenzae b			
Non beta lactamase	Amoxycillin	50 i.v. 4 h	7
Beta lactamase producer	Cefotaxime*	50 mg/kg i.v. 6 h	7
Unknown	Cefotaxime*	50 i.v. 6 h	7

*Ceftriaxone 50 mg/kg 12 h can be substituted for cefotaxime.

dehydration or shock has been corrected, overhydration is avoided by moderate fluid restriction, for example to 50% of calculated maintenance fluid requirements. This reduces the risk of cerebral oedema and hyponatraemic seizures (for discussion, see Chs 20, 22). Fluid administration is then adjusted according to the serum sodium levels, adequacy of circulation and improvement in the clinical state.

Corticosteroids

As inflammatory mediators contribute to the pathophysiology of bacterial meningitis, a role for dexamethasone when treating meningitis has been advocated. Most experience, however, has been with Hib meningitis and any benefit for either pneumococcal or meningococcal meningitis remains unproven. There are also concerns over dexamethasone's effectiveness for treating β-lactam resistant pneumococcal meningitis. Until this is resolved, dexamethasone should probably not be considered part of standard therapy for bacterial meningitis.

Acute complications

During meningitis, complications from central nervous system infection or systemic effects of infection are common. Children with frequent or protracted seizures, circulatory instability or signs of cerebral oedema should be managed in an intensive care unit.

Convulsions

About 20–30% of children with bacterial meningitis have convulsions before admission to hospital. Lorazepam will control most convulsions, but if these recur or are prolonged they raise intracranial pressure, worsening the cerebral ischaemic injury. Administration of phenytoin or phenobarbitone and mechanical ventilation is often indicated. It is important to suspect hyponatraemia or hypoglycaemia as a cause of convulsions in any child with meningitis.

Cerebral oedema

Careful observations for signs of increased intracranial pressure are essential. These include:
- progressive loss of consciousness
- irregular breathing
- pinpoint pupils
- respiratory arrest.

Management involves fluid restriction and circulatory and respiratory support.

The syndrome of inappropriate antidiuretic hormone secretion (SIADH) occurs often in meningitis. This results in dilution of the extracellular fluid compartment and fluid shift into cells. When it involves the brain, cerebral oedema develops. Careful fluid management with regular monitoring of the serum sodium concentration can usually avoid cerebral oedema in meningitis. The diagnosis of SIADH is made when the serum sodium concentration is less than 130 mmol/l and is accompanied by urine sodium concentrations greater than 20 mmol/l. When SIADH is present and is complicated by cerebral oedema, the treatment is fluid restriction, but intravenous hypertonic saline, mannitol or frusemide are used in an emergency.

Circulatory shock

Approximately 5–10% of children with bacterial meningitis present in shock and initially require large volume fluid resuscitation to maintain tissue perfusion and blood pressure. Care is required to avoid worsening cerebral oedema and provoking hyponatraemic seizures. Inotropic agents are used to support the circulation.

Neurological lesions

Neurological deficits, such as hemiparesis, persistent hypotonia, ataxia and isolated cranial nerve palsies are present in 10–20% of children during the acute illness, but are often reversible.

Subdural effusions

These are accumulations in the subdural space, usually of sterile fluid with a high protein content. Generally asymptomatic, subdural effusions can be associated with:
• persistent or recurring high fever
• focal or generalised convulsions
• persistent vomiting
• increasing head circumference or fontanelle tension
• development of a focal neurological deficit.

Cerebral CT (Fig. 39.3) establishes the diagnosis of subdural effusion. Most subdural effusions resolve spontaneously, but a very large symptomatic effusion may require surgical drainage.

Persistent (> 7 days) or secondary fever

Frequently this results from:
• viral nosocomial infection

• subdural effusion
• thrombophlebitis
• other suppurative lesions
• immune mediated disease — reactive arthritis or pericarditis.

Uncommonly, fever may also result from:
• inadequately treated meningitis
• a parameningeal focus
• drugs.

Cerebral imaging

Cranial CT or MRI are useful in identifying:
• subdural collections
• brain abscess
• cerebral vascular thrombosis
• hydrocephalus.

These tests are considered for patients with:
• prolonged coma
• persistent irritability or seizures
• persistent focal neurological deficits
• enlarging head circumference
• recurrent disease.

Outcome

• Mortality 2–5%.
• Intellectual disability, spasticity, seizures, hydrocephalus, deafness 10–15%.
• Subsequent learning and behaviour disorders 25–30%.

Meningitis in infancy, delayed diagnosis, persistent or late onset seizures and focal neurological signs are independent risk factors for long term complications.

All children should have their hearing tested following meningitis, either by brainstem (auditory) evoked potentials or formal audiometry. Regular review should be continued in children with persisting auditory and neurological abnormalities.

Primary prevention

Protein conjugated vaccines have made Hib meningitis uncommon in countries where the vaccines are available as part of the routine immunisation schedule (Ch. 8). Similar technology has been used for the development of new meningococcal and pneumococcal vaccines. However, the multiple serotypes of these organisms and their variable immunogenicity mean that they are unlikely to be as successful overall as the Hib vaccines. The important, but poorly immunogenic, meningococcal serogroup B strain poses additional challenges for safe and effective vaccine development.

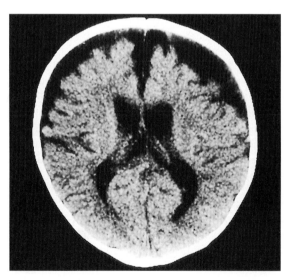

Fig. 39.3 Cranial CT of a 5 month old boy with pneumococcal meningitis who developed secondary fever and generalised seizures on his 7th day in hospital. It shows subdural effusions over both frontal lobes. He received anticonvulsant therapy only and the effusion resolved spontaneously.

Chemoprophylaxis

Transmission of *N. meningitidis* and Hib is by oral and respiratory secretions. Those at increased risk of infection are:
- household members
- childcare contacts
- persons intimately exposed to oral secretions.

Each should immediately receive rifampicin, 20 mg/kg (maximum 600 mg) as a single daily dose for 2 days. Alternatively a single dose of intramuscular ceftriaxone (125 mg for children, 250 mg for adults) is given, or adults may receive 500 mg of ciprofloxacin. The index case does not require further prophylaxis if treatment has included a third generation cephalosporin. Parents must be warned that, if they or their children are unwell, immediate medical attention should be sought.

Because of the increased risk of Hib infection in young contacts, rifampicin 20 mg/kg (maximum 600 mg) as a single daily dose for 4 days is prescribed for the index case of Hib meningitis and all household contacts, if the child is aged less than 2 years or if the household contacts include unimmunised children younger than 4 years. Unlike *N. meningitidis*, single doses of ceftriaxone do not eradicate Hib from the nasopharynx. In contrast, chemoprophylaxis is not required in cases of pneumococcal meningitis.

Special circumstances

Neonatal meningitis

Neonates, particularly if premature, are at increased risk of meningitis (Ch. 35). The responsible pathogens are mainly:
- *Streptococcus agalactiae*
- *Escherichia coli*
- *Listeria monocytogenes*

As in infants, the symptoms and signs of meningitis are subtle. Approximately 5–20% of septic neonates have concomitant meningitis. Initial therapy is with amoxycillin and cefotaxime until culture and antibiotic sensitivities are available. Antibiotic treatment is 2 weeks for Gram positive meningitis, and 3 weeks for Gram negative bacillary cases.

Infants aged 1–3 months and the immunocompromised

These patients may have meningitis from pathogens common to both neonates and older children. Empiric therapy (usually with amoxycillin and cefotaxime) must be capable of treating a wide range of pathogens. When the CSF Gram stain or antigen testing suggests *S. pneumoniae* as the causative agent, vancomycin should replace amoxycillin.

Meningococcaemia

While *N. meningitidis* serogroup A is associated with epidemics in parts of subSaharan Africa, serogroups B and C are endemic in industrialised countries. Large increases in disease caused by meningococcal clones have been observed in several European and other countries in recent years. New Zealand is currently experiencing near epidemic disease caused by a clonal serogroup B strain.

Approximately 60% of invasive meningococcal disease is acute meningococcaemia. Although nearly 70% have concomitant meningitis, signs of sepsis dominate the clinical course. Half the cases occur in children aged less than 5 years. Most patients present critically ill with a petechial or purpuric rash (Fig. 39.2). The clinical course is rapidly progressive, with the time from onset of fever until death as short as 12 hours. While overall mortality for invasive meningococcal disease is 5%, case fatality reaches 10–20% for the fulminant form of the disease.

> ### Clinical example
>
> Kenisia, aged 18 months, awoke with fever and vomiting. During the next 2 hours she became more lethargic and developed a faint red macular rash over her buttocks and legs. Her doctor noted the rash had spread, becoming darker and non blanching. He diagnosed meningococcaemia and gave 600 mg of penicillin intramuscularly before transferring her immediately to hospital. Six hours after the onset of symptoms, Kenisia was pale and shocked. She received aggressive fluid resuscitation, inotropes and assisted ventilation. Although blood cultures were sterile, polymerase chain reaction (PCR) testing for the *porA* DNA sequence in her peripheral white blood cells confirmed the diagnosis of meningococcal infection. During the following 4 days she gradually improved and a delayed lumbar puncture showed 20 white blood cells only. Subsequently skin grafting was required for a large necrotic area over the abdominal wall.

The clinical features of meningococcaemia are initiated by the release of cell wall products, which activate proinflammatory cytokines and complement leading to endothelial injury with capillary leak and loss of vasomotor tone. The major cause of death in meningococcaemia is circulatory collapse from capillary leak, intravascular volume depletion, vasodilatation and myocardial failure. Haemodynamic collapse in combination with DIC leads to multiorgan dysfunction.

Treatment is urgent and is commenced immediately the diagnosis is suspected, and ideally after taking blood cultures. Penicillin G is the drug of choice, the recommended dose being 60 mg/kg i.v. 4 hourly. The patient is managed in respiratory isolation during the first 24 hours of treatment. Management should be in an intensive care unit and includes plasma expanders and circulatory and respiratory support. While prehospital treatment with penicillin has reduced the number of culture confirmed cases, the use of molecular techniques to detect meningococcal DNA in sterile fluids has greatly aided diagnosis.

Tuberculous meningitis

This is most common in children younger than 5 years. The onset is gradual, with malaise, fever and irritability, progressing over 1–2 weeks to drowsiness, neck stiffness, seizures, cranial nerve palsies and coma. Typical CSF changes are listed in Table 39.1. There may be no history of infectious contacts. Mantoux testing is often normal and a chest X ray abnormality is present in only half of the cases. Gastric lavage, urine and CSF are sent for culture, while some centres offer PCR testing for *Mycobacterium tuberculosis* DNA. Cranial CT may detect hydrocephalus and basilar meningeal inflammation. Treatment is with isoniazid, rifampicin and pyrazinamide. A fourth drug is added if there are concerns over potential drug resistance. Steroids are also used during the first weeks of therapy.

Recurrent meningitis

This is uncommon and underlying causes should be sought:
- immunodeficiency (Ch. 43)
- neuroanatomical defects — intracranial or lumbosacral.

Consider neuroanatomical defects when enteric bacteria or *Staphylococcus aureus* are cultured from the CSF. Cranial and spinal MRI, or high resolution CT of the temporal and frontal bones, may be indicated.

Viral meningitis and encephalitis

Many viruses are capable of invading the central nervous system and, depending upon the primary site of involvement, the clinical designations used are meningitis and encephalitis (Table 39.3).

Viral meningitis

Non polio enteroviruses cause 80–90% of identifiable cases. The onset is acute with:
- fever
- headache
- vomiting
- neck or spine stiffness.

Abdominal pain is common and occasionally a macular rash appears, suggesting an enterovirus as the causative agent. Parotid or mandibular swellings implicate mumps. Signs of meningism indicate the need for lumbar puncture. Typical CSF findings in viral meningitis are presented in Table 39.1.

PCR testing of CSF specimens for enterovirus genetic material has become an important diagnostic tool. Other disorders that may present in a similar fashion and need to be considered include:
- partially treated bacterial meningitis
- tuberculous meningitis
- cryptococcal meningitis
- cerebral abscesses
- cerebral tumour.

A repeat lumbar puncture or cerebral imaging may be required to further clarify the diagnosis.

Viral meningitis is a benign disease, and requires symptomatic treatment only. Complete recovery without sequelae is expected within a few days. An antiviral

Table 39.3 Viruses and non bacterial infecting agents which may commonly cause meningitis and encephalitis

Postinfectious encephalomyelitis without direct invasion of CNS
Measles, rubella, varicella, Epstein–Barr virus, mumps, influenza, *Mycoplasma pneumoniae*

Meningitis and/or encephalitis with viral CNS infection
Enteroviruses — ECHO, coxsackie and polio viruses. These usually cause meningitis but encephalitis can occur
Mumps — usually meningitis, less often meningoencephalitis
Herpes simplex virus type 1 can cause focal (usually temporoparietal) encephalitis (HSV-1 or -2 can cause encephalitis in neonates)
Other herpes group viruses — HH-6 and -7, EBV, varicella
Arbovirus (arthropod borne virus) for example Japanese encephalitis virus or Australian encephalitis virus

Progressive encephalitis
For example subacute sclerosing panencephalitis due to measles virus infection, or human prion disease

agent, pleconaril, with activity against enteroviruses is undergoing investigation.

Viral encephalitis and myelitis

Encephalitis means inflammation of the brain. Acute viral encephalitis includes either direct infection of neural tissue involving predominantly grey matter, or postinfectious encephalomyelitis that follows a variety of viral and bacterial infections. Postinfectious encephalomyelitis most often presents after a non specific respiratory illness, and is characterised by widespread asymmetric white matter demyelination in the absence of direct invasion. Clinically the distinction is difficult unless the demyelinating illness complicates an exanthem.

Encephalitis presents with an array of neurological signs:
- fever
- behaviour disturbance
- altered consciousness
- seizures
- ataxia or other movement disorders
- focal neurological deficits.

Meningism is frequently absent. The involvement of the spinal cord (transverse myelitis) may develop in isolation and can lead to flaccid paralysis, loss of tendon reflexes, neurogenic bladder and a definable sensory level. When it occurs, acute cord compression from a spinal extradural abscess or some other cause must also be considered and urgently excluded by MRI or CT myelogram.

Causes of acute encephalitis may be suggested by:
- the season
- recent travel history
- family illness
- animal exposures
- drug and immunisation history
- presence of lymphadenopathy, parotitis, rash or pneumonia.

Investigations to identify the aetiological agent include:
- PCR and viral culture of CSF, blood, respiratory secretions, faeces and urine
- serology.

The CSF profile of encephalitis is outlined in Table 39.1, but almost 50% of patients have normal CSF parameters. However PCR analysis provides a rapid and accurate diagnosis for a wide range of pathogens. Electroencephalographic (EEG) abnormalities are seldom specific but may be helpful in herpes simplex virus (HSV) encephalitis. MRI is more sensitive than cranial CT and helps differentiate postinfectious encephalomyelitis from encephalitis. Other treatable causes of acute encephalopathy should be sought.

Initially, aciclovir is given until a diagnosis of HSV encephalitis can be excluded by clinical, radiological and PCR criteria. Treatment is supportive, involving:
- careful fluid management
- seizure control
- assisted ventilation for respiratory failure
- maintenance of nutrition.

Corticosteroids should be considered when the MRI shows striking enhancement of multifocal white matter lesions consistent with postinfectious encephalomyelitis.

Almost 10% of children with encephalitis die and long term studies suggest that nearly half of the survivors have neurological or educational disabilities. Young age, coma, delayed presentation, high CSF protein and infection with HSV or *M. pneumoniae* are associated with a poor prognosis. However, patients can make excellent recoveries, even after prolonged coma.

Herpes simplex encephalitis

Herpes simplex virus causes a severe, sporadic localised encephalitis. Unlike other causes of encephalitis it is amenable to treatment with the antiviral agent, aciclovir, which reduces the mortality to below 20%. However, many survivors still have severe neurological or behavioural sequelae. More than 95% of postneonatal cases are caused by HSV-1 and one third result from a primary infection.

The course described in the clinical example is typical of HSV encephalitis. PCR is the diagnostic test of choice. While frontal and temporal lobe localisation is characteristic, PCR and MRI testing have shown that the

---

Clinical example

Jack, aged 10 years, was admitted to hospital with a 3 day history of fever, headache, intermittent delirium and progressive lethargy. On presentation he had several left sided focal seizures. His temperature was 39.8°C; he was drowsy, with neck stiffness, and had a left hemiparesis.

His CSF had $180 \times 10^6/l$ lymphocytes and $100 \times 10^6/l$ red cells. The protein content of the CSF was mildly elevated and the glucose concentration was normal. HSV encephalitis was suspected and aciclovir (500 mg/m^2 i.v. 8 hourly) was started. Phenytoin controlled his seizures. An EEG demonstrated periodic discharges localised to the right temporal lobe and an MRI scan showed increased signal in T2 weighted images of this region (Fig. 39.4). PCR of the CSF was positive for HSV-1 DNA.

He gradually improved over several days, but was still febrile after 2 weeks of treatment. A repeat lumbar puncture revealed persisting HSV-1 DNA and increased intrathecal HSV antibodies. Aciclovir was continued for another week. His fever settled and the hemiparesis resolved, but he was left with major behaviour and learning disabilities.

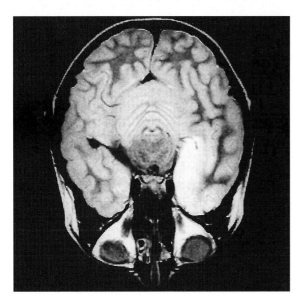

Fig. 39.4 MRI of a 10 year old boy with HSV encephalitis (see text for clinical details) which shows an increased signal in T2 weighted images of the left temporal lobe.

disease can be diffuse in neonates who have mainly HSV-2 disease (Ch. 35) and in young children.

Slow virus infection

Some viruses can cause a subacute or chronic neurodegenerative disorder. The major example in childhood is subacute sclerosing panencephalitis, a rare late compli-cation of measles, especially if measles occurs early in life. Rubella is a less common cause. The disorder is manifest by:

- deterioration of behaviour, personality and intellect
- myoclonic seizures
- motor disturbance.

The onset is usually several years after measles. As the disease progresses, spastic paresis, tremors, athetosis and ataxia develop. The disease runs a variable but progressive course and is usually fatal within 2 years. Initially, the EEG shows a typical 'suppression-burst pattern'. The typical clinical picture and high titre CSF measles antibody establish the diagnosis.

Transmissible spongiform encephalopathies

Transmissible spongiform encephalopathies (TSEs) are a group of clinical syndromes in animals and humans characterised by a slowly progressive neurodegenerative course. All are caused by toxic accumulation within the CNS of an abnormal cell surface protein, the prion protein. New variant Creutzfeldt–Jakob disease has attracted considerable attention as it represents the first instance where an animal TSE has jumped the species barrier to infect humans. Several cases have been reported in adolescents. The first symptoms are those of depression and dysaethesia, then ataxia, involuntary movements and spasticity quickly follow, leading to death within 3 years. The EEG recording remains a useful diagnostic test. Distinctive amyloid plaques are seen on brain biopsy.

Infections in tropical and developing countries

40

M. J. Robinson, D. R. Brewster

More than 50% of the world's population lives within the latitudes of 30°N and 20°S, commonly referred to as the tropics and subtropics. The majority of tropical inhabitants are in developing countries where health outcomes tend to be much poorer (Table 40.1) than in developed countries such as Australia. In addition, educational standards are lower with a high rate of illiteracy, particularly for women, which is an important determinant of child survival. Personal hygiene, water and sanitation standards are also poor in the developing world, placing individuals at higher risk of infectious diseases, particularly enteric infections in a tropical climate. In addition, poor developing countries are characterised by high fertility and child mortality rates, with under 5 child mortality rates of up to 316 per 1000 in Sierra Leone (compared with 5 per 1000 in Australia).

Rather than exotic tropical diseases, the main causes of morbidity and mortality are common conditions such as malaria, diarrhoeal diseases, acute respiratory infections, malnutrition and now AIDS (Table 40.2). Paediatric practice is probably more influenced by economic factors than by geography or climate, so paediatrics in the developing world is above all a medicine of poverty. It deals with children from poor families with heavy burdens of disease, and health care resources for the task are very limited.

Twelve million children under 5 years of age die each year, mostly from diarrhoea, pneumonia, malaria or malnutrition. Half of deaths in children in hospital occur within 24 hours of admission. The World Health Organization has developed treatment protocols for these diseases, based upon simple clinical indicators such as fast breathing, chest wall retractions, inability to drink, drowsiness, convulsions, pallor, etc., which could be assessed by health workers with minimal training. However, the acute respiratory infection (ARI) programme found that counting respiratory rates was not

Table 40.1   Major reasons for low health standards in tropical and developing countries

Poverty
Overcrowding
Political corruption
Droughts
Famines
Civil wars
Low educational standards
Poor personal hygiene
Poor water and sanitation
Low vaccination rates
Unregulated fertility

Table 40.2   Paediatric admissions* in five African and Pacific Island countries: percentage of cases (% case fatality)

Disease	% Cases (% mortality)				
	Malawi[1]	Gambia[2]	Zimbabwe[3]	Solomon Islands[4]	Papua New Guinea[5]
Malaria	32.5 (5.5)	35.3 (11.9)	<1.0 (0)	18.1 (0)	7.3 (0.7)
Severe anaemia	8.3 (18.1)	15.9 (10.8)	<1.0 (0)	7.6 (2.0)	4.0 (4.8)
Pneumonia	13.3 (17.6)	16.8 (10.8)	11.3 (2.1)	22.8 (1.6)	32.2 (4.9)
Diarrhoeal disease	20.8 (14.4)	11.6 (13.0)	16.7 (2.3)	11.3 (2.1)	13.4 (3.6)
Severe malnutrition	10.9 (31.4)	11.2 (19.6)	8.9 (31.3)	5.9 (<1)	4.2 (11.1)
Meningitis	2.5 (40.0)	3.0 (35.3)	1.0 (46.2)	2.9 (3.8)	2.9 (16.1)
Measles	0.2 (0)	0.1 (0)	7.1 (31.9)	0 (0)	7.2 (11.5)
Total admissions (% mortality)	7871 (14.6)	9584 (13.3)	2147 (6.1)	2696 (1.9)	4106 (5.8)

*Using the same diagnostic criteria, but with multiple diagnoses allowed (HIV prevalence low except in Malawi).
[1]Queen Elizabeth Central Hospital, Blantyre, Malawi, Central Africa, 1993 (with high rate of HIV infection).
[2]Royal Victoria Hospital, Banjul, The Gambia, West Africa, 1988–1990.
[3]Masvingo Provincial Hospital, Masvingo, Zimbabwe, 1984–1985.
[4]Central Hospital, Honiara, Solomon Islands, Pacific Islands, 1986–1987.
[5]Port Moresby General Hospital, Port Moresby, Papua New Guinea, Pacific Islands, 1986.

always easy and that malaria also causes fast breathing, making it difficult to differentiate from pneumonia on this basis. This led to the Integrated Management of Childhood Illness (IMCI) initiative, which aimed to reduce child morbidity and mortality in developing countries by improved management of common illnesses (Table 40.3). A study of emergency management at district hospitals, however, found major deficiencies in triage, emergency care, monitoring, drug availability, staffing levels and the use of protocols. This suggests that more emphasis needs to be placed upon on site supervision of health workers in the developing world. Although protocols may be useful, they are no substitute for clinical experience in a supervised setting. In addition to acute care protocols, there are a number of important child health programmes such as GOBI-FFF):

- **g**rowth monitoring
- **o**ral rehydration therapy
- **b**reastfeeding promotion
- **i**mmunisations
- **f**amily planning
- supplementary **f**eeding
- **f**emale literacy.

These programmes are part of primary health care services. Poor nutrition is an important contributor to the high childhood mortality from infectious diseases in the developing world. Over half of child deaths are due to the potentiating effects of malnutrition on infections, most of which are due to mild to moderate malnutrition.

The ease of air travel and the frequency of people of all ages visiting the tropics has made it essential for the student and practising doctor to have an appreciation of tropical medicine. Migration, for both personal and humanitarian reasons (refugees), makes it almost certain that some will carry disease undetected by the medical screening process. It is of the greatest importance in any unusual illness, particularly a febrile one, that a history of overseas travel is sought. The purpose of this chapter is to give an overview of health problems in tropical regions of Australia and developing countries. It is not possible to discuss in detail all of the many disorders endemic to these areas, so readers are urged to look elsewhere for specific advice on treatment. Only bacterial infections, HIV infection, malaria, dengue fever, schistosomiasis, parasitic infestations, and infections of tropical Australia will be briefly discussed.

Bacterial infections

Serious bacterial infections are much more common in children in tropical and developing countries than in temperate and developed countries. *Haemophilus influenzae* type b (Hib) and *Streptococcus pneumoniae* (pneumococcus) have been the main causes of bacterial sepsis in children, but the new conjugate vaccines are changing this pattern in developed countries. They are still too expensive for developing countries, where in addition to Hib and pneumococcus, *Staphylococcus aureus*,

---

Table 40.3 Diagnostic classifications and clinical signs for referral to hospital. (Adapted from Integrated Management of Childhood Illness (IMCI))

Young infants (0–2 months)
1. **Possible serious bacterial infection**
   Seizures, tachypnoea (≥ 60 breaths/minute), severe chest indrawing, nasal flaring, grunting, bulging fontanelle, perforated eardrum, omphalitis, fever or hypothermia (≥38°C or <30°C), many or severe skin pustules, difficult to wake up or cannot be calmed within 1 hour.
2. Diarrhoea with severe dehydration
   Lethargic or unconscious, sunken eyes and skin pinch goes back very slowly
3. Severe persistent diarrhoea (≥ 14 days)
4. Not able to feed

Children (2 months–5 years)
1. **General danger signs**
   Not able to drink or breastfeed, vomits everything, convulsions, or lethargic or unconscious
2. **Severe febrile disease**
   Fever (rectal temperature ≥38°C) and any general danger sign, or stiff neck
3. **Severe pneumonia**
   Cough or difficult breathing and any general danger sign, chest indrawing, or stridor when calm
4. **Diarrhoea with severe dehydration**
   Abnormally sleepy or difficult to wake up, sunken eyes, not able to drink or drinking poorly, skin pinch goes back very slowly
5. **Severe persistent diarrhoea (≥14 days) with dehydration**
   Restless/irritable, sunken eyes and skin pinch goes back slowly
6. **Severe malnutrition or severe anaemia**
   Visible severe wasting, oedema of both feet, or severe palmar pallor

Salmonella species and meningococcus (in some areas) are also important causes of sepsis. In infants under 3 months, the commonest causes of bacteraemia are the pneumococcus, *Staph. aureus, Strep. pyogenes, Escherichia coli* and *Salmonella* species. In contrast to developed countries, neonatal sepsis from group B streptococcus is still uncommon in most of the developing world.

In recent years there has been a resurgence of tuberculosis in tropical and developing countries, with the epidemic of HIV infection, which has been accompanied by the emergence of resistant strains of the tubercle bacillus. The accurate diagnosis of tuberculosis in young children in the developing world is often difficult because of the unavailability of sputum, the unreliability of gastric as–pirates and Mantoux testing, and the overlap in clinical presentation with malnutrition, respiratory infections and AIDS. Treatment is expensive, with even short course chemotherapy taking 6 months and requiring drug combinations (e.g. isoniazid, rifampicin, pyrazinamide) making compliance problematic.

Salmonella infections

Salmonella infections occur worldwide, but are particularly important in tropical and developing countries. Over 200 species of salmonella bacteria are known to exist. Common sources of human infection include shellfish, poultry, fish, meat and dairy products. Three clinical syndromes are associated with salmonella infection:

- acute gastroenteritis (e.g. *S. enteritidis)*
- septicaemia (e.g. *S. choleraesuis)*
- enteric fever (e.g. *S. typhi* and *paratyphi).*

A systematic review of antibiotics in non typhoidal *Salmonella* infections found no evidence of a clinical benefit in non severe cases, and it appeared to increase adverse effects and prolong the period of stool carriage.

Typhoid fever is confined to humans and occurs where standards of hygiene and sanitation are poor and a clean water supply is unavailable. Carriers of *S. typhi*, particularly those working in the food industry, are an important reservoir of infection. The typical presentation is fever, malaise, headache, abdominal discomfort and sometimes vomiting and diarrhoea. In severe disease, toxaemia is profound and complications such as small bowel perforation occur in older children. Although typhoid fever was widely considered a disease of school age, it may also affect younger children, with a clinical picture of sepsis and milder and atypical manifestations compared with older children. The diagnosis is established from blood cultures in the first or second week or positive serology, bearing in mind previous vaccination. Antibiotic resistance to ampicillin and co-trimoxazole is common, so chloramphenicol is the drug of choice in the developing world. Third generation cephalosporins (e.g. ceftriaxone) or quinolones (e.g. ciprofloxacin) are highly effective and the drugs of choice if affordable.

HIV infection

The HIV epidemic has transformed the face of paediatrics in Africa and the same is true in Asia. The prognosis of children presenting with malnutrition, chronic diarrhoea, lymphadenopathy, pneumonia and tuberculosis is clouded by the spectre of HIV. It is also causing profound disruption to families due to death and disease of parents and hence increasing number of children orphaned by AIDS.

The rates of mother to child transmission of HIV-1 without treatment are about 20–30% in the developing world, with the risk in individual infants proportionate to the mother's viral load. Antiviral prophylaxis in pregnancy and elective caesarean delivery have reduced vertical transmission rates of HIV positive mothers in developed countries to <2%, but these antiretroviral prophylaxis and treatment regimens are too expensive for developing countries. A less expensive regimen of antiviral prophylaxis such as two-doses of nevirapine (to mother in labour and the infant at 72 hours, drug cost US$4) has been shown to reduce transmission by 47% compared with zidovudine. Other regimens are under evaluation. Breastfeeding increases the risk of postpartum HIV transmission by about 3.2% per year of breastfeeding after the age of 2.5 months, but the risk is likely to be higher during the early postpartum period. Since breastfeeding offers considerable protection in developing countries against mortality from diarrhoeal disease, it is still recommended in spite of the additional risk of HIV transmission.

The common presentations of HIV infection in hospitalised children under 2 years are:

- interstitial pneumonia in well nourished infants of 3–9 months, often with marked tachypnoea and frothy sputum, but no wheezes or crackles in the chest, and usually no hepatosplenomegaly or lymphadenopathy (*Pneumocystis carinii* pneumonia).
- failure to thrive in late infancy, with severe wasting and stunting, and often with chronic diarrhoea.
- marasmus or marasmic kwashiorkor (but not kwashiorkor) in a breastfed child.
- An increase in serious bacterial infections in infancy, particularly meningitis, pneumonia and soft tissue infections.

Other suggestive diagnostic features of HIV include lymphadenopathy (especially axillary), non suppurative parotitis, pericardial effusion, myocarditis, pericarditis and chronic papular dermatitis. When HIV is common, it needs to be excluded in virtually any unusual clinical presentation, as atypical HIV infection is still more likely than typical features of a rare disease.

Malaria

Malaria is a major global health problem, with over 40% of the world's population exposed to various degrees of risk, almost exclusively in tropical regions. Severe and complicated malaria is caused by *Plasmodium falciparum* infection. The two main forms of severe malaria in children are cerebral malaria and severe anaemia. Cerebral malaria tends to be in older children (mean age 3–4 years) in areas with seasonal and moderate transmission, compared with severe anaemia, which is most frequent in younger children (mean 1–2 years) with high malarial transmission. The interval between symptom onset and death is short, averaging less than 3 days. Unlike adults, renal failure, pulmonary oedema, shock, jaundice and disseminated intravascular coagulation (DIC) are uncommon in childhood malaria, as are the classical malaria paroxysms with cold shivers, burning heat and drenching sweats.

Parasites are not synonymous with disease, so in 1000 children bitten by an infected mosquito there might be 400 asymptomatic infections, 200 cases of clinical malaria, 12 cases of severe malaria and 1 death. Not only do many children have parasitaemia without disease, but the density of peripheral blood parasitaemia bears little relationship to mortality, as infected red cells cytoadhere and sequester in the microvasculature. Thick blood film microscopy remains the gold standard for malaria diagnosis, but new rapid diagnostic tests are available using immunochromatographic methods to detect *Plasmodium*-specific antigens. Their main disadvantages at present are cost, inability to quantify parasite density, persistently positive tests after adequate treatment, and lack of species and sexual–asexual (e.g. gametocytes) stage differentiation. Tests under development are likely to improve further on rapid malarial diagnosis and may be able to detect sequestered parasites.

Cerebral malaria has been defined as unrousable coma not attributable to any other cause in a patient with falciparum malaria. The level of consciousness is confounded by convulsions and the postictal state, so coma must persist for 30 minutes after a convulsion for a diagnosis of cerebral malaria to be made. In Africa, cerebral malaria has a mortality of around 15%; neurological sequelae occur in 23% of survivors with profound coma on admission. However, all except 4% have fully recovered 6 months after admission. The main features of severe disease are:
- deep and prolonged coma
- decerebrate posturing
- hypoglycaemia
- status epilepticus
- brain swelling
- lactic acidosis.

Other features that may increase mortality are dehydration, bacteraemia, an abnormal breathing pattern due to metabolic acidosis, seizures or cerebral oedema.

Severe malarial anaemia presents to hospital with respiratory distress due to heart failure from an abrupt drop in haemoglobin or lactic acidosis. The need for blood transfusion can be confirmed on blood film by heavy parasitaemia and lack of reticulocyte response. On the other hand, in a child with malaria pigment with few or no parasites and many reticulocytes and nucleated red cells (marrow response), but without overt cardiac failure, it may be possible defer transfusion, as rapid clinical improvement can usually be expected within 24 hours. Excessive transfusion is a significant risk, particularly in infants, so it is important to monitor volumes, give packed cells where possible and limit transfusions to 10–15 ml/kg over not less than 4 hours.

Viral haemorrhagic fevers

A number of viruses are capable of producing haemorrhagic disease in humans (Table 40.4). They are mainly arthropod borne, the most common vectors being ticks and mosquitoes. The clinical features of these infections are generally similar to those of dengue haemorrhagic fever, which is described below.

Dengue virus infection

This is the commonest arbovirus infection in the world, being particularly common in tropical countries. Most cases are sporadic, but it is endemic in South East Asia and epidemics have occurred in the Americas. It is transmitted by mosquitoes, mainly *Aedes aegypti*, which is also the vector for yellow fever. The incubation period is 2–7 days and asymptomatic infections are common. The clinical features are abrupt onset of high fever with generalised aches and pains and a macular skin eruption. The flu-like illness lasts 2–6 days and then may relapse a day or two later with fever and rash, followed by fatigue for several weeks.

Table 40.4 Agents causing viral haemorrhagic fever

Disease	Viral agent
Yellow fever	Flavivirus
Dengue	Flavivirus
Chikungunya	Alphavirus
Rift Valley fever	Bunyavirus
Kyasanur virus disease	Flavivirus
Hantaan virus disease	Bunyavirus
Lassa fever	Arenavirus
Marburg virus disease	Filovirus
Ebola virus disease	Filovirus

Severe dengue is characterised by the two syndromes:
- dengue haemorrhagic fever
- dengue shock syndrome.

In the former, a petechial rash appears on about the third day, with bleeding from the gums, nose, gastrointestinal tract and venepuncture sites. After the initial phase, when the fever is beginning to subside, signs of circulatory failure appear, with restlessness, pallor, diaphoresis and cool peripheries. Pleural effusion, characteristically on the right side, and ascites may develop. Typical laboratory findings include thrombocytopenia, elevated haematocrit, abnormal liver enzymes and coagulation tests (e.g. PTT and tourniquet test). Dengue shock syndrome results from marked plasma leakage due to a diffuse vasculitis, often with features of DIC. Dengue shock syndrome usually progresses from haemorrhagic fever, but some children present in circulatory difficulties after a period of only 1–2 days.

The management of dengue fever is symptomatic and supportive. This means an adequate fluid intake, the use of plasma expanders, the replacement of coagulation factors, paracetamol (not aspirin) and careful clinical observation. Most children will recover with adequate treatment, but a mortality of 2% remains even in sophisticated centres. It is still not clear why about 6% of children with dengue progress to shock or haemorrhagic syndromes. Epidemics can only be contained by vector control until there is a vaccine.

Schistosomiasis (bilharzia)

This infection with one of the three trematodes of *Schistosoma,* namely *haematobium, mansoni* and *japonicum,* afflicts about 200 million people worldwide. With increasing tourism to and migration from Africa, the Middle East, Brazil and parts of Asia (China, Japan, Philippines) where the disease is endemic, cases are now being seen in Australia. Although children are often the most heavily infected in endemic areas because of their contact with fresh water where the intermediate molluscan (snail) host lives, they do not often present with disease until later in life. The early symptoms, apart from red itchy papules at the site of entry, may occur 4–10 weeks after exposure, with fever, urticaria, arthralgia and eosinophilia due to an immune complex disease (Katayama fever), which is more common in tourists and rare in children. The clinical features of established disease depend on the species involved.

With *S. haematobium* the key early feature is terminal haematuria due to the granulomatous response in the bladder, which untreated may progress over years of heavy exposure to obstructive uropathy, hydronephrosis and pyelonephritis. With *S. mansoni,* diarrhoea with blood and mucus and abdominal discomfort may be occasional presenting features, but most infected children have few specific symptoms and complain only of tiredness, lack of energy, anorexia and weight loss. This can present later in life after chronic exposure as hypersplenism, portal hypertension and bleeding oesophageal varices from hepatic granulomas with fibrotic changes.

It is important that schistosomiasis be considered in any child who is chronically unwell and who comes from or has visited a country where the disease is endemic. The diagnosis is made by finding characteristic ova in urine or faeces. An ELISA serological test is useful in a developed country setting. Praziquantel is the drug of choice, and is highly effective and relatively free of side effects. Prevention involves various control measures in endemic areas and education of parents about the risks of swimming in still fresh water (lakes, ponds and streams) in endemic areas, where there is often an even greater risk posed by hippopotamuses and crocodiles.

Parasitic infestations of the gastrointestinal tract

These are extremely common in some areas where almost 100% of children carry one or more parasite species. For details of the structure of these parasites, their ova and life cycles, the reader is referred elsewhere. Symptoms (Table 40.5) and modes of presentation vary and multiple infestations may occur simultaneously.

Diagnosis of parasitic infections is established by finding the organism, or more commonly the specific ova, in a fresh stool specimen. Drug treatment is available and is in general effective and well tolerated. However, it is emphasised that the major factors promoting parasite colonisation of the gut are poor hygiene through ignorance, overcrowding and malnutrition.

Entamoeba histolytica

This is the commonest intestinal parasite affecting children in the tropics and is often associated with other bowel infections, for example, *Salmonella* spp. and *Trichuris trichuria.* Children with E. *histolytica* are often symptomless despite carrying and excreting large numbers of cysts each day.

Abdominal discomfort may be the only symptom. In an acute attack of amoebiasis there is severe diarrhoea with stools containing blood and mucus but little pus. Other symptoms are abdominal cramps, tenesmus and toxaemia. In chronis amoebiasis, alternating periods of diarrhoea and constipation are present in association with tenderness over the large bowel and at times hepatomegaly. Amoebic liver abscess, a well known complication in adults, is rare in childhood.

Table 40.5 Symptoms of parasitic gastrointestinal and other infections

Symptom	Parasite
Chronic blood loss	Ankylostomiasis *Entamoeba histolytica* *Trichuris trichiurua*
Chronic diarrhoea	Ankylostomiasis *Entamoeba histolytica* *Trichuris trichiura* *Giardia lamblia*
Malabsorption	*Giardia lamblia* but to a lesser extent With most parasites
Protein loss	With almost all parasites
Local irritation	*Trichuris trichiura* *Enterobius vermicularis (pinworm)*
Intestinal obstruction	A heavy load of *Ascaris lumbricoides*
Invasion of specific organs	*Ascaris lumbricoides* Anklyostomiasis (hookworm) *Toxocara* species
Mass lesion	Hydatid disease

Table 40.6 Common infections in Aboriginal community children in tropical Australia

Respiratory infections
Otitis media — especially chronic suppurative otitis media
Acute bronchiolitis, *chronic mucopurulent bronchitis progressing to bronchiectasis
Bacterial pneumonia, often *Streptococcus pneumoniae*

Infectious diarrhoea
*Enteropathogenic *Escherichia coli* (EPEC) and enteroaggregative *E. coli* (EAEC)
Rotavirus
Strongyloides stercoralis and cryptosporidium
Salmonella (but clinical dysentery uncommon)

Intestinal nematodes
*Whipworm — *Trichuris trichiura*
*Strongyloides, which causes diarrhoea and occasionally disseminated infection
*Hookworm — *Ancylostoma duodenale* (less common now due to widespread use of albendazole)

Skin infections
Impetigo and cellulitis — usually *Streptococcus pyogenes*
Boils and abscesses — usually *Staphylococcus aureus*
*Scabies, often with pyoderma
Tinea corporis — usually *Trichophyton rubrum*

Bone, joint and muscle infections
Septic arthritis, often *Staphylococcus aureus*
Osteomyelitis and *pyomyositis, usually *Staphylococcus aureus*

Other
*Rheumatic fever (group A *streptococcus*)
*Poststreptococcal glomerulonephritis (group A *streptococcus*)
*Epidemic gonococcal conjunctivitis (occasionally)
*Trachoma (*Chlamydia trachomatis*)
Hepatitis A (usually anicteric)

*Predominantly occurs in Aboriginal children.

The diagnosis is established by demonstrating motile *E. histolytica* from a fresh specimen of stool or from the ulcerated mucosa seen at endoscopy. Serology is useful in invasive disease.

Specific infections of the Australian tropics

Table 40.6 lists the common infections in hospitalised children in the Top End of Australia. Murray Valley encephalitis (MVE) is endemic in northwest Australia, with significant rates of exposure but a low clinical attack rate of about 0.1% of those infected. However, those who develop clinical illness develop a devastating encephalitis with fever, coma, seizures and neurological signs of cerebellar, spinal cord and brainstem involvement, with a mortality of 20% and neurological sequelae in up to 40% of survivors. While more common in the tropical north of Australia, Ross River and Barmah Forest viruses cause outbreaks throughout Australia. Infection in children is usually asymptomatic and it is likely that infection in childhood accounts for the very low incidence of clinical disease in Aboriginal communities in northern Australia despite high rates of seropositivity.

Melioidosis is caused by the bacterium *Burkholderia pseudomallei*, which is ubiquitous in soil and water in northern Australia and is even more common in Thailand. Disease in children is relatively uncommon compared with adults (e.g. only 4% of cases at Royal Darwin Hospital are in children) because predisposing chronic disease risk factors, such as diabetes and alcoholism, are less common. Although pneumonia is the commonest presentation of melioidosis, there is a wide spectrum of manifestations from mild cutaneous lesions to fulminant disease with multiple visceral abscesses. Prolonged treatment is required, usually with the antibiotics ceftazidime and co-trimoxazole.

HIV infection in childhood

R. Doherty

Human immunodeficiency virus (HIV) infection of children is a complex and changing area of clinical practice that has application in virtually all parts of the world. Recent advances in treatment have reduced mortality in Western communities, but HIV infection remains a major problem. Clinical features of HIV infection appear as a continuum, although the case definition of the acquired immune deficiency syndrome (AIDS) continues to be useful in global surveillance. Around the world, vertical transmission of HIV from mother to infant is the most important route of transmission in the paediatric age group.

Epidemiology

HIV has become an enormous problem globally since its emergence in 1981, and has been described by the World Health Organization (WHO) as a combined threat to global health as well as to development and security in many countries of the world. While the dominant impact remains in Africa, the impact of HIV and AIDS has spread into Europe, Central and South East Asia and into South America.

Global epidemiology

WHO estimates for the end of 1999 suggest that some 35 million people (1.3 million children) worldwide were living with HIV infection, and that some 19 million people, including 4 million children, had died from AIDS. An estimated 2.8 million deaths (280 000 children) and 5.4 million new infections (620 000 children) occurred in 1999 alone. Cumulatively, 13.2 million children had been orphaned by AIDS by that time. Of 15 000 new infections daily, 95% occur in developing countries and 1700 are in children. Half of the remaining 13 000 occur in the 15–24 year age group, and half occur in women. The dominant risk factor for HIV infection globally remains heterosexual sex, although local epidemiological factors, especially the incidence of drug use and prostitution, can have profound regional effects as well. Almost all children with HIV infection have acquired it from their mothers at delivery or in the postnatal period.

HIV in Western communities

In Western communities, the incidence of HIV infection in children is correlated most strongly with the rates of infection in young women who use injected drugs or who are partners of injecting drug users. Transmission of HIV between men who have sex with men and via shared injecting equipment remain the dominant modes of transmission. The introduction of screening of blood supplies has been very effective in reducing transmission associated with blood products, but episodes still occur on rare occasions. Improvements to screening questionnaires and technical methods are important steps for the future. Transmission via needle stick injury, especially in an occupational setting, remains a very small but significant component of the epidemiology of HIV.

HIV in Australia

The epidemiology of HIV in Australia follows a pattern similar to that of most Western communities, although the low incidence of HIV infection in injecting drug users up to mid 2001 has meant that there have been relatively few children with HIV infection in Australia. At the end of 2000, surveillance data for Australia suggested that some 12 400 people currently had HIV infection, with over 18 000 cases of HIV infection recorded cumulatively. New diagnoses of HIV infection and of AIDS have declined in Australia since 1994, presumably as a result of preventive strategies and the impact of clinical care. Only a small number of children have been reported meeting criteria for AIDS in Australia, although these numbers may not reflect the impact of contaminated blood products in boys with haemophilia and other recipients of transfusions who remained asymptomatic until after reaching 15 years of age.

Mother to infant transmission of HIV

To the end of 1999, 204 children were known to have been exposed at birth to HIV infection in Australia, and of these, between 19% and 25% became infected. The rate of transmission from mother to infant in Australia seems higher than in similar countries, and the reasons for this are not entirely clear. In half of these cases, the mother's infection was not diagnosed antenatally, suggesting that improved recognition of infection in women is an important step towards recognition and prevention of infection in children. With application of appropriate strategies, an infection rate of about 2% of exposed infants should be possible.

Recent evidence suggests that breastfeeding does contribute substantially to the overall risk of mother to infant transmission of HIV in communities where breastfeeding cannot be avoided. However, the overall increase in HIV transmission is still not sufficient to abolish the beneficial effects of breastfeeding in countries where safe and readily affordable alternative forms of milk feeding are not available. Transmission may be lessened if feeding is exclusive and does not continue past 6 months.

Clinical example

Kim presented at 6 months of age with refractory wheezing associated with parainfluenza virus type 3. He had an unusual papular rash on his trunk, which on biopsy showed features suggestive of Gianotti–Crosti syndrome, an uncommon manifestation of hepatitis B and other virus infections. He did not have hepatitis Bs antigen in his plasma. He had splenomegaly, and generalised lymphadenopathy, which had been present since birth. At his mother's request, he was tested for evidence of HIV infection and antibodies were demonstrated in his serum. HIV was isolated from peripheral blood lymphocytes, and viral DNA was found in these cells by PCR assay. He was fully breastfed and had been immunised normally with standard vaccines including oral polio vaccine (OPV). His mother was also tested and was found to have HIV infection.

Therapy was begun with zidovudine alone, and serial measurement of plasma virus load showed a decline followed shortly by a steady rise. Lamivudine was added and therapy was complicated by the appearance of anaemia and thrombocytopenia requiring frequent interruptions to therapy. He presented at 9 months of age with fever and apparent pain in his right hip. A bone scan suggested pelvic osteomyelitis and Kim required prolonged therapy in hospital with intravenous antibiotics. The splenomegaly persisted and despite withdrawal of antiretroviral therapy his platelet count remained low. Repeated measurement of plasma virus load showed levels as high as 1 000 000 copies/ml and the protease inhibitor ritonavir was added to zidovudine and lamivudine with a good but transient effect on plasma viral load. The spleen became massive and persistent thrombocytopenia became severe. He developed recurrent gastrointestinal haemorrhages and had several episodes of bacteraemia and cellulitis. Active therapy was eventually withdrawn with his mother's full consent, and he died at home aged 18 months following a presumed intracranial haemorrhage.

This infant had clinical features evident at birth and most likely had intrauterine infection in the setting of undiagnosed maternal infection. He experienced very early onset of severe clinical manifestations, and severe adverse effects from therapy which were compounded by the effects of progressive disease. His illness occurred during the period in which children had far less access to antiretroviral agents than adults with less severe disease and his early course was undoubtedly compromised by the use of inadequate therapy. Nevertheless, it is unlikely he would have tolerated full combination therapy and his clinical course was characteristic of infants with early onset of disease.

Virology, immunology and pathogenesis

HIV is a member of the lentivirus family of retroviruses. The hallmark of retroviruses is their use of an RNA dependent DNA polymerase (reverse transcriptase, RT) to produce a double stranded DNA proviral genome from the single stranded RNA of the particle genome. The proviral DNA is integrated into the host cell genome and thereafter behaves much like a region of cellular DNA. Lentiviruses have the ability to cause acute infection of some cells, followed by a life long chronic infection of other cells and thus the host. The virus family includes viruses of many mammalian species, including other primates, sheep, horses, cats and goats. The organisation of the virus genome and the electron microscopic morphology of the virus is similar in family members. The genome of HIV is extremely elegant in that at least nine genes are encoded in only 9300 bases. There are several important regulatory genes and the virus has a common gene promoter region which appears responsive to cellular as well as virus encoded signals.

Following initial infection, the virus load in the infected child increases rapidly (over a few weeks) to very high levels, then declines spontaneously, partly due to an immune response and perhaps partly due to the disappearance of susceptible target cells. After a variable period, which may be as much as 10 years or more, the numbers of virus circulating in plasma begin to rise and a concomitant decline in immune function appears (circulating CD4+ cell numbers particularly). Following this, the infected child becomes susceptible to opportunistic infections and the non specific symptoms attributable directly to HIV infection may emerge.

There is good evidence for an early and strong cellular and antibody mediated immune response to HIV in infected children and it appears that the cytotoxic T cell response is very important in control of virus replication, leading to an initial phase of low circulating numbers of virus. In a small number of children, the presence of cytotoxic T cell activity against HIV without other evidence of infection suggests the possibility that an aborted infection may have occurred.

The predominant target cell for HIV is the CD4+ T lymphocyte (helper T cell), although cells of monocytic lineage (macrophages), neural tissue cells and other cell types are also permissive for infection. The long term effect of infection of CD4+ lymphocytes is a steady, eventually complete, depletion of this cell type from lymph nodes and from the peripheral blood, leading to loss of immune functions normally regulated by CD4+ T cells. One of the key effects is susceptibility to viral and parasitic infection, evident particularly when the CD4+ cell count is below 25% of total lymphocyte numbers (or below 200 in adolescents). Reactivation of latent viruses of the herpes group including Epstein–Barr virus, cytomegalovirus and varicella zoster virus is a characteristic feature. In addition, the lack of helper function in maturation of B cell responses leads, even at early stages, to a dysgammaglobulinaemia in which total immunglobulin concentrations may be very high but where the response to novel antigens is inadequate. Children with HIV infection commonly acquire infections with bacteria similar to those seen with classical hypogammaglobulinaemia.

The neurotropism of HIV has been a serious problem in paediatric HIV management, with onset of neurological manifestations earlier in children than is generally seen in adults. There are several direct and indirect effects by which HIV may cause neuronal death and the brain tends to function as a sanctuary site for HIV. Progressive involvement of the brain in children most commonly manifests as developmental delay and ultimately severe regression; and imaging studies may show severe cerebral atrophy.

The factors influencing mother to infant transmission are not fully understood, but several important conclusions regarding events can be drawn from studies of prevention. While placental cells are probably at least partly permissive for HIV infection, only a small proportion of infants appear to have intrauterine infection as distinct from perinatal infection. The load of virus circulating in maternal plasma at the time of delivery appears to be strongly associated with the risk of transmission but, even so, transmission has occurred from women with undetectable levels of plasma viraemia. The mode of delivery and use of invasive monitoring are also associated with risk of infection and it is now evident that elective caesarean delivery before onset of labour reduces the risk of infection by a factor of about four. Perhaps curiously, in twin pregnancies the second twin is at lower risk of infection even when delivered by lower uterine segment caesarean section (LUSCS).

Clinical features

The clinical features of HIV infection are numerous and extremely diverse. They reflect:
- the direct effects of HIV itself (diarrhoea, fevers, lymphadenopathy, weight loss)
- the result of impaired immunity (opportunistic infections)
- the effect of indirect damage to important organs (neurological effects, nephropathy).

Infants infected perinatally rarely show clinical features which assist diagnosis, although the presence of lymphadenopathy and hepatosplenomegaly at birth suggests established infection *in utero* rather than infection at delivery. Other features, such as growth failure and developmental delay or regression, are characteristic of progressive infection even though they may be apparent in the first 12 months of life. The classical clinical features of HIV infection are presented in Fig 41.1. Perhaps paradoxically, some clinical features appear to have no adverse implications (lymphadenopathy) or may even be associated with increased survival times (pulmonary lymphoid hyperplasia). Malignancies are less common in HIV infected children than in infected adults, but Kaposi sarcoma and even squamous cell carcinomas have been reported.

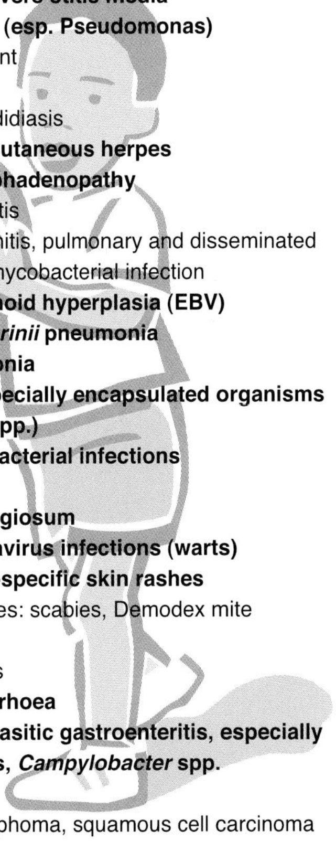

HIV encephalopathy
Toxoplasma encephalitis
CMV retinitis and encephalitis
Progressive multifocal leucoencephalopathy
(polyomavirus infection)
Recurrent and severe otitis media
Chronic sinusitis (esp. Pseudomonas)
Parotid enlargement
Oral candidiasis
Oesophageal candidiasis
Recurrent mucocutaneous herpes
Generalised lymphadenopathy
Necrotising gingivitis
Tuberculosis: adenitis, pulmonary and disseminated
Non-tuberculous mycobacterial infection
Pulmonary lymphoid hyperplasia (EBV)
Pneumocystis carinii **pneumonia**
Bacterial pneumonia
Bacteraemia (especially encapsulated organisms
and *Salmonella* spp.)
Other systemic bacterial infections
Herpes zoster
Molluscum contagiosum
Human papillomavirus infections (warts)
Eczema and non-specific skin rashes
Ectoparasitic rashes: scabies, Demodex mite
Splenomegaly
Interstitial nephritis
Non specific diarrhoea
Bacterial and parasitic gastroenteritis, especially
cryptosporidiosis, *Campylobacter* spp.
Failure to thrive
Malignancies: lymphoma, squamous cell carcinoma
esp genital tract, Kaposi sarcoma

Manifestations in bold typeface are common
and important features

Fig. 41.1 Clinical features of HIV infection in childhood.

Clinical classification

The revised HIV paediatric classification system is shown in Table 41.1. This classification has little clinical utility as a means of determining the timing of antiretroviral therapy, but it provides an important framework for staging diseases in the absence of other markers. An immunological classification based on the number or proportion of lymphocytes expressing CD4 also has been developed, and is shown in Table 41.2. Young children, especially those under 6 years, have higher levels of circulating lymphocytes than adults and the relative degree of immune impairment is best determined by the proportions rather than absolute numbers. The simple immune classification allows planning for introduction of both prophylactic and antiretroviral therapy.

Diagnosis and monitoring

Diagnosis of HIV infection in a child requires:
- demonstration of antibodies which are unequivocally those of the child, or
- direct evidence of the presence of the virus itself (viral antigen or RNA in plasma, proviral DNA in cells or isolation of HIV from cultured lymphocytes).

Serological testing requires careful conduct of a screening assay (usually a rapid ELISA assay), followed by a confirmatory test (usually an immunoblot assay). In children old enough to have lost all detectable antibodies transferred across the placenta, the requirements for diagnosis are the same as for adults. Formal diagnosis of

---

Table 41.1   Revised classification system for paediatric HIV infection. (From CDC 1994 Morbidity and Mortality Weekly Report, Vol. 43)

Category N: not symptomatic
Children who have no signs or symptoms considered to be the result of HIV infection or who have only one of the conditions listed in category A

Category A: mildly symptomatic
Children with two or more of the conditions listed below but none of the conditions listed in categories B and C:
- lymphadenopathy (≥0.5 cm at more than two sites; bilateral = one site)
- hepatomegaly
- splenomegaly
- dermatitis
- parotitis
- recurrent or persistent upper respiratory infection, sinusitis, or otitis media

Category B: moderately symptomatic
Children who have symptomatic conditions other than those listed for category A or C that are attributed to HIV infection. Examples of conditions in clinical category B include but are not limited to:
- anaemia (<8 g/dl), neutropenia (<1000/mm^3) or thrombocytopenia (<100 000/mm^3) persisting ≥30 days
- bacterial meningitis, pneumonia or sepsis (single episode)
- candidiasis, oropharyngeal (thrush), persisting (>2 months) in children >6 months of age
- cardiomyopathy
- cytomegalovirus infection, with onset before 1 month of age
- diarrhoea, recurrent or chronic
- hepatitis
- herpes simplex virus (HSV) stomatitis, recurrent (more than two episodes within 1 year)
- HSV bronchitis, pneumonitis, or oesophagitis with onset before 1 month of age
- herpes zoster (shingles) involving at least two distinct episodes or more than one dermatome
- leiomyosarcoma
- lymphoid interstitial pneumonia or pulmonary lymphoid hyperplasia complex
- nephropathy
- nocardiosis
- persistent fever (lasting >1 month)
- toxoplasmosis, onset before 1 month of age
- varicella, disseminated (complicated chickenpox)

Category C: severely symptomatic
Children who have any condition listed in the 1987 surveillance case definition for acquired immunodeficiency syndrome
(CDC 1987 Revision of the CDC surveillance case definition for acquired immunodeficiency syndrome, MMWR 36 (suppl): 1–155), with the exception of lipoid interstitial pneumonia

Table 41.2 Immunological classification system for HIV infection, based on age-specific CD4+ T lymphocyte counts and per cent of total lymphocyctes. (From CDC 1994 Morbidity and Mortality Weekly Report Vol. 43)

Immunological category	Age of child					
	<12 months		1–5 years		6–12 years	
	µl	(%)	µl	(%)	µl	(%)
1. No evidence of suppression	≥1500	(≥25)	≥1000	(≥25)	≥500	(≥25)
2. Evidence of moderate suppression	750–1499	(15–24)	500–999	(15–24)	200–499	(15–24)
3. Severe suppression	<750	(<15)	<500	(<15)	<200	(<15)

infection should be confirmed where possible by two complementary methods, but in many cases repeat serological testing on two different samples is sufficient. The availability of rapid and sensitive molecular assays which detect HIV nucleic acid in lymphocytes or plasma has greatly improved the evaluation of infants of mothers with HIV infection. If no HIV nucleic acid is detected in several samples during the first 4–6 months of life, it is highly likely that HIV infection has not occurred, regardless of the continued presence of antibodies to HIV in the serum.

Where sophisticated laboratories are not available, the diagnosis of HIV infection is much more difficult. In some settings, the use of two different screening test kits allows presumptive identification of infection, but for much of the world diagnostic testing is not possible and diagnoses are made on clinical grounds alone.

Where laboratory facilities permit, HIV infection can be monitored by serial (usually every 3 months in otherwise well children) estimation of plasma virus load and of circulating numbers of CD4+ lymphocytes. Less sensitive but less expensive methods include measuring serum levels of HIV p24 antigen (one of the core structural proteins of the virus particle). Other assays which provide indirect information about immune function have not been widely used in monitoring paediatric patients.

Management

Prevention of mother to infant transmission

Mother to infant transmission can be reduced by about two thirds by use of antiretroviral therapy in pregnant women and treatment of the infants with low dose zidovudine for 6 weeks after birth. The now famous ACTG 076 study recruited only women who had never received treatment before, but subsequent experience has shown that previously treated women can benefit from such intervention as well. The best predictor of success is complete suppression of the mother's plasma virus load at the time of delivery. In addition to therapy, the routine use of elective caesarean delivery at 38 weeks of gesta-tion, and avoidance of breastfeeding where possible, has led to a reduction in the transmission rate from about 25% overall to about 2%.

Because routine use of prolonged antiretroviral therapy in women is not possible in many countries, the recognition that a single dose of nevirapine for mother and baby also reduced transmission by about 50%

Clinical example

Simon was born at 38 weeks of gestation by elective LUSCS to his 31 year old G2P1 mother, Christine. She had discovered her HIV infection during the pregnancy when offered testing as part of antenatal assessment. Christine had begun therapy with zidovudine, lamivudine and nevirapine soon after diagnosis, and monitoring of treatment had shown a decline in plasma viral load to fewer than 400 copies/ml (below the threshold of detection for the assay).

Examination of Simon after delivery showed no evidence of lymphadenopathy, rashes or splenomegaly. Treatment with zidovudine (2 mg/kg every 6 hours) was commenced after a few hours and, after a careful bath, he was treated as a normal infant. He received formula feeds and his mother's lactation was suppressed with supportive treatment. The zidovudine therapy was continued for 6 weeks and at that time co-trimoxazole therapy was introduced to prevent primary infection with *Pneumocystis carinii*.

Blood collected at 2 days and at 1, 3 and 6 months of age was tested for proviral DNA by PCR assay. All of these tests were negative and, despite clear evidence of serum antibodies to HIV, co-trimoxazole was discontinued. Simon received routine immunisations other than OPV, and after his last negative PCR test he commenced his course of OPV to catch up to his peers.

This infant and his mother were managed by the optimal protocol for reduction of mother to infant transmission: effective prenatal antiviral therapy, elective caesarean delivery prior to onset of labour, avoidance of breastfeeding, postnatal zidovudine and subsequent co-trimoxazole. Sequential assays failed to detect HIV nucleic acid in lymphocytes and he remains well. His older sister was tested twice and showed no evidence of HIV infection.

provides considerable hope. This 1999 Ugandan study suggests that relatively cheap and practical plans for reducing transmission are possible. Even if the cost can be managed, access to such programmes for women in many countries may be impossible geographically. In addition, in most communities of the developing world, breastfeeding adds more benefit in terms of infant survival than is lost in transmission of HIV via breast milk, and breastfeeding remains an important child health issue in these communities. As a result, vertical transmission will remain a significant problem in global terms.

Antiretroviral therapy

Antiretroviral therapy became part of standard management of HIV infection in children during the late 1980s, and some of the first evidence for the effect of therapy on survival and of the clinical impact of resistance mutations came from paediatric studies. In the mid 1990s, several new classes of drugs (protease inhibitors and non nucleoside reverse transcriptase inhibitors) became available for treatment of HIV infection in patients older than 12 years. This led to a new era in which researchers and the community began to view HIV infection as more like a chronic, manageable problem for which very long term therapy would be effective in control rather than cure. The initial lack of availability of these agents for children created a serious anomaly that was finally resolved by a combination of research and changes to policy.

One of the key issues relevant to the use of long term, highly active antiretroviral therapy (HAART) now is the lack of information regarding the very long term safety of antiretroviral agents, an issue of particular relevance to children who may need treatment from soon after birth. At this stage, these issues do not in any way preclude use of therapy in infected children.

Because the development of antiretroviral agents has become a major pursuit for many large pharmaceutical companies and a steady stream of new agents is entering clinical trials, the basic principles of antiretroviral therapy are more important than the details of individual drugs. Physicians caring for HIV infected children have an important role as advocates to ensure that safe and effective treatments and formulations are available for the paediatric cohort and that appropriate studies of these agents are undertaken as efficiently as possible.

Agents in use

There are about 15 antiretroviral agents available in Australia (mid 2001) for use in HIV infected children (Table 41.3). These agents fall into three main categories based on their mechanism of action, and between them they target two key steps in virus replication:
- reverse transcription of viral RNA into proviral DNA
- proteolytic processing of a large viral precursor protein into the structural proteins which form the skeleton of the viral capsid.

Table 41.3   Antiretroviral agents available for use in children

Drug class	Mechanism of action	Representative agents	Important adverse effects	Important drug interactions
Nucleoside analogue inhibitors of RT	Inhibit RT via incorporation into growing DNA chain and via competitive effect	Zidovudine (AZT), lamivudine (3TC), stavudine (d4T), didanosine (ddI), abacavir	Anaemia, neutropenia, nausea, headache, pancreatitis, peripheral neuropathy, severe rash	May interact with drugs to potentiate adverse events such as pancreatitis and peripheral neuropathy
Non nucleoside RT inhibitors (NNRTs)	Direct inhibition of RT via binding to active site	Nevirapine, delavirdine, efavirenz	Hepatitis, elevated transaminases, rash (8%), CNS effects	Phenytoin, protease inhibitors, cisapride, oral contraceptive pills, proton pump inhibitors, calcium channel blockers, rifampicin
Protease inhibitors	Reversible inhibition of HIV protease: block cleavage of gag polyprotein into capsid components	Indinavir, ritonavir, saquinavir, nelfinavir, amprenavir, lopinavir	Nausea, vomiting, anorexia, diarrhoea, circumoral paraesthesiae, insulin resistance, lipodystrophy, hepatitis, photosensitive rash	Cisapride*, some antihistamines*, ergot derivatives, rifampicin and rifabutin, metronidazole, ketoconazole, non nucleoside reverse transcriptase inhibitors, clarithromycin

* Potentially fatal.

Careful clinical trials of antiretroviral agents in children are important and allow determination of drug pharmacokinetics, appropriate dosages, efficacy and safety so that paediatric therapy is not simply done using extrapolation from adult trials.

Efficacy

Effective antiretroviral therapy reduces the circulating plasma virus load in treated patients and, in most cases, combination (three or four drug) therapy results in the virus load dropping to undetectable numbers (currently less than 50 copies/ml). The duration of this effect is variable but can be prolonged, particularly where adverse effects of the treatment are absent. The reappearance of viral RNA in plasma is usually associated with the appearance of mutations conferring resistance to at least one of the agents in the current regimen.

Suppression of the plasma (and, by inference, tissue) virus load is associated with improved immune function, measured by rising circulating CD4+ lymphocyte counts and by assays of T cell function. In some cases, CD4+ cell numbers rise to levels well above those seen in normal children. It is still not clear that T cell function is entirely normal even with such high CD4+ cell numbers, although it appears that prophylactic antibiotic therapy is not required after numbers have risen to these levels.

The efficacy of HAART is also evident in the dramatic decline in deaths and hospital admissions due to HIV and AIDS in communities where this therapy is available. These effects have been evident in paediatric cohorts as well and correlate strongly with the time of introduction of routine use of combination therapy

Timing introduction and changes to therapy

There remains some uncertainty about the exact time at which antiretroviral therapy is best introduced, but at a practical level it seems reasonable to recommend that any child with:
- clinical symptoms
- an increasing viral load, or
- immune impairment irrespective of virus load or the presence of symptoms

should be offered therapy with one of the recognised active combinations (in 2002, usually two nucleoside analogue agents (zidovudine and lamivudine) and either nevirapine, efavirenz or a protease inhibitor). The effect of this therapy should be monitored about every 3 months by measuring:
- CD4+ lymphocyte numbers
- plasma virus load
- specific biochemical and haematological markers of drug toxicity.

A special case has been argued for early treatment of any infant known to be infected before 12 months of age irrespective of immune or virological monitoring results, but there are few data which actually show that this approach is linked to improved survival.

Irrespective of the indications, the most important prerequisite for introduction of therapy is the commitment of the family (and wherever possible the child) to the treatment. The regimens are complex and require considerable effort on the part of the child and family. Incomplete adherence to treatment allows plasma levels of drugs to fall below suppressive levels and creates the ideal environment for emergence of resistant strains of HIV and clinical failure, and deferred introduction is preferable to early failure through poor adherence.

Changes to the treatment regimen should be considered if clinical progression occurs, if T cell numbers fall or if viral load increases significantly during therapy. The choice of agents for the new regimen is heavily dependent on those in the failing programme, particularly where protease inhibitors are being used. Considerable cross resistance between these agents has been recognised and use of one agent may preclude the use of several others in subsequent therapy. The precise level (especially virus load) at which to recommend changing therapy cannot be defined with certainty, and depends on the tempo of changes, clinical features and particularly the patient's history of previous treatment. In some children, the range of available agents may be limited by the lack of suitable paediatric formulations.

Future challenges

Contemporary antiretroviral therapy is still only suppressive, and evidence suggests that, even at undetectable levels of plasma virus load, there is virus replication evident in tissues such as regional lymph nodes. The hallmark of HIV's function as an efficient parasite is the integration of viral genetic information into the host cell chromosome, and there does not as yet seem to be a clear pathway by which this process could be arrested or reversed. The pharmacological properties of many antiretroviral agents make them relatively unsuitable for use in children and many compromises are needed in current practice. If lifelong suppressive therapy over a normal life span is the most likely approach to therapy for the foreseeable future, the safety of antiretroviral agents over 50 years or more is of great importance.

Supportive and prophylactic therapy

At the time that the immune deficiency becomes moderately severe (CD4+ cell count <25% or <200 in older children), prophylactic therapy for prevention of *Pneumocystis carinii* pneumonia is indicated. In most settings, oral co-trimoxazole (trimethoprim plus sulphamethoxazole) is effective and well tolerated, but allergic reactions may arise on occasions. At about the same level of immune function, prophylaxis against bacterial infections, especially, *Streptococcus pneumoniae,* should be considered, and oral penicillin twice daily is probably as effective as monthly infusions of immunoglobulin. At more advanced levels of immune deficiency, prophylaxis against fungal infections (especially Candida) and *Mycobacterium avium-intracellulare* may be needed.

Infants treated for perinatal exposure to HIV should receive co-trimoxazole prophylaxis from the end of the 6 weeks of antiretroviral therapy until HIV infection has been excluded. If infection is confirmed, the co-trimoxazole should be continued until 12 months of age and thereafter if immune function warrants.

Nutritional aspects

HIV infection is associated with substantial metabolic and nutritional demands in children and careful records of linear growth and weight gain are an important part of routine clinical care. An initial decline in growth may be an early sign of increased viral replication and the first introduction of antiretroviral therapy is often accompanied by impressive catch up growth. In early phases of infection and where effective therapy is in place, no additional nutritional requirements are apparent, but with clinical progression a child may find it very difficult to maintain adequate intake, especially where oral infections or ulceration are a problem. Nutritional supplements added to formula or delivered by nasogastric and even gastrostomy tube may be necessary to maintain weight in more advanced stages of infection. The nutritional challenge may be compounded by the adverse effects of medications that induce anorexia or diarrhoea. In addition, enteric opportunistic infections may cause malabsorption in a variety of ways.

Immunisation issues

Children who have suspected or proven HIV infection are able to respond to normal childhood vaccines (Ch. 8) for at least the period until immune dysfunction is evident, but, as in other cellular immunodeficiency states, live poliovirus vaccine should be avoided. Responses to polysaccharide bacterial vaccines may be suboptimal, although the extent of this is not clear. A normal immunisation schedule should be used and inactivated (killed) polio vaccine administered at appropriate points in the schedule. Perhaps surprisingly, evidence on both efficacy and safety supports the use of measles, mumps and rubella (MMR) vaccine in HIV infected children without severe immunodeficiency. HIV infected children should receive the conjugate pneumococcal vaccine where possible. At this stage, the varicella (live attenuated virus) vaccine should not be administered to HIV infected children, although it may transpire that this vaccine is safe in this group. Bacille Calmette–Guérin (BCG) vaccine (live attenuated mycobacterium) is not recommended for infected children in areas of low tuberculosis prevalence, such as Australia and New Zealand, and should be deferred in infants of indeterminate status until HIV infection has been excluded. The WHO recommends, however, that BCG be administered routinely to infants in countries with a high prevalence of tuberculosis, irrespective of their HIV infection status.

Social issues

Children with HIV infection represent a community group that is particularly likely to experience social difficulty and hardship. An infant infected by vertical transmission is likely to represent the third infection in the family, and even where an infant does not acquire infection perinatally the circumstances of a family where both parents have HIV infection are likely to be fragile. Despite recent improvements in survival of adults with HIV infection, the uninfected children of couples with HIV have special challenges ahead of them and the global phenomenon of 'AIDS orphans' is well recognised. Family circumstances are even more challenging where a parent (or both parents) is an active injecting drug user. Even without additional challenges arising from social disadvantage, families of HIV infected children face significant challenges and may be badly affected by community responses driven by unfounded fears.

Issues of confidentiality are of vital importance to most families with an HIV infected child. Where parents of an infected child choose to reveal the child's infection status to a school or other agency, special care needs to be taken to ensure that these issues are understood and that the groups receiving the information are well aware of their responsibilities to the child.

Questions

1. Which of the following viruses can cause a morbilliform rash?
   (A) Enteroviruses
   (B) Influenza
   (C) Measles
   (D) Parainfluenza
   (E) Rubella

2. Which of the following childhood infections can be prevented by vaccination?
   (A) Chickenpox
   (B) Glandular fever (EBV infection)
   (C) Mumps
   (D) Parvovirus B19 infection
   (E) Rubella

3. In a 2 year old child which of the following are likely causes of exudative tonsillitis?
   (A) Adenovirus
   (B) Coxsackie A virus
   (C) Epstein–Barr virus
   (D) Group A streptococcus
   (E) Herpes simplex virus

4. Jessie, a previously well 8 year old girl, presents with an acute febrile illness and painful movement of her left hip. On examination, hip movement is severely restricted and painful. Should you:
   (A) Send her home for bed rest with review the following day
   (B) Admit her to hospital and place her leg in skin traction only
   (C) Admit her, collect blood for culture, and commence intravenous antibiotics
   (D) Admit her, collect blood cultures, drain her hip under general anaesthesia and commence intravenous antibiotics

5. Michael is aged 15 months and has been walking for 2 months. Not long after waking in the morning he became irritable and began crying. He refused to walk, but would crawl. He seemed better later that day and would take a few tentative steps, but the same pattern of events occurred the next day. His mother noted that he seemed to have tenderness over his lower back when she bathed him that evening. He developed a mild fever and his mother took him to see the local medical officer. The doctor confirmed that he was tender over his lower thoracic spine, and referred him urgently to the children's hospital

with a provisional diagnosis of discitis. Which of the following are correct?
   (A) He should have a bone scan
   (B) He should have blood cultures taken
   (C) X rays of his spine should be done but are unlikely to show abnormalities at this stage
   (D) He will probably have severe arthritis of his spine in later life if he has discitis
   (E) There is a major risk of a cord compression syndrome developing acutely in discitis

6. Dean, aged 7 months, presented with 18 hours of fever and poor feeding. He was drowsy and became very irritable when aroused. His limbs and trunk were mottled, his fontanelle was tense and he resisted neck flexion. A lumbar puncture was performed. This revealed 1500×10^6/l neutrophils, a raised protein, low glucose and numerous Gram positive diplococci. Should you:
   (A) Add vancomycin to the third generation cephalosporin you have already prescribed
   (B) Give dexamethasone after the second antibiotic dose
   (C) Immediately restrict fluids to 10% of calculated maintenance requirements
   (D) Administer rifampicin as prophylaxis to all household contacts
   (E) Order a CT scan if he developed focal seizures on the fourth day of treatment

7. Olivia, aged 4 years, presented to a rural medical centre with a 12 hour history of fever, headache, neck stiffness and vomiting. A macular truncal rash that blanches under pressure is seen. Meningococcal meningitis is suspected. Which of the following is true?
   (A) The rash is characteristic of meningococcal disease
   (B) Early administration of intramuscular penicillin may reduce mortality
   (C) Prehospital antibiotics reduce the chances of a microbiological diagnosis
   (D) The risk of mortality exceeds 20%
   (E) Protein conjugated serogroup C vaccines have been successfully introduced into Britain

8. Jasmine, a previously healthy 12 year old girl, presented with a 2 day history of fever, headache, photophobia, vomiting and neck stiffness. She had received two doses of amoxycillin for tonsillitis and a faint maculopapular rash was appearing over the upper trunk. Despite obvious meningism she did not look unwell. A lumbar puncture produced cloudy CSF with 500×10^6/L white cells,

which were predominantly lymphocytes. The CSF protein was slightly elevated, glucose was normal and the Gram stain was negative for organisms. Her headache improved following the lumbar puncture. Which of the following is correct?

(A) The CSF findings indicate a partially treated bacterial meningitis

(B) *Neisseria meningitidis* is the most likely causative agent

(C) Viral meningitis is more common during summer and autumn

(D) Aciclovir is the empiric treatment of choice

(E) Throat and stool swabs may help identify the organism

9. **In malaria, which of the following is/are true?**

(A) The disease is contracted from the bite of an infected anopheline mosquito

(B) The causative mosquito vector typically feeds at dusk and early evening

(C) In prevention, adequate clothing cover, mosquito repellant, flywire screening and mosquito proof netting are important

(D) All children going to countries where malaria is endemic should be vaccinated against malaria

(E) *Plasmodium falciparum* malaria is highly resistant to chloroquine

10. **Which of the following is/are correct?**

(A) Dengue fever is a disease of the tropics only

(B) The severe form is associated with purpura, thrombocytopenia and a rising haematocrit level

(C) Dengue haemorrhagic fever is very uncommon in adult life

(D) There are four serotypes of the dengue virus

(E) Dengue infection may be asymptomatic in the very young

11. **Which of the following is/are correct?**

(A) The commonest febrile illness of children in the tropics is malaria

(B) Dengue fever is the commonest arthropod borne virus infection in the world

(C) Diarrhoea is the commonest presenting symptom in typhoid infection

(D) Haematuria is the presenting symptom in a child with *Schistosoma haematobium* infection

(E) *Entamoeba histolytica* infection is often associated with other parasitic bowel parasites

12. **In the prophylaxis of malaria for travellers, which of the following is/are important?**

(A) Chloroquine prophylaxis

(B) The use of mosquito repellents

(C) Wearing clothing that covers most of the body during the daytime

(D) Sleeping under mosquito bed nets impregnated with permethrin

(E) Continuing appropriate drug prophylaxis for a month after returning home

13. **Which of the following is/are true of malaria?**

(A) Splenomegaly occurs in 90% of attacks in non immunes

(B) Hypoglycaemia is a common complication of severe cerebral malaria

(C) Lactic acidosis is a common complication of severe malarial anaemia

(D) Corticosteroids are beneficial in cerebral malaria

(E) Homozygous sickle cell disease protects against severe malarial infection

14. **The following is/are true of Aboriginal children in northern Australia?**

(A) They have poor compliance with immunisations

(B) Epidemics of melioidosis occur every wet season

(C) Scabies is endemic

(D) Most have tropical enteropathy syndrome due to poor hygiene

(E) They have high rates of group A streptococcal infections

Answers and explanations

1. (A), (B), (C) and (D) are correct.

2. (A), (C) and (E) are correct.

3. (A), (B), (C) and (E) are correct.

4. The correct answer is (D). The clinical features are of an acute synovitis of the hip. The severe pain and markedly restricted motion of the hip are indicative of suppurative arthritis due to a bacterial infection. Transient synovitis usually produces milder synovitis. As the clinical features are those of suppurative arthritis, it is important to decompress the hip joint by aspiration and arthrotomy. Release of the pressure within the hip minimises the likelihood of avascular necrosis of the femoral head and damage to the articular cartilage. The joint fluid, as well as blood, is collected for culture. At the age of 8 years, the most likely organism is *Staphylococcus aureus* and intravenous flucloxacillin is an appropriate initial form of treatment while awaiting the culture results. Early arthrotomy and intravenous antibiotics can be expected to cure the infection rapidly and prevent permanent damage to the joint. Delay in implementing this treatment, (A) and (B), will result in permanent damage to the joint. Antibiotic therapy (C) is not adequate when used alone.

5. The correct answers are (A), (B) and (C). This clinical presentation is consistent with discitis. Children at this age will not be able to indicate where the pain is occurring, but careful assessment and examination

will reveal loss of back movement and local tenderness in discitis. A bone scan will show an inflammatory focus (A), and MRI may also be useful, although this will require anaesthesia at this age. Blood cultures should be taken (B) in order to detect a vertebral osteomyelitis, although generally no organism will be isolated in discitis. X rays also should be done, but will be unlikely to show changes at this early stage (C). There is no evidence that discitis leads to later inflammatory arthritis or osteoarthritis (D). Cord compression is not a complication of discitis (E), although it can occur if there is a vertebral osteomyelitis and formation of an extradural abscess.

6. The correct answers are **(A)** and **(E)**. (A) Antibiotic resistance in some countries has resulted in 10% or more of pneumococcal isolates becoming resistant to both penicillin and cephalosporins. Whenever pneumococcal meningitis is suspected, the synergistic combination of vancomycin and a third generation cephalosporin is administered until antibiotic susceptibility results are available. (B) Whether dexamethasone should be administered with the first dose of antibiotics in children with pneumococcal meningitis is controversial. There are no good data demonstrating clinical benefit and in experimental models steroids delay CSF sterilisation. (C) The mottled limbs and trunk suggest hypovolaemia. Priority is given to restoring the circulating blood volume. (D) The risk of household transmission and meningitis from *Staphylococcus pneumoniae* is much lower than with *Neisseria meningitidis* and Hib. Chemoprophylaxis is not recommended. (E) Children with focal seizures are more likely to have neurological sequelae. While seizures developing late in the course of management may indicate SIADH and hyponatraemia, causes that can be identified by cerebral imaging include subdural effusion, cerebritis, vascular thrombosis and abscess formation.

7. The correct answers are **(B)**, **(C)** and **(E)**. (A) Between 50 and 80% of children with meningococcal disease will have a rash at the time of their first presentation. In only half the cases is the rash initially non blanching and haemorrhagic. Some never develop a rash and in 10% the rash does not evolve beyond the macular stage. (B) Uncontrolled observations in New Zealand and the United Kingdom suggest that prehospital antibiotics reduce case fatality rates. Public health authorities in both countries and in Australia recommend that antibiotics be given when meningococcal disease is suspected. (C) Prehospital antibiotics reduce the rate of positive cultures from blood and CSF from approximately 60% to 25%. PCR testing for meningococcal DNA from sterile sites has partially addressed this problem. (D) Mortality from meningococcal meningitis is 2–3%, which is lower than other causes of bacterial meningitis and significantly lower than in cases of fulminant meningococcaemia. (E) Following a hyperendemic period of meningococcal disease from a virulent clone of serogroup C in Britain lasting several years, a MenC conjugate vaccine was introduced in late 1999. This was followed by a reduction in meningococcal serogroup C disease in the target age groups.

8. The correct answers are **(C)** and **(E)**. (A) The CSF findings are typical of viral meningitis. In meningitis caused by enteroviruses or mumps there may be a predominance of neutrophils and the CSF glucose may be as low as 1.5–2.0 mmol/l. A repeat CSF examination 12–24 hours later may help clarify the diagnosis. Although prior antibiotics reduce the chances of identifying a bacterial pathogen by culture or Gram stain, the CSF cell count and biochemistry change very little. TB meningitis should always be considered when there are roughly equal proportions of neutrophils and mononuclear cells, especially when the CSF protein is elevated and the glucose is reduced. (B) While antibiotics might mask the clinical diagnosis of meningococcal meningitis, especially when a rash is present, the patients are usually much sicker, the illness progresses rapidly and the CSF examination is characteristic of bacterial meningitis. (C) Enteroviruses are the most common cause of viral meningitis and in temperate climates infection from these agents peaks during late summer and autumn. (D) Aciclovir is used to treat herpes simplex encephalitis. Herpes simplex is an uncommon cause of viral meningitis in children. The investigational drug, pleconaril, is being evaluated for its role in viral meningitis. (E) Throat and stool cultures may detect pathogens implicated in viral meningitis. The more sensitive PCR tests give an opportunity for early identification of a broad range of viruses in the CSF that previously went undetected by traditional culture techniques.

9. The correct answers are **(A)**, **(B)**, **(C)** and **(E)**. (A) *Anopheles* is the only species of mosquito carrying the malarial parasite. (B) is correct but infection can be acquired at any time of day or night. The preventive measures in (C) are at least as important as malarial prophylaxis with drugs. It is also important to restrict breeding grounds by proper drainage and preventing water from collecting in jars, automobile tyres and other household utensils where the mosquito breeds. (D) At this time a proven malarial vaccine does not exist, although research towards one continues. (E) The *Plasmodium falciparum* parasite is highly resistant to chloroquine so that drug prophylaxis combinations are often necessary (e.g. pyrimethamine with dapsone, mefloquine and doxycycline, proguanil and chloroquine).

401

Resistance of *P. vivax* or *P. malariae* to chloroquine is much less common.

10. The correct answers are **(B)**, **(C)**, **(D)** and **(E)**. (A) Although the disease is essentially a disorder of tropical countries where it is usually carried by the mosquito vector *Aedes aegypti*, which cannot tolerate low temperatures, other *Aedes* species, and in particular *Aedes albopictus*, can survive in cold regions and cause dengue. (B) The onset is non specific, with fever, rash, headache and limb and joint pains. After several days the child may become very ill with a purpuric rash, thrombocytopenia and a rising haematocrit level, the result of a generalised vasculitis. (C) The reasons for this are poorly understood. It is likely that young infants may carry protective antibodies from the mother and that adults are immune from previous infections. (D) This is correct and has hampered the development of an effective vaccine. (E) Dengue infections vary from asymptomatic infection, particularly in the very young, to an unpleasant febrile illness (most common), through to the severe forms of dengue haemorrhagic fever and dengue shock syndrome.

11. The correct answers are **(B)**, **(D)** and **(E)**. (A) The commonest infections in children from tropical countries are respiratory tract infections and diarrhoeal disease. (B) It is estimated that 100 million new infections occur worldwide each year. The incidence of dengue virus infection is increasing in tropical regions of Asia, Africa and Central and South America. (C) By far the commonest presenting symptom is fever, which is not initially associated with other clinical signs or symptoms. It needs to be considered in any child with a high fever who has recently returned from a country where typhoid is endemic. (D) This needs to be considered in any child coming from a country where schistosomiasis is endemic (e.g. Africa, Central and South America). (E) Multiple bowel infections and infestations are common in poor tropical populations (e.g. *Trichuris trichuria*, salmonella, giardiasis and *Ascaris lumbricoides*).

12. **(B)**, **(D)** and **(E)** are correct. Most *falciparum* infections are resistant to chloroquine, so prophylaxis generally involves other drugs such as mefloquine, proguanil or doxycycline, and sometimes combinations (including with chloroquine for vivax or malariae infections). Protection against mosquito bites is important but protective clothing is most useful at dusk when the anopheles mosquitos feed.

13. **(B)** and **(C)** are correct. Splenomegaly occurs in <50% of cases but splenomegaly rates in children may be high in hyperendemic or holoendemic malarial regions. Hypoglycaemia and lactic acidosis are common complications of severe malaria. Although cerebral oedema may occur in cerebral malaria, steroids have not been shown to be beneficial. Heterozygote children with a sickle trait have some protection against severe malaria but not homozygote children with sickle cell disease.

14. **(C)**, **(D)** and **(E)** are correct. Aboriginal children in the Northern Territory have higher immunisation rates than non Aboriginal children, with >90% fully vaccinated. Melioidosis is much more common in adults and there are only a few sporadic cases in children. Although scabies usually occurs in 7 year epidemics, it has been endemic for many years in northern Australian Aboriginal children, with many adults suffering severe crusted (Norwegian) scabies. Aboriginal children in tropical Australia have high intestinal permeability ratios indicative of subclinical mucosal damage, and overseas studies indicate that this is associated with poor hygiene and overcrowding. Group A streptococcal infections are associated with acute glomerulonephritis and rheumatic fever, which are common in Aboriginal children in northern Australia.

PART 12   FURTHER READING

Anonymous 1997 Integrated management of childhood illness: a WHO/UNICEF initiative. Bulletin of the World Health Organization 75 (Supplement 1): 7–128

Baker M, McNicholas A, Garrett N et al 2000 Household crowding: a major risk factor for epidemic meningococcal disease in Auckland children. Pediatric Infectious Disease Journal 19: 983–990

Bale J F Jr 1999 Human herpesviruses and neurological disorders of childhood. Seminars in Pediatric Neurology 6: 278–287

Cabellos C, Martinez-Lacas J, Tubau F et al 2000 Evaluation of combined ceftriaxone and dexamethasone therapy in experimental cephalosporin-resistant pneumococal meningitis. Journal of Antimicrobial Chemotherapy 45: 315–320

Carr A J, Cole W G, Roberton D M, Chow C W 1993 Chronic multifocal osteomyelitis. Journal of Bone and Joint Surgery 75B: 582–591

Cherry J D 1999 Parvovirus infections in children and adults. Advances in Pediatrics 46: 245–269

Cole W G 1991 The management of chronic osteomyelitis. Clinical Orthopaedics and Related Research 264: 84–89

Cutts F T, Robertson S E, Diaz-Orlega J L, Samuel R 1997 Control of rubella and congenital rubella syndrome (CRS) in developing countries, part I: Burden of disease from CRS. Bulletin of the World Health Organization 75: 55–68

Cutts F T, Henao-Restrepo A, Olive J M 1999 Measles elimination: progress and challenges. Vaccine 17 (Supplement 3): S47–52

Davis L E, Kennedy P G E 2000 Infectious diseases of the nervous system. Butterworth-Heinemann, Oxford

Do T T 2000 Transient synovitis as a cause of painful limps in children. Current Opinions in Pediatrics 12: 48–51

Edmond K, Currie B, Brewster D, Kilburn C 1998 Pediatric melioidosis in tropical Australia. Pediatric Infectious Disease Journal 17: 77–80

Eich G F; Superti Furga A, Umbricht F S, Willi U V 1999 The painful hip: evaluation of criteria for clinical decision-making. European Journal of Pediatrics 158: 923–928

English M, Waruiru C, Amukoye E 1996 Deep breathing of children with severe malaria: indicators of metabolic acidosis and poor outcome. American Journal of Tropical Medicine and Hygiene 55: 521–524

Fernandez M, Carrol C L, Baker C J 2000 Discitis and vertebral osteomyelitis in children: an 18-year review. Pediatrics 105: 1299–104

Grimwood K, Anderson P, Anderson V, Tan L, Nolan T 2000 Twelve year outcomes following bacterial meningitis: further evidence for persisting effects. Archives of Disease in Childhood 83: 111–116

Hoffner R J, Slaven E, Perez J, Magana R N, Henderson S O 2000 Emergency department presentations of typhoid fever. Journal of Emergency Medicine 19: 317–321

Infection and Immunisation Committee, New Zealand Paediatric Society 1999 Penicillin- and cephalosporin-resistant pneumococcal meningitis: the future is now. New Zealand Medical Journal 112: 14–15

Jenson H B 2000 Acute complications of Epstein–Barr virus infectious mononucleosis. Current Opinion in Pediatrics 12: 263–268

Jodar L, Feavers I M, Salisbury D, Granoff D M 2002 Development of vaccines against meningococcal disease. Lancet 359: 1499–1508

Kalter H D, Schillinger J A, Hossain M 1997 Identifying sick children requiring referral to hospital in Bangladesh. Bulletin of the World Health Organization 75 (Supplement) 1: 65–75

Kautner I, Robinson M, Kuhnle U 1997 Dengue virus infection: epidemiology, pathogenesis, clinical presentation, diagnosis and prevention. Journal of Pediatrics 131: 516–524

Kocher M S, Zurakowski D, Kasser J R1999 Differentiating between septic arthritis and transient synovitis of the hip in children: an evidence-based clinical prediction algorithm. Journal of Bone and Joint Surgery American Volume 81: 1662–1670

Leach C T 2000 Human herpesvirus -6 and -7 infections in children: agents of roseola and other syndromes. Current Opinion in Pediatrics 12: 269–274

Mahle W T, Levine M M 1993 *Salmonella typhi* infection in children younger than five years of age. Pediatric Infectious Disease Journal 12: 627–631

Mancini A J 1998 Exanthems in childhood: an update. Pediatric Annals 27: 163–170

Marsh K, Forster D, Waruiri C et al 1995 Indicators of life-threatening malaria in African children. New England Journal of Medicine 332: 1399–1404

Negrini B, Kelleher K J, Wald E R 2000 Cerebrospinal fluid findings in aseptic versus bacterial meningitis. Pediatrics 105: 316–319

Pelletier D L 1994 The potentiating effects of malnutrition on child mortality: epidemiologic evidence and policy implications. Nutrition Reviews 52: 409–415

Read R C, Camp C J, di Giovine F S 2000 An interleukin-1 genotype is associated with fatal outcome of meningococcal disease. Journal of Infectious Diseases 182: 1557–1560

Sirinavin S, Garner P 2000 Antibiotics for treating salmonella gut infections. Cochrane Database System Reviews (2): CD001167

Sonnen G H, Henry N K 1996 Pediatric bone and joint infections: diagnosis and antimicrobial management. Pediatric Clinics of North America 43: 933–947

US Department of Health and Human Services 1994 Revised classification system for human immunodeficiency virus infection in children less than 13 years of age. Morbidity and Mortality Weekly Report 43: 1–19

Van Deuren M, Brandtzaeg P, van der Meer J W M 2000 Update on meningococcal disease with emphasis on pathogenesis and clinical management. Clinical Microbiology Reviews 13: 144–166

Whitely R J, MacDonald N, Asher D M and the Committee on Infectious Diseases 2000 American Academy of Pediatrics technical report. Transmissible spongiform encephalopathies: a review for pediatricians. Pediatrics 106: 1160–1165

Whiteley RJ, Gnann J W 2002 Viral encephalitis: familiar infections and emerging pathogens. Lancet 359: 507–514

Whitty C J, Mabey D C, Armstrong M, Wright S G, Chiodini P L 2000 Presentation and outcome of 1107 cases of schistosomiasis from Africa diagnosed in a non-endemic country. Transactions of the Royal Society of Tropical Medicine and Hygiene 94: 531–534

World Health Organization, Division of Control of Tropical Diseases 1990 Severe and complicated malaria, 2nd edn. Transactions of the Royal Society of Tropical Medicine and Hygiene, London

Useful links

http://www.aap.org (American Academy of Pediatrics)

http://www.cdc.gov (Centers for Disease Control (CDC) Atalanta, GA, USA)

http://www.cdc.gov/ncidod/dbmd/diseaseinfo/meningococcal_g.htm (Meningococcal disease)

http://www.cdc.gov/ncidod/dvrd/virlmen.htm (Viral meningitis)

http://www.cdc.gov/nip (US national immunisation programme)

http://www.idsociety.org (Infectious Diseases Society of America)

http://www.meningitis-trust.org.uk/ (Information on meningitis from the Meningitis Trust)

http://www.mic.ki.se:80/Physicians.html (List of Karolinska Institute's web resources)

http://www.musa.org/ (Meningitis Foundation of America: support and information)

http://www.ncbi.nlm.nih.gov:80/entrez/query/static/clinical.html (PubMed clinical search)

http://www.phls.co.uk (Public Health Laboratory Service (PHLS) UK)

http://www.tropmed.org (Australasian Society of Tropical Medicine)

http://www.unicef.org:80/sowc00/ (State of the world's children)

PART 13

ALLERGY, IMMUNITY AND INFLAMMATION

The atopic child

M. Gold

General principles

Definition, prevalence and burden of disease

Atopy is defined as the ability of an individual to form specific IgE antibodies to one or more common inhaled aeroallergens such as animal dander, pollen, mould or house dust mite. The clinical expression associated with this immune dysregulation may be an atopic disease which includes:

- atopic dermatitis
- asthma or
- allergic rhinoconjunctivitis.

Interestingly, some atopic individuals do not express clinical disease and the reasons for this variable disease expression are not known. For example, 30–40% of individuals in developed countries can be shown to be atopic yet only 5–20% may manifest an atopic disease.

There is a marked variation in the global prevalence of atopic disease. This variation occurs not only between countries but also regionally within countries. The prevalence is highest in countries that are westernised, industrialised and/or urbanised. In these countries atopic diseases are now the commonest ailments of childhood, and Australian and New Zealand children have the fifth highest global rates of atopic disease (Table 42.1). The prevalence of atopic disease has been increasing in most communities for reasons that are not yet apparent. Environmental factors are thought to account for the variable and increasing prevalence of atopic disease. A commonly cited hypothesis is that the lack of early childhood exposure to recurrent infections, possibly gastrointestinal infections and viral infections, may predispose to atopy in genetically susceptible individuals. Such a hypothesis can be supported by epidemiological and possibly immunological evidence.

Because atopic diseases are common, often chronic and usually begin in early childhood, the burden to the community, family and individual is considerable. The cost burden of asthma to the Australian community is estimated to range from $585–720 million per annum, with the cost of allergic rhinitis being only marginally less. Importantly, the impact of severe atopic disease such as atopic dermatitis, on a family may exceed that of other chronic childhood disorders such as diabetes mellitus.

Pathogenesis

Although atopy is defined by an excessive production of IgE, this is only one of many immunological changes that characterise the condition, which is associated with a complex dysregulation of the humoral and cellular immune systems (Fig. 42.1). For this to occur, both a genetic predisposition and early life environmental allergen exposure are important. Central to this understanding is that naive T helper lymphocytes respond in a particular way to an allergen by secreting specific cytokines which regulate the production of IgE. Continued allergen exposure initiates the allergy cascade, in which there is an early and late response. This occurs in cells located in the skin, respiratory tract, gastrointestinal tract and the vascular system; the end result in some individuals is an atopic disease.

Approach to diagnosis, investigation and management

An assessment of the atopic child should include:
- history and examination, including
  - the presenting and associated atopic disease
  - the differential diagnoses
  - any extrinsic triggers, including allergens
  - any complications and associated conditions
- investigations
  - allergen specific IgE
- management
  - avoidance of any extrinsic triggers, including allergens

Table 42.1 Prevalence (%) of atopic disorders among Australian children. (Data obtained from the International Study of Asthma and Allergy in Childhood questionnaire based survey of 10 914 children in Melbourne, Sydney, Adelaide and Perth (see Further Reading))

Disorder	6–7 year olds (%)	13–14 year olds (%)
Eczema ever (current eczema)	23 (11)	16 (10)
Asthma ever (current wheeze)	27 (25)	28 (29)
Hayfever ever (current rhinitis)	18 (12)	43 (20)

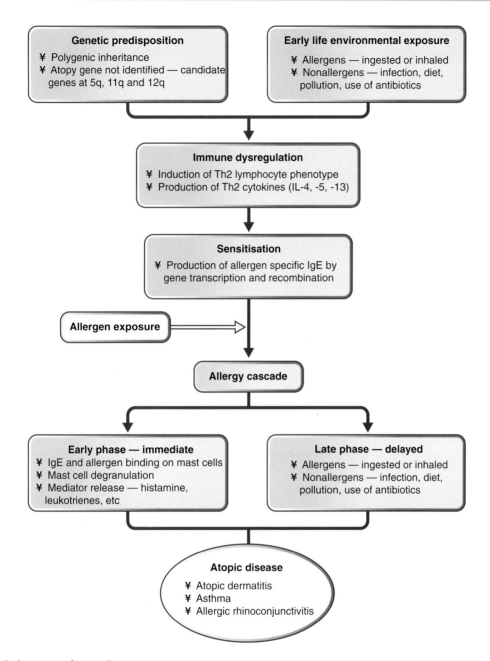

Fig. 42.1 Pathogenesis of atopic disease.

— symptomatic treatment
— additional interventions: referral, prevention, immunotherapy.

History and examination

The history and examination should cover the following aspects:
• Specific symptoms
— Nature, timing (seasonal, perennial, episodic), situational (specific site or circumstance).
• Severity of symptoms and degree of disability

— Medication required to control symptoms, medical visits and hospitalisation, school absenteeism, interference with sleep, sport or play.
• Use of medication
— Current and past medications, efficacy, compliance, technique of use and side effects.
• Environmental history — identification of triggers
— Exposure to common allergens (Table 42.2) and non allergen (for example, cigarette smoke) triggers should be considered.
— A trigger may be easily identified if the onset of symptoms is acute and occurs soon after exposure,

407

Table 42.2   Allergens that may trigger symptoms in atopic children

Inhaled allergens
Animal dander — cat, dog, horse, rabbit
Pollen — grass (rye, couch, timothy), weed (plantain), tree (olive, plane)
Mould — *Alternaria, Aspergillus, Cladosporium, Pencillium* spp.
House dust mite — *Dermatophyagoides pteronyssinus, D. farinae*
Cockroach

Ingested allergens
Food — cows' milk, egg, nuts, fish, shellfish, soy, wheat, fruit
Medication — antibiotics (penicillin) and non antibiotic medication

Miscellaneous
Latex contained in balloons and surgical gloves

Table 42.3   Examination of the atopic child

Growth	Weight
	Height
Facies	Facial pallor
	Allergic shiners — infraorbital dark circles due to venous congestion
	Dennie–Morgan lines — wrinkles under both eyes
	Mouth breathing
	Dental malocclusion — from longstanding upper airway obstruction
	Sinus tenderness
Skin	Atopic dermatitis
	White dermatographism — white discoloration of skin after scratching
	Xerosis — dry skin
	Urticaria and/or angio-oedema
Nose	Horizontal nasal crease
	Inferior nasal turbinates — pale and swollen
	Clear nasal discharge
Respiratory	Chest deformity — Harrison sulcus, increase in AP diameter
	Respiratory distress
	Wheeze and/or stridor
Eyes	Conjunctivitis
	Subcapsular cataracts associated with conjunctivitis
Ears	Tympanic membrane dull and retracted
Throat	Tonsillar enlargement
	Postpharyngeal secretions and cobblestoning of mucosa
Cardiovascular	Blood pressure

if symptoms occur in a specific geographic location, are seasonal, or occur repeatedly following similar exposures.
— A trigger may be difficult to identify when continuous exposure results in chronic symptoms.
— Identification of possible triggers requires knowledge of the likely circumstances of allergen exposure.
• On examination atopic children may have a typical appearance (Table 42.3).

Assessment

Once the history and examination are completed there is seldom difficulty in diagnosing the presenting atopic disease. However, since many children manifest more than one atopic disease, it is important to consider whether any other of the atopic conditions is present. A differential diagnosis should be considered, as uncommon disorders may be missed and may assumed to be due to an atopic disease (Table 42.4).

Investigations

Investigations in the atopic child are limited. Total IgE is elevated in the majority of children with atopic disease but there is substantial overlap with non atopic children. Measurement of total IgE is seldom indicated. Allergen specific IgE (ASE) is more useful and can be determined using both in vivo (skin testing) and in vitro (serological) methods (Table 42.5). Measurement of ASE may be helpful in identifying a specific allergen trigger. However, interpretation of the ASE result is critical:
• The presence of specific IgE to an allergen is only one factor in establishing if the allergen is a clinically significant trigger.

• The predictive value of a negative result is higher than the predictive value of a positive result.
• The result should always be correlated with the history and/or a trial of allergen avoidance with or without subsequent challenge.
• An ASE result should always be discussed with the parent or caregiver to avoid misinterpretation. Failure to do this often leads to inappropriate avoidance measures, which is particularly important when foods are excluded from the diets of children solely on the basis of a positive ASE result.

Management

The aims of management in atopic disease may vary depending on the clinical context.

Table 42.4	Differential diagnosis of atopic disease
Atopic disease	Differential diagnosis
Atopic dermatitis	Seborrheic dermatitis Psoriasis Wiskott–Aldrich syndrome* Hyper IgE syndrome*

Asthma	Infection — viral, bacterial, mycobacterial
	Congenital anomaly, e.g. vascular ring
	Cystic fibrosis
	Immunodeficiency disease
	Aspiration syndrome secondary to
	    gastro-oesophageal reflux,
	    incoordinate swallowing, or
	    tracheo-oesophageal fistula
	Inhaled foreign body
	Cardiac failure

Allergic rhinitis	Infective rhinitis Non allergic rhinitis Vasomotor rhinitis Rhinitis medicamentosa Sinusitis Adenoidal hyperatrophy Nasal polyps Nasal foreign body Choanal atresia (unilateral, bilateral)

* These immunodeficiency diseases may have atopic dermatitis as a component.

Table 42.5	Determination of allergen specific IgE	
	Skin testing	Serology
Method	Skin puncture test	RAST
Availability	Limited	Widely
Expense	Cheap	Expensive
Results	Immediate	Delayed
Risk of anaphylaxis	Rare	Nil
Interference	Antihistamines Extensive atopic dermatitis Dermatographism	High total IgE
Sensitivity	++++	++
Specific	++++	++

Prevention of atopic disease

The offspring of families at high risk because either or both parents and/or siblings have an atopic disease have been targeted for the primary prevention of atopy. Current primary preventative strategies have recommended reduced exposure to environmental allergens and irritants perinatally, during infancy and in early childhood. The hypothesis is that reduced exposure during this critical period will prevent (or delay) the onset of atopic disease in genetically susceptible individuals.

Prenatal exposure to tobacco smoke is a risk factor for wheezing in infancy and postnatal exposure is associated with an increased incidence of asthma and allergic rhinitis. The effect of exposure to inhalant allergens in early life is important. Exposure to indoor allergens, particularly house dust mite, is also an important risk factor for the development of asthma. Dietary manipulation in the first months of life has been used in attempts to prevent atopic dermatitis and associated food allergy. Although further studies are awaited to assess the role of early avoidance of allergens in the prevention of atopic disease, it would appear sensible to advise families who have infants at high risk of atopy to:

- avoid exposing the infant to tobacco smoke.
- prolong breastfeeding (12 months if possible).
- delay the introduction of solids (4–6 months).
- consider use of a hypoallergenic formula if breastfeeding is not possible.
- restrict the maternal intake of allergenic proteins (such as nuts, eggs, cows' milk) during breastfeeding. This measure is controversial and if this is prescribed it should be done in conjunction with a dietician.

Since approximately 50% of infants with atopic dermatitis may progress to develop asthma and allergic rhinoconjunctivitis, strategies are being considered to prevent the progression of atopic disease. A recent double blind placebo controlled study has shown that the daily use of a non sedating antihistamine may prevent the development of asthma in infants with atopic dermatitis who have been sensitised to either house dust mite or to grass pollen.

Management of symptomatic atopic disease

Once the child has developed symptomatic atopic disease, management involves allergen identification and avoidance, and symptomatic treatment. Immunotherapy may be appropriate for selected children.

Allergen identification and avoidance. When possible, this remains an important component of management. Avoidance measures may involve considerable parental education, effort and expense. Note that:

- With ingested allergens these measures are particularly important when atopic disease is associated with a food allergy, as this is the only means of therapy.
- With inhalant allergens, methods have been evaluated to reduce exposure to indoor allergens, most importantly the house dust mite (Table 42.6). A number of studies in sensitised individuals have demonstrated improvements in atopic dermatitis and allergic rhinitis following house dust mite reduction measures. The benefits of house dust mite avoidance in asthma is much more controversial.

Table 42.6 Methods to reduce house dust mite exposure

Definitely useful
Encase bedding in impermeable covers (dust mite covers):
  most important measure since the bed is the major source
Hot water washing of bedding and clothes (>56°C): will
  destroy house dust mite and remove allergens

Probably useful
Replacement of fitted carpets with smooth flooring
Hard surface cleaning with a damp cloth, at least once a
  week

Possibly useful
Air filtration, ionisers and air conditioning

Unlikely to be useful
Acaricides (dust mite sprays) for the carpet and mattress

• Other indoor allergens (cat, cockroach, mould) and outdoor allergens are less easily avoided and alternative forms of therapy may be required.

Symptomatic treatment. When allergen avoidance is difficult, the response is partial or the allergen cannot be identified, symptomatic treatment is indicated. A number of medications are available, including antihistamines, sympathomimetics, mast cell stabilisers, corticosteroids and leukotriene antagonists (Table 42.7).

Induction of tolerance: immunotherapy. Allergen immunotherapy was first used for grass pollen induced allergic rhinitis almost 100 years ago and is only effective for IgE mediated inhalant allergic disease. Although the exact mechanism is not known, the induced state of tolerance to an allergen is associated with the production of block-

Table 42.7 Medications for the symptomatic treatment of allergic disease

	Important mechanisms of action in allergic disease	Examples
Antihistamines	**1st and 2nd generation** H_1-receptor antagonism **2nd generation** Above plus antiallergic effects Decrease mediator release Decreased migration and activation of inflammatory cells Reduced adhesion molecule expression	Diphenhydramine Promethazine Hydroxyzine Cetirizene Loratadine Terfenadine
Sympathomimetics	**Beta agonists** Bronchial smooth muscle relaxation Reduce mast cell secretion **Alpha and beta agonists** Bronchial smooth muscle relaxation Vasoconstriction — skin and gut Inotropic and chronotropic effects Reduce mast cell secretions Glycogenolysis	Salbutamol Albuterol Terbutaline Adrenaline
Theophylline	Phosphodiesterase inhibition Improved respiratory muscle function Respiratory stimulant Improved ciliary function Anti inflammatory effects	Theophylline
Cromolyn	Mast cell stabiliser Inhibits chemotaxis of eosinophils Inhibits pulmonary neuronal reflexes	Cromolyn sodium Nedocromil sodium
Corticosteroids	Reduce T cell cytokine production Reduce eosinophil adhesion, chemotaxis Reduce mast cell proliferation Reduce vascular permeability Reverse adrenoreceptor downregulation	Hydrocortisone Beclomethasone Budesonide Fluticasone/fluisolide Triamcinolone acetonide
Leukotriene antagonists	5-Lipoxygenase enzyme inhibition or LTD4 receptor antagonist	Zileuton Montelukast Zafirlukast

ing antibodies, downregulation of Th2 lymphocytes and a decrease in ASE.

Immunotherapy should be initiated and supervised by an experienced allergist. Pollen induced allergic rhinoconjunctivitis remains the main indication for immunotherapy and should be considered in children who have intractable and disabling symptoms that have failed to respond to allergen avoidance and to symptomatic treatment. Immunotherapy for children who present primarily with asthma is controversial. Not only is the risk of an adverse reaction higher in these children but they are often sensitised to both seasonal and perennial allergens. No form of immunotherapy is currently available for atopic dermatitis.

Future prevention and management of atopic disease

A number of novel approaches and therapies may become available to prevent and manage atopic disease in the future:

- Specific methods of allergen avoidance are being studied in large prospective studies for the primary prevention of atopic disease.
- An alternative approach is to expose high risk infants to an 'allergy vaccine' which would induce a Th1 rather than Th2 lymphocyte response. Measures under current laboratory investigation include the use of novel vaccines and adjuvants.
- For those children with symptomatic atopic disease a number of trials are investigating ways to prevent disease progression or to reduce the long term consequences, such as airway remodelling in chronic asthma. Of particular interest is the role of pharmacotherapy (antihistamines, cromolyn and corticosteroids) or immunotherapy.
- A number of novel immunopharmacological agents are under investigation for symptomatic disease. These include an anti-IgE monoclonal antibody which binds IgE thereby preventing IgE, binding to mast cell receptors. Other agents under investigation include cytokines and cytokine antagonists.
- There is renewed interest in immunotherapy, as a number of new developments are likely to enhance this form of therapy for symptomatic disease. These measures include the use of recombinant allergens, novel adjuvants, combinations of allergens and modulatory cytokines, naked plasmid DNA vaccines, and peptide vaccines.

Specific atopic disorders

The majority of children who develop atopic dermatitis or asthma present by 6 years of age, with most individuals manifesting symptoms of allergic rhinoconjunc-

tivitis by 20 years of age. However, there is a predictable pattern of disease expression which is called the 'allergic march':

- Expression of atopy usually starts with atopic dermatitis, which presents in the first 6 months of life and improves in the second year of life.
- Approximately 50% of children with atopic dermatitis will then develop asthma in early childhood.
- With resolution of asthma in late childhood some children then develop allergic rhinitis, which may be life long.
- Importantly, in a number of children all forms of atopic disease may be expressed concurrently. For this reason, although one atopic disease maybe predominant at a particular age, it is always important to consider which other atopic conditions may be present.

Atopic dermatitis (Ch. 73)

Definition and clinical presentation

Atopic dermatitis is a chronic inflammatory skin disorder that is associated with overproduction of IgE and eosinophils due to a systemic Th2 cytokine response. Histamine, neuropeptides, proinflammatory cytokines, mast cells, eosinophils and antigen presenting cells are all increased in skin affected by atopic dermatitis. The cardinal features of atopic dermatitis include:

- intense pruritus
- a relapsing course
- a typical distribution of skin rash
- a personal or family history of an atopic disease
- additional features which may be present
  — dry skin (xerosis), skin infection, white dermatographism
  — other atopic diseases and atopic facies (Table 42.3)
  — food allergy and intolerance.

The main symptom of atopic dermatitis is intense pruritus, which when severe may be associated with disruption of sleep, school and social interactions and can profoundly affect the quality of life. In older children and adolescents, disfigurement and teasing may be important. The appearance of the skin in atopic dermatitis may be variable:

- In infants with an acute presentation the lesions are erythematous, papulovesicular and mostly occur on the face, scalp, extensor surfaces of the limbs and trunk.
- With increasing age the lesions localise to the hands, feet and the antecubital and popliteal flexures.
- Chronic changes include lichenification of the skin, which is a skin thickening resulting from persistent rubbing and scratching.
- The skin is almost invariably dry and the appearance of the skin may be altered by intense excoriation and secondary bacterial infection.

Investigations

Determination of specific IgE to inhaled or ingested allergens should be considered if the atopic dermatitis is extensive and has not responded to measures of general skin care and symptomatic treatment.

Most affected children above 2 years of age have a raised total IgE concentration and have measurable specific IgE to common inhaled and ingested allergens. This is a marker of atopic status rather than indicating that a specific allergen may be a trigger for atopic dermatitis. Response to withdrawal of the allergen is currently the only way to determine the significance of these results.

Management

A number of triggers may exacerbate atopic dermatitis, including:
- skin irritants (for example, soap, heat)
- viral infection
- food
- allergens such as house dust mite, animal dander, mould and pollen
- bacterial (*Staphylococcus aureus*) or viral (herpes simplex type I) skin infection
- stress.

The aim of management is to reduce as many of these triggers as possible and to provide symptomatic relief until the disorder improves, which fortunately occurs in most children.

The majority of children respond to general measures of skin care, which include:
- avoidance of skin irritants — soaps, shampoo, woollen clothing, hot baths
- frequent use of topical moisturisers (at least twice daily)
- antiseptic measures — antiseptic bath oil, topical antiseptic cream (intermittent)
- wet wraps — wet dressings (bandages) applied to the affected skin.

If symptoms persist despite these general measures then medication should be considered:
- Topical corticosteroids are used commonly:
  - The least potent steroid should always be used for maintenance therapy.
  - If possible steroids should be used intermittently.
  - Potent steroids must be avoided on the face and creases.
- Sedating antihistamines may be useful intermittently particularly for night time itch.
- Antibiotics may also be useful for secondary bacterial infection of the skin.

If symptoms persist and are severe despite general measures of skin care and topical steroids, an allergy review would be appropriate; the aim would be to identify allergens that could be significant triggers. Allergen avoidance is particularly important in infants and children who have associated food allergies and those who have been sensitised to house dust mite.

Unfortunately, there are a small number of children who, despite all these measures, have severe and disabling atopic dermatitis and these children may require intermittent hospitalisation for intensive topical therapy, phototherapy and immunosuppressive medication.

Asthma (Ch. 47)

Definition and clinical presentation

Asthma is defined as a chronic inflammatory lung disorder that is usually associated with bronchial hyperactivity and presents as a symptom complex of cough, wheeze and shortness of breath. Since asthma is discussed elsewhere (Ch. 47), this chapter will review asthma in the context of the atopic child.

Although the exact cause of asthma is not known, the two most significant risk factors are a family history and atopy. Specifically, between 60 and 80% of asthmatic children are atopic. Furthermore, sensitisation to indoor allergens (house dust mite and cockroach) combined with exposure to high levels of these allergens is an important risk factor associated with symptomatic asthma. The implication is that exposure to indoor allergens may contribute to the development of asthma and that ongoing exposure or intermittent exposure may be a trigger factor for asthma.

Role of inhaled allergens in the development of asthma. One of the important features of asthma is airway inflammation, which is characterised by infiltration of the airways with mast cells, lymphocytes and eosinophils. It is postulated that this chronic inflammatory response may be initiated by allergen exposure in a genetically susceptible individual.

Allergen triggers and asthma. Asthma has multiple triggers, the most important of these being viral infections and physical factors such as cold air and exercise. However, in individuals who have become sensitised to inhaled allergens, further allergen exposure may act as a trigger for asthma:
- Bronchial challenge studies show that acute bronchospasm can be induced in atopic asthmatics by inhalation of aeroallergens.
- Epidemics of asthma have been documented in association with airborne allergens.
- The level of exposure to indoor allergens has been correlated with the extent of asthma severity.
- In controlled settings asthmatic symptoms, peak expiratory flow rate and bronchial hyperresponsiveness improve when individuals avoid allergens to which they are allergic.

Investigations

Demonstration of ASE may be useful in children who:
- Present with the symptom complex of cough and/or wheeze and in whom the diagnosis of asthma may not be clear, as atopy is commonly associated with asthma.
- Have persistent asthma. Determination of ASE to inhaled allergens could be considered part of routine asthma management in children with persistent asthma. Identification of those individuals sensitised to animal dander and house dust mite may be useful.
- Determination of ASE is not indicated in episodic asthma because viral infection is the most frequent trigger. However, if a specific inhaled allergen trigger is suspected from the history, ASE may be helpful.

Management

The management of asthma depends on the frequency and severity of the condition. Episodic asthma may require intermittent treatment, while persistent asthma may require continuous treatment (Ch. 47). Asthma education is critical and includes an explanation of the disease, education about techniques of using the inhalers and spacers, home monitoring, an explanation of the side effects of medications, an action plan for home treatment, and education about allergen avoidance.

Allergen identification and avoidance in asthma

Studies of dust mite reduction in atopic asthmatics with persistent asthma have had variable results. It is clear that studies that have markedly reduced the exposure of asthmatics to house dust mite (for example by hospitalisation) have shown an improvement in asthma. However, clinical trials that have aimed to reduce dust mite exposure in patients' homes have had more variable results, which probably correlate with the effectiveness of dust mite reduction methods. Although effective methods have been evaluated to reduce house dust mite levels, these are expensive and time consuming and often not adhered to by patients (Table 42.6). Removal of pets from the homes of sensitised asthmatics should be recommended but occurs uncommonly.

Ingested allergens rarely trigger asthma as a sole manifestation. Other features in relation to episodes of asthma are:
- Acute bronchospasm, which may be part of anaphylaxis in asthmatic children but occurs with other manifestations of anaphylaxis, such as skin rash or vomiting.
- Cows' milk ingestion, which is not uncommonly implicated by parents as a cause of upper respiratory tract symptoms, including asthma; however, empiric removal of cows milk from the diets of children with asthma is not justified.
- In some asthmatics, ingestion of metabisulphite, which can result in an immediate bronchospasm. This is because of a pharmacological intolerance to metabisulphite, possibly as a result of direct irritation of the airway. Metabisulphite is a commonly used preservative in a number of food substances including meat, dried fruit, fruit juices and hot chips.

Allergic rhinoconjunctivitis (Ch. 75)

Definition and clinical presentation

Allergic rhinoconjuctivitis is rare in infants under 6 months old. Perennial allergic rhinoconjuctivitis may occur at any age in childhood and seasonal allergic rhinoconjuctivitis often develops in older children.

The primary functions of the nose are olfaction and air filtration and humidification. This is achieved by the nasal structure, which ensures that inhaled air is in contact with an extensive and highly vascular mucosal membrane. In sensitised individuals, mucosal contact with inhaled allergens in the nose and conjunctiva elicits IgE mediated mast cell degranulation and a chronic inflammatory response.

The history should determine the specific symptoms, as the presentation is quite variable, with either rhinitis or conjunctival symptoms predominating:
- The symptoms of rhinitis are nasal obstruction, itch, sneezing and rhinorroea.
- Conjunctival symptoms include itching and an increase in tear fluid.

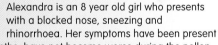

Clinical example

Alexandra is an 8 year old girl who presents with a blocked nose, sneezing and rhinorrhoea. Her symptoms have been present for 12 months, have not become worse during the pollen season and are worse at night. She has been snoring. Nasal decongestants have been used for the past month and have not relieved her symptoms.

The symptoms suggest perennial allergic rhinitis. A complete history should be obtained, including possible exposure to indoor allergens, including animal dander. Skin or radioallergosorbent test (RAST) to indoor allergens would be indicated and, if positive, a trial of allergen avoidance measures would be indicated. Symptomatic treatment with topical nasal steroids should be commenced if there is no response to allergen avoidance. Nasal steroids are more effective than antihistamines for nasal obstruction. Nasal decongestants should not be used for longer than 5 days because of the risk of mucosal damage. With the snoring it would be important to exclude obstructive sleep apnoea (OSA), which is suggested by daytime symptoms such as sleepiness, headache and poor concentration. Continued snoring or symptoms of OSA would necessitate further review to exclude adenoidal hypertrophy.

- The timing of symptoms provides important information concerning possible triggers. Symptoms may be seasonal, perennial, a combination of perennial and seasonal or episodic:
- Symptoms during spring, summer or autumn indicate seasonal allergic rhinoconjunctivitis, which may be triggered by pollen (grass, weed or tree) or mould.
- Perennial symptoms may be due to indoor allergens (house dust mite, animal dander, cockroach).
- Episodic symptoms are most often due to exposure to animal dander but may occur in response to other allergens.

Examination of the nose and eyes is important (Table 42.3):

- The inferior nasal turbinates can be visualised with a light source (using an otoscope), with the diagnostic features being pallor and swelling. When severe, the swollen nasal turbinates may extend to the nasal septum and may be mistaken for nasal polyps, which are uncommon in children. Typical findings may not be present.
- Conjunctival injection and oedema affect both the bulbar and tarsal conjunctiva and appear as redness and swelling.

Rhinitis symptoms may occur without evidence of an allergic cause (Table 42.4). If nasal obstruction is the main symptom, it is important to exclude an anatomical cause. If symptoms such as sneezing, rhinorrhoea and/or obstruction are predominant, alternative diagnoses such as vasomotor or infective rhinitis need to be considered.

Investigations

Determination of ASE is not indicated in seasonal allergic rhinitis unless symptoms are intractable and immunotherapy is being contemplated. ASE is indicated in perennial allergic rhinitis if symptoms are troublesome because, if specific IgE to an indoor allergen(s) can be demonstrated, a trial of allergen avoidance measures would be justified.

Management

In children sensitised to indoor allergens a trial of avoidance measures should be instituted. The choice of symptomatic treatment depends on the nature, severity and timing of symptoms. Intermittent and infrequent symptoms can be treated with antihistamines. Prolonged symptoms are best treated with topical steroids combined with antihistamines if control is inadequate. For seasonal allergic rhinoconjunctivits treatment should be commenced prior to the onset of spring:

- Topical nasal corticosteroids are most effective for nasal obstructive symptoms but also reduce rhinorrhoea, sneezing and conjunctival symptoms. Steroids may take up to a week to work and may require prior use of a decongestant to allow adequate nasal delivery. In general, nasal steroids have been shown to be safe in children but epistaxis may be a problem in some children. This can be reduced by directing the nasal spray away from the nasal septum.
- Cromolyn is a safe alternative for both nasal and conjuctival application but needs to be given frequently because of the short duration of action.
- Antihistamines (oral or topical) are useful for symptoms of rhinorrhoea and nasal itch but are not effective for nasal obstruction. When given orally, non sedating and long acting antihistamines are preferred but often are more expensive.
- Use of nasal decongestants (vasoconstrictors), either topical or oral, for longer than 5 days should be discouraged.

Immunotherapy should be considered in children with pollen induced seasonal allergic rhinoconjuctivitis who have failed to respond to symptomatic treatment, provided the selection criteria have been fulfilled.

Complications of atopic disease and important associated conditions

Food allergy and intolerances

Adverse reactions to food are often reported in children with atopic disease. The important reactions to consider are food allergies and intolerances, particularly in infants and young children with atopic dermatitis (Table 42.8). Conversely, food is an uncommon trigger for asthma and

Table 42.8   Food allergy versus food intolerance

	Food allergy	Food intolerance
Mechanism	Immune mediated IgE mediated Non IgE mediated — cell mediated	Non immune mediated Pharmacological
Food triggers	**Food proteins** Cows' milk Egg Nuts Fish and shell fish Soy Wheat Fruits	**Food chemicals** Food additives Preservatives Food colourings Monosodium glutamate Natural constituents Salicylates Amines Monosodium glutamate

allergic rhinitis. Food allergy and intolerance may occur in children without any atopic disease.

Food allergy

IgE mediated food allergy

It is important to recognise IgE mediated food allergy in children with atopic disease:

- The condition is more common in infants and children with atopic dermatitis. In some studies of children presenting with atopic dermatitis up to one third may have an IgE mediated food allergy.
- Those children who have asthma and IgE mediated food allergy are at greater risk of experiencing more severe reactions, and rarely mortality from anaphylaxis may occur in this group of children.

Diagnosis. The diagnostic hallmark of IgE mediated food allergy is that symptoms usually occur immediately (minutes to hours) after ingestion of the food. Although the most severe manifestation of IgE mediated food allergy is anaphylaxis, a generalised skin rash may be the sole manifestation. Anaphylaxis is a multisystem disorder characterised by involvement of the following systems:

- skin — generalised skin erythema, urticaria or angio-oedema
- respiratory system — rhinorrhoea, sneezing, cough, wheeze, stridor, respiratory distress
- gastrointestinal system — abdominal pain, vomiting, diarrhoea
- cardiovascular system — hypotension if severe collapse with loss of consciousness.

Up to 60% of children who have an IgE mediated allergy to one food protein may have an allergy to another, with the majority having reactions to cows' milk, egg, nuts, soy, fish and wheat. Hence, if an infant presents with reaction to one food it is always important to exclude others.

Non IgE mediated food allergies. Delayed food allergies are thought to be mediated by cellular mechanisms, probably involving T lymphocytes. Cow or soy milk protein is the usual trigger but other food proteins may be involved:

- The most common reaction is an exacerbation of underlying atopic dermatitis, which usually presents as a delayed reaction 1–2 days after exposure to the offending food.
- A number of gastrointestinal manifestation of non IgE mediated food allergy may occur:
  - Cows' milk protein induced colitis presents as a well infant with fresh blood in the stools, which resolves once cows' milk is excluded from the infant's diet or from the diet of the mother if breastfeeding.
  - Food protein induced enterocolitis may present as sudden vomiting, dehydration and collapse, which may be mistaken for a gastroenteritis or bowel obstruction and occurs within hours of exposure to the food trigger.
  - Other manifestations include an enteropathy, which may present as failure to thrive, irritability, chronic diarrhoea and anaemia or recurrent vomiting, which may be mistaken for gastro-oesophageal reflux.

Food intolerances

Food intolerances are thought to be pharmacological in nature. Important food intolerances in atopic children include:

- Metabisulphite, a commonly used preservative, which may trigger acute wheeze in selected children with asthma.
- Facial skin rashes due to contact irritation from foods such as tomato and citrus are common in children with atopic dermatitis.
- Generalised exacerbations of eczema may occur in children with atopic dermatitis due to a food intolerance.

Investigations of food allergy and intolerance

The investigation of food allergy and intolerance is limited:

- If an adverse food reaction is thought to be IgE mediated, determination of ASE is indicated. However,

Clinical example

Michaela is a 12 year old girl with severe persistent asthma. She presents for follow up after a recent admission to the intensive care unit for acute respiratory symptoms diagnosed as status asthmaticus. In passing, her mother mentions that immediately prior to her most recent episode she had inadvertently eaten a chocolate containing peanuts. She does not eat peanuts because she reports that it makes her mouth 'feel funny'. Her mother recalls that as an infant she experienced two episodes of generalised skin rash immediately following peanut ingestion.

The history is suggestive of an IgE mediated peanut anaphylaxis. Children with asthma are at increased risk of mortality from anaphylaxis. Additional questions in the history should ascertain whether she experienced any urticaria, angio-oedema, abdominal pain, or vomiting with the most recent episode, as this would confirm the recent presentation as being due to anaphylaxis rather than status asthmaticus. A skin or RAST test to peanut should be obtained. Management should include the complete dietary exclusion of all nuts, an anaphylaxis action plan, adrenaline for first aid use (Epipen), and a Medic Alert bracelet. Her parents and other carers (including those at school) should be trained to use the anaphylaxis action plan. At this age nut allergy is likely to be life long.

foods should not be excluded from the diet based solely on a skin or RAST test.

- There are no validated tests for non IgE mediated food allergy or food intolerances. The only investigation is to demonstrate an improvement of symptoms following withdrawal of the food trigger and recurrence of symptoms with rechallenge. Double blind and placebo controlled challenges are preferable but are seldom available except in specialised facilities. An open and non blind challenge is more practical but is less accurate.
- Empiric use of a diet which eliminates a number of naturally occurring food substances should never be instituted for more than 4 weeks and should be used as a diagnostic trial. If the child responds this should be followed by appropriate challenges to identify food triggers.
- Use of unsubstantiated tests, for example 'Vega' or 'Cytotoxic' tests, should never be used to diagnose food allergy or intolerance.

Clinical example

Justine is 6 months old and is known to have atopic dermatitis. She has been otherwise well and her current weight is 10.0 kg. She is breastfed and because her mother is about to return to work she is offered her first bottle feed containing a cows' milk protein formula. Immediately after drinking a small amount she becomes irritable, vomits and then develops generalised urticaria, a persistent cough, difficulty breathing and stridor.

This infant has experienced an anaphylactic reaction to cows' milk protein. Although this is the first apparent exposure, she is likely to have been exposed to cows' milk protein in maternal breast milk. Adrenaline is required for the emergency management and is most easily administered by deep intramuscular injection (0.01 ml/kg of 1:1000, that is, 0.1 ml at Justine's weight of 10.0 kg). The response is usually rapid but the dose can be repeated until a clinical response is obtained. It is important to ensure that the family is educated regarding subsequent exclusion of cows' milk from her diet. In addition, other allergenic food proteins including egg, nut, soy, fish, shellfish and wheat should be excluded if these have not yet been ingested and tolerated. Determination of specific IgE to these food proteins and an allergy review would be indicated. Tolerance to cows' milk develops in the majority of children by school age.

Management

The only management available for food allergy or intolerance is exclusion of these foods from the childs diet. Additionally:

- Education of the parents and other carers, particularly when young children attend child care and kinder-

garten, is essential and may require the advice of a dietician.

- In breastfed infants with atopic dermatitis and food allergy, exclusion of food triggers from the maternal diet may also be tried but this is best done with the support of a dietician.
- With any exclusion diet it is important to ensure that the diet is nutritionally adequate. This is particularly important as regards calcium intake when milk products are excluded.
- In atopic children who have had food anaphylaxis the following points are important:
  — Anaphylaxis is a medical emergency and requires prompt recognition and treatment (Table 42.9).
  — All children should undergo subsequent specialist review.
  — Appropriate dietary advice is essential to avoid recurrent episodes.
  — Adrenaline for first aid use by parents and other carers should be considered. This is most conveniently prescribed in the form of an autoinjector device (Epipen). Appropriate training and documentation in the form of an anaphylaxis action plan is essential.

Prognosis

The natural history of food allergy and intolerances is to improve with increasing age. IgE mediated nut, fish and shellfish allergies are an exception since these allergies may be life long, although tolerance may develop in up to 10% of children. Therefore carefully supervised challenge with the implicated food at 6 month intervals is recommended with the exception of food anaphylaxis.

Table 42.9   Emergency management of anaphylaxis

1. Remove the trigger
2. Administer adrenaline by deep intramuscular injection: 0.01 ml/kg of 1:1000 adrenaline (max. dose 0.5 ml)
3. Establish an airway if required and administer oxygen
4. Assess circulation. If hypotensive: administer i.v. adrenaline dose 0.1 ml/kg of 1:10 000 (max. dose — 3 ml); administer i.v. fluids, normal saline 10–20 ml/kg as a bolus
5. Repeat doses of adrenaline can be administered every 5 minutes until clinical improvement occurs
6. Antihistamines and steroids are not administered for the initial management but should be given as second line therapy

Recurrent or chronic sinusitis in allergic rhinitis

Allergic rhinitis should be considered as a possible predisposing factor in children who:

- Have recurrent or chronic sinusitis. The orifices of the frontal, ethmoid and maxillary sinuses are located in close proximity to the nasal turbinates and rhinitis may predispose to ostial obstruction. Symptoms of sinusitis in older children and adults are typical and include facial pain, toothache, headache and fever (Ch. 75); however, young children may present with rhinorrhoea, cough, postnasal discharge, periorbital swelling, and otitis media.
- Have secretory otitis media, in whom the incidence of atopy is increased. However, it remains unclear whether allergic rhinitis is a significant underlying factor because of eustachian tube obstruction. If indicated, allergic rhinitis should be treated in such children but this may not improve the secretory otitis media.

Obstructive sleep apnoea in allergic rhinitis

Nasopharygeal obstruction in children may present with snoring and, if severe obstructive sleep apnoea (OSA). OSA may present in children with early morning headache, daytime sleepiness and poor concentration. Children who present with allergic rhinitis should be questioned about these symptoms and those children presenting with upper airway obstruction should be evaluated and, if needed, treated for allergic rhinitis.

Skin infection in atopic dermatitis

Bacterial, viral and fungal skin infection is an important complication of atopic dermatitis:

- *Staphylococcus aureus* is detected almost universally in atopic dermatitis. The organism produces exotoxins which may potentiate the inflammatory process. Topical antiseptic measures are important but oral antibiotics may be required.
- Herpes simplex virus (HSV) type I may infect lesions and present as vesicular lesions which soon ulcerate. Generalised HSV skin infection may be severe and would be an indication for hospitalisation and parenteral aciclovir.
- Dermatophyte infections may occur in atopic dermatitis and should be considered in resistant lesions.

Spasmodic croup

Spasmodic croup is a condition of recurrent sudden upper airway obstruction which presents as stridor and cough, usually in the early hours of the morning (Ch. 46). Typically the condition is short lived and there are no features to suggest an infective laryngotracheobronchitis such as fever or coryza. Approximately 50% of these children have an atopic disease. The condition is managed symptomatically and there is no evidence to suggest that measures such as allergen avoidance or symptomatic treatment with antihistamines are useful.

Immunodeficiency and its investigation

D. M. Roberton

Infections are part of normal childhood, but some children have unusual susceptibility to infection because of deficiencies in their immune defences.

Resistance to infection

Resistance to infection is provided by two major mechanisms: non specific defences, and specific immune responses. Components of the non specific immune responses are:

- intact epithelial barriers, for example skin and mucosal surfaces
- normal production and flow of secretions and body fluids, for example respiratory tract secretions, tears and urine
- normal microbial flora, for example the skin and gastrointestinal tract
- normal numbers and function of phagocytic cells (polymorphonuclear cells, macrophages) and normal complement function.

These non specific immune defences provide varying degrees of protection against any pathogen. In contrast, the adaptive immune response provides specific immune responses unique to the antigens of the agents causing the infection. This is associated with the development of immunological memory. Important components of the adaptive or specific immune response are:

- Antigen processing and presentation. This may be by macrophages, epithelial cells, B cells or T cells.
- B cells, which are responsible for the production of antibody.
- Specific antibody of varying isotypes in serum, tissues and secretions, including breast milk.
- T cells, which are activated by presentation of antigen, interactions with other cells and by the actions of cytokines.

The adaptive immune response is an integral part of the inflammatory response and is controlled by a complex series of interactions. Defects in the immune response may be due to:

- immaturity, as in prematurity and early childhood
- failure of development of components of the immune response, as seen in the primary immunodeficiency disorders

- acquired disorders, as in HIV or other infections, immunosuppression, and loss of mediators of the immune response.

Development of the immune response

Fetus

Components of the adaptive immune response appear during the first trimester of pregnancy. However, the fetus exists in an environment which is effectively free of extrinsic antigen. Therefore no specific immune responses develop until exposure to the microbiological environment occurs at the time of birth. To afford some protection in the early neonatal period, there is active transport of IgG from the maternal circulation to the fetus during the latter part of the second trimester and the third trimester. There is no transfer of IgA or IgM. Infants born prematurely may fail to acquire some of this maternally derived antibody.

Neonate

Some components of the immune response at birth remain immature. T lymphocytes respond to mitogens satisfactorily, but have a phenotype which is representative of naive cells (CD45RA) and are deficient in their ability to produce or express some cytokines, particularly interferon γ.

T cell help for some B cell responses is diminished. The neonate has almost no IgA or IgM at birth, and B cells are slower in their ability to produce these immunoglobulin isotypes than adult B cells. The development of antibody of high affinity for antigen also may be deficient. There is very little antibody in secretions in the neonatal period and in infancy. Breastfeeding provides secretory IgA and specific antibody as a form of passive immunity.

Some complement components are present in only low concentrations at birth, and neutrophil migration may be deficient in the newborn.

Infancy and later childhood

Maternally acquired IgG is catabolised during the first months of life and IgG concentrations in serum reach their lowest levels at 3 months of age. Endogenous immunoglobulin production commences at birth, with serum IgM concentrations becoming equivalent to adult levels by about 3 years, IgG by 5–6 years and IgA by 9–12 years. Antibody formation to polysaccharide antigens, such as pneumococcal or haemophilus outer membrane polysaccharides, is T cell dependent and is poor during the first 2 years of life.

Cytokine production and T cell help become more mature during the first 2 years of life, and memory lymphocyte development occurs rapidly during the first few months after birth. Complement concentrations rise relatively early, and neutrophil migration matures rapidly.

Consequences of immaturity of the immune response in early childhood

Whereas there is a relative immunodeficiency at birth, it is the immunological naivety of infancy and early childhood that is responsible for the increased incidence of infection seen in early childhood in comparison with later life.

During childhood, the immune system encounters many infecting agents for the first time and specific primary immunological responses develop with each new infection. Therefore childhood is a period during which the overall frequency of infections is increased. Reinfection is prevented on subsequent challenge by the rapid recruitment of secondary responses, a function of memory lymphocytes. The number of infections per year of life is maximal between the second and fourth years, with half of all children experiencing nine or more infections between their third and fourth birthdays. During the first 12 years of life, the mean number of infections experienced per child in a cohort study of Australian children was 67.

Primary immunodeficiency disorders

The primary immunodeficiency disorders are relatively rare disorders which are often congenital and sometimes familial. In these disorders the defect in the immune system usually is a functional defect of one component of the immune response. The World Health Organization Working Party classification of the major primary immunodeficiency disorders is given in Table 43.1.

Table 43.1   WHO classification of primary immunodeficiency disorders

Disorder	Inheritance
1. Predominantly antibody deficiency	
X linked agammaglobulinaemia (XLA)	XL
Common variable immunodeficiency (CVID)	Unknown, some AR
Hyper IgM syndrome (HIM)	XL (sometimes AR)
IgA deficiency	Unknown
Selective IgG subclass deficiency	Unknown
Transient hypogammaglobulinaemia of infancy	Unknown
Antibody deficiency with normal immunoglobulins	Unknown
2. Combined immunodeficiencies	
Severe combined immunodeficiency (SCID)	AR, some XL, some unknown
ADA deficiency	AR
PNP deficiency	AR
3. Other well defined immunodeficiency syndromes	
Wiskott–Aldrich syndrome (WAS)	XL
Ataxia telangiectasia (AT)	AR
DiGeorge anomalad	None
4. Defects of phagocytic cell function	
Chronic granulomatous disease (CGD)	XL, some AR
Leucocyte adhesion defects	AR
G6PD deficiency	XL
Myeloperoxidase deficiency	AR
Shwachman syndrome	AR

Table 43.1 (continued)

Disorder	Inheritance
5. Complement deficiencies	
C1 inhibitor deficiency	AD
Deficiencies of individual complement components or control proteins	Usually AR
6. Other	
Chronic mucocutaneous candidiasis	Variable
Hyper IgE syndrome	Variable, some AD

XL, X linked; AR, autosomal recessive; AD, autosomal dominant; ADA, adenosine deaminase; PNP, purine nucleoside phosphorylase; G6PD, glucose 6 phosphate deficiency.

In recent years the gene localisation and the molecular nature of the defects in many of these disorders have been elucidated (Table 43.2).

A common feature of these disorders is susceptibility to recurrent and/or unusual infections. Investigation for the detection for a primary immunodeficiency is undertaken when:
- there is an unusually high frequency of infections
- infections recur repeatedly after appropriate antibiotic treatment
- infections occur with organisms which usually are of low pathogenicity
- there is family history of a primary immunodeficiency disorder
- there are clinical or phenotypic features which frequently are associated with a primary immunodeficiency.

Investigation

Initial screening for many of the primary immunodeficiency disorders can be undertaken very simply by doing tests on a 1 ml blood sample, as shown in

Table 43.2 Gene localization and molecular defects in some of the primary immunodeficiency disorders

Disorder	Location	Molecular defect
Autosomal		
DiGeorge	22q11	Submicroscopic deletions
ADA def	20q3.1	ADA
PNP def	14q3.1	PNP
Ataxia telangiectasia	11q22–23	
CVID	?6p21.3	
IgA deficiency	?6p21.3	
IgG subclass def	2p11; 14q32.3	
LAD1 and 2 def	21q22.3	CD18(b chain) of 11a(LFA1) 11b(CR3) 11c(150/95) Sialyl Lewis X ligand of E selectin
AR CGD	7q11.23	p47-phox
	1q25	p67-phox
	16q24	p22-phox
X linked		
XLA	Xq21.3–q22	btk
XLHIM	Xq26–27	CD40L
XCGD	Xp21.1	gp91-phox
XSCID	Xq13.1–q21.1	IL2Rγ chain
Wiskott–Aldrich	Xp11–p11.2	WASP

phox, phagocyte oxidase.

Table 43.3 Laboratory tests used in the investigation of primary immunodeficiency disorders

Test	Relevant information
Initial screening tests	
Complete blood count	Neutrophil, lymphocyte and platelet numbers
Immunoglobulins	IgG, A and M concentrations
Antibody formation	Antitetanus and antidiphtheria antibody to vaccine antigens
More complex investigations	
Lymphocyte phenotypes	Presence of lymphocytes expressing particular cell surface receptors (for example, CD3: T cells; CD19: B cells)
Lymphocyte proliferation	Ability of lymphocytes to respond to proliferative stimuli (for example, phytohaemagglutinin or anti-CD3 antibody)
Immunoglobulin subclasses	Age related concentrations of IgG 1, 2, 3 and 4
Neutrophil function	Neutrophil oxidative function, microbial killing capacity and chemotaxis
Complement studies	Quantitative and functional analyses
Chromosomal and molecular studies	Definitive studies to determine specific defects and for genetic counselling and antenatal diagnosis

Table 43.3. These tests are available in most laboratory services. More complex tests, some of which are also shown in Table 43.3, should be undertaken in more specialised immunology service laboratories.

Treatment

The principles of treatment of the primary immunodeficiency disorders are the following:

- awareness of the high susceptibility to infection and the early use of appropriate antibiotics
- prophylactic use of antibiotics in some conditions — for example, cotrimoxazole in chronic granulomatous disease (CGD) and for pneumocystis prophylaxis in severe combined immunodeficiency (SCID); intermittent ketoconazole in chronic mucocutaneous candidiasis
- replacement therapy where possible — for example, intravenous immunoglobulin in hypogammaglobulinaemia; bone marrow transplantation in SCID and Wiskott–Aldrich syndrome; purified C1 inhibitor in acute episodes in C1 inhibitor deficiency
- avoidance of immunisation in, for example, SCID and panhypogammaglobulinaemia.

Brief details of some of the primary immunodeficiency disorders are given below.

Predominantly antibody deficiencies

X linked agammaglobulinaemia (XLA)

Boys with this disorder experience recurrent bacterial infections from the age of 3–6 months as passively acquired maternal IgG concentrations fall. Nose, middle ear and lower respiratory tract infections are common. Recurrent or chronic lower respiratory tract infections lead eventually to bronchiectasis. The usual infecting organisms are *Streptococcus pneumoniae*, *Haemophilus influenzae* and *Staphylococcus aureus*. Bacterial meningitis, septicaemia, septic arthritis and osteomyelitis occur with increased frequency.

Immunological abnormalities are:

- absent B cells
- markedly low IgG concentrations and absent IgA and IgM
- absence of functional antibody.

The defect is due to btk gene mutations. The gene product is a kinase that is an important component of B cell intracellular signalling after activation of the B cell receptor. Many different mutations of btk have been described following study of affected kindreds.

The treatment of XLA is:

- replacement therapy with intravenous immunoglobulin at 4 weekly intervals
- antibiotic treatment of specific infections.

Specific therapy to replace the defective btk gene product is not yet available. Identification of the specific mutation in affected kindreds allows effective genetic counselling, carrier detection and antenatal diagnosis.

Common variable immunodeficiency (CVID)

Patients with this disorder develop an acquired panhypogammaglobulinaemia, often in adult life but sometimes in early childhood. They experience recurrent upper and lower respiratory tract and other infections, including giardiasis. Affected individuals have a higher incidence of lymphoid and other malignancies, this being more marked in affected females.

Immunological abnormalities are:

- variable decrease in immunoglobulin isotypes
- poor antibody formation.

The aetiology of the disorder is not yet known, although it is likely that there are abnormalities of T cell regulation of B cell function.

The treatment of CVID is:

- replacement immunoglobulin
- antibiotic treatment of specific infections.

The disorder appears to be sporadic with no inheritance pattern, although there is a higher than expected incidence of selective IgA deficiency in affected kindreds.

Selective IgA deficiency

This is the most common of the primary immunodeficiency disorders (1:500–1:700 of the normal population). IgA is absent from serum and secretions. Most individuals with selective IgA deficiency are asymptomatic, although some have recurrent sinopulmonary infections. These are more common if there is an associated deficiency of IgG2 and/or IgG4 immunoglobulin subclasses. Some infants and young children have delayed maturation of their ability to produce IgA (transient IgA deficiency). Selective IgA deficiency is not an inherited disorder: the underlying defect is not yet known.

IgG subclass deficiencies

Some children with recurrent infections, usually sinopulmonary infections, have deficient concentrations of one or more IgG subclasses. The most common deficiencies are of IgG4 and IgG2. However, there is no clear relationship between susceptibility to infections and specific IgG subclass concentrations in many children.

At age 18 months, Luke was attending a creche 4 days a week while both of his parents worked. He was the youngest of three children in the family. His sister had just started school, at the age of 5 years 5 months, and his older brother who was 4 years old was at kindergarten 4 days a week. All of the children seemed to have frequent colds, and Luke had also had a discharging ear recently. Luke's parents were worried about his recent infections, and his general practitioner arranged for a complete blood count (CBC) and serum immunoglobulin measurements.

The CBC was normal, although his MCV was at the lower limit of the normal range. Lymphocyte and neutrophil numbers were normal for his age. His IgG and IgM concentrations were also normal for his age, but his serum IgA concentration was 0.11 g/l (normal range for 18 months 0.30–1.73 g/l.) IgG subclass concentrations were normal for age. He appeared to have a partial IgA deficiency, which was unlikely to be related to his infections. The infections were more likely to be related to his increased exposure both by attending a creche, and also because of infections transmitted from his older siblings. No specific treatment was required apart from treating each infection appropriately. By the age of 4 years the frequency of infections had decreased, and his serum IgA concentrations had risen to the normal range.

Combined immunodeficiency disorders

Severe combined immunodeficiency (SCID) (Fig. 43.1)

These disorders form a heterogeneous group. A common feature is dysfunction of T cells, leading to poor recognition of antigen and to defective antibody formation. Affected children are extremely susceptible to infection, and most die before the age of 1 year if untreated.

There are several recognisable variants of SCID. Pneumocystis pneumonia is frequent (Fig. 43.2). Infections due to measles and chickenpox usually are fatal. Failure to thrive is due to repeated infections and persistent diarrhoea. Persistent candidiasis is common.

Immunological abnormalities are:

- very low numbers of T cells
- absent B cell function, although in some forms B cell numbers are normal
- absent or non functional immunoglobulin.

The primary defect has been determined in some forms of SCID. Examples are deficiency of the IL-2 receptor γ chain in X linked SCID, and defects of recombination activating genes (RAG) and intracellular kinases such as zap 70 in others. Defects of enzymes necessary for purine metabolic pathways (adenosine deaminase, ADA; purine nucleoside phosphorylase, PNP) are associated with some autosomally recessively inherited forms of SCID. Elucidation of the causative defect in SCID is important for genetic counselling and antenatal diagnosis.

The treatment of the various forms of SCID is:

- antibiotics for specific infections
- cotrimoxazole for pneumocystis prophylaxis
- replacement immunoglobulin
- bone marrow transplantation or stem cell transplantation.

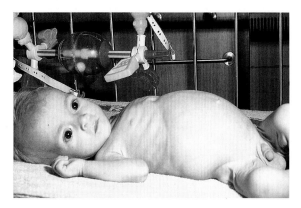

Fig. 43.1 A child with severe combined immunodeficiency. The poor nutrition is due to a chronic diarrhoeal illness and he also has had pneumocystis pneumonia.

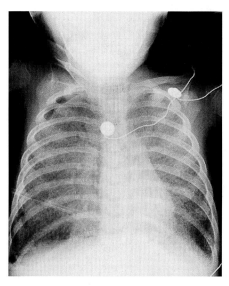

Fig. 43.2 Chest X ray of a 7 month old child with severe combined immunodeficiency and pneumocystis pneumonia. There is diffuse pulmonary consolidation and a pneumothorax is present on the right. There is no thymic shadow.

Severe combined immunodeficiency with ADA deficiency may respond to ADA replacement therapy. Some patients have received experimental gene replacement therapy.

Other well defined immunodeficiency disorders

Children with these disorders have recognisable phenotypic features which lead to the diagnosis.

Wiskott–Aldrich syndrome (WAS)

Affected boys have recurrent infections, eczema and bleeding problems due to platelet abnormalities (thrombocytopenia and small platelet size). Treatment of this disorder is bone marrow transplantation.

Ataxia telangiectasia

This is an autosomal recessive disorder. Affected children often present with progressive ataxia during the first few years of life. Telangiectases are seen on the bulbar conjunctivae, pinnae and elsewhere.

DiGeorge anomalad

This disorder arises from interference with development of structures derived from the third and fourth pharyngeal arches during embryogenesis. It consists of thymic hypoplasia, hypoparathyrodism presenting as symptomatic hypocalcaemia, and congenital heart disease (frequently an interrupted aortic arch or truncus arteriosus). The expression of the disorder is variable; laboratory features are low numbers of CD3 positive cells and hypocalcaemia. Microdeletions of the long arm of chromosome 22 are common in this disorder (Ch. 27).

Defects of phagocytic cell function

Chronic granulomatous disease (CGD)

Abnormalities of NADPH oxidase function in phagocytic cells in CGD cause deficient killing of microorganisms. Most affected children are boys, with X linked inheritance, but some forms have autosomal recessive inheritance. Affected children commonly present with recurrent staphylococcal infections, and also have a high incidence of infection with *Aspergillus* sp.

Immunological abnormalities are:
- deficient killing of staphylococci in vitro
- deficient neutrophil oxidative metabolism.

Clinical example

At age 18 months, Vikram developed an enlarged, painful and fluctuant cervical lymph node. This was drained and *Staphylococcus aureus* was isolated. He had two similar cervical abscesses during the next 18 months. At the age of 4 years he developed a staphylococcal pneumonia, associated with an empyema. Careful enquiry with respect to his family history revealed that a maternal great uncle had died in infancy after presenting with osteomyelitis.

The immunology laboratory reported that Vikram had an abnormal nitroblue tetrazolium test (NBT), a screening test of neutrophil oxidative metabolism. Subsequent tests of neutrophil oxidative function (chemilluminescence and iodination) were deficient, as was neutrophil microbial killing. His mother's neutrophil tests showed partial deficiencies, consistent with a carrier state. Western blotting studies confirmed a gp91 NADPH oxidase abnormality, which is known to be inherited as an X linked abnormality. These results confirmed that Vikram had chronic granulomatous disease (CGD).

After recovery from his pneumonia, Vikram was treated with prophylactic cotrimoxazole daily and interferon γ subcutaneously three times weekly. He was given itraconazole daily in an attempt to prevent infection with *Aspergillus* sp., a common and serious pathogen in CGD. He received a bone marrow transplant from his HLA matched non carrier sister 1 year later, and his neutrophil function after engraftment was normal.

Treatment is:
- prophylactic antibiotics
- interferon γ given subcutaneously
- bone marrow transplantation in some patients.

There is the potential for gene therapy.

Leucocyte adhesion defects (LADs)

Abnormalities of expression of cell surface structures responsible for adhesion and emigration of phagocytic cells lead to failure to respond to infections adequately, with early death. Examples are deficiencies of the CD11a,11b,11c/CD18 adhesion molecule complex.

Complement disorders

These are relatively rare disorders. Deficiency of C2 sometimes is associated with systemic lupus erythematosus. C3 deficiency leads to severe and often fatal infections. Recurrent neisserial infections are seen with deficiencies of the terminal components of the complement pathway (C6–8). Assay of haemolytic complement (CH50) activity is a useful test of the integrity of the classical pathway of complement. C1 inhibitor deficiency is an autosomal dominant disorder which causes intermittent episodes of angio-oedema. These can be life threatening if the airway is involved; urgent treatment with purified or recombinant C1 inhibitor is required.

Secondary immunodeficiency disorders

The immune system is affected secondarily by many other disorders in childhood. The secondary immunodeficiencies are much more common than the primary immuno-deficiency disorders. Secondary immunodeficiency may be due to:
- suppression of the immune system
- loss of immunological mediators.

These may occur as part of the disease process or may be due to treatment.

Table 43.4 lists some disorders which lead to secondary immunodeficiency.

Table 43.4   Disorders leading to secondary immunodeficiency

Disorder	Type of secondary immunodeficiency
Malnutrition	Deficient cell mediated immune responses Zinc deficiency
Loss of mediators	IgG loss in nephrotic syndrome Protein loss in burns Splenectomy
Malignancy	Bone marrow infiltration Lymphoid system malignancies
Immunosuppressive therapy	Corticosteroids (lymphopenia, altered lymphocyte function) High dose cytotoxic therapy Irradiation
Infection	Neutropenia after some infections Depressed cell mediated immunity after measles, disseminated tuberculosis HIV infection (Ch. 41)

Connective tissue disorders

D. M. Roberton, M. J. Robinson

The term connective tissue disorder is used to describe an inflammatory process, usually chronic and of unknown aetiology, which involves non organ specific tissues or tissue components. The events which initiate and sustain the inflammation are unknown. The development of one of these disorders can occur at any time in childhood, and they are not inherited.

Table 44.1 lists some of the important connective tissue disorders of childhood.

Pathology and laboratory findings

The histological features of the various connective tissue disorders differ, but have in common evidence of active inflammation and repair processes. Common findings on investigation in a child with one of the connective tissue disorders are:

- hypochromic microcytic anaemia
- elevated ESR and CRP
- autoantibodies, for example, antinuclear antibody (ANA)
- histological evidence of inflammation in tissues such as synovium, kidney, blood vessels or muscle.

Incidence

The connective tissue disorders in childhood generally are rare. The most common are the various forms of childhood chronic inflammatory arthritis. In some population studies, chronic arthritis of childhood has been found to occur at a rate that suggests an incidence of 1 new case per year per 10 000 children under the age of 16 years. As these forms of arthritis have a duration of

Table 44.1   Inflammatory connective tissue disorders of childhood

Juvenile arthritis
Systemic lupus erythematosus
Juvenile dermatomyositis
Scleroderma
Overlap syndromes
Vasculitides

several years, there may be as many as 1 in every 1000 children with some form of persisting inflammatory arthritis, and mild forms may be even more common.

Other connective tissue disorders are much more rare. Systemic lupus erythematosus (SLE) is uncommon, but is seen more frequently in some ethnic groups, for example in those from some Asian countries, and it is more common in females. In Australia, SLE is up to four times more common in indigenous people than in those of Caucasian origin. Juvenile dermatomyositis and scleroderma are rare in childhood.

Arthritis in children

The term arthritis means inflammation in a joint. Symptoms of arthritis include:

- pain in or around the joint
- warmth
- swelling
- occasionally redness
- loss of function, particularly loss of range of movement.

The acute onset of inflammation in a joint in any child must be considered to be due to infection or trauma until proven otherwise. Infection may occur as a primary septic arthritis, or as extension of infection into the joint space from a nearby osteomyelitis (Ch. 38). Infection in a joint may be seen also in association with other systemic infections. Meningococcal and *Haemophilus influenzae* type b meningitis may be followed by joint infection with these organisms, or by sterile effusions in joints. Trauma may be responsible for joint symptoms in association with a fracture, or disruption of soft tissue elements in or near to the joint. Inflammation in a joint may occur as a result of bleeding into the joint in haemophilia (Ch. 54), or rarely may be due to foreign body penetration.

Chronic or idiopathic arthritis in children

Inflammation in a joint for which no infective or other cause is found, and which persists for more than 6 weeks, is known as juvenile arthritis. Stiffness of joint movement, particularly in the mornings and in cold weather, is common in inflammatory arthritis.

Table 44.2   **Criteria for the diagnosis of juvenile arthritis**

Arthritis of one or more joints, defined as swelling or effusion or two of:

- joint warmth
- pain on motion or joint tenderness
- limitation of motion

Duration of 6 weeks or longer
Age of onset less than 16 years
Absence of other rheumatic disease, mechanical causes or other identifiable joint disorder

The clinical criteria for the definition of chronic arthritis in a child are listed in Table 44.2. Juvenile arthritis differs from adult rheumatoid arthritis, as in almost all instances it is rheumatoid factor (RF) negative. Further, the active inflammation in juvenile arthritis often remits with time.

There are three major categories of juvenile arthritis. These categories are defined according to the characteristics of disease during the first 6 months after onset, even if the pattern changes subsequently. The three major categories in order of prevalence are:

- oligoarthritis
- polyarthritis
- systemic arthritis.

Oligoarthritis

Clinical example

Teresa was 2 years and 4 months old when she developed a painful left knee and began to limp. Her knee repidly became swollen and felt warm to touch. There was no history of any preceding injury, and she had not had any recent infections. Her doctor was worried that Teresa may have had a septic arthritis, or an osteomyelitis in bone close to the joint. She referred Teresa urgently to a children's hospital orthopaedic unit. However, a joint aspirate, blood cultures and a bone scan did not suggest infection, and the knee swelling became less in subsequent days.

A few weeks later Teresa still complained of soreness in her left knee, and had difficulty straightening it in the mornings when she woke. Her right ankle then became swollen and painful. Careful examination of all of her joints showed that she also had some swelling and restriction of range of movement of her right wrist. It appeared likely that she had an oligoarthritic form of juvenile arthritis. Blood tests showed that she was strongly ANA positive (titre 1:1280), and slit lamp examination of her eyes confirmed the presence of anterior uveitis in her right eye. She was treated with night time splinting for her left knee and her right wrist, physiotherapy to improve the range of movement of the affected joints, anti-inflammatory medications, and steroid drops and mydriatics to her affected eye.

This is the most common form of chronic arthritis in childhood and accounts for over half of all cases. By definition, four or fewer joints are involved during the first 6 months after onset. Oligoarthritis is more common in early childhood, with onset being seen most often between the ages of 1 and 4 years. Girls are affected nearly twice as often as boys. Joint involvement almost always is asymmetrical. The joints affected most commonly are the knee joints (Fig. 44.1), followed in frequency by the ankle joints, wrists and elbows. Onset usually is with pain, loss of function and swelling of the involved joint or joints.

The diagnosis of oligoarthritis is one of exclusion. The child presenting with an acute monoarthritis must initially be evaluated carefully for infective or other causes (Ch. 38). Hip disease is rare in this early onset form of oligoarthritis, and a child presenting with hip involvement as the initial manifestation of an arthritis must be investigated carefully for disorders such as

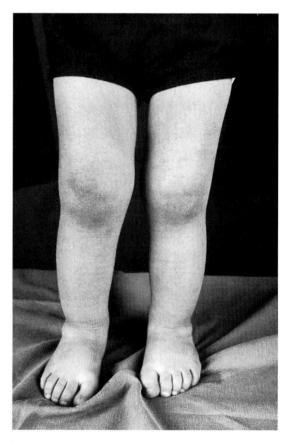

Fig. 44.1   Oligoarthritis involving the right knee joint in a 3 year old boy. There is swelling of the knee due to an effusion in association with synovial proliferation. There is also increased growth of the right leg. This is the result of epiphyseal overgrowth secondary to the increased vascular supply to the area of inflammation.

septic arthritis or osteomyelitis, and, in the appropriate age groups, avascular necrosis of the femoral head (Perthe disease) and slipped femoral capital epiphysis (Ch. 25).

There is little or no systemic disturbance in oligoarthritis. X rays of involved joints show soft tissue swelling, and sometimes effusions and widening of the joint space, but erosions are not present. Epiphyseal overgrowth and lengthening of the involved limb is common as a result of the increased blood supply in the presence of chronic inflammation. Rheumatoid factor is not present, but approximately half of all children with oligoarthritis have a positive serological test for ANA. This group is at higher risk for anterior uveitis (see below).

Polyarthritis

Polyarthritis is less common than oligoarthritis. By definition, five or more joints are involved in the first 6 months after onset. Polyarthritis accounts for approximately one quarter to one third of cases of chronic arthritis in childhood. Girls are affected almost twice as often as boys, and, although the presentation may be at any age in childhood, onset is more common between the ages of 2 and 4 years.

Young children with polyarthritis have asymmetrical large joint involvement, with any of the large joints being susceptible. Asymmetrical small joint involvement is also common (Fig. 44.2). Hip disease may occur, particularly later in the disease course. The degree of disability with polyarthritis can be considerable. Joint deformities are common.

Rheumatoid factor is absent in almost all children with polyarthritis, although a small subgroup may be RF positive (see below). Tests for ANA are positive in some children but less frequently than in oligoarthritis. X rays show similar changes to those in oligoarthritis, although erosions may be seen, particularly in those with severe disease, and may imply a less good prognosis.

Systemic arthritis

Systemic arthritis may have its onset at any age in childhood, and also has been described as a rare occurrence in adults. Extra-articular manifestations are the predominant features at onset, and affected children may not develop evidence for joint disease for many months, making diagnosis difficult.

Systemic arthritis affects both sexes equally, and accounts for about 10% of cases of chronic arthritis in childhood. The initial presentation is with a daily recurrent fever above 39°C, returning to or below 37°C between spikes (quotidian fever). The fever spikes may occur once or twice daily. At the time of the fever, affected children are very irritable and movement appears painful. Individual joints may have no or

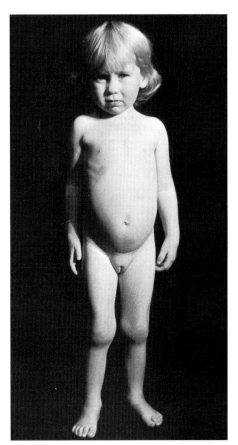

Fig. 44.2 Polyarthritis. This young girl has polyathritis. There is involvement of the ankles, knees, wrists and fingers and swelling of the right shoulder. Both temperomandibular joints are involved, as are her hips and cervical spine.

minimal evidence of inflammation in the early phases of the illness, although muscle tenderness may be present. Spikes of fever may be associated with a classical rash which consists of small salmon pink macules. The macules usually are less than 5 mm in diameter and appear and fade rapidly. The rash commonly is seen on the upper trunk, around the neck and in the axillae. It may be induced by a warm bath or by gently rubbing the skin (Koebner phenomenon).

Generalised lymphadenopathy is frequent, and there may be significant enlargement of the liver and spleen. Serositis occurs, with abdominal pain and pericarditis. Pericardial effusions may be detected by cardiac ultrasound.

Diagnosis often is difficult in the early stages of disease because of the absence of apparent joint involvement. Many of the features of the presentation are consistent with an infective process, and investigations undertaken are those for fever of unknown origin, including serial blood cultures, urine and other cultures. Some malignancies also can present with similar features. Most children will require admission to hospital for further observation and extensive investigation initially. In many cases, the diagnosis is confirmed only later in the course of the disorder when other causes have been excluded and arthritis becomes evident.

Joint involvement can be in large and small joints. Although the course of the arthritis may be prolonged, with exacerbations after many years free of symptoms, most children with systemic arthritis eventually recover with little or no residual disability; however, some may progress to severe and disabling joint deformity.

Other forms of idiopathic arthritis of childhood

There are a number of forms of juvenile arthritis.

Rheumatoid factor (RF) positive polyarthritis

Some children, particularly girls, may present in later childhood or in adolescence with an arthritis associated with persistently positive blood tests for RF. The arthritis usually is symmetrical and involves predominantly small joints. There may be erosions on X ray of involved joints. This disorder appears to be early onset adult type rheumatoid arthritis, and may have a poor outlook in terms of eventual joint deformity and function.

Extended oligoarthritis

A small number of children with onset of arthritis as an oligoarthritis later have involvement of more than four joints, and in particular may develop persisting asymmetrical involvement of small joints of the hands and feet. This is known as extended oligoarthritis.

Psoriatic arthritis

Some children with oligoarthritis or polyarthritis have features suggestive of an association with psoriasis, although the skin rash of psoriasis may not appear for many years. Dactylitis (sausage like swelling of one or more fingers or toes) may be seen (Fig. 44.3), and nail abnormalities (pitting or onycholysis) or the presence of a family history of psoriasis may provide clues to the likelihood of psoriasis.

Enthesitis related arthritis

Enthesitis means inflammation of tendon insertions and fascia. This may be associated with the later development of a spondyloarthropathy, particularly ankylosing spondylitis. The axial skeleton features of restricted spinal movement and sacroiliitis may not appear for some years. Children with enthesitis related arthritis are more likely to be B27 positive. Some children may

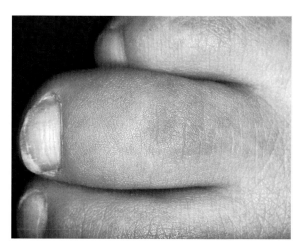

Fig. 44.3 Dactylitis in a child with psoriatic arthritis.

Clinical example

At age 14 years, Tyson had pain at the posterior aspect of his heels, particularly after playing competitive basketball. Physical examination showed tenderness at the insertion of the tendo Achilles bilaterally, and he was also tender over the soles of his feet at the sites of origin and insertion of the plantar fascia. There was slight swelling of his left ankle. He had a normal range of spinal movement, but there was slight tenderness over his right sacroiliac joint on direct palpation, as well as over the sternoclavicular joints bilaterally. He was found to be HLA B27 positive, and his father had a history of back stiffness from early adult life.

Tyson's presentation was of an enthesitis and arthritis, and being B27 positive suggested a higher relative risk of a spondyloarthropathy. It was recommended that he be seen by an orthotist for fitting of heel cup orthoses in his shoes, and he trialled a non steroidal anti-inflammatory drug for 2 months. However, he continued to have significant foot pain and began to complain of low back discomfort, so he commenced sulphasalazine in gradually increasing doses.

---

present with enthesitis related arthritis associated with occult or unrecognised inflammatory bowel disease.

Arthritis in association with other connective tissue disorders

Persisting arthritis occasionally may be seen in some of the other connective tissue disorders such as systemic SLE.

Eye disease in juvenile arthritis

Inflammatory changes of the uveal tract of the eye (uveitis) are a very important associated abnormality in children with almost all forms of chronic arthritis. The highest incidence is in those with oligoarthritis, especially those who are ANA positive, of whom the majority will develop uveitis in one or both eyes at some stage during the course of the disease. However, it may occur in ANA negative children with arthritis, and in children with polyarthritis, systemic arthritis and in those with psoriatic arthritis.

The inflammatory changes of anterior uveitis usually are entirely asymptomatic. Therefore regular examination of the eyes by an ophthalmologist using a slit lamp is essential. This needs to be performed at 4 monthly intervals in many children, particularly those with oligoarthritis. Less frequent assessment may be needed in systemic arthritis. The degree of inflammation in the eye does not relate to the severity or duration of the arthritis: some children may have minimal joint involvement and severe uveitis. Treatment is with mydriatics and topical steroid preparations. Untreated eye disease may lead to severe impairment of vision due to cataract formation and the development of adhesions of the iris (synechiae). An acute symptomatic iritis may occur in the spondyloarthropathy syndromes, and a granulomatous posterior uveitis may be present in sarcoidosis.

Investigation of chronic arthritis in childhood

Useful initial investigations are listed in Table 44.3. A microcytic anaemia may be present secondary to the chronic inflammatory state. The ESR usually is elevated, but may be normal. The ANA pattern, when positive, usually is homogeneous. Rheumatoid factor (IgM antibody against IgG) is persistently positive only rarely, but may indicate RF positive polyarthritis. It may be useful to look for the presence of the HLA B27 antigen if a spondyloarthropathy is suspected or in the presence of an enthesitis related arthropathy. The B27 antigen is demonstrable on blood lymphocytes in approximately 8% of the normal Caucasian population, but is present in at least 90% of those with ankylosing spondylitis.

X rays

X rays of involved joints in the early stages usually show no abnormalities or only soft tissue changes. Changes seen later in the course of the disorder may include bone overgrowth, progressive joint damage, and ultimately joint ankylosis. Ankylosis may be seen in the cervical spine particularly. In very severe disease, and in RF positive disease, there may be joint erosions but these are a relatively unusual finding. X rays also are important in excluding some other disorders which may mimic idiopathic arthritis, for example, bone tumours, unsuspected fractures and radiopaque foreign bodies.

Management of idiopathic arthritis

Management of chronic arthritis of childhood involves management of:
- the disease process
- the resulting disability for the child and his or her family
- associated abnormalities, such as growth effects and uveitis if present.

As for all chronic disorders in childhood a team management programme is important. Members of the team are the family doctor, paediatric rheumatologist, physiotherapist, occupational therapist, social worker, schoolteacher and ophthalmologist. Others who have a role are the orthotist, psychologist, psychiatrist, and support group coordinators or similar patient and family interest group supporters.

Management of the disease process

The principles of management of the disease process are:
- maintenance of joint function
- relief of pain
- anti-inflammatory therapy.

Maintenance of joint function

Joint function is maintained by rest, physiotherapy, and joint splinting when necessary. When a joint is acutely inflamed and painful, rest is necessary to relieve pain. However, gentle passive movement is still important to maintain the full range of joint movement. As inflammation improves, an active exercise programme is introduced as soon as it is tolerated to further improve the range of joint movement and to strengthen muscles around the involved joint. This is done with the guidance of an experienced physiotherapist. Hydrotherapy is an important adjunct to therapy, and usually involves a regular exercise programme in a heated pool.

Splinting is used to maintain involved joints in a good functional position when at rest. This is used most commonly as knee extension splints in bed at night. Other joints where splints are used frequently are the ankle and the wrist.

Table 44.3   Initial investigations in suspected juvenile arthritis

Complete blood examination (CBC)
Erythrocyte sedimentation rate (ESR) and C reactive protein (CRP)
Rheumatoid factor (RF)
Antinuclear antibody (ANA)
X ray of involved joints (may X ray contralateral joints for comparison)
Ophthalmological assessment using a slit lamp

Relief of pain

Persisting pain in the involved joints is a major burden for many children. Pain in the joints of the lower limbs interferes with walking. Pain in any joint can lead to poor sleeping, irritability and a decreased appetite. Inability to do simple activities because of specific joint pain has a marked effect on the child and family. For example, children with painful wrists and fingers may no longer be able to dress themselves or feed themselves. Resting of joints in a functional position may assist in pain control. Warmth may relieve the discomfort of stiff joints, whereas the hot and acutely inflamed joint may be made more comfortable with ice packs. Simple analgesics such as paracetamol are important. The non steroidal anti-inflammatory agents can help with pain control by relieving inflammation, although they do not have primary analgesic activity.

Anti-inflammatory therapy

Non steroidal anti-inflammatory drugs (NSAIDs). The aim of anti-inflammatory therapy in chronic arthritis in childhood is to use the most effective medications with the least possible adverse effects. In the majority of children this can be achieved by use of a non steroidal anti-inflammatory medication. Aspirin is no longer used. An important consideration in young children is that the NSAID be available in syrup form so that it can be taken easily and so that the dose can be titrated accurately. Naproxen is available in syrup form (125 mg/5 ml), as is ibuprofen. Piroxicam is available in a dispersible tablet form. All NSAID medications can cause gastrointestinal irritation, vomiting or bleeding, although these effects seem to be less common in children than in adults. Medications should be taken with meals. The dose of naproxen is 15 mg/kg/day, in two doses. It may be 6 weeks or more before a full anti-inflammatory effect is seen.

Renal dsyfunction has been reported only rarely in children receiving non steroidal anti-inflammatory medications. Some children may develop a scarring porphyria-like rash, particularly on sun exposed areas of skin: the forehead, bridge of the nose, cheeks and dorsum of the hands (Fig. 44.4).

Methotrexate. In children in whom joint inflammation is not controlled adequately with NSAID medications, methotrexate therapy, given as a single weekly dose, has been shown in randomised controlled trials to be beneficial. This should be undertaken only under the supervision of a paediatric rheumatology service. The dose can be increased gradually, with careful monitoring of hepatic and haematological function. It may be several months before improvement in joint inflammation and function is apparent. Methotrexate is the only one of the 'second line' agents shown in controlled trials to have a significant effect on outcome in childhood chronic arthritis.

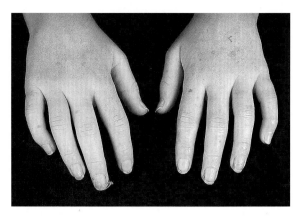

Fig. 44.4 Skin rash associated with the use of a non steroidal anti-inflammatory medication. The rash in this child was due to the use of naproxen, and occurred in sun exposed areas of the skin. It resolved gradually over several years after cessation of the naproxen.

Leflunomide. Leflunomide is a further second line agent which is used frequently in adult arthritis, but it has not yet been trialled formally in childhood arthritis. It is not recommended for use in young children, but may have a place in treatment in adolescents with active arthritis who are unable to tolerate methotrexate.

Sulphasalazine. Sulphasalazine may be of benefit in some children, particularly in those with enthesitis related arthritis and in those with spondyloarthropathy.

Corticosteroids. Corticosteroids may be given orally in severe systemic arthritis to control fever and serositis. In some children with very severe or resistant arthritis, steroids may be necessary to allow reasonable joint function. However, they are likely to be needed long term and have major side effects, particularly on growth; therefore oral steroids are avoided wherever possible.

Intra-articular instillation of triamcinolone acetonide or hexacetonide can be very helpful for control of arthritis in isolated joints resistant to usual therapy, for example in a persistently inflamed knee joint which has not responded to an adequate dose and duration of NSAID therapy. Corticosteroid eye drops are an important part of therapy for uveitis.

Anti TNF therapy. Anti TNF therapies (etanercept, infliximab) are now being used for some children with severe arthritis not controlled by other agents.

Prevention and management of disability

The mainstay of treatment of chronic arthritis in children is the physiotherapy programme to maintain joint function. The physiotherapy programme needs to be tailored to the needs of each joint and to be appropriate to the level of activity and needs of the child and his or her family. Appropriate seating at home and at school, encouragement and assistance with activities of daily living, and information for other caregivers, for example schoolteachers, are all important.

Surgical intervention is needed only rarely, but is appropriate when joints have become severely deformed and when joint replacement is necessary, for example for severe and long standing hip disease.

Disability support allowances paid by government are an important part of assistance for parents to provide the extra care needed. Patient travel allowances and pharmaceutical benefits are also available. Parent and patient support groups are valued greatly by families with affected children.

Management of associated abnormalities

The management of uveitis has been described above. Growth may be impaired in any chronic inflammatory state, and nutritional assessment and advice is important. In children with severe disease and with significant disability, psychological support is also needed.

Outcome of juvenile arthritis

In spite of the significant joint disease seen during the active phases of arthritis, the long term outcome is good when appropriate therapy is provided. Approximately 80% of affected children will have minimal residual joint dysfunction 15 years after onset. The best outlook is for those with oligoarticular disease with onset in early childhood. Long term disability is seen most frequently in those with severe polyarticular onset disease and in those whose systemic disease progresses rapidly to widespread and progressive polyarticular involvement.

Severe impairment of vision with synechiae and cataract formation may occur with aggressive uveitis.

Other disorders associated with arthritis in childhood

Reactive arthritis may occur after gastrointestinal tract infection with *Salmonella*, *Yersinia* and *Campylobacter* species. Usually there is an oligoarthritis which lasts for a few weeks only. Treatment with NSAIDs is usually effective. The Reiter triad of conjunctivitis, urethritis and arthritis is rare in childhood.

Some viral infections may be associated with arthralgia or arthritis. These include rubella, Ross River virus, Epstein–Barr virus and hepatitis virus infections. Some bacterial infections may cause a persistent arthritis: tuberculosis is still an important cause of chronic joint infection in some countries. Tuberculosis may also be associated with a reactive arthritis (Poncet disease).

Lyme disease is rare in Australia but is an important cause of arthritis in some parts of the world. Infection with tick borne *Borrelia* species leads to a rash known as

Table 44.4   Miscellaneous conditions that may be associated with joint pain or dysfunction in childhood

Legg–Calvé–Perthes disease
Slipped upper femoral epiphysis
Transient synovitis (for example, irritable hip)
Foreign body synovitis (for example, plant thorn synovitis)
Chondromalacia patellae and anterior knee pain syndromes
Unrecognised trauma
Some metabolic and inherited disorders and syndromes
Hypermobility conditions
'Overuse' conditions, especially in elite child athletes and
    gymnasts
Reflex neurovascular dystrophy
Conversion symptoms and hysterical gait abnormalities

erythema chronicum migrans, neurological signs and a relapsing arthritis, usually of one or more large joints. It is responsive to penicillin.

Rheumatic fever (Ch. 52) and Henoch–Schönlein purpura (Chs. 54, 62)) have an associated arthritis which is transient in nature. Haemophilia (Ch. 54) with recurrent intra-articular joint bleeding leads to destructive changes in joints, particularly in the knee and the ankle.

Miscellaneous disorders which may present as joint pain or dysfunction in childhood

Other conditions which may present with joint pain or dysfunction are listed in Table 44.4.

Systemic lupus erythematosus

Systemic lupus erythematosus (SLE) is a persistent multisystem disorder of unknown aetiology. Autoantibodies are seen in serum and in tissue biopsy samples but their role in the manifestations of disease remains unknown. The disorder is relatively rare in childhood but probably is more common than scleroderma or dermatomyositis. Presentation under the age of 4–5 years is rare. Girls are affected more commonly than boys, although the female: male ratio is lower than in adult life. Although SLE is often a mild and slowly progressive disorder when it has its onset in adult life, in childhood it is usually severe and often presents acutely. There is a high incidence of severe renal involvement and significant morbidity and mortality.

Clinical features

The onset of SLE is often associated with non specific symptoms of lethargy, low grade fever, loss of appetite, and oral and nasal ulceration. The Raynaud phenomenon may be present and patchy alopecia may occur. By the time of presentation a rash is usually present. This is

Angela developed bruises and recurrent nose bleeds at the age of 13 years. She had been increasingly lethargic and pale for 4 weeks, with weight loss and recurring mouth ulcers. She had complained of aching knees and elbows. She also noted some hair loss. Blood tests showed a haemoglobin of 86 g/l, with 3200 white cells/mm³ and 18 000 platelets/mm³. She was referred to hospital with a provisional diagnosis of leukaemia; however, there were no blast cells in her peripheral blood film.

Further clinical examination showed vasculitic lesions on the tips of her fingers and toes, a faint malar rash, intranasal ulcers, and proteinuria and microscopic haematuria on dipstick testing of her urine. Her ESR was 95 mm/h; she had a positive ANA (titre 1:1280 with a homogeneous pattern); a positive direct Coombs test; low C4 and C3, and a DNA binding assay result of 53 IU/ml (normal range <7 IU/ml). Phase contrast microscopy of the urine red cells showed them to be of glomerular origin. A diagnosis of SLE was made. On high dose prednisolone therapy, given as twice daily therapy initially, her symptoms, haemoglobin, white cell count and platelet count improved. A later renal biopsy revealed diffuse proliferative glomerulonephritis.

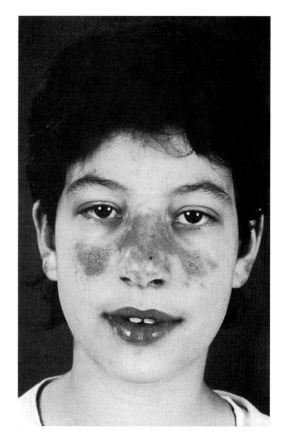

Fig. 44.5 Systemic lupus erythematosus: facial rash in a girl with active lupus vasculitis. There are also vasculitic lesions on both ears.

characteristically a photosensitive vasculitic rash with scaling and erythema over the malar area (Fig. 44.5). Other areas of involvement are the scalp, ears, arms, thighs and the base of the neck. Often there are also vasculitic lesions on the pulp of the digits (Fig. 44.6), extensor surfaces of the arms and legs, and the palate. Purpura or ecchymoses may be present as a result of thrombocytopenia.

Arthralgia and joint symptoms are common, but resolve rapidly when treatment is commenced. Renal involvement causes microscopic haematuria and proteinuria. Some children will present with macroscopic haematuria, a mixed nephritic–nephrotic picture, or with hypertension.

Approximately one third of children with SLE will have central nervous system manifestations. These may be in the form of convulsions, psychoses, headache, chorea or a polyneuropathy. These features are usually secondary to central nervous system vascular involvement. Lung and cardiac abnormalities may also be present.

Laboratory findings

Common laboratory findings are:

- elevated ESR
- leucopenia and Coombs positive haemolytic anaemia
- thrombocytopenia
- low C4
- microscopic haematuria, and altered renal function.

Important diagnostic findings in SLE are the presence of autoantibodies. ANA is present, often in very high titre.

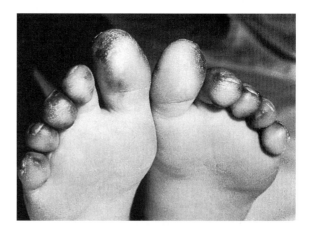

Fig. 44.6 Systemic lupus erythematosus: vasculitic lesions on the toes of a 9 year old girl with active disease. She also had a diffuse proliferative glomerulonephritis and anaemia in association with thrombocytopenia.

The ANA may be directed against extractable nuclear antigens (ENA) and therefore may show specificity against Sm, Ro (SSA) and La (SSB). Antibody against native or double stranded DNA is assessed using the DNA binding radioimmunoassay. High concentrations of antibody against native DNA are associated with more severe renal disease. Anticardiolipin antibody may be present.

Biopsy of involved tissues such as skin and kidney shows evidence of inflammation and immunoglobulin and complement deposition in blood vessels and tissues.

Management

It is often necessary to use high dose prednisone initially in SLE in childhood to control the disease process rapidly after diagnosis. Doses of 2 mg/kg/day up to 60–75 mg per day may be needed, sometimes in split daily doses. In very severe disease, pulses of intravenous methylprednisolone at a dose of 25–30 mg/kg up to a maximum of 1 g per dose may be required for up to 3 consecutive days. The doses of steroids required often lead to significant side effects, including increased susceptibility to infection. SLE itself increases susceptibility to infection; infection is an important cause of morbidity and mortality in SLE.

Other drugs which have a place in the management of SLE are hydroxychloroquine, azathioprine, methotrexate, cyclophosphamide, and cyclosporin A.

Treatment of SLE requires careful and expert supervision. Renal biopsy is necessary in many patients to determine the extent of renal disease and to monitor progress.

The outcome for children with SLE has improved markedly in recent decades. With careful therapy, renal function is maintained. There must always be a high index of suspicion for infection. Side effects of steroid therapy, including avascular necrosis of the femoral heads, decreased spinal mineralisation and growth suppression, are difficult areas of management. The aim of therapy is to allow a normal life expectancy with minimal disease and treatment morbidity.

Neonatal lupus syndrome

Some infants born to mothers with serological evidence of lupus will have transient manifestations of the disorder. These are due to transplacental passage of maternal IgG autoantibody, particularly anti-Ro and anti-La antibody. The most common abnormality is a discoid lupus-like skin rash, which gradually fades as maternally acquired antibody titres decrease. The most important complication is congenital heart block, which persists throughout life and may require placement of a cardiac pacemaker.

Juvenile dermatomyositis

Dermatomyositis in children can occur at any age, but is seen most commonly between the ages of 4 and 10 years. Weakness and tenderness of proximal muscle groups in the limbs is a major component of the disorder and a presenting feature may be a gait abnormality or even an inability to walk. Weakness of muscles may progress to involve the trunk and respiratory muscles in severe disease. In some children onset may be rapid and life threatening; in others progression may be insidious.

A typical feature of juvenile dermatomyositis is swelling and a rash around the eyes. The areas of involvement, particularly of the upper eyelids, are described as having a violaceous colour. There is often also evidence of erythema and vasculitis over the malar areas, V region of the anterior neck and upper trunk, and over the extensor surfaces of the elbows and the anterior aspects of the knees.

Muscle enzymes in serum are often elevated and there may be abnormalities on electromyography and muscle biopsy. Treatment is with corticosteroids in high dose and with very gradual reduction over a period of approximately 18 months. Some children have persistent disease activity or multiple relapses; other treatments used in these situations have been azathioprine, cyclophosphamide, methotrexate and cyclosporin. Complications are muscle contractures, calcinosis of areas of skin and subcutaneous tissue, and rarely a lipodystrophy syndrome. However, many children have a very good outcome after a number of years with appropriate treatment.

Scleroderma

The major feature of scleroderma is thickening and atrophy of the skin and subcutaneous tissues. This may occur in several forms. Localised scleroderma, either morphea or linear scleroderma, is the more common presentation in childhood. Morphea is the development of isolated patches of scleroderma, often over the trunk, where the involved skin becomes thickened, deeply tethered, and has patches of depigmentation and also areas often of excess pigmentation. There are no associated systemic features. Systemic sclerosis is uncommon in childhood.

Scleroderma is particularly difficult to treat, and there is little evidence that immunosuppressive agents are effective in modifying the disease course.

Overlap syndromes

Some children with connective tissue disorders appear to have features of several of the disorders described above. An example is mixed connective tissue disease (MCTD), in which there is the Raynaud phenomenon, nodules, arthralgia or arthritis, and sometimes muscle tenderness and weakness. Patients with MCTD characteristically have a speckled pattern ANA with specificity for U1RNP. Some children with MCTD later develop manifestations of SLE.

Vasculitis syndromes

Table 44.5 provides a classification of primary vasculitic disorders in childhood. The commonest are Henoch– Schönlein purpura (Chs 54, 62) and Kawasaki disease.

Table 44.5	Primary vasculitic disorders in childhood
Category	Example
Polyarteritis	Polyarteritis nodosa
	Microscopic polyarteritis nodosa
	Kawasaki disease
Leucocytoclastic vasculitis	Henoch–Schönlein purpura
Granulomatous vasculitis	Wegener granulomatosis
Giant cell arteritis	Takayasu arteritis
Other vasculitides	

> ### Clinical example
>
> David was 2 years old and had been well previously when he developed a high fever. He became very irritable, refused to eat, and developed marked swelling of his cervical nodes. His mouth and throat were reddened, and he was thought to have a viral infection. Two days later he had marked conjunctival reddening, a measles-like rash on his trunk, and swelling of his hands and feet. A diagnosis of Kawasaki disease was made on the basis of the clinical features. He was admitted to a children's hospital and was given 2 g/kg of intravenous immunoglobulin as an infusion over 10 hours. The fever, rash and irritability resolved rapidly. Echocardiograms were performed on admission, at 6 weeks and at 3 months, but no coronary artery aneurysms were seen. Low dose aspirin (5 mg/kg/day) was given as a single daily dose until the echocardiogram at 3 months after onset was shown to be normal.

Kawasaki disease

Kawasaki disease has been described worldwide, but is more common in children of Japanese descent. It is seen most often between the ages of 1 and 4 years. The diagnostic criteria are a fever of >38.5°C for 5 or more days in the absence of evidence of a streptococcal infection and with at least four of the following five manifestations:

- bilateral non purulent conjunctival injection
- oral mucosal changes (erythema or dry cracked lips or strawberry tongue)
- cervical lymphadenopathy with one node 1.5 cm or more in diameter
- changes in the extremities (swelling of hands or feet, or erythema of palms or soles, or membrane-like peeling of the skin; Fig. 44.7)
- a generalised rash, which often is morbilliform in appearance.

A major complication of this disorder, reflecting its vasculitic nature, is a propensity to develop proximal arterial aneurysms. This is seen in the coronary arteries particularly and is found in approximately 20% of untreated patients on echocardiography. The incidence of coronary artery aneurysm formation can be reduced greatly by treatment with intravenous immunoglobulin during the early phase of the acute illness.

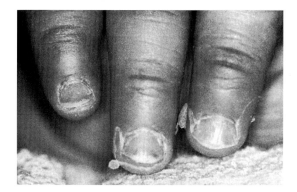

Fig. 44.7 Kawasaki disease. Peeling of the hands or feet later in the course of this disorder may begin in a characteristic periungual distribution, as seen in this 2 year old boy, who also had cervical lymphadenopathy, a rash, non purulent conjunctivitis and intense erythema of the oral mucosa.

PART 13 SELF-ASSESSMENT

Questions

1. A 12 year old with a weight of 40 kg has a persistent asthma. He is stung by a bee and develops the immediate onset of generalised urticaria and angio-oedema. He presents to his general practitioner shortly after the sting and at this stage is noted to have a persistent cough and wheeze. While being assessed he complains of feeling light headed. Which interventions are indicated in the immediate management of this child?
   (A) Intravenous hydrocortisone
   (B) Inhaled ventolin
   (C) Oral antihistamines
   (D) Intramuscular adrenaline
   (E) Normal saline (20 ml/kg)

2. Hannah is 12 months of age and has generalised and severe atopic dermatitis. She was weaned to a cow's milk protein formula at 6 months of age without apparent worsening of her eczema. At 8 months she had generalised urticaria immediately after ingestion of a hard boiled egg. Which of the following should be part of her management?
   (A) Dietary exclusion of cow's milk protein
   (B) Prolonged topical use of potent corticosteroids
   (C) Exclusion of egg from the diet
   (D) Skin or RAST testing to house dust mite
   (E) Daily use of skin moisturisers

3. Sam, a 7 year old boy, has infrequent episodic asthma. Past episodes have always occurred while he is in his own home, and there are no indoor pets. His parents have consulted a naturopath and a 'Vega' test has been performed. This 'shows' that he has had reactions to cow's milk and wheat and these foods have been excluded from his diet. No milk alternative has been added to his diet. Which of the following statements is/are true?
   (A) The 'Vega' test has been validated scientifically
   (B) Skin or RAST testing to indoor allergens is indicated
   (C) He should be commenced on preventer treatment
   (D) His intake of calcium is likely to be deficient

4. Timothy is aged 24 months and has recently had bacterial meningitis due to *Haemophilus influenzae* type b, in spite of having received all of his childhood immunisations, including Hib vaccine. Further enquiry reveals that he has had a persistent cough for about 6 months, and he has had several episodes of otitis media, two of these episodes later being associated with discharge of pus from his ears. Which of the following are appropriate?
   (A) Take a careful family history, with particular emphasis on deaths in early life of male children on the maternal side of the family
   (B) Arrange for blood tests to measure his immunoglobulin concentrations
   (C) Give further Hib immunisation
   (D) Do a chest X ray
   (E) Measure the immunoglobulin concentrations of his 6 month old brother

5. At birth, Jennifer was found to have severe congenital heart disease. She had an interrupted aortic arch, and required early cardiac surgery. She had brief convulsions after the corrective surgery and was found to have a low ionised serum calcium concentration. Immune function tests showed low numbers of CD3 positive cells. Which of the following are correct?
   (A) Fluorescent in situ hybridisation (FISH) chromosomal analysis for a chromosome 22 microdeletion should be done
   (B) Her low calcium concentrations are likely to be due to poor parathyroid function
   (C) She should be assessed for HIV infection
   (D) If a chromosome 22 abnormality is found, other children in the family are highly likely to have the same abmormalities
   (E) The hepatitis B vaccine given to her at birth may have resulted in a hepatitis-like disease because of viral replication in association with an immunodeficiency

6. Cory developed nephrotic syndrome at the age of 4 years. He had marked oedema, including periorbital swelling and ascites, marked proteinuria, and pleural effusions. He was admitted to hospital, and after the diagnosis was confirmed he was treated with high dose prednisolone. Which of the following are correct?
   (A) The major immunoglobulin isotype lost in the urine with his proteinuria will be IgM
   (B) When he recovers, he will need to restart all his childhood immunisations
   (C) He is at significant risk of streptococcal infections while he is proteinuric
   (D) The prednisolone therapy will make him more susceptible to infection
   (E) He should have intravenous immunoglobulin therapy in the acute stage

7. Felicity is aged 18 months and has suddenly stopped walking, preferring to crawl. She cries

435

when she attempts to put weight on her right leg. Her mother has also noted that Felicity has preferred to use her left hand to hold her cup when drinking during the last 8 weeks, having previously usually used her right hand. Examination shows that Felicity has swelling of her right knee, and it is painful to straighten fully. Her knee is only slightly warm to touch. Her right wrist is swollen, and there is significant restriction of movement of her wrist because of pain. She does not have a fever. Which of the following are correct?

(A) Felicity is likely to have osteomyelitis of her right knee and wrist
(B) She should have an ASOT (antistreptolysin O test) performed to exclude rheumatic fever
(C) A finding of a negative rheumatoid factor excludes juvenile arthritis
(D) She should have clotting studies performed to exclude a bleeding disorder
(E) She is only likely to have uveitis if she has more than four joints involved

8. At age 4 years, Zak developed a high swinging fever, marked irritability when his temperature rose above 38.5°C, and seemed very unwell. Extensive investigation did not find any evidence of infection. He was found to have generalised lymphadenopathy and splenomegaly, and he was anaemic clinically. His symptoms persisted for 3 weeks and eventually he was admitted to hospital for further assessment. Which of the following are correct?

(A) His symptoms and signs could be indicative of an underlying malignancy such as a non Hodgkin's lymphoma
(B) He could have systemic onset juvenile arthritis
(C) Echocardiography looking for evidence of a pericardial effusion is indicated
(D) The absence of arthritis on examination would not exclude a diagnosis of systemic onset juvenile arthritis
(E) A fine macular rash apparent around his upper trunk and in the axillae would be consistent with systemic onset juvenile arthritis

9. Yvette had a swollen ring finger for several months at age 7 years. She then developed swelling in one knee and, 10 weeks later, in an ankle. Which of the following are correct?

(A) The swollen ring finger could have been dactylitis
(B) Her presenting history is suggestive of a psoriatic arthropathy
(C) Examination for nail pitting should be undertaken
(D) The silvery scaling skin lesions of psoriasis are often seen over the extensor aspects of the

elbows, in the periumbilical region and at the upper end of the natal cleft
(E) Prednisolone should be used to control her arthritis

10. In childhood systemic lupus erythematosus (SLE) which of the following are common?

(A) A homogenous pattern of ANA antibody
(B) Low C4 concentrations in active disease
(C) Microscopic haematuria at presentation due to red cells of renal origin being present in the urine
(D) A strong family history of individuals with SLE
(E) Chorea due to the CNS vasculitic effects of the disorder

11. In juvenile dermatomyositis:

(A) Weakness is seen mainly in distal muscle groups in the limbs
(B) A malar rash suggests that the disorder will progress to SLE
(C) Measurement of muscle enzymes such as creatine kinase (CK) is indicated
(D) Prednisolone therapy is the main treatment
(E) Subcutaneous calcification may be seen in the later stages of disease

Answers and explanations

1. The correct answer is **(D)**. Anaphylaxis is an acute and severe IgE mediated allergic reaction which results from mast cell degranulation and the release of mediators (histamine, leukotrienes). The clinical manifestation of this is a multisystem reaction characterised by generalised skin rash (urticaria, angio-oedema), airway tract obstruction (stridor, wheeze), and hypotension (loss of conciousness). Anaphylaxis may be more severe in asthmatic children. Adrenaline is the drug of choice in the initial management of anaphylaxis (D). Without severe hypotension, absorption from the deep intramuscular route is adequate. Adrenaline has both positive inotrophic and chronotropic properties; it is a bronchodilator as well as reducing mediator release. There is evidence to indicate that adrenaline is most effective when given soon after the onset of anaphylactic symptoms. Adrenaline can be repeated every 5 minutes until there is clinical improvement. Intravenous fluids may also be required if the patient is hypotensive (E). Steroids, antihistamines and inhaled ventolin are used as secondary medications and can be administered once cardiovascular and respiratory compromise has been corrected (A,B,C).

2. The correct answers are **(C)**, **(D)** and **(E)**. The most important aspect of management in atopic dermatitis is basic skin care, which includes the avoidance of skin irritants (such as soaps and wool), the frequent

use of topical application of skin moisturisers (E) and control of skin staphylococcal infection (intermittent antiseptic bath oil). If these measures fail to control atopic dermatitis then topical steroids may be required. The least potent steroid which controls symptoms should be used and prolonged use of potent steroids should be avoided because they may cause skin damage (B). Some infants with atopic dermatitis have IgE mediated food allergy and these foods when ingested may be a trigger for atopic dermatitis. Dietary exclusion of these proteins is important in management. Exclusion of egg is appropriate here because of the immediate urticarial reaction (C); other foods, especially milk, should not be removed empirically from the diets of children with atopic dermatitis (A). This may lead to nutritional deficiencies, particularly calcium and protein. Allergens, in particular house dust mite, may be significant triggers for atopic dermatitis. Skin or RAST testing to identify those children who have been sensitised to house dust mite and a trial of house dust mite reduction methods would be appropriate in generalised atopic dermatitis (D). In those infants with atopic dermatitis who have been sensitised to house dust mite the daily use of non sedating anthistamines has been shown to delay (or prevent) the onset of asthma.

3. The correct answer is **(D)**. The most frequent trigger for episodic asthma is upper respiratory tract viral infections. The 'Vega' test is not validated scientifically and cannot be used to diagnose food allergy (A) (or anything else). Food allergy and intolerance is an uncommon cause of episodic asthma. The exceptions are with metabisulphite intolerance and when acute bronchospasm is part of a generalised anaphylactic reaction. Metabisulphite is a commonly used food preservative which can cause local irritation of the respiratory tract in some asthmatics resulting in both upper and lower airway obstruction. Food anaphylaxis often is associated with bronchospasm in asthmatics but usually is accompanied by other symptoms such as skin rash and gastrointestinal symptoms. Skin or RAST testing to indoor allergens is seldom indicated in episodic asthma and exposure to these allergens is usually continuous and would be unlikely to give rise to episodic symptoms (B). Preventer treatment is only indicated in persistent asthma and would not be indicated in infrequent episodic asthma (C). Cow's milk and cow's milk products are an important source of dietary calcium and diets which have excluded milk products are unlikely to meet the daily calcium requirements of growing children (D).

4. The correct answers are **(A)**, **(B)**, **(D)** and **(E)**. This history is suggestive of an unusual susceptibility to bacterial infections, possibly agammaglobulinaemia.

This may be X linked, and therefore a careful family history looking for evidence of an inherited susceptibility to infection in males on the maternal side of the family is important (A). If he does have X linked agammaglobulinaemia (XLA), his IgG, IgA and IgM concentrations will be very low or absent (B), and B cells will be absent on more extensive testing of immunological function. This will mean that he cannot make functional antibody, and will not be able to respond to vaccines (C). The only way for him to acquire functional antibody if he has XLA is to receive regular intravenous immunoglobulin infusions. A chest X ray will be useful to determine if there is any evidence of bronchiectasis (D). If he does have XLA, his mother may be a carrier, and his brother could also have inherited the disorder (E).

5. The correct answers are **(A)**, **(B)** and **(C)**. This history is consistent with the DiGeorge anomalad, which is part of the spectrum of chromosome 22 microdeletion disorders (A). In DiGeorge anomalad, there are abnormalities of structures arising from the third and fourth pharyngeal arches, including the great vessels, the thymus and the parathyroids. Therefore hypocalcaemia is common (B). Her low CD3 numbers suggest an immunodeficiency, and all children with an immunodeficiency should have HIV infection excluded (C). The 22 microdeletion syndromes have variable expression and inheritance: although there may be a risk for other children in the family having a 22 microdeletion, this is not very high (D). If Jennifer did receive hepatitis B vaccine at birth, as recommended in the standard immunisation schedule, this will not have been harmful as it is an inactive recombinant vaccine (E). However, it is appropriate for children with primary immunodeficiency disorders not to receive further vaccines of any type after diagnosis until expert opinion has been sought.

6. The correct answers are **(C)** and **(D)**. The protein lost in the urine is largely albumin, but other proteins are also lost, including IgG. Patients with nephrotic syndrome may have very low serum IgG concentrations as a result. IgM is of much higher molecular weight than IgG, and therefore is much less likely to be lost in the urine (A). Immunological memory is not impaired in nephrotic syndrome, and, when he recovers, his ability to respond appropriately to vaccine associated antigens will not be altered, so reimmuinisation will not be needed (B). However, during the acute stage he is at significant risk of infection, due to loss of IgG, the oedematous tissues, and the prednisolone therapy (D). There is a particular risk of systemic streptococcal infections, which can be rapidly progressive and can cause death (C): prophylactic penicillin therapy should be considered during the acute stage. Intravenous

437

immunoglobulin, however, will not be effective (E). It consists of IgG and will be lost almost immediately in the urine while the proteinuria continues.

7. None of the answers is correct. Osteomyelitis is unlikely, in that there is clinical evidence from the history that she has had at least wrist joint involvement for several weeks, and although her knee involvement is recent, osteomyelitis at two sites is rare (A). Persistent inflammation in a joint is not a feature of rheumatic fever (B), and an elevated ASOT in itself is not diagnostic of rheumatic fever. Most children with juvenile arthritis are negative for rheumatoid factor (C). If she has not had a history of bruising or bleeding, haemarthroses are unlikely, and the most common form of clotting disorder leading to haemarthroses is haemophilia A, which is sex linked (D). Her history and findings are most consistent with juvenile arthritis with an oligoarthritis. Uveitis may occur in any child with juvenile arthritis, and is most common in children with oligoarthritis. There is no relationship between the number of joints involved and the development of uveitis (E).

8. **All answers are correct**. The history and findings suggest a systemic inflammatory response, which could be associated with occult infection, a malignancy (A), or other systemic disorder such as systemic onset arthritis (B). Investigations in this situation must look for a wide range of possible disorders. Systemic onset arthritis frequently is associated with a serositis, and evidence of a pericardial effusion would be consistent with this diagnosis (C). Children who develop systemic onset arthritis often do not have arthritis at presentation (D); the arthritis usually becomes apparent after several weeks or months. The salmon pink fine macular rash around the upper trunk and in the axillae at the times of high temperature, or when warm, such as in a warm bath, are typical of the active systemic phase of systemic onset arthritis (E).

9. The correct answers are **(A)**, **(B)**, **(C)** and **(D)**. Her presentation is suggestive of a psoriatic arthritis, in that her finger swelling, if it involved the whole finger and not just the joints, would be consistent with dactylitis (A), which is typical of a psoriatic arthropathy (B). Nail pitting is often seen in individuals with psoriasis (C), even in the absence of the typical skin lesions and distribution of psoriasis (D). Prednisolone is not used in arthritis unless it is severe and cannot be controlled with other anti-inflammatory agents (E).

10. The correct answers are **(A)**, **(B)** and **(C)**. It is very rare to have SLE in childhood in the absence of a positive immunofluorescence test for ANA, and the pattern is usually homogeneous (A), although it also commonly is speckled. Active SLE is associated with circulating immune complexes, and a low C4 is seen as complement is consumed by the immune complexes (B). Most children and adolescents with SLE have significant renal involvement and inflammatory glomerulonephritis, leading to haematuria (C). Phase contrast microscopy of the red cells in the urine will show them to be of renal origin. Although there is a somewhat increased incidence in families of connective tissue disorders, in general, if one family member is affected, it is unusual for several individuals in one family to have SLE if a child has SLE (D). Chorea may represent cerebral manifestations of SLE but it is relatively uncommon (E).

11. The correct answers are **(C)**, **(D)** and **(E)**. In juvenile dermatomyositis, the weakness is in the proximal muscle groups (A). A facial rash is common, and is often seen over the malar area, the margins of the upper eye lids, and over the dorsum of the interphalangeal joints of the hands and the dorsum of the metacarpophalangeal joints. However, the rash has no relationship with SLE (B). Serum concentrations of muscle enzymes such as CK are often elevated in juvenile dermatomyositis, particularly in active disease (C). The most effective treatment is high dose prednisolone orally (D), and intravenous pulse prednisolone therapy may be used in severe or resistant cases. Some children develop cutaneous calcinosis later in the course of the disease (E), and it can be very difficult to treat.

PART 13   FURTHER READING

Boros T, Kay D, Gold M 2000 Parent reported allergy and anaphylaxis in 4173 South Australian children. Journal of Paediatrics and Child Health 36: 36–40

Conley M E 2000 Genetics of primary immunodeficiency diseases. Reviews in Immunogenetics 2: 231–242

Ewan P 1998 Anaphylaxis. ABC of allergies. BMJ 316: 1442–1445

Fireman P 2000 Therapeutic approaches to allergic rhinitis: treating the child. Journal of Allergy and Clinical Immunology 105: S616–621

Fischer A 2001 Primary immunodeficiency diseases: an experimental model for molecular medicine. Lancet 357: 1863–1869

Fischer A, Hacein-Bey S, Le Deist F et al 2000 Gene therapy of severe combined immunodeficiencies. Immunological Reviews 178: 13–20

ISAAC Steering Committee 1998 Worldwide variation in prevalence of symptoms of asthma, allergic rhinoconjunctivitis, and atopic eczema: ISAAC. Lancet 351: 1225–1232

Leung A 2000 Atopic dermatitis: new insights and opportunities for therapeutic intervention. Journal of Allergy and Clinical Immunology 105: 860–876

Myers T R, Chatburn R L 2000 Pediatric asthma disease management. Respiratory Care Clinics of North America 6: 57–74

Onel K B 2000 Advances in the medical treatment of juvenile rheumatoid arthritis. Current Opinions in Pediatrics 12: 72–75

Peak J, Roberton D M 2000 Advances in the diagnosis of primary immunodeficiency disorders in childhood. Current Paediatrics 11: 149–157

Petty R E, Cassidy J 2001 Textbook of pediatric rheumatology, 4th edn. W B Saunders, Philadelphia

Schwartz S A 2000 Intravenous immunoglobulin treatment of immunodeficiency disorders. Pediatric Clinics of North America 47: 1355–1369

Segal B H, Holland S M 2000 Primary phagocytic disorders of childhood. Pediatric Clinics of North America 47:1311–1338

Sherry D D 2000 What's new in the diagnosis and treatment of juvenile rheumatoid arthritis. Journal of Pediatric Orthopedics 20: 419–420

Smith C I 2000 Experiments of nature: primary immune defects deciphered and defeated. Immunological Reviews 178:5–7

Tovey E, Marks G 1999 Methods and effectiveness of environmental control. Journal of Allergy and Clinical Immunology 103: 179–191

Vihinen M, Arredondo-Vega F X, Casanova J L et al 2001 Primary immunodeficiency mutation databases. Advances in Genetics 43: 103–188

Woo P, Wedderburn L R 1998. Juvenile chronic arthritis. Lancet 35: 969–973

Wulffraat N M, Kuis W 2001 Treatment of refractory juvenile idiopathic arthritis. Journal of Rheumatology 28: 929–931

Useful links

http://www.aaaai.org (American Academy of Allergy Asthma and Immunology)

http://www.allergy.org.au (Australasian Society of Clinical Immunology and Allergy)

http://www.allergyfacts.org.au (Australian anaphylaxis support group)

http://www.arthritis.org/communities/about_AJAO.asp (The web site of the American Juvenile Arthritis Organization, a Council of the Arthritis Foundation of the US. Follow the links to a large variety of resources)

http://www.f.webring.com/hub?ring=pidring&index (A web page giving links to a good selection of other web sites on primary immunodeficiency disorders)

http://www.goldscout.com/ (A user friendly site for children, their families, and for paediatricians and other health professionals. The site is updated regularly by Dr Thomas Lehman of the Division of Pediatric Rheumatology, Hospital for Special Surgery, New York. There are many links to other sites, and there are listings of patient education material)

http://www.harcourthealth.com (Follow path to the Journal of Allergy and Clinical Immunology)

http://www.ipopi.org/ (Web site of the International Patient Organisation for Patients with Primary Immunodeficiency Diseases. There are related organisations in many countries, including Australia and New Zealand)

http://www.jmfworld.org/html/primary_immunodeficiency.html (A useful web site written from a family's perspective, with a good section on the various types of primary immunodeficiency disorders in easy to understand terms)

http://www.pia.org.uk/ (Web site of the Primary Immunodeficiency Association of the UK. Good list of publications available to patients and their families)

RESPIRATORY DISORDERS

45 Acute upper respiratory tract infections in childhood

C. Mellis

Upper respiratory tract infections (URTIs) are the scourge of young children and their parents. In the first 5 years of life children average 6–8 episodes per annum. The timing and frequency of these infections depends largely on the level of exposure; therefore they occur earlier and more often in those with older siblings and those who attend daycare (Fig. 45.1). By far the majority of URTIs are viral in origin, are of mild severity, and are of short duration (5–7 days). These illnesses are self-limiting and require no specific pharmacological intervention (Tables 45.1 and 45.2). The age of the child is the major predictor of type, severity and extent of a viral respiratory tract infection (Table 45.2).

Nevertheless, these recurring URTIs of early childhood are important, particularly when they occur repeatedly during the winter months. Local complications of viral URTIs do occur in a significant percentage, especially acute otitis media and acute sinusitis (Fig. 45.2). Progression of the infection into the lower respiratory tract is a risk, particularly with some of the more potent respiratory viruses such as parainfluenza (viral 'croup') and respiratory syncytial virus (RSV; acute viral bronchiolitis). The proportion who develop these complications depends largely upon the child's age and the specific infecting virus, plus other host and environmental factors as outlined in Figure 45.3.

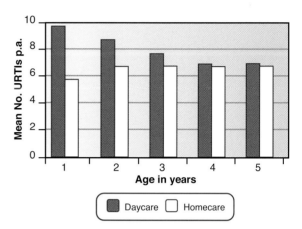

Fig. 45.1 Number of respiratory tract infections per year in infants and preschoolers (daycare versus homecare). From data in Isaacs D, Moxon E R, 1996.

Table 45.1   Infecting agents in upper respiratory tract infections

	Usual	Common	Uncommon
Common cold	Rhinoviruses	Coronaviruses Enteroviruses	Adenovirus Influenza A + B Respiratory syncytial virus (RSV)* Parainfluenza[†]
Pharyngitis	Adenovirus[a]	Epstein–Barr virus[b] Streptococcus[f]	Herpes simplex[c] Coxsackie/ECHO[d,e] Parainfluenza Influenze A+B Coronaviruses Streptococcus[f]

* School age children (infants and preschoolers commonly develop lower respiratory tract infection with RSV).
[†] The major cause of 'croup' in preschool children.
a–f see text for details:
[a] Ulcerative pharyngotonsillitis.
[b] Epstein–Barr viral pharyngitis.
[c] Herpes stomatitis.
[d] Herpangina.
[e] Hand, foot and mouth disease.
[f] Streptococcal tonsillitis.

Table 45.2 Age of child and type of respiratory tract infection

Age	Type of infection
Newborn	Risk of acute, more generalised systemic illness with respiratory viruses (looks 'septic')
Infant	High risk of lower respiratory tract involvement with respiratory viruses (particularly acute viral bronchiolitis with RSV)
Toddler/preschooler	High risk of viral laryngotracheobronchitis ('croup') with respiratory viruses (especially parainfluenza viruses) Very frequent viral respiratory tract infections, mostly confined to upper respiratory tract
School age (5–15 years)	Lower rates of viral respiratory tract infections Suspect bacterial tonsillitis (streptococcal) Suspect Epstein–Barr viral pharyngitis/tonsillitis Suspect *Mycoplasma pneumoniae* if lower respiratory tract involvement (bronchitis and bronchopneumonia)

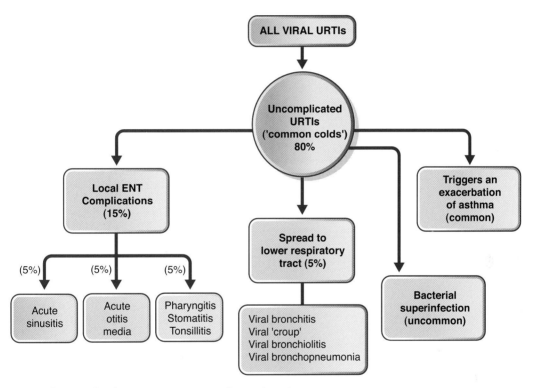

Fig. 45.2 Complications of viral upper respiratory tract infections (URTIs).

Additional issues with URTIs are: the clinical problem of differentiating common viral pharyngitis from uncommon streptococcal pharyngitis; viral URTIs can lead to significant systemic illnesses (such as Henoch–Schönlein purpura); and the most common trigger of severe acute exacerbations of asthma in young children is a viral URTI.

An obvious difficulty with URTIs is the arbitrary definitions used to describe them, such as rhinitis, pharyngitis, tonsillitis and stomatitis. There is clearly substantial overlap with these syndromes as the viral infection will cross anatomical boundaries. Indeed, viral inflammation of the respiratory tract is usually diffuse rather than focal, while bacterial infections of the respiratory tract (such as streptococcal tonsillitis) are more anatomically localised.

By far the most common form of URTI is the 'common cold', which is also known as viral nasopharyngitis, acute coryzal illness or viral catarrh, but overall it is probably best described as an uncomplicated viral URTI.

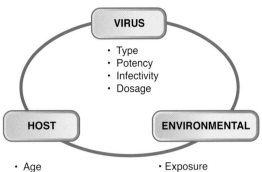

Fig. 45.3 Frequency and severity of viral URTIs depends on complex interaction of virus, host and environment. *Aboriginal or Torres Strait Islander; †environmental tobacco smoke.

Common cold (uncomplicated viral URTI)

This is defined as an acute illness where the major symptoms are:

- nasal (snuffliness, sneezing and rhinorrhoea)
- sore throat
- conjunctival irritation (red, watery eyes).

The symptoms are mild, fever is minimal or absent and all symptoms resolve between 5 and 7 days.

The usual pathogen responsible for an uncomplicated viral URTI is rhinovirus, of which there are numerous specific strains. However, there are a large number of potential respiratory viruses which can produce this syndrome (Table 45.1). These viruses are highly infectious and spread via both droplets (particularly by sneezing) and nasal secretions on hands and fomites (clothing, handkerchiefs, toys, cot sides). Viral shedding is maximal in the 7 days after inoculation and most have a short incubation period (2–3 days). Therefore, close proximity such as household contacts with older schoolage siblings, daycare attendance, overcrowding, lower socioeconomic status and poor personal hygiene are all associated with high rates of URTI (Fig. 45.3).

Local ENT complications of the common cold include otitis media and acute sinusitis (Fig. 45.2), and a small proportion progress to involve the lower respiratory tract.

Oropharyngitis/tonsillitis

This is a clinical syndrome in which the major complaint is acute sore throat and/or discomfort on swallowing (dysphagia). The illness is generally mild and self-limiting, with three quarters of patients free of pain within 2–3 days of onset, whether due to a respiratory virus or β-haemolytic streptococcus.

There are a number of specific, recognisable syndromes of oropharyngitis/tonsillitis.

Ulcerative pharyngotonsillitis

This is due to an adenovirus infection and typically occurs in infants and toddlers. It produces an isolated exudative tonsillitis resembling streptococcal tonsillitis or Epstein–Barr pharyngitis. Other respiratory viruses (including RSV and parainfluenza) usually cause a more diffuse nasopharyngitis rather than this focal tonsillar inflammation. The enteroviruses (coxsackie and echovirus) and herpes simplex virus can also produce ulcerative pharyngotonsillitis.

Clinical example

Adam, 3 years old, presented with fever, sore throat and difficulty swallowing during the previous 24 hours. When first seen he had an axillary temperature of 38.2°C, and both tonsils were swollen and inflamed with a visible yellow exudate scattered over both tonsils. There was bilateral enlargement of the lymph nodes in the anterior cervical chain. A clinical diagnosis of acute streptococcal tonsillitis was made, a throat swab taken for culture, and oral penicillin prescribed. However, he represented several days later because of ongoing fever, and the development of a clear nasal discharge and watery eyes. He had a mild dry cough but was now drinking well and not complaining of a sore throat. His throat culture was sterile. The illness was almost certainly due to a respiratory virus (such as parainfluenza adenovirus). Several days later his mother rang to say that he was now virtually back to his normal self. This case clearly demonstrates the major clinical difficulty in distinguishing a bacterial from a viral tonsillitis/pharyngitis.

Epstein–Barr virus pharyngitis/tonsillitis

Although this typically occurs in older, schoolage children it can cause an exudative tonsillitis in the very young. The tonsillitis is associated with a membrane and marked cervical lymphadenopathy plus generalised symptoms, including fever, lethargy, anorexia and headache.

Primary herpes simplex stomatitis

This has a peak incidence in children aged 1–3 years and typically causes multiple discrete ulcers on the *anterior* regions of the oropharynx — tongue, gums and palate. It is generally accompanied by 'cold sore' vesicles on the lips or circumoral region, significant fever and lymphadenopathy (especially submental and anterior cervical lymph glands). The ulcers generally persist for 5–7 days and can cause considerable pain, feeding difficulty and irritability.

The usual treatment is analgesics, such as paracetamol or soothing, topical gels, which are best given immediately before feeding. Aciclovir should only be used in the immunocompromised child.

Clinical example

At the age of 18 months, Jennifer developed a high fever, and became very irritable. She cried loudly when given cordial to drink, and spat it out. She could not swallow her saliva, and was dribbling constantly. Her mouth looked red and inflamed, and her mother took her urgently to see her general practitioner.

Jennifer was difficult to examine, but her mouth seemed very painful. She had submental and cervical lymphadenopathy. With gentle persuasion, her general practitioner encouraged her to open her mouth. The gingivae and anterior oropharynx were bright red, and there were many small ulcers on her gums and on the tongue and hard palate, many of which were covered by a grey-white exudate.

Jennifer had an acute gingivostomatitis due to herpes simplex virus. She was given small frequent sips of water and milk to maintain her hydration. She could not take paracetamol because she had difficulty swallowing in the first 24 hours, and it was difficult to apply a topical analgesic gel because of pain. The first night, a paracetomol suppository was used to provide some analgesia. The ulcers healed after 4 days and did not leave any scars.

Herpangina

This typically occurs in preschool children and is due to one of the enteroviruses (coxsackie or echoviruses). It results in a number of discrete mouth ulcers, localised to the *posterior* portion of the oropharynx — tonsillar pillars, pharyngeal wall, uvula and palate. This is in contrast to the anterior ulcers of herpes simplex virus.

Hand, foot and mouth disease

This illness of young children is due to enteroviruses and results in lesions similar to herpes simplex virus. The usual symptoms are sore throat and refusal to eat and drink. This is usually accompanied by a vesicular or macular papular rash on the hands, feet, buttocks or trunk. The mouth ulcers are generally on the tongue, palate and buccal mucosa. The illness classically occurs in miniepidemics, making recognition somewhat easier.

Acute bacterial tonsillitis (group a β-haemolytic streptococcal pharyngitis)
(Table 45.3)

While it is important to distinguish viral pharyngitis from streptococcal pharyngitis, unfortunately this is not easy on clinical grounds; however, if three or more of the following characteristics are present then it is likely to be streptococcal infection:
- fever
- tonsillar exudate
- tender, enlarged anterior cervical lymph nodes
- absence of cough.

This clinical dilemma can be overcome by use of rapid laboratory tests to confirm the presence of streptococcal pharyngitis, thus rationalising the use of antibiotics and doubts about efficacy.

While it would appear logical to give antibiotics in the presence of an apparent streptococcal pharyngitis, current evidence casts doubts on efficacy. A Cochrane review of randomised control trials concluded that antibiotics confer little benefit in the treatment of sore throat, irrespective of whether the infection is due to a virus or streptococcus. Despite this, in children known to be at high risk of complications of streptococcal infection (poststreptococcal glomerulonephritis and rheumatic fever), the threshold for giving antibiotics should be considerably lower. Populations at particular risk include Aboriginal and Torres Strait Islanders, and Pacific Islander children.

Table 45.3 Clinical features of group A β-haemolytic streptococcal tonsillitis

History
Age 5–15 yrs
Abrupt onset
Severe sore throat (pain and difficulty swallowing)
Systemic symptoms
  headache
  abdominal pain/nausea/vomiting
No cough or coryzal/nasal symptoms

Examination
Tonsillar exudate, purulent and patchy (rather than a
  membrane); marked inflammation of throat and tonsils
Enlarged, tender bilateral anterior cervical lymph nodes
No nasal discharge

Acute sinusitis (rhinosinusitis)

This complication occurs in approximately 5% of viral URTIs and generally involves the maxillary sinuses. The usual manifestation is a profuse, mucopurulent nasal discharge with nasal obstruction. Uncomplicated acute viral sinusitis normally resolves without specific treatment in 7–10 days. Thus, if the child has a mucopurulent nasal discharge continuing beyond 10 days the possibility of secondary bacterial sinusitis needs to be considered.

A Cochrane review of five randomised control trials involving over 400 children found 10 days of antibiotics will reduce the probability of persistence of nasal discharge in the short to medium term; however, the benefits are modest and no long term benefits have been documented. The reviewers concluded that larger, well designed studies are indicated before the question about antibiotics for acute sinusitis in children can be dogmatically answered. The usual organisms responsible for acute bacterial sinusitis are pneumococcus, *Haemophilus influenzae*, and *Moraxella catarrhalis*. Amoxicillin is therefore generally considered the antibiotic of choice.

Acute otitis media (Ch. 75)

This local complication of viral URTIs is characterised by earache, fever, reduced hearing, and non specific discomfort and irritability in the very young child. Examination shows a red tympanic membrane with loss of the normal anatomical landmarks on the tympanic membrane. Less commonly the eardrum is visibly bulging.

This complication of viral URTI most commonly occurs in the very young, particularly between 6 months and 2 years of age. Virtually all children will have at least one episode of otitis media and some are particularly prone to this complication. The microbiology of otitis media has been accurately documented in a recent large study from Finland. In this study, middle ear fluid was obtained (by myringotomy) in over 90% of 2500 episodes of clinical acute otitis media during the first 2 years of life. A bacterial pathogen, particularly pneumococcus, *M. catarrhalis* and *H. influenzae*, was cultured in over 80%.

Although this suggests that young children with acute otitis media should be treated with an antibiotic, such as amoxicillin plus clavulanic acid (Augmentin), the evidence is unimpressive. A Cochrane Review of seven randomised control trials (over 2000 children) found no reduction in earache at 24 hours between antibiotics and placebo, and only a 6% absolute reduction in pain at 2–7 days. The authors found approximately 80% of all children with acute otitis media, irrespective of treatment, will be pain free by 2–7 days. Thus, the benefit of antibiotics is small and is possibly outweighed by the 5% risk of adverse effects (rash, diarrhoea and/or vomiting). Consequently, simple oral topical analgesics (anaesthetic ear drops) may be the best option. However, as with streptococcal pharyngitis, in patients at increased risk of suppurative complications of otitis media (particularly Aboriginal, Torres Strait Islanders and Pacific Islanders) the threshold for prescribing antibiotics should be substantially lower.

The duration of antibiotic administration has also been addressed in a Cochrane Review, which concluded that 5 days antibiotics is adequate treatment for uncomplicated ear infections in children. This review considered those randomised control trials which compared short course antibiotics (less than 7 days) to longer course (7 or more days) and found no difference in outcome.

Streptococcus pneumoniae is the most common reported bacterial cause of acute otitis media (between one third and one half of all cases) and initial trials of multivalant conjugate vaccines against the serotypes responsible for otitis media have been shown to be effective.

Approach to management of respiratory tract infections

Uncomplicated viral URTIs (common cold)

It should be evident that antibiotics are not indicated in this condition. A Cochrane Review has demonstrated that antibiotics offer no advantage over placebo; further, antibiotics were associated with a 6% rate of adverse events (rashes and gastrointestinal symptoms).

The possible role of nasal decongestants has been addressed in three randomised control trials in children. A combined 'antihistamine with decongestant' in all three studies failed to show efficacy in young children. The most recent was a single dose study which resulted in temporary relief of nasal congestion but was associated with a high rate of adverse events, particularly sedation. Almost 50% of the children receiving the 'antihistamine and nasal decongestant' were asleep within 2 hours of the medication, compared to 27% in the placebo. Obviously, from the parents' viewpoint this 'adverse' event may be seen as desirable. Nevertheless, antihistamines have been associated with paradoxical excitability, hallucinations, agitation and seizures. Furthermore, 10% of all poison centre calls are related to overdose with various cough and cold medications.

Use of alternative treatments such as echinaecia have been popularised over recent years. The use of echinaecea for preventing and treating the common cold has been the subject of a Cochrane Review. These reviewers concluded that, although the majority of available studies report positive results, the quality of the trials is poor and the results are inconclusive, due to heterogeneity of both the preparations used and the outcome measures employed. Obviously, further high quality multicentre randomised control trials are indicated to address this question appropriately.

Prevention of URTIs (Table 45.4)

Reduce exposure

Reducing exposure to respiratory viruses is extremely difficult. In daycare settings, cohorting of children into smaller and age specific groups is of benefit. While the cohorting, or exclusion, of children suffering from URTIs may help, unfortunately person to person spread often occurs *before* the child has obvious symptoms of an URTI.

Simple measures such as hand washing by both staff and children, improving ventilation and reducing overcrowding are all of value.

Reduced exposure to environmental tobacco smoke

While the evidence relating to respiratory infections and passive smoking relates predominantly to lower respiratory infections, there is also evidence that URTIs in young children are increased in those exposed to environmental tobacco smoke.

Vaccination

The effect of vaccination against the serotypes responsible for pneumococcal otitis media has now been demonstrated, although further trials are essential.

The use of influenza A and B vaccine in infants and young children remains controversial. Recent American studies found that, during years when influenza viruses predominate, the rates of hospitalisation with acute respiratory disease in children under 2 years of age (without specific risk factors) were as high as 2% per annum. Consequently, it has been suggested that routine influenza vaccination be considered in all young children. A recent Japanese study found routine vaccination of schoolchildren caused a major reduction in mortality from influenza in the elderly. This confirms that children are the major disseminators of influenza, and routine annual influenza vaccination for children could become policy in the near future.

In children over the age of 1 year, it is possible to use the potent, selective inhibitors of influenza A and B virus neuraminidase. These agents, which can be taken either by inhalation or orally, have proven effective both in the treatment and prevention of household spread of influenza. These agents appear to be free of major adverse effects, and emergence of drug resistant strains of viruses has not been a problem. The role of these agents in the treatment and prevention of influenza virus infection will soon be clarified.

Table 45.4   Prevention of upper respiratory tract infections

Reduction of exposure in daycare
Cohorting (both age and symptomatic of respiratory tract infection)
Reducing overcrowding
Improving ventilation
Individual use of personal items (such as toothbrushes and facecloths)
Strict hand washing by both staff and children

Education of parents re spread of respiratory viruses and appropriate care
Similar issues to those outlined above for daycare
Education re no antibiotics for URTIs
Symptomatic treatment should be minimal

Reduced exposure to environmental tobacco smoke
Especially in homes and cars

Vaccination
Influenza vaccine
  to prevent serious influenza A + B infections in young children
  to reduce the pool of infection to protect the elderly community
Pneumococcal conjugate vaccine (to reduce rates of acute otitis media)

Summary

The vast majority of respiratory tract infections in young children are uncomplicated 'common colds' that require no specific treatment. Although local ENT complications are not uncommon, antibiotic treatment for acute sinusitis and acute otitis media offers very limited benefit but does cause adverse effects (particularly rashes and gastrointestinal symptoms). A very small proportion of URTIs are bacterial. Streptococcal tonsillitis resolves quickly without complication in the majority of children and without antibiotics. When treating populations known to be at high risk of suppurative complications, high rates of poststreptococcal glomerulonephritis or rheumatic fever, there must be a substantially lower threshold for antibiotic treatment.

The age of the child, the specific infective agent and other host and environmental factors have a major bearing on the nature of the respiratory infections, including the timing, frequency, severity and likelihood of either local or distant complications.

Key learning points

- Young children experience 6–8 viral URTIs per year. A large variety of respiratory viruses can cause URTIs in young children.
- The vast majority (approx 80%) of respiratory tract infections in young children are mild, self-limiting viral URTIs ('common colds') which require no treatment.
- The child's age and the specific type of virus are the most powerful predictors of the type of respiratory infection the child will experience.

- Local ENT complications of viral URTIs (for example acute sinusitis, acute otitis media, pharyngitis) occur in approximately 15% of URTIs. These may benefit from symptomatic therapy (such as analgesics); antibiotics are not generally necessary.
- A very small proportion of URTIs are bacterial (and may benefit from antibiotics). The most common is streptococcal pharyngitis ('tonsillitis'), especially in school age children.
- Both spread of the viral infection into the lower respiratory tract and secondary bacterial infection are uncommon complications.

Stridor and croup 46

P. D. Sly

Stridor and croup are both disorders that have obstruction of the middle airways as an underlying cause of the symptoms with which they present.

Stridor

Physiological principles

Stridor is defined in *Dorland's Illustrated Medical Dictionary* (28th edition) as 'a harsh, high-pitched respiratory sound such as the inspiratory sound often heard in acute laryngeal obstruction'. While this definition is strictly correct, it is not all that helpful and gives no information about how and why stridor comes about. Stridor is a harsh, high pitched noise heard predominantly during inspiration. Consideration of the physiological principles underlying this fact gives some clue as to the site of the lesion causing the stridor. The presence of an added respiratory sound implies an obstruction to the free flow of gas through the airway tree. This obstruction is usually known as flow limitation. Flow limitation in a compliant tube, such as the airways, is accompanied by fluttering of the walls, which occurs to conserve energy when driving pressure exceeds the pressure required to produce the maximal flow. The fluttering of the walls produces a respiratory noise. When this phenomenon occurs during inspiration, the resultant noise is known as stridor, and when it occurs during expiration, the noise is known as wheeze.

During breathing, there are pressure gradients between the airway opening and the alveoli. Inspiration occurs when alveolar pressure is lowered below atmospheric pressure and air flows in to equalise the pressures. At the onset of expiration, alveolar pressure exceeds atmospheric pressure and air flows out. There are also pressure gradients across the airway wall and these tend to alter airway calibre. The pressure around the extrathoracic airways, that is, those above the thoracic inlet, is atmospheric, while the pressure around the intrathoracic airways essentially is equal to the pleural pressure. As illustrated in Figure 46.1, the pressure gradients across the airway wall during inspiration means that there is a net force tending to narrow the extrathoracic airways and to dilate the intrathoracic airways (Fig. 46.1A). During expiration, the direction of the forces is opposite, resulting in a tendency to narrow intrathoracic airways and dilate extrathoracic airways (Fig. 46.1B).

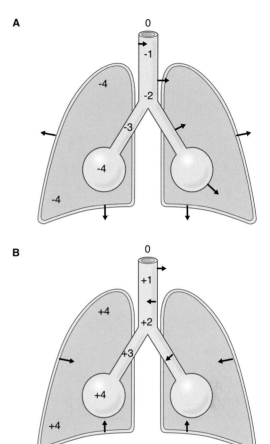

Fig. 46.1 The distribution of pressures throughout the respiratory system during **A** inspiration and **B** expiration. Atmospheric pressure is shown as zero. During inspiration, the expansion of the thorax results in pleural pressure falling below atmospheric. This relatively negative pressure is transmitted to the alveoli and a pressure gradient is established between the airway opening and the alveoli. Gas flows into the lungs along this pressure gradient. The pressure outside the airways is essentially pleural pressure and results in net forces that tend to expand intrathoracic airways and to collapse the extrathoracic trachea. As shown in B, the pressure gradients are opposite during expiration.

As stridor is an inspiratory noise, the predominant site of obstruction (the site responsible for the flow limitation) is generally in the extrathoracic airways. Stridor with an expiratory component, that is, where the noise can also be heard at the beginning of expiration, can result from either a severe obstruction producing flow limitation during expiration as well, or from a lesion that extends into the intrathoracic airways.

Differential diagnosis

When considering the differential diagnosis, several factors need to be taken into consideration. These include:

- *Age of onset.* A stridor present from the first few days of life suggests a congenital or structural cause.
- *Speed of onset of symptoms.* Infective causes such as croup tend to come on quickly; however, most cases of congenital or structural stridor initially present following a viral upper respiratory illness.
- *Progression of stridor.* Stridor increasing in severity over weeks to months suggests a progressive lesion, such as subglottic haemangioma.
- *Effect of body position.* Stridor which is worse when lying supine is seen commonly with laryngomalacia.
- *Presence of an expiratory component.* This suggests a more severe obstruction which limits flow during expiration as well as during inspiration.
- *Quality of voice.* While the voice frequently is normal, a hoarse voice would suggest a vocal cord lesion.
- *Other medical conditions that could contribute to the pathogenesis or presentation:* febrile illness, ex premature infant, gastro-oesophageal reflux, cutaneous haemangiomas, Möbius syndrome.

Classification

1. Acute stridor
   a. Common causes
      — laryngotracheobronchitis (croup)
   b. Rare causes (in developed countries)
      — laryngeal trauma
      — acute angioneurotic oedema
      — retropharyngeal abscess
      — peritonsillar absess (quinsy)
      — acute epiglottitis (typically a low pitched rumbling noise coming from the supraglottic area)
      — diphtheria
2. Persistent stridor
   a. Common causes
      — laryngomalacia (infantile larynx)
      — congenital subglottic stenosis
      — acquired subglottic stenosis in a premature infant who required intubation
   b. Uncommon causes
      — subglottic haemangioma
      — vocal cord palsy (unilateral or bilateral)
      — laryngeal webs
      — cysts of the posterior tongue or aryepiglottic folds
      — subglottic mucus retention cysts in a premature infant who required intubation
      — Vascular ring (note this usually presents with a predominantly expiratory noise)
   c. Rare causes
      — laryngocoele
      — laryngeal cleft
      — tracheal stenosis (note this usually presents with a predominantly expiratory noise).

Characteristics of the more important causes of stridor

Laryngomalacia

Laryngomalacia, which is sometimes known as infantile larynx, is the most common cause of persistent stridor. It is not well named, as the larynx and vocal cords are actually normal. The supraglottic tissues appear as if they are too large for the size of the glottis and narrow the glottic aperture during inspiration instead of the more normal widening during inspiration. This can occur in a number of ways, the most common being:

- a long curled (sometimes called omega shaped) epiglottis collapsing during inspiration so that the lateral walls touch, restricting the free passage of air
- floppy arytenoid processes prolapsing into the glottic aperture during inspiration
- a long epiglottis collapsing against the posterior pharyngeal wall during inspiration.

In more severe cases combinations of these mechanisms may be responsible for the inspiratory obstruction.

Laryngomalacia classically produces a cog wheel stridor, with no expiratory component. The cog wheel nature to the stridor is likely to come from vibrations of the supraglottic tissues as the degree of obstruction varies during the inspiratory effort. The stridor may be worse when the infant is lying supine, although this feature is not always seen. More severe obstruction may be associated with suprasternal and sternal retraction during inspiration.

Laryngomalacia is usually a benign condition that does not require any treatment, except to reassure the parents that this is the case. Severe laryngomalacia may be associated with failure to thrive and gastro-oesophageal reflux. The importance of parental reassurance should not be underestimated, as the stridor is likely to last for 2–3 years. Frequently parents find the most distressing part of having a child with laryngomalacia are the looks from people when they take the child out in public and the well intentioned advice received from relatives.

Subglottic stenosis

Subglottic stenosis refers to a narrowing in the upper part of the trachea, immediately below the glottis. This narrowing may be congenital or acquired. ***Congenital*** *subglottic stenosis* occurs typically at the level of, and involves, the cricoid cartilage. The tracheal epithelium typically appears normal but the cross-sectional area of the lumen is reduced and typically does not vary with respiration. *Acquired subglottic stenosis* usually results from trauma and is most commonly seen in premature infants who required intubation. Older infants and children who require prolonged intubation are also at risk. Here the tracheal epithelium is more likely to be replaced by scar tissue.

Subglottic stenosis may present soon after birth or the presentation may be delayed. The stenosis, either congenital or acquired, is usually not progressive but the degree of obstruction may increase, for example as the child's activity levels increase or at times of respiratory infection. The typical presentation is with stridor, particularly at times of respiratory infection. If the obstruction is severe enough, the stridor may have an expiratory component and be associated with suprasternal and sternal retractions.

Many cases of subglottic stenosis do not require treatment and most will improve with growth. Laser and dilatation treatments generally are disappointing. More severe obstruction may require surgery, usually involving a procedure in which the cricoid cartilage is split and reconstructed.

Subglottic haemangioma

The subglottic area can also be narrowed by a haemangioma occurring in this area. These are typical haemangiomas occurring in the submucosal layer of the tracheal wall. As with other haemangiomas, they enlarge during the first year of life and typically present with increasing stridor and inspiratory obstruction. The stridor is rarely present at birth and most come to attention around 4–6 months of age. As the obstruction become worse, the stridor develops an expiratory component and is associated with sternal and suprasternal retractions. Approximately 50% of subglottic haemangiomas are associated with cutaneous haemangiomas, although the converse association is much less frequent.

The earlier a subglottic haemangioma presents, the more likely that surgical treatment will be necessary. Tracheostomy remains the definitive treatment, although some cases do respond to medical treatment with corticosteroids or interferon.

Investigations

The most important investigations in elucidating the cause of a stridor are a thorough history and physical examination. As discussed above, the characteristics of the stridor, the time of onset, the progression, and whether or not an expiratory component is present will clarify the cause of the stridor on many occasions.

Persistent stridor with an expiratory component always warrants further investigation. The definitive investigation for stridor is a bronchoscopy, preferably performed with a flexible, fibreoptic bronchoscope. Laryngoscopy is not sufficient as the subglottic area and lower trachea cannot be safely and adequately assessed. Frequently the trachea can be visualized on penetrated radiographs of the chest and lateral neck; however, these X rays rarely replace the need for bronchoscopy.

Clinical example

Tran is a 3 month old infant who has been referred to the respiratory medicine clinic for assessment of persistent stridor. She was born at term following an uneventful antenatal course and normal vaginal delivery. The stridor was not present at birth and was noticed for the first time at the age of 2 months when she caught a cold from her older brother. Her mother is extremely concerned that something is seriously wrong with her baby as several relatives have told her it is not normal for a baby, to make these types of noises.

Since that time the stridor has been present on most days but is less commonly heard when she is sleeping. Her mother is concerned that the stridor is becoming louder and, on questioning, reports that sometimes an expiratory component can be heard. The stridor is typically worse when she is crying or when lying supine for nappy changes.

Examination reveals a female infant who looks scrawny. Her height is on the 50% percentile but her weight is just below the 10% percentile. She has two typical strawberry naevi on her trunk. While being held in her mother's arms, a cog wheel stridor with no expiratory component can be clearly heard. When she is lying supine, the stridor is associated with a soft, but definite, expiratory component and mild suprasternal retraction.

Discussion points
- What is the most likely diagnosis?
- What investigations are warranted?

A flexible bronchoscopy was performed under general anaesthesia and revealed laryngomalacia, with a tightly coiled epiglottis and prolapsing arytenoid processes. The subglottic area and lower airways were normal.

Discussion points
- Is any treatment warranted?
- Is the fact that her weight percentile is lower than her height percentile of concern?
- Is the laryngomalacia likely to be responsible for her relative failure to thrive (lower weight percentile than height percentile). How could this come about?

The bronchoscopic findings are diagnostic of laryngomalacia and one can be confident that the symptoms will resolve spontaneously with time. The relative failure to thrive may be related to the increased work of breathing required to overcome the obstruction. However, a dietary assessment is warranted before attributing the failure to thrive to this mechanism. As the obstruction decreases with time, her work of breathing will also decrease and the failure to thrive should resolve.

Croup (Laryngotracheobronchitis)

Croup is usually considered to exist in two forms:
- acute viral croup
- recurrent (or spasmodic) croup.

While these two conditions have a number of similarities, they are likely to be distinct entities. They have in common that they involve the larynx, trachea and bronchi and present with a typically barking cough. The cough is so typical it is usually referred to as a 'croupy' cough.

Acute viral croup

Acute viral croup is typically a disease of toddlers, being rare in the first 6 months of life and reaching a peak incidence of 5 cases per 100 children per year during the second year of life. Boys are affected more commonly than girls. Most children who get acute viral croup will only ever have one or two episodes. These episodes typically begin with the symptoms of an upper respiratory infection and progress to typical croup over 1–2 days. The most common viruses isolated from children with croup are parainfluenza virus type 1 (up to 50% in some series), parainfluenza virus type 3 (up to 20%) and respiratory syncytial virus (approximately 10%).

Clinical manifestations

As mentioned above, croup usually begins with signs and symptoms of an upper respiratory infection, including fever and rhinitis. A cough may be present. The typical barking croupy cough usually begins during the night or the early hours of the morning. As the disease progresses, stridor may be heard on exertion initally. If the subglottic obstruction progresses further, stridor may be heard at rest and an expiratory component may be heard. The typical cough continues to be heard.

If the degree of obstruction continues to worsen, the stridor may become more difficult to hear and the child may become distressed and restless. Cough may be absent at this stage. The lack of stridor comes about because the amount of air moving through the obstructed airway is not sufficient to generate the noise (see above). The distress and restlessness are most likely to be due to hypoxia and signal impending complete respiratory obstruction.

The viral illness generally lasts 7–10 days, but the typical croupy cough usually only occurs on the first 2–3 nights.

Investigations

Most children with croup do not warrant any investigations. Viral diagnosis on nasal secretions, usually obtained by per nasal aspiration, can be helpful from an epidemiological point of view but will not alter management. Chest X rays are not helpful for children with typical croup.

Children less than 6 months old who present with croup or those whose croup runs an atypical course warrant investigation. The most useful investigations are likely to be a lateral neck X ray and flexible bronchoscopy.

Management

The majority of children with croup do not require any treatment. Symptomatic treatment for fever and cold symptoms may be warranted. Children with a croupy cough and stridor on exertion (but not at rest) can usually be managed with supportive treatment only. There is a widespread belief that exposing these children to steam, especially by steaming up the home bathroom, helps relieve stridor. There is no evidence to support this treatment. The only benefit that is likely to come from sitting with the child in a steamy bathroom is from sitting quietly with the child and not from the steam.

Children with stridor at rest warrant medical assessment. The most useful treatment for croup that has reached this severity is corticosteroids. These can be give orally in syrup form or inhaled (nebuliser or metered dose inhaler and spacer). The mechanism of action is not known but is likely to be via a topical action. A single dose of steroids decreases the risk of hospitalisation dramatically.

More severe obstruction can be relieved by nebulised adrenaline. This is usually give as a 50:50 mix of the L- and D-isoforms (known as racemic adrenaline). This relieves obstruction by causing a topical vasoconstriction, which wears off in 1–4 hours, depending on the severity of the underlying obstruction.

Severe obstruction may require intubation or even tracheostomy, although the need for these types of treatment have become much less with the widespread use of oral corticosteroids in the emergency departments of paediatric hospitals in Australia.

Recurrent (spasmodic) croup

Some children suffer recurrent episodes of croup, frequently without the preceding viral prodrome usually seen in acute viral croup. Typically these children are well when they go to bed and wake in the early hours of the morning with a barking cough and stridor. Fever is unusual in this form of croup. The same viruses as found in acute viral croup may be found in the upper airways of children with spasmodic croup, although the relationship between the viruses and the symptoms is less clear. Frequently children with recurrent croup have a family history of atopy and asthma or have asthma themselves.

This, together with the uncertain relationship between the clinical symptoms and the presence of a virus, have led to the concept that spasmodic croup maybe a manifestation of upper airway hyperresponsiveness. There are no direct data to support or refute this hypothesis.

Spasmodic croup may be severe enough to require treatment with oral corticosteroids, nebulised adrenaline or even intubation; however, the episodes are frequently short lived and often settle by the time the child presents to the emergency department.

While controlled trials have not been carried out, there is a substantial body of anecdotal evidence that frequent bouts of recurrent croup can be prevented by maintenance therapy with inhaled corticosteroids via a spacer.

47 Asthma

R. Henry

Asthma is the most common chronic illness in children. It is the major acute illness requiring admission to hospital in most developed countries, including Australia and New Zealand, and is the major chronic condition associated with absence from school. In spite of its frequency, there is no definition of asthma that encapsulates its features and is of practical value in making the diagnosis in an individual child.

For the clinician, asthma is recurrent episodes of cough, wheeze and breathlessness. This is an oversimplification because it is possible to have asthma without the triad of cough, wheeze and breathlessness. Furthermore, a minority of children with these symptoms will have other conditions.

For the physiologist, asthma is a condition associated with airway hyperreactivity (loosely referred to as 'twitchy airways') and with reversible airways obstruction. Objective measurement of airway hyperresponsiveness can be obtained by measuring lung function such as peak expiratory flow (PEF) or forced expiratory volume in 1 second (FEV_1) in a bronchial challenge test. Airway hyperreactivity is defined as a significant fall (usually about 20%) in lung function after inhalation of chemicals (such as methacholine or histamine), after inhalation of hypertonic saline, after cold, dry air, or following exercise. Airway hyperreactvity and reversible (or variable) airways obstruction also may be demonstrated by an increase in PEF or FEV_1 of more than 10% following a bronchodilator, or by fluctuations in PEF measurements obtained on a regular basis at home. There are limitations to this physiological definition of asthma. These include the fact that most children are unable to cooperate with challenge tests to measure airway hyperresponsiveness (AHR) until they are 5 or 6 years old, and that there is an imperfect correlation between children with AHR and clinical features of asthma.

For the pathologist, the definition of asthma relates to mucosal oedema, mucous hypersecretion and smooth muscle spasm in the small airways. Airway inflammation is prominent. A limitation of this definition is that airway specimens have been difficult to obtain before death. In recent years non invasive methods, such as induction of sputum with hypertonic saline, or invasive methods, such as bronchoalveolar lavage (BAL) at bronchoscopy, have enabled research into airway inflammation.

For the immunologist, the focus for asthma is on the atopic state. In an allergic response, degranulation of mast cells occurs, with the release of chemical mediators into the airways and a resultant asthmatic response (Ch. 42). Our understanding of the cytokines that are important in asthma remains incomplete. Indeed, the mast cell, the eosinophil and the neutrophil all seem to have important roles in the pathogenesis of asthma.

What causes asthma?

The causes of asthma may be thought of at a number of different levels (Table 47.1). Genetic factors are important in predisposition. If one identical twin has asthma, the other twin has a 60% chance of developing asthma. Genetic markers for asthma have been reported on different chromosomes, including 5, 6, 11 and 12. It may be that there is genetic heterogeneity or that different components of heredity are being described, such as inheritance of atopy in contrast to inheritance of airway hyperresponsiveness. Even when an individual is born with a genetic predisposition to asthma, environmental stimuli are necessary to induce (or sensitise to) the asthmatic state. Identification of inducers of asthma is difficult but they may include allergens and cigarette

Table 47.1 Causes of asthma

Predisposing
Genetic: ? chromosomes 5, 6, 11, 12

Inducers (sensitisers)
Hygiene hypothesis
Allergens
Cigarette smoke
Other irritants, such as ozone
Occupational (rare in children)

Triggers
Infections, for example viral, mycoplasma, pertussis
Exercise, especially in cold, dry air
Allergens, for example house dust mite, pollen, animal dander, foods
Environment, for example cigarette smoke, ozone, SO_2
Emotional, such as laughing
Chemicals, for example salicylates, metabisulphite

Sustainers (maintainers)
Allergens
Viruses
Environmental irritants

smoke (particularly in the early months of life). One explanation for the observed increase in asthma incidence is the 'hygiene hypothesis'. The hypothesis is that early exposure to infection stimulates a Th1 lymphocyte response, whereas absence of infection stimulates a Th2 lymphocyte response, with production of IgE. If there are few infections in early life, the Th2 response may persist for longer in childhood. In developed countries with advantaged living standards, the frequency of infections in early life, particularly severe infections, is less than in disadvantaged countries. This is an explanation for the observations that asthma is more common in developed than developing countries, and that older siblings and attendance at day care are protective against asthma.

Once asthma has developed, a variety of triggers may precipitate individual attacks. Viral respiratory infections are by far the most important, with approximately 80% of admissions to hospital with asthma being associated with viral infections. Other triggers are listed in Table 47.1. Once asthma is established, ongoing environmental factors are necessary to sustain (or maintain) the asthmatic state. Allergens, viruses and non specific irritants have all been shown to increase airway hyperresponsiveness.

Diagnosis

The diagnosis of asthma is easy to make in the child who has:
- recurrent episodes of cough
- wheeze
- breathlessness, and who is
- completely well between attacks.

Other clinical presentations may be less classical, such as:
- nocturnal cough
- persistent cough in association with acute respiratory infections, or
- a history of 'rattly breathing' in the absence of a definite history of wheeze.

In each of these scenarios asthma is possible. One approach is a therapeutic trial of asthma medications, such as a bronchodilator at the time of symptoms. In other cases, investigations may be necessary to support the diagnosis of asthma or to suggest another diagnosis. Useful tests may be:
- chest X ray (abnormalities will suggest another diagnosis)
- measurement of FEV_1 before and after a bronchodilator (reversible airways obstruction would confirm asthma)
- a bronchial provocation test (a significant fall in FEV_1 or PEF after inhalation of hypertonic saline would support asthma)
- allergen skin prick tests (demonstration of atopy would support asthma).

Clinical example

John was a 12 year old boy who presented with a history of breathlessness and chest pain which occurred towards the end of an 800 m run. Neither cough nor wheeze was present. He had received bronchodilators and sodium cromoglycate before exercise without benefit. A trial of inhaled corticosteroids for 6 weeks had also been ineffective. His parents were both keen athletes and hoped that John would become a champion athlete.

Physical examination was normal. FEV_1 was normal and a hypertonic saline challenge test was negative, with no evidence of airway hyperresponsiveness. He was non atopic on allergen skin tests. After an explanation to John and his parents that he did not have asthma, John indicated that he was not interested in competitive athletics. He was discharged on no treatment. One year later he was completely well. He could play regular sport with no difficulties.

The tests used were helpful in confirming that John did not have asthma.

Investigations

The majority of children with asthma, especially those with infrequent episodic symptoms, do not require any investigations. As indicated above, tests such as a chest X ray or tests of airway hyperresponsiveness have more of a role in making the diagnosis or suggesting another cause than in assessing the asthma.

Lung function

Spirometry to measure FEV_1 and forced vital capacity before and after a bronchodilator may help assess severity and response to therapy. Children with episodic disease will have normal lung function and no response to bronchodilators between exacerbations. Children with persistent symptoms may show airways obstruction with improvement after inhalation of a bronchodilator. Fixed airways obstruction suggests either severe asthma or an alternative diagnosis such as cystic fibrosis.

Portable peak flow meters can be used at home on a regular basis to measure PEF. Children with well controlled disease will have normal values with little variability between readings. Poorly controlled asthma is associated with both decreased PEF and wide fluctuations in PEF over days or weeks. In most cases regular PEF measurement will be unnecessary.

Allergy tests

The role of allergen skin prick testing in asthma is controversial. Some paediatricians believe that allergen testing does not result in information that is of any clinical relevance; others believe it is an essential part of assessment of the child with asthma. Most children with asthma are atopic but allergen avoidance measures have not been shown to have a major role in management (Ch. 42).

Pattern of asthma

There is a wide spectrum of severity of asthma. This is relevant in terms of management and prognosis. Some children have episodic symptoms, with extended periods when they are totally symptom free. Others have persistent asthma, with symptoms present on most days. One way to classify the spectrum of severity of asthma is:
- *infrequent episodic*
- *frequent episodic*
- *persistent asthma.*

The distinctions between these three categories are somewhat arbitrary. Children with infrequent episodic symptoms may be typified as those who have 3–5 exacerbations of asthma a year and are well clinically and have normal lung function in the symptom free intervals. About 75% of children with asthma have infrequent episodic disease. About 20% of children with asthma have frequent episodic asthma. They may have six or more attacks per year but are well between exacerbations. Those with persistent asthma (about 5%) will have symptoms on most days.

Questions that are particularly helpful in clarifying the pattern of asthma include:
- Are there nocturnal symptoms?
- Are there symptoms on waking in the morning?
- Is there normal exercise tolerance?
- How much school is missed due to asthma?
- How frequent is the use of bronchodilator medication?

Management

Drugs used to treat asthma

There are two main strategies in the drug treatment of asthma. The first is the use of ***reliever*** medications to reverse acute airway obstruction. The main drugs are:
- bronchodilators (beta-2 sympathomimetic agents, anticholinergic agents and theophyllines)
- corticosteroids.

The second is preventing symptoms by decreasing airway inflammation and bronchial hyperreactivity. The main ***preventer*** medications are:
- corticosteroids (inhaled and oral)
- sodium cromoglycate
- nedocromil sodium
- leukotriene antagonists.

Symptom controllers (long acting beta-2 sympathomimetic agents) are used in combination with inhaled corticosteroids to augment asthma preventer therapy.

Beta-2 sympathomimetics (beta-2 agonists) are the most widely used reliever medications. They are available as metered dose aerosols, powder inhaler devices, nebuliser solutions, oral and injectable preparations. The preferred route of administration is by inhalation. Most children can use a powder inhaler device effectively from 5–6 years of age and a standard metered dose aerosol from 7–8 years. Spacer attachments, with a flexible facemask or with a one way mouthpiece, will allow younger children to use a metered aerosol and are also very valuable in acute attacks of asthma when the child's technique may deteriorate. The beta-2 agonists can be nebulised with a compressed air pump or using oxygen as the driving gas. This has become the first line therapy in acute severe asthma.

Beta-2 agonists can be used immediately prior to exercise to help prevent exercise triggered asthma.

Ipratropium bromide is an anticholinergic agent which is available as a nebuliser solution or as a metered aerosol. Its main use is in combination with beta-2 agonists in acute severe asthma.

Theophyllines are available as oral, rectal and intravenous preparations. Intravenous aminophylline used to be a first line therapy in acute asthma but has been replaced by beta-2 agonists, ipratropium bromide and the early use of oral corticosteroids. The absorption of the rectal form is erratic and this preparation is not recommended. Long acting oral preparations have been popular, especially to control nocturnal symptoms, but the emphasis on preventive therapy has led to decreased use.

Sodium cromoglycate and nedocromil sodium are preventer therapies available as dry powder inhaler, metered aerosol or nebuliser solution. The main target population is children with frequent episodic asthma in whom the aim is to prevent asthma symptoms. They are used on a regular basis over a number of months. In addition, either may be taken immediately before exercise to block asthma provoked by exercise.

Corticosteroids are available as oral or injectable forms, metered dose aerosols, dry powder inhaler devices and nebulised preparations. Oral corticosteroids are required by a minority of children for the treatment of acute exacerbations, and by a small proportion of children with persistent asthma to optimise control. Inhaled corticosteroids are effective preventers. They are the therapy of choice for persistent asthma and for children with frequent episodic disease not controlled by sodium cromoglycate or nedocromil sodium. The use of spacer devices, especially in children receiving higher doses of inhaled corticosteroids (more than 400 μg daily) is recommended to minimise the possibility of side effects from oropharyngeal deposition.

Leukotriene antagonists are preventer therapy available in oral form. They are effective but their position in the therapeutic armamentarium is still being established.

Acute exacerbations of asthma

The focus of management of acute attacks of asthma is assessment of severity of the episode and treatment to restore baseline lung function. The initial assessment attempts to identify those whose asthma is mild and will be managed at home, those who may require admission to hospital and those who will definitely require admission and may need management in an intensive care unit.

- *Mild asthma* usually involves coughing, a soft wheeze, minor difficulty in breathing, no difficulty in speaking in sentences, initial PEF at least 60% of predicted and oxygen saturation (SaO_2) of at least 94%.
- *Moderate asthma* involves persistent cough, loud wheeze, obvious difficulty in breathing with use of accessory muscles, able to speak in phrases, PEF 40–60% of predicted and SaO_2 91–93%.
- *Severe asthma* involves a very distressed and anxious child, gasping for breath, unable to speak more than a few words in one breath, pale and sweaty, possibly cyanosed, palpable pulsus paradoxus and poor air entry with a silent chest. The PEF will be <40% of predicted and SaO_2 90% or less.

One protocol for the management of acute asthma would be to begin with a beta-2 agonist agent such as salbutamol or terbutaline. In mild and moderate cases this may be given by inhalation using a metered dose aerosol and spacer device. In more severe cases it is delivered via a nebuliser with oxygen as the driving gas.

If the bronchodilator does not provide relief for at least 3–4 hours, further beta agonist may be given together with oral corticosteroids. Children who are expected to require inhaled beta agonist more frequently than 3–4 hourly should be managed in hospital. When there is an inadequate response to therapy with beta agonists, oxygen and corticosteroids, inhaled ipratropium bromide has been shown to have a small additive effect.

Intravenous aminophylline is an effective bronchodilator but there is little evidence that it has an effect additive to that achieved with maximal doses of beta agonists. Many paediatric units have not used aminophylline for asthma for many years.

The resolution of an acute attack of asthma is not the end of treatment and should be used as an opportunity to consider the background control and management of the child's asthma.

Episodic and persistent asthma

Drug therapy for infrequent episodic asthma is a beta agonist as required. A 35 year follow up of Melbourne schoolchildren showed that those with infrequent episodic asthma who were not treated with preventer medication had an excellent prognosis, with no evidence of long term abnormalities in lung function. Children with frequent episodic asthma should receive preventer medication. One approach has been to use sodium cromoglycate initially and to replace it with inhaled corticosteroids if there is an inadequate clinical response. Some clinicians use inhaled corticosteroids as the first line preventer. Persistent asthma is unlikely to respond to sodium cromoglycate; inhaled corticosteroids are the preventers of choice in persistent asthma.

Clinical example

Jill was a 4 year old who had persistent asthma. She had been admitted to hospital at the age of 3 months with bronchiolitis. Since then she had 6–8 episodes of wheezing each year, usually triggered by colds. Even at her best, she tended to wheeze after a few minutes of exercise and had about two nights each week when her sleep was disturbed by cough and wheeze. Her treatment had been with a beta agonist as required. This relieved her symptoms but she tended to have it most days.

She was started on inhaled steroids administered via a spacer device. Within 2 weeks, there was dramatic improvement, with cessation of nocturnal symptoms and marked improvement in exercise tolerance. Her dose of inhaled steroids was decreased, with continued benefit. Over the next 6 months she did not require beta agonists more than once a month.

The management of asthma is more than drug treatment. Some of the issues are shown in Table 47.2. The child and family need education about asthma and its management. Avoidable factors such as cigarette smoke should be eliminated from the child's environment. Allergen avoidance measures have a role for some children but the clinician needs to be wary about creating false expectations that allergen avoidance is likely to have a major beneficial impact for most children. Explanation of the difference between reliever and preventer therapy is vital (many patients find it useful to remember that most reliever medications are blue, metered dose inhalers). Demonstration of correct inhaler technique and reinforcing the need for good compliance are essential. An appropriate ***crisis management plan*** should be developed by the doctor and implemented by the family. In particular a *written action plan* should be provided, together with arrangements for follow up.

Table 47.2   Asthma management

Education
Natural history
Medications
Inhaler technique
Compliance
Exercise
Family concerns and expectations
Crisis care

Assess severity with lung function

Aim for optimal control of symptoms and normal life style

Drugs
Beta-2 sympathomimetics
Sodium cromoglycate and nedocromil sodium
Inhaled corticosteroids
Oral corticosteroids
Ipratropium bromide
Theophyllines
Leukotriene antagonists

Control trigger factors if possible

Review regularly

Clinical example

Amy is a 4 year old girl who has had four admissions to hospital with asthma in the past year. She has also had disturbed sleep due to wheeze 3–4 times a week. After a few minutes exercise she has to stop because of wheeze and breathlessness. She has been treated with salbutamol on an 'as necessary' basis. On average she has salbutamol at least once a day. You decide to start her on inhaled corticosteroids on a regular basis.

Write down a modified asthma management plan for Amy's parents, including day to day management and how to treat an acute exacerbation.

Prognosis

Approximately 60% of those children with infrequent episodic asthma will cease wheezing by early adult life, but only 20% of those with frequent episodic asthma and less than 5% of those with persistent asthma become wheeze free in adult life. Nevertheless, with appropriate therapy asthma can be controlled. For children with frequent episodic and persistent asthma the price of a normal life will be taking regular preventive medication and avoiding smoking.

Wheezing disorders other than asthma
48

R. Henry

The child who wheezes

Although asthma is by far the most common cause of a recurrent wheeze, the term 'wheeze' should not be used interchangeably with asthma, as there are many other possible causes. It is difficult to describe a sound and this makes a definition of wheeze imprecise. Wheeze is typically a high pitched, musical whistle heard during expiration. The term wheeze refers to the noise heard either with or without a stethoscope.

In the normal situation, a child's breathing is inaudible without a stethoscope because the velocity of airflow in the airways is too low to produce a sound. When the airways narrow, turbulence occurs. Wheeze may occur when the velocity of airflow increases as a consequence of the airways narrowing. In diseases such as asthma and bronchiolitis, the pathology is in the small airways. This sometimes leads to the erroneous impression that the wheeze is due to air whistling through narrowed small airways. Theoretically, the velocity of airflow in the smaller airways is far too low to cause a wheeze, even when there is significant narrowing. The wheeze is generated in the trachea and major bronchi, which are made narrower by secondary compression during expiration. The physiological explanation is that the small airways obstruction leads to a forced expiration with positive (rather than the usual negative) intrapleural pressure. This positive intrapleural pressure exceeds the pressure within the lumen of the trachea and other large airways, resulting in compression of these airways during expiration and producing a wheeze in these dynamically narrowed larger airways. Examples are demonstrated in Figures 48.1 and 48.2.

Although obstruction in the small airways is the usual reason for wheeze generated in the large airways, obstructive lesions in the trachea or main bronchi can also cause wheeze. In this case, the wheeze may be generated by the increase in velocity of airflow at the level of the obstruction. Thus, foreign bodies in the intrathoracic part of the large airways or large airway compression from tuberculous lymph notes may manifest themselves as wheeze.

Since wheeze can develop because of narrowing of either the small or large airways, there are many potential causes. One way of classifying the likely causes of wheeze in an individual child is to consider wheeze in different age categories.

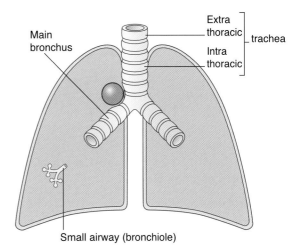

Fig. 48.1 An obstructive lesion in the region of the right main bronchus and carina producing an audible wheeze.

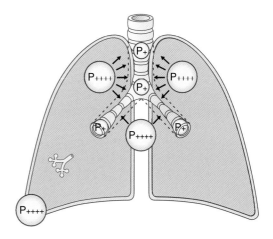

Fig. 48.2 Widespread narrowing of the small bronchioles — for example, in viral bronchiolitis.

Wheezing in infants, toddlers and the preschool child

Table 48.1 lists potential causes of wheezing in younger children.

Table 48.1 Causes of wheeze in infants, toddlers and the preschool child

Obstruction of small airways
Acute viral bronchiolitis
Transient infant wheeze
Asthma
Aspiration
Chronic lung disease of prematurity
Bronchiectasis

Obstruction of large airways
Airway malformations
Vascular malformations
Mediastinal cysts/masses
Inhaled foreign body
Ingested foreign body

Clinical example

Edward was 10 months old when he was referred to a paediatrician because of an 8 month history of wheeze. His mother reported that he wheezed all the time. She was embarrassed to take him out in public because people would stop her and tell her to take Edward to see a doctor. She indicated that he did not ever seem to be in discomfort with his wheeze. Neither cough nor breathlessness had been present. He had been treated with inhaled corticosteroids and salbutamol for 3 months, both without apparent clinical benefit. There was no family history of asthma. He was thriving, with a weight of 10.5 kg. He was smiling and playing contentedly but had a loud wheeze. The diagnosis of transient infant wheeze was suspected. The nature of this entity was explained to his mother and his medications were ceased. During the next 12 months his wheezing resolved gradually.

Obstruction of small airways

Acute viral bronchiolitis

This is the most common cause of wheeze in the first year of life and is usually due to respiratory syncytial virus (RSV). The clinical features of acute viral bronchiolitis are described in detail in Chapter 49.

Transient infant wheeze versus asthma

The natural history of wheezing in the first 6 years of life has been studied to try to assess the factors that determine whether children wheeze and whether they outgrow the symptoms. One cohort study found that about 50% of children had no wheezing in the first 6 years of life; 20% had at least one lower respiratory tract illness with wheezing during the first 3 years of life but no wheezing by 6 years (transient infant wheezing); about 15% had persistent wheezing; and 15% developed wheezing after the age of 3 years.

Children with transient infant wheeze appear to have airways that are of relatively small calibre and may be floppy. Maternal smoking is a risk factor but neither a personal nor family history of atopy is more common than in children who do not wheeze. Transient infant wheezing is a benign condition.

Children who continue to wheeze at 6 years of age are more likely to have had wheezing without colds, to be atopic, to have a first degree relative with asthma, to be male and to have a mother who smokes.

It is often difficult to distinguish which infants with wheezing have or will develop asthma from those with a transient problem. For this reason the appropriate management of individual infants with wheeze may require the input of a consultant paediatrician.

Aspiration bronchitis/bronchiolitis/pneumonia

This possibility should always be considered in small infants with recurrent or persistent lower respiratory symptoms, including cough and wheeze. Aspiration is usually due to gastro-oesophageal reflex or incoordinate swallowing, or a combination of the two. Incoordinate swallowing will lead to aspiration occurring during feeds, whereas there will be a delay between feeding and coughing with reflux. Some children have incoordinate swallowing due to delayed maturation of the normal mechanisms for swallowing, while others have problems secondary to disease of the central nervous system (such as cerebral palsy). Less commonly, aspiration may be due to an anatomical communication such as a tracheo-oesophageal fistula.

Chronic lung disease of prematurity (bronchopulmonary dysplasia)

The preterm infant who develops hyaline membrane disease and requires ventilation and high concentrations of supplemental oxygen may go on to develop chronic lung disease (Ch. 34). This is thought to result from the interaction of immaturity of the lung, oxygen toxicity, mechanical ventilation and possibly repeated aspiration. This is now a common condition seen in tertiary referral paediatric centres, and persistent cough and wheeze for the first year or two of life is common. When these children develop acute viral bronchiolitis, it is likely to be a particularly severe disease.

Suppurative lung disease

Familial reasons for suppurative lung disease (bronchiectasis) are important. Cystic fibrosis occurs in 1 in 2500 live births in the Caucasian population (Ch. 50). Infants with cystic fibrosis may have lower respiratory tract symptoms such as cough, wheeze and manifestations of repeated lower respiratory infections. The wheeze in this situation is usually due to bronchiolitis, sometimes viral and sometimes bacterial.

Other familial forms of suppurative lung disease which may present in infancy with cough and wheeze include immunodeficiencies such as X linked hypogammaglobulinaemia (Ch. 43) and primary ciliary dyskinesia (immotile cilia syndrome).

Acquired bronchiectasis may occur after bronchiolitis or pneumonia. Well recognised causes include adenovirus infection (especially types 7 and 21) and measles (Ch. 37). Ongoing aspiration may also lead to bronchiectasis. Often the aetiology is unknown.

Obstruction of large airways

Congenital airway malformations

Tracheomalacia/bronchomalacia. This is a primary malformation of either tracheal or bronchial cartilage resulting in excessive floppiness of the central airways. This causes wheeze and a brassy cough, likened to the 'bark' of a seal. Children who have had a repaired tracheo-oesophageal fistula (TOF) have tracheomalacia. Their cough is referred to as a 'TOF cough'. Tracheomalacia may be complicated by sudden, very severe obstructive episodes knowing as 'dying spells'. These are due to transient total apposition of the anterior and posterior tracheal walls.

Congenital lobar emphysema. This is a result of a congenital deficiency of cartilage in a lobar bronchus, which causes obstruction to the bronchus, overdistension of that lobe, and subsequent displacement of the adjacent lung and mediastinum. Generally, these infants present in the neonatal period with respiratory distress accompanied by wheeze and overdistension of the chest. Treatment is surgical removal of the affected lobe, and the long term prognosis is excellent.

Subglottic/tracheal haemangioma. These lesions are absent at birth (as are haemangiomas of the skin), but appear during the first few months of life. The symptoms of expiratory wheeze, inspiratory stridor and respiratory distress typically occur between the ages of 6 weeks and 6 months. The actual noise produced depends upon the anatomical site of the mass. Laryngeal or subglottic lesions cause inspiratory stridor; and intrathoracic tracheal lesions cause expiratory wheeze. Approximately half of these infants will also have cutaneous haemangiomas in the head and neck region. The diagnosis can only be made reliably by bronchoscopy under general anaesthesia. Spontaneous resolution of the haemangioma may take a few years and intervention (such as laser therapy) may be necessary.

Congenital tracheal/bronchial stenosis. This may occur anywhere in the central tracheobronchial tree, resulting in varying degrees of obstruction. Normally, these infants will present with breathlessness, expiratory wheeze and/or inspiratory stridor, depending upon the site and extent of the narrowing.

Vascular malformations

Vascular ring. The true vascular ring is usually due to a double aortic arch malformation. This results in early onset of wheeze and stridor, cough and recurring lower respiratory tract infection. Diagnosis can be made on barium swallow, which demonstrates an abnormal indentation of the oesophagus posteriorly plus an indentation of the anterior wall of the tracheal air column on lateral views. Diagnosis is confirmed at bronchoscopy and surgical excision of the smaller arch is indicated after delineation of the anatomy by angiography. Other vascular malformations that may cause symptoms include innominate artery compression of the trachea (often associated with localised tracheomalacia), aberrant subclavian artery and rare forms of pulmonary artery sling.

Large left to right cardiac shunt. External compression of the bronchi can occur in the presence of enlarged, hypertensive pulmonary arteries, particularly when there is associated left atrial enlargement. The left atrium lies immediately adjacent to the tracheal bifurcation and infants with this combination seem particularly prone to bronchial compression; for example, ventricular septal defect and persistent ductus arteriosus. Clinically, this obstruction results in overdistension of one or both lung fields with associated wheeze and breathlessness.

Mediastinal cysts and tumours

Cystic hygroma/lymphangioma. Usually these contain elements of both cystic hygroma (cavernous lymphangioma) and capillary lymphangioma within the same lesion. Although the majority of these are in the neck, they can involve the mediastinum, where they tend to be more cystic and can cause compression of the central airways. In this site surgical removal may be indicated.

Bronchogenic cysts. These are usually adjacent to the lower trachea, carina or main bronchi. Although embryological in origin, they can present quite late in childhood, or even in adult life; however, if large, they will present with wheeze and breathlessness, and an obvious middle mediastinal mass will be noted on chest X ray. Treatment is surgical excision.

Oesopageal duplication cysts, neurenteric and gastroenteric cysts. These are usually in the posterior mediastinum and therefore are less likely to impinge upon the airway; however, duplication cysts may be in the middle mediastinum and may result in wheeze and respiratory difficulty. Treatment is by surgical excision.

Teratomas. These are the most common of the germ cell tumours and, while most are in the sacrococcygeal region, between 10 and 15% are found in the anterior mediastinum and frequently cause compression of adjacent structures, particularly the trachea or main bronchi. These tumours may be benign (dermoid cysts) or malignant. Malignancy can be determined only after histological evaluation; excision is mandatory.

Mediastinal lymphadenopathy. Extrinsic compression of the main bronchi may occur due to enlarged hilar lymph nodes secondary to primary tuberculosis. Classic features are recent weight loss, cough, fever, wheeze and breathlessness. The chest X ray will show hilar lymphadenopathy, narrowing of the adjacent mainstem bronchus and frequently a parenchymal lesion, representing the primary complex (Fig. 48.3). Other causes of enlarged hilar lymph nodes in this age group may be lymphomas.

Inhaled foreign body

The majority of children presenting with an inhaled foreign body are toddlers and preschool children. The most common foreign bodies are nuts (especially peanuts), but other food material and small objects (for example, plastic toys, grass seeds, leaves) can be inhaled into the airways. One third of children present with the classic diagnostic triad of choking, asymmetrical air entry and abnormal chest X ray. Many children present with acute onset of wheeze, accompanied by cough and breathlessness. Chest X rays may show air trapping from a ball valve obstruction, particularly if both inspiratory

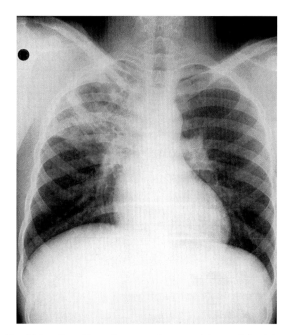

Fig. 48.3 Chest X ray demonstrating consolidation of the right upper lobe; this child had a strongly positive Mantoux test. Diagnosis — primary pulmonary tuberculosis.

and expiratory views are taken (Fig. 48.4). Other X ray findings include atelectasis and radiopaque foreign bodies; however, about one third of children with an inhaled foreign body have a perfectly normal chest X ray. Similarly, although there may be diminished breath sounds over one side of the chest, or localised high pitched expiratory wheeze, physical signs may be absent. If a foreign body is suspected, then bronchoscopy should be considered.

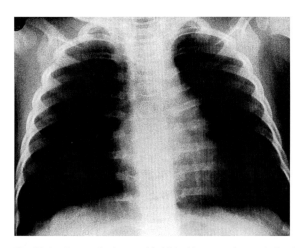

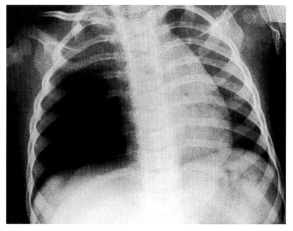

Fig. 48.4 X rays of a 3 year old child with acute wheeze during inspiration (left) and expiration (right). The inspiratory film is normal. The expiratory film shows marked trapping in the right lower zone, consistent with a ball valve (partial obstruction) in the right main bronchus. At bronchoscopy a peanut was removed from the right main bronchus.

Pablo, a 3 year old boy, had no past history of chest problems. Ten days previously he had been to a friend's birthday party and was observed to have a choking episode while laughing. Shortly beforehand he was seen emptying a bowl full of salted peanuts into his mouth. During the choking episode he was blue around the lips and he coughed uncontrollably for 2–3 minutes. Following this episode, he appeared to be normal and continued playing at the party. Since the party, however, his mother had noted a troublesome cough and a soft, but persistent, wheeze. On examination, the only abnormal finding was localised expiratory wheezing and softer inspiratory breath sounds over the right chest, both front and back. A chest X ray (inspiratory film) was normal; an expiratory film showed right sided hyperinflation and mediastinal shift to the left.

Because of the history and physical signs, a foreign body inhalation was suspected and he was admitted to hospital for a bronchoscopy. Two large fragments of peanut were removed from the right main bronchus. There were no abnormal chest findings following this procedure, and at follow up 2 weeks later he was perfectly well.

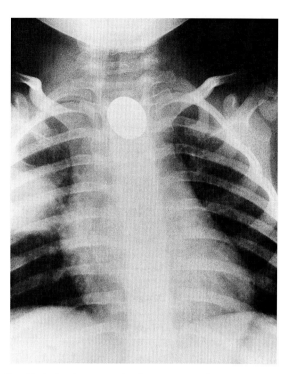

Fig. 48.5 A coin impacted in the upper oesophagus has distorted the adjacent trachea causing wheeze and consolidation — collapse of the right upper lobe.

Ingested foreign body

Quite large foreign bodies (coins, toys, bones) may be swallowed and may fail to pass through the relatively narrow upper oesophagus. If these foreign bodies are large (Fig. 48.5), or irregularly shaped, they may cause significant obstruction to the adjacent extrathoracic trachea. In most cases this will produce inspiratory stridor, but expiratory wheeze may also be audible. These children will have difficulty swallowing of recent onset, plus persisting fever and malaise as a consequence of inflammation of the oesophagus from the large foreign body. Radiopaque foreign bodies will be visible on X ray providing the upper portion of the airways is present on the chest film. Management is by removal of the foreign body by oesphagoscopy under general anaesthesia.

Wheeze in school aged children/adolescents

Causes of wheezing in older children are listed in Table 48.2.

Obstruction of small airways

As well as the conditions mentioned previously, *Mycoplasma pneumoniae* is a common cause of wheezing in school aged children. This organism is an important trigger for asthma and will often be seen as one of the causes of an exacerbation of asthma. Other children,

without a history of previous wheezing, may develop symptoms with mycoplasma infections. Suggestive clinical features include protracted cough and fever, combined with widespread crackles on chest auscultation and extensive radiological changes (especially parahilar and peribronchial) in a child who looks well. Oral erythromycin is the appropriate antibiotic.

Obstruction of large airways

Bronchial adenomas

These are rare and usually present with wheeze and breathlessness due to the mechanical effects of the

---

Table 48.2   Causes of wheeze in school aged children/ adolescents (5–15 years)

Obstruction of small airways
Asthma
Mycoplasma pneumoniae infection
Bronchiectasis

Obstruction of large airways
Inhaled/ingested foreign bodies
Mediastinal masses/tumours
Bronchial adenoma
Alpha 1-antitrypsin deficiency
Hysterical wheeze/stridor

tumour. A persistent irritating cough and failure to respond to asthma therapy are typical.

Alpha 1 antitrypsin deficiency

Most children and adolescents will present with neonatal hepatitis or a known family history of this disorder. Respiratory symptoms usually develop in the third or fourth decade but cough, wheeze and breathlessness may begin in childhood.

Hysterical wheeze/stridor

Fictitious asthma is sometimes seen, particularly in young females. It is more common for there to be inspiratory stridor rather than wheeze. The noise is generated by the vocal cords, which are held in apposition during exhalation, and by dynamic compression of central airways due to the violent expiratory effort. Usually there is considerable emotional turmoil involving the child and family, and the possibility of sexual abuse needs to be considered.

Lower respiratory tract infections and abnormalities in childhood

P. N. Le Souëf

Infection in the lower respiratory tract is very common in childhood, as many infections that are appear to be located in the upper respiratory tract include a lower respiratory tract component. A lower respiratory tract infection can be considered to be present when there are symptoms or signs that arise from below the thoracic inlet. In developing countries, acute lower respiratory infections remain the greatest cause of mortality in children under the age of 5 years.

Pneumonia

Pneumonia is a major cause of morbidity and mortality in children and is characterised by consolidation of the alveoli with or without interstitial involvement. There are many different causes of pneumonia, including inflammation related to:
- aspiration
- viral infection
- bacterial infection
- atypical infections.

Symptoms of acute infective pneumonia include dyspnoea, fever and associated malaise. Cough may be dry or moist. Pleuritic chest pain may be present. If the pneumonia involves the apices, neck pain may be present and can be confused with the stiff neck of meningism. If the diaphragmatic pleural surface is involved, pain can be referred to the shoulder tip.

Signs include tachypnoea and respiratory distress, dullness to percussion, and, on auscultation, localised crackles and bronchial breathing. None of these symptoms or signs is specific for pneumonia and the clinical diagnosis is suspected when the history and examination are consistent. Signs of established pneumonia or complications of the condition include those related to:
- pleural effusion — shifting of mediastinum or trachea, dullness to percussion (with stony dullness in large effusions), reduced or absent breath sounds, and bronchial breathing above the effusion
- pneumothorax — uncommon, shifting of mediastinum or trachea, reduced breath sounds.

Investigations assist in establishing the diagnosis:
- *Chest radiography* is the most reliable investigation for this purpose. In a sense, the chest radiograph is

definitive, as if it is clear the diagnosis is ruled out at that time. In general, lobar consolidation is suggestive of bacterial pneumonia, a more central peribronchial infiltrate may indicate *Mycoplasma* infection, and patchy or peripheral consolidation may be more in keeping with a viral infection, but the specificity of these observations is relatively poor. Importantly, all these radiological features can be seen on occasion with asthma.
- *Blood culture* may be performed if clinically indicated, but bacteraemia is not common in the majority of bacterial pneumonias.
- *Antigen examination of a pernasal aspirate* can be helpful in detecting the presence of causative respiratory viruses.
- *Sputum* is often difficult to obtain and its usefulness in diagnosis is poor due to contamination by upper airway bacteria.
- *Bacterial antigen detection in the peripheral blood* is of limited use.

Staphylococcal pneumonia

Pneumonia caused by *Staphylococcus aureus* is usually a severe form of pneumonia and is more common in younger children, especially those under 2 years of age. Its prevalence is increased in children from a socially disadvantaged background, and in developed countries, particularly in indigenous people.

The child with staphylococcal pneumonia usually appears more unwell than with other forms of pneumonia, and high fever, pallor, tachypnoea and respiratory distress are all more common. The onset is usually acute and the course is more rapid. Signs on chest auscultation are non specific, but chest X rays are more likely to show marked abnormalities. Early in the course of the illness, staphylococcal pneumonia may have radiological features in common with other forms of bacterial pneumonia, including lobar consolidation, patchy shadowing and a small pleural effusion. Within days, however, more serious findings may be evident, including widespread opacifications, large pleural effusions and displacement of intrathoracic structures. More specific to staphylococcal pneumonia are abscesses, either single or multiple, and large or encysted pleural effusions with thick walls. Air leaks, including pneumothorax, pneumomediastinum,

465

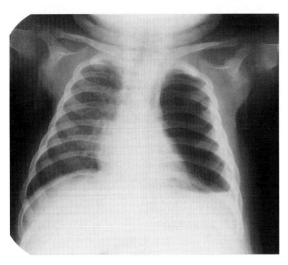

Fig. 49.1 Staphylococcal pneumonia showing a large left sided pneumatocoele.

pneumopericardium and, in particular, pneumatoceles are highly specific for staphylococcal pneumonia (Fig. 49.1). However they are not pathognomonic of this condition as air leaks including pneumatoceles can be found in pneumonia caused by *E.coli, klebsiella, pseudomonas,* group A streptococci and pneumococci. These more serious problems may be defined most accurately using chest computerised (CT) scans.

Investigations

Blood cultures may be positive in the acute phase of the illness. Aspiration of pleural effusions may be undertaken to assist with diagnosis, but the fluid from an empyema may be sterile if sufficient antibiotic treatment has been given.

Management

Infants in whom staphylococcal pneumonia is suspected should be hospitalised to allow adequate observation during the acute phase of the illness and rapid treatment of air leaks. Antibiotics need to be broad spectrum until an accurate diagnosis can be made. The combination of a beta-lactamase resistant penicillin such as flucloxacillin and a third generation cephalosporin, both given intravenously, is commonly used, as it combines direct treatment of staphylococci as well as coverage of other common respiratory pathogens. In children under approximately 2 years of age, flucloxacillin should be considered for addition to the treatment regimen of any child with clinically significant pneumonia, due to the much higher prevalence of staphylococcal pneumonia in this age group. In some communities, resistance to beta-lactamase resistant penicillins (so called methicillin resistant *Staphylococcus aureus* (MRSA)) may occur, so

other drugs such as clindamycin should be considered. Nosocomial MRSA infections are more likely to show multiple drug resistances than community acquired MRSA infections. The duration of antibiotic treatment needs to be at least 2–3 weeks, but 6 weeks of treatment is now commonly undertaken to reduce the risk of relapses.

Surgical intervention

As noted, surgery may be undertaken early in the course of the illness to assist in diagnosis or to reduce the mechanical effects of large effusions. Whether or not surgery reduces the duration of illness is less clear, although the decision to drain an effusion is often taken with the expectation that drainage will reduce the space occupying and pressure effects of a large effusion as well as reducing the recovery time. The decision to drain an effusion also needs to take into account the availability and expertise of a suitably experienced and technically skilled paediatric surgeon.

Long term outcome

The long term outcome of staphylococcal pneumonia is remarkable as there is a very high likelihood of a complete return to normality. Children examined radiologically some years after recovery generally show no evidence of previous problems, despite extensive, serious abnormalities in chest X rays at the time of the illness.

> ### Clinical example
>
> Jasmine, a 9 month old girl, was brought to the local doctor by her mother. She had been unwell for 2 days, with increasing fever, lethargy and difficulty feeding. The doctor noticed that she was pale, listless and tachypnoeic and scattered coarse crackles were heard over her lung fields on auscultation. She was transferred by ambulance to hospital where a chest X ray showed opacification in the right upper and left lower lobes. She was treated with oxygen and intravenous flucloxacillin and cefotaxime. Blood culture was positive for *S. aureus* and treatment with flucloxacillin was continued for 6 weeks. She slowly improved and she was fully recovered when seen after the antibiotic treatment had been completed.

Pneumococcal pneumonia

Streptococcus pneumoniae is the most common cause of bacterial pneumonia in children at any age. Pneumococcal pneumonia is most common in children under 3 years of age. Risk factors include male gender, indigenous race, day care attendance, frequent upper respiratory tract infections, preterm delivery and otitis media.

The onset of pneumonia may be preceded by symptoms of a mild upper respiratory infection. Symptoms of pneumonia then appear and include fever, tachypnoea, nasal flaring and grunting. Pleuritic chest pain is often present, but cough can be absent. Signs include reduced movement of the chest wall on the affected side, dullness to percussion, reduced breath sounds and bronchial breathing over the area involved. Dullness to percussion may indicate the presence of an empyema. If the upper lobes are involved, neck stiffness may be present, and the child may be misdiagnosed as having meningitis.

Chest X ray findings vary widely, but common findings are a well defined round opacification, lobar involvement (Fig. 49.2) or patchy changes. Empyema, abscesses and pneumatoceles are less common than in staphylococcal pneumonia. Blood culture may be positive and an increased white cell count in peripheral blood is common.

Current treatment is to make the diagnosis as early as possible and administer penicillin and a third generation cephalosporin. The response to treatment is usually rapid and complete recovery can be expected.

Clinical example

Ben, a 3 year old boy, presented with a 4 day history of cough, and fever. He was noted to be mildly unwell, to have a respiratory rate of 50 breaths per minute and bronchial breathing over the left base posteriorly. A chest X ray showed opacification confined to the left lower lobe. He was treated with parenteral then oral penicillin and was afebrile within 8 hours. The bronchial breathing had disappeared the next day and he was back to normal health within a week. A repeat X ray 1 month later was normal.

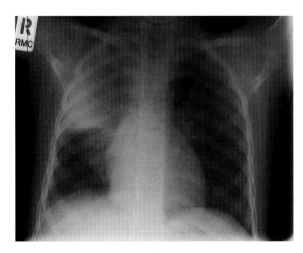

Fig. 49.2 Pneumococcal pneumonia showing lobar consolidation of the right upper lobe.

Haemophilus influenzae **type b pneumonia**

Pneumonia due to *H. influenzae* has become less frequent since the introduction of immunisation against this organism. *H. influenzae* is a Gram negative, pleomorphic coccobacillus. The organism is surrounded by a polysaccharide capsule and is found in the upper respiratory tract of the majority of normal, non immunised children, and less commonly in those who have been immunised. Three quarters of invasive infections occur in children aged under 2 years. Apart from age, risks factors for *H. influenzae* infection include indigenous race, lower socioeconomic group, male gender and immunodeficiencies.

The signs and symptoms of *H. influenzae* pneumonia are not distinguishable from those found in other pneumonias. Similarly, the radiological features are not specific to this organism. For children who are ill, treatment with a parenteral third generation cephalosporin is recommended, and for children who are less unwell, oral amoxicillin/clavulanic acid is appropriate. Other children in the family do not require prophylactic treatment if they are adequately immunised.

Mycoplasma pneumonia

Mycoplasma pneumoniae is a frequent causative organism of pneumonia in children. The clinical course is characterised by the gradual development of fever, malaise, upper respiratory symptoms and cough. Signs can include widespread sparse fine crackles or coarse crackles. In children with a tendency to asthma, wheeze is commonly present. The chest X ray often shows changes that are more striking than expected for the degree of clinical illness. The findings themselves are usually non specific, but can include perihilar opacification and involvement of the lower lobes. The diagnosis is supported by positive serology. Treatment with erythromycin is indicated, but the response to treatment may be restricted to a reduction in general symptoms, as the clinical course of the pneumonia itself may not be affected by treatment.

Other causes of bacterial pneumonia

Other bacteria that can cause pneumonia in the community include:

- *Group A beta-haemolytic streptococci (S. pyogenes)*. Although a common cause of bacterial pharyngitis, this organism is not a common cause of pneumonia. Its incidence is highest after 5 years of age and it occurs more commonly in winter. When it does cause pneumonia, the disease tends to be rapidly progressive, severe, and poorly responsive to antibiotic therapy. The symptoms of fever, chest pain and haemoptysis are more common than in other forms of pneumonia,

467

and a higher percentage of cases will have large pleural effusions and empyema. If proven by culture, the treatment of choice is high dose intravenous penicillin G.

- *Group B beta-haemolytic streptococci.* This organism is a common and important cause of neonatal pneumonia, which occurs soon after birth and has a rapidly progressive course, can mimic respiratory distress of prematurity and has a high mortality. *Group B streptococci* rarely cause pneumonia after the neonatal period and in these 'late onset' cases, the course of the disease is usually not as acute as in the neonatal cases.
- *Klebsiella pneumoniae.* This organism causes pneumonia in neonates and in the immunocompromised host. It is a rare cause of pneumonia in children. In the latter, bacteraemia is more common than pneumonia. The clinical picture of *Klebsiella* pneumonia initially is not distinguishable from other forms of pneumonia, but the complications of lung abscess and pneumatocele may occur. Treatment with an aminoglycoside, a third generation cephalosporin or both of these drugs is usually recommended. Prior to the antibiotic era, mortality was high.
- *Other bacterial organisms* that can cause pneumonia in children include anthrax, *Bordetella pertussis*, brucella, *Burkholderia cepacia*, *Citrobacter* sp., *Corynebacterium sp., Escherichia coli, Listeria monocytogenes, Mycobacterium* sp., *Neisseria meningitidis*, *Pasteurella* sp., *Proteus sp., Pseudomonas aeruginosa*, *Salmonella* sp., and *Yersinia* sp.

Viral pneumonia

Viruses are common causes of pneumonia in children of all ages and the spectrum of disease varies widely. Risk factors for viral pneumonia are:

- *Age.* Children under 5 years of age are at greatest risk of viral pneumonia, but the risk remains high throughout the first decade of life.
- *Season.* Peak seasonal incidence is in winter.
- *Passive smoke exposure.* Maternal smoking increases the risk, and the influence is greatest in the first year of life.
- *Poor socioeconomic status.* This is a risk factor in both the developing and the developed worlds.
- *Pre-existing chronic problems.* The risk of developing viral pneumonia is also increased if a chronic chest problem such as cystic fibrosis, congenital heart disease or chronic postneonatal lung disease is present.

The most important causative viruses are parainfluenza viruses, influenza viruses, respiratory syncytial virus and adenoviruses. All of these can cause other respiratory illnesses apart from pneumonia, including acute upper respiratory tract infection, acute laryngotracheitis, bronchitis and bronchiolitis. Symptoms of these illnesses can coexist with those of pneumonia. Other viruses that can cause

> ### Clinical example
>
> Dana, an 8 year old girl, was brought to her general practitioner with a 3 day history of fever, increasing dry cough and loss of appetite. Her 12 year old brother had also been unwell with a cough and a fever. On examination, her doctor noted a temperature of 37.8°C, a respiratory rate of 28 breaths per minute, mild soft tissue recession, and the presence of sparse, coarse crackles bilaterally on auscultation. A chest X ray showed scattered areas of patchy opacification. No other investigations were done. She was treated symptomatically and recovered uneventfully over the next few days, having had a viral pneumonia.

pneumonia include rhinoviruses, cytomegalovirus and measles. The radiological features of viral pneumonias are non specific, but patchy infiltrates are more characteristic than lobar involvement (Fig. 49.3). Treatment with antiviral agents can be worthwhile, but supportive measures alone are most commonly used.

Fungal pneumonia

Fungal causes of pneumonia or pneumonia-like illnesses occur most commonly in immunocompromised children and include *Actinomyces, Aspergillus, Candida, Cryptococcus, Histoplasma* and *Nocardia* spp.

Protozoal pneumonia

Protozoa that are causes of pneumonia or pneumonia-like illnesses also occur most commonly in immunocompromised children and include *Cryptosporidium* spp., *Pneumocystis carinii* and *Toxoplasma* spp.

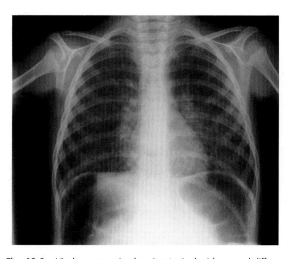

Fig. 49.3 Viral pneumonia showing typical widespread diffuse opacification.

Pulmonary tuberculosis

Tuberculosis (TB) is a disease caused by infection with *Mycobacterium tuberculosis*. Pulmonary TB remains an important cause of morbidity and mortality in children worldwide. The tubercle bacillus was discovered by Koch in 1822, and in the 20th century the spread of the disease was reduced in developed countries by effective public health and therapeutic approaches. However, late in the century the incidence began to increase due to the dismantling of control measures and the contribution of the AIDS epidemic. In the 21st century, the incidence of the disease is likely to increase and the Centers for Disease Control predict that there will be 12 million new cases of tuberculosis per year by 2005.

Children usually acquire the infective agent from an adult or adolescent rather than from other children. Most children with TB are under 5 years of age, with a lower incidence between 5 and 15 years. Other risk factors are low socioeconomic conditions and an indigenous racial background. The organism is transmitted mainly by inhalation in the indoor environment and only a small percentage of those infected will develop disease. The disease does not appear for weeks, months or years after infection. The initial lesion is often subpleural, occurring with an associated lymph node response that comprises a primary complex. The disease does not progress further in most patients but, when it does, the lung may be damaged by extensive caseation, effusions may occur and lymph nodes may enlarge and obstruct major airways. The disease may then disseminate and produce miliary, meningeal or renal tuberculosis.

Early in the course of the disease there are often few symptoms or signs of pulmonary disease, and in many cases pulmonary disease is manifest by non specific symptoms, including weight loss, malaise and fever. In time, most patients will develop a cough, and if there is airway compression wheeze may result.

Diagnosis is established by:
- suggestive chest X ray findings
- a positive tuberculin skin test (>15 mm skin induration from 5 TU of PPD-S is taken as evidence of disease; 10–15 mm suggests that infection has occurred, but disease may not be present; false negatives can occur in early or severe disease)
- culture of the organism from early morning gastric lavage
- light microscopic identification of bacilli from sputum, bronchoalveolar lavage fluid or pleural fluid.

Treatment has traditionally been with triple therapy which consists of 6 months treatment. Rifampicin, isoniazid and pyrazinamide are given for 2 months, then rifampicin and isoniazid for a further 4 months. A positive skin test without any evidence of pulmonary disease is treated with isoniazid alone for 6–9 months.

Atypical mycobacterial infection

Atypical mycobacteria (*M. avium, intracellulare, scrofulaceum*) can, on rare occasions, cause pulmonary disease in immunocompetent children, particularly in Australia. Pulmonary lymphadenopathy can be so marked as to obstruct airways. Diagnosis is made by specific skin testing and by identification of bacilli from fluid or tissue. Response to treatment is slow and therapy may need to be continued for 12–24 months, but prognosis for full recovery appears to be excellent.

Congenital disorders of the lower respiratory tract

Congenital lung abnormalities

Congenital anomalies of the lung are rare, but they may present well into childhood and their symptoms can be non specific; most can be detected on chest X ray:
- *Lung cysts* can vary from being simple and solitary to multiple and complex. Cysts can become infected if they communicate with the airway. They can also cause symptoms if they become enlarged and compress surrounding structures. Cystic adenomatoid malformation is rare and consists of multiple cysts and abnormal proliferation of lung elements. If sufficient lung is involved, it can result in chronic respiratory insufficiency.
- *Congenital lobar emphysema* is characterised by overinflation of a lung lobe and commonly presents before 6 months of age with respiratory distress or tachypnoea. It can require surgical intervention if the emphysematous lobe causes significant compression of neighbouring lung.
- *Sequestration* of the lung refers to an abnormality of the lung where a part of the lung is discontinuous with the rest of the lung. It can be intra pulmonary or extrapulmonary. The former is much more common and is more likely to become infected and require surgical removal. The latter is found most frequently on the left side, has an aberrant systemic blood supply and may be asymptomatic.

Congenital chest wall abnormalities

- *Pectus excavatum* is a midline concave depression of the lower sternum. It is very common, is not usually associated with any underlying respiratory abnormality and does not affect rib cage or lung function in most cases.
- *Thoracic dystrophies* are characterised by impaired development of the chest wall and are associated with pulmonary hypoplasia.

- *Scoliosis* can cause a restrictive functional defect in chest wall function if the angle of the curve is great enough.
- *Congenital diaphragmatic hernia* can present with early onset respiratory distress and can be difficult to diagnose if the gut above the level of the diaphragm on the chest X ray is misinterpreted as opacified or cystic lung.

Congenital lower airway abnormalities

- *Tracheomalacia and bronchomalacia* produce the symptoms of wheeze or stridor. If the airway above the thoracic inlet is affected by malacia, these symptoms are heard during inspiration, whereas if the tracheomalacia is below the thoracic inlet, the noises are heard on expiration. Malacia refers to the softening of the airway and its cause is usually unknown.
- *Oesophageal atresia and tracheo-oesophageal fistula* present at birth with drooling and respiratory distress from aspiration. The diagnosis is confirmed by failure to be able to pass a nasogastric tube; treatment is surgical. The rare H-type tracheo-oesophageal fistula has an aberrant connection between the oesophagus and the trachea and eventually presents with symptoms and signs suggestive of aspiration.
- *Bronchogenic cysts* are usually single and can be very large. Signs vary from nil to severe problems produced by compression of adjacent structures

Primary ciliary dyskinesia (PCD)

Primary ciliary dyskinesia is an inherited disorder and is caused by a series of ultrastructural abnormalities of cilia that inhibit cilial beating. The incidence is approximately one in 16 000 births and usually it is inherited as an autosomal recessive condition. Half the cases have dextrocardia and these cases are said to have Kartagener syndrome, which was originally diagnosed on the basis of the presence of the triad of bronchiectasis, chronic sinusitis and dextrocardia. Symptoms are related to the sites where cilial function is important in moving fluid along mucosal surfaces. The tracheobronchial tree is lined with ciliated epithelium and cilia are also found in the nose, sinuses, middle ear, eustachian tubes and reproductive tract. Most children with PCD have a chronic moist cough, and physiotherapy and the liberal use of antibiotics are important to prevent bronchiectasis.

Cystic fibrosis and other causes of chronic cough

50

A. B. Chang, S. M. Sawyer

Cough is the most common symptom of respiratory disease and is one of the most common reasons parents seek medical attention in young children. Cough can indicate the entire spectrum of childhood illness, ranging from being a symptom of the 'common cold' to a symptom of severe, life limiting disorders such as cystic fibrosis. Most cough in children is acute and resolves promptly. Prolonged or chronic cough is defined as cough lasting longer than 4–6 weeks. It is always abnormal and deserves careful consideration of the cause.

Pathophysiology

Cough involves a complex series of reflexes. It is a forceful expiration after a buildup of pressure in the thorax (up to 300 mmHg) and by contraction of expiratory muscles against a closed glottis. This leads to expulsion of air at high velocity, and sweeps material within the airways towards the mouth. Inspiration of a variable volume of air occurs when cough is stimulated. Successive coughs may or may not be preceded by inspiration.

Cough is an important component of normal respiratory function through two mechanisms. Firstly, mechanical stimulation of the larynx causes immediate expiratory efforts through the expiratory reflex, a primary defensive mechanism that is stimulated when foreign objects (such as food or fluid) are inhaled. Secondly, cough enhances mucociliary clearance. The absence of a forceful cough (for example, generalised muscular weakness) has important clinical repercussions, such as difficulty clearing secretions, atelectasis, lobar collapse and recurrent pneumonia.

When the presenting symptom is cough, the following issues should be considered:
- Cough, especially nocturnal cough, is not reported reliably when compared to objective measures of cough.
- Cough usually resolves spontaneously, which makes evaluation of therapeutic interventions difficult.
- Many cough treatments are not based on the results of randomised controlled trials.

- As the aetiology and management of cough in childhood is quite different from that for adults, extrapolation of the adult cough literature to children can be harmful.

Approach to diagnosis and management

Figure 50.1 outlines a schematic approach to the diagnosis and management of chronic cough. The key questions are presented in Table 50.1. Initial categorisation of cough into acute cough, subacute cough and chronic cough, according to duration, is helpful. There is, however, no strict definition of chronic cough. Most acute cough arises from respiratory viruses and settles within 2 weeks. Subacute cough commonly lasts 2–4 weeks, while chronic cough is cough lasting longer than 4–6 weeks.

The key point in the assessment of chronic cough is whether it is specific or non specific, according to the presence or absence of particular features (Table 50.2). Children younger than 6 years do not generally expectorate sputum. Thus the productive cough of older children and adults manifests as a moist or 'rattling' cough in younger children. The presence of any of these symptoms or signs raises the possibility of an underlying disorder.

The choice of investigation depends on the clinical findings. However, minimum investigation of chronic cough in children is a chest radiograph and lung spirometry (if the child is over 6 years old). Diagnoses to be considered include:
- bronchiectasis
- cystic fibrosis
- asthma
- retained foreign body
- aspiration lung disease
- atypical respiratory infections
- cardiac anomalies
- interstitial lung disease.

If basic investigations are not helpful, referral to a general or respiratory paediatrician is indicated rather than further investigations.

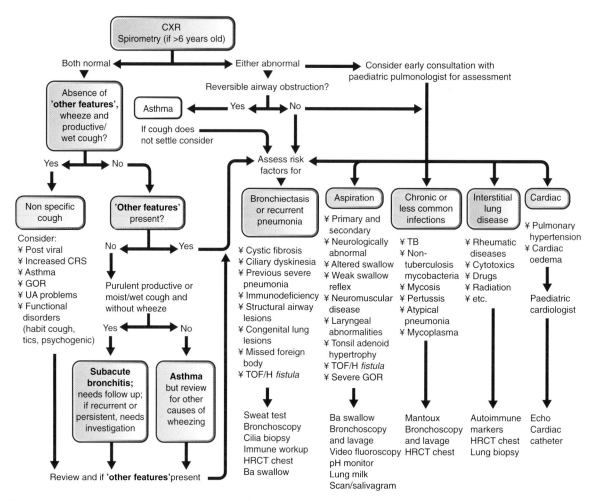

Fig. 50.1 A guide for management of the child with a chronic/persistent cough (> 4 weeks). Symptoms and signs vary according to age and illness severity. CRS, cough receptor sensitivity; CXR, chest X ray; GOR, gastro-oesophageal reflux; HRCT, high resolution computed tomography; TOF/H, tracheo-oesophageal fistula, H-type; TB, tuberculosis; UA, upper airway. Adapted with permission from Journal of Asthma 2001 38: 299–399.

Table 50.1 Key questions to consider

- Is the cough representative of an underlying respiratory disorder?
- Are any of the symptoms and signs in Table 50.2 present?
- Are exacerbating environmental factors present (passive or active tobacco smoking, other lung toxicants)?
- Should the child be referred promptly?

Clinical example

Anita, a 13 year old girl, was referred to a respiratory physician for a chronic cough. She had been managed incorrectly as an asthmatic for more than 10 years. On specific questioning, Anita indicated that she had been coughing for as long as she could remember and that her cough was worse in

the mornings and she often expectorated sputum. Her cough had been stable and she had not noticed any exertional dyspnoea. She had no growth failure and did not have digital clubbing. Given that she had some features of bronchiectasis, high resolution CT of her chest was performed and it revealed focal changes in the right basal segment (Fig. 50.2). Her immunoglobulin profile was normal and she was Mantoux and sweat test negative. On flexible bronchoscopy, a retained foreign body (piece of shell) was visualised and removed from the right medial segment of her right lower lobe. The foreign body had caused prolonged partial bronchial obstruction and was the aetiology for Anita's localised bronchiectasis.

It is important to define the aetiology of any child's chronic cough. This child had features, listed in Table 50.2, which indicated that she had specific cough and further investigations were indicated. In children it is best for investigations to be performed in a children's facility.

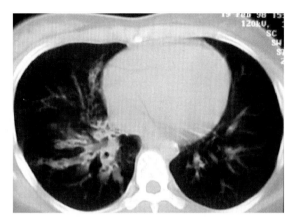

Fig. 50.2 High resolution CT (HRCT) scan of Anita (as described in the clinical example), a 13 year old child with a moist cough for more than 10 years. This child had been incorrectly managed as an asthmatic for 10 years until referred for another opinion. The HRCT scan shows focal bronchiectasis of the right basal segment. Flexible bronchoscopy was undertaken. A foreign body (piece of shell) was removed from the right basal medial bronchus.

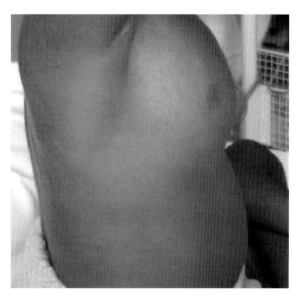

Fig. 50.4 Severe pectus carinatum. This can be present in children with any chronic lung diease.

Table 50.2 Symptoms and signs alerting to the presence of an underlying disorder

- Moist or productive cough
- Recurrent sinopulmonary infections
- Dyspnoea or exertional dyspnoea
- Wheeze
- Stridor
- Feeding or swallowing difficulties
- Failure to thrive
- Clubbing (Fig. 50.3)
- Haemoptysis
- Chest wall deformity (Fig. 50.4)
- Adventitious sounds on auscultation
- Cardiac abnormalities

Management of non specific cough

The majority of children with non specific cough have postviral cough and/or increased cough receptor sensitivity. There is no serious underlying cause of non specific cough and reassurance is a large part of management. Understanding and listening to parental concerns and expectations is important. There is no evidence that 'over the counter' (non prescription) medications reduce cough in young children.

Identification of exposure to enviromental tobacco smoke (ETS) in children, and active smoking in adolescents, is an important part of respiratory history taking. Environmental tobacco smoke exposure can cause non specific cough and can exacerbate a variety of respiratory disorders, including otitis media, asthma and pneumonia. Non specific cough is a reason to encourage parents to stop smoking. If smoking cessation cannot be achieved, aim to reduce smoking in enclosed spaces such as the house and car.

Habit cough is a cause of non specific cough, especially in older children and younger adolescents. The age of diagnosis is broad, but is commonly 4–15 years. Severe cases are more common in adolescents than children. The cough is classically 'honking' or 'croup-like'. It is generally absent in sleep and is worse at times where attention is focused on the cough. Habit cough generally settles promptly once parents are aware that there is no underlying respiratory problem. Mental health expertise is required for those with more severe or prolonged

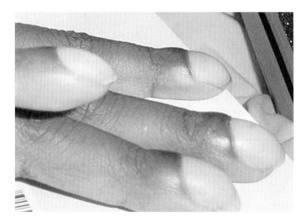

Fig. 50.3 Digital clubbing in a boy with bronchiectasis.

symptoms, especially if there are other features of somatisation or concerns of underlying psychopathology.

Cough, asthma and allergy

There is little doubt that children with asthma can present with cough. However, most children with chronic cough do not have asthma. Furthermore, while nocturnal cough is a feature of children with asthma, nocturnal cough alone is uncommonly due to asthma. In a randomised placebo controlled trial of inhaled salbutamol or corticosteroids in children with recurrent cough, the presence of airway hyperresponsiveness did not predict the efficacy of these medications for cough. If preventer medication is used, it should be introduced on a trial basis, with early review and cessation of medication if the cough does not respond to asthma therapy. Failure to do so will result in escalation of medication dose with the risk of significant side effects.

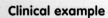

Clinical example

Gino was first seen by a paediatric respiratory physician when aged 8 years. He had been receiving 2000 μg/day of inhaled corticosteroids for the last 6 years for a chronic dry cough and had been managed as an 'asthmatic'. His medications were escalated when his cough did not respond to the steroids. When seen, his chest X ray and spirometry were normal, he was cushingoid and earlier pictures of him showed a normal sized 3 year old boy (Fig. 50.5). His 6 year old brother's body habitus was also normal. He had been exposed to tobacco smoke and had an element of habitual cough. His asthma medications were subsequently withdrawn and his cough eventually subsided when he was no longer exposed to tobacco smoke and received appropriate counselling.

This example illustrates the importance of obtaining a history of smoke exposure. Also, it is crucial not to 'overdiagnose' asthma based on the presence of isolated cough. In children, when cough is representative of asthma, the cough should subside within 2 weeks of appropriate asthma treatment. If the cough does not subside, the asthma therapy should be withdrawn and should not escalated.

A longitudinal population study of cough in infants and children revealed that recurrent cough (rather than chronic cough) presenting in the first year of life resolved over time in the majority of children. The group of children with recurrent cough without wheeze had neither airway hyperresponsiveness nor atopy, and differed significantly from those with classical asthma, with or without cough, in the persistence of symptoms over time. It is believed that these infants may have more narrow airways and that airway growth leads to symp-

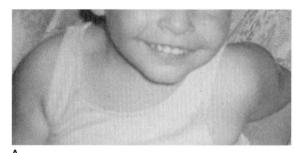

A

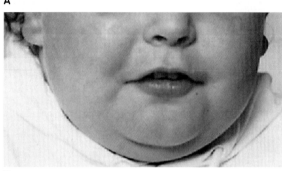

B

Fig. 50.5 This previously normal child had a chronic dry cough, which was incorrectly treated with escalating doses of inhaled corticosteroids, as described in the clinical example. **A** The boy before he commenced steroids. **B** After years of treatment with inhaled steroids, he was cushingoid in appearance; however, there had not been any change in his cough.

tomatic improvement. This group of infants is hard to differentiate clinically from those who continue to have recurrent cough due to asthma, making predictions of future illness difficult in infancy.

Cough, gastro-oesophageal reflux (GOR) and aspiration lung disease

Gastro-oesophageal reflux can be associated with cough. However, while GOR can cause cough, cough can also cause GOR and causative links are hard to identify. The view that GOR is a frequent cause of cough is now challenged. Gastro-oesophageal reflux is neither a specific nor frequent cause of chronic cough in children. As cough is very common in children and respiratory symptoms may exacerbate GOR, it is difficult to delineate cause and effect. Infants regularly regurgitate, yet few, if any, well infants cough with these episodes.

Aspiration lung disease can result from severe GOR and from laryngopalatal discoordination or discoordinated swallowing. These children present with chronic cough but usually in the context of severe developmental or neurological disturbance. The investigational evidence for aspiration lung disease can be difficult. Ambulatory oesophageal pH studies can identify GOR. However, a positive result does not confirm that aspiration has occurred. Similarly, primary aspiration (from swallowing discoordination) is also difficult to confirm as current standard tests, such as a nuclear medicine milk scan or a barium swallow, provide only a 'single moment' test which may not be representative of the child's routine feeding pattern.

Cough, sinusitis and postnasal drip

Although it is widely stated that sinusitis/postnasal drip is a common cause of cough, there is little supportive evidence. There are no cough receptors in the pharynx or postnasal space. Although sinusitis is common in childhood, it is not associated with asthma or cough once allergic rhinitis, a common association, is treated. The relationship between nasal secretions and cough is more likely to be linked by common aetiology (infection and/or inflammation causing both) or due to throat clearing of secretions reaching the larynx.

Bronchiectasis

Bronchiectasis can be the end result of a number of different respiratory disorders. In contrast to earlier times, it is now an uncommon disorder in non indigenous Australians. Bronchiectasis can be diffuse or focal. Diffuse disease usually develops secondary to an underlying disorder, such as cystic fibrosis, immunodeficiency or primary ciliary dyskinesia, although it can be idiopathic. Focal bronchiectasis more commonly reflects airway narrowing, either congenital (for example, bronchial stenosis) or acquired (for example, retained foreign body). In indigenous Australians, bronchiectasis is not uncommon and is thought to result from earlier childhood respiratory infections (postinfectious bronchiolitis obliterans). Congenital forms of bronchiectasis (such as in Williams–Campbell syndrome) are rare.

The spectrum of bronchiectasis varies from mild to severe. Symptoms and signs reflect the extent of the disease. Children with bronchiectasis have a chronic moist or productive cough and typically are clubbed. The cough is characteristically worse in the mornings. Physical findings are non specific: clubbing, pectus carinatum, coarse crepitations and localised wheeze may or may not be present.

Plain X rays will show suggestive features in severe disease (dilated and thickened bronchi may appear as 'tramtracks') but are insensitive in mild disease. Confirmation is by high resolution CT scan of the chest (routine CT provides insufficient detail).

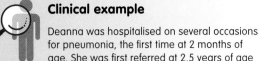

Clinical example

Deanna was hospitalised on several occasions for pneumonia, the first time at 2 months of age. She was first referred at 2.5 years of age and had a prolonged moist cough. She had a hyperinflated chest wall, early digital clubbing and growth failure. Her weight was below the third percentile and her height was at the third percentile. Her chest high resolution CT showed postinfectious bronchiolitis obliterans and bronchiectasis. Other investigations were normal. Her parents were taught home physiotherapy and she was admitted for a prolonged course of intravenous antibiotics. Following discharge, she remained on maintenance co-trimoxazole. Deanna's daily moist cough disappeared when her bronchiectasis was aggressively treated with antibiotics and physiotherapy.

A child with suspected bronchiectasis should be referred for investigation of a specific cause, and specific treatment instituted when indicated, for example in cystic fibrosis and immunodeficiency. The general approach to managing chronic respiratory infection in bronchiectasis is similar to that described for cystic fibrosis, using physiotherapy techniques to promote airway clearance, and antibiotics to treat associated infection. Pooled immunoglobulin replacement is indicated for those with identified immunodeficiency syndromes. Surgery is very rarely indicated, and only for those with focal disease.

Primary ciliary dyskinesia

Primary ciliary dysknesia syndromes encompass several congenital disorders, all of which affect the ciliary function of several organs, including the upper and lower respiratory tracts and genitourinary tract. The term includes Kartagener syndrome (situs invertus associated with bronchiectasis), immotile cilia syndrome, ciliary dysmotility and primary orientation defects of ciliary components. Primary ciliary dyskinesia has a prevalence of 1:20 000, is mostly autosomal recessive in inheritance and probably is genetically heterogenous.

Cilial ultrastructure consists of a 9 + 2 arrangement: the axoneme consists of nine peripheral microtubular doublets surrounding a central pair of microtubules. Abnormality in cilial function is due to alteration of cilial ultrastucture associated with change in the ciliary beat frequency. Secondary abnormalities in both ultrastructure and function can also occur as a result of infection, smoking or pollutants. Cilial dysfunction markedly reduces mucociliary clearance and results in recurrent infections of both the upper and lower respiratory tract (middle ear infections, pneumonia, bronchitis, bronchiectasis). In the genitourinary tract, ciliary dysfunction can lead to infertility in males and ectopic pregnancies in females.

The severity of primary ciliary dyskinesia varies widely. Presentation can be early in life with neonatal respiratory illness. In infants and older children, the diagnosis should be considered in those with chronic cough, bronchiectasis, recurrent pneumonia, atypical asthma, recurrent rhinosinusitus and chronic secretory otitis media. Specific investigations for primary ciliary dyskinesia include assessment of mucociliary clearance, measurement of ciliary beat frequency and electronic microscopic identification of cilial ultrastructure.

Cystic fibrosis

Cystic fibrosis (CF) is the most common life threatening autosomal recessive disorder in Australians, affecting approximately 1 in every 2500 births. It is caused by a defect in the CF transmembrane conductance regulator gene (CFTR). The CFTR gene encodes a protein for a cyclic AMP regulated chloride channel present on many epithelial cells, including those of the conducting airways, gut and genital tract. The commonest mutation, Δ508, accounts for approximately 70% of mutant alleles, and more than 700 mutations have been described.

Diagnosis

All infants are now screened at birth for CF. A two stage screening procedure is widely used. Initially, immuno-reactive trypsin (IRT) is measured in Guthrie blood spot samples. Samples with an IRT level above the 99th percentile are then tested for the common mutation (additional mutations are tested in some states).

Most Australian children with CF are identified by neonatal screening, with the diagnosis being confirmed with a sweat test (pilocarpine iontophoresis) at 6–10 weeks. Newborn screening does not detect all children with CF. A sweat test should be arranged if there are phenotypic features suggestive of CF. An elevated sweat chloride (>60 mmol/l) and sweat sodium (>60 mmol/l) is diagnostic. To minimise the multiple errors that can occur (especially false negatives), sweat testing should be undertaken in a laboratory that routinely does sweat tests. A diagnostic complication is that, very infrequently, patients have been identified with an abnormal CF genotype yet have a normal sweat test result. A borderline sweat test result is more commonly seen in those with retained pancreatic function.

Between 15 and 20% of Australian infants with CF present with meconium ileus, a form of neonatal intestinal obstruction, before results of screening are known. Antenatal diagnosis for CF is available when both parents are known carriers of the CF gene due to the birth of a previous child with CF or a family history. Community screening is not currently undertaken in Australia.

Clinical features

Cystic fibrosis affects multiple organ systems, causing a range of clinical problems of varying severity (Table 50.3). It is a severe disorder, although the occasional child has mild disease. Rarely, it is so mild that it is not diagnosed until adult life, following a presentation of pseudomonas pneumonia or male infertility.

Cystic fibrosis has a major impact on the lungs, where the altered physicochemical properties of the airway epithelium result in abnormally viscid mucus and bacterial colonisation of the respiratory tract. The lungs of a child with CF are normal at birth but, with time, chronic airway infection develops, causing progressive obstructive lung disease. Clinically, chronic productive cough develops as bronchiectasis progresses and lung function deteriorates. Clubbing is a feature.

Malabsorption is present in approximately 90% of children with CF from failure of the exocrine pancreas. Additionally, there are various degrees of gastric and duodenal hyperacidity, impaired bile salt activity and mucosal dysfunction. Stools are abnormal, being typically frequent and bulky. Growth failure may result from many reasons, including inadequate energy intake, malabsorption and chronic bacterial infection. Long term retention of pancreatic function is associated with better survival.

As survival of patients with CF improves, a range of CF related diseases becomes more important. This includes impaired growth and nutrition, diabetes mellitus and liver disease (both seen in approximately 15–20% of adolescents and adults), arthropathy and arthritis, and

Table 50.3 Common manifestations of cystic fibrosis
Respiratory Chronic productive or moist cough Features of bronchiectasis Clubbing
ENT Nasal polyps
Gastrointestinal Meconium ileus Features of malabsorption Distal intestinal obstruction syndrome Liver disease Endocrine pancreatic insufficiency (diabetes mellitus)
Reproductive Male infertility
General Growth delay
Metabolic Salt depletion

osteoporosis. Men are generally infertile due to bilateral absence of the vas deferens. Women are fertile, although pregnancy presents a range of health risks to both the fetus and mother. Women have increased rates of vaginal yeast infections and stress incontinence.

Principles of management of a child with CF

The median age of survival has improved dramatically as a range of clinical improvements has developed over time. Thirty years ago, median survival was less than 10 years. The current median survival is approximately 30 years, although there is a marked gender difference, with males surviving significantly longer than females. A range of improvements has contributed to these improved health outcomes, including:
- a stronger focus on nutrition
- the development of more specific and potent antibiotics.

However, a key intervention has been the development of specialised CF centres, characterised by a multidisciplinary team of health professionals including respiratory physicians, gastroenterologists, physiotherapists, nutritionists, nurses, surgeons and social workers. The goal of treatment is to maintain as high a quality of life as possible for as long as possible in order to slow the relentless progression of lung disease that occurs in CF.

The key elements of respiratory management of CF consist of:
- prompt use of antibiotics to delay the onset of bacterial colonisation
- aggressive treatment of recurrent respiratory infections
- promotion of mucociliary clearance by daily physiotherapy
- minimisation of other causes of lung damage (for example, smoking, aspiration)
- promotion of normal growth through high energy diet and pancreatic supplementation
- identification and treatment of complications as they arise (haemoptysis, pneumothorax, etc.).

Respiratory infections should be treated aggressively, as recurrent infection and the accompanying inflammation promotes loss of lung function. The most common respiratory bacteria are *Staphylococcus aureus* and *Haemophilus influenzae* in the early years, followed by *Pseudomonas aeruginosa* and *Burkholderia cepacia*.

Gastroenterological and nutritional management consists of:
- pancreatic enzyme replacement (lipase, protease, amylase) at each meal
- high energy diet
- vitamin supplementation with vitamin A, D, E and K, and salt tablets
- early identification of liver disease
- early identification of distal intestinal obstruction syndrome.

Cystic fibrosis is a life long chronic condition. As children grow and mature into adolescents and young adults, the psychosocial aspects of the disease take on different dimensions for individuals, siblings and parents. In adolescence, attention to body image issues and feelings of difference due to chronic disease can help maintain young people's adherence with the health care regimen. Declining health despite good adherence can, however, be especially demoralising.

Lung transplantation is increasingly undertaken to treat end stage lung disease. Gene therapy is still in the experimental phase.

Summary

Cough is the most common manifestation of respiratory problems in children. Although it can be a distressing symptom, its presence is vital for respiratory health. A chest X ray and spirometry (if aged more than 6 years) are the minimal investigations in a child with a chronic cough, i.e. a cough that has been present for more than 4 weeks. When cough is associated with other symptoms (specific cough), investigations and/or referral are required to identify the cause. Non specific cough is largely managed expectantly, trying to explore parent anxieties, and minimise investigations and environmental triggers such as tobacco smoke. There is little evidence that the common causes of persistent, isolated cough in adults (asthma, gastro-oesophageal reflux, sinusitis and nasal disease) cause chronic cough in children and adolescents.

PART 14   SELF-ASSESSMENT

Questions

1. **Brett is a 7 year old boy who woke this morning with fever, sore throat and difficulty swallowing. His parents said he seemed quite well when he went to bed the previous night. Brett is now also complaining of nausea, loss of appetite and headache. He is the only child of a middle class family. On examination he has an axillary temperature of 38.1°C. Examination of the throat reveals purulent patches on red, inflamed tonsils and the whole of the posterior pharynx is red and oedematous. He also has bilateral, tender enlarged cervical lymph nodes but no obvious coryza, rhinitis or cough. Which of the following is/are true:**
   (A) The painful sore throat will resolve within 2–3 days with or without antibiotics
   (B) Adenoviral infection is more likely than group A β-haemolytic streptococcal infection
   (C) There is a high probability this is group A β-haemolytic streptococcal pharyngitis
   (D) Antibiotics are not necessary because Brett does not belong to a group at risk of either poststreptococcal glomerulonephritis or rheumatic fever
   (E) A throat culture and delaying antibiotics for 24–48 hours (depending upon the result) is appropriate and will not increase the risk of poststreptococcal glomerulonephritis or rheumatic fever

2. **Mary is 18 months old and presents with a 24 hour history of fever and irritability and is now refusing feeds. On examination there are a number of small, discrete mouth ulcers on the posterior pharyngeal wall, tonsillar pillars, uvula and adjacent regions of the soft palate. There is no obvious cervical lymph adenopathy and no cutaneous rash. Which of the following is/are true:**
   (A) This is likely to be herpangina secondary to coxsackie virus
   (B) The absence of rash makes herpes simplex virus and hand, foot and mouth disease unlikely
   (C) Epstein–Barr viral pharyngitis is the most likely cause.
   (D) The most likely cause is group A β-haemolytic Streptococcus
   (E) Antibiotics are indicated to reduce the likelihood of a secondary bacterial infection of these mouth ulcers

3. **Which of the following statements about stridor in children are correct?**
   (A) Stridor is most likely to be generated from an obstruction to the extrathoracic airways
   (B) The severity of the upper airway obstruction can be determined by how loud the stridor is
   (C) An expiratory component to a stridor indicates an obstruction to airways below the thoracic inlet
   (D) Stridor with an expiratory component warrants further investigation, whereas a purely inspiratory stridor may not

4. **Which of the following physical signs may give a clue as to the cause of stridor in an 8 month old infant?**
   (A) Stridor is worse during the day and may be very soft or absent when the child is asleep
   (B) Stridor is worse when the child is lying supine, such as during bathing and changing
   (C) The child has a typical cutaneous haemangioma on the anterior chest wall
   (D) The child's voice and cry are normal

5. **Which of the following statements about croup are correct?**
   (A) The most common viruses associated with acute viral croup in toddlers are parainfluenza viruses
   (B) Hot steam and cold mist are both of proven benefit in treating acute viral croup
   (C) Corticosteroids, either oral or inhaled, are the treatment of choice for children with moderate to severe croup
   (D) Recurrent (spasmodic) croup is frequently associated with a family history of asthma or atopy

6. **John is a 2 year old boy with persistent asthma. You decide to start him on regular preventer therapy with inhaled steroids. Which of the following is/are true about drug delivery?**
   (A) A metered dose inhaler, volume spacer device and a face mask attachment would be an appropriate consideration
   (B) A powder inhaler device would be very convenient
   (C) Use of a nebuliser and compressor pump to administer regular inhaled steroids is unlikely to be necessary
   (D) Use of a spacer device decreases the likelihood of oral candidiasis
   (E) He needs to take big breaths to inhale the medication

7. **Clare is a 14 year old girl whose asthma has worsened during the previous year. Which of the following is/are likely explanations?**

(A) She has started smoking

(B) Her asthma has become resistant to the preventer therapy

(C) She is not taking her medication regularly

(D) Her inhaler technique is poor

(E) She has a pet cat to which she is allergic

8. **Amanda is a 3 year old girl who presents to the emergency department with an acute attack of asthma. She receives salbutamol via a metered dose inhaler and spacer device. Her wheeze improves markedly but after 2 hours she is wheezing and breathless again. Which of the following is/are true?**

(A) She should have further salbutamol

(B) Oral prednisolone will decrease her risk of admission to hospital

(C) Her $P\text{CO}_2$ is likely to be raised

(D) Spirometry will help to assess the severity of her asthma

(E) If the $S\text{aO}_2$ is 94%, she can be sent home immediately

9. **A 2 year old child is suspected of inhaling a foreign body. Which of the following is/are true?**

(A) It is unlikely to have lodged in the left side of the tracheobronchial tree

(B) The X ray will be abnormal in 30% of cases

(C) Choking, asymmetrical air entry and an abnormal chest X ray occur in most cases

(D) A peanut is the most likely foreign body

(E) Flexible bronchoscopy is indicated for removal

10. **Which of the following increases the likelihood that wheezing in infancy will be associated with asthma in later childhood?**

(A) Eczema

(B) Diminished lung function soon after birth

(C) Male gender

(D) Maternal asthma

(E) Positive serology to respiratory syncytial virus at 2 years of age

11. **A 6 year old girl presents with a 3 day history of cough, wheeze and fever, She looks well but has widespread crackles on auscultation and extensive changes on chest X ray. Which of the following is/are true?**

(A) Erythromycin is an appropriate antibiotic

(B) The most likely organism will be identified on blood culture

(C) Asthma is a likely diagnosis

(D) She can probably be managed at home

(E) Serology may be useful in establishing the diagnosis

12. **Symptoms that can be expected with tracheomalacia that involves the intrathoracic trachea are:**

(A) Tachypnoea

(B) Wheeze

(C) Cough on swallowing

(D) Inspiratory stridor

(E) Expiratory stridor

13. **Staphylococcal pneumonia:**

(A) Is more common in infants

(B) Is typically associated with lobar pneumonia

(C) Is associated with markedly abnormal chest X ray findings

(D) Commonly causes long term lung damage

(E) Is a common cause of air leaks in the lung

14. **Pulmonary tuberculosis in children is:**

(A) Most commonly spread from other children

(B) Most common in those under 5 years of age

(C) Associated with a tuberculin skin test of 10–15 mm

(D) Best treated with triple therapy for the first 6 months

(E) Not caused by atypical mycobacteria

15. **Children with the following diseases usually first present to their doctors with a chronic cough**

(A) Asthma

(B) Bronchiectasis

(C) Gastro-oesophageal reflux

(D) Cystic fibrosis

(E) Primary ciliary dyskinesia

16. **Children with bronchiectasis:**

(A) Should be investigated to exclude associated diseases

(B) Should be regularly reviewed

(C) Should receive mucolytics

(D) Can be confidently diagnosed on a chest X ray

(E) Require an HRCT scan of the chest for accurate diagnosis

17. **A child with chronic cough:**

(A) Should always be referred

(B) Should be investigated if either the chest X ray or spirometry is abnormal

(C) Can have a habit cough

(D) The cough is always associated with a serious underlying respiratory disease

(E) The cough can be caused by exposure to tobacco smoke

18. **Clubbing can result from which of the following conditions?**

(A) Primary ciliary dyskinesia

(B) Asthma

(C) Idiopathic bronchiectasis

(D) Habit cough

(E) Cystic fibrosis

Answers and explanations

1. The correct answers are **(A)**, **(C)**, **(D)** and **(E)**. Whether the tonsillitis is due to a virus or streptococcus the pain subsides in approximately 80% of children within 48–72 hours (A). Antibiotics have minimal impact on the duration or severity of sore throat. Adenoviral tonsillitis is more common in infants and toddlers (B). The illness has characteristic features of streptpococcal pharyngitis and he is in the age group where this is a common causative agent (C). Antibiotics are only indicated if the patient belongs to groups within high risk of suppurative complications or poststreptococcal complications (D). (E) is currently seen as the most scientific option, although the cost effectiveness needs to be evaluated.

2. The correct answers are **(A)** and **(B)**. This is the typical age group and classic distribution of the mouth ulcers of herpangina (A). Both HSV and hand, foot and mouth disease usually present with a skin rash or skin lesions as well as the stomatitis (B). Epstein–Barr viral pharyngitis is a common cause of similar illness in older children but is uncommon in infants and toddlers (C). Group A haemolytic streptococcal infection is only common in school age children, and the lesions here are not typical of streptococcal infection (D). (E) is incorrect. Bacterial complications are rare and antibiotics do not influence the natural history of herpangina.

3. The correct answers are **(A)** and **(D)**. Stridor is a noise made predominantly during inspiration and is usually generated by an obstruction in the extrathoracic airways because, as the pressure outside the extrathoracic airways is greater than that inside during inspiration, the airways tend to narrow during inspiration (A). (B) is incorrect as the loudness of the stridor relates to the magnitude of the inspiratory flow. As the obstruction becomes more marked or the child becomes more exhausted, less inspiratory flow is likely and the stridor may become softer. (C) is incorrect as an expiratory component to a stridor is most likely to be due to an obstruction in the extrathoracic airways that is severe enough to cause obstruction to airflow during expiration as well as during inspiration. (D) is correct because the presence of an expiratory component signifies more significant obstruction and warrants further investigation. A purely inspiratory stridor with the typical characteristics of laryngomalacia may not warrant further investigation.

4. The correct answers are **(B)** and **(C)**. (A) is incorrect as the loudness of the stridor is more related to the volume of inspiratory flow than to the degree of obstruction. Infants have higher inspiratory flows when active during the day than they do when sleeping. This does not help distinguish the cause of the stridor. (B) is correct. Stridor resulting from the glottic tissues, such as laryngomalacia, is typically worse with the infant supine. (C) is correct. Approximately 50% of subglottic haemangiomas are accompanied by a cutaneous haemangioma. (D) is incorrect because the voice and cry are frequently normal, even with abnormalities of the vocal cords.

5. The correct answers are **(A)**, **(C)** and **(D)**. (A) is correct as parainfluenza viruses, especially types 1 and 3, are the most common causes of croup at all ages. (B) is incorrect. While there is a strong belief in the community, and among some physicians, that steam and mist help relieve the airway obstruction associated with croup, there is no evidence that this is the case. Hot steam is dangerous and cold mist delivered in mist tents (thankfully a blast from the past!) complicates nursing management and monitoring of the child. (C) is correct. Low dose oral or inhaled (usually nebulised) corticosteroids have been shown to be beneficial in double blind trials in reducing the severity of the croup and decreasing the need for admission to hospital. (D) is correct. Recurrent or spasmodic croup is frequently associated with a family history or asthma or atopy and is less clearly related to an upper respiratory tract viral infection.

6. The correct answers are **(A)**, **(C)** and **(D)**. A metered dose inhaler with spacer device and a face mask to enable delivery would be appropriate at this age (A). He would not be able to use a powder inhaler device at this age as he would not be able to coordinate his breathing sufficiently to activate the device; children are not usually able to use these until the age of 5–6 years (B). Although a nebuliser driven by a compressor is effective it is likely to be more difficult to administer (how many 2 year olds have the patience to sit still for 5 minutes to have a nebuliser?) and it is no more efficacious (C). Spacer devices do decrease the incidence of oral candidiasis when using inhaled steroid medications (D). Tidal breathing through the spacer device is adequate for delivery of the medication at this age (E).

7. The correct answers are **(A)**, **(C)** and **(D)**. Starting smoking is a very common cause of worsening of asthma in teenage years, and teenagers need to be strongly encouraged not to smoke (A). 'Resistance' to preventer therapies in a pharmacological sense does not develop (B). It is much more likely that compliance has decreased (C). Again, this is common in the adolescent years. Another common reason for poor efficacy of therapy with inhaled medications is that inhaler technique is poor (D). Allergic responses to new pets may lead to exacerbations of asthma, but this is much less likely than other causes (E).

8. The correct answers are **(A)** and **(B)**. The mainstay of therapy of her acute episode of asthma is inhaled beta-2 sympathomimetic, at a frequency sufficient to give airway dilatation (A). Early introduction of oral corticosteroids will decrease the accompanying airway inflammatory response: several hours are needed for steroids given orally to be effective, but timely administration will lead to early control of inflammation, and hopefully admission to hospital because of worsening uncontrolled asthma will not occur (B). PCO_2 is not likely to be raised in asthma unless there is respiratory failure. Amanda's PCO_2 is likely to be low because she is tachypnoeic (C). She will be too young to be able to do spirometry (D). (E) is incorrect: although oxygen saturation is a guide to severity, a normal saturation needs to be considered in the overall context. Until it is known whether or not the frequency of her requirement for a reliever will be no more frequent than 3–4 hourly, she should not be sent home.

9. The correct answers are **(B)** and **(D)**. (A) is false because, contrary to popular belief, foreign bodies are evenly distributed between the two sides. X rays are abnormal in approximately 30% of cases (B), but this also means that in about two thirds of cases X rays are normal. Choking and asymmetrical air entry and typical X ray findings are seen in about one third of cases overall (C). Peanuts are common as foreign bodies in airways in this age group (D), and have significant implications because of their propensity to initiate an inflammatory response. Rigid bronchoscopy is needed for adequate removal (E).

10. The correct answers are **(A)**, **(C)** and **(D)**. Eczema and later asthma are associated (A). Diminished lung function soon after birth is associated with transient infant wheezing, but not with asthma in later childhood (B). Males are more likely to have asthma (C), and a maternal history of asthma also confers a greater risk of later asthma (D). (E) is incorrect. Almost all children will have evidence of RSV infection by this age.

11. The correct answers are **(A)**, **(D)** and **(E)**. This is likely to be infection with *Mycoplasma pneumoniae*. Erythromycin is the antibiotic of choice (A). However, the organism is difficult to grow, and does not cause bacteraemia (B). The clinical features are not consistent with asthma (C). Although the illness is distressing, it is not usually severe and does not usually require hospital admission (D). A positive IgM titre to mycoplasma would be diagnostic (E).

12. The correct answers are **(B)**, **(D)** and **(E)**. Tracheomalacia does not normally cause tachypnoea (A). Wheeze is heard (B), and is expiratory if the malacia is intrathoracic. Stridor is also present in tracheomalacia, and is also heard in expiration if the malacia is intrathoracic (D), (E). Coughing on swallowing is not a symptom of tracheomalacia (C).

13. The correct answers are **(A)**, **(C)** and **(E)**. Staphylococcal pneumonia is more common in children under the age of 2 years overall, and is more common in infants than in the second year of life (A). The X ray findings are often dramatic (C), but are less likely to be lobar than widespread, often with the later development of abcesses, empyema or pleural effusions, and pneumatoceles (B), (E). Surprisingly, with treatment the long term outlook for normal radiological appearances and normal lung function is good (D).

14. The correct answers are **(B)** and **(D)**. Most children with pulmonary tuberculosis acquire it from an infected adult or adolescent (A). Younger children are more susceptible (B). Disease associated with tuberculosis will normally result in a tuberculin skin test (using 5 TU) result of >15 mm diameter induration (C). Six months of triple therapy is required (D), using rifampicin, isoniazid and pyrazinamide. Rarely, atypical mycobacteria may cause pulmonary disease in childhood (E).

15. **(B)** and **(E)** are correct. Although children with asthma and gastro-oesophageal reflux may have a cough, most children with asthma and gastro-oesophageal reflux do not have chronic cough. The presentation for asthma is usually wheeze and dyspnoea, with or without an acute or subacute cough. In Australia, most children with cystic fibrosis are diagnosed on neonatal screening and sweat test. Children with bronchiectasis and primary ciliary dyskinesia are usually diagnosed following a presentation with chronic cough or recurrent chest infections.

16. **(A)**, **(B)** and **(E)** are correct. Associated diseases must be excluded in children with bronchiectasis, as the management can differ markedly. Chest radiographs are too insensitive to diagnose bronchiectasis and an HRCT scan is required. Children with bronchiectasis should be seen regularly to review treatments that optimise lung health.

17. **(B)**, **(C)** and **(E)** are correct. Some causes of chronic cough can be benign and are easily managed by general practitioners. If either of the minimum investigations are abnormal, the child with a chronic cough deserves investigations to assess for the presence of a serious underlying disorder. Tobacco smoke exposure can cause bronchitis and thus chronic cough. This must always be explored, especially in adolescence.

18. **(A)**, **(C)**, **(E)** are correct. Cystic fibrosis, idiopathic bronchieactasis and primary ciliary dyskinesia are causes of suppurative lung disease where the end result is generalised bronchiectasis, and thus clubbing can be present in children with these diseases.

481

PART 14 FURTHER READING

Adegbola R A, Obaro S K 2000 Diagnosis of childhood pneumonia in the tropics. Annals of Tropical Medicine and Parasitology 94: 197–207

American Thoracic Society Official Statement 2001 Targeted tuberculin testing and treatment of latent tuberculosis infection. American Journal of Respiratory and Critical Care Medicine 161: S221–247

Arroll B, Kenealy T 2001 Antibiotics for the common cold (Cochrane review). Issue 1, Cochrane library. Update Software, Oxford

Asher M I 1999 Infections of the upper respiratory tract. In: Taussig L M Landau L I, Le Souef P N, Morgan W J, Martinez F D, Sly P D (eds) Pediatric respiratory medicine. Mosby, St Louis, pp 530–546

Ausejo M, Saenz A, Pham B et al 1999 The effectiveness of glucocorticoids in treating croup: meta-analysis. BMJ 319: 595–600

Callaghan C W 2000 Wet nebulization in acute asthma: the last refrain? Chest 117: 1226–1228

Chang A B 1999 State of the art: cough, cough receptors, and asthma in children. Pediatric Pulmonology 28: 59–70

Chang A B, Asher M I 2001 A review of cough in children. Journal of Asthma 38: 299–301

Christiansen S C 2000 Day care, siblings, and asthma — please, sneeze on my child. New England Journal of Medicine 343: 574–575

Clemens C J et al 1997 Is an antihistamine decongestant combination effective in temporarily relieving symptoms of the common cold in preschool children? Journal of Pediatrics 130: 463–466

Del Mar C B et al 2001 Antibiotics for sore throat (Cochrane review). Issue 1, Cochrane library. Update Software, Oxford

Eskola J et al 2001 Efficacy of a pneumococcal conjugate vaccine against acute otitis media. New England Journal of Medicine 344: 403–409

Geelhoed G C 1997 Croup. Pediatric Pulmonology 23: 370–374

Glasziou P P 2001 Antibiotics for acute otitis media in children (Cochrane review). Issue 1, Cochrane library. Update Software, Oxford

Goel A, Bamford L, Hanslo D, Hussey G 1999 Primary staphylococcal pneumonia in young children: a review of 100 cases. Journal of Tropical Pediatrics 45: 233–236

Hayden F G et al 2000 Inhaled zanamivir for the prevention of influenza in families. New England Journal of Medicine 343: 1282–1289

Isaacs D, Moxon E R (eds) 1996 A practical approach to paediatric infections. Churchill Livingstone, New York

Izurieta H S et al 2000 Influenza and the rates of hospitalisation for respiratory disease among infants and young children. New England Journal of Medicine 342: 232–239

Juven T, Mertsola J, Toikka P, Virkki R, Leinonen M, Ruuskanen O 2001 Clinical profile of serologically diagnosed pneumococcal pneumonia. Pediatric Infectious Diseases Journal 20: 1028–1033

Kozyrskyj A L et al 2001 Short course antibiotics for acute otitis media (Cochrane review). Issue 1, Cochrane library. Update Software, Oxford

Lau K F, Jayaram R, Fitzgerald D A 2001 Diagnosing inhaled foreign bodies in children. Medical Journal of Australia 174: 194–196

Martinez F D, Wright A L, Taussig L M et al 1995 Asthma and wheezing in the first six years of life. New England Journal of Medicine 332: 133–138

Massie R J, Robertson C F, Berkowitz R G 2000 Long-term outcome of surgically trerated acquired subglottic stenosis in infancy. Pediatric Pulmonology 30: 125–130

Melchart D 2001 Echinacea for preventing and treating the common cold (Cochrane review). Issue 1, Cochrane library. Update Software, Oxford

Morris P 2001 Antibiotics for persistent nasal discharge (rhinosinusitis) in children (Cochrane review). Issue 1, Cochrane library. Upgrade Software, Oxford

Phelan P D, Olinsky A, Robertson C F 1994 Respiratory illness in children, 4th edn. Blackwell Scientific, Oxford

Powell C V, Stokell R A 2000 Changing hospital management for croup. What does this mean for general practice? Australian Family Physician 29: 915–919

Principi N, Esposito S, Blasi F, Allegra L 2001 Mowgli study group. Role of *Mycoplasma pneumoniae* and *Chlamydia pneumoniae* in children with community-acquired lower respiratory tract infections. Clinical Infectious Diseases 32: 1281–1289

Reichert T A et al 2001 The Japanese experience with vaccinating schoolchildren against influenza. New England Journal of Medicine 344: 889–896

Smith K C 2001 Tuberculosis in children. Current Problems in Pediatrics 31: 1–30

Suissa S, Ernst P, Benayoun S, Baltzan M, Cai B 2000 Low-dose inhaled corticosteroids and the prevention of death from asthma. New England Journal of Medicine 343: 332–336

Taussig L M, Landau L I 1999 Pediatric respiratory medicine. Mosby, St Louis

Wald E R 1992 Sinusitis in children. New England Journal of Medicine, 326: 319–323

Useful links

http://www.asthmaaustralia.org.au (Asthma Australia)

http://www.cdc.gov/nchstp/tb/ (Information service on tuberculosis from the Division of Tuberculosis Elimination, Centers for Disease Control, Atlanta, USA)

http://www.cf-web.org (For cystic fibrosis)

http://www.childrenshospital.org/cfapps/A2ZtopicDisplay.cfm?Topic=Croup (Children's Hospital Boston: child health A–Z — croup)

http://www.cochrane.org (The Cochrane Collaboration. Go to the Cochrane Airways Group in the Cochrane Library)

http://www.cyh.com/cyh/parentopics/usr_index0.stm?topic_id=149 (Parenting and child health: croup)

http://immuneweb.xxmc.edu.cn/infection%20and%20immune/Primary%20Ciliary%20Dyskinesia.htm (Information on primary ciliary dyskinesia from Prof C. O'Callaghan, Leicester, UK)

http://www.merck.com/pubs/mmanual/section6/chapter70/70a.htm (For bronchiectasis)

http://www.NationalAsthma.org.au (National Asthma Campaign (Australia))

http://www.nch.edu.au/parents/factsheets/rescrouj.htm (The Children's Hospital, Westmead: factsheets — croup)

http://www.pier.shef.ac.uk/home.htm (For cough and general paediatrics)

http://www.thoracic.org/adobe/statements/latenttb1-27.pdf (American Thoracic Society official statement. Targeted tuberculin testing and treatment of latent tuberculosis infection)

http://www.who.int/inf-fs/en/fact178.html (World Health Organization web site providing information on approaches to reducing mortality from respiratory diseases)

CARDIAC DISORDERS

51 Assessment of the infant and child with suspected heart disease

J. Wilkinson

Cardiac abnormalities or disease affect approximately 1% of children in the developed world and 2–3% in developing countries, the difference largely being related to rheumatic heart disease in such areas.

The prevalence of congenital malformations of the heart is approximately 8 in 1000 newborn infants. Acquired heart disease in developed countries includes:

- myocarditis
- septic pericarditis
- cardiomyopathies.

Transient involvement of the heart may occur in viral illnesses such as mumps and measles, but this seldom leads to long term problems. Acute myocarditis may follow viral infections (especially coxsackie B) and often appears to be immunologically mediated. Coronary arteritis with the formation of multiple coronary aneurysms is an important feature of Kawasaki disease (Ch. 44).

Manifestations

Heart disease may manifest itself with symptoms, either due to congestive heart failure or to cyanosis. Many patients are asymptomatic and their heart defect comes to light with the discovery of a heart murmur at a routine examination.

Evaluation in symptomatic patients

A careful note needs to be made of the onset of symptoms. In babies, breathlessness, feeding difficulties, inability to complete feeds, and poor weight gain are important (Fig. 51.1). Is cyanosis persistent or intermittent? Its relationship to feeding, crying or other activities or precipitating factors should be sought. Normal infants

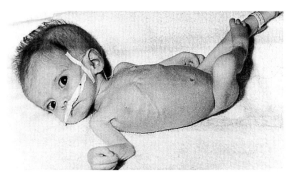

Fig. 51.1 Infant with evidence of severe failure to thrive, dyspnoea and feeding difficulties (note nasogastric tube) due to a large ventricular septal defect.

and children may manifest peripheral cyanosis when cold (often noted after a bath) or when running a fever; cyanosis may also be associated with breath holding in children with normal hearts.

Particular attention should be paid to the palpation of peripheral pulses and auscultation.

Pulses

Examination of pulses should include both left and right arms and femoral pulses, best felt simultaneously to make comparison easy. Reduced lower limb pulses suggest coarctation but apparently normal lower limb pulses do not exclude this diagnosis. Bounding pulses may be associated with persistent ductus. Pulses (especially lower limb pulses) may be difficult to feel in the early newborn period, even in normal babies, and require practice. The pulse rate in children varies markedly with activity and the resting rate is the only rate that needs to be noted (Table 51.1).

Table 51.1 Approximate normal upper limit for pulse, respiratory rate and systolic blood pressure, at rest; resting measurements consistently above these values should arouse suspicion

Age group	Pulse rate (beats/min)	Respiratory rate (breathe/min)	Systolic BP (mmHg)
0–8 weeks	160	50	70
Older infant	145	40	85
Toddler	130	30	100
Older child	115	20	115

Blood pressure

Measurement of blood pressure should be a routine part of examination in children. Use of an appropriate cuff is vital. The balloon should be of sufficient length to encircle at least two thirds of the arm, be centred over the artery, and should be wide enough to cover two thirds of the distance from the antecubital fossa to the acromium of the scapula. In practice, the largest cuff that can be fitted to the upper arm without covering the antecubital fossa is appropriate. Blood pressure should normally be recorded by auscultation of Korotkoff sounds, as in adults, although palpation (of the brachial or radial pulse) may be employed to assess systolic pressure in young children and infants if auscultation proves to be difficult. Significant errors in blood pressure are more likely to result from the use of a cuff which is too small than one which is overlarge.

For measurement of leg pressure a cuff may be placed on the thigh. Again the balloon should encircle at least two thirds of the limb and be centred over the artery. An adult arm cuff may be large enough for young children but larger children or adolescents will require a 'thigh cuff'.

Normal blood pressure varies at different ages (Table 51.1).

Palpation of the cardiac impulse

Location of the apex beat and documentation of any abnormal/forceful impulse is important, as is palpation for thrills.

Auscultatory findings

Splitting of the second sound should be noted (Fig. 51.2). Splitting is normally only audible during inspiration. A wide split is present when splitting is heard during both phases of respiration. Fixed splitting, a feature of atrial septal defect, implies absence of variation between inspiration and expiration (Fig. 51.3).

Accentuation of the pulmonary component of the second sound tends to be associated with a loud second sound, which may be palpable, often with no definite splitting, and implies the presence of pulmonary hypertension. However, it should be noted that the normal aortic closure sound may be loud in children with a thin chest wall and is sometimes palpable at the upper left sternal border. The presence of an ejection click (Fig. 51.2) is a useful ancillary auscultatory finding. Such sounds are heard shortly after the first heart sound and tend to be high frequency and discrete in character. If heard at the apex, it usually implies a bicuspid aortic valve or aortic stenosis. When originating from the pulmonary valve, it is heard at the left sternal edge and varies with respiration, being louder on expiration. This finding is characteristic of pulmonary valve stenosis.

Murmurs

When a heart murmur is heard, a process of 'murmur analysis' needs to be applied. This involves:

- timing
- localisation
- amplitude (grading)
- characterisation
- radiation.

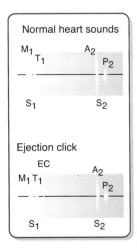

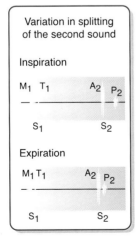

Fig. 51.2   Illustration of normal heart sounds, normal splitting of the second sound and ejection click (EC).

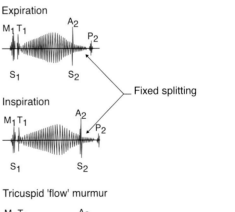

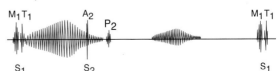

Fig. 51.3   Auscultatory signs associated with an atrial septal defect (ASD) showing ejection systolic murmur, fixed splitting of S_2 and tricuspid flow murmur (Ch. 52).

Timing

Murmurs may be systolic (limited to systole), diastolic (limited to diastole) or continuous (extending from systole into diastole). Murmurs should be timed against the carotid pulse or apical impulse. Distal pulses, such as the radial pulse, can produce incorrect assessment of timing.

Localisation

The point of maximum intensity of the murmur should be identified.

Amplitude

Murmurs may be graded according to the scale in Table 51.2.

Characterisation

Ejection murmurs (Fig. 51.4) are systolic and are crescendo–decrescendo in character, starting shortly after the first sound. Good examples are the murmurs of pulmonary or aortic valve stenosis.

Pansystolic murmurs (Fig. 51.4) are murmurs which commence at the first sound and continue to the second sound. They may be due to atrioventricular valve incompetence (for example, mitral incompetence) or a ventricular septal defect (VSD).

Diastolic murmurs may be *early diastolic* (Fig. 51.5) (commencing at the second sound) or *mid diastolic* (Fig. 51.3). The former reflect either aortic or pulmonary incompetence, whereas mid diastolic murmurs are due to turbulence during ventricular filling and reflect stenosis of or increased flow through the mitral (or tricuspid) valve.

Other characteristic murmurs include *early* (Fig. 51.5) and *late systolic* murmurs (reflecting a tiny muscular VSD or mitral valve prolapse, respectively) and the *late diastolic* murmur associated with mitral stenosis.

Characterisation of murmurs also includes assessment of the pitch of the murmur and its quality, for example, 'harsh', 'musical' or 'vibratory'.

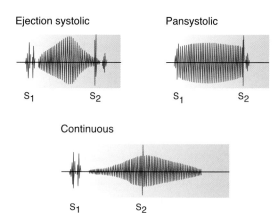

Fig. 51.4 Common murmurs and their relationship to the heart sounds S_1 and S_2.

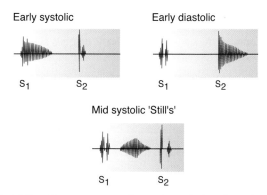

Fig. 51.5 Other murmurs: early systolic, early diastolic and Still's murmur.

Radiation

A murmur that is easily audible/loud away from the precordial area (for example, the neck or axilla) is said to 'radiate' towards the area in question.

Innocent murmurs

There are four characteristic types of innocent murmurs:
- Still's murmur
- pulmonary flow murmur
- carotid bruit
- venous hum.

Table 51.2	Grading of murmurs		
Grade	Amplitude	Thrill	Comments
1	Very soft	Absent	Scarcely audible
2	Soft	Absent	Easily audible
3	Loud	Absent	Very easily audible
4	Loud	Faint/localised	Very easily audible
5	Very loud	Easily felt/widespread	Very easily audible
6	Very loud	Easily felt/widespread	Heard with stethoscope off chest wall

Still's murmur

This is a short mid systolic murmur best heard at the left sternal border or between the apex and left sternal edge. This murmur is sometimes referred to as 'Still's' murmur (Fig. 51.5) or a 'vibratory' murmur. The murmur is of medium frequency and has a vibratory or slightly musical quality. It tends to become softer if the patient stands and is louder when the patient is squatting or lying supine.

Pulmonary flow murmur

This is a soft blowing ejection murmur, maximal in the pulmonary area. Murmurs of this kind are frequently heard in early infancy and may radiate softly to the axillae, when they may be labelled as innocent with a high degree of confidence, and are less common later in childhood. In older children, distinction from an atrial septal defect or mild pulmonary stenosis can be difficult, and usually requires an electrocardiogram (ECG) and X ray and in many cases an echocardiogram.

Carotid bruit

This medium frequency, rough ejection systolic murmur heard over the carotid artery (right or left or bilateral) at the root of the neck is very common in children, being usually softer or inaudible below the clavicle.

Venous hum

A high pitched, blowing, rather variable, continuous murmur, heard over the sternoclavicular junctions or over the neck and changing with the position of the head, is frequently heard in children. This murmur almost always disappears completely when the patient lies flat and may be eliminated by gentle compression of the neck veins.

It should be appreciated that innocent murmurs may be heard in around 50% of normal school aged children and adolescents. In early infancy, the frequency of soft murmurs is probably around 80%. Because of the very high frequency of soft heart murmurs, it is essential that all doctors involved in caring for infants and children become familiar with the common innocent murmurs and should be able to recognise them with confidence and be able to exclude organic heart disease (Fig. 51.6). Simple ancillary investigations (e.g. ECG, chest X ray) may be helpful. Echocardiography is not usually necessary. Where doubt exists, patients should be referred for formal cardiological assessment.

Cyanosis

The distinction between peripheral and central cyanosis is important. The terms are often thought to describe the site at which cyanosis is seen, whereas they reflect the *site of origin* of cyanosis. Peripheral cyanosis, originating in areas of poor tissue perfusion, is not seen in areas of good perfusion. By contrast, central cyanosis is generalised. Examination of the tongue and mucous membranes will usually exclude central cyanosis. In the presence of central cyanosis the arterial Po_2 will be depressed, with the rare exception of cyanosis associated with methaemoglobinaemia. Where doubt exists about the presence of cyanosis the use of pulse oximetry is frequently very helpful.

Clinical example

Malcum, aged 14, is referred with a history of cough, breathlessness and wheeze on exertion and a heart murmur that was noticed for the first time recently. His mother comments that he has always tended to be blue when exposed to cold and after swimming. He has been diagnosed in the past as having mild asthma and used to have regular treatment with Ventolin. Examination reveals a small, thin adolescent with a slightly forceful cardiac impulse at the left sternal edge. He has a soft (grade 2/6) ejection systolic murmur, best heard in the pulmonary area and the 2nd sound is widely split. His chest X ray shows a cardiothoracic ratio of approximately 0.5 and his ECG shows no abnormality.

These features are not typical of an innocent murmur and he requires further investigation with an echocardiogram. This shows an atrial septal defect (ASD) — a condition that can easily be missed, as the clinical signs may be subtle and the X ray and ECG do not necessarily provide clues to the presence of a structural abnormality. His symptoms are related to asthma and to peripheral cyanosis with exposure to cold. His small stature and thin body build may be related to his ASD and he may have a growth spurt after this is closed.

Manifestations of heart failure

Cardiac failure in infancy tends to be dominated by pulmonary congestion, which leads to dyspnoea/tachypnoea.

Dyspnoea contributes to feeding difficulties, reduced intake and increased metabolic rate. Failure to thrive often results. Chronic dyspnoea may lead to the appearance of Harrison's sulci, which are deformations of the ribcage at the site of the diaphragmatic attachments. Crepitations at the lung bases are usually a manifestation of superimposed infection rather than heart failure in infants.

Systemic venous congestion is manifest by liver enlargement and/or oedema. Liver engorgement results in an enlarged, abnormally firm liver with its edge palpable 2.5–5 cm below the costal margin. In infants, oedema is often diffuse and difficult to detect. Elevated jugular venous pressure cannot be assessed easily in infancy.

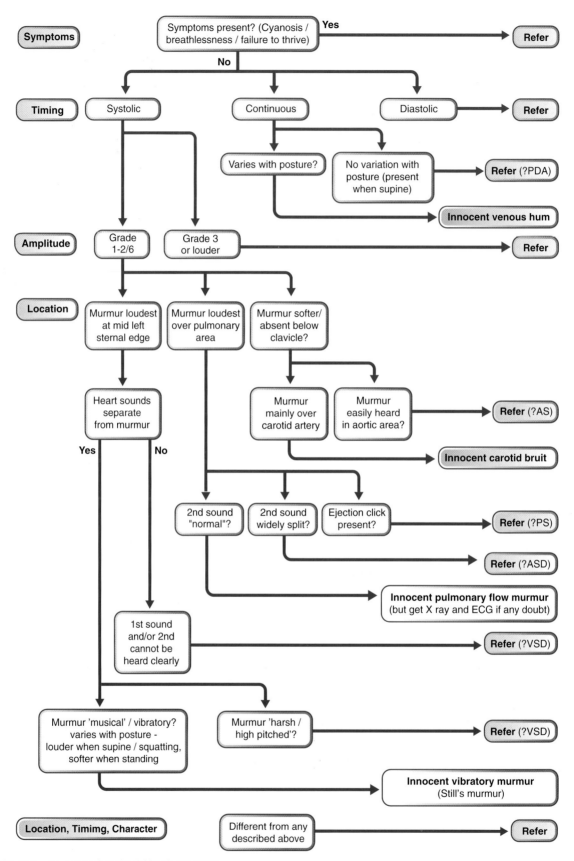

Fig. 51.6 An approach to the child with a murmur.

Other evidence of cardiac failure may include persistent tachycardia, a chronic dry cough, and profuse sweating, especially of the forehead and scalp (Fig. 51.1).

Clinical example

Amy, an infant of 4 weeks, presented with poor feeding. Her paediatrician had previously seen her in the perinatal period when examination was normal with no heart murmur, and normal pulses. Over the past 2 weeks she had been increasingly breathless with feeds and had not gained any weight. Examination showed a tachypnoeic infant (respiratory rate 80/min) with easily felt radial and brachial pulses but absent femoral pulses. The cardiac impulse was forceful to palpation and the liver edge was palpable 4 cm below the right costal margin.

These features suggested congestive heart failure (tachypnoea and liver enlargement) associated with a coarctation of the aorta. Investigations included a chest X ray, which showed cardiomegaly and pulmonary congestion, and an ECG, which showed evidence of right ventricular hypertrophy (a finding that is very common with coarctation presenting in early infancy). An echocardiogram was organised and confirmed the diagnosis.

Early surgical repair was recommended

Note that the lower limb pulses may be palpable in the early newborn period before the ductus closes. For this reason the fact that initial cardiac examination appears normal does not exclude coarctation!

Investigations

Chest X ray

The chest X ray provides information about heart size, shape and lung vascularity. The heart is enlarged when, on a PA chest film, the cardiothoracic ratio exceeds 0.5 in an adult or 0.55 in a child. In infancy the cardiothoracic ratio may be as large as 0.6 (Fig. 51.7). If vascular shadows in the hilum are increased, this implies high pulmonary flow (pulmonary plethora; Fig. 51.7) or pulmonary venous congestion. Diminished vascular marking (pulmonary oligaemia) is associated with the decreased pulmonary flow occurring in some forms of cyanotic heart disease: for example, tetralogy of Fallot. Individual cardiac chamber size is often difficult to assess on plain chest X rays, though variations in cardiac contour may provide useful clues.

Electrocardiogram

The electrocardiogram (ECG) provides information about heart rate and rhythm and about atrial or ventricular hypertrophy or hypoplasia.

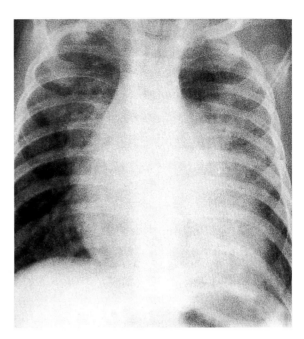

Fig. 51.7 Chest X ray showing cardiomegaly and pulmonary plethora in a child with a large VSD (Ch. 52).

In the newborn infant, right ventricular forces tend to dominate, whereas by the end of the first year of life left ventricular forces predominate. This evolution reflects changes in ventricular wall thickness, and evaluation of ventricular hypertrophy needs to take into account the normal values for children of each age group. Additionally, normal values for heart rate, PR interval, QRS duration, QT interval and T wave axis vary at different ages.

Echocardiography

Current echocardiographic instruments allow the sectional anatomy of the heart, as it beats in 'real time', to be displayed on a television monitor. This is referred to as cross sectional echocardiography (Fig. 51.8).

Doppler echocardiography allows quantitation of the direction and flow velocity at individual sites. This can provide useful quantitative information about the presence and severity of valvar stenoses, regurgitation and septal defects.

Colour flow Doppler is a modality in which the lines of information are split, with Doppler sampling at different sites being displayed as colour on the television monitor. Computerised image processing generally allows good quality imaging along with colour flow maps, which provides a visual display of flow in the areas being examined.

Cardiac catheterisation

Cardiac catheterisation allows measurement of intracardiac pressures and shunts. It also allows for angiographic

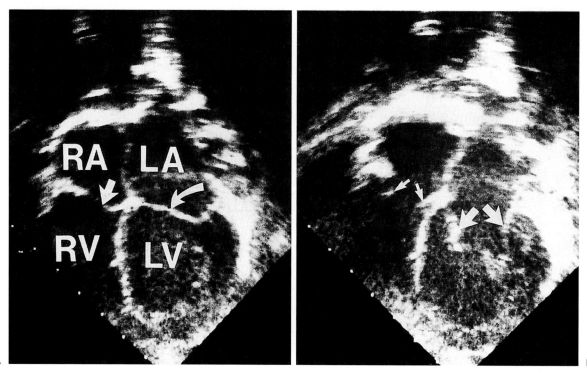

Fig. 51.8 Echocardiogram: 'four chambers view'. **A** Four chambers with the mitral valve (curved arrow) and tricuspid valve (straight arrow) closed during ventricular systole. **B** Same anatomy during diastole with the mitral (large arrows) and tricuspid (small arrows) valves open. The atrial and ventricular septa can be seen separating the left heart chambers (LA and LV) from the right sided chambers (RA and RV).

demonstration of abnormal anatomy. As much of this can be obtained using echocardiography, the requirement for catheterisation has diminished substantially. It may also be used for therapeutic purposes, such as balloon valvuloplasty (for pulmonary or aortic valve stenosis) or placement of a device to close a persistent ductus arteriosus or atrial septal defect.

In the vast majority of cases, a diagnosis can be made and treatment instituted on the basis of non invasive investigations without cardiac catheterisation. However, catherisation may be necessary for planning surgical treatment, especially in more complicated heart defects.

Treatment

Cardiac failure

The development of heart failure in infancy should be regarded as an emergency requiring urgent hospitalisation, usually at a major cardiac centre. The transportation of such infants can present a major challenge and may well be best achieved by arranging for the patient to be accompanied by well trained medical and/or nursing personnel with appropriate resuscitation equipment.

Circulatory support

Intravenous dobutamine or dopamine may be life saving. Digoxin should usually be avoided in such cases as renal impairment leads to rapid accumulation and toxicity.

Prostaglandin

In infants developing symptoms in the newborn period, due to congenital heart disease, a 'ductus dependent congenital defect' is often responsible. Infants with such defects (coarctation of the aorta, pulmonary atresia, transposition) may benefit from infusion of prostaglandin E_1 to reopen the ductus.

Respiratory support

In the presence of severe cardiac and/or respiratory failure, positive pressure ventilation may be helpful in allowing stabilisation of the child's condition.

Correction of acidosis

Where respiratory or metabolic acidosis are present, these should be corrected by ventilatory support and/or intravenous sodium bicarbonate.

Diuretics

Frusemide (furosemide) is usually the diuretic of choice. This may be given parenterally initially. If diuretics are required for more than a limited period, potassium depletion may develop and potassium supplements or coadministration of a potassium sparing diuretic such as spironolactone (Aldactone) should be considered.

Oxygen

Oxygen should be administered if significant hypoxia is detectable, although in the presence of significant cyanotic congenital heart disease the administration of oxygen will seldom produce much improvement in oxygenation.

Feeding

Gavage feeding via nasogastric tube may be helpful if the infant is too breathless to feed adequately. Introduction of high calorie feeds may be helpful. Infants with heart failure tend to tolerate small frequent feeds better than larger feeds. In the presence of more severe congestive failure feed volume should be reduced to 120 ml/kg/24 h to avoid fluid overload.

Surgery

In many cases, surgical treatment offers the best means of alleviating the problem which has produced heart failure, and medical treatment should only be pursued in an effort to achieve stabilisation of the infant's condition and allow a diagnosis to be reached so that planning of surgical management may proceed.

52 Common heart defects and diseases in infancy and childhood

J. Wilkinson

Congenital malformations affecting the heart and/or great vessels occur in a little under 1% of newborn infants. Eight defects are relatively frequent and together make up approximately 80% of all congenital heart disease (Table 52.1).

Presenting features

The major presenting features are:
- the presence of an abnormal murmur
- development of symptoms or signs of congestive heart failure
- central cyanosis
- any combination of the above.

Acyanotic defects

These comprise approximately 75% of all congenital heart defects and can be subdivided into (1) those that are associated with an isolated left to right shunt, and (2) those that are not associated with any shunting, in which no septal defect is present.

Defects with a left to right shunt are the following:
- ventricular septal defect (VSD)
- persistent ductus arteriosus (PDA)
- atrial septal defect (ASD)
- atrioventricular septal defect (AVSD).

Ventricular septal defect

These comprise around 30% of all cardiac defects. They vary from tiny defects, of pinhole size, to huge defects. Small defects are more common than large ones and are usually asymptomatic. Defects are frequently situated in the region of the membranous septum, but VSDs involving the muscular septum are also common (Fig. 52.1). Very tiny muscular defects may be demonstrated by echocardiography in infants with no clinical signs to suggest a septal defect.

With a small VSD, there is usually a loud, harsh high pitched systolic murmur audible at the left sternal border, frequently associated with a thrill. The heart sounds otherwise may be normal and there are often no other abnormal findings. The murmur is most often 'pansystolic' in timing, but this is not invariably so. Another very characteristic finding is that of an early systolic (decrescendo) murmur, which is often well localised at the mid left sternal border and reflects a very small muscular defect which is functionally closing with each systolic contraction.

With a larger VSD, signs of cardiac failure may be present and the physical signs are different. These may include a parasternal heave, a displaced apex and the systolic murmur may be considerably softer. An additional diastolic murmur may be heard at the apex, due to increased flow through the mitral valve. Infants with a large VSD often thrive poorly, suffer dyspnoea with feeds

Table 52.1 Relative frequency of common congenital heart defects

Defect	Approximate frequency %
Ventricular septal defect (VSD)	30
Persistent arterial duct (ductus arteriosus; PDA)	12
Atrial septal defect (ASD)	8
Pulmonary stenosis (PS)	8
Aortic stenosis (AS)	5
Coarctation of the aorta	5
Tetralogy of Fallot	5
Transposition of the great arteries (TGA)	5

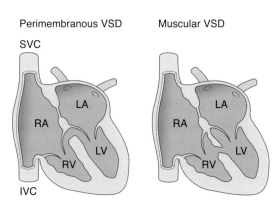

Fig. 52.1 Sites of ventricular septal defect (VSD). In the left panel, the defect is close to the membranous part of the ventricular septum (perimembranous VSD). In the right panel, the defect is in the muscular septum.

and are prone to recurrent chest infections. Tachypnoea, dyspnoea, sweating and hepatomegaly are frequent findings.

With small defects, the chest X ray and electrocardiogram (ECG) are frequently normal. With larger defects, the X ray shows cardiomegaly and increased pulmonary vascular markings (pulmonary plethora) (see Fig. 51.7). The ECG often shows biventricular hypertrophy. The site and size of the defect can be documented well with echocardiography.

The natural history of a VSD varies. Small defects frequently undergo spontaneous closure, which may occur in 50% or more. Some moderate defects may also diminish in size and the shunt becomes minor. Important complications include progressive aortic incompetence, when one leaflet of the aortic valve prolapses into an adjacent VSD, or the development of infundibular pulmonary stenosis. Small isolated defects may be left alone if the evidence shows no significant haemodynamic disturbance and the patient remains symptom free.

Large VSDs are associated with a variable degree of pulmonary hypertension which is related to transmission of systemic pressure through the defect into the right ventricle. In the presence of a large (non restrictive) defect pulmonary artery systolic pressure may be 'systemic' (similar to that in the aorta). This is present from birth and may lead to the development of pulmonary vascular obliterative disease. Progression of pulmonary vascular damage will eventually result in the appearance of cyanosis (Eisenmenger syndrome), developing in adolescence or early adult life.

Early surgical repair (before age 6 months) of a VSD is indicated if congestive heart failure appears in infancy, or if pulmonary hypertension is present. Surgery can be carried out at any age from the newborn period. However, most affected infants with a large VSD do not become symptomatic until the second or third month of life. Repair at a later age may be indicated if the defect fails to close and continues to cause a significant shunt, or if complications such as aortic valve prolapse develop. In practice only around 25% of children with a VSD will need surgery for it.

Persistent ductus arteriosus

Failure of the ductus arteriosus to close in the newborn period may be due to a congenital abnormality or to severe prematurity. The clinical findings depend on the size of the ductus. Patients with a small PDA frequently remain asymptomatic and the only abnormal finding may be a continuous murmur audible at the upper left sternal border (in or above the pulmonary area). Such murmurs may be present throughout the cardiac cycle ('machinery murmur') but sometimes disappear during diastole and may be sufficiently short to be mistaken for a purely systolic murmur.

In the presence of a large ductus, collapsing pulses are frequently apparent. The apex may be displaced and forceful and an apical mid diastolic murmur may be heard (due to increased blood flow across the mitral valve).

Symptoms such as failure to thrive, dyspnoea and recurrent chest infections are similar to those of a large VSD.

The presence of cardiomegaly and pulmonary plethora on the chest X ray indicates a large shunt and left ventricular hypertrophy will, if present, usually be seen on the ECG. The diagnosis can be confirmed by echocardiography; cardiac catheterisation is not usually necessary.

In symptomatic premature infants, specific medical treatment with indomethacin, which inhibits prostaglandin synthesis, may be effective in promoting ductal constriction. Unfortunately, drug treatment is not effective in mature infants with a persistent ductus and in such patients intervention to close the ductus is indicated. This should be carried out at an early stage in symptomatic patients (including premature infants if indomethacin is ineffective) but may be delayed until the second year of life or subsequently in asymptomatic patients with a small ductus. In such infants surgery is indicated to eliminate the risk of infective endocarditis, rather than to treat cardiac failure or pulmonary hypertension. An alternative to surgical ligation is device closure, either by introduction of one or more embolisation coils or by placement of an occlusion device via a cardiac catheter.

Atrial septal defect

Defects of the atrial septum are usually situated in the region of the fossa ovale and are termed secundum ASD (Fig. 52.2). Unlike small VSDs and PDAs (which tend to be associated with loud murmurs), small ASDs may go completely undetected. With larger defects, a significant shunt is present, but this is not associated with pulmonary

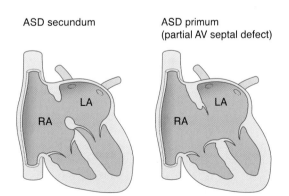

Fig. 52.2 Common types of atrial septal defect (ASD). Secundum defects are in the fossa ovale (mid atrial septum). Primum defects are low in the atrial septum and abut on the atrioventricular valves, which are abnormal and often incompetent.

hypertension (with rare exceptions) and seldom leads to symptoms during infancy. Isolated ASDs hardly ever lead to the Eisenmenger syndrome.

The characteristic findings in children with an ASD are related to the increased blood flow through the right side of the heart. An ejection systolic murmur, due to high pulmonary flow, is present in the pulmonary area, and a soft mid diastolic murmur may be heard at the lower end of the sternum, secondary to increased tricuspid flow. A parasternal heave related to a dilated right ventricle may be palpable. The aortic and pulmonary components of the second heart sound are widely separated and frequently remain equally separated during both phases of respiration (fixed splitting) (see Fig. 51.3).

While most children are free of any major symptoms, their growth is often mildly impaired compared with siblings, and exercise tolerance may be slightly reduced. If they reach adult life without surgery, those with a significant shunt are liable to the development of atrial flutter or fibrillation in middle adult life and frequently become increasingly handicapped by exertional dyspnoea and effort intolerance at the age of 40–50 years, even if arrhythmias are not a problem.

The chest X ray characteristically shows an increase in transverse cardiac diameter with pulmonary plethora. The electrocardiogram tends to show features of partial right bundle branch block. The diagnosis may be confirmed by echocardiography; cardiac catheterisation is usually not required.

Closure should be recommended in cases where there is evidence of a significant shunt. Surgical repair may usually be achieved by direct suture, but may require insertion of a patch. A recently introduced alternative is device closure: a procedure carried out at cardiac catheterisation whereby a self-expanding 'double umbrella device' is placed in the defect. This is an appropriate non surgical option for many patients with central defects of small to moderate size with good margins, but is not applicable very large defects or those with poorly formed margins.

Atrioventricular septal defect

This category of defect, which accounts for approximately 3% of all congenital cardiac defects, includes a group of ASDs low in the atrial septum which abut on the atrioventricular valves and may involve the upper part of the ventricular septum. When the ventricular septum is intact (partial AVSD), only an atrial communication is present. This is referred to as an ostium primum ASD (Fig. 52.2) and is almost invariably associated with malformations of the mitral and tricuspid valves, which are often incompetent, for example, cleft mitral valve.

Children with this type of defect may, if mitral incompetence is severe, become symptomatic in infancy or early childhood. In the absence of significant mitral regurgitation, however, the features resemble those of a secundum ASD.

When a significant VSD coexists (complete AVSD — common atrioventricular canal; (Fig. 52.3)), the presentation resembles that of an isolated large VSD and most infants become symptomatic with difficulty feeding and failure to thrive in the early months of life. This defect is commonly associated with Down syndrome.

The chest X ray usually shows quite marked cardiomegaly and pulmonary plethora, especially in the complete form of the defect. The ECG characteristically shows left axis deviation accompanied by partial right bundle branch block. The presence of left axis deviation distinguishes ostium primum ASDs from secundum defects. Echocardiography confirms the diagnosis and will differentiate partial from complete atrioventricular defects. Cardiac catheterisation is not usually required.

Surgical repair is almost always required. When pulmonary hypertension is present this is generally recommended in the early months of life (3–6 months) in order to obviate the risk of pulmonary vascular disease. In patients with an isolated ostium primum ASD, when pulmonary hypertension is absent, surgery may be delayed until the age of around 4 years. Operation involves placement of a patch to close the ASD and repair of the mitral valve cleft to eliminate mitral incompetence, if present.

The following defects have no shunt, and are obstructive lesions:

- pulmonary stenosis
- aortic stenosis
- coarctation of the aorta.

Pulmonary stenosis

Pulmonary stenosis, usually valvar in site, is the commonest of the pure obstructive malformations. The pulmonary valve is abnormal, with thickened leaflets and partially fused commissures. In some cases the valve may be bicuspid.

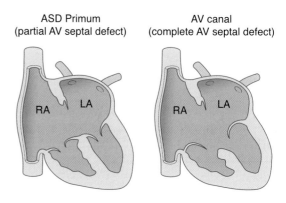

ASD Primum
(partial AV septal defect)

AV canal
(complete AV septal defect)

Fig. 52.3 Atrioventricular (AV) septal defect. The complete form is associated with a common AV valve and the septal defect allows communication between all four cardiac chambers.

Other sites of pulmonary stenosis, occurring as isolated abnormalities, are less frequent. These include muscular subpulmonary obstruction involving the right ventricular outflow tract (infundibular stenosis) and supravalve or branch pulmonary stenosis.

Most patients are asymptomatic in infancy and childhood. An ejection systolic murmur, best heard in the pulmonary area and radiating through to the back, is the characteristic finding. The murmur occasionally may be associated with a thrill. The pulmonary component of the second sound is often abnormally soft or inaudible, although in mild cases it may be heard and the degree of splitting is often increased. An early ejection sound (ejection click) is usually audible at the left sternal border (Fig. 52.4) with valvar stenosis. Characteristically the click is louder during expiration and fades on inspiration.

The chest X ray usually demonstrates a normal heart size, but the main pulmonary artery is often unusually prominent (poststenotic dilatation). This produces an abnormal convexity on the upper left heart border just below the aortic knuckle. The ECG may be normal with mild obstruction, but shows right ventricular hypertrophy in more severe cases.

Mild pulmonary stenosis is generally a benign condition and often is non progressive. More severe pulmonary stenosis leads eventually to effort intolerance, angina on exertion and cardiac failure. Rarely, severe pulmonary stenosis may present in early infancy with cyanosis due to right to left shunting through the foramen ovale or an associated ASD.

The diagnosis may be confirmed by echocardiography, but cardiac catheterisation is usually required to assess the severity more precisely. Traditionally, treatment involved surgical valvotomy but in recent years this has usually been replaced by a catheter technique involving inflation of a balloon in the valve orifice to separate the fused commissures (balloon pulmonary valvotomy or valvuloplasty). This procedure is simple and effective in most cases, requires only a very short hospital stay, and saves the patient an open heart operation.

Aortic stenosis

As in pulmonary stenosis, the valve is abnormal with thickened leaflets and fused commissures. In most cases with aortic stenosis the valve is bicuspid. Subaortic stenosis with a fibrous stricture or with muscular obstruction (hypertrophic subaortic stenosis) also occurs but is less common. Stenosis in the ascending aorta, above the aortic valve, also may be encountered (supra-aortic stenosis).

With rare exceptions, affected children are symptom free in infancy and early childhood and present with the chance finding of an ejection systolic murmur over the precordium and in the aortic area. Characteristically, with valvar stenosis the murmur is best heard to the right of the sternum and radiates to the carotids. A thrill is commonly present over the carotids and may also be felt in the aortic area. An ejection click is usually heard with valvar stenosis (Fig. 52.4) and is often most easily audible at the apex or lower left sternal border. In mild and moderate cases there may be no other abnormal finding. In more severe cases a forceful apical impulse due to left ventricular hypertrophy may be apparent. In subaortic stenosis the murmur is best heard at the left sternal edge and a click is not heard. Conversely, the murmur of supravalve stenosis often is best heard over the carotid artery.

The natural history of aortic stenosis is generally one of gradual progression. Symptoms include dizziness and syncope on exertion, angina pectoris, effort intolerance and sudden death. In a small minority of cases, with 'critical' stenosis, severe congestive heart failure may appear in early infancy.

In mild and even moderate aortic stenosis, the chest X ray and ECG may show little abnormality. In more severe cases the ECG tends to show left ventricular hypertrophy, but this is often late in appearing. Echocardiography allows assessment of the site and severity of the obstruction.

Treatment should be recommended if significant stenosis is present, even in the absence of symptoms. Balloon aortic valvotomy is feasible as an alternative to surgery and currently is the preferred treatment option for most cases, but may lead to worsening aortic incompetence. Operation involves aortic valvotomy on heart lung bypass.

Mild pulmonary stenosis

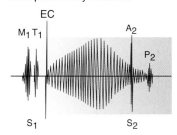

Mild aortic stenosis

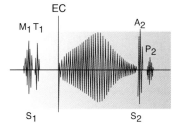

Fig. 52.4 Auscultatory findings in pulmonary and aortic stenosis. The ejection click (EC) is earlier in pulmonary stenosis and the second sound is widely split. In aortic stenosis the click is best heard at the apex.

Coarctation of the aorta

In this condition a discrete stricture is present in the distal part of the aortic arch close to the site of the ductus arteriosus. The maximal site of obstruction is usually opposite to or just proximal to the aortic end of the ductus arteriosus or ligamentum arteriosum (Fig. 52.5).

Coarctation of the aorta is often associated with other cardiac defects, including aortic stenosis, ventricular septal defect and mitral valve abnormalities. A bicuspid aortic valve is present in 40% of cases even in the absence of other malformations.

Coarctation usually leads to the development of severe cardiac failure in the newborn period, often in the second or third week of life. Alternatively, in around 30% of cases, presentation may be delayed until late in childhood or even adolescence or adult life.

The characteristic physical findings are of diminished or absent femoral pulses. Simultaneous palpation of the right brachial pulse and a femoral pulse frequently shows quite obvious delay in the appearance of the latter. Upper limb blood pressure often is elevated, sometimes severely so, and there is a marked discrepancy between arm and leg blood pressure, usually greater than 20 mmHg.

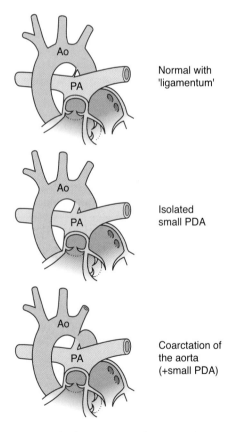

Normal with 'ligamentum'

Isolated small PDA

Coarctation of the aorta (+small PDA)

Fig. 52.5 Aorta and pulmonary artery showing persistent ductus and site of coarctation (often associated with persistent ductus arteriosus, PDA).

The chest X ray and ECG findings vary according to the age of presentation. In symptomatic infants cardiomegaly and pulmonary congestion are usually seen on the chest X ray, and the ECG shows right ventricular hypertrophy. In later childhood the X ray may show an abnormal appearance of the aortic knuckle and rib notching due to the presence of enlarged intercostal arteries which act as collateral routes for flow of blood into the lower systemic segment. This is seldom seen before the age of 8 years. The ECG may show left ventricular hypertrophy.

Treatment

In infancy the onset of congestive heart failure is often related to closure of the ductus arteriosus. Before closure of the ductus, the pulmonary artery pressure is usually sufficient to allow adequate flow of blood into the descending aorta via the ductus, but after the ductus starts to close the flow of blood in the lower part of the circulation becomes inadequate. For this reason infusion of prostaglandin E_1 intravenously may palliate symptoms by causing the ductus to reopen. Other medical measures may help to ameliorate heart failure and improve the condition of the infant before operation. Early surgery, as soon as the diagnosis is established, is always indicated in symptomatic cases. Patients who remain free of symptoms should be assessed carefully for the development of hypertension and, if this is present, surgery should be carried out during early childhood. In other patients intervention may be deferred until later in childhood. In selected cases, with a localised coarctation shelf, balloon angioplasty may be employed as an alternative to surgical repair. Patients who have required surgical relief of coarctation (especially those operated in early infancy) and those who have had balloon angioplasty may develop restenosis at the coarctation site, although this is less common with newer surgical techniques.

Unoperated patients with coarctation (that is, those who escape detection during childhood) are at a high risk from serious complications or death during adolescence or early adult life. Complications include left ventricular failure, aortic dissection and subarachnoid haemorrhage due to ruptured berry aneurysm.

Hypoplastic left heart syndrome

A small subgroup of infants with both severe aortic stenosis and coarctation may present with associated gross hypoplasia of the left ventricle. In some cases the aortic valve and/or mitral valve are atretic (Fig. 52.6).

Such infants present with severe cardiac failure or shock in the early days of life. All peripheral pulses are diminished or absent and manifestations of cardiac failure are severe.

The condition is invariably lethal without surgery. Medical treatment including infusion of prostaglandin

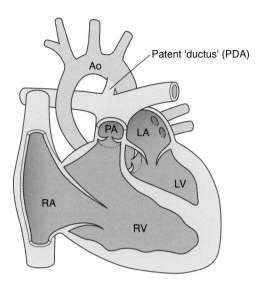

Fig. 52.6 Hypoplastic left heart syndrome showing hypoplasia of: left ventricle, mitral valve, aortic valve, ascending aorta. The ductus provides the only effective route through which the systemic circulation can be maintained from the right ventricle with right-to-left shunting across the duct.

and other measures may lead to improvement. Palliative surgery (the Norwood procedure) is possible and can produce long term survival. Heart transplantation, even in the newborn period, is offered to some infants, mainly in a small number of centres in the USA.

Cyanotic defects

The presence of cyanosis in a child with congenital heart disease indicates that deoxygenated blood from the systemic venous system is being directed back into the systemic circulation without transiting the pulmonary vascular bed. Cyanotic defects account for approximately 25% of all congenital heart malformations. All such defects are associated with the presence of a septal defect coupled with additional abnormalities which alter the pressure relationship between the two sides of the heart so that, instead of pure left to right shunting, right to left or bidirectional shunting occurs, producing cyanosis.

Three major subgroups exist. In the first group (exemplified by the tetralogy of Fallot) pulmonary blood flow is reduced due to a combination of obstruction to normal flow into the lung circulation and a septal defect behind the obstruction through which blood may shunt from right to left. In the tetralogy of Fallot the shunt is almost completely right to left, whereas in some other defects associated with low pulmonary flow the physiology is more complex, with right to left shunting at one level and left to right shunting at another, for example, tricuspid atresia, and pulmonary atresia.

In the second group of cyanotic defects bidirectional shunting is associated with very large communications between the left and right sides of the heart with free mixing of blood, for example, 'single ventricle', and truncus arteriosus. In such defects pulmonary blood flow is usually high and pulmonary hypertension is a feature. Cyanosis is generally very mild and may pass unnoticed.

A third group of cyanotic defects, best exemplified by transposition of the great arteries, may be considered as a 'plumbing problem'. In transposition, the aorta and pulmonary artery are connected to the wrong side of the heart and as a result systemic venous blood is directed straight through into the systemic circulation again (see below).

Tetralogy of Fallot

Of the four components which comprise Fallot tetralogy (VSD, pulmonary stenosis, right ventricular hypertrophy, overriding aorta) the important ones are pulmonary stenosis and the VSD (Fig. 52.7). The presence of severe pulmonary stenosis, which characteristically is associated with infundibular muscular obstruction coupled frequently with valvar hypoplasia and commissural fusion, leads to elevation of right ventricular pressure. In most patients, the systolic pressure in the left and right ventricles is equal, but the marked resistance to ejection into the pulmonary circulation, due to the stenosis, produces right to left shunting into the aorta. The degree of right to left shunting is not influenced much by the overriding aorta.

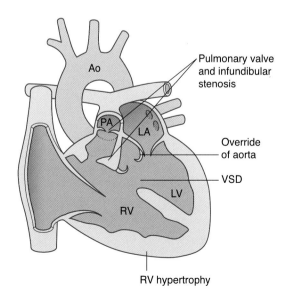

Fig. 52.7 Fallot's tetralogy, showing infundibular and valvar pulmonary stenosis and hypoplasia of the branch pulmonary arteries, all of which are frequent.

Clinical features

Cyanosis is not usually obvious in the newborn period, but appears later in infancy in most affected children. Oxygan staturations (with pulse oximetry) may be normal or mildly depressed in the early weeks of life. A harsh ejection systolic murmur is audible at the left sternal edge and/or in the pulmonary area (infundibular stenosis) and radiates through to the back. The second heart sound is often quite loud but single because the pulmonary closure sound is inaudible (Fig. 52.8).

Cyanosis appears gradually during the first 6–12 months of life or rarely in later childhood, and characteristically is more obvious on crying or on exertion. A characteristic feature is the development of intermittent episodes of severe hypoxia and cyanosis (hypoxic spells), which may appear spontaneously but quite commonly are precipitated by stress or exercise. Such spells are characterised by marked pallor or cyanosis with dyspnoea and distress. Loss of consciousness may occur. Hypoxic spells are associated with increased right to left shunting and a sharp reduction in pulmonary flow. In the past these have been attributed to infundibular 'spasm', although in practice the physiology is more complex and spasm does not occur. First aid treatment of these spells, which are potentially dangerous, involves soothing and pacifying the distressed infant with a view to trying to induce sleep. In severe cases intramuscular morphine may be helpful. Older infants and children have reduced exercise tolerance and often adopt a squatting posture at regular intervals during exertion. This manoeuvre, in which the child squats down on the haunches with knees up to the chest, increases systemic venous return and systemic vascular resistance. The latter reduces right to left shunting and the increased venous return produces a significant transient rise in pulmonary blood flow with improved oxygenation.

Course and prognosis

Cyanosis generally progresses gradually, with diminishing exercise tolerance, finger clubbing and in severe cases growth retardation. Development of cardiac failure is unusual but the severe cyanosis leads to compensatory polycythaemia, and cerebral thromboembolic complications, for example, stroke, may occur. Infective endocarditis and cerebral abscess also are important complications.

Investigations

The chest X ray shows the heart size to be normal with an uptilted apex and concave pulmonary segment associated with reduced lung vascularity (oligaemia). In severe cases the cardiac contour may resemble the shape of a wooden clog — *coeur en sabot* — often referred to as 'boot shaped'. The ECG usually shows right ventricular hypertrophy. Echocardiography is diagnostic, but cardiac catheterisation may be required before surgical correction.

Differential diagnosis

In infancy, before the onset of cyanosis, the murmur often is mistaken for that of a small VSD. Other cyanotic defects, such as tricuspid atresia, may be differentiated by ancillary investigations, such as ECG, X ray and echocardiogram.

Treatment

Total correction involving repair of the VSD and relief of the infundibular and pulmonary valve stenosis can be carried out even in early infancy if the anatomy is suitable. However, many affected children have quite marked hypoplasia of the branch pulmonary arteries and this may make it desirable to delay repair and to carry out one or more palliative shunt operations first. These involve creating a communication between the aorta and a pulmonary artery to increase pulmonary blood flow, allowing better growth of the branch pulmonary arteries. The earliest systemic to pulmonary shunt operation (Blalock operation) involved anastomosis of one subclavian artery with the ipsilateral branch pulmonary artery. Currently, most surgeons use a modification of the operation, employing a prosthetic tube graft to create the anastomosis.

Infants who are having significant hypoxic spells can be treated medically in the short term with beta adrenergic blocking drugs, for example, propranolol, to prevent spells while the child is awaiting surgery.

Transposition of the great arteries

In this condition the aorta and pulmonary arteries arise from the incorrect ventricles. This is described as ventriculoarterial discordance (Fig. 52.9). Systemic venous blood is directed through the right side of the heart back into the aorta and pulmonary venous blood through the left side of the heart and back into the pulmonary circula-

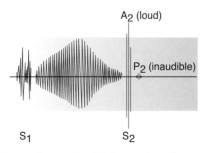

A₂ (loud)

P₂ (inaudible)

S₁   S₂

Fig. 52.8 Auscultatory signs in Fallot tetralogy. The systolic murmur is 'ejection', due to the pulmonary stenosis. The aortic closure sound is accentuated and pulmonary closure is so soft as to be inaudible. The second sound appears to be 'single'.

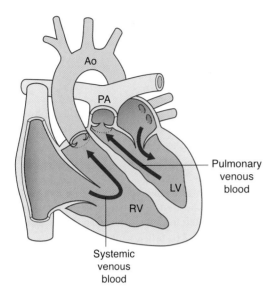

Fig. 52.9 Transposition of the great arteries. Systemic venous blood is ejected from the right ventricle to the aorta, while pulmonary venous blood passes from the left ventricle to the pulmonary artery.

tion. Survival is dependent on transfer of blood across from each circuit into the other via a foramen ovale, ductus arteriosus or a septal defect. Affected infants generally survive for several days or even weeks due to shunting through the foramen ovale and/or ductus arteriosus, but few live longer than a month without help, unless they have a coexisting septal defect, for example, a large VSD.

Clinical features

Cyanosis is present from the early hours of life and usually progresses gradually over the next few days. Metabolic acidosis also may develop due to the tissue hypoxia if the situation persists untreated. Apart from the cyanosis the infant may appear completely normal. Palpation reveals a forceful right ventricular impulse at the left sternal edge, but on auscultation there is frequently no murmur audible.

Investigations

The chest X ray shows a normal sized or mildly enlarged heart with a contour which sometimes resembles an 'egg on its side'. Pulmonary vascular markings are usually increased. The ECG shows normal ventricular complexes, but may manifest T wave abnormalities. The diagnosis may be established rapidly by echocardiography.

Treatment

Cardiac catheterisation is performed as an emergency procedure and a catheter with an inflatable balloon at the tip is passed into the left atrium via the foramen ovale. After inflation of the balloon the catheter is withdrawn with force into the right atrium, producing a tear in the atrial septum and hence creating an atrial septal defect (balloon atrial septostomy). This allows more effective interatrial shunting with amelioration of the cyanosis and hypoxia.

Surgery

After successful balloon septostomy most infants will manage comfortably for many weeks or months. Surgical correction can now be performed in the newborn period by transferring the pulmonary artery and the aorta back to their appropriate ventricles. It is also necessary to transfer the tiny coronary arteries across from the aortic root (above the right ventricle) to the new aortic origin from the left ventricle. The operation is technically difficult and needs to be performed in early infancy, usually the first month of life, before the left ventricle has adapted to feeding the low pressure pulmonary circulation.

An alternative approach which has been used widely in the past, and is still used occasionally, involves waiting until the infant is 3–6 months old or older and then rerouting blood at atrial level by insertion of a complex intra-atrial patch or baffle (Mustard operation) or by repositioning the patient's own atrial septum and infolding of part of the right atrium (Senning operation). These operations, although conceptually difficult to understand, are relatively straightforward to perform and carry low surgical mortality. For this reason, they were preferred by many surgeons to the arterial switch procedure described above, which is technically more difficult to perform, but which has now almost completely replaced the atrial redirection operations.

Tricuspid atresia

In this malformation the tricuspid valve is blocked completely and there is no communication between the right atrium and ventricle. Systemic venous blood passes via the foramen ovale or an ASD into the left side of the heart, and at ventricular or arterial level a left to right shunt exists (via a VSD or PDA). This allows blood to perfuse the pulmonary circulation, usually in reduced amounts.

Clinical features

Cyanosis develops early. A systolic murmur is audible along the left sternal border.

Diagnosis

The diagnosis may be suspected on the characteristic ECG pattern of left axis deviation, right atrial hypertrophy, left ventricular hypertrophy and right ventricular hypoplasia. Echocardiography confirms the diagnosis.

Treatment

A palliative shunt operation may be performed in infancy (see above under tetralogy of Fallot). Later in childhood reconstructive cardiac surgery is usually feasible and involves the creation of an anastomosis/connection between the systemic veins (SVC and IVC) and the pulmonary arteries, allowing systemic venous blood to pass directly into the pulmonary circulation (Fontan operation).

Pulmonary atresia

In this condition the origin of the pulmonary artery from the right ventricle is completely obstructed or absent. Blood in the right side of the heart passes via an ASD, foramen ovale or VSD into the left ventricle and aorta. The pulmonary circulation depends on collateral flow from the aorta via a PDA or other collateral channels.

Clinical features

Cyanosis develops early and many infants have an easily audible continuous murmur due to the associated PDA or other collaterals feeding the pulmonary circulation from the aorta.

Diagnosis

The diagnosis is usually confirmed by echocardiography, although it may be suspected strongly on clinical grounds coupled with ECG and X ray findings.

Treatment

Initial medical therapy may involve prostaglandin infusion to maintain patency of the ductus. Early surgical treatment usually involves a systemic to pulmonary shunt procedure. At a later stage, which depends on the associated defects, surgical correction may be performed by opening up a way through from the right ventricle into the pulmonary arteries, often by insertion of a 'valved conduit'.

Persistent truncus arteriosus

This defect is associated with the presence of a single artery which branches shortly after arising from the heart to give rise to the pulmonary artery and aorta. The truncal valve usually sits astride a large VSD and receives blood from both right and left ventricles.

Clinical features

Cyanosis is usually mild or absent and congestive heart failure often appears in the newborn period. Most infants will have a systolic murmur and in some cases a diastolic murmur may be heard due to incompetence of the abnormal truncal valve.

Diagnosis

The diagnosis can be made by echocardiography. Chest X ray and ECG findings are usually non specific.

Treatment

The only effective treatment is surgical correction, which needs to be carried out in early infancy. The pulmonary artery is separated from the truncus and, after closure of the VSD leaving the aorta arising from the left ventricle, a valved conduit is placed to connect the right ventricle to the pulmonary arteries.

Clinical example

Kylie, a 10 month old infant, has been known to have a murmur since the age of 3 months but is growing normally and is asymptomatic apart from intercurrent respiratory infections.

Examination shows her to be acyanotic with normal pulses and a normal cardiac impulse with no thrill. On auscultation she has a harsh, high-pitched murmur (grade 2/6) in the pulmonary area, which is present during systole and extends into early diastole. The murmur is also audible in the back. Her chest X ray is normal, as is her ECG.

The fact that her murmur extends into diastole means that it is a 'continuous murmur'. The normal X ray and ECG suggest that there is no major haemodynamic disturbance and the defect is likely to be minor. The respiratory infections are therefore unlikely to be related to the cardiac abnormality.

The diagnosis is a small patent ductus arteriosus.

Acquired heart disease in children

There are several forms of acquired heart disease in children.

Myocarditis

This condition follows a viral infection, although the aetiological mechanism may well be, in part, immunologically mediated. The disease quite frequently follows coxsackie B infection, but may be associated with a wide variety of other viruses. Congestive heart failure may develop rapidly or insidiously and the condition is accompanied by ECG, X ray and echocardiographic evidence of extensive myocardial damage, ventricular dilatation and depressed myocardial function. In the past, the condition was frequently fatal, although some patients recovered. Use of immunoglobulin or immunosuppressive drug therapy (for example, steroids, azathioprine, cyclosporin) may improve the prospects for recovery.

Cardiomyopathy

This term encompasses a group of conditions with heart muscle disease and myocardial dysfunction, often associated with heart failure. In most cases the aetiology is unknown and no specific treatment is available. In those patients where the condition progresses to end stage heart failure, cardiac transplantation offers the only prospect of survival.

Rheumatic heart disease

Rheumatic heart disease is now very uncommon in the developed world. The condition follows acute rheumatic fever, although a clear history of rheumatic fever may be absent in some cases. It probably is the result of an abnormal immune response on the part of the host to certain streptococcal antigens, which results in an autoimmune disorder affecting the heart, synovial membranes and other tissues.

The main sequelae of rheumatic fever are the development of damage to the cardiac valves, resulting in the development of mitral stenosis and/or incompetence and aortic stenosis/incompetence.

Clinical manifestations

Rheumatic fever follows a streptococcal infection, usually tonsillitis.

Major criteria for diagnosis include:
- migratory polyarthritis mainly affecting large joints
- evidence of carditis with tachycardia, cardiac enlargement, the development of new murmurs and, in severe cases, cardiac failure
- choreiform limb movements: Sydenham chorea
- a transient demarcated skin rash on the trunk: erythema marginatum
- the development of nodules over bony prominences.

Minor criteria are:
- fever
- arthralgia
- previous history of rheumatic fever
- raised ESR or C reactive protein
- prolonged PR interval on ECG.

All patients with suspected rheumatic fever should have throat cultures and be tested for evidence of streptococcal antibodies (ASO titre, anti-DNAase titre).

Diagnosis

The diagnosis cannot usually be regarded as established unless evidence of a recent streptococcal infection is demonstrable, i.e. a positive throat culture or positive antibody titres. If such evidence is found, however, the presence of two minor and one major criteria as listed above, or the presence of two or more major criteria, may be regarded as indicative of the presence of rheumatic fever.

Treatment

Treatment involves bedrest and administration of aspirin in full anti-inflammatory doses. Steroids may also be administered in the presence of more severe carditis and will usually reduce the duration of the acute episode, although they probably do not affect the development of chronic valve disease.

Infective endocarditis

The presence of structural cardiac abnormalities associated with turbulent blood flow within the heart or major arteries predisposes to seeding of bacteria into endothelial erosions associated with jet lesions. The development of a transient bacteraemia is usually the precursor of such infection, although the source of the bacteraemia is often not clear.

Symptoms include fever, rigors, anorexia and weight loss. Physical signs may include evidence of anaemia, sometimes with petechial haemorrhages, splinter haemorrhages in the nailbeds, splenomegaly and finger clubbing. In many cases the manifestations are relatively subtle and a high index of suspicion is required if the diagnosis is to be reached. Any child with known structural heart disease, whether operated or not, is at risk (with the exception of a PDA or a secundum ASD that has been closed surgically or with a device more than 6 months previously). Should such a patient become chronically unwell or have prolonged unexplained fever, he or she should be investigated with a view to excluding infective endocarditis. Investigations should include a full blood count and ESR, multiple blood cultures and careful echocardiography, including, if necessary, transoesophageal echocardiography to identify vegetations.

Occasionally infective endocarditis may develop in a patient with no previously known cardiac defect.

The responsible organism is most commonly *Streptococcus viridans* or staphylococci (both *aureus* and *albus*). Other organisms include enterococci, *Escherichia coli*, and fungi, especially *Candida albicans*.

Treatment involves intravenous antibiotic therapy, usually for a period of 6 weeks. Bactericidal drugs should be used and the choice of antibiotic(s) should be made on the basis of sensitivity testing of the infecting organism from cultures. Rarely, where severe valve damage develops during the acute illness, or with large vegetations in the heart, surgery may be required to remove vegetations and/or repair or replace damaged valves.

Prophylaxis against endocarditis should be advised in all patients who are considered to be at risk and should be administered on occasions when a bacteraemia is likely to result from surgical or dental procedures. Such procedures include dental extractions and other dental procedures involving significant gingival trauma, other oropharyngeal instrumentation and surgery on the bowel and genitourinary tract. Effective cover can usually be achieved with amoxycillin (with an aminoglycoside, in addition, to cover procedures on the genitourinary or gastrointestinal tract). In the main a single dose of antibiotic, administered an hour prior to the procedure (oral dose) or at induction of anaesthesia (intravenous dose), is adequate as the bacteraemia induced by such procedures is very transient.

Cardiac arrhythmias

Phasic variation in heart rate (*sinus arrhythmia*) is a normal phenomenon in children. It is usually related to respiration, although not invariably so.

Paroxysmal supraventricular tachycardia (SVT)

This condition is characterised by the sudden onset of very rapid tachycardia, usually with a rate of 200–300 beats per minute. Affected infants usually become pale and appear mildly distressed with tachypnoea and poor feeding. Heart failure may develop and the appearance of SVT in an infant requires urgent treatment. Older children are often aware of their rapid heart rate and adult observers may notice pulsation in the neck.

The acute episode may sometimes be terminated by vagal manoeuvres, such as the application of ice packs to the face, or the Valsalva manoeuvre. Intravenous adenosine, or in older children verapamil, will usually terminate the episode, or alternatively a DC shock may be applied.

The ECG between episodes will often show evidence of pre-excitation with Wolff–Parkinson–White syndrome.

Some patients have recurring attacks over many years and need chronic antiarrhythmic drug treatment or definitive intervention to ablate the source of the arrhythmia, although this is seldom needed in early childhood.

Heart block

Congenital heart block is an uncommon problem in the newborn period. It may present with fetal bradycardia, which can be misinterpreted as indicating fetal distress. Of affected infants, 50% have no structural cardiac abnormality but a range of congenital anomalies may be associated with heart block. Infants with otherwise normal hearts may develop heart block due to the presence of maternal autoimmune antibodies, which should be looked for in the mother of all affected children. Some mothers will have evidence of systemic lupus erythematosus or other collagen disease. Others are asymptomatic but have autoimmune antibodies, which are probably responsible for damage to the conduction system of the fetus.

The heart rate is usually in the range of 40–70 beats per minute. Infants with heart rates above 55 beats per minute are often asymptomatic and will tolerate the bradycardia well. Slower heart rates and/or the presence of associated structural cardiac defects often lead to the development of heart failure and the need for implantation of a permanent pacemaker.

Ventricular arrhythmias

Sustained ventricular arrhythmias are uncommon during childhood; however, the presence of ventricular premature beats may be detected as irregularities in the pulse on routine examination or on a chance ECG. The presence of such premature beats in an otherwise normal child with no other evidence of heart disease may be regarded as benign, and even when premature beats occur frequently they very rarely lead to any symptoms or require treatment.

Long QT syndrome

A small number of families or individual children manifest electrocardiographic evidence of prolonged repolarisation with increase in the corrected QT interval on the ECG. Such patients are vulnerable to development of paroxysmal ventricular tachycardia or ventricular fibrillation, usually associated with a sudden emotion (for example, fright) or with exertion. Any patient developing dizziness or syncope on exertion should therefore be assessed with a view to excluding this condition, which often is familial and may lead to sudden death.

Treatment may involve antiarrhythmic medication, implantation of a pacemaker or surgical stellate ganglionectomy.

PART 15   SELF-ASSESSMENT

Questions

1. The following may be true of 'innocent' murmurs:
(A) The murmur may be 'continuous' and vary with position of the head and neck
(B) Such murmurs are often early systolic in timing
(C) A systolic murmur, well heard at the left sternal border, may soften or disappear when the patient stands
(D) May be heard over the carotid artery
(E) The diagnosis can only be made confidently after an echocardiogram has excluded structural defects

2. A 3 month old infant with tetralogy of Fallot may manifest the following:
(A) An oxygen saturation on pulse oximetry of 96%
(B) An ejection systolic murmur best heard in the pulmonary area
(C) A single second heart sound
(D) Episodic cyanosis/hypoxia when crying
(E) A 'pansystolic' murmur (due to the associated VSD)

3. Infective endocarditis:
(A) May present with fever and rigors in a patient with no previous history of cardiac disease/defect
(B) Is always associated with splenomegaly and clubbing
(C) May be suspected on echocardiography, in the absence of other clinical signs or major symptoms
(D) Is usually treated with a 6 week course of intravenous antibiotics
(E) May require urgent surgery

4. Paroxysmal supraventricular tachycardia, in a 1 month old infant
(A) May present with pallor, breathlessness and poor feeding
(B) Is frequently associated with Wolff–Parkinson–White syndrome
(C) May respond to a facial ice bag
(D) Should be treated as a medical emergency
(E) Is likely to require radiofrequency ablation to eliminate the arrhythmia substrate

5. When examining peripheral pulses:
(A) Both arm pulses should be examined simultaneously
(B) Normal femoral pulses in a newborn infant exclude a diagnosis of coarctation
(C) The right radial pulse in a neonate is usually easier to feel than the left

(D) Femoral pulses may be hard to detect in normal newborn babies
(E) A collapsing pulse is likely to be present in a child with a VSD

6. The following are true of VSD:
(A) A VSD is present in more than 25% of children with congenital heart defects
(B) The Eisenmenger syndrome will develop if the defect is not operated on before the age of 2 years
(C) A VSD may be found on echocardiography in the absence of any abnormal clinical signs
(D) Most defects will require surgical repair during infancy or early childhood
(E) Most affected children are asymptomatic

Answers and explanations

1. (A) True (this is characteristic of a 'venous hum'). **(B)** False (early systolic murmurs, which start at the first sound, are characteristic of small muscular VSD). **(C)** True (this is frequently the case with a Still (vibratory) murmur). **(D)** True (true of innocent carotid bruits). **(E)** False (echocardiography is not required unless the murmur is atypical or there are other suspicious features).

2. (A) True (in the early months there may be very little desaturation at rest). **(B)** True (the murmur is due to pulmonary stenosis). **(C)** True (the pulmonary closure sound may be inaudible so the 2nd sound is perceived as being single). **(D)** True (hypoxia becomes much more pronounced with distress/activity). **(E)** False (the VSD is large and ventricular pressures are equal, so the VSD does not generate a 'pansystolic' murmur).

3. (A) True (underlying heart disease may have been overlooked previously or (rarely) may be absent). **(B)** False. (splenomegaly and clubbing are late developments and may not develop if treated early). **(C)** True (vegetations may be found occasionally, even when the patient has little symptomatology). **(D)** True. **(E)** True (if severe valve incompetence results acutely, surgery to replace or repair the valve may be needed).

4. (A) True (in infants symptoms are often non specific). **(B)** True (but some accessory pathways may not manifest WPW). **(C)** True (a simple way of producing vagal stimulation). **(D)** True (infants can decompensate quite rapidly and need urgent treatment to correct the arrhythmia). **(E)** False (RF ablation is seldom used in early childhood and many patients will cease to have episodes spontaneously).

503

5. **(A)** True (it is useful to compare the arm pulses with each other as well as with the lower limb pulses). **(B)** False (while the ductus is open lower limb pulses may be palpable; the diagnosis may be missed until it closes). **(C)** False. **(D)** True (it is very common to find that the femoral pulses are of small volume in the first 2–3 days). **(E)** False (characteristic of patent ductus rather than VSD).

6. **(A)** True (as an isolated defect, or as the main abnormality, VSD occurs in around 30% of infants with heart defects). (B) False (Pulmonary vascular disease and shunt reversal usually develops gradually over 10–20 years or longer. Many children, even with large defects, may have reversible pulmonary hypertension until later in childhood; however, surgery is recommended during infancy to reduce the risk of pulmonary vascular disease). **(C)** True (tiny VSDs can be seen on echocardiography in some apparently normal babies). (D) False (only around 25% of VSDs need surgery; many close spontaneously or are very small and unimportant). **(E)** True (most children with VSDs have small defects and are symptom free).

PART 15 FURTHER READING

Archer N, Burch M 1998 Paediatric cardiology: an introduction. Chapman and Hall, London

Moller J H, Hoffman J I E 2000 Pediatric cardiovascular medicine. Churchill Livingstone, New York

Useful links

http://www.americanheart.org/children/ (American Heart Association — heart disease in children)

http://www.paediatrics.unimelb.edu.au/5th%20year/Lecture%20Notes/N-Cardiac.doc (University of Melbourne — lecture notes/case examples in paediatric cardiology)

http://www.rch.unimelb.edu.au/cardiology/website/Glossary/glossary.html (Glossary of terms used in paediatric cardiology)

http://www.rch.unimelb.edu.au/cardiology/website/Library/library.html (Diagrams and handouts on congenital heart defects)

HAEMATOLOGICAL DISORDERS AND MALIGNANCIES

53 Anaemias of childhood

K. Tiedemann, G. Tauro

Pallor is a common presenting symptom in childhood. It may reflect conditions as diverse as anxiety, pain, acute severe infection, cardiovascular insufficiency due to cardiac disease, blood loss, or anaemia due to a variety of causes. Anaemia, or the presence of a haemoglobin below the lower limit of normal for age, is the end result of:

- inadequate production of erythrocytes
- abnormal erythrocyte nuclear maturation
- defective haemoglobinisation, or
- an increased rate of red cell loss or destruction.

The onset may be rapid, resulting in acute symptoms and signs such as profound lethargy, hypotension, air hunger and cardiac failure. Alternatively the onset of anaemia may be very gradual over months, producing few symptoms until cardiovascular decompensation occurs. Pallor, because of its gradual development, is often not observed by parents until profound and may be brought to attention by someone who has not seen the child for some time.

Diagnostic approach

A careful history and physical examination will usually allow a provisional diagnosis as to the cause of anaemia and will distinguish pallor secondary to acute severe infection, cardiac disease, pain or anxiety from that due to acute blood loss or anaemia.

History

In the history particular attention should be paid to the following.

Duration and speed of onset of pallor

Very rapid onset of pallor occurs when there is acute blood loss, severe haemolysis, or acute severe infection. Gradual development of increasing pallor suggests a progressive cause of anaemia or systemic disease with secondary anaemia.

Associated symptoms

Lethargy and irritability are often a feature of anaemia. Fever with acute pallor and lethargy, however, may suggest severe infection, such as septicaemia, pneumonia or meningitis, rather than anaemia.

A history of recent trauma, overt blood loss or abnormal bruising should be sought. Relatively minor trauma may cause rupture and inapparent intraperitoneal bleeding from an abnormally enlarged viscus such as spleen or a Wilms tumour.

A long history of bruising is suggestive of a congenital bleeding disorder, thrombocytopenia or platelet dysfunction. Recurrent epistaxes are a feature of some of these conditions and may lead to iron deficiency and anaemia.

Joint and bone pains may suggest chronic arthritic disorders but are also common in leukaemia and metastatic tumours with marrow infiltration.

Pallor associated with dark urine and jaundice suggests haemolysis. A history of recurrent jaundice in the past suggests that there may be a hereditary haemolytic anaemia.

Birth and neonatal history

Low birth weight, prematurity, neonatal blood loss, exchange transfusion, twin pregnancy and prolonged neonatal illness predispose to iron deficiency during infancy.

Onset of jaundice within 24 hours of birth suggests a haemolytic process. ABO or Rh blood group incompatibility between mother and infant, inherited enzyme abnormalities (glucose-6-phosphate dehydrogenase (G6PD), pyruvate kinase and glucose phosphate isomerase deficiencies) and inherited red cell membrane disorders such as hereditary spherocytosis (HS) should be excluded.

Dietary history

Inadequate dietary intake of iron, folate and vitamin B_{12}, all necessary for normal erythropoiesis, may be the cause of anaemia, particularly in infancy and early childhood. Enquiry should be made about the type and volume of milk feeding, the age of introduction and type of solid feedings, iron supplementation and folate content of the foods given. Children with food fads and infants of vegans are at risk of multiple vitamin deficiencies, including folate, vitamin B_{12} and iron.

History of drug or toxin exposure

Many drugs and toxins have been associated with marrow failure, either in a dose dependent fashion or by an idiosyncratic mechanism. Careful enquiry should be made about maternal drug ingestion during pregnancy, drugs prescribed for the child in preceding months and other potentially harmful drugs and toxins to which the child may have had access in the home.

The family history

Many haematological disorders have an inherited basis. G6PD deficiency is X linked, and hereditary spherocytosis usually is dominantly but occasionally recessively inherited. One parent or another near relative may have a relevant haematological disorder, but may not be aware of the genetic implications and how the disorder may be manifest in a child. In common recessively inherited conditions such as thalassaemia, the parents may not be aware of their carrier status, or, knowing that they have heterozygous disease, may not be aware of the consequences of homozygous inheritance.

General features

History of past illnesses should be reviewed and symptoms of non haematological disease, particularly those suggestive of chronic inflammatory joint disease, chronic inflammatory bowel disease and chronic renal disease, should be sought. Severe allergic manifestations may be associated with chronic occult blood loss from the bowel. Emotional and behavioural disorders may be associated with eating disorders, leading to an inadequate dietary intake of haematinics.

Examination

An overall assessment of the child presenting with pallor is important. A pale child who is restless, lethargic and irritable may be manifesting symptoms of hypoxia or cardiac decompensation and requires prompt assessment and treatment. Volume depletion in children, whether from blood loss or secondary to dehydration, generally is well compensated for by vasoconstriction and tachycardia. Hypotension is a late sign of decompensation and is an indication that urgent treatment is required. Children tolerate gradually progressive anaemia well, but the development of an intercurrent acute febrile illness may lead to cardiac decompensation and presentation with severe anaemia.

Specific features to be sought in the examination are evidence of:

- infective illness: fever, tachypnoea, grunting, neck stiffness or rash.
- blood loss: trauma, telangiectasis or melaena.
- haemolysis: jaundice, splenomegaly and dark urine.
- marrow failure: bruising, petechiae, and infection.
- malignancy: weight loss, lymphadenopathy, hepatosplenomegaly, abdominal or other mass.
- chronic illness: growth failure, poor nutritional status, severe eczema, joint swelling or deformity, hypertension or urinary abnormalities suggestive of renal disease, cardiomegaly, murmurs or signs of heart failure.

Initial investigation

Progressive selective investigation, guided by the history, clinical findings and the result of the blood count, is recommended. The first investigation will be a blood count (full blood examination (FBE) or complete blood count (FBC)), with red cell indices, a reticulocyte count and examination of the blood film. Care must be taken to relate the findings to the normal values for the age of the child (Table 53.1). In most instances the size and shape of the red cells, together with platelet and leucocyte parameters, will suggest a probable aetiology and the direction of further investigations.

The following should be noted.

Haemoglobin concentration (Hb g/l)

There is considerable variation in the normal haemoglobin with age (Table 53.1).

Mean cell volume (MCV fl)

This is highest in the neonate (98–118 fl), falls to its lowest value between 6 and 24 months of age (79–86 fl), then increases progressively throughout childhood (75–92 fl). A low MCV indicates microcytosis, and a high MCV indicates macrocytosis.

Table 53.1 Normal haemoglobin values for age

Age	Hb (g/l)
Birth	135–200
1 month	100–180
2 months	90–140
6 months	95–135
1 year	105–135
2–6 years	110–145
6–12 years	115–155
> 12 years (female)	120–160
> 12 years (male)	130–180

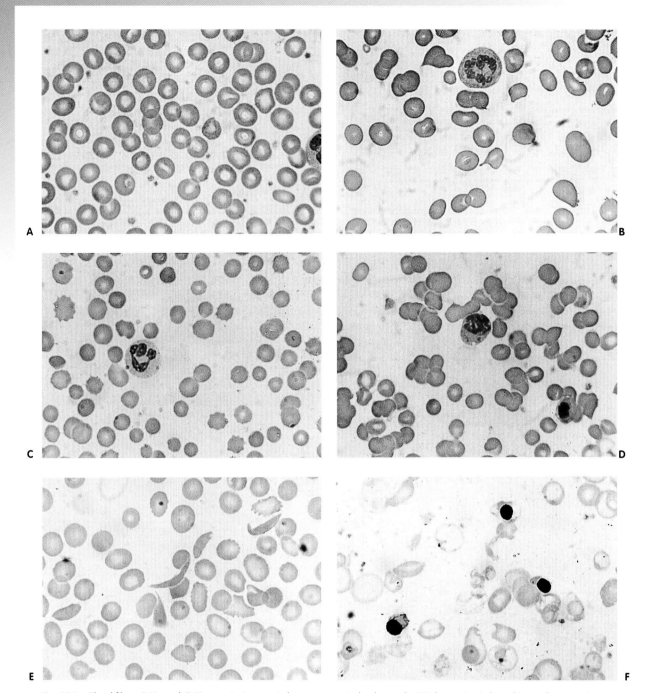

Fig. 53.1 Blood films. **A** Normal. **B** Macrocytosis — note hypersegmented polymorph. **C** Spherocytes in hereditary spherocytosis. **D** Autoimmune haemolytic anaemia showing red cell agglutination. **E** Sickle cell disease. **F** Thalassaemia major showing hypochromic microcytes and macrocytes, with nucleated red cells.

Reticulocyte count

This may be expressed as a percentage of the total red cell count (3–7% in the neonate, thereafter 0–1%), or more usually as an absolute count 20–100 × 10⁹/l). An increased reticulocyte count indicates active regeneration of red cells, seen after blood loss, haemolysis or in response to correct haematinic therapy. A low reticulocyte response in the presence of anaemia indicates a lack of marrow response, because of a deficiency of the necessary iron or vitamins or inappropriate therapy for the anaemia, or inability to respond, such as marrow aplasia or infiltration.

Leucocyte count (total white cell count, WCC) and differential

The WCC is elevated in the neonatal period with a neutrophil predominance. Lymphocytes predominate from 2 weeks of age until about 6 years, after which the neutrophil count gradually rises to become the predominant cell line. Neutrophilia after the neonatal period usually indicates bacterial infection. Lymphocytosis is seen in viral infections; aplasia is associated with leucopenia and blasts are generally seen in leukaemia.

Platelet count

The normal range is $150–450 \times 10^9$/l. Spontaneous bruising rarely occurs until the platelet count falls to less than 30×10^9/l. In association with anaemia the count may be normal as in early nutritional deficiencies, high in regenerative states, or low in immune thrombocytopenia, severe nutritional anaemia, aplasia, leukaemia or marrow infiltration with metastatic tumour.

Examination of the blood film

This is as important as the evaluation of the red cell indices, leucocyte count and platelets. The presence of abnormal red cell size, shape, inclusions, haemoglobin content, and evidence of regeneration usually will suggest the cause of the anaemia, and direct the next stage of investigation. The presence of abnormal leucocytes, or abnormal platelet numbers, may suggest a specific diagnosis such as leukaemia. Examples of a normal blood film and blood films in some conditions associated with anaemia are shown in Figure 53.1.

Additional investigations

Further investigations are guided by the provisional diagnosis formulated on the basis of history, examination and assessment of the FBE and film. An understanding of normal erythroid development (Fig. 53.2) and the pathophysiology leading to the development of specific changes in red cell morphology is helpful in understanding the resultant disease states. These are detailed in Tables 53.2–53.4. Further investigations which may be indicated after assessment of the FBE and film are listed below.

Microcytic anaemias

In these anaemias there is defective 'haem' or globin chain synthesis.

Dietary deficiency or increased losses suspected

Measure:
- serum iron, transferrin concentration
- serum ferritin
- serum proteins.

Family history/ethnicity suggestive of thalassaemia

Do:
- Hb electrophoresis
- test for Hb H inclusions
- DNA studies for alpha thalassaemia
- Family studies.

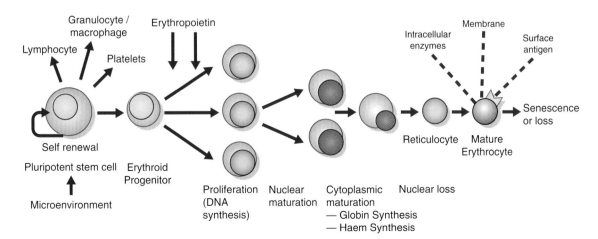

Fig. 53.2 The normal development of the red cell. Pathological processes at each stage of development may lead to altered production, red cell size, haemoglobin content or red cell survival.

Anaemias with oval macrocytes

In these anaemias there is impaired DNA synthesis. Do:

- red cell and serum folate
- serum vitamin B_{12} level
- Schilling test for B_{12} absorption
- transcobalamin II assay.

Anaemia with round macrocytes

Do:
- liver function tests
- thyroid function tests (hypothyroid).

Regenerative normocytic anaemia

This is associated with haemolysis or recovering aplasia. Do:
- urinalysis for urobilinogen, urobilin and haemoglobin
- serum bilirubin
- serum haptoglobin concentration (binds free Hb)
- Coombs test (direct antiglobulin test) (autoimmune haemolytic anaemia, AIHA)
- red cell enzyme assays (G6PD; pyruvate kinase, PK).
- osmotic fragility studies, autohaemolysis studies, glycerol lysis test (HS)
- haemoglobin electrophoresis (HbSS, unstable Hb)
- Family studies.

Aregenerative normocytic anaemia

This is associated with marrow failure or replacement. Do:
- bone marrow aspirate (BMA)/trephine.

This is frequently the best test to assess the cause of anaemia as it allows an assessment of the amount and quality of production and maturation of erythrocytes, leucocytes and platelets as well as the detection of abnormal cells. Bone marrow aspiration is performed easily from the posterior iliac crest, with local anaesthesia and sedation as required. Occasionally a trephine biopsy may be required to assess marrow cellularity, or to look for metastatic tumour deposits. In children this requires general anaesthesia.

Disorders of stem cell proliferation

Pluripotential stem cell failure (aplastic anaemia)

Normal marrow function is dependent on stem cell renewal and maturation of all cell lines. Failure of stem cell proliferation and differentiation results in aplastic anaemia. Both genetically determined and acquired forms occur (Table 53.2).

Fanconi anaemia

Fanconi anaemia, the commonest of the genetic forms of aplastic anaemia, is recessively inherited and is

---

Table 53.2 Causes of anaemia due to defective stem cell proliferation

Pathological process	Aetiology	Disease entity	Usual age of presentation

Pluripotential stem cell failure	Congenital
	Acquired
	  Drugs
	  Infection
	  Idiopathic
		Fanconi anaemia
		Aplastic anaemia
			Variable, majority <10 years
			Any age

Erythroid stem cell failure	Congenital
	Acquired
	  Idiopathic
	
	  Erythropoietin deficiency
	
	  Unknown
		Blackfan–Diamond syndrome
		
		Transient erythoblastopenia of childhood (TEC)
		Chronic renal failure
		Hypothyroidism
		Chronic infection
		Chronic inflammatory disease
			Neonate–6 months
			
			<5 years

Bone marrow replacement	Malignant transformation of progenitors Marrow infiltration Abnormal accumulation of metabolic substrates	Leukaemia Disseminated malignancy Lipid 'storage' disease	Infant–adult Infant–adult

characterised by a variable phenotype, progressive marrow failure and an increased risk of malignancy. There appear to be multiple gene defects in this condition which explains the diversity of clinical manifestations.

Approximately 75% of children have congenital abnormalities, with a wide range of defects. The commonest are café au lait spots, short stature, microcephaly and skeletal anomalies, with thumb and radial hypoplasia or aplasia being most characteristic. Renal anomalies, stenosis of auditory canals, micro-ophthalmia, hypogenitalism and a variety of anomalies of the gastrointestinal tract may also occur. The child shown in Figure 53.3 shows many features of this disorder.

The diagnosis may be suspected at birth if there are congenital abnormalities. Haematological abnormalities are rare at birth. Pancytopenia develops gradually, usually by the age of 10 years. Onset is earlier in boys than girls. Macrocytosis is followed by thrombocyto-

penia, neutropenia, then anaemia. Bone marrow aspirate and trephine show hypoplasia or aplasia.

In contrast, infants with the thrombocytopenia–absent radii (TAR) syndrome are severely thrombocytopenic at birth and have radial anomalies without thumb abnormalities.

The diagnosis of Fanconi anaemia is established by special chromosome studies of lymphocytes. Chromosomes from patients with Fanconi anaemia show markedly increased spontaneous and alkylating agent (cells incubated with mitomycin C or diepoxybutane) induced chromosomal breaks, gaps, rearrangements, exchanges and endoreduplication. Antenatal diagnosis is possible.

Androgen therapy may produce long remissions of the anaemia, but has little effect on thrombocytopenia and neutropenia. Its use is associated with masculinisation and therefore is undesirable in young children, particularly girls. Granulocyte macrophage colony stimulating factor has been used with some success. Bone marrow transplantation offers the only possibility of cure of the aplasia. Supportive care with transfusions and antibiotics is required for patients without a marrow donor, but death from infection, bleeding or the development of leukaemia usually occurs within a decade of diagnosis.

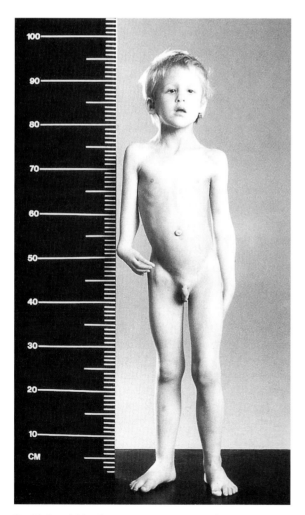

Fig. 53.3 Child with Fanconi anaemia. Note short stature, absent right radius and thumb, micro-ophthalmia and the presence of a hearing aid.

> ### Clinical example
>
> John, aged 5 years, presented with pallor and bruising of several months duration. He had a past history of tracheo-oesophageal fistula, and had always been small, with his height and weight on the 3rd centile for age. His teacher had expressed concern about his hearing. On examination he was pale, had multiple bruises, and several café au lait spots. He had a convergent squint and his external auditory canals were narrow. There was no hepatosplenomegaly or lymphadenopathy. A blood test showed a macrocytic anaemia with an Hb of 80 g/l, and a white cell count of 1.4×10^9/l with neutrophils 0.7×10^9/l. The platelet count was 25×10^9/l. A bone marrow aspirate showed hypocellular fragments, and trephine biopsies confirmed marrow aplasia. Cytogenetic studies on peripheral blood lymphocytes confirmed that he had Fanconi anaemia by showing an increased rate of spontaneous and mitomycin C induced chromosome breaks. His sister was found to be HLA identical with normal cytogenetic studies, and plans were made for elective bone marrow transplantation within the next few months.

Acquired aplastic anaemia

A number of agents may cause marrow failure, either in a dose dependent fashion (irradiation and cytotoxic drugs) or in an idiosyncratic fashion. Some viral infections are associated with marrow suppression. No cause is identified in about 50% of children with marrow failure. Fanconi anaemia must be excluded by cytogenetic studies as not all affected individuals have congenital abnormalities.

Common causes are:

- drugs: chloramphenicol, anticonvulsants, non steroidal anti-inflammatory agents and cytotoxic drugs
- chemicals: benzene, organic solvents, insecticides
- viral hepatitis: usually non A, non B, non C hepatitis, less commonly Epstein–Barr virus, cytomegalovirus, parvovirus or HIV
- preleukaemic: acute lymphoblastic leukaemia occasionally has a transient period of aplasia before the onset of the disease
- paroxysmal nocturnal haemoglobinuria.

Presentation is with the gradual onset of pallor, lethargy and bruising. There may be a history of recent infection. Physical examination reveals little other than pallor, bruising, petechiae and oral mucosal bleeding. Importantly there is no enlargement of liver, spleen or lymph nodes, but there may be fever and focal infection associated with the neutropenia.

The blood shows a pancytopenia with a normocytic anaemia without regeneration. Bone marrow aspirate and trephine biopsies reveal absent or decreased haemopoiesis.

Initial management depends on the severity and clinical manifestations of the aplasia. Potentially causative agents must be removed. Infections are treated vigorously. Supportive red cell and platelet transfusions are given as required. Early referral to a tertiary centre is vital. Although a small number of children will recover within a few weeks, bone marrow transplantation from an HLA compatible sibling is generally regarded as the treatment of choice for severe aplastic anaemia, particularly in the under 5 years old age group. Only 30% of children will have a matched sibling donor. For the remainder, antithymocyte globulin, together with granulocyte colony stimulating factor and cyclosporin, produces improvement or complete recovery in about two thirds of children. Onset of response may not occur for 2–3 months after initiation of therapy and supportive care during this time is vital. For those failing to respond, unrelated donor transplantation is an option and a donor search should be initiated early.

Red cell aplasia (erythroid stem cell failure)

Isolated aplasia of red cells results in a normocytic normochromic anaemia without reticulocytosis. The platelets and WCC are normal. Congenital and acquired forms occur.

Congenital red cell aplasia (Diamond–Blackfan syndrome)

This disorder is almost certainly heterogenous, with sporadic, dominant and recessive forms occurring. The defect has not been determined, but is possibly due to a defect in the erythroid progenitor cell.

Normocytic anaemia may be present at birth and usually is evident by 2–3 months of age. Early treatment with steroids results in a reticulocytosis and increase in haemoglobin in about two thirds of patients. Some steroid responsive patients are successfully weaned off steroids but many remain steroid dependent. Those failing to respond to steroids or requiring large doses will need regular blood transfusion and chelation therapy. Bone marrow transplantation has corrected the condition in steroid resistant patients.

Acquired red cell aplasia

Pure red cell aplasia (PRCA) is primarily a disease of adults but cases have been documented in teenagers. A large number of disorders, including thymoma, malignancy, autoimmune disease, viral infection and drug administration, have been implicated. Therapy is directed primarily toward the cause but may include immunosuppression, plasmapheresis, thymectomy and splenectomy.

Transient erythroblastopenia of childhood (TEC)

This self limited, aregenerative anaemia occurs typically in children between 1 and 3 years of age. The aetiology remains unclear, but antibodies directed against early red cell precursors have been documented in some children. Parvovirus B19 has not been consistently isolated.

The typical presentation is with pallor of gradual onset in an otherwise well child. The only abnormal clinical finding is pallor. The anaemia may be marked, without evidence of regeneration. A bone marrow aspirate generally will show absent or diminished erythropoiesis, but if spontaneous recovery is already occurring at the time of presentation there may be many early erythroid progenitors present.

As the onset of the anaemia is gradual, most children will have compensated well and tolerate quite marked degrees of anaemia. If, however, there is no evidence of recovery occurring by the time the Hb falls to levels below 50 g/l, transfusion is likely to be required. Folic acid supplements should be given during the recovery phase. Spontaneous recovery usually occurs within 1–2 months, and it is unusual for more than one transfusion to be required. Steroids have no role in the management of this disorder.

Transient erythroid aplasia in chronic haemolytic anaemias

An aplastic crisis may occur in patients with one of the chronic haemolytic anaemias, such as sickle cell disease, hereditary spherocytosis and autoimmune haemolytic anaemia. Infection with human parvovirus B19 has been documented as the usual cause. Folic acid deficiency may be a further precipitating factor.

Because of the shortened red cell survival, there is a precipitous fall in haemoglobin when erythroid proliferation ceases. Pallor and lethargy develop relatively quickly. The absence of jaundice, lack of increase in the degree of splenomegaly, and the absence of a reticulocyte response enables one to distinguish an aplastic crisis from increased haemolysis. Blood transfusion is likely to be required. Spontaneous recovery usually begins within 10–14 days.

Marrow replacement

Infiltration with neoplasia, particularly leukaemia, is the commonest cause of marrow failure in childhood. Several other childhood malignancies (neuroblastoma, non Hodgkin lymphoma, Ewing sarcoma and rhabdomyosarcoma) metastasise to the bone marrow. Progressive pancytopenia with a normocytic anaemia and an associated shift to the left in the erythroid and myeloid series develops. Nucleated red cells and immature granulocytes (left shift) may be seen in the peripheral blood (leucoerythroblastic blood picture).

Replacement of marrow with storage cells (for example, Gaucher disease), fibrous tissue (myelofibrosis) or bone (osteopetrosis) will have a similar result. Careful examination of the blood film looking for leukaemic blasts, and a bone marrow examination which will identify abnormal cells, is required in any child with pancytopenia.

Dyserythropoietic/ineffective erythropoiesis

Congenital dyserythropoietic anaemias

This group of rare hereditary disorders of erythropoiesis is characterised by ineffective erythropoiesis resulting in shortened red cell survival with associated jaundice, a variable degree of anaemia, with normocytic to macrocytic red cell morphology, and anisopoikilocytosis and fragmentation in some types (Table 53.3). Bone marrow findings are characterised by erythroid hyperplasia, multinuclearity and internuclear bridging. The aetiology is unknown. Some patients in whom haemolysis is severe require regular transfusions.

Table 53.3   Anaemias that are due to ineffective erythropoiesis and dyserythropoiesis

Pathological process	Aetiology	Disease entity	Usual age of presentation
Impaired DNA synthesis (megaloblastosis)	Unknown	Congenital dyserythropoietic anaemia	Infancy to adulthood
	Vitamin B^{12} deficiency		
	Congenital	Transcobalamin II deficiency	Neonates–3 months
		Congenital pernicious anaemia	<3 years
	Acquired	Maternal B$_{12}$ deficiency	3–12 months
		Juvenile pernicious anaemia	>10 years
		Ileal resection	
		Regional ileitis	Any age
		Blind loop syndrome	
	Folate deficiency		
	Congenital	Rare metabolic abnormalities	Infancy
	Acquired	Dietary deficiency	Any age
		Malabsorption (coeliac disease)	
		Increased utilisation (haemolysis)	
Defective haem synthesis (microcytosis)	Iron deficiency	Dietary deficiency	Infancy, adolescence
		Malabsorption	Any age
		Blood loss	Any age
		Occult	
		Overt	
Reduced/absent globin chain synthesis	Gene deletion/mutation	Beta thalassaemia major	6 months–5 years
		HbH disease (alpha thalassaemia)	Any age
		Thalassaemia traits	Any age
Abnormal globin chain production	Gene mutation/ amino acid substitution	Haemoglobinopathies	Any age
		Sickle cell disease	1–4 years

Megaloblastic anaemia

Megaloblastic anaemias in childhood are rare, but prompt diagnosis of the cause is important to prevent potentially irreversible neurological damage which may result from deficiencies of vitamin B_{12} or its transport protein transcobalamin II.

Vitamin B_{12} deficiency

Because the daily requirement for vitamin B_{12} is low and body stores generally are high, dietary deficiency of vitamin B_{12} is rare, occurring only after prolonged inadequate intake, as may occur in vegans. Breast fed infants of vitamin B_{12}, deficient vegans are also at risk and may present with anaemia, in the first year of life. The majority of children with vitamin B_{12} deficiency have a malabsorptive problem, either specific to vitamin B_{12} as in pernicious anaemia, or secondary to inflammation or loss of the ileum, the portion of the small bowel in which vitamin B_{12} absorption occurs.

Vitamin B_{12} deficiency results in an anaemia with oval macrocytosis, hypersegmentation of neutrophils and thrombocytopenia (Fig. 53.1B). Bone marrow examination shows erythroid hyperplasia with megaloblastosis characterised by abnormally large erythroid and myeloid progenitors, in which nuclear maturation is delayed as compared to cytoplasmic maturation. Intramedullary destruction of erythroid precursors leads to a mild unconjugated hyperbilirubinaemia.

Therapy depends on the cause of the vitamin B_{12} deficiency. Dietary deficiency is treated by an initial dose of parenteral vitamin B_{12}, followed by dietary correction. Abnormalities of absorption, whether due to pernicious anaemia, ileal malabsorption or resection, require long term intramuscular injection of the vitamin (hydroxycobalamin) at 1–3 month intervals according to the severity of the malabsorption.

Folate deficiency

Daily folate requirements are low, but body stores are small. Folate is heat labile and, although ubiquitous in food, it is often destroyed by cooking.

Extra folate is required at times of rapid growth, during pregnancy, and in patients with haemolytic anaemias. Deficiency is most likely to occur under these circumstances. Dietary deficiency most commonly occurs in infants fed exclusively on goat's milk, which is deficient in the vitamin. Malabsorption occurs in generalised malabsorptive syndromes such as coeliac disease and Crohn disease.

Some anticonvulsant drugs, for example, phenytoin, may interfere with folate absorption, and megaloblastic changes are common among patients taking these drugs.

Inherited disorders of folate metabolism are rare, and may present diagnostic difficulty.

Folate deficiency presents with a macrocytic anaemia, without neurological abnormality. Oral administration of folic acid is effective in reversing deficiencies. Doses required are small, as 0.1 mg daily produces an optimal haematological response. In patients with increased requirements or malabsorption, higher doses of 0.5–5 mg daily are given. It is essential to exclude coexistent vitamin B_{12} deficiency before treatment as the haematological picture may improve initially with folate therapy but progression of the neurological effects of vitamin B_{12} deficiency will still occur.

Defective haem synthesis

Iron deficiency

Iron deficiency is the commonest cause of anaemia in childhood, being particularly common in the first 2 years of life when iron requirements are increased because of rapid growth and dietary intake often is inadequate. Early adolescence is another risk period for development of iron deficiency because of rapid growth.

Low birth weight infants and infants having exchange transfusions or frequent blood sampling have low total body iron stores and are at high risk of early development of iron deficiency anaemia, as iron stores and dietary intake are inadequate to keep up with rapid postnatal growth. Breast milk and cow's milk have a similar iron content but iron bioavailability from breast milk is approximately 50%, compared with 10% from cow's milk. Breast fed term babies therefore are rarely iron deficient in the first 6 months of life but iron concentrations in breast milk decline postnatally and the iron content of breast milk is insufficient to meet the needs of the infant over the age of 6 months.

Oral iron supplementation (2 mg/kg/day) is given to low birth weight infants, generally from approximately 3 months of age. Iron containing foods should be introduced by 6 months of age to all term babies. Most infant formulae are iron fortified. Infants weaned early onto cow's milk (before 12 months of age), particularly those in whom milk continues to be the major component of the diet without the appropriate introduction of mixed solid feedings, are the group presenting most commonly with gross iron deficiency. In some, iron deficiency is exacerbated by the development of cow's milk protein enteropathy, leading to peripheral oedema secondary to hypoalbuminaemia in addition to anaemia.

Older children with diets poor in iron containing foods (red meat, white meats, legumes, green vegetables, egg yolk) are also at risk. Blood loss must always be considered in an iron deficient child or adolescent without an appropriate dietary history. Menorrhagia is an important cause of iron deficiency in adolescent girls. Occult blood loss is usually gastrointestinal in origin, from such diverse causes as cow's milk enteropathy, polyps, hae-mangiomas, Meckel diverticulum and hereditary telang-iectasia, but repeated epistaxes and chronic blood loss from the renal tract must be excluded.

Iron malabsorption is uncommon and usually is as-sociated with malabsorption syndromes such as coeliac disease or chronic inflammatory bowel disease.

Iron deficiency initially leads to depletion of marrow iron stores, without any haematological abnormality. When iron stores are exhausted, serum iron concentration and transferrin binding falls and there is reduced intra-cellular iron availability for haem synthesis, with a con-sequent reduction in haemoglobin production, leading to microcytosis and the development of anaemia.

Symptoms of early iron deficiency with no or minimal anaemia may include poor attention span and irritability. As anaemia develops, cognitive deficits may increase and lethargy and pallor become apparent. Some chronically iron deficient children exhibit pica (the ingestion of non food items such as dirt, clay, and chewing of ice).

Examination reveals pallor, most easily detected in the palmar creases and conjunctivae. Signs of cardiac decompensation will occasionally be present if the anaemia is severe. Mild splenomegaly is found occa-sionally but is more common in thalassaemia minor, from which iron deficiency must be distinguished.

Investigations

The haemoglobin will range from normal to very low, relative to the normal for age. The MCV and MCHC fall before the haemoglobin level drops. Microcytosis and hypochromia are seen on the blood film. A low serum fer-ritin confirms iron deficiency but normal to high levels are seen in acute liver disease, acute infection and chronic inflammatory disease and do not rule out iron deficiency. The serum iron concentration is low in both iron deficiency and chronic disease, but the transferrin concentration is increased in iron deficiency and decreased in chronic disease. Although usually not required to make the diagnosis of iron deficiency, bone marrow aspiration will confirm the diagnosis by demon-strating the absence of stainable iron.

Lead poisoning also is associated with a microcytic, hypochromic anaemia. Lead absorption is enhanced in iron deficiency and the two may coexist.

Therapy of iron deficiency involves correction of the underlying cause and replenishment of iron stores. Improvement in the dietary intake of iron containing foods is the most important strategy in the majority of iron deficient children. Reduction in the total milk content of the diet may be necessary to allow the child to develop an appropriate appetite. If a source of blood loss is identified, appropriate therapy is undertaken and iron supplements given until the deficiency is corrected.

Therapeutic iron is optimally given orally in two to three divided doses daily in a dose of 6 mg/kg/day of elemental iron. Absorption is enhanced when iron is taken with orange juice, and between meals, but the side effects of abdominal discomfort are reduced when iron is taken with food. Ferrous sulphate is cheaper and better absorbed than ferrous gluconate, but the gluconate is better tolerated. A reticulocyte response to iron should be seen within 7–10 days, but iron therapy should continue for 4–6 weeks after the haemoglobin level returns to normal, to replenish iron stores. The stools are grey-black in individuals on iron.

It is rarely necessary to use the parenteral route for iron administration, but in occasional children with poor absorption or poor compliance, intravenous infusions of iron may be required.

> ### Clinical example
>
> Tan, a 15 month old boy, had been breast fed for 10 months and then was given cow's milk. He had occasional solid foods only, and rarely had any foods with a significant iron content. He had become irritable, seemed to be low in energy and slept more than his parents thought was usual. When he was seen by his doctor because of an upper respiratory tract infection, he was noted to have pale conjunctivae and pale palmar creases.
>
> His Hb was 51 g/l, his MCV was 51 fl, and his MCHC was 15 pg. The total WBC was normal and his platelet count was 432×10^9/l. The blood film showed microcytic and hypochromic red cells; there was no reticulocytosis and no basophilic stippling. The serum ferritin was 4 μg/l (normal range 16–300), the serum iron was 5 μmol/l (normal range 9–27), and the iron binding capacity was 83 μmol/l (normal range 45–72).
>
> His anaemia had all the features of an iron deficiency anaemia due to a deficient iron intake in his diet. A dietician assisted in instructing his mother in ways to improve his diet by including foods such as red and white meats, green vegetables, legumes and egg yolks. He was given ferrous gluconate mixture at a dose of 6 mg/kg of expected weight/day, to be taken as two doses daily. His parents were asked to give this with orange juice to improve absorption. They were warned that the mixture could make his stools a grey-black colour but that this was not of concern. They were asked to brush his teeth after each dose to prevent any minor staining. They were warned of the toxic effects of iron if taken in overdose accidentally by an inquisitive toddler; the mixture was provided in limited amounts only in a bottle with a safety top, and they were asked to keep it in a secure place, preferably a locked cupboard.
>
> The iron mixture was continued for 3 months. His reticulocyte count rose in a few days, and his Hb began to rise in 10 days. By 6 weeks of therapy his Hb was normal; the iron mixture was continued for another 6 weeks to ensure that his iron stores were replenished.

Haemoglobinopathies

Haemoglobin is a compound protein made up of two pairs of globin chains with a haem molecule inserted into each. One of these globin chains is designated as the alpha chain, the other variably being termed beta, delta, epsilon (ϵ), gamma and zeta (ζ). Zeta and epsilon chains are expressed only in early embryonic life, with zeta chain production switching to alpha chain production and gamma chain production replacing epsilon chain synthesis in the early weeks of gestation. In the perinatal period there is a further switch from gamma to beta chain production. The predominant fetal haemoglobin is HbF ($\alpha_2\gamma_2$). In children beyond 6 months of age and adults, the major haemoglobins are HbA ($\alpha_2\beta_2$) and HbA2 ($\alpha_2\delta_2$). A number of abnormalities of globin chain production or point mutations within globin genes may result in significant disease.

Thalassaemias

These are genetic disorders characterised by reduced or absent production of one or more of the globin chains of haemoglobin.

The thalassaemias are found commonly in people originating from the Mediterranean region, Middle East, the Indian subcontinent, South Asia and Africa. The inheritance is in a mendelian recessive manner.

Beta thalassaemia

Beta thalassaemia occurs as a result of point mutations or deletions within one or both of the two beta globin genes, resulting in reduced or absent production of beta globin chains. The heterozygous state is termed thalassaemia minor and the homozygous state thalassaemia major.

Beta thalassaemia minor

Affected individuals usually are asymptomatic, with mild anaemia detected either during investigation of another illness or as a result of family screening. Mild pallor and splenomegaly may be noted but the examination often is unremarkable. There is a mild microcytic hypochromic anaemia with occasional target cells. The differential diagnosis is iron deficiency, although both may coexist. The HbA2 level is elevated. If present, iron deficiency may mask the thalassaemia minor, preventing diagnosis until the iron deficiency is corrected.

Beta thalassaemia major (Cooley anaemia)

This is caused by the inheritence of two abnormal beta genes. At birth the haemoglobin is normal, but as the γ–β

switch occurs, there are no (β^0) or insufficient (β^+) beta chains to balance alpha chains. Excess alpha chains precipitate, causing shortened red cell survival with destruction within the bone marrow (ineffective erythropoiesis) and spleen. HbA production is inadequate to compensate for the gradual fall in HbF as gamma chain production switches to inadequate beta chain production.

Children with thalassaemia major usually present between 3 months and 1 year of life with pallor and hepatosplenomegaly. There may be mild jaundice. Occasionally presentation is delayed to 4–5 years, with these children having increased skin pigmentation, frontal bossing and malar prominence due to chronic marrow expansion. The Hb may be very low, with blood examination revealing hypochromia, red cell stippling, microcytosis, macrocytes, target cells and nucleated red cells (Fig. 53.1F). An elevated HbF level (usually 50–100%) confirms the diagnosis. Globin chain synthesis studies can differentiate between β^+ and β^0 thalassaemia.

Without treatment, the severe chronic anaemia leads to growth retardation, poor musculoskeletal development and increased iron absorption, resulting in skin pigmentation. Extramedullary haemopoiesis in liver and spleen together with hypersplenism result in organ enlargement and abdominal distension. Marrow expansion produces the characteristic facial appearance with frontal bossing, maxillary hypertrophy with exposure of the upper teeth, prominence of the malar eminences and a flattened nasal bridge. Skull X rays show expansion of the diploic space, and the subperiostial bone has a typical 'hair on end' appearance. There is cortical thinning of long bones and fractures may occur. Death usually occurs within 10 years from cardiac failure, cardiac arrythmias or infection.

Current treatment is with regular transfusion at 3–4 weekly intervals, aiming to suppress endogenous haemopoiesis (preventing marrow expansion) and keep the Hb level above 100 g/l. Regular transfusion results in iron loading and chelation therapy must accompany transfusion support to prevent the toxic effects of iron on the myocardium, liver, pancreas and gonads (cardiac arrythmias, cardiac failure, diabetes mellitus, hepatic fibrosis, infertility). The chelator desferrioxamine is currently given by subcutaneous infusion via a syringe pump over 10 hours nightly. Compliance, particularly during adolescence, is often a problem. A safe, effective oral chelator is awaited eagerly. All patients receive folic acid supplements and hepatitis B vaccination and are encouraged to participate in all normal activities. Splenectomy preceded by pneumovax immunisation is still required occasionally.

Bone marrow transplantation from matched siblings is producing high cure rates provided it is carried out before hepatic dysfunction develops, but long term results are still to be evaluated.

With improvements in therapy some patients are now surviving into the fifth decade. A proportion of adults have preservation of gonadal function and have had children.

Haemoglobin E/β thalassaemia

Haemoglobin E ($\beta^{26Glu-Ly}$) occurs extensively throughout South East Asia. Neither the heterozygous nor homozygous state produce clinical abnormalities. The doubly heterozygous state of HbE with beta thalassaemia results in a clinical condition similar to thalassaemia major. Diagnosis is confirmed by blood examination and haemoglobin electrophoresis. Clinical presentation and management are similar to a moderately severe beta thalassaemia.

Alpha thalassaemia

There are four alpha globin genes and alpha thalassaemia results from the loss of one or more of these. The loss of one gene produces neither haematological nor clinical abnormality (silent carrier). Loss of two genes results in hypochromia and microcytosis, but no anaemia, and is known as alpha thalassaemia trait. Alpha thalassaemia occurs with a very high incidence in Asian populations and is assuming increasing importance in our community.

Haemoglobin H disease

The loss of three alpha genes results in the formation of excess beta chains which form an unstable tetramer (β_4), accounting for 30–40% of the total haemoglobin. The clinical picture is similar to beta thalassaemia intermedia with pallor, jaundice and moderate hepatosplenomegaly. There is a moderate anaemia (Hb 80–100 g/l) and persistent reticulocytosis. The anaemia is aggravated by infections, pregnancy and oxidant drugs (for example, phenacetin or primaquine), which should be avoided. No specific treatment other than folic acid supplements are necessary.

Haemoglobin Barts (hydrops fetalis syndrome)

All four alpha genes are deleted and no alpha chains are produced. The haemoglobins present are Hb Barts (γ_4) 70%, and HbH (β_4) 0–20% and Hb Portland ($\zeta_2 \gamma_2$). Severe fetal anaemia develops, resulting in cardiac failure, hepatosplenomegaly and generalised oedema. The infants generally are stillborn or die shortly after birth. In utero transfusions may result in a liveborn infant, and exchange transfusion followed by ongoing transfusion support has led to the survival of a few patients. Bone marrow transplantation should cure these patients.

Sickle cell disease

Haemoglobin S (HbS) results from a single amino acid substitution in the beta globin chain ($\beta^{6\ Glu-Val}$). Under hypoxic conditions, deoxyhaemoglobin S polymerises into fibre bundles which distort the cell into a sickle shape. Sickling may be reversible on reoxygenation or may become irreversible. The sickle cell gene occurs in people from Africa, the Middle East and the Mediterranean region as well as in the Afro-American population.

The heterozygous carrier (*sickle trait*) is asymptomatic with normal Hb and red cell morphology. Haemoglobin electrophoresis reveals an HbA of approximately 60% and an HbS level of 30–40%.

In the homozygous state (*sickle cell anaemia*) there is a normochromic normocytic haemolytic anaemia with target cells, sickle cells, nucleated red cells, fragments and spherocytes (Fig. 53.1E). The diagnosis is confirmed by finding an elevated HbS (60–90%) on electrophoresis with approximately 2% HbA$_2$, the remainder being HbF. The higher the level of HbF the less severe the symptoms of the disease.

The doubly heterozygous *sickle trait–beta thalassaemia* is expressed with clinical features very similar to those of homozygous sickle cell disease. In contrast to sickle cell anaemia, the red cells are microcytic and hypochromic and target cells are present. Sickling can be demonstrated and both HbS and HbA$_2$ are elevated. Examination of the parents' blood confirms sickle cell trait in one and thalassaemia minor in the other. The management of this condition is similar to that for sickle cell anaemia.

The clinical course of the patient with sickle cell disease, or doubly heterozygous sickle/thalassaemia, is characterised by 'crises' as a result of sickling of red cells which obstruct the lumen of capillaries and small venules, causing infarction of surrounding tissues. Haemolytic 'crises' may also occur during infective illness.

Presentation is usually between the ages of 6 months and 4 years with pallor, jaundice, abdominal or limb pain and/or swelling of the hands and feet. Haemolytic crises are characterised by increased pallor and jaundice, infarctive 'crises' with acute pain generally of limbs or back, and aplastic crises with an aregenerative anaemia. Splenic sequestration crises occur in young children predominantly under the age of 5 years. In this potentially life threatening complication, red cells are trapped in splenic sinusoids, resulting in hypovolaemia, a rapid increase in splenic size, and profound anaemia. Patients with sickle cell disease have an increased risk of infection, particularly pneumococcal infection. Functional asplenia secondary to repeated splenic infarction occurs in most patients.

The emphasis in management is on avoidance of enviromental factors known to precipitate a crisis. The following protective measures are recommended:

- Good nutrition with regular folic acid supplements.
- Penicillin prophylaxis from infancy, with prompt treatment of infections.
- Maintenance of adequate hydration, particularly during hot weather.

- Prevention of vascular stasis. This may occur with tight clothing, the use of tourniquets applied during an operative procedure and exposure to cold.

Vaso-occlusive crises require prompt control of pain, the maintenance of hydration and treatment of underlying infection. Severe crises (pulmonary syndrome or cerebral infarction) require blood transfusion to reduce the HbS concentration. Occasionally exchange transfusion may be required.

Patients with splenic sequestration require prompt restoration of intravascular volume and correction of acidosis.

Patients with frequent crises may be managed with regular blood transfusions to suppress endogenous HbS production. These patients also require iron chelation. Successful bone marrow transplantation has been reported.

Genetic counselling

Current DNA techniques allow prenatal diagnosis of the thalassaemias and sickle cell disease. With increased community awareness and education, many couples who carry either a thalassaemia or sickle trait are now seeking antenatal counselling and prenatal diagnosis. This will have significant effects on the incidence of newly diagnosed homozygotes in the future.

Anaemia due to increased red cell destruction (haemolysis)

Anaemia secondary to haemolysis (Table 53.4) occurs when bone marrow replacement does not keep pace with the rate of destruction.

Haemolysis may be intravascular or may occur by phagocytosis within the spleen or liver. Intravascular haemolysis occurs in some autoimmune haemolytic anaemias, acute haemolysis in G6PD deficiency, and acute transfusion reactions. Free haemoglobin is released and combines with haptoglobin. The complex is cleared by the reticuloendothelial system of the liver and spleen. If the free plasma haemoglobin concentration exceeds the haptoglobin binding capacity, haemoglobinuria occurs. The colour of the urine may vary from pink through brown to almost black, depending on the amount of free haemoglobin excreted.

If haemolysis occurs predominantly in the reticulo-endothelial system (autoimmune haemolytic anaemia, membrane abnormalities), there is little free haemoglobin in plasma. Haemoglobin is converted to bilirubin within phagocytes, transported to the liver bound to albumin, then conjugated and excreted into the bile. Jaundice is variable, depending on the rate of haemolysis and hepatic conjugation. To compensate for the reduced red cell survival the bone marrow increases its output of red cells,

Table 53.4 Anaemias that are due to increased red cell destruction

Pathological process	Aetiology	Disease entity	Usual age of presentation
Oxidative cell damage	Enzyme defects of the glycolytic pathway	G6PD deficiency PK deficiency	Neonate–10 years Neonate–adult
Membrane abnormality (decreased red cell deformability)	Congenital — splenic destruction	Hereditary spherocytosis Hereditary elliptocytosis	Neonate–adult
Antibody mediated membrane damage	Fetomaternal Rh and ABO incompatibility	Haemolytic disease of newborn	In utero–24 hours
	Autoantibodies ± complement reacting with red cell membrane Infection Drugs Autoimmune disease	Autoimmune haemolytic anaemia	Any age
Toxic membrane damage	Infection Heavy metals	*Clostridium perfringens* Wilson disease	Any age Late childhood–adult
Mechanical membrane damage	Membrane damage	Disseminated intravascular coagulopathy Haemolytic uraemic syndrome Cardiac prosthesis	Any age Childhood

releasing immature reticulocytes and, in acute severe haemolysis, nucleated red cells into the peripheral blood.

Intracellular enzyme defects

Mature red cells lack a nucleus and intracellular organelles necessary for synthesis of proteins and generation of ATP via oxidative pathways. Energy production for maintenance of the integrity of the red cell is via one of the two glycolytic metabolic pathways within it. About 95% of glucose metabolism is via the anaerobic Embden–Myerhof pathway and 5% through the hexose monophosphate shunt (pentose phosphate pathway). Enzyme defects in either pathway result in oxidative damage and haemolysis. Deficiencies or abnormalities of G6PD, the first enzyme in the hexose monophosphate shunt, are extremely common worldwide. All the documented enzyme deficiencies of the Embden–Myerhof pathway resulting in haemolytic anaemias are rare. Examples are pyruvate kinase deficiency and glucose phosphate isomerase deficiency.

G6PD deficiency

This X linked enzyme deficiency is the commonest inherited disorder of the red cell. It is fully expressed in hemizygous males and in homozygous females. Heterozygous females show a variable level of enzyme activity due to variation in X chromosome inactivation. There are over 200 variant enzymes and the clinical expression of the disorder is variable, with four major clinical syndromes. Neonatal jaundice is common in the Chinese and Mediterranean variants; favism (acute haemolysis after ingestion of broad beans or inhalation of pollen) is a feature of the Mediterranean variant; while oxidative stress induced haemolysis (drugs, infection), although common to all variants, is the predominant feature in affected individuals of African descent. Individuals of northern European descent have chronic moderate haemolysis, while other variants only experience haemolysis with appropriate stress. Patients typically present severely anaemic with dark urine, having been well until 1–2 days days prior to presentation. The precipitating factor usually is identifiable on history. Because of the rapidity of the fall in haemoglobin there often is profound lethargy and restlessness at presentation.

Examination of the blood film shows polychromasia and anisocytosis and typically 'blister' cells. The diagnosis is established by enzyme assay in mature red cells. Enzyme levels are higher in reticulocytes in some variants and a normal enzyme level at the time of an acute haemolytic episode does not exclude the diagnosis. Management is to avoid precipitating factors. Patients having acute crises may require blood transfusion, although a brisk reticulocyte response may result in rapid spontaneous recovery.

Clinical example

Thomas is an 8 year old boy from Hong Kong. He presented with the onset of pallor over 24 hours and was passing very dark urine. He had recently been treated for tonsillitis. He had no past history of serious illness. On examination, apart from marked pallor, splenomegaly was present. His urine contained haemoglobin. Blood tests revealed a haemoglobin of 40 g/l with an elevated reticulocyte response. Blister cells were evident on the blood film. The G6PD assay was borderline normal and assays on the parents showed his mother was heterozygous for G6PD deficiency. One month after this episode, Thomas was shown to have a severe deficiency of G6PD activity. The earlier borderline result was caused by the presence of many young red cells with high G6PD activity.

Intrinsic membrane defects

Abnormalities of the red cell membrane result in alterations of cell shape, usually due to changes in transmembrane electrolyte flux. Changes in cell shape cause decreased deformability, splenic trapping and destruction within the spleen, resulting in chronic haemolytic anaemia. The commonest membrane abnormality is hereditary spherocytosis, a dominantly inherited condition.

Hereditary spherocytosis

There is a marked variability in the severity of haemolysis in this condition. Neonatal jaundice is common. Some children present with anaemia in infancy, while others remain asymptomatic until a haemolytic or aplastic crisis occurs in association with a viral infection. Hypersplenism or gallstones may result in the presentation of a previously asymptomatic patient with well compensated haemolysis. A positive family history is often obtained.

Examination reveals pallor, often mild jaundice and a variable degree of splenomegaly. The diagnosis is suggested by the presence of spherocytes in the peripheral blood (Fig. 53.1C). Increased osmotic fragility, autohaemolysis and a positive glycerol lysis test confirms the diagnosis.

Folic acid supplements should be given. Blood transfusion may be required for anaemia resulting from inadequately compensated haemolysis and for aplastic crises during which the haemoglobin may fall precipitously. Aplastic crises usually are associated with parvovirus B19 infection. Haemolysis is abolished by splenectomy. Overwhelming postsplenectomy infection may occur, particularly in children less than 5 years of age. Pneumococcal, meningococcal and *Haemophilus influenzae* b immunisations should be given presplenectomy, and penicillin prophylaxis continued indefinitely postsplenectomy.

Decisions about splenectomy should be based on the following:

- degree of haemolysis and anaemia
- age
- size of spleen
- presence of gallstones.

> ### Clinical example
>
> Angela is 9 years of age. In the neonatal period she required exchange transfusion for severe jaundice. She had always been pale and had a small appetite. With upper respiratory tract infections, her pallor had increased and jaundice had appeared. At 2 years of age hereditary spherocytosis was diagnosed and folic acid supplements were commenced. Angela's father also has this condition. She presented with abdominal pain, pallor, icterus and splenomegaly of 6 cm. Ultrasound examination confirmed the presence of gallstones. Following pneumococcal and *Haemophilus influenzae* b vaccination, splenectomy and cholecystotomy with removal of gallstones was undertaken. Prophylactic penicillin was commenced after the surgery and continued indefinitely.

Extrinsic membrane damage

Acquired membrane damage leading to haemolysis can result from antibody–antigen reactions, mechanical insults (for example, intravascular prosthetic patches), burns, toxins (for example, copper) and infective agents (for example, *Clostridium perfringens*).

Antibody mediated haemolysis

The binding of immunoglobulin or complement, or a combination of the two, to the red cell membrane may result in premature cell destruction or immune haemolysis. The antibody involved may be IgG (warm antibody) or IgM (cold antibody). Immune haemolytic anaemias may be classified as follows.

Isoimmune haemolysis in the newborn (Ch. 33)
- Rh incompatibility (mother Rh –ve; baby Rh +ve).
- ABO incompatibility (mother group O: baby group A or B).

Idiopathic. In many instances of IgG warm antibody mediated haemolysis, no definite aetiological agent is identified.

Post infectious. Many common infectious diseases, such as measles (IgG), infectious mononucleosis (IgM) and mycoplasma infection (IgM) may be associated with acute haemolysis.

Drug related. This is very uncommon in children. Some drugs stimulate the production of antibodies which are directed against red cell antigens, but not against the drug, for example, α-methyl dopa. A second mechanism involves a drug, such as penicillin, binding to the red cell membrane, with antibody to the drug being formed and attaching to the drug. The antibody coated red cells then undergo destruction in the spleen. The third mechanism of drug related haemolysis involves the deposition of antibody–antigen complexes on the red cell surface with activation of complement and brisk intravascular haemolysis.

Associated with connective tissue disease or malignancy. This is rare in childhood but may be associated with systemic lupus erythematosus in adolescence.

Presentation of a child with immune mediated haemolysis is usually acute with rapid onset of pallor, severe anaemia and dark urine. Jaundice may be present. Life threatening anaemia may develop rapidly, with vaso-constriction, cardiac failure and hypoxia. Modest splenomegaly is often present.

The peripheral blood shows a predominantly normocytic anaemia with spherocytes, fragmented red cells and rouleaux formation (Fig. 53.1D). In cold agglutinin disease, agglutination is seen on the blood film. As a compensating reticulocytosis develops, polychromasia and macrocytosis are seen. A positive Coombs test confirms the diagnosis. The specificity of the Coombs reagent used classifies the type of antibody involved. The commonest are warm IgG antibodies, but cold IgM antibodies are found in association with mycoplasma infection and infectious mononucleosis.

Urgent blood transfusion may be required. Compatible blood usually cannot be obtained and the 'least incompatible' blood should be used. Transfused cells may be haemolysed rapidly and careful observation is required. Repeated transfusions may be necessary. Adequate hydration must be maintained to avoid renal tubular damage from haemoglobinuria. Where a warm antibody is identified, steroid therapy is instituted and maintained until the Hb stabilises, then tapered gradually. Children with cold antibodies require warming of the blood to 37°C before transfusion.

Haemolysis is usually self limiting over the course of days to weeks. Occasional patients may have severe ongoing haemolysis, or frequent relapses. Plasma exchange, exchange transfusion or high dose immunoglobulin may be useful, but if these measures fail, splenectomy may be life saving.

Blood loss

Blood loss, if acute, results in vasoconstriction, then tachycardia and finally hypotension. The haemoglobin, if measured very early in the course of a bleeding episode, will be normal or only slightly reduced. When there has been time for haemodilution to occur, the haemoglobin falls. A compensatory reticulocytosis occurs after approximately 48 hours. Chronic blood loss results in iron deficiency anaemia.

Abnormal bleeding and clotting

B. Saxon

Bleeding disorders range from those that are severe and potentially life threatening, through to mild disorders that may be difficult to distinguish from normal. Some characteristics of abnormal bleeding include:
- spontaneous bruising or petechiae
- deep tissue bleeding and haemarthrosis
- prolonged bleeding following trauma, surgery or dental procedures.

Abnormal bleeding is the result of a disorder of one of the following:
- the blood vessel or its supporting tissue
- the platelet
- the coagulation mechanism.

Clinical approach to diagnosis

As a general rule, history taking, physical examination and a small number of relatively simple laboratory tests will find most causes of abnormal bleeding. The history, with particular reference to the past and family history will usually provide the most valuable information.

History

Onset of bleeding

The phase of life during which the onset of bleeding occurs gives important information about the likely cause.

Prenatal and neonatal

- Congenital infection may result in a bleeding disorder.
- Mucosal bleeding occurs with haemorrhagic disease of the newborn (HDN).
- Umbilical stump bleeding is associated with factor XIII deficiency and dysfibrinogenaemias.
- Intracranial haemorrhage may occur with factor deficiencies and with neonatal thrombocytopenia.
- Prolonged bleeding following circumcision is suggestive of haemophilia.

Early childhood

- Often implies a congenital defect.

- Bruising, muscle and joint bleeding is strongly suggestive of haemophilia.
- Petechiae and mucosal bleeding suggests a platelet problem or von Willebrand disorder.

Sudden onset

- Usually an acute problem such as immune thrombocytopenic purpura (ITP).
- Non accidental injury (NAI) may have a haemorrhagic presentation with inadequate explanations for each specific bruise, which may have an unusual distribution (Ch. 12). Skeletal trauma and other stigmata of NAI may be present.

Family history

A proper family tree must be constructed which will aid in determining whether the inherited disorder is X linked (haemophilia A and B (Christmas disease)), recessive (most types of von Willebrand disorder and haemorrhagic hereditary telangiectasia) or dominant (most platelet function disorders). Clinical penetrance in haemophilia carriers and von Willebrand disorder may be variable.

Past history

A past history of easy bruising, bruising at abnormal sites, prolonged bleeding following trivial trauma, or bleeding following surgery and dental extractions are all indications for investigation.

Site of bleeding

Specific bleeding sites have characteristic associations:
- Joint bleeding: haemophilia A and B
- Nasal mucosa: Local irritation; von Willebrand disorder and platelet dysfunction
- Gums, periosteum, skin: Scurvy
- Gastrointestinal: HDN in babies; liver disease in older children
- Retro-orbital: haematological malignancy or disseminated solid tumour
- Shins only: often an integral part of being a preschooler or junior primary child; not pathological on its own.

Associated diseases

In the presence of disorders such as systemic lupus erythematosus, liver disease, extrahepatic portal hypertension, gross splenomegaly, giant haemangiomas, reticuloendothelial malignancies and leukaemia, bleeding is anticipated and is readily explicable. Bleeding is a feature of a number of less common systemic disorders.

Drug ingestion

Drugs may produce abnormal bleeding through:
- depression of clotting factors: anticoagulants, liver toxins
- bone marrow depression: chloramphenicol, cytoxic agents, radiation
- antigen–antibody reactions with platelet membranes: quinine group of drugs
- direct inhibition of enzymes in platelets: aspirin effects on platelet cyclo-oxygenase.

Physical examination

The following should be noted on physical examination.

The type of skin bleeding

Petechiae alone strongly suggest a platelet or vessel problem, while ecchymoses alone suggest a factor deficiency. Combined petechiae and ecchymoses suggest a severe disorder, often of platelet origin.

The site of the bleeding

Confirmation of history, defining the number of all different bleeding sites and assessment of severity of bleed and functional implications are all important aspects for both diagnosis and management.

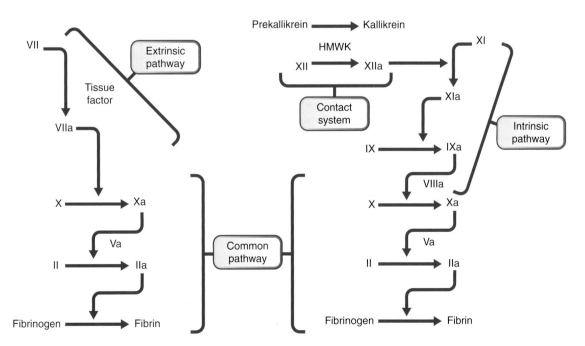

Fig. 54.1 The coagulation system as measured by initial blood tests: prothrombin time (INR; left) and aPTT (right). HMWK, high molecular weight kininogen; 'a' indicates activated factor. This figure does not represent in vivo coagulation, rather the coagulation factors (in test tubes) which influence the prothrombin time and aPTT.

Splenomegaly

Hypersplenism occurs when a large spleen removes platelets from the circulation, which leads to bleeding. The problem is the underlying cause of the splenomegaly. Hepatomegaly, splenomegaly, lymphadenopathy and/or anaemia, in association with bleeding, strongly suggest leukaemia.

Miscellaneous

Bleeding in association with eczema is a feature of Wiskott–Aldrich syndrome; telangiectasia and mucosal bleeding are typical of hereditary haemorrhagic telangiectasia. Hyperelastic skin, hyperextensible joints and bruising are associated with Ehlers–Danlos syndrome.

Investigation of bleeding in childhood

The tests in Table 54.1 are the most important.

Other tests

Measurement of von Willebrand factor level (antigen), activity (ristocetin cofactor) and factor VIII level are required to diagnose von Willebrand disorder. The bleeding time is losing favour because of its scarring potential and newer platelet function analyser testing. The bleeding time is characteristically prolonged in thrombocytopenia (normal 2–7 minutes), von Willebrand disorder and platelet function disorders but will be normal in all other coagulation disorders.

Disorders of bleeding due to vascular defects

The commonest vascular defects seen in childhood are:
- anaphylactoid purpura
- infective states
- nutritional deficiency.

Table 54.1 Interpretation of initial blood tests in children with abnormal bleeding

Test	Result	Common causes	Less common causes
Blood count	Isolated thrombocytopenia	ITP NAIT	Congenital anomaly Early SAA
	Pancytopenia	Leukaemia SAA DIC	Myelodysplasia Osteopetrosis
	High white cell count and thrombocytopenia	Leukaemia Infections	Myeloproliferative disorders
Blood film	Thrombocytopenia and red cell fragmentation	Microangiopathic anaemia, e.g. HUS	
	Small platelets		Wiscott–Aldrich syndrome
	Giant platelets		Bernard–Soulier syndrome
Prothrombin time (PT/INR)	Isolated prolongation	Vitamin K deficiency Warfarin therapy	Congenital FVII deficiency
	Prolonged PT and aPTT	DIC Septicaemia Liver disease	FX, FV, prothrombin or fibrinogen deficiency
aPTT	Isolated prolongation	Unfractionated heparin therapy Haemophilia A or B 'Lupus anticoagulant'	FXI deficiency Contact system deficiency
All tests	Normal	NAI	

aPTT, Activated partial thromboplastin time; Contact system refers to factor XII, prekallikrein and high molecular weight kininogen; DIC, Disseminated intravascular coagulation; HUS, Haemolytic uraemic syndrome; INR, International normalised ratio; ITP, Immune thrombocytopenic purpura; NAI, Non-accidental injury; NAIT, Neonatal alloimmune thrombocytopenia; SAA, Severe aplastic anaemia.

Anaphylactoid purpura (Henoch–Schönlein purpura, HSP)

The aetiology of this disorder is still not clear. It is readily recognised by the characteristic distribution of the rash over the buttocks, legs and backs of the elbows (Fig. 54.2). Frequently it is accompanied by abdominal pain, melaena, joint swellings and occasionally a glomerulonephritis. In anaphylactoid purpura the bleeding time, INR, aPTT and platelet counts are normal; the Hess test is positive in only 25% of cases. Thus, diagnosis must be made on the clinical picture alone. The outlook is excellent except for an occasional child who develops a progressive renal lesion (Ch. 62). No specific therapy exists, although in children with severe abdominal pain corticosteroids may be helpful.

Infective states

The purpura associated with such disorders as meningococcaemia, other septicaemias and dengue haemorrhagic fever are the result of a severe angiitis caused by antigen–antibody complexes. Severe bleeding which may accompany these states is the result of activation of the coagulation mechanism producing disseminated intravascular coagulation. Management involves that of the infection and of the associated vascular collapse.

Nutritional deficiency

Scurvy occurs in the artificially fed infant with inadequate vitamin C supplementation. The child is often pale with skin bruises; immobile in the frog position due to painful subperiosteal haemorrhages; and has gingival bleeding. A wrist X ray will demonstrate the characteristic dense lines in the metaphyses of the radius and ulna and the 'eggshell' like epiphyses. Treatment with vitamin C (100–200 mg/day) reverses the clinical features within a week.

Purpura fulminans

This is a life threatening and rare form of non thrombocytopenic purpura that may follow such infections as scarlet fever, varicella, measles and some other viral infections. Typically there are rapidly spreading skin haemorrhages involving the buttocks and lower extremities. Congenital deficiencies of either protein C or S are the cause of neonatal purpura fulminans.

Miscellaneous

Bleeding from vascular wall defects is a feature of a group of rare disorders. These include hereditary haemorrhagic telangiectasia, polyarteritis nodosa, other vasculitides and uraemia. Anoxia, and thus damage to the capillary wall, may cause purpura in the asphyxiated newborn. The bleeding that accompanies Cushing syndrome, the Ehlers–Danlos syndrome and in cutis laxa is the result of defects in vascular supporting issue.

Bleeding due to platelet disorders

Bleeding disorders due to platelet abnormalities are usually due to thrombocytopenia but may be due to qualitative platelet defects. The various types of inherited and acquired thrombocytopenias are listed in Table 54.2.

Immune thrombocytopenic purpura (ITP)

Immune thrombocytopenic purpura is the most common acquired bleeding disorder in children. It may be acute or chronic (defined as lasting longer than 6 months), episodic or continuous. Common to all clinical variations is the marked reduction in platelet life span due to immune mediated splenic sequestration.

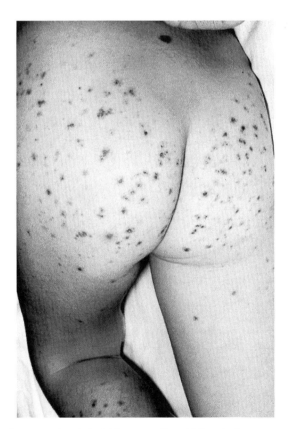

Fig. 54.2 Anaphylactoid purpura. The rash is typically distributed over the buttocks and backs of the legs.

Table 54.2 Inherited and acquired thrombocytopenias

	Disorder	Key information
Inherited		
With platelet dysfunction	Bernard–Soulier syndrome	GpIb-V-IX adhesion receptor defect — inability to bind with vWF
	Wiscott–Aldrich syndrome	Small platelets, eczema, infections, X linked, *WASP* mutations
	X linked thrombocytopenia	Small platelets, X linked, *WASP* mutations
	Grey platelet syndrome	Granule defect, bone marrow fibrosis
Without platelet dysfunction	May–Hegglin anomaly	Large platelets, Dohle bodies in neutrophils
	Alport syndrome	Large platelets, nephritis, deafness, cataracts, several variants
	Thrombocytopenia with absent radii (TAR)	Decreased megakaryocytes, typical bone anomalies
	Mediterranean macrothrombocytopenia	Large platelets, autosomal dominant
	Fanconi anaemia	Thrombocytopenia often precedes other cytopenias
Acquired		
Neonatal	Immune thrombocytopenia	Neonatal alloimmune or maternal autoimmune
	Intrauterine infection	TORCH
	Pre-eclampsia	
	Birth asphyxia	
	Giant haemangioma	'Kasabach–Merritt syndrome' features platelet consumption
Any age	Immune thrombocytopenia	ITP is the most common acquired thrombocytopenia
	Autoimmune disorders	Antiphospholipid antibodies may be present (SLE)
	DIC	Sepsis or other cause evident. Low coagulation factors
	HUS	Microangiopathic haemolysis, usually normal INR and aPTT
	Bone marrow infiltration	Leukaemia, lymphoma, disseminated solid tumours, HLH
	Bone marrow failure	Severe aplastic anaemia
	Drug induced	Cytotoxic therapy, chloramphenicol
	Hypersplenism	Platelets trapped in spleen, as in portal hypertension

DIC, disseminated intravascular coagulation; HUS, haemolytic uraemic syndrome; HLH, Haemophagocytic lymphohistiocytosis; ITP, immune (idiopathic) thrombocytopenic purpura; SLE, systemic lupus erythematosus; TORCH, **T**oxoplasmosis, **O**ther (e.g. HIV and parvovirus B19), **R**ubella, **C**ytomegalovirus, **H**erpes Simplex; vWF, von Willebrand factor.

Features of typical acute ITP

- 80–90% of paediatric ITP cases.
- Preceding viral illness is common.
- Peak age 2–5 years.
- Abrupt onset of bleeding.
- Mucosal and skin bleeding.
- Petechiae common.
- Otherwise normal examination; that is, there is no lymphadenopathy or hepatosplenomegaly.
- Platelet count usually $<20 \times 10^9$/l.
- Normal red cell and white cell parameters.
- No need for other investigations if these 'typical' features are present.
- Differential diagnosis is predominantly that of evolving aplastic anaemia.

Chronic ITP occurs in 10–20% of cases and often has an insidious onset in children aged over 7 years; it affects girls more commonly than boys. *Recurrent ITP* is rare

and is characterised by thrombocytopenia at more than 3 month intervals.

Treatment approaches to ITP are shown in Table 54.3.

Clinical example

Chloe presented at the age of 4 years, 2 weeks after a viral upper respiratory infection, with a 3 day history of a petechial rash on her face and gum bleeding with toothbrushing. Examination revealed several fresh skin bruises along with the petechiae. There was no hepatosplenomegaly and the only palpable lymph nodes were slightly tender 2 cm diameter tonsillar nodes. The only abnormality on full blood examination was a platelet count of 9×10^9/l. She was treated with prednisolone 4 mg/kg daily in three divided doses for 4 days as an outpatient, with daily platelet counts. On the second day of treatment her platelet count was 65×10^9/l and the count became normal within 5 days. She had no further episodes of thrombocytopenia.

Table 54.3   Treatment options for acute ITP with either bleeding problems or if the platelet count is <20 × 10⁹/l

Treatment option	Advantages	Disadvantages	Time course to resolution
First line therapy			
Conservative	No drug side effects	Longest time to platelet >20 × 10⁹/l ~1% risk of ICH while awaiting platelet recovery	75% remission in 4–6 weeks 15% take 4–6 months
Corticosteroids (standard dose)	No blood product exposure	Steroid side effects common	1 week
Corticosteroids (high dose)	No blood product exposure Rapid rise in platelets	Steroid side effects less common	Platelets >20 × 10⁹/l: 2 days Platelets >50 × 10⁹/l: 3–4 days
IVIG	Rapid rise in platelets	Pooled blood product with one or less viral inactivation steps	Platelets >20 × 10⁹/l: 1–2 days Platelets >50 × 10⁹/l: 3 days
Second line therapy			
Anti-Rh(D) antibody		Only useful in Rh positive children Less effective than steroid or IVIG	
Splenectomy	Most useful in children >5 years old with chronic ITP	Immunisations for meningococcus, *Haemophilus influenzae* and pneumococcus are mandatory Lifelong antibiotic prophylaxis	Rapid in the majority

ICH, intracranial haemorrhage.
Standard dose: prednisolone 2 mg/kg body weight daily for 21 days.
High dose: prednisolone 4 mg/kg body weight daily for 4–7 days.
Steroid side effects include gastric irritation, transient diabetes and other metabolic derrangements, immune suppression, cushingoid body fat distribution, growth delay, osteopenia and rarely avascular necrosis of the femoral head.
IVIG: intravenous gammaglobulin 0.8 g/kg body weight, repeat within 1–3 days if platelets <20 × 10⁹/l.
IVIG side effects include flu-like symptoms and rarely transient aseptic meningitis. Blood products theoretically may transmit viral and prion particles.

Bleeding due to qualitative platelet defects

The child with a functional platelet defect will have a normal platelet count but abnormal platelet function tests. These tests analyse aggregation of platelets in response to several stimuli. The more common disorders in this group are the 'aspirin like' syndrome and platelet storage pool disorders. The most severe disorder is Glanzmann disease. Before undertaking platelet function studies one must ensure that there has been no ingestion of aspirin for at least 7 days.

Bleeding due to coagulation disorders

Physiology of coagulation

Following the formation of a platelet plug at the site of vessel injury, fibrin is laid down and is crosslinked to form a protein mesh. This process (coagulation) is usually initiated by factor VIIa binding to exposed tissue factor. This complex activates factors IX and X. Activated factor X recruits a cofactor, factor Va, to activate prothrombin (factor II). This process takes place on a phospholipid surface such as a platelet. Thrombin is a powerful procoagulant, activating factors V, VIII and XI, and cleaving fibrinogen to form fibrin. The activation of 'upstream' coagulation factor causes more thrombin generation (Fig. 54.3). Fortunately, thrombin also activates key inhibitors of coagulation to prevent excessive clot formation. Clearly a defect in any major protein could lead to significant bleeding problems.

Haemophilia

Prevalence

- Haemophilia A (factor VIII deficiency): 5–10 males per 100 000.
- Haemophilia B (Christmas disease, factor IX deficiency): 0.5–1 per 100 000.
- Factor XI deficiency: rare.
- Other factor deficiencies: exceedingly rare.

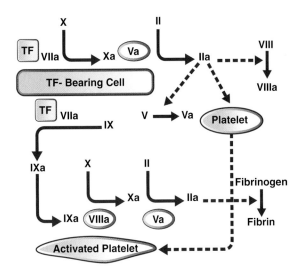

Figure 54.3 Initiation of coagulation and the production of a fibrin clot. TF, tissue factor.

Clinical example

Albert was born at term, received intramuscular vitamin K and developed a large bruise in his thigh. No circumcision was performed. He always seemed to have fingerprint bruises under his arms from being picked up. When he began sitting unaided he developed buttock bruising and when he began walking he presented to the accident and emergency department with a swollen, hot right ankle. The joint had virtually no movement and an ultrasound confirmed a fluid filled joint. The history was highly suggestive of haemophilia. The INR was normal, the aPTT was 90 seconds and the factor VIII level was <1%. Haemophila A was diagnosed and prophylaxis with 30 U/kg recombinant factor VIII three times per week was commenced. At the age of 4 years he fell from a chair onto his occiput after missing a dose of prophylaxis. Within 2 hours he had a falling level of consciousness and respiratory depression. A CT scan diagnosed a subdural haematoma. Treatment with high dose factor VIII and neurosurgical intervention led to an uneventful recovery.

Genetics

Haemophilia A and B are both X linked. Up to one third of all new cases of haemophilia are due to new mutations. Female carriers sometimes have low levels of factor VIII or IX and have a mild bleeding disorder.

Severity

Defined by plasma factor level and correlates with clinical severity:

severe: <2%, frequent spontaneous deep tissue bleeding
moderate: 2–5%, infrequent spontaneous bleeding
mild: 6–30%, bleeding with trauma and surgery, not spontaneously.

Clinical manifestations

Neonatal. A positive family history or known carrier status allows for definitive diagnosis in the newborn period. Cord blood genetics are most reliable. Some laboratories will perform factor VIII or IX assays on cord blood but technical difficulties may arise and results should be interpreted with caution. There is prolonged bleeding following circumcision. Intracranial haemorrhage is suspicious of a bleeding disorder in the term neonate.

Early childhood. Skin and soft tissue bleeds are common in the first year and beyond. Haemarthroses usually only occur once the child is walking. The ankles are common bleeding sites in young children; elbow and knee bleeding (Fig. 54.4) occur more commonly in older children.

Specific bleeds. Bleeding into the forearm may occlude the neurovascular bundle and cause a Volkmann ischaemic contracture. Bleeding into the posterior pharyngeal wall may interfere with respiration and cause dysphagia. Iliopsoas bleeding may be complicated by femoral nerve compression. Intracranial vascular accident is the cause of death in 7% of haemophiliacs. Haematuria is common in adolescents and is seldom serious.

Chronic illness. There is synovial hypertrophy and arthritis. HIV/AIDS occurred in >50% of patients receiving blood products in the years 1980–1985. Hepatitis C

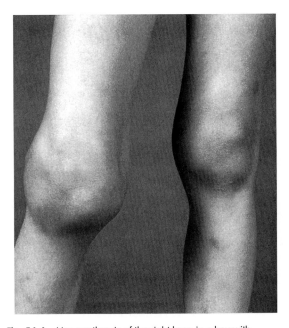

Fig. 54.4 Haemarthrosis of the right knee in a boy with haemophilia.

infection is also common prior to viral identification, screening and viral inactivation of plasma products. Variant Creutzfeld–Jakob disease (vCJD) is a prion disease. It is possibly transmitted in blood products and is not removed by current viral inactivation processes. There are no cases described in children with haemophilia. Psychosocial problems arise due to chronic illness, life style restrictions and the need for injections.

Complications. Inhibitors are anti-FVIII or anti-FIX antibodies which prevent regular doses of factor concentrate from working. Therapeutic options include high dose human factor, porcine factor or recombinant factor VIIa — a factor VIII and IX bypass agent. Central lines may be required to ensure venous access in young children. These may be complicated by infection or large vein thrombosis.

Management

Correct or prevent the bleeding tendency
- Mild and moderate haemophilia A often responds to DDAVP infusions to elevate plasma factor VIII.
- One unit of factor VIII/kg bodyweight given intravenously increases the factor VIII by approximately 2%.
- Life threatening bleeds require plasma factor levels of >80%.
- Most other bleeds require plasma factor levels of 30–60%.
- Prophylactic infusions of 25–40 U/kg three times a week 'converts' severe disease into moderate disease, thereby decreasing the risk of spontaneous bleeding.

Choice of product
- Plasma derived and recombinant factor VIII and XI are available.
- Recombinant factor is usually preferred due to the smaller risk of infectious agent transmission but is costly.
- Plasma derived factor products are screened for HIV and hepatitis B and C and then have viral inactivation step(s) in the processing.

Orthopaedic
- Rest, immobilisation, ice, compression and elevation (RICE) are usually sufficient to control pain.
- Splinting followed by exercises when pain has settled preserves function.

Haemophilia centres
- Focus of education and training for patient and family.
- Multidisciplinary group with expertise in haemophilia management.

Inhibitors
- Occur in up to 20% of patients.
- Low titre inhibitors can be treated by high dose factor VIII

- High titre inhibitors require 'immune tolerance' therapy for eradication of inhibitor, and infusions of the factor VIII and IX bypass agent, recombinant factor VIIa, to treat bleeds.

> ### Clinical example
>
> Vanessa is a 13 year old girl with menorrhagia since menarche. She has always had 'easy bruising' and required a transfusion after tonsillectomy due to excessive bleeding. She often bleeds from her gums after brushing her teeth. Her older sister and her mother both have heavy periods but neither has had severe postsurgical bleeding. Platelet count, INR and aPTT were all normal. von Willebrand antigen was 30%, activity (ristocetin cofactor) 25% and factor VIII 35%. She was diagnosed with mild von Willebrand disorder.

von Willebrand disorder

This disorder has the following features:
- Quantitative (types 1 and 3) or qualitative (type 2) defect in von Willebrand factor (vWF), a molecule which assists platelet adhesion to the subendothelium.
- Common: 125 per million population.
- Type 1 is inherited as autosomal dominant, is mild and is the most common.
- Types 2 and 3 are rare.
- Mucosal bleeding, excessive bruising and postoperative or post-traumatic bleeding.
- Prolonged bleeding time but normal INR and aPTT, unless severe disease is present.
- Abnormal vWF antigen and activity (ristocetin cofactor).
- Treatment for type 1 vWF is DDAVP which releases stored vWF/factor VIII.
- DDAVP may be repeated once stores have reaccumulated, usually after 12–24 hours.
- Plasma derived factor VIII products often contain vWF and may be used in those unresponsive to DDAVP.
- Cryoprecipitate should be avoided due to lack of viral inactivation.

Haemorrhagic disease of the newborn (HDN)

Haemorrhagic disease of the newborn fortunately is now rare, since the introduction of routine vitamin K administration for all babies at the time of delivery. Features of HDN:
- Coagulation factors requiring vitamin K for post-transcriptional modification:
  — factor II (prothrombin)
  — factor VII
  — factor IX
  — factor X
  — protein C and S
- These fall in neonates as a result of nutritional deficiency.

- Bleeding is usually from the gastrointestinal tract.
- Occurs early, often day 2–3.
- Prophylactic vitamin K eliminates this disease.
- Vitamin K 1 mg given by the intramuscular route stops bleeding rapidly.

Clotting due to coagulation disorders

Physiology of anticoagulation

The formation of a fibrin clot is tightly regulated in its local environment by anticoagulants. Local thrombin binds thrombomodulin located on normal endothelium which activates protein C. Activated protein C (APC) with the cofactor, protein S, inhibits factors Va and VIIIa by cleaving the molecules. A mutation of factor V at one cleavage point prevents the APC inhibitory effect and is termed APC resistance. The mutation is called factor V Leiden. The other key coagulation inhibitor is antithrombin, a direct inhibitor of thrombin and also factors Xa, IXa, XIa and XIIa. Heparins potentiate the effect of antithrombin greatly. The largest risk factor for paediatric thrombosis is not a protein deficiency but the presence of a central venous catheter.

Table 54.4 lists the causes and features of thrombosis in childhood.

Table 54.4   Major causes of thrombosis in childhood

Cause	Clinical features	Diagnostic tests	Treatment
Venous access device	Blocked access/emboli, limb swelling	Echocardiography and contrast radiography	Heparin. Removal of device
Phospholipid antibodies	Superficial/deep vein thrombosis	Prolonged INR/aPTT, not corrected by normal plasma	Often no therapy, may require corticosteroids or heparin
Protein C and S homozygous	Purpura fulminans	Very low protein C or S	Protein C replacement + heparin
Protein C and S heterozygous	Superficial/deep vein thrombosis; rare cerebral, mesenteric and renal vein thrombosis	Low protein C or S	Heparin followed by long term warfarin
Factor V mutation, (Arg506 to Gln), 'FV Leiden'	Early onset vascular disease in family	Activated protein C resistance test	Heparin and long term warfarin
Antithrombin deficiency	Venous thrombosis in adolescence	Decreased level of antithrombin	Antithombin replacement, heparin and warfarin
Dysfibrinogenaemia	Rare thrombosis in childhood	Prolonged thrombin time and snake venom times	Replacement therapy
Homocysteinaemia	Arterial and venous thrombosis	Biochemical tests	Diet and short term anticoagulants

Leukaemia and other cancers in childhood

55

K. Waters, P. Smith

Childhood malignancy, with an incidence of 1 in 600 in children aged between 1 and 15 years, has an overall cure rate of 80%, which means by 2010, 1 in 1000 young adults will be survivors of childhood cancers. The incidence is shown in Table 55.1. While uncommon, malignancy must be suspected in any child who presents with a mass and non specific systemic symptoms such as fever, weight loss, malaise, pain and night sweats. Prompt referral by the general practitioner to a tertiary centre for diagnostic workup and multidisciplinary care is essential. Central to the management of malignant disease is the provision of appropriate emotional support to the child and family. Parents must be informed in a manner that they can fully understand of the nature of the disease, its course, treatment and prognosis. The older child and teenager also must be informed honestly about the disease and its treatment, but always in a manner that is optimistic and stresses that long term gains far outweigh any short term side effects.

Aetiology of childhood cancer

Childhood cancer results from abnormal gene function within replicating cells. Commonly, this is the result of mutations involving inactivation of tumour suppressor genes such as RB1, p53 or WT1, or activation of cellular proto-oncogenes such as MYC or ABL. The classical mechanisms of mutational activation or inactivation of

genes include point mutation (for example, RB1 inactivation or RAS activation) and translocation (for example, BCR-ABL translocation in chronic myeloid and Philadelphia positive acute leukaemia). It is clear that an inactivating event occurring at each RB1 allele ('two hits') is sufficient to initiate the oncogenesis of retinoblastoma. For most other tumours a more complex cascade of events is required. Newer information implicates classes of genes that modulate DNA repair, such as the Fanconi anaemia class of genes (FACA, C, D), and the fact that epigenetic phenomena such as inappropriate genomic imprinting may play a role in oncogenesis (for example, loss of imprinting at the IGF2 locus in Wilms tumour). The role of inappropriate telomerase activity in oncogenesis is currently being explored.

Most oncogenic genetic events occur in dividing somatic cells. However, it is clear that, especially when dealing with tumour suppressor genes and less commonly with oncogenes, it is possible to inherit an abnormal allele so that only a single event is required at the other allele to set the scene for initiation of oncogenesis. This explains the tumour associated syndromes such as familial retinoblastoma (RB1) and Li–Fraumeni syndrome (p53), where an inactive tumour suppressor allele is inherited, and multiple endocrine neoplasia type 2 (RET), where an active oncogene is inherited.

There are numerous environmental agents that are associated with childhood malignancy. These include viral infection (Epstein–Barr virus associated with epidemic Burkitt lymphoma), ionising radiation (with leukaemia) and certain chemicals and drugs (benzene, alkylating agents, etoposide with leukaemia).

Table 55.1 Frequency of malignancy in childhood

Malignant disease	Frequency (%)
Leukaemia	35
Primary CNS tumours	20
Lymphoma: non Hodgkin and Hodgkin	10
Wilms tumour	6–8
Neuroblastoma	6–8
Rhabdomyosarcoma, soft tissue sarcoma	5
Sarcoma of bone: Ewing and osteosarcoma	4
Histiocytosis	5
Teratoma	2
Retinoblastoma	1
Hepatic	1
Others	5

Acute leukaemia in childhood

Leukaemia is characterised by abnormal proliferation of lymphoblasts or myeloblasts in the bone marrow, secondarily involving the blood, reticuloendothelial system leading to lymphadenopathy and hepatosplenomegaly, bones, joints and rarely CNS, testes and skin.

In children, 80% is acute lymphoblastic (ALL), 20% acute myeloid (AML) and 1% chronic myeloid (CML), being more common in males and in the 2–5 year age group.

531

Aetiology

While irradiation, chemical carcinogens (benzene, chlorambucil, epipodophyllotoxins) and oncogenic viruses induce leukaemia in animal models, the cause in children is unknown but is probably multifactorial. There is an increased incidence in Down syndrome, and in certain rare genetic diseases such as ataxia telangiectasia, Wiskott–Aldrich syndrome and Fanconi anaemia.

Clinical example

Sally is a 3 year old girl who has had intermittent fever for 3 weeks, followed by pallor and lethargy and recent easy bruising. Reluctance to walk and irritability have been present for 4 weeks. Examination reveals a pale child with truncal petechiae, limb bruising, mild cervical adenopathy and 3–4 cm of splenomegaly. What is the differential diagnosis?

The presence of fever suggests infection, pallor suggests anaemia and petaechiae and bruising, thrombocytopenia. A full blood count would confirm this. Adenopathy and splenomegaly suggest reticuloendothelial involvement or infection. Again, blood count and film examination are warranted. Bone marrow aspirate is then required for diagnosis of ALL, even if the white cell count is elevated and blast cells are present on the peripheral film.

Clinical and laboratory manifestations

- Pallor, lethargy, decreased exercise tolerance in 60% due to anaemia with red cell morphology being normal.
- Easy bruising and petaechiae, usually of brief onset over some days due to thrombocytopenia in 50%.
- Low grade fever, mouth ulcers or infection due to neutropenia in 50%.

- Total white cell count $<10 \times 10^9/l$ in 25%, $10–50 \times 10^9/l$ in 50% and $>50 \times 10^9/l$ in 25% with blast cells usually present.
- Vague skeletal symptoms of bone and joint pain, sore legs, poor sleeping, decreased play and activities in 25% for days to weeks.
- Lymphadenopathy, hepatosplenomegaly in 60–70%.
- Marrow examination showing 70–100% leukaemic blast cells with cytochemistry; immunophenotype; cytogenetics and molecular genetic analyses confirming subtype of ALL. AML is also subtyped by these tests. Precursor B cell ALL accounts for 80%, T cell ALL for 20%, mature B cell for 1% of ALL.

Table 55.2 illustrates current prognostic features with traditional clinical prognostic features of ALL (age <2 or >10 years and white cell count $>50 \times 10^9/l$) becoming less significant with improved treatment and molecular/genetic features more important. With current therapy, 75–80% of children with ALL and 60–70% with AML can be expected to be cured if managed at a tertiary centre.

Features predicting a poor prognosis in ALL include slow clearing of blasts with induction therapy; hypodiploidy or DNA index <1.00; t(9;22), t(4;11), 11q23 abnormalities and t(1;19). Hyperdiploidy (>55 chromosomes) and t(12;21) predict for a good prognosis.

Treatment of acute lymphoblastic leukaemia

- Induction therapy with vincristine, daunorubicin, asparaginase, prednisolone, intrathecal methotrexate has a 98% remission induction rate.
- Presymptomatic CNS therapy with intrathecal methotrexate and later intensification therapy with high dose intravenous methotrexate reduces the CNS

Table 55.2 Risk group classification for acute lymphoblastic leukaemia

Risk group	Clinical features	Molecular/genetic features

Low risk	1. Age 2–10 years
	   WCC $< 50 \times 10^9/l$
	2. Not T cell phenotype
	3. No CNS or testicular disease
	4. Rapid response to induction therapy
		1. DNA index > 1.16
		2. Absence of: t(9;22) BCR?ABL
		   t(4;11) MLL/AF$_4$
		   t(1;19)
		   MLL rearrangement
		3. t(12;21) TEL/AML1
		4. t(8;14) t(2;8) or t(8;22) (with short-term intensive therapy)

High risk	Those not in low or very high risk groups	
Very high risk	1. Induction failure 2. Age <12 months	1. t(9;22), t(4;11) 2. MLL rearrangements

relapse rate to less than 2–3%. Cranial irradiation is avoided because of its deleterious effects on cognitive function.

- Consolidation chemotherapy with cyclophosphamide, Ara-C and 6-thioguanine and Ara-C/VP-16 in high risk patients.
- Reinduction and reconsolidation therapy.
- Continuation therapy with monthly vincristine and 5 day steroid pulses together with oral 6-mercaptopurine and methotrexate to complete 2 years of therapy in total.
- Use of sulphamethoxazole/trimethoprim prophylaxis to prevent *Pneumocystis carinii* infection throughout treatment.

During remission, the child is well and should be encouraged to lead normal activities for age, even during expected periods of myelosuppression. Adequate and prompt antibiotic treatment of febrile neutropenia is essential.

Relapse

- Usually detected on routine full blood count or occasionally recurrence of initial symptoms.
- 80–90% second remission induction rate.
- Poor results with further chemotherapy: <20% able to cease therapy.
- Stem cell transplantation from an HLA compatible sibling or volunteer unrelated marrow or umbilical cord donor leads to cure in 50–60% but graft versus host disease, opportunistic infection and leukaemic relapse remain major obstacles to cure.
- 20–25% of patients with ALL will still fail treatment and die with infections, bleeding and bone pain being common terminal manifestations. Disabling infection must be adequately treated together with judicious use of blood and platelet transfusions. Pain relief is paramount, with morphine mixture or slow release morphine preparations usually effective. Most families prefer terminal care in their home with the support of palliative care and district nursing services and their family practitioner.

Acute myeloid leukaemia

- Remission achieved in 85–90% of cases but only with intensive chemotherapy, which produces severe marrow hypoplasia.
- Intensive supportive care with nutrition, antibiotics, blood and platelet transfusions during hypoplastic phase is required.
- Stem cell transplantation depending upon prognostic factors — morphological subtype, cytogenetics, rate of remission.
- Expected cure rate of 60–70%.

Lymphoma

Non Hodgkin and Hodgkin lymphoma (disease) manifest different clinical patterns of behaviour in children compared with adults.

Non-Hodgkin lymphoma (NHL)

- More common in boys than girls, with a high frequency of marrow and/or central nervous system involvement.
- A classification suitable for paediatric use is:
  — poorly differentiated diffuse lymphoblastic — T cell
  — small non cleaved undifferentiated non Burkitt or Burkitt — B-cell
  — large cell lymphoma — rare in children.
- Presents with painless enlargement of lymph nodes, either local or generalised.
- Clinical staging is followed by pathological staging with organ imaging, bone marrow and CSF examination.

Clinical example

William is a 10 year old boy with a 2–3 week history of cough, difficulty in sleeping flat, some wheeze and sudden onset of faint stridor. Examination reveals supraclavicular adenopathy, a mass palpable in the suprasternal notch, decreased air entry and percussion note at the right base. His face is suffused with venous distension.

Symptoms and signs suggest superior vena caval syndrome with airway obstruction. Chest X ray confirms large mediastinal mass and a right pleural effusion. CT chest to assess airway. Urgent diagnosis and therapy is required to prevent complete airway obstruction. Most likely diagnosis is T cell non Hodgkin lymphoma. Precautionary admission to ICU is recommended.

Mediastinal primary of T cell immunophenotype accounts for 25% of non Hodgkin lymphoma and often presents with acute superior vena caval and/or airway obstruction (a medical emergency) producing stridor and cough, usually with an associated pleural effusion and characteristically occurring in preteen or early teenage males. Diagnosis, immunophenotyping and cytogenetics may be made on pleural aspirate, suprasternal or supraclavicular node biopsy or rarely direct biopsy of mediastinal mass.

Abdominal lymphoma accounts for 35–40% and is of B cell immunophenotype and characteristically presents as either local tumour causing intussusception and readily removable or with massive diffuse abdominal disease, often with ascites.

A t(8;14) translocation is characteristic of Burkitt lymphoma.

Following pathological diagnosis and staging, multiagent chemotherapy is started, the intensity and duration depending upon stage and immunophenotype. Irradiation therapy has no role. Stages I and II have a >90%, and stages III and IV a 70–80%, cure rate.

Hodgkin disease

- Uncommon in children, boys affected more frequently than girls.
- Painless lymph node enlargement, most commonly cervical and often of many months duration, is the common presentation.
- Open biopsy confirms the diagnosis and pathological staging with chest X ray, CT of lung and abdomen, gallium scan and marrow aspirate and/or trephine completes workup.
- Chemotherapy is the mainstay of treatment, with irradiation therapy having no role or a supplemental role only in patients with massive mediastinal involvement.
- MOPP (nitrogen mustard, vincristine, prednisolone, procarbazine) is a potent cause of infertility in both boys and girls and is myelosuppressive and immunosuppressive. Less toxic regimens are being investigated.
- Cure rate is excellent: 90–95% irrespective of stage.

Langherhans cell histiocytosis

- Previously called histiocytosis X and divided into eosinophilic granuloma (bony disease only); Hand–Schüller–Christian disease (bone involvement with exophthalmus and diabetes insipidus); Letterer–Siwe disease (skin, liver, spleen, marrow involvement).
- Not a true neoplasm but a disorder of immune regulation or cytokine production.
- Bone involvement, particularly skull, with associated soft tissue swelling and radiologically discrete punched out lesions.
- Skin involvement with refractory seborrhoea or nappy rash.
- Chronic otitis media.
- Premature eruption of teeth or four quadrant mouth ulcers.
- Diabetes insipidus secondary to posterior pituitary involvement.
- Rarely chronic diarrhoea.
- Diffuse disease with fever, hepatosplenomegaly, rash, diarrhoea, weight loss, lung involvement in children younger than 5 years.

Treatment varies according to the extent of the disease. Single bone lesions are treated with curettage only;

multiple bony lesions with prednisolone, methotrexate or vinblastine. Bony recurrence is not uncommon and retreatment may be necessary on more than one occasion. DDAVP is required if diabetes insipidus is present, when it is usually lifelong. Diffuse disease is treated with combinations of vinblastine, prednisolone, methotrexate or etoposide, with excellent results.

Other histiocytic disorders in childhood, such as familial haemophagocytic reticulosis and true malignant histiocytosis, are very rare.

Solid tumours in childhood

While rare, malignancy must be considered in any child who presents with a lump or non specific systemic symptoms such as weight loss, fever, pain, night sweats — the so called malignant malaise. A multidisciplinary approach to diagnosis and treatment is mandatory and is responsible for the high cure rate now attainable. While cure is the first priority, cure without cost — be that physical, emotional, scholastic, financial — is now of prime importance. Accurate diagnosis is the first step, either by needle biopsy, incisional or excisional biopsy or complete removal of the affected organ. In many instances, definitive surgery will be delayed until primary chemotherapy has caused tumour shrinkage, making the tumour more readily resectable.

Staging appropriate to tumour type follows and determines the treatment required. Chemotherapy is the mainstay of treatment, with irradiation therapy having a supplemental or no role due to its effects on growth and development. For most tumours:
- Stage I refers to tumour confined to the organ of origin and totally resectable.
- Stage II to extension beyond the organ of origin but totally resectable.
- Stage III to surgically irremovable tumour or residual local tumour after resection.
- Stage IV to metastatic disease.

At presentation, treatment should begin with curative intent, even for those with widely disseminated disease.

Wilms tumour (nephroblastoma)

- Most common before 5 years of age.
- Association with the Wilms aniridia, genitourinary abnormalities, mental retardation syndrome (WAGR); Denys–Drash and Beckwith–Wiedemann syndromes.
- Presentation is with abdominal mass, occasionally associated with pain. Haematuria is uncommon. Hypertension may be present.
- Differential diagnosis includes polycystic kidney, hydronephrosis, neuroblastoma, hepatoblastoma and rarely splenomegaly.

- Diagnosis is established by abdominal ultrasound or CT, with biopsy if very large and difficult to resect.
- Surgical removal of involved kidney, biopsy of regional nodes and inspection of other kidney and liver are performed.
- Chest X ray and CT of lung complete staging.
- Frequency and intensity of chemotherapy depend upon stage and histological subtype (anaplastic, clear cell sarcoma and rhabdoid are rare variants) with vincristine, actinomycin, doxorubicin, cyclophosphamide, etoposide being used.
- Irradiation therapy for certain stage III and IV patients.
- Cure rate for stage I is 95–100%, stage II> 95%, stage III 80–90% and stage IV 80%.

Neuroblastoma

A tumour of the sympathetic nervous system or adrenal medulla, most common in children under 5 years; 50% are adrenal and 30% abdominal. Thoracic primaries may be discovered on an incidental chest X ray or may be massive before producing symptoms.

Presentation is with abdominal mass, usually with pain, weight loss, pallor. Paraplegia due to dumb-bell intervertebral extension as the only sympton often occurs and retention of urine with pelvic primaries is common. In 70–75% initial symptoms are due to metastases: bone pain, limp, reluctance to walk, proptosis, bruising around the eyelids. Opsomyoclonus and ataxia are rare paraneoplastic symptoms.

Histologically, neuroblastoma is a small blue round cell tumour which may contain rosettes and neurofibrils and stain positively with neurone specific enolase. Elevated urinary catecholamines are usually present. Marrow infiltration is frequent and may resemble ALL. Biopsy is required for histological diagnosis and molecular studies to confirm prognosis. *MYCN* amplification and allelic loss from chromosome 1p predict for a poor prognosis (as do bony metastases). Isotope bone scan and MIBG scan complete staging.

Age and stage are closely related, with stage I and II tumours tending to occur in children under 1 year old. Treatment is with surgical resection alone, with a >90% cure rate. Chemotherapy with vincristine, doxorubicin, cisplatinum, cyclophosphamide and etoposide is used in stage III and IV disease and then surgery if possible, with irradiation to the primary site if residual tumour is present or irresectable. Very high dose chemotherapy with stem cell rescue is increasingly used for poor prognosis patients (*MYCN* amplified). Cure rates for stage III and IV disease are only 20–30%.

Stage IV represents patients under 12 months of age with a small primary (inferring resectability) and a specific pattern of metastases to the skin (the 'blueberry muffin' baby) and/or liver and/or bone marrow but not bone, where spontaneous regression may occur in up to

60%. Local irradiation to the liver may be required. Mass screening of infants has not lived up to its promise.

Soft tissue sarcoma

Most are rhabdomyosarcoma, with orbital and head and neck primaries accounting for 30%, extremities 25%, genitourinary 20% and trunk 10%. Presenting signs and symptoms (e.g. proptosis or urinary retention) vary according to site of origin. Tissue diagnosis and staging determine therapy, which is primarily chemotherapy. Surgery should be non mutilating, with irradiation therapy often necessary. Survival rates are 80–90% in stages I and II, 30–50% in stage III and 10–20% in stage IV.

Bone sarcoma

Clinical example

Mark, aged 14, has a 6–9 month history of a dull ache in his right lower thigh becoming more severe and constant over the past 2–3 weeks. Vague history of injury at onset of symptoms. Now swelling of lateral aspect of thigh above knee. Clinically diffuse, firm non tender mass present.

The most likely diagnosis is a bone or soft tissue sarcoma. Plain X ray of femur confirms a soft tissue mass overlying a lytic area in the lower femur, with periosteal elevation. CT and MRI scan required to delineate anatomy, followed by biopsy which revealed Ewing sarcoma. Staging with CT lung, bone scan and marrow aspirate to determine extent of disease and thus prognosis and therapy required.

Ache subsequently leading to pain over weeks to months, with ultimately appearance of a mass, is the usual presentation. CT and MRI scan of the involved area followed by biopsy confirm the diagnosis. Chest X ray, CT lung and bone scan and marrow aspirate complete staging. Over 50% of osteosarcomas occur around the knee. Ewing sarcoma of the pelvis is usually very large at diagnosis.

Initial intensive chemotherapy to shrink the primary and control micrometastases is followed by limb preserving surgery or excision of the affected bone. Resection of pulmonary metastases in osteosarcoma may lead to cure. Irradiation is avoided wherever possible. Cure is expected in 60–70%.

Hepatoblastoma

Usually presents as a painless large right upper quadrant mass with an elevated serum alpha fetoprotein level. Needle biopsy confirms diagnosis. Intensive chemotherapy to control the primary makes definitive surgery easier. Cure rate of 70–80% even with metastatic disease.

Teratoma

Most commonly arise in the sacrococcygeal area but also in ovary, testis, mediastinum and CNS. Most are benign and cured with surgery. Usually have an elevated alpha-fetoprotein. Malignant teratomas (yolk sac carcinoma) have a high cure rate with cisplatinum and etoposide pre- or post- surgical excision.

Central nervous system tumours

Second in frequency after leukaemia. Clinical presentation depends upon site. Meningiomas and metastatic cerebral tumours are rare. Table 55.3 shows a working classification of CNS tumours.

Presentation

Early symptoms and signs of CNS tumours may be few and difficult to elicit. Evidence of raised intracranial pressure is the most common because posterior fossa and deep midline tumours usually obstruct CSF pathways.

Signs and symptoms of raised intracranial pressure

- Headache, usually early morning, gradually increasing in frequency and severity
- Vomiting which often relieves headache
- Drowsiness, bradycardia and hypertension (late signs)
- Tense fontanelle and 'cracked pot' percussion note indicating hydrocephalus
- Papilloedema.

Table 55.3   CNS tumours

1. Supratentorial
   a. Hemisphere: astrocytoma; glioblastoma; primitive neuroectodermal tumour
   b. Midline: craniopharyngioma; optic nerve glioma; pineal

2. Infratentorial
   a. Cerebellar and fourth ventricle: astrocytoma; medulloblastoma; ependymoma
   b. Brainstem: brainstem glioma

3. Spinal cord
   Astrocytoma; ependymoma

Signs and symptoms of involvement of the posterior fossa:

- Truncal ataxia due to central cerebellar tumours
- Incoordination and tremor due to lateral lesions
- Cranial nerve palsies, suggest a brainstem lesion
- Defective upward gaze with tumours of the pineal region.

Signs and symptoms of deep midline tumours around the third ventricle:

- Impaired visual acuity and visual field defects due to craniopharyngioma or optic nerve glioma
- Diabetes insipidus and growth failure
- Severe wasting and anorexia due to the 'diencephalic syndrome' of a hypothalamic tumour.

Epilepsy

- Uncommon presentation as a sole symptom.
- Consider tumour with focal epilepsy or progressively more difficult to control epilepsy.
- Investigations should include CT and MRI scan of brain and spinal cord.

Treatment

- Low grade astrocytoma: surgery alone, occasionally chemotherapy (carboplatin)
- High grade astrocytoma: surgery and chemotherapy
- Brain stem glioma: irradiation therapy
- Medulloblastoma: surgery and chemotherapy if less than 4 years; irradiation added if older than 4 years
- High grade tumours: surgery, chemotherapy and irradiation therapy.

Late effects

- Learning disorders due to effect of irradiation on cognitive functions in children younger than 4 years
- Growth failure due to growth hormone deficiency and/or spinal irradiation.

Retinoblastoma

- Leukocoria (cat's eye reflex) and/or squint.
- Exophthalmus and/or metastases rare in developed countries.
- Regular EUA or genetic screening in those with positive family history.
- Enucleation of affected eye (unilateral cases) and more affected eye in bilateral cases.

- Cryotherapy, laser coagulation, thermochemotherapy in an attempt to avoid enucleation.
- Irradiation therapy.
- Patients with germline RB1 mutation have increased risk of osteosarcoma (spontaneous or irradiation induced) in later life.

Late effects

Recognition of the late effects of treatment, be it surgery, irradiation or chemotherapy, is increasingly important. Our aim is for cured children to have a normal quality of life, educational and employment prospects, normal marriage prospects and normal offspring.

Terminal phase

When death from progressive disease is inevitable, full support must be provided to the child and family. Emotional and physical loneliness must be avoided. Most children will be aware they are dying but may continue to 'deny' this to the last moment. Honesty is particularly important with adolescents. Most families prefer their child to die in the familiar surroundings of their own home. The help of a supportive family physician and palliative care service is essential. Bereavement support should be available after death. Similar help must be available to all staff involved in the child's care.

PART 16   SELF-ASSESSMENT

Questions

1. Nicholas is a 12 year old boy with sickle thalassaemia. He presents with a 24 hour history of pain in his right leg below the knee and is having difficulty walking. He is slightly jaundiced, and his spleen is palpable 3 cm below the left costal margin. His temperature is 38°C. Which of the following statements are correct?
   - (A) He should be admitted to hospital
   - (B) Analgesia should be delayed until the haemoglobin is known
   - (C) Immediate radiological examination of the leg bones will diagnose bone infarction
   - (D) Blood cultures should be taken

2. Effie, a 13 month old girl, presents with a 2 day history of increasing pallor, lethargy and irritability. She has been febrile and jaundiced for 24 hours and her urine is noted to be very dark. She had neonatal jaundice for which no treatment was required. She has a temperature of 38.5°C and the spleen is palpable 2 cm below the lower costal margin. The Hb is 60 g/l with 20% reticulocytes and the white cell count is 14.0×10^9/l with 10% neutrophils and bands. Which of the following statements are correct?
   - (A) The fact that she is jaundiced with dark urine indicates biliary obstruction
   - (B) A blood culture should be performed
   - (C) There may be difficulty in crossmatching blood for transfusion
   - (D) The G6PD screen is likely to be positive

3. Paul, an 11 month old boy who was born at 35 weeks gestation, presents with poor weight gain over the preceding 3–4 months, pallor, irritability and intermittent diarrhoea. He is breast fed but cereal, fruit and vegetables were introduced from 6 months of age. He is on the 10th centile for weight and 50th centile for length. There are no specific findings other than pallor. Blood count shows an Hb of 70 g/l with an MCV of 102 fl, and oval macrocytes. The platelet count is 95×10^9/l and neutrophils show hypersegmentation. Which of the following statements is true?
   - (A) A bone marrow aspirate (BMA) should be performed
   - (B) The most likely diagnosis is dietary folate deficiency
   - (C) His mother should have a blood test performed
   - (D) Treatment should not be instituted until results of serum vitamin B_{12} and serum and RBC folate are available

4. Iron deficiency is very common. It is most reliably detected by:
   - (A) Taking a good social history
   - (B) Physical examination
   - (C) Looking for signs of blood loss
   - (D) Having a blood count and film examination performed
   - (E) Performing a bone marrow aspiration and staining for iron stores

5. The following are risk factors for iron deficiency anaemia in a 12 month old infant:
   - (A) Prematurity
   - (B) Being small for gestational age (SGA) at birth
   - (C) Maternal anaemia during pregnancy
   - (D) Multiple pregnancy
   - (E) Exchange transfusion requirements in the neonatal period

6. **A moderately severe iron deficiency in a child requiring surgery within 1 week is best treated by:**
   (A) Oral iron
   (B) Intramuscular iron
   (C) Transfusion
   (D) Exchange transfusion

7. **Rachel is a 5 year old girl with severe recurrent tonsillitis, and tonsillectomy is planned. She has multiple bruises of variable ages on her shins and several bruises over bony prominences. She experiences epistaxes almost monthly; sometimes these last over 20 minutes. Is her surgical risk increased?**
   (A) No, bleeding history is not abnormal
   (B) No, platelet count, INR and APTT are normal
   (C) Yes, history suspicious of a bleeding disorder
   (D) Unable to determine

8. **Regarding thrombosis in children, which of the following are true?**
   (A) Presence of a central venous line is the greatest risk factor
   (B) 'Lupus anticoagulants' commonly cause thrombosis
   (C) Thromboses are usually venous and involve the superior vena cava drainage system
   (D) Should be treated with heparin, then warfarin

9. **Typical features of acute immune thrombocytopenic purpura (ITP) are:**
   (A) Age of onset is usually greater than 12 years
   (B) Lymphadenopathy
   (C) Isolated thrombocytopenia on blood count
   (D) Rapid response to steroid therapy
   (E) Splenomegaly

10. **Nancy, a 2 year old girl, has refractory seborrhoea and nappy rash. She is also irritable, feeding poorly and is noted to have gum ulceration in the molar area. Examination confirms these findings and shows a petechial-like rash behind both ears and on her trunk. To diagnose, should you:**
    (A) Do platelet function studies
    (B) Biopsy the seborrhoeic lesions
    (C) Stage extent of disease with skeletal survey, LFTs, chest X ray, marrow aspirate
    (D) Treat with intensive multidrug chemotherapy

11. **Vince, a 3 year old boy, has developed an area of faint bruising around his upper eyelid. He has been irritable and reluctant to walk and has had a poor appetite and weight loss. Physical examination confirms very firm right sided cervical adenopathy and a distended abdomen. Would you?**
    (A) X ray the orbits
    (B) Perform a bone marrow aspirate

(C) Biopsy the cervical glands
(D) Collect urine for catecholamine and metabolite levels

12. **In the presence of Wilms tumour:**
    (A) Most children present with abdominal distension due to an abdominal mass
    (B) Haematuria is a common presentation
    (C) There is a higher incidence of Wilms tumour in some syndromes such as the Beckwith–Wiedmann syndrome and the Denny–Drash syndrome
    (D) Dissemination of Wilms tumour usually is to the lungs
    (E) The cure rate for Wilms tumour with a coordinated treatment programme is approximately 30%

Answers and explanations

1. The correct answers are **(A)** and **(D)**. (A) He should be admitted to hospital as he probably has an infarctive crisis involving either soft tissue or bone and will need to be adequately hydrated. (D) If the bone is involved this time, bone infarction can be complicated by osteomyelitis so blood culture is indicated. (B) Analgesia should be given immediately, but not using opiates which may depress respiration and cause further hypoxia if the haemoglobin is low. The jaundice and splenomegaly are features of chronic haemolysis but may be aggravated by the infarctive crisis. (C) X ray in the acute stage is unlikely to demonstrate bone infarction.

2. The correct answers are **(B)** and **(C)**. The story of increased pallor associated with jaundice and dark urine suggests acute haemolysis with haemoglobinuria. (A) Acute obstructive jaundice would be uncommon at this age and not associated with gross anaemia. (B) The fever and high white cell count may reflect infection, which could be a precipitating cause of haemolysis. Fever may, however, be secondary to intravascular haemolysis and the elevated white count reflect increased marrow activity in response to haemolysis. (C) The Coombs test is likely to be positive, in which case the antibody is likely to crossreact and make a 'compatible' crossmatch unlikely. (D) G6PD deficiency is X linked and a girl is unlikely to present with acute haemolysis.

3. The correct answers are **(A)** and **(C)**. (A) This infant has a macrocytic anaemia which may be due to vitamin B_{12} or folate deficiency, or a congenital dyserythropoietic anaemia. The latter is rare but will be diagnosed on the BMA performed to confirm megaloblastosis. (B) Folate deficiency would be unlikely in a breast fed baby eating vegetables,

although his requirements will have been increased because of his prematurity. The failure to thrive and diarrhoea could be secondary to malabsorption from coeliac disease, in which case folate deficiency is possible. At this age a megaloblastic anaemia due to vitamin B_{12} deficiency would reflect either malabsorption from congenital pernicious anaemia or low stores at birth with (C) subsequent inadequate intake in breast milk and diet because of maternal deficiency. (D) As soon as the diagnosis of megaloblastosis has been confirmed by BMA, treatment with both vitamin B_{12} and folate should be commenced. Delaying may result in neurological damage if the deficiency is vitamin B_{12}.

4. The correct answer is **(D)**. The most reliable method is demonstration of a low Hb, MCV and MCH, associated with a microcytic hypochromic blood film. (A) A history is important but not totally reliable. (B) Physical examination may miss anaemia unless care is taken to look for pallor in the obvious sites (palmar creases, nail beds, conjunctiva, and so on), and is not reliably detected unless the Hb is less than 70 g/l. (C) Evidence of blood loss often is difficult to detect. (E) Bone marrow aspiration is not warranted for iron deficiency, even to differentiate it from thalassaemia — the rare case of sideroblastic anemia in childhood is an exception.

5. The correct answers are **(A)**, **(B)**, **(D)** and **(E)**. The fetus absorbs iron across the placenta, particularly in the last 3 months of pregnancy. If premature delivery occurs, this process is interrupted and premature infants usually require supplemental iron to replenish their iron stores (A). Infants who are SGA at birth often have a period of rapid catchup growth, and also may need supplemental iron to meet their growth needs (B). Iron transport across the placenta is an active process and the fetal needs are met in preference to those of the mother (C). Most multiple pregnancies do not go to term, so that the babies are preterm and are at risk of later iron deficiency (D). Although haemolytic anaemias, which are the usual reason for exchange transfusions in the neonatal period, do not result in a net loss of iron to the body, the blood used for the exchange transfusion is from adult donors, and has a lower haemoglobin content (typically 120–140 g/l) than the blood of the newborn (140–180 g/l), resulting in loss of available iron (E).

6. Much will depend on the age of the child, the degree of anaemia, which operation is to be performed, and the degree of decompensation present. The correct answer in this situation would be **(C)**. Iron deficiency is invariably slow to develop, so that many children are able to compensate over a period. Decompensation may occur with severe anaemia if a further blood loss occurs in a short time. Treatment with oral iron avoids the risks inherent with all blood transfusions, but return to a safe level of Hb would be too slow in this instance (A). This also applies to intramuscular iron (B), which is also very painful to administer. (C) Careful transfusion several days before operation would be the treatment choice in this instance, with the possibility of a directed donation in some circumstances. There are no indications for exchange transfusion in this situation (D).

7. The correct answer is **(C)**. Bruising on shins only is very common in young children but generalised bruising or petechiae are suggestive of a bleeding disorder, most commonly von Willebrand disorder. (A) is an unsafe assumption, particularly when an operation with relatively high bleeding risk is being contemplated. Answer (B) indicates that initial tests have been performed and are normal. While thrombocytopenia and significant coagulation factor deficiencies have been assessed, neither von Willebrand disorder nor congenital platelet dysfunctions have been excluded. Finally, (D) is incorrect as history alone is a strong indicator of bleeding risk even without a diagnosis.

8. The true answers are **(A)**, **(C)** and **(D)**. Deep vein thrombosis in the absence of a central venous line is rare in children (A). Most central lines are placed in the large veins at the base of the neck and clots in the upper venous system are much more common than lower limb and inferior vena cava clots (C). Heparin, either unfractionated or low molecular weight, is the current standard therapy for clots, followed by maintenance warfarin (D). Direct thrombin inhibitors are becoming more available but their role is yet to be defined in paediatrics. Lupus anticoagulants (B) are antibodies which interfere with the APTT and sometimes the INR. These are usually benign and transient in children.

9. The correct answers are **(C)** and **(D)**. ITP occurs at any age: ITP in older children (A) has an increased risk of being a chronic form. Neither lymphadenopathy (B) nor splenomegaly (E) occur in typical ITP and if these are present they may be associated with leukaemia, infections and other causes of thrombocytopenia. Typical ITP must have isolated thrombocytopenia on the blood film (C): the presence of other anomalies is an indication for bone marrow examination. Acute ITP responds well to steroids (D) or immunoglobulin infusions.

10. The correct answers are **(B)** and **(C)**. The diagnosis of Langerhans cell histiocytosis is usually confirmed by biopsy of the skin or bony lesions. (A) Platelet function studies are not appropriate in view of the other

features. (D) Treatment with multidrug chemotherapy has greatly improved the prognosis but is inappropriate before the diagnosis has been confirmed and (C) staging of the disease performed.

11. The correct answers are **(B)** and **(D)**. The clinical diagnosis is stage IV neuroblastoma. (B) Diagnosis could be made on marrow aspirate and (D) positive urine results, obviating the need for node biopsy (C). Further staging would be with an abdominal ultrasound and isotope bone scan, which would detect orbital involvement (A). Rarely, acute myeloid leukaemia may present with orbital involvement.

12. The correct answers are **(A)**, **(C)** and **(D)**. Most children with Wilms tumour are noted to have an asymptomatic abdominal mass as the presenting problem (A). Haematuria is a relatively uncommon presentation, being seen in 10–20% (B). The tumour has a higher frequency of occurrence in these two syndromes, and is seen with a high frequency in children with aniridia and in children with the aniridia, genitourinary abnormality, mental retardation abnormality (W(ilms)AGR) (C). Dissemination will occur mainly to the lungs if relapse occurs (D). Treatment of Wilms tumour has a high success rate, with a cure rate of over 80%.

PART 16   FURTHER READING

Abshire T C 1996 The anemia of inflammation: a common cause of childhood anemia. Pediatric Clinics of North America, 43: 623–637

Ashley-Koch A, Yang Q, Olney R S 2000 Sickle hemoglobin (HbS) allele and sickle cell disease: a HuGE review. American Journal of Epidemiology 151: 839–845

Fiorillo A, Farina V, D'Amore R, Scippa L, Cortese P, DeChiara C 2000 Longitudinal assessment of cardiac status by echocardiographic evaluation of left ventricular diastolic function in thalassaemic children. Acta Paediatrica 89: 436–441

Fosburg M T, Nathan D G 1990 Treatment of Cooley's anemia. Blood 76: 435–444

Gallagher P G, Ehrenkranz R A 1995 Nutritional anemias in infancy. Clinics in Perinatology 22: 671–692

Gaynon P S, Trigg M E, Heerma N A et al 2000 Children's Cancer Group Trials in childhood acute lymphoblastic leukaemia:1983–1995. Leukaemia 14: 2223–2233

George J N, Woolf S H, Raskob G E et al 1996 Idiopathic thrombocytopenic purpura: a practice guideline developed by explicit methods for the American Society of Hematology. Blood 83: 3–40

Hedner U 2000 Recombinant coagulation factor VIIa: from the concept to clinical application in hemophilia treatment in 2000. Seminars in Thrombosis and Hemostasis 26: 363–366

Hilden J M, Emmanuel E J, Fairclough D L et al 2001 Attitudes and practices among paediatric oncologists regarding end-of-life care: results of the 1998 American Society of Clinical Oncology Survey. Journal of Clinical Oncology 19: 205–212

Kulkarni R, Lusher J 2001 Perinatal management of newborns with hemophilia. British Journal of Haematology 112: 264–274

Lillyman J, Hann, I, Blanchette V 1999 Pediatric hematology, 2nd edn. Churchill Livingstone, London

Mannucci P M 2001 How I treat patients with von Willebrand disease. Blood 97: 1915–1919

Matsunaga A T, Lubin B H 1995 Hemolytic anemia in newborn. Clinics in Perinatology 22: 803–828

Miller D R, Baehner R L 1995 Blood diseases of infancy and childhood, 7th edn. C V Mosby, St Louis

Modell B, Harris R, Lane B et al 2000 Informed choice in genetic screening for thalassaemia during pregnancy: audit from a national confidential inquiry. British Medical Journal 320: 337–41

Modell B, Khan M, Darlison M 2000 Survival in beta-thalassaemia major in the UK: data from the UK thalassaemia register. Lancet 355: 2051–2052

Monagle P, Adams M, Mahoney M et al 2000 Outcome of pediatric thromboembolic disease: a report from the Canadian Childhood Thrombophilia Registry. Pediatric Research 47: 763–766

Monagle P, Michelson A D, Bovill E, Andrew M 2001 Antithrombotic therapy in children. Chest 119(1 Supplement): 344S–370S

Nathan D G, Orkin S H 1998 Nathan and Oski's hematology of infancy and childhood, 5th edn. W B Saunders, Philadelphia

Oberlin O, Rey A, Anderson J et al 2001 Treatment of orbital rhabdomyosarcoma: survival and late effects of treatment. Results of an international workshop. Journal of Clinical Oncology 19: 197–204

Oski FA 1993 Iron deficiencies in infancy and childhood. New England Journal of Medicine 329: 190–193

Packer R J, Boyett J M, Janss A J et al 2001 Growth hormone replacement therapy in children with medulloblastoma: use and effect on tumour control. Journal of Clinical Oncology 19: 480–487

Petrou M, Modell B, Shetty S, Khan M, Ward RH 2000 Long-term effect of prospective detection of high genetic risk on couples' reproductive life: data for thalassaemia. Prenatal Diagnosis 20: 469–474

Piu C-H 1999 Childhood leukaemias. Cambridge University Press, Cambridge

Pizzo P A, Poplack D G 1997 Prinicples and practice of paediatric oncology, 3rd edn. Lippincott-Raven, Philadelphia

Smith H 1996 Diagnosis in paediatric haematology. Churchill Livingstone, London

Wethers DL 2000 Sickle cell disease in childhood: part II. Diagnosis and treatment of major complications and recent advances in treatment. American Family Physician 62: 1309–1314

Young N S, Maciejewski J 1997 The pathophysiology of acquired aplastic anemia. New England Journal of Medicine 336: 1365–1372

Useful links

http://www.aabb.org (American Association of Blood Banks)

http://www.anzccsg.nch.edu.au (Australia and New Zealand Children's Cancer Study Group)

http://www.arcbs.redcross.org.au (Australian Red Cross blood service) http://www.childrensoncologygroup.org (Children's Oncology Group (USA))

http://www.haemophilia.org.au (Hemophilia Foundation Australia)

http://www.haemophilia-forum.org (Hemophilia forum)

http://www.md.ucl.ac.be/siop (International Society for Paediatric Oncology)

http://www.med.unc.edu/isth (International Society on Thrombosis and Haemostasis)

http://www.ncbi.nlm.nih.gov/entrez (PubMed — one of the faster and more efficient free Medline services)

http://www.nhlbi.nih.gov/health/prof/blood/sickle/sick-mt.htm (A health care worker information site published by the National Heart, Blood and Lung Institute of the NIH in the USA)

http://www.sicklecellsociety.org/ (A UK based charity site for patient information on sickle cell disease)

http://www.text.nlm.nih.gov/ftrs/tocview (Clinical guidelines for managing sickle cell disease from the Agency for Health Care Research and Quality)

http://www.ukts.org/ (Web site of the UK Thalassaemia Society. The organisation was started in 1976 by parents of children with thalassaemia, and the site has information for parents and children)

http://www.wfh.org (World Federation of Hemophilia)

SEIZURE DISORDERS AND DISORDERS OF THE NERVOUS SYSTEM

56 Seizures and epilepsies

A. S. Harvey

Few events are more alarming to parents than their child having a breath holding attack, febrile convulsion or first epileptic seizure. Seizures of some type occur in 5% of children. Most are single episodes occurring in the context of acute neurological insults or intercurrent illnesses. Epilepsy, defined as recurrent, unprovoked afebrile seizures, occurs with a prevalence of 0.5–1.0% during childhood.

The International League Against Epilepsy classification of seizures, based on clinical and EEG features (1981), recognises two major categories: partial seizures and generalised seizures (Table 56.1). Partial seizures originate in a localised part of the cerebral cortex, whereas generalised seizures commence synchronously in both hemispheres. Partial seizures are further classified as either simple partial (with preserved consciousness), complex partial (with impaired consciousness) or partial with secondary generalisation, although consideration of partial seizures by their site of origin in the brain is sometimes more useful.

Complementary to the classification of seizure types is a classification of epilepsies or epileptic syndromes (Table 56.2), the conditions which predispose to epileptic seizures. An epilepsy syndrome encompasses seizure type, possible aetiology, associated clinical features, EEG and imaging findings, and prognosis. Epileptic syndromes are often classified according to presumed

aetiology. Idiopathic (primary) epilepsies are those seizure disorders with no identifiable aetiology other than a genetic predisposition to seizures. These epilepsies are usually manifest by characteristic partial or generalised seizures, predictable age at seizure onset, stereotypic EEG patterns, absence of other neurological problems, good response to treatment, and favourable outcome. Idiopathic epilepsies are being gradually understood as abnormalities of ion channels and neurotransmitter receptors of neuronal membranes. Symptomatic (secondary) epilepsies are those seizure disorders which are the result of known or presumed (cryptogenic) cerebral abnormalities, such as structural brain lesions or metabolic disturbances. These epilepsies have variable clinical and EEG characteristics depending on the underlying aetiology and age at onset, are often associated with other neurological problems, and often have a poor prognosis for seizure control.

Table 56.2   Common epilepsy syndromes in childhood, by age

Neonate
Symptomatic neonatal seizures
Benign neonatal convulsions (familial and non familial)

Infancy
Febrile convulsions
Infantile spasms
Benign and severe myoclonic epilepsies of infancy
Benign infantile convulsions (familial and non familial)

Childhood
Typical absence epilepsy of childhood
Benign (idiopathic) partial epilepsies of childhood (rolandic, occipital, others)
Primary generalised epilepsy with tonic–clonic seizures
Myoclonic epilepsies, including Lennox–Gastaut syndrome
Temporal lobe epilepsy and other symptomatic partial epilepsies

Adolescence
Juvenile absence epilepsy
Juvenile myoclonic epilepsy
Temporal lobe epilepsy and other symptomatic partial epilepsies

---

Table 56.1   Classification of epileptic seizure type, based on clinical and EEG features

Partial (focal)
Simple partial: consciousness preserved, e.g. focal motor or sensory disturbances
Complex partial: consciousness impaired, e.g. staring with automatisms
Secondarily generalised

Generalised
Tonic–clonic
Absence
Myoclonic
Clonic
Tonic
Atonic

Common epilepsies of infancy, childhood and adolescence

Neonatal seizures

Neonatal seizures differ from seizures in older children because of special aetiological and developmental factors. Clonic jerking and tonic stiffening, which may be generalised, focal or multifocal, are the common seizure manifestations. Causes of neonatal seizures include hypoxic-ischaemic encephalopathy following fetal distress or intrapartum asphyxia, metabolic disturbances such as hypoglycaemia, hypocalcaemia and inborn errors of metabolism, and infections such as intrauterine cytomegalovirus and toxoplasmosis or postnatally acquired bacterial meningitis and herpes encephalitis. Cerebral malformations are important causes of seizures in infancy and childhood, but may occasionally cause seizures in the newborn period. Benign familial neonatal convulsions is a rare, dominantly inherited, seizure disorder with familial seizures occurring in otherwise normal neonates.

Treatment

Treatment depends on the diagnosis, arrived at after blood glucose, calcium and magnesium estimations, CSF examination, and sometimes brain imaging. Pending the results of investigations, a therapeutic trial of intravenous glucose, intravenous calcium, and pyridoxine should be considered. Phenobarbitone in an initial dose of 15 mg/kg is the anticonvulsant of choice but phenytoin is also effective. Blood level monitoring of anticonvulsants is essential in the maintenance therapy of newborns.

Febrile convulsions

Fever and convulsions may coexist with infections of the central nervous system, such as meningitis and encephalitis, and with intercurrent infection in children with epilepsy. However, fever and convulsions most commonly occur together in the condition called febrile convulsions, in which, during infancy and early childhood, there is a predisposition to convulse in the presence of fever. Although not considered epilepsy, the syndrome of febrile convulsions does represent an age dependent predisposition to seizures with an identifiable precipitant, like many idiopathic epilepsies. Genetic factors are important, as a family history of febrile convulsions or epilepsy is present in more than 30% of children. As for many idiopathic epilepsies, febrile convulsions are being understood as disorders of ion channels.

A febrile convulsion is defined as a seizure in which there is neither clinical nor laboratory evidence of central nervous system infection, temperature is 38°C or higher, and the child has not had previous afebrile convulsions. Convulsions are of generalised tonic-clonic type and brief duration in most cases, although infants may have predominantly tonic, clonic, atonic or sometimes focal manifestations and occasionally seizures are prolonged. Most febrile convulsions are associated with upper respiratory tract infections and viraemias.

Febrile convulsions occur in approximately 3% of the population, commencing between age 5 months to 5 years, with most manifesting in the first 2 years of life. In approximately one third of cases the febrile convulsions are recurrent, the risk increasing to one half if there is onset in infancy or a family history of febrile convulsions. Approximately 3% of children with febrile convulsions go on to have later afebrile convulsions, that is epilepsy, the risk being increased further if there is evidence of abnormal development or neurological problems, the child has a family history of epilepsy, or the convulsions are prolonged, focal or multiple within a febrile illness. When epilepsy follows febrile convulsions it is invariably a later manifestation of the same underlying seizure predisposition; rarely are later epileptic seizures the result of brain injury from prolonged or focal febrile convulsions. Febrile convulsions are not associated with later intellectual impairment.

Treatment

The cause of the febrile illness is treated on its own merits. There is debate about the role of antipyretics and gentle cooling, but most paediatricians would recommend such measures. The convulsion will usually have ceased before medical help is obtained; however, if a febrile convulsion has not ceased after 3–5 minutes, it is a matter of urgency to terminate the seizure, usually with rectal or intravenous diazepam. Meningitis should be seriously considered if the child has a history of vomiting, is younger than 6 months, has repeated seizures following presentation, has been treated with antibiotics or seems more seriously ill than would be expected following a simple febrile convulsion.

Anticonvulsant medication does not diminish the likelihood of later epilepsy, and given the benign nature of febrile convulsions and the potential adverse effects of antiepileptic drug treatment in infancy, treatment is very rarely prescribed for febrile convulsions. Parents and carers need explanation and reassurance about the likelihood of further febrile seizures, the benign nature of the disorder in most children, and the management of subsequent febrile illnesses. Some children with recurrent or prolonged febrile convulsions may be prescribed oral or rectal diazepam, respectively, although these remain controversial issues.

Infantile spasms

This syndrome presents in the first year of life and is often of sinister significance because seizures may be difficult to control and development disability often follows. The onset is usually between 3 and 8 months of age and males are affected twice as commonly as females. The common type of flexor or salaam spasm, which is essentially a massive myoclonic jerk or brief tonic seizure, consists of sudden drawing up of the legs, hunching forward of the neck and shoulders, and flinging out of the arms in extension. Opisthotonic or extensor spasms are less common. Spasms characteristically occur in clusters of several over a minute or two, clusters repeated many times a day. The EEG usually shows a very disorganised pattern called hypsarrhythmia, with high voltage, multifocal epileptic activity (Fig. 56.1). Development is often delayed in these infants prior to the onset of spasms, or there may be loss of visual attention and arrest of developmental progress at onset. The triad of infantile spasms, developmental delay and hypsarrhythmia is referred to as West syndrome. Differential diagnosis includes a variety of normal infant behaviours, such as sleep jerks and colic, and less sinister myoclonic epilepsies in infancy.

Infantile spasms have many different causes and the common factor is probably the timing and diffuse nature of a severe disturbance of the immature central nervous system. A cause is identified in about two thirds of infants, causes including cerebral injury from prior prenatal or perinatal ischaemia or infection, brain malformation, neurocutaneous syndromes such as tuberous sclerosis, or inborn errors of metabolism such as vitamin B_6 deficiency or phenylketonuria. In these symptomatic cases, outcome for seizures and development is usually poor. In the cryptogenic cases where no cause is apparent from history, examination, brain imaging and metabolic screening, outcome is more variable; if there is a prior history of developmental delay and spasms are not quickly controlled with treatment, outcome is again poor. Overall, 70–80% infants develop some degree of intellectual disability and, although spasms often cease promptly with treatment, in 30–50% children there is the later appearance or gradual transformation to a partial or generalised epilepsy after 2–4 years of age.

Treatment

The treatment of infantile spasms is controversial an differs around the world. Treatment choices include corticosteroids (e.g. prednisolone 2 mg/kg/day orally or ACTH 40 units/day intramuscularly for 1–2 months with slow withdrawal thereafter), vigabatrin at 50–150 mg/kg/day or sodium valproate at 50–100 mg/kg/day for 6–12 months, or a benzodiazepine such as clonazepam or nitrazepam. Pryidoxine should always be given as a trial, prior to commencement of anticonvulsants or steroids.

Absence epilepsies

Absence epilepsies are idiopathic generalised epilepsies manifest predominantly by absence seizures. Absence seizures usually commence between 4 and 12 years of age. Absence seizures are manifest by sudden cessation of activity with staring, usually lasting only 5–15 seconds. Blinking, upward deviation of the eyes, slight mouthing movements and some fidgeting hand movements may

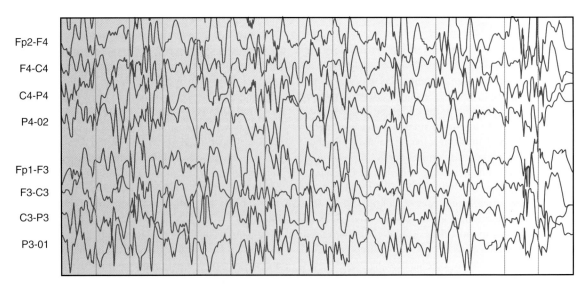

Fig. 56.1 The EEG pattern of hypoarrhythmia showing diffuse, continuous, high amplitude, irregular sharp waves, spikes and slow waves on a disorganised background, typical of that seen in infantile spasms.

Clinical example

Baby Jonathan presented at age 5 months with episodes of stiffening and drawing up of his legs, thought to be colic. The attacks lasted a few seconds only and occurred up to 10 times each day. During the attacks, his eyes were noted to roll up and he appeared unaware, often ending with a brief cry. His parents were also concerned that he seemed irritable, less interested in toys, and was not smiling as responsively as previously. Pregnancy, birth and early developmental histories were unremarkable. On examination he fixed and followed poorly and his motor abilities were at a 3 month old level. Examination of the skin revealed several depigmented patches on the legs, trunk and back. A cluster of typical infantile spasms occurred during the assessment, with there being stronger arm and leg stiffening on the right and eye deviation to the right side. EEG showed irregular sharp waves and spikes on a disorganised background, approaching a hypsarrhythmic pattern, the epileptic activity being more prominent on the left. CT of the brain showed calcified nodules around the lateral ventricles anteriorly and several faintly calcified lesions in the cortex. A diagnosis of infantile spasms secondary to tuberous sclerosis was made and he was commenced on vigabatrin, the spasms ceasing after the second dose, and improved visual attention apparent in the week following.

occur. The child does not fall, is rarely incontinent and returns to normal activity promptly at the offset of the absence. Many attacks occur in a day. Attacks can usually be precipitated in the clinic room and during EEG with hyperventilation. Attacks are characterised by generalised spike-wave activity on an otherwise normal EEG background (Fig. 56.2). The two common types of absence

epilepsy are ***typical childhood absence epilepsy*** (so called petit mal epilepsy), which manifests in preschool and young primary school age children with usually just absence seizures and spike-wave activity at 3 Hz on EEG, and ***juvenile absence epilepsy***, which presents in the peripubertal years with typical absence seizures but a faster spike-wave pattern on EEG and a greater chance of associated generalised tonic-clonic and myoclonic seizures. Differential diagnosis of absence seizures includes day dreaming and complex partial seizures.

Treatment

Sodium valproate, ethosuximide and lamotrigine are the medications used commonly to treat absence seizures. Ethosuximide is ineffective in controlling tonic–clonic seizures, so is not used in children with juvenile absence epilepsy. Treatment is usually for 2 years only in typical childhood absence epilepsy, with an expectation of seizure remission, and through puberty in juvenile absence epilepsy, with later appearance of tonic–clonic seizures being a risk. Intellectual development is usually normal.

Benign partial (focal) epilepsies of childhood

The benign partial epilepsies of childhood are some of the most common forms of epilepsy in children, these being idiopathic epilepsies in which otherwise normal preschool and primary school age children have sleep related partial seizures, EEG showing prominent focal epileptic patterns and brain imaging revealing no abnormality. The two most common varieties are ***benign rolandic epilepsy*** (***benign partial epilepsy with centro-temporal spikes***), in which the seizure focus is low in the

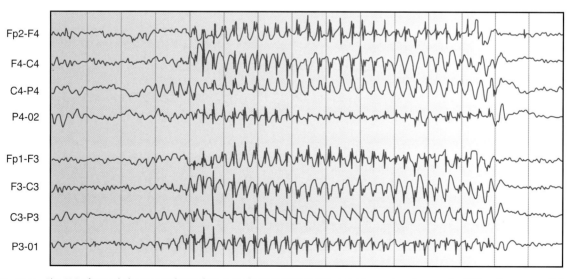

Fig. 56.2   The EEG of typical absence epilepsy during an absence seizure showing a paroxysm of generalised 3Hz spike-wave activity.

central sulcus (rolandic) region on one or both sides, and **benign occipital epilepsy**, in which the seizure focus is over the occipital region.

In benign rolandic epilepsy, seizure onset is usually between 5 and 10 years of age and there is a male predominance. Partial seizures manifest with a spectrum of sensorimotor features. The mildest seizures may be simple partial with tingling and/or twitching of the cheek, tongue and face, drooling of saliva, gurgling or choking noises, and preservation of consciousness but with inability to speak. The attacks may progress to include jerking of the arm or one half of the body with impairment of consciousness, and some children have secondarily generalised seizures where focal onset is not appreciated. Attacks are most commonly in sleep or immediately on

waking, such that parents are often unable to give a good description of their onset. In benign occipital epilepsy, presentation is often in slightly younger children with complex partial seizures manifest by staring, eye deviation and vomiting, or daytime attacks in which unusual visual symptoms are described and migraine-like headache may follow. In both varieties of benign focal epilepsy, EEG recording which includes sleep always demonstrates the characteristic focal epileptiform pattern (Fig. 56.3). In typical cases, brain imaging is usually unnecessary.

Treatment

Seizures are usually infrequent in the benign partial epilepsies, many children having only one or two seizures, and because of their usually brief nature and nocturnal occurrence, treatment with antiepileptic medications is not always necessary. If warranted, treatment with low dose carbamazepine or sodium valproate for a 1–2 year period is usually adequate. Prognosis is usually excellent, with absence of cognitive and behavioural problems, and remission of seizures by the teen years, hence the term 'benign'.

Primary (idiopathic) generalised epilepsies with tonic–clonic seizures

The primary generalised epilepsies with tonic–clonic seizures are a somewhat heterogenous group of idiopathic epilepsies with generalised tonic–clonic seizures, sometimes associated with absence and myoclonic seizures. As for other idiopathic epilepsies, there is no demonstrable brain or metabolic abnormality, normal

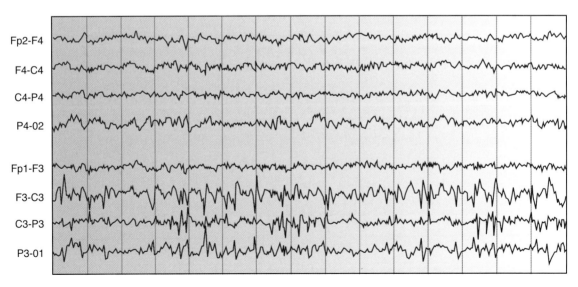

Fig. 56.3 The EEG of benign partial epilepsy of childhood with centrotemporal spikes (benign rolandic epilepsy) showing focal epileptiform activity in the left central region (lower three channels).

Michael, a developmentally normal 8 year old boy, presented to the emergency department of a regional hospital after being found fitting in bed at 5 a.m. while holidaying with his family. The seizure was brief, seemingly generalised tonic–clonic, associated with prominent gurgling noises, and followed by a 10–15 minute period where his speech was slurred and his right arm appeared weak. The parents recalled hearing similar noises from Michael's bedroom once or twice previously and finding the pillow wet with saliva in the morning. Michael described waking from his sleep in this seizure, having an electricity feeling in his mouth, and being unable to call out to his brother who was sleeping in the room with him. A paternal uncle had febrile convulsions in infancy and a maternal cousin had absence epilepsy. An EEG arranged subsequently showed left centrotemporal spikes which increased dramatically in sleep and a diagnosis of benign rolandic epilepsy was made. CT of the brain was not performed. Following much parental counselling and reassurance about this type of epilepsy, they decided to postpone treatment until another definite seizure occurred. General safety and lifestyle advice was given about seizures, although it was appreciated that seizure occurrence in the day was unlikely in this syndrome.

indicate a partial seizure with secondary generalisation. Generalised tonic–clonic seizures often occur during intercurrent febrile illnesses in young children with primary generalised epilepsy, and either during sleep or following periods of sleep deprivation or stress in older children and adolescents. The differential diagnosis of generalised tonic–clonic seizures includes partial seizures with secondary generalisation and convulsive features associated with syncope or breath holding spells.

Treatment

Sodium valproate is the drug of choice for generalised tonic–clonic seizures, especially when there is documented generalised spike wave on EEG and/or presence of absence or myoclonic seizures. Carbamazepine is sometimes used for 'indeterminate' generalised tonic–clonic seizures when other features of primary generalised epilepsy are lacking. Lamotrigine, phenytoin and benzodiazepines are also effective for generalised tonic–clonic seizures. Seizure control is usually possible with medication and lifestyle adjustments (e.g. avoiding sleep deprivation). In juvenile myoclonic epilepsy, treatment into adult life is recommended, as a seizure predisposition frequently persists.

intellect, often a family history of seizures, and the EEG shows characteristic epileptiform patterns, in these epilepsies those being generalised spike-wave and polyspike-wave discharges on a normal background. Seizures may begin at any time in childhood and adolescence, with onset around the time of puberty being common. Sometimes there is a past history of febrile convulsions or absence seizures with different EEG findings; in these cases, the later occurrence of tonic–clonic seizures and change in the EEG merely represents an age dependent, evolving expression of the same underlying, genetically determined seizure disorder. The syndrome of *juvenile myoclonic epilepsy* is recognised by the association of generalised tonic–clonic seizures, early morning myoclonic jerks and sometimes brief absence seizures in adolescence, the tonic–clonic seizure often having occurred in the setting of sleep deprivation. The EEG shows 4–7 Hz generalised spike-wave activity.

Initially in tonic–clonic seizures there is generalised (tonic) stiffening in extension, with temporary cessation of respiration and falling if standing. The tonic phase gradually progresses to a phase with generalised, rhythmic (clonic) jerking. Tonic–clonic seizures invariably cease spontaneously, usually within a few minutes, and are followed by a postictal period with depressed consciousness in which the child usually sleeps. On awakening there may be a headache, but there is no memory for the event. There are no warning symptoms (aura) nor any focal features in generalised tonic–clonic seizures of primary generalised epilepsy; if present, they would

Stephanie, a 13 year old girl with a history of a single febrile convulsion in infancy, presented to a regional hospital emergency department after having a generalised tonic–clonic seizure at year 7 school camp. The seizure occurred in the shower at 7 a.m., the morning after girls in her dormitory had stayed awake until 4 a.m.! Stephanie was heard to fall in the shower and was found by a friend convulsing on the shower floor. She sustained a forehead bruise and hot water scalding on her back. There was no history of prior (unrecognised) staring episodes. When asked specifically about jerking of the arms, Stephanie said that she had on occasions dropped things in the kitchen at breakfast time and on one occasion had to walk away from looking at a computer game her brother was playing because she felt sick and her head was jerking. There was no family history of epilepsy. Subsequent EEG recording showed frequent bursts of generalised fast spike-wave activity, amplified by hyperventilation and photic stimulation. A diagnosis of primary generalised epilepsy with tonic-clonic seizures and photic sensitivity was made, with the clinical picture being highly suggestive of juvenile myoclonic epilepsy specifically. Long discussions were held with Stephanie and her parents over the initial and subsequent consultations, highlighting safety and lifestyle factors. Sodium valproate was commenced after discussion of potential weight gain and mild hair loss side effects, these concerning Stephanie more than the risk of subsequent seizures. The family were given a guarded prognosis for seizure remission in later teen years and regular review was arranged.

Temporal lobe epilepsy

Temporal lobe epilepsy is a partial epilepsy syndrome in which seizures arise in the temporal lobe on one or both sides, due commonly to either scarring or a developmental lesion in the temporal lobe. Such symptomatic partial epilepsies can arise in any part of the brain as a result of tumours, cysts, scars and developmental malformations. When no cause is found on brain imaging, an idiopathic partial epilepsy may be suspected but will be difficult to diagnose without the characteristic EEG pattern. There is a predilection for 'epileptogenic lesions' to occur in the temporal lobe to some extent, and temporal lobe epilepsy is certainly the most common type of uncontrolled partial epilepsy in adults.

Partial seizures of temporal lobe origin may be simple partial (auras), complex partial or secondarily generalised. They may commence at any age, but commonly begin in the middle of the first decade. Complex partial seizures of temporal lobe origin are characteristically manifest by motionless staring, changed facial expression suggesting fear or bewilderment, and fidgeting hand movements called automatisms. In some there may be head turning and stiffening of the limbs on one side. Autonomic disturbances such as facial flushing or pallor, lip smacking, salivation, chewing and swallowing, and sometimes vomiting are common; apnoea may be the predominant manifestation of complex partial seizures in infancy. Warning of an impending seizure is often present, but may not be easily described by a young or developmentally delayed child. Fear, unusual smells or tastes, abdominal discomfort, and psychic or perceptual disturbances such as dreamy states and feelings of familiarity (déjà vu) may be described. Complex partial seizures last longer than absence seizures, generally 30–60 seconds, are usually infrequent and commonly occur in clusters over several days, alternating with seizure-free periods.

The EEG may be normal, show non specific abnormalities or show focal epileptic patterns over the temporal lobe of origin. Video EEG monitoring is sometimes necessary to characterise attacks and confirm the diagnosis, the differential diagnosis including day dreaming, absence seizures, behavioural problems and migraine. Brain imaging with MRI is needed to search for an underlying cerebral lesion, although not always present. These principles apply also to frontal, parietal and occipital lobe epilepsies in which the child does not have a recognisable idiopathic partial epilepsy.

Treatment

Carbamazepine is the drug of choice for seizures in temporal lobe epilepsy. Seizures are often resistant to treatment over time and the patient is tried on various medications. Cognitive and behavioural problems may be present in children with temporal lobe epilepsy, as non epileptic manifestations of the underlying temporal lobe disturbance or lesion, and often require psychological assessment and intervention. Spontaneous remission occurs in some patients but when seizures remain uncontrolled and impact significantly on the child's lifestyle, temporal lobectomy may be considered.

Clinical example

Steven, a 13 year old boy with a history of learning problems and aggressive behavioural outbursts, was referred for management of refractory absence seizures and tonic–clonic seizures. Seizures began at about 5 years of age and there was a prior history of bacterial meningitis at 13 months, complicated by seizures and transient right sided weakness at presentation. His current seizures occurred in clusters and consisted of an aura of fear and abdominal discomfort, followed by cessation of activity, loss of responsiveness and unusual posturing of his right hand. These were clearly of complex partial type and the tonic–clonic seizures seemed to begin in this manner, presumably being secondarily generalised. None of the three antiepileptic medications used in the past had controlled his seizures. Because of increasing school difficulties and uncontrolled epilepsy he was further evaluated, with MRI showing scarring of the hippocampus in the left temporal lobe, video EEG recording of seizures showing electrical onset in the left temporal lobe region, and cognitive testing showing normal intellect but decreased language and verbal memory abilities. Left temporal lobectomy was subsequently performed and after a 2 year period free of seizures his medications were gradually weaned. Learning and behavioural difficulties persisted but were better managed with understanding of their cause, abolition of seizures, and institution of specific behavioural and educational strategies.

Non epileptic episodic disorders

Not all episodes of neurological dysfunction in infancy and childhood are epileptic. Sleep disorders, movement disorders, circulatory disturbances, migraine and some normal behaviours may mimic epileptic seizures (Table

Table 56.3 Differential diagnosis of epileptic seizures

Normal infant and child behaviours, e.g. sleep jerks, day dreaming
Parasomnias, e.g. night terrors, sleep walking
Breath holding spells
Syncope
Migraine
Movement disorders, e.g. tics, tremor, clonus
Miscellaneous, e.g. benign paroxysmal vertigo, shuddering attacks, psychogenic seizures

56.3). Disorders frequently misdiagnosed as seizures are breath holding attacks in infancy and syncope in children and adolescents, because of their sudden and seemingly unprovoked occurrence with loss of consciousness and sometimes associated convulsive movements.

Breath holding attacks (reflex hypoxic syncope)

Attacks usually commence in the first or second year of life. Crucial to the diagnosis is recognition that attacks are precipitated by either physical trauma, such as a knock or a fall, or emotional trauma such as fright, anger or frustration, the precipitants not always being significant and noticed. Attacks usually commence with crying, but this may be brief or absent. Apnoea then occurs with cyanosis or pallor, and may then either terminate without apparent loss of consciousness, or progress with the child becoming unconscious, limp and sometimes briefly stiffening or jerking in response to the cerebral hypoxia. Incontinence may occur with such convulsive features. Recovery is usually rapid, although some children are drowsy and lethargic after an attack with convulsive features. Attacks usually cease by the third or fourth year of life. They are not a cause of death, epilepsy, intellectual disability or cerebral damage in later life.

The pathophysiology of breath holding attacks is not well understood, but in the pallid variety the infants seem to have exaggerated vagal responses to noxious stimuli, often with profound bradycardia and even brief asystole. Iron deficiency anaemia seems to be an exacerbating factor in some children with frequent attacks or prominent convulsive features.

Syncope

Syncope or fainting is not uncommon in infants, children and adolescents. As in adults, it is the result of decreased cardiac output and cerebral perfusion leading to loss of consciousness and falling. As with breath holding attacks, brief tonic stiffening, clonic jerking or incontinence can follow the loss of consciousness and lead to misdiagnosis as an epileptic seizure. Recovery is usually prompt following syncope. Light headedness or visual loss prior to loss of consciousness, and sweating and tachycardia during recovery, are suggestive of syncope. However, the most important clue to syncope is the situation in which the episode occurred. Syncope should be suspected as the basis of loss of consciousness or apparent epileptic seizures when attacks occur during or following vomiting illnesses, prolonged standing, venepuncture, injury, or watching medical or veterinary procedures. Syncope without an obvious precipitant or syncope during exercise or in water should prompt concern about a cardiac cause, such as prolonged QTc syndrome or aortic stenosis.

General principles of management of seizures

Three important and successive steps in the assessment of a child with suspected seizures are to:

- distinguish epileptic seizures from non epileptic attacks
- determine the type(s) of epileptic seizures the child is having, most importantly whether they are generalised or partial
- determine the type of epilepsy or epilepsy syndrome in the child having recurrent seizures, or at least try and determine whether the epilepsy is likely to be idiopathic or symptomatic.

The diagnosis of epileptic seizures should be made on clinical grounds with investigations used to confirm the diagnosis, help characterise the seizure disorder and determine the underlying cause. Metabolic disturbance, especially hypoglycaemia and hypocalcaemia should always be considered, especially with convulsions in infancy. An EEG is seldom of value in the assessment of febrile convulsions. The role of the EEG is mainly in distinguishing partial from generalised seizures and in aiding diagnosis of specific epilepsy syndromes. In this way, the EEG may assist in making the correct choice of anticonvulsant medication and determining the need for brain imaging. In children with undiagnosed recurrent attacks, or children with epileptic seizures of uncertain type, simultaneous video EEG monitoring may be of benefit.

Brain imaging, usually with MRI, is indicated in children with partial seizures and focal EEG abnormalities not characteristic of an idiopathic partial (benign focal) epilepsy syndrome, in children with evidence of neurological impairment or abnormal physical findings suggesting an underlying cerebral abnormality, and in children with progressive or uncontrolled seizures. Brain imaging is unnecessary in typical cases of idiopathic epilepsy such as absence epilepsy, benign partial epilepsy of childhood with centrotemporal spikes, and primary generalised epilepsies with tonic–clonic seizures.

Antiepileptic medications reduce the likelihood of seizures but do not alter the course of epilepsy, that is, seizures do not remit any sooner on treatment. The decision to treat a child with epilepsy with anticonvulsant medication depends on the epilepsy syndrome diagnosis and several other patient and family factors. The appropriate anticonvulsant is usually indicated by the seizure type (Table 56.4).

Seizures can usually be controlled with one medication at an optimal dose. Children vary greatly in their dosage requirements and tolerance of anticonvulsants, age and associated comorbidities being the main determinants. Except in status epilepsy and severe convulsions, appro-

Table 56.4 Antiepileptic medications most effective in different seizure types

Seizure type	Anticonvulsant
Partial	Carbamazepine, lamotrigine, sodium valproate, gabapentin, topiramate
Generalised tonic–clonic	Sodium valproate, carbamazepine, lamotrigine, topiramate, phenytoin
Absence	Sodium valproate, ethosuximide, lamotrigine
Myoclonic, atonic, tonic	Sodium valproate, lamotrigine, benzodiazepines
Neonatal seizures	Phenobarbitone, phenytoin, clonazepam
Infantile spasms	Vigabatrin, prednisolone/ACTH, benzodiazepines, sodium valproate

Table 56.5 Side effects of antiepileptic medications

Medication	Side effects
Toxicity	
Common to most antiepileptic medications	Drowsiness, ataxia, tremor, nystagmus, dysarthria, confusion, nausea, vomiting, weight gain
Idiosyncratic	
Carbamazepine	Rash, leucopenia, hyponatraemia, irritability, depression
Sodium valproate	Alopecia, acute hepatic failure, pancreatitis
Lamotrigine	Rash, severe hypersensitivity syndrome
Clonazepam	Severe behavioural changes, increased bronchial and salivary secretions
Phenytoin	Rash, serum sickness type illness
Phenobarbitone	Behaviour disturbance
Topiramate	Kidney stones, weight loss, speech disturbance
Vigabatrin	Peripheral vision impairment, psychosis, behaviour disturbance

priate drugs are commenced singly and in low dosage and then increased gradually to a dose where seizure control is obtained, side effects appear or maximum dosage and serum levels are surpassed. The duration of therapy depends on the epilepsy syndrome diagnosis, the degree of seizure control and the patient's lifestyle. Several years of freedom from seizures are desirable before anticonvulsants are ceased, and this is best done slowly over a period of months.

Almost all anticonvulsants produce side effects such as drowsiness and unsteadiness if given in excess (Table 56.5). These effects are common when medications are commenced and the dose increased, but they often wear off after the maintenance dose is reached. Some antiepileptic medications have side effects of an idiosyncratic type.

Use of serum levels for monitoring some antiepileptic medications is particularly useful if seizure control is inadequate, side effects attributable to toxicity are suspected or if compliance is uncertain. Barbiturate and phenytoin levels correlate well with both seizure control and side effects, a lesser correlation being present with carbamazepine and sodium valproate. There is little role for blood level monitoring with ethosuximide, benzodiazepines and the newer antiepileptic agents. Blood level monitoring is of particular value in young infants, in children with intellectual disability and in patients with impaired consciousness, that is, patients who are not able to describe side effects. Blood levels are also useful in checking compliance.

For children with uncontrolled epilepsy, in whom seizures continue despite correct diagnosis and correct prescription of antiepileptic medications, specialised treatments such as epilepsy surgery, a ketogenic diet and vagal nerve stimulation may be considered. Surgical treatment is reserved for children with well characterised and refractory partial epilepsy in whom seizures are impacting greatly on quality of life, and, preferably, the region of seizure origin is away from critical functional cortex and an identifiable lesion is present on MRI. Epilepsy surgery is only carried out after detailed evaluation in a centre with special experience in paediatric epileptology.

It is necessary to consider a child and his or her total environment, and not only the seizures, when treating epilepsy. Problems pertaining to education and vocation and the management of emotional disorders associated with epilepsy may be more difficult to manage than the actual convulsions. Safety issues, such as supervision while bathing and swimming, preventing injuries from falls, traffic safety, and the first aid treatment of seizures need to be discussed with parents and carers.

Cerebral palsy and neurodegenerative disorders 57

D. Reddihough, K. Collins

Cerebral palsy

Cerebral palsy is the term used for a persistent but not unchanging disorder of movement and posture due to a defect or lesion of the developing brain. It is generally applied to children with permanent motor impairment due to non progressive brain disorders occurring before the age of 5 years. There are many different causes, a wide range of manifestations of the motor disorder, and various associated problems.

Cerebral palsy is not a single disorder, but a group of disorders with diverse implications for children and their families. For some young people with mild cerebral palsy, the only motor deficit may be a minimal hemiplegia, causing clumsiness with certain movements. In other children with severe cerebral palsy, the motor deficit may be spastic quadriplegia with little or no independent movement. Because each child with cerebral palsy is different, individual assessment and treatment are essential.

Prevalence

Cerebral palsy is the commonest physical disability in childhood. Studies from several parts of the world, including Western Australia, Sweden and the United Kingdom, have shown that the prevalence of cerebral palsy is between 2.0 and 2.5 per 1000 live births. While the overall prevalence of cerebral palsy has remained fairly stable since 1970, there has been a change in the relative contribution of the various subtypes. In particular, there has been a consistent rise in the prevalence of cerebral palsy among low birth weight infants (Fig. 57.1).

Aetiology

The cause of cerebral palsy is unknown in many children. There is a significant association with prematurity and low birth weight but *it is important to remember that most low birth weight infants do not develop cerebral palsy.*

In a significant proportion of children who have cerebral palsy, there appears to have been no single event but rather a sequence of events responsible for the motor damage. This has led to the concept of 'causal pathways', a sequence of interdependent events that culminate in disease. It is likely that interdependent events are responsible for many cases of cerebral palsy.

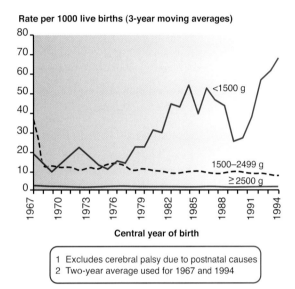

Rate per 1000 live births (3-year moving averages)

Central year of birth

1. Excludes cerebral palsy due to postnatal causes
2. Two-year average used for 1967 and 1994

Fig. 57.1 Birth weight specific cerebral palsy rates per 1000 live births (3 year moving averages) in Western Australia, 1967–1994. From Watson L, Stanley FJ, Blair E 1999 Report of the Western Australia Cerebral Palsy Register to Birth Year 1994. TVWTelethon Institute for Child Health Research, Perth, with permission.

Historical aspects

There has been a fundamental change in our understanding of aetiological factors during the past 15 years. Before this time, most cases of cerebral palsy were thought to be caused by lack of oxygen during either labour or the perinatal period and it was expected that improvement in obstetrics and neonatal care would result in lower rates of cerebral palsy. There was an increased use of interventions such as caesarean section and electronic fetal monitoring but, although the stillbirth and neonatal death rates declined, the cerebral palsy rate remained constant.

In the past, minor obstetric and neonatal events were used as an explanation for cerebral palsy. Current research suggests that about 8–10% of cases are associated with perinatal asphyxia. The term 'birth asphyxia' should not be used to imply that a lack of oxygen during labour or delivery has caused detrimental effects, as it is often impossible to ascribe clinical signs and symptoms in the newborn to an event during birth. Perinatal asphyxia is the preferred term to describe a situation in which there have been perinatal events likely to reduce oxygen supply, evidenced by significant acidosis, followed by a failure of function in at least two organs (usually the brain and kidney). It is important to remember that perinatal asphyxia may not necessarily be the primary cause of the cerebral palsy and is generally not preventable.

Current knowledge about aetiology

It is helpful to consider the timing of the brain insult:
- Prenatal events are thought to be responsible for approximately 75% of all cases of cerebral palsy.
- Perinatal events contribute 10–15%.
- Postnatal causes account for about 10% of all cases.

A prenatal cause is assumed in the absence of clear evidence for a perinatal or postnatal cause.

Prenatal causes

Malformations. Disturbances of brain development result in a variety of malformations, including neuronal migration disorders. These malformations are identified by imaging techniques, particularly magnetic resonance imaging (MRI), and information about the timing of possible adverse events is provided. While the presence of malformations provides a cause for the motor impairment, the cause of the malformation itself generally remains unexplained.

Vascular. Brain imaging provides evidence of previous vascular events such as middle cerebral artery occlusion (Fig. 57.2).

Infective. Maternal infections during the first and second trimesters of pregnancy, including the TORCH group of organisms (*t*oxoplasmosis, *r*ubella, *c*ytomegalovirus and *h*erpes simplex virus), may cause cerebral palsy. It has also been suggested that maternal infections in the perinatal period may form part of the causal pathway to cerebral palsy in some children.

Genetic. There are some uncommon genetic syndromes associated with cerebral palsy.

Metabolic. Iodine deficiency in early pregnancy is an important cause of cerebral palsy in many parts of the world. Maternal thyroid disease has also been implicated.

Toxic. There have been reported cases associated with lead and methylmercury ingestion.

Perinatal causes

Problems during labour and delivery. Obstetric emergencies such as obstructed labour, antepartum haemorrhage or cord prolapse may compromise the fetus.

Neonatal problems. Conditions such as severe hypoglycemia or untreated jaundice may be responsible.

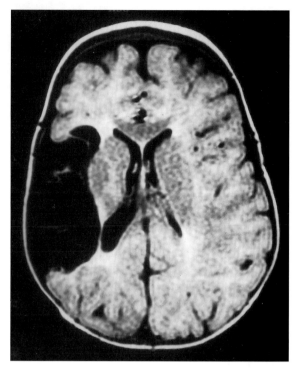

Fig. 57.2 MRI brain scan on 2 year old boy with left spastic hemiparesis, showing loss of brain tissue in right temporal and frontal lobes, consistent with an old (prenatal) right middle cerebral artery territory infarct.

Premature and low birth weight infants

Premature and low birth weight children differ from those born at term in their higher risk of cerebral palsy. The rate of cerebral palsy in infants born below 33 weeks is up to 30 times higher than those born at term. Some premature infants develop brain damage from complications of their immaturity, such as intraventricular haemorrhage, while others are damaged earlier in pregnancy. Intrauterine growth retardation is associated with cerebral palsy in both term and preterm infants.

Periventricular leucomalacia is a common radiological finding in premature children with cerebral palsy. It is caused by an ischaemic process, usually occurring between 28 and 34 weeks of gestation, in the watershed zone that exists in the periventricular white matter of the immature brain. Periventricular leucomalacia may also be found in infants born at term, suggesting that the insult occurred early in the third trimester even though the pregnancy progressed to term.

Multiple pregnancy

There is an increased risk of both mortality and cerebral palsy in multiple births that are associated with preterm delivery, poor intrauterine growth, birth defects and intrapartum complications. The increased risk to twins of cerebral palsy is not entirely explained by their increased risk of prematurity and low birth weight. Intrauterine death of a co-twin is a factor unique to multiple pregnancies and is associated with a 6-fold increase in rate of cerebral palsy per twin confinement, or an 11-fold increase in rate per child.

Postnatal cerebral palsy

Infection and injuries are responsible for most cases of postnatal cerebral palsy in developed countries:
- The introduction of vaccines against *Haemophilus influenzae* type b has had a significant effect on an important cause of bacterial meningitis but other organisms such as meningococcus and pneumococcus remain.
- Injuries are an important group as there are clear prospects for prevention. Injuries may be accidental (such as motor vehicle accidents and near drowning episodes), or due to physical abuse. Important preventive measures include improved road safety and mandatory fencing around home swimming pools.

Other causes of postnatal cerebral palsy include apparent life threatening events and cerebrovascular accidents. Meningitis, septicaemia and infections such as malaria are important causes of cerebral palsy in developing countries.

> ### Clinical example
>
> Mary is aged 2 years 6 months. Her mother went into labour at 33 weeks gestation after an uneventful pregnancy. The delivery was rapid and Mary's Apgar scores were 6 at 1 minute and 8 at 5 minutes. Her parents remember some panic in the labour ward and felt that more could have been done to slow the labour. Mary developed hyaline membrane disease and mild jaundice. In the early neonatal period she had difficulty sucking, which was attributed to her prematurity. She was slow in her motor development and did not sit until the age of 15 months. A diagnosis of cerebral palsy was made at that time.
> When Mary was 2 years old, her parents requested an opinion as to whether subsequent children were likely to have cerebral palsy, believing that her prematurity and problems at birth were responsible for her condition. MRI of the brain demonstrated a brain malformation with bilateral clefts in the cerebral cortex, dating the problems to early pregnancy rather than the perinatal period.

Key learning point

- *It is important to establish the cause of cerebral palsy if at all possible. It is helpful for families and essential for genetic counselling.*

Table 57.1 Investigation of possible causes of cerebral palsy

History of pregnancy, birth and neonatal period, together with physical examination:
- Cause clear, for example, massive antepartum haemorrhage followed by neonatal encephalopathy: no further investigation
- cause not clear: urine/plasma metabolic screen
  consider infections
  chromosome analysis
  radiological investigation — MRI
  (provides information about the timing of the damaging event)

An approach to investigation of possible causes for cerebral palsy is shown in Table 57.1

Classification

There are three major ways in which cerebral palsy is classified — by the type, the topographical distribution and the severity of the motor disorder.

Type of motor disorder

Cerebral palsy is a disorder of movement (difficulties with voluntary movement and/or abnormal movements), posture and muscle tone (hypertonus and hypotonus). As a result there are various types of movement disorder.

Spastic cerebral palsy (70%). This is the commonest type. Spasticity involves increased muscle tone with characteristic clasp knife quality. Children with spasticity often have underlying weakness. In spastic cerebral palsy, there is damage to the motor cortex or corticospinal tracts, in contrast to dyskinetic and ataxic cerebral palsy which are associated with abnormalities of the basal ganglia and cerebellum, respectively.

Dyskinetic cerebral palsy (10–15%). This refers to a group of cerebral palsies with involuntary movements and is characterised by abnormalities of tone involving the whole body. Several terms are used within this group:
- **Dystonia** is an involuntary increase in extensor tone.
- **Athetosis** refers to slow writhing movements involving the distal parts of the limbs.
- **Chorea** is the term for rapid jerky movements.

Ataxic cerebral palsy (less than 5%). Children have a fine tremor, more noticeable when movements are initiated, and often have poor balance and hypotonia. Ataxia is associated with other neurological conditions that must be excluded before this diagnosis is made. Some children have a mixed motor disorder.

The topographical distribution

The terms diplegia, hemiplegia and quadriplegia are used and apply to children with spastic cerebral palsy as the extrapyramidal type usually involves four limbs:

- The term **diplegia** describes the distribution where the predominant problem is in the lower limbs. There is usually some upper limb involvement, which may be subtle. This is the pattern most commonly seen in premature infants who have the radiological finding of periventricular leucomalacia.
- Children with **spastic hemiplegia** usually have normal intelligence, frequently have epilepsy (50–70%), may have sensory impairments in the upper limb and may have visual deficits (homonymous hemianopsia).
- Children with **spastic quadriplegia** frequently have problems such as intellectual disability, epilepsy and visual difficulties. There is often poor trunk control and oromotor difficulties in addition to four limb involvement.

Severity of the motor disorder

Children who walk independently are described as having mild cerebral palsy, those ambulating with sticks or frames as moderate cerebral palsy, and those that are wheelchair dependent are classified as having severe cerebral palsy. These terms do not take into account the severity of individual motor problems, nor do they consider cognitive and other deficits, which may have a profound impact on the eventual outcome. Recently a Gross Motor Function Classification System has been introduced; this groups children into various age ranges and provides five levels of severity. It is a useful research tool.

Presentation

The diagnosis of cerebral palsy is not always easy, particularly in children born prematurely. Signs may evolve during the first year of life. For example, spasticity is not usually present in the early weeks of life and, conversely, abnormal neurological signs may disappear. Cerebral palsy may present as follows:

- Follow up of 'at risk' infants, such as those born prematurely or those with a history of neonatal encephalopathy.
- Delayed motor milestones, particularly delay in learning to sit, stand and walk.
- Development of asymmetric movement patterns, for example, strong preference for one hand in the early months of life.
- Abnormalities of muscle tone, particularly spasticity or hypotonia. The latter in isolation should always be treated with caution as it may be an early sign of global developmental delay rather than cerebral palsy.
- Management problems, for example, severe feeding difficulties, abnormalities of behaviour such as unexplained irritability. These problems should be interpreted carefully as many other conditions can present with these features.

Examination involves a search for abnormalities in muscle tone and deep tendon reflexes, along with persistence of primitive reflexes.

Key learning point

- *Observation of the child often provides more information than 'hands on' examination. It will provide information about the presence or absence of age appropriate motor skills and their quality.*

Associated disorders

- Visual problems occur in about 40% of children with cerebral palsy, and include strabismus, refractive errors, visual field defects and cortical visual impairment.
- Hearing deficits occur in 3–10% of children with cerebral palsy. High frequency hearing loss may be found in children with congenital rubella or other viral syndromes.
- Speech and language problems: receptive and expressive language delays and articulation problems occur.
- Epilepsy occurs in up to 50% of children with cerebral palsy, most commonly in those with severe motor problems.
- Cognitive impairments: while intellectual disabilities and learning problems are common, there is a wide range of intellectual ability in children with cerebral palsy and children with severe physical disabilities may have normal intelligence. Perceptual difficulties are also frequent.

Some children with cerebral palsy have only a motor disorder.

Management

A team approach is essential, involving a range of health professionals and teachers, with input from the family of paramount importance. Management of the child with cerebral palsy involves:

- management of the associated disabilities, health problems, and consequences of the motor disorder
- assessment of the child's capabilities and referral to appropriate services for the child and family.

Management of the associated disabilities, health problems and consequences of the motor disorder

Associated disabilities

- All children require a **hearing** and **visual** assessment.
- Assessment, advice and review of anticonvulsants for **epilepsy**.
- Children may benefit from formal **cognitive** assessment and may need help with their educational programme. Assessment of cognitive abilities can be difficult when children have severe physical disabilities.

Health problems

- **Growth** should be monitored and dietary advice sought to ensure that nutrient and calorie intake is adequate. Failure to thrive and undernutrition are frequent problems, caused by eating difficulties due to oromotor dysfunction. Nasogastric or gastrostomy feeds should be considered if there is difficulty in achieving satisfactory weight gains, or if the length of time taken to feed the child interferes with other activities. Conversely, **obesity** is a significant problem and may interfere with progress in motor skills.
- Investigation and management of **gastro-oesophageal reflux**, which occurs commonly in cerebral palsy. It can result in oesophagitis or gastritis, causing pain and poor appetite, and if severe, aspiration can result.
- Dietary and laxative advice regarding the frequent problem of **constipation**. Immobility, low fibre diet and poor fluid intake are contributory factors.
- Lung disease. Some children with severe cerebral palsy develop chronic **lung disease**, due to aspiration from oromotor dysfunction or severe gastro-oesophageal reflux occurring over a period of time. The presence of coughing or choking during meal times, or wheeze during or after meals, may signal the possibility of aspiration, but it may also occur without clinical symptoms or signs. There is no 'gold standard' test for aspiration but barium videofluoroscopy may be helpful. Alternative feeding regimens, such as the use of a gastrostomy, should be considered if aspiration is present.
- Many children with cerebral palsy, particularly those born prematurely, have **ventriculoperitoneal shunts**.
- **Dental health**. Children are at risk for dental problems and should be regularly monitored.
- **Osteoporosis.** Pathological fractures may occur in children with severe cerebral palsy.
- Most importantly, **emotional problems** can be overlooked and may be responsible for suboptimal performance, either with academic tasks or in the self-care area.

Consequences of the motor disorder

- Management of **drooling** (poor saliva control). Speech pathologists can assist with behavioural approaches and methods to improve oromotor control. Medication (anticholinergics) and surgery are helpful in some children.
- **Incontinence**. Children may be late in achieving bowel and bladder control due to cognitive deficits or lack of opportunity to access toileting facilities because of physical disability and/or inability to communicate. Sometimes children have detrusor over-activity causing urgency, frequency and incontinence.
- **Orthopaedic problems**. Children may develop contractures which require orthopaedic intervention. Surgery is mainly undertaken on the lower limb, but is occasionally helpful in the upper limb. Physiotherapists are essential in the postoperative rehabilitation phase.
  - The hip. Non walkers and those partially ambulant are at risk for hip subluxation and dislocation. Early detection is vital and hip X rays should be performed at yearly intervals. If there is evidence of subluxation or dislocation, children should be referred for an orthopaedic opinion. Dislocation causes pain and difficulty with perineal hygiene. Ambulant children occasionally develop hip problems.
  - The knee. Flexion contractures at the knee may require hamstring surgery.
  - The ankle. Equinus deformity at the ankle is the commonest orthopaedic problem in children with cerebral palsy. Toe walking is treated conservatively in young children with orthoses, inhibitory casts, and botulinum toxin A therapy. Older children benefit from surgery for a definitive correction of the deformity.
  - Multilevel surgery. Sometimes children require surgery at several different levels (for example, hip, knee and ankle). This involves a single hospitalisation and is called 'single event multilevel surgery'. It is of most benefit to children who walk independently or with the assistance of crutches. The usual age is between 8 and 12 years. The aims of surgery are to correct deformities and to improve both the appearance and efficiency of walking. An accurate assessment of the walking problems is undertaken in a gait laboratory. A carefully planned intensive rehabilitation physiotherapy programme lasting up to 1 year is required to maximise the benefits.
  - The upper limb. Procedures can be offered following careful assessment.
  - Scoliosis. Correction is sometimes necessary.
- Spasticity management is aimed at improving function, comfort and care and requires a team approach. Options include:
  - **Oral medications**, for example, diazepam, dantrolene sodium and baclofen. These medications may not be effective or may cause unwanted effects.
  - **Inhibitory casts** aim to increase joint range and facilitate improved quality of movement. The main

application is below knee casts for equinus but occasionally casts are used in the upper limb.

— **Botulinum toxin A** is injected into muscles and reduces localised spasticity.

— **Intrathecal baclofen** is administered by a pump implanted under the skin. This treatment is suitable for a small number of children with severe spasticity and may enhance quality of life.

— **Selective dorsal rhizotomy** is a neurosurgical procedure whereby anterior spinal roots are sectioned to reduce spasticity. Randomised trials have provided conflicting evidence of its usefulness, and an intensive rehabilitation period is required.

Assessment of the child's capabilities and referral to appropriate services for the child and family

The role of the team. Careful assessment in conjunction with a multidisciplinary team is essential to enable children to achieve their optimal physical potential and independence:

* Physiotherapists give practical advice to parents on positioning, handling and play, to minimise the effects of abnormal muscle tone and encourage the development of movement skills. They also give advice regarding the use of orthoses, special seating, wheelchairs and other mobility aids.
* Occupational therapists help parents to develop their child's upper limb and self-care skills, and also recommend suitable toys, equipment and home adaptations.
* Speech pathologists assist in the development of communication skills, including advising about augmentative communication systems for children with limited verbal skills. They provide guidance about feeding difficulties and saliva control problems.
* Orthotists, medical social workers, psychologists, special education teachers and nurses are helpful.

Therapy approaches. Therapy to address movement problems and to optimise children's progress in all areas of development is incorporated into early intervention and school programmes. The two most commonly used approaches by therapists in Australia are:

1. *Neurodevelopmental therapy (NDT).* This is a therapeutic approach to the assessment and management of movement problems with the goal of maximising the child's functional ability. This therapy was developed by Dr and Mrs Bobath and hence is sometimes known as 'Bobath therapy'. Family members receive education in NDT principles so that they can implement the programme at home, preschool and school.
2. *Programmes based on the principles of Conductive Education.* Conductive Education is a Hungarian system for educating children and adults with movement disorders. It provides an integrated group programme where children and parents learn to develop skills in all areas of life, for example, daily living, physical, social, emotional, cognitive and communication skills.

Assistive technology. Appropriate equipment tailored for the individual child can enhance communication, mobility, learning and socialisation. Examples include powered wheelchairs, electronic communication devices, and computers for educational and recreational purposes.

Trends in service provision. Services are best provided within local communities. Therapists and special education teachers work with children at home and later in childcare centres, kindergartens and schools. Most children attend regular preschools and schools but others benefit from attendance at centre based early intervention programmes and special schools. It is essential that parents are made aware of all available options.

Alternative therapies. There are many non mainstream (or 'alternative') treatments available. Sometimes great claims are made for alternative approaches that usually are not justified. Families can be reassured that any new treatment that is of value will be assessed and incorporated into mainstream practice. There is no evidence to suggest that alternative methods are superior to conventional treatments and some may do harm. It is important that professionals are aware of alternative approaches and are prepared to critically examine their claims.

Working with families. Care of the child with cerebral palsy involves developing a trusting and cooperative relationship with the parents. The child is part of a family unit, and concerns in parents or siblings must be addressed. As with all children, a supportive home environment builds self-esteem and confidence. Parents may need practical support, such as provision of respite care, and may be helped by meeting other families in similar circumstances, or by attending parent support groups. Provision of information about financial allowances is an important aspect of care.

Life expectancy

Children with mild and moderate cerebral palsy have a normal life span. Those with severe motor impairment, particularly those who are wheelchair dependent and require tube feeding, have a reduced life expectancy. Chronic lung disease is the most common cause of morbidity and mortality in this group.

Neurodegenerative disorders

This section addresses the problem of the child who presents because of concern about regression in development that has been normal previously, or with

Clinical example

Tom was born at 26 weeks gestation. He had many neonatal problems, including a grade IV intraventricular haemorrhage. The parents were informed that some degree of cerebral palsy was likely. At 4 months corrected age, his mother noted that his right hand was fisted. The diagnosis of cerebral palsy was confirmed and a physiotherapy programme was commenced.

When he began to walk independently at 24 months corrected age, his gait was noted to be asymmetrical with a tendency to walk on his toes on the right side. This problem was more apparent by 30 months and he fell more than would be expected for his age. Inhibitory casts were applied for 4 weeks and he was fitted with an ankle–foot orthosis (AFO). His walking pattern was much improved after this treatment, but after a further 10 months the problem had recurred. This time Tom appeared not only to walk in equinus, but he also was flexed at the knee. Hamstrings as well as calf muscles were tight. Botulinum toxin A injections were given to both muscle groups with an excellent result. A new AFO was made as he had grown considerably over this time. When Tom was 5 years old, he required further botulinum toxin A injections. At 6 years of age, surgery was undertaken by the same orthopaedic surgeon who had been monitoring him since the age of 24 months. Now he is 10 years old and no treatment is currently planned, although the family has been advised that further surgery may be required following his adolescent growth spurt.

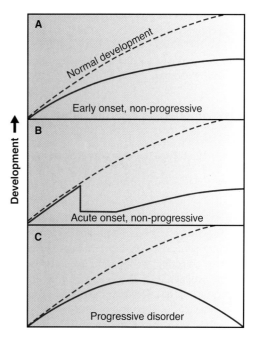

Fig. 57.3 Curves demonstrating the course of development over time in a child with static (**A** and **B**) and progressive neurological disease (**C**) compared with expected normal development. The actual age scale will vary, and a different curve may apply to each aspect of development in each child or disease process.

apparent worsening of a pre-existing neurological disorder. In infants and young children, concern may arise because of loss of gross and fine motor, personal social and language skills, as introduced in Chapter 4. Declining school performance may lead to referral of the older child.

An approach to this problem will be outlined, with examples of the many disorders that may present in this way. Some of these disorders are mentioned in Chapter 31. Broader management issues are covered in Chapter 11. The suggested reference texts listed at the end of this part provide a more detailed account of the wide range of neurodegenerative conditions. The diagnostic process is presented here as a series of questions.

Is there evidence of regression or lack of progress in any area of development?

This is sought in a sequential history of progress in each area of development, supplemented by questions such as 'How is your child's speech now, compared with this time last year? Is there any area where your child has gone backward or shown no progress at all?'

A clear ongoing loss of former skills, as shown in the latter part of curve C in Figure 57.3, raises obvious concern about a progressive disorder, but this may be less certain during the earlier 'plateau' phase before actual regression appears.

This is to be distinguished from the pattern of abnormally slow, but consistent, progress shown in curve A. This is often found in children with an intellectual disability or cerebral palsy, who may be seen to fall behind other children in abilities, while in fact continuing to acquire new skills, but at a slower pace, due to a static brain disorder arising in the prenatal or perinatal period.

A variation on this pattern, seen in curve B, occurs in the child whose initially normal progress is interrupted by an acute injury or illness (for example, meningitis) causing brain damage with later slower development.

Could the apparently progressive symptoms be due to a static disorder complicated by other factors?

Such factors are often amenable to treatment, and include the following:

- Frequent seizures, especially subtle myoclonic and atonic episodes, which may severely impair alertness and coordination.
- Drug toxicity, particularly from antiepileptic drugs.
- Psychological or emotional factors, including depression, withdrawal and psychosis. A particular problem is the tendency for autistic children to show arrest or

regression in social and language skills during the second year of life.

- Joint deformities due to soft tissue contractures in spastic 'cerebral palsy', leading to worsening of postural stability and gait.

If this is a progressive disorder, what is its distribution in terms of brain anatomy?

Important anatomical patterns to consider are as follows.

One lesion

Progressive hemiparesis, perhaps associated with focal seizures, suggests a cerebral hemisphere tumour, while spinal cord tumours may produce progressive weakness and spasticity affecting the lower limbs, either alone or with variable upper limb involvement, thus imitating diplegic cerebral palsy. This clinical pattern, sometimes with associated ataxia, is also seen in slowly progressive hydrocephalus, even in the absence of a cerebral neoplasm. The triad of cranial nerve palsies, corticospinal tract signs and ataxia suggests a brainstem glioma. Most other childhood tumours of the nervous system raise clear concern because of symptoms of raised intracranial pressure, but the insidious visual loss associated with optic nerve glioma and craniopharyngioma often is not recognised as a progressive problem until late in its course.

One functional system or group of systems

The prototype of 'system degenerations' is Friedreich ataxia. In this disorder, abnormalities of spinocerebellar, corticospinal and sensory tracts arise in the second decade of life. In other cerebellar ataxia syndromes there is involvement not only of neural pathways but of other body organs, as with ataxia telangiectasia, in which chromosomal breaks, immunological defects and skin lesions occur. A system disorder involving basal ganglia or extrapyramidal motor function may be inferred from the signs of dystonia, rigidity and choreoathetosis. An important example in this category is Wilson disease, which is treatable with penicillamine. Peripheral neuromuscular diseases, which also may be regarded as system disorders, are discussed separately in Chapter 58.

A multifocal process, with several discrete lesions in the brain

This is exemplified by recurrent cerebral infarctions associated with cyanotic congenital heart disease. In the absence of cardiac disease, repeated cerebral vascular occlusions are suggestive of moya-moya disease, a well recognised but poorly understood syndrome. Angiography here shows progressive occlusion of the major cerebral arteries, with a curious network of fine collateral vessels in the basal ganglia.

Among a recently defined group of disorders, known collectively as mitochondrial encephalomyelopathies, one form (MELAS) may present with repeated stroke-like episodes and multifocal brain lesions, associated with abnormal mitochondria in muscle, increased lactate levels in blood and cerebrospinal fluid, and deletions of the nuclear or mitochondrial DNA controlling mitochondrial enzyme activity.

Homocystinuria, an inborn error of amino acid metabolism, may present with recurrent cerebral venous or arterial thromboses. While multiple sclerosis is a major cause of multifocal lesions in young adults, it seldom begins in childhood.

A diffuse degenerative disorder of the nervous system

Diseases causing widespread loss of neurological function are generally separated into those that begin by affecting predominantly cortical grey matter, or nerve cell bodies, and those in which white matter, or nerve sheath myelin, is primarily involved. While this distinction is of clinical value, many disorders are not easily classified in this way.

Diffuse disorders of grey matter. These tend to cause seizures (often myoclonic) and early loss of intellectual function, with progressive impairment of language, comprehension and memory. In addition, involvement of nerve cells in the retina leads to a variable pattern of visual loss. This clinical syndrome is seen in several of the lipid storage disorders, of which Tay–Sachs disease is the best known. Subacute sclerosing panencephalitis is an infrequent complication of measles and evolves as a sequence of behavioural change, intellectual decline, myoclonic jerks and later rigidity.

Diffuse disorders of white matter. By involving corticospinal tracts, these tend to present with early motor impairment and spasticity, and may masquerade initially as 'cerebral palsy'. Impaired vision, when present, reflects optic pathways disease. Peripheral nerve myelin also may be involved, with clinical effects, as in Krabbe disease and metachromatic leucodystrophy, both of which are lipid storage disorders.

The above three questions can generally be answered after a careful clinical history and examination, but the remaining steps in diagnosis require knowledge of a growing number of recognised but rare diseases. In practice, this will involve specialist consultation.

Which disorders are known to occur in children of this age, and to produce the other clinical features present in this child?

Individual neurodegenerative diseases tend to have a characteristic age of onset. It is useful to consider broad age ranges (early infancy, late infancy and later childhood) in narrowing the diagnostic field. Next, by matching possible diagnoses against associated clinical findings, such as enlargement of liver and spleen, ocular abnormalities or unusual facial features, the physician may further refine the search and select the most relevant diagnostic tests.

Clinical example

Vincent, age 6 years, was referred to a paediatric neurologist because the teachers at his special school were concerned about his deterioration over several months, with loss of speech and comprehension of language, impaired coordination and increasingly hyperactive, aggressive behaviour. He had been diagnosed as having developmental delay at age 3 years because of limited speech and overactive behaviour. On examination, in addition to the developmental and behavioural findings, he had slightly coarse facial features with thickened eyebrows, a palpably enlarged liver and a mild thoracic kyphosis. These features raised the clinical suspicion that he had **Sanfilippo disease**, one of a group of disorders in which a deficiency of lysosomal enzymes leads to an accumulation of mucopolysaccharides in the tissues and excretion in the urine. The diagnosis was confirmed on specific blood and urine tests. Much professional support was needed by Vincent's parents, confronted with the prospect of their son's progressive dementia and immobility as well as the autosomal recessive inheritance of his condition.

A diagnosis is often reached merely by answering these questions. If not, it is useful next to turn from clinical features to pathophysiology.

Are any other, less evident diagnoses suggested by a systematic review of known mechanisms of disease?

The previous selective clinical correlations can be investigated further by considering in turn the major categories of:

- disease process, including metabolic errors, neurocutaneous disorders, slow virus infections and chronic intoxications
- biochemical substrates, such as lipids, vitamins and minerals,
- cellular organelles, that is lysosomes, peroxisomes and mitochondria, with their respective disorders.

This search may yield a further short list of possible diagnoses, known to the clinician but not considered, usually because of limited recent experience with them.

Are there any treatable disorders among the diagnoses being considered in this child?

This important question may alter the priority of investigation, as a potentially treatable disorder, however unlikely, must be rigorously excluded at an early stage. The major groups to recognise are the following:

- Neoplasms and other space occupying lesions involving the brain, and especially the spinal cord or optic nerves, where they are often not suspected until late, after irreversible damage.
- Subacute and chronic infections of the nervous system, such as tuberculous and cryptococcal meningitis and HIV infection.
- Intoxications: lead poisoning, glue sniffing, prescribed medications and, occasionally, chronic drug administration by a disturbed parent.
- Inborn errors of metabolism. The use of a modified diet in phenylketonuria is well known, but may also be of value in rarer disorders. Removal of toxic agents, for example, copper chelation in Wilson disease, may be possible. In seizures due to pyridoxine dependency and in other vitamin dependency syndromes, large doses of vitamins may effectively compensate for the metabolic defect.
- Deficiency states, especially of vitamins required for normal growth and function of the nervous system.

Effective treatment is not yet available for most degenerative neurological disorders of childhood, but accurate diagnosis remains the basis for genetic counselling, and for offering a realistic prognosis. A specific diagnosis or 'answer' is of great value to parents in coping with the distress of having a disabled child.

58 Neuromuscular disorders

A. Kornberg

Neuromuscular disease in childhood has until recently received little attention. This is not surprising given that many of the conditions were difficult to diagnose without sophisticated investigations and they were generally untreatable. However, this group of disorders cannot be ignored because of the significant morbidity and mortality associated with them, the genetic implications, and the arrival of potential therapies. The establishment of an early diagnosis is important in the rational management of these disorders as it allows prognostic and genetic information to be provided. Accurate diagnosis in this wide array of disorders is dependent on a careful clinical assessment followed by confirmatory and appropriate investigations. While recent advances have unravelled the molecular biology of many neuromuscular conditions, the clinical assessment of patients remains the cornerstone of the diagnosis and management. If clinical assessment is found wanting, the use of even the best technology may not supply the required diagnostic information.

The management of peripheral neuromuscular disease requires recognition, diagnosis, therapy and counselling.

Recognition that a child's presenting symptoms or signs may be due to peripheral neuromuscular disease

Please listen to the patient, he's trying to tell you what disease he has.

Dr Michael H. Brooke *The Clinician's View of Neuromuscular Disease*

Although the hallmark of neuromuscular disease is weakness, parents do not come into the consulting room saying 'I'm worried because my child is weak'. The physician needs to recognise that the presenting symptoms or signs relate to the peripheral neuromuscular system before the diagnostic process begins. The failure of recognition results in diagnostic delay with frequent presentations to a doctor, be it the family doctor or other specialist. While this failure does not usually affect the ultimate prognosis, it adds considerably to patient and parental frustration. The main tragedy occurs when opportunities for preventive strategies are missed and a second affected child is born in the immediate or even extended family.

Common presenting complaints include:
- difficulty walking and running
- poor at sports
- clumsy or poorly coordinated
- not able to keep up with peers
- frequent falls
- tires easily.

Another trap in the recognition of neuromuscular disease in childhood is that classical neurological signs, readily demonstrated at the end of a disease process in adult patients, are expected to be present in children at the beginning of the disease process. For example, in Charcot–Marie–Tooth (CMT) disease, adult patients will have gross pes cavus, areflexia and the so called 'inverted champagne bottle legs'. In children, the early features are commonly an abnormal walk or run, clumsiness, frequent falls, with foot deformity as a presenting symptom in a minority. In addition, although areflexia is the rule in adult patients, about 10% of children with Charcot–Marie–Tooth disease have normal reflexes at presentation. Not understanding the age dependent symptoms and signs of various neuromuscular disorders will lead to the failure of recognition of a neuromuscular disease in childhood.

Other modes of presentation include a family history of neuromuscular disease; weakness, hypotonia, respiratory or feeding difficulty in the neonatal period; delayed motor milestones; abnormal gait (particularly toe walking), and orthopaedic abnormality, such as foot deformity or scoliosis. Some patients present with non neuromuscular problems, such as mental retardation or delayed language development, as, for example, in Duchenne muscular dystrophy.

Diagnosis of neuromuscular disease based on anatomical, electrophysiological, biochemical, histopathological or DNA identification

After recognising that the symptoms are due to neuromuscular disease, the differential diagnosis is usually based on a logical anatomical approach. Although this may appear to be simplistic, as some disorders may affect more than one anatomical area or be multisystem, this approach will provide a broad differential diagnosis that will lead to a definitive diagnosis.

The anatomical localisation is based on the clinical findings listed in Table 58.1 and includes disorders affecting the:
- anterior horn cell
- anterior and posterior nerve roots

Table 58.1 Clinical clues helpful in establishing the site of the lesion in neuromuscular disease

Clinical feature	Anterior horn cell	Peripheral nerve	Neuromuscular junction	Muscle
Weakness	Proximal	Distal	Cranial/proximal	Proximal
Hypotonia	++	+	+/−	++
Hyporeflexia	+/−	Early	+/−	Late
Fasciculations	+++	+	−	−
Sensory abnormalities	−	+/−	−	−
Myotonia	−	−	−	+/−
Autonomic dysfunction	−	+/−	−	−
Muscle enlargement	−	−	−	+/−

- peripheral nerve (motor, sensory, autonomic)
- neuromuscular junction
- muscle.

The use of a time frame of symptoms, such as acute, subacute or chronic, may also provide an important filter for the differential diagnosis.

The definitive diagnosis rests on a combination of:
- clinical history and examination
- family history
- serum enzymes, particularly creatine kinase (CK)
- electrophysiology (for example, nerve conduction studies, electromyography, repetitive nerve stimulation)
- histology of muscle and/or nerve
- metabolic studies (for example, muscle glycogen, carnitine assay)
- DNA studies.

With only few exceptions, electrophysiological, biopsy and/or DNA studies should be undertaken as the implications of a neuromuscular disease diagnosis are so great for the child and immediate family, and sometimes the extended family.

Anterior horn cell disorders

Acute

Poliomyelitis

This disorder is rare in developed countries. It should still be considered where there is acute onset of lower motor neurone flaccid paralysis of a single limb, or with patchy asymmetrical distribution, particularly if associated with fever, vomiting, neck or spine stiffness and muscle pain or spasm.

Hopkins syndrome

A clinical syndrome of asthma with flaccid paralysis of a limb resembling poliomyelitis has been recognised (Hopkins syndrome). Anterior horn cell dysfunction has been identified with magnetic resonance imaging through the clinically affected segments of the spinal cord. Coxsackie and echovirus infections have occasionally produced weakness thought to be of anterior horn cell origin.

Chronic

In childhood the chronic disorders, characterised pathologically by degeneration of anterior horn cells and associated clinically with progressive muscle weakness (at least for a time), are called the spinal muscular atrophies (SMAs). The important clinical syndromes and their classification are listed in Table 58.2.

SMA type I (Werdnig–Hoffmann disease)

This autosomal recessive disorder occurs in approximately 1 in 25 000 live births, making it one of the commonest fatal autosomal recessive disorders humans. The earliest symptom may be decreased fetal movements in late pregnancy. Presentation is invariably before 6 months of age and is either at birth, with hypotonia, weakness, joint deformity and respiratory difficulty, or more commonly later with marked hypotonia and limb weakness,

Table 58.2 Clinical classification of childhood onset proximal SMA

Designation	Symptom onset (months)	Course	Death (years)
I (severe)	0–6	Never sits without support	<2
II (intermediate)	<18	Never stands without aid	>2
III (mild)	>18	Stands alone	Adult

poor feeding, poor cough, and cry. The onset is sometimes relatively rapid and when first seen the child usually is severely weak (Fig. 58.1). Weakness, although generalised, is maximal in the shoulder and hip girdle muscles. Intercostal muscle weakness leads to chest deformity, a poor cough and a weak cry. The respiratory pattern becomes diaphragmatic. Deep tendon reflexes are absent. Fasciculations of the tongue are an important clinical clue, but this can be an exceedingly difficult sign to be certain about and one can only be confident if the baby is relaxed and there are no 'voluntary' movements of the tongue. Facial weakness is only mild and extraocular movements remain full, giving the baby an alert appearance. Death, usually from pneumonia and respiratory failure, occurs by 18 months of age in 95% of patients, with those with onset in the first 2 months of life having the shortest survival.

The genetic abnormality has been mapped to chromosome 5q13.3 and involves several different genes (SMN and NAIP). Prenatal diagnosis is available.

Key learning points

- **A positive diagnosis of fasciculations of the tongue should not be made unless the tongue has no voluntary movement, i.e. is not protruded, the child is not crying or actively moving the tongue.**
- **The presence of deep tendon reflexes makes it extremely unlikely that the child has type I SMA and an alternative diagnosis should be considered.**

SMA type II (chronic childhood spinal muscular atrophy)

Clinical onset is almost invariably before 3 years of age, with SMA type II at least as common as Werdnig–Hoffmann disease. About one half of children affected by this disorder never walk, and only 5% are still walking by 20 years of age. Survival varies from 18 months through to adult life.

The clinical picture is one of severe generalised weakness and wasting, with proximal predominance. Deep tendon reflexes are decreased or absent and often there are fasciculations of the tongue. The facial muscles may be mildly weak, but eye movements remain normal and the patient usually is normal intellectually. Some patients have a fine, rapid tremor of the hands. Major management problems include the prevention of orthopaedic deformity, especially scoliosis, and the management of the respiratory complications of muscle weakness. The genetic abnormality is allelic to that for SMA type I.

SMA type III (Kugelberg–Welander syndrome)

Patients with late onset and a moderately benign clinical course are classified as SMA type III (Kugelberg–Welander syndrome). Most have onset in the first 2 decades with only a few in the third decade and survival is usually for many decades. While many remain ambulant over many years, particularly those with later onset, some do lose the ability to walk during childhood years. The genetic abnormality is allelic to that for SMA types I and II.

Peripheral nerve disorders

A number of peripheral neuropathies occur in childhood, with various time courses (acute, subacute or chronic). They may be inherited or acquired; they may involve motor, sensory or autonomic fibres, or commonly mixtures of all three. Pathologically, they may be associated with combinations of demyelination and axonal degeneration. Some central nervous system degenerative disorders, such as Krabbe disease and metachromatic leucodystrophy, may also have a peripheral neuropathy component. The commonest disorders in childhood are Guillain–Barré syndrome and peroneal muscular atrophy or Charcot–Marie–Tooth disease. Chronic inflammatory demyelinating peripheral neuropathy (CIDP), while uncommon, is important because it is responsive to immunotherapies.

Acute neuropathies

Guillain–Barré syndrome

Guillain-Barré syndrome (GBS) is the most common acute neuropathy in clinical practice and can occur at any

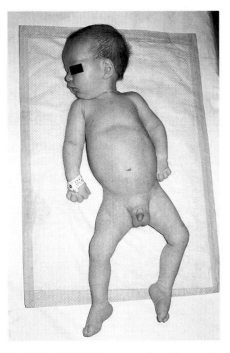

Fig. 58.1 Child with SMA I showing profound hypotonia and weakness.

age, although it is rare in infancy. An infection, commonly of the upper respiratory tract or gastrointestinal tract (*Campylobacter jejuni*), precedes the neurological syndrome in at least 50% of cases. Typical GBS is a monophasic illness with symmetric, ascending weakness involving proximal and distal muscles. Paraesthesia and muscle pain may be presenting complaints but sensory impairment is usually minimal. Severe back pain and stiffness may occur, especially in young children. Tendon reflexes are lost early in the course of the illness. Cranial nerve involvement, particularly the facial nerve, is relatively common. Autonomic involvement can cause wide fluctuations of the blood pressure as well as cardiac arrhythmias and bladder dysfunction. Respiratory failure occurs in about 30% of patients and in addition may be associated with pharyngeal dysfunction. GBS typically progresses over a period of less than 4 weeks, with most patients reaching their maximal deficit within 2 weeks of onset. Artificial ventilation for periods of up to 8 weeks occasionally may be required. Recovery continues over weeks to many months, with most children returning to normal function. Some more severely affected children may have residual weakness.

Diagnosis is based on the clinical features, with elevation of the CSF protein with only a few, if any, cells. A nerve conduction study may be useful in difficult diagnostic situations. Intravenous gamma globulin or plasmapheresis, if used early, may hasten recovery but otherwise treatment is supportive.

Management of GBS requires special expertise in medical and nursing care and children should be referred to centres used to dealing with this condition. Monitor blood pressure and cardiac rhythm, as autonomic dysfunction is one of the potentially serious complications. In severely affected individuals who are ventilated and with little movement, it may appear that the patient is unresponsive. The patient can see, hear and think. It is important to explain what is happening at all times and reassure them that they will get better.

Chronic neuropathies

Chronic inflammatory demyelinating peripheral neuropathy

This condition is rare but treatable and is thought to be an autoimmune disorder. It usually presents as a subacute or chronic neuropathy. The course can be monophasic but is usually relapsing and remitting over many weeks or months duration. Acute presentations can occur and may cause confusion with Guillain–Barré syndrome. Symptoms and signs of weakness, often most prominent proximally, bring the child to medical attention. The diagnosis is confirmed by nerve conduction studies, elevated CSF protein and pathological abnormalities in a nerve biopsy.

Intravenous immunoglobulin, corticosteroids, other immunosuppressive agents and plasmapheresis have all been used with varying degrees of success. Many children regain normal strength, although some are left with muscle weakness.

Peroneal muscular atrophy (Charcot–Marie–Tooth; hereditary motor and sensory neuropathy) syndrome

This is the commonest chronic inherited neuropathy syndrome in childhood. Various forms of it are known and are based on electrophysiological and DNA criteria. Most families show autosomal dominant inheritance, but autosomal recessive and X linked forms can occur. Approximately 60% have onset of symptoms in the first decade of life.

Pes cavus, loss of foot dorsiflexion and eversion, hyporeflexia and sensory loss are typical clinical features in childhood. However, relatively asymptomatic children may present because of a family history, while others present with gait disturbance, particularly toe walking, frequent falling or poor coordination. Weakness and wasting in the legs may progress slowly and distal weakness in the arms is sometimes seen. Thickened peripheral nerves can occasionally be palpated.

The diagnosis can be confirmed by a nerve conduction study but readily available DNA studies are the usual first step in diagnosis. The DNA studies show a duplicated region on chromosome 17p (PMP-22 gene). Parents of children with suspected PMA should be examined.

No cure is available but ankle–foot orthoses or orthopaedic procedures to correct foot deformity are often required and helpful. Progression is only relatively slow, with patients leading a fairly full life.

Clinical example

Claudine, a 5 year old girl, was seen by her paediatrician because of frequent falling. He found mild ataxia of gait and areflexia, but no other abnormality. There was an extensive family history (autosomal dominant inheritance pattern) of a chronic neuropathy consistent with PMA. Her mother was asymptomatic.

Examination of Claudine's mother revealed minor sensory loss in the feet and hyporeflexia. Both mother and child had DNA evidence of the PMP-22 gene duplication, confirming the diagnosis of PMA.

Children with neuromuscular disease often do not have all the clinical features seen in adults and sometimes it is the family history that gives the vital clue. The clinical severity of PMA varies considerably and some adults can be asymptomatic. Careful clinical examination of a parent and further diagnostic studies sometimes unmask the apparent missing link. The absence of foot deformity or sensory disturbance in a child does not exclude PMA.

Neuromuscular junction disorders

Acute

Infant botulism

Infant botulism results from the production of *Clostridium botulinum* exotoxin in the gastrointestinal tract. It differs from botulism associated with food poisoning, in which there is ingestion of preformed toxin from contaminated food. In infant botulism, botulinum spores are ingested, with honey implicated in many cases. The disease usually occurs in infants under 9 months of age.

Constipation for days or weeks typically precedes the onset of symptoms of floppiness, weakness and ptosis, which occur over hours or 1–2 days at most. Feeding and swallowing difficulty, a poor cough, weak cry, hyporeflexia and respiratory insufficiency are typical. Extraocular movements may be impaired and dilated, sluggishly reacting pupils are often seen and can be helpful diagnostically. Deterioration may be rapid, with many patients requiring artificial ventilation for up to 2 months while the neuromuscular junctions regrow.

Diagnosis is clinical, supported by isolation of the organism and its toxin from faeces. Treatment is supportive. Botulinum antitoxin has been used but has not been shown to be helpful. The prognosis is excellent, with full recovery unless complications from cerebral hypoxia intervene. Prompt recognition and transfer to a facility capable of long term ventilatory support is essential.

Chronic

Autoimmune myasthenia gravis

Myasthenia in most children has an autoimmune basis with antibody directed against neuromuscular junction postsynaptic acetylcholine receptors. Onset occurs at any time from the second year of life onwards. Symptoms are present for less than 1 month in the majority of patients and many have an episode of respiratory failure if untreated. Symptoms and signs are similar to those in adults, although relatively more prepubertal patients have only ocular problems. Ptosis, eye movement disorder, diplopia, difficulty chewing and swallowing, and slurred speech with or without predominantly proximal limb muscle weakness of recent onset should raise the suspicion of myasthenia gravis. Fatigability, the hallmark of myasthenia, is usually prominent, but this is not invariable.

Suspicion of myasthenia gravis should trigger an urgent diagnostic assessment. Diagnosis is based on clinical observation of fatigability, often best seen in the upper eyelid, response to intravenous or intramuscular anticholinesterase agents such as edrophonium or neostigmine, repetitive nerve stimulation and assay of acetylcholine receptor antibodies. Symptomatic relief may be obtained by oral administration of an anticholinesterase, commonly pyridostigmine. Corticosteroids, thymectomy and plasmapheresis have a role in selected circumstances. Although myasthenia gravis is a serious long term and potentially fatal disorder, the disease remits in some children.

Transient neonatal myasthenia gravis

Transient neonatal myasthenia gravis occurs in about 10% of offspring of mothers with myasthenia gravis. It is due to placental transfer of antiacetylcholine receptor antibodies from a myasthenic mother to her fetus during pregnancy. This was one of the reasons why a humoral mechanism for myasthenia gravis was considered highly likely, prior to proof of this mechanism by passive transfer of myasthenia from human to mouse accomplished in the mid 1970s.

Onset of symptoms is not immediately after birth but is usually in the first 96 hours; feeding difficulty, respiratory difficulty and weakness or hypotonia are the main features. Myasthenic symptoms in the mother may be minimal. Appropriate supportive measures and anticholinesterase medication are used until the syndrome resolves over the ensuing weeks. This correlates with the expected diminution of passively transferred IgG antiacetylcholine antibodies that had been transferred from mother to infant. The infant returns to normal and does not subsequently have myasthenia gravis.

Congenital myasthenic syndromes

Congenital myasthenic syndromes are not one disease but many different rare genetic–biochemical disorders of the neuromuscular junction encompassing both the pre- and postsynaptic regions. They are not autoimmune disorders. Detailed electrophysiological and morphological testing, available in only a few laboratories, is usually required to diagnose and characterise these disorders definitively. Hypotonia, limb weakness, facial weakness, ptosis, ophthalmoplegia and apnoeic episodes, particularly with infections, may be seen but the emphasis varies with the particular syndrome. Some show improvement with time despite life threatening episodic apnoea in infancy, while others have more persistent problems. Individuals do not have acetylcholine receptor antibodies. Some respond to antianticholinesterase preparations while others do not or worsen. As these are not autoimmune disorders, immunomodulatory therapies normally used in myasthenia gravis are without benefit.

Muscle disorders

Acute myopathies

Myopathic disorders with acute onset of weakness are uncommon. Snake bite or drugs may rarely trigger rhabdomyolysis, or acute muscle breakdown. The dominantly inherited, sometimes fatal, syndrome of malignant hyperthermia during anaesthesia causes muscle necrosis and myoglobinuria. This disorder is associated with central core disease (see below). Rhabdomyolysis with myoglobinuria appears occasionally after an upper respiratory tract infection or after exercise and is probably related to an underlying metabolic disorder of muscle.

Chronic myopathies

Congenital myopathies

The congenital myopathies are a group of inherited disorders clinically relatively non specific, but with specific or distinctive findings on morphological analysis of the muscle biopsy. Advances in histochemical and electron microscopy techniques over the last 30–40 years have enabled characterisation of patients into well defined myopathies, whereas previously they were given non specific diagnoses such as 'floppy infant syndrome'. The identification of these disorders allows important genetic and prognostic information to be given to the family.

These myopathies, usually inherited, are characterised by onset of weakness and hypotonia at or shortly after birth, or occasionally later in childhood or adulthood. Weakness may be mild or severe and usually is only slowly progressive. Pathologically there are structural changes in individual muscle fibres or variations in the number or size of the muscle fibre types.

Some of the well recognised disorders are central core myopathy (Fig. 58.2) and nemaline myopathy.

Key learning point

- **In a family exhibiting autosomal dominant inheritance of a muscle disorder consistent with a congenital myopathy, central core disease should be considered a possibility and precautions taken against malignant hyperthermia if an anaesthetic is given (e.g. for a muscle biopsy).**

Progressive muscular dystrophies

The muscular dystrophies are a group of inherited disorders of muscle characterised by weakness presenting from birth to late adulthood, with the common feature being the pathological appearance of dystrophic muscle (Fig. 58.3). These disorders primarily affect skeletal muscle but other tissues may be involved; for example, congenital muscular dystrophy may be associated with white matter abnormalities in the brain. The dystrophies are the commonest serious muscle diseases and as a group place a significant burden on the patient, the family and the community in medical, social and economic terms.

The various forms of muscular dystrophy share a common pathogenesis of muscle plasma membrane instability secondary to the lack of, or abnormality of, proteins and glycoproteins linking the subsarcolemmal cytoskeleton to the extracellular matrix (Fig. 58.4). Not all dystrophies have had the absent or abnormal protein characterised. Absence or dysfunction of these structural proteins makes the muscle fibre more prone to damage.

Many of the muscular dystrophies share common clinical features although the severity varies. The age of onset, pattern of weakness, family history and relatively specific findings on examination are important in diagnosing the type of muscular dystrophy. Some of the muscular dystrophies are named because of their pattern of weakness but these labels will probably change with the identification of protein defects.

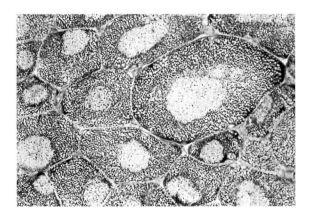

Fig. 58.2 Muscle biopsy in central core disease.

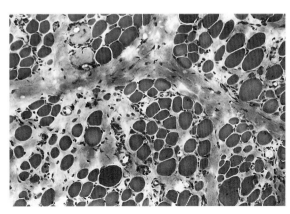

Fig. 58.3 Dystrophic muscle biopsy.

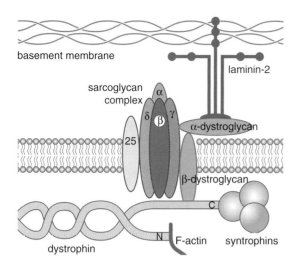

Fig. 58.4 Subsarcolemmal cytoskeleton.

The clinical features of some muscular dystrophies are described below.

Duchenne muscular dystrophy. DMD is the most common muscular dystrophy, occurring in 1 in 3500–5000 live male births. It is an X linked disorder and occurs nearly exclusively in males. It is a disease of devastating proportions as it is progressive, has significant genetic implications, there are no curative treatments available, and it has serious medical complications. It causes death in the second or third decade and ranks high on the list of devastating diseases as judged by its effect on the person, the family and the requirements for community resources.

DMD is caused by a mutation at the Xp21 chromosome site. This causes a lack of dystrophin, a muscle protein that is thought to be important in the stability of the muscle membrane. Two thirds of patients have a family history of muscular dystrophy or are isolated cases with an unsuspecting female carrier in the family, while one third appear to arise as spontaneous mutations.

Development in the first year of life is usually normal. The first symptoms are usually recognised from 18 months to 4 years of age, with delayed walking being the most common presenting complaint. Approximately 50% of children with DMD do not walk before 18 months of age. Abnormal walking or running, toe walking, difficulty in climbing, difficulty in getting up from the floor or chair, and frequent falls are other prominent early features. A significant percentage of children will also have developmental problems other than motor delay, such as intellectual impairment or delayed language development. The intellectual impairment and language delay are non progressive and mean IQ is approximately 85. While many are intellectually normal, some children are moderately intellectually disabled. The dual problems of motor and intellectual disabilities are severely incapacitating socially and educationally.

Proximal muscle weakness accounts for the motor difficulties. This can be demonstrated on formal testing or alternatively by functional testing, such as getting the child to rise from the floor. Typically, with this action the Gower sign is exhibited (Fig. 58.5). A Gower sign is not specific for DMD and is seen in other disorders with proximal muscle weakness. Enlargement (pseudohypertrophy) and firmness of the calf, quadriceps and triceps muscles is commonly seen (Fig. 58.6).

Some variability in course is exhibited from child to child, although the following generalisations encompass most children with DMD. Between the ages of 4 and 6 years there is an apparent improvement in mobility, with the children typically performing new motor activities. This is because normal muscle development (and regeneration) outstrips the degenerative process. After this period of improvement, relentless decline in function occurs, with increasing proximal and distal weakness in the limbs. Trunk muscles are also weakened. This leads to a worsening waddling gait, increasing lumbar lordosis and increasing equinovarus foot deformities. Independent mobility is lost, usually between 8 and 13 years of age, with the child becoming wheelchair bound, after which scoliosis generally develops. During the second decade of life there is a gradual decline in pulmonary function, related to the scoliosis and progressive muscle weakness. Death is usually due to respiratory complications, although cardiac failure secondary to a cardiomyopathy can occur. Cardiac arrhythmias may be a terminal event.

The diagnosis of DMD should be based on the family history (if any), clinical features, serum creatine kinase test, DNA deletion testing and muscle biopsy. Pathological confirmation of the diagnosis is essential except where the diagnosis has been confirmed in another family member or by a DNA deletion. The creatine kinase is a reliable screening test and invariably is grossly elevated in a child with DMD, even from the neonatal period. Conversely, a normal creatine kinase test after the neonatal period excludes the later development of DMD.

Key learning point

- **The commonest reason for the late diagnosis of DMD is to not think of the diagnosis in a young male with delayed motor, mental or language development.**

Effective genetic counselling can be offered only if the first case in the family is diagnosed before other affected males are born. The early diagnosis of DMD can be facilitated by using the following criteria for ordering serum creatine kinase estimations in males:
- known or suspected family history of dystrophy
- male not walking before 18 months of age without obvious cause
- unexplained gait disturbance (particularly toe walking)
- unexplained mental retardation
- unexplained language delay.

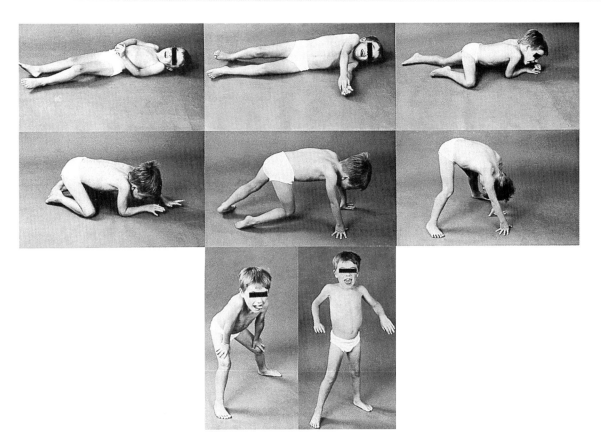

Fig. 58.5 The Gower sign in a patient with Duchenne dystrophy, illustrating the sequence of manoeuvres required to rise from the supine position. (From Williams 1982, with permission.)

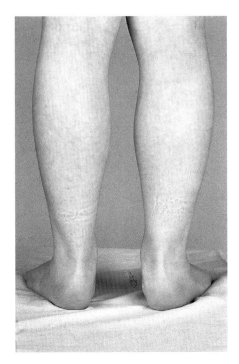

Fig. 58.6 Pseudohypertrophy of muscles.

Detection and counselling of female carriers is a most important aspect of family management. The male offspring of a known carrier have a 50% risk of having Duchenne dystrophy, while 50% of female offspring will be carriers. Females may still be carriers even though there is no other family history. Only 60% of known carriers have an elevated creatine kinase level and hence a normal level does not exclude the carrier state. DNA technology can now be applied to offer antenatal diagnosis by detecting deletions from the X chromosome or by linkage analysis.

Currently there is no cure for muscular dystrophy. Corticosteroids may provide symptomatic improvement in strength but they do not change the natural history of the disorder.

Management involves a very positive approach to satisfying the emotional, social and educational needs of the child and his family, togther with judicious use of physiotherapy, orthotic devices and surgery for orthopaedic deformity.

Becker muscular dystrophy. Becker muscular dystrophy is a disorder allelic to DMD but much less common. It is less severe than DMD and has a variable age of presentation.

Facioscapulohumeral (FSH) syndrome. Facioscapulo-humeral (FSH) muscular dystrophy is a relatively common autosomal dominant disorder which predominantly affects the shoulder girdle, in particular the periscapular, humeral and facial muscles. It is a relatively mild disorder with very slow progression. Onset is commonly in adolescence or early adult life, although occasionally it may be very early childhood.

In a typical case, facial muscle weakness is one of the first symptoms. Patients have difficulty closing the eyes, blowing out the cheeks, whistling or sucking through a straw. The shoulder girdle weakness usually begins at the same time as the facial weakness is noted and can be quite asymmetric. Symptoms include difficulty lifting the arms above the head. There is obvious winging of the scapulae in adult patients, but this may not be so obvious in children. On abduction of the shoulders, the scapulae move upwards and give the shoulders a characteristic appearance. Foot drop is not uncommon. An infantile form has been described which presents with more severe weakness. The infantile form of FSH dystrophy is associated with deafness and visual loss.

The locus for autosomal dominant FSH has been mapped to the distal arm of chromosome 4.

Sensorineuronal hearing loss and Coats disease, a proliferative retinopathy, are associated with early onset FSH dystrophy. Aggressive treatment of these associated disorders is important.

Myotonic disorders

These are a clinically heterogeneous group, with myotonia being the characteristic clinical feature. Myotonia is the inability of muscles to relax after voluntary contraction or stimulation. Myotonia can be detected during attempted relaxation of a voluntary contraction, such as after shaking hands or eyelid closure, by percussion of a muscle, or by electromyography. Older children may describe myotonia as stiffness or cramping.

Many of these disorders have been shown to be due to defects of muscle ion channels. In some instances different mutations within the one gene can cause myotonia and/or periodic paralysis.

Myotonia congenita (Thomsen disease)

Autosomal dominant and autosomal recessive forms occur. Onset is in infancy or early childhood with symptoms due to myotonia, such as stiffness, difficulty initiating rapid movements and sometimes feeding difficulties. Muscle hypertrophy is common. The myotonia decreases with continued activity and may be aggravated by cold. Improvement occurs with increasing age. Symptomatic relief of myotonia with quinine or mexiletine may be useful.

Myotonic dystrophy (Steinert disease)

Myotonic dystrophy is an autosomal dominant disorder, but an affected parent may be relatively asymptomatic and not diagnosed until detailed examination and investigation is undertaken. The disease is due to an excessive number of repeats of the sequence CTG on the long arm of chromosome 19 and this can be used for diagnostic testing in difficult cases and for antenatal diagnosis. The spectrum of clinical severity in myotonic dystrophy is extremely broad, requiring genetic testing to help clarify the diagnosis in minimally affected patients.

Juvenile type. The clinical features are similar to those seen in adults, with distal muscle weakness, wasting and myotonia, an expressionless face due to facial muscle weakness and ptosis. Cataracts, frontal alopecia, testicular atrophy, cardiopulmonary insufficiency and dementia may occur in adult life.

Congenital type. A syndrome of hypotonia, weakness, arthrogryposis, feeding difficulty, respiratory difficulty and marked facial weakness all present at birth, along with other dysmorphic features, has been recognised. Invariably the mother has myotonic dystrophy. Mental retardation is common if the child survives the neonatal period.

Clinical example

Mrs McGill, aged 25 years, had myotonic dystrophy, as did her father, sister and brother. She had a son and twin daughters who were normal at birth and who remained asymptomatic. Her next child, Tessa, was 4 weeks premature and at birth was very hypotonic, had some respiratory difficulty and required gavage feeding. There was marked bilateral facial weakness, talipes equinovarus and mild flexion deformity at the knees. The respiratory and feeding difficulties gradually resolved, but the facial muscle weakness remained and she later showed delay in motor and language milestones. There was no clinical myotonia when Tessa was seen at 3 years of age.

Tessa had typical features of the congenital form of myotonic dystrophy, which typically occurs if it is the mother who is the affected parent. Some babies are stillborn, while others do not survive the neonatal period. She was only moderately affected and will survive into adult life, but will almost certainly require special schooling. The dominant inheritance is clear from the family history. Mrs McGill and her husband wanted to know if the other children might develop the disease. Although they were asymptomatic at the time, there was still a chance that they had inherited the abnormal gene. DNA testing for the triplet expansion on chromosome 19 could be used to allow antenatal diagnosis.

Key leaning point

- **Facial diplegia with respiratory difficulty or pharyngeal incoordination in a neonate should raise the suspicion of congenital myotonic dystrophy.**

Inflammatory myopathy

Acute viral myositis

Acute viral myositis is a clinically recognisable syndrome of acute onset of pain and tenderness of the gastrocnemius and soleus muscles several days after an upper respiratory tract infection, often with influenza B virus. Recovery occurs in a few days.

Chronic inflammatory myopathy

This may occur as 'idiopathic' disorders, such as dermatomyositis or polymyositis, or as part of a recognised collagen vascular disease. The clinical features are discussed in Chapter 44.

Metabolic myopathies

A large number of individually uncommon metabolic disorders may produce episodic, acute or chronic muscle weakness, hypotonia, stiffness or cramping, exercise intolerance or myoglobinuria. Symptoms are sometimes accentuated or precipitated by exercise, rest after exercise, fasting or excessive carbohydrate intake.

The underlying metabolic defects usually are in glycogen metabolism (for example, Pompe disease), lipid metabolism (for example, carnitine deficiency, carnitine palmityltransferase deficiency), potassium metabolism (for example, the periodic paralyses associated with hyper-, hypo- or normokalaemia), or a variety of mitochondrial functions (for example, myopathies with cytochrome oxidase deficiency and Kearns–Sayre syndrome of progressive external ophthalmoplegia).

Knowledge of the underlying metabolic causes of many of these disorders is increasing and the hope is that, once the underlying pathophysiological processes are elucidated, more specific and effective therapies will become available.

The 'floppy' infant syndrome

Hypotonia, or floppiness, is a common observation in infancy and has many different causes. Normal muscle tone depends not only on the peripheral neuromuscular system, but also on spinal cord and higher centres. Indeed, disorders affecting the central nervous system are more frequently the cause of the floppy infant syndrome than peripheral neuromuscular causes (Ch. 57). Muscle tone is assessed by observation of posture, assessment of the resistance of joints to passive movements and of range of movement.

When an infant or young child is found to be significantly hypotonic, an important question is whether the hypotonia is 'central' or 'peripheral' in origin. Hypotonia of peripheral neuromuscular origin usually is associated with significant weakness (for example, Werdnig–Hoffmann disease), while central hypotonia usually is not associated with significant weakness (for example, Down syndrome or Prader–Willi syndrome). In practice, the differentiation in early childhood can sometimes be quite difficult. Apart from the absence of significant weakness, clues to a central cause of hypotonia may be:

- a history of adverse perinatal events
- abnormal behaviour in the neonatal period
- delayed mental development
- seizures
- abnormality of head size or shape
- the presence of normal or brisk deep tendon reflexes.

Hypotonia of peripheral neuromuscular origin is usually, but not invariably, accompanied by hyporeflexia in an alert baby with normal mental development.

Acknowledgements

I would like to thank Dr Lloyd K. Shield who has been my mentor and the person who kindled my interest in neuromuscular disease. Dr Shield's previous contributions to this textbook form the major part of this chapter.

Large heads, hydrocephalus and neural tube defects

P. Flett, R. Russo

Large heads

A large head may be due to enlargement of the brain substance or the fluid filled spaces of the brain. The more common causes include:

- a large cerebrum
- an oversized, overweight brain (as in megalencephaly)
- a dilated cerebrum (as in hydrocephalus)
- a tiny cerebrum (as with large chronic subdural hygromas)
- no cerebrum (as in hydranencephaly).

The two major categories of aetiology responsible for megalencephaly are anatomic and metabolic. A large head with normal sized ventricles and normal neurodevelopmental examination may be related to familial factors, as in benign familial anatomic megalencephaly or macrocephaly. However, the large dolichocephalic head in cerebral gigantism will have large ventricles, but normal ventricular pressure, and associated limited intellect, poor coordination and coarse facial features.

Head enlargement in metabolic megalencephaly is a late manifestation of many cerebral degenerative disorders, such as lysosomal storage diseases. Megalencephaly occurs in a wide variety of clinical disorders and syndromes, can be unilateral or bilateral, and is associated with a wide spectrum of developmental symptoms and signs. An acute increase in intracranial pressure should prompt consideration of the possibility of drug intoxication (tetracycline, vitamin A, nalidixic acid), lead encephalopathy, subdural haematoma and Reye syndrome.

Hydranencephaly is a condition of uncertain aetiology. The cerebral cortex is represented by a thin membrane composed of glial cells, with islands of cerebral cortex sometimes scattered in this tissue. The third ventricle, basal ganglia, brainstem and cerebellum are present but may reveal morphological abnormalities. The head size is usually normal at birth but increases rapidly within a few weeks of life. Neurological function initially may be normal, but shortly after gross neurological abnormality is evident (rigid muscle tone, tremors and persistent and exaggerated primitive reflexes). Optic atrophy is common and the head transilluminates readily. The child sleeps excessively, is irritable, feeds poorly and has unstable thermoregulation. Electroencephalography reveals a flat tracing or a few low voltages over islands of cerebral cortex.

Hydrocephalus

Hydrocephalus (Greek: *hydro* meaning water, and *cephale*, head) refers to a group of conditions characterised by:

- an increase in cerebrospinal fluid (CSF) volume
- ventricular dilatation
- elevation of intraventricular pressure.

Hydrocephalus occurs when there is an imbalance between the formation and absorption of CSF. Impaired absorption is almost always due to some degree of obstruction along the CSF pathways. If the passage of CSF is obstructed within the ventricular system, the resultant hydrocephalus is labelled *non communicating*, while if obstruction exists in the surface pathways, the hydrocephalus is described as being *communicating*. The rate of this volume change varies from patient to patient, and depends in large part on the degree of obstruction. The lesions that commonly produce hydrocephalus are listed in Table 59.1.

In supratentorial lesions, CSF obstruction is a late event so that neurological or endocrinological abnormalities often precede symptoms of raised intracranial pressure. Less commonly, cerebral tuberculoma, torular

Clinical example

Ivan, a 5 year old boy, presented with a 2 month history of early morning headache and vomiting. This was associated with a decline in his school performance and he was noted to be increasingly unsteady on his feet. The significant findings on examination included a wide based unsteady gait, horizontal nystagmus and severe bilateral papilloedema. CT revealed the presence of a large mass in the cerebellar vermis that was distorting the fourth ventricle.

He underwent a craniotomy and the tumour arising in the cerebellar vermis was excised. Following operation the symptoms of raised intracranial pressure subsided and serial CT showed a resolution of the dilated lateral and third ventricles.

With this patient, excision of the obstructing mass was an effective form of treatment for a significant degree of non communicating hydrocephalus.

The presenting symptoms were due in part to raised intracranial pressure and in part to interference with cerebellar function.

Table 59.1 Lesions producing hydrocephalus

Non communicating	Communicating

Aqueduct stenosis or atresia
  Commonest site of intraventricular obstruction in infants with congenital hydrocephalus
  May occur as an isolated anomaly or may be associated with myelomeningocele and the Arnold–Chiari malformation
  Histologically, subependymal gliosis around the aqueduct is demonstrable
  May be slowly progressive in some, not being clinically apparent for several years before obstructive symptoms appear
  Sporadic
  Familial
  – inherited as a sex linked trait, features include a short flexed thumb, mental retardation and other cerebral abnormalities
 	
Obstruction at the fourth ventricle
  Dandy–Walker syndrome
  – cystic dilatation of the fourth ventricle, with cerebellar hypoplasia; other structural brain anomalies may also occur
  – associated with atresia of the exit foramina of the fourth ventricle
  – hydrocephalus may be present at birth or may develop subsequently
  – diagnosis is suggested in typical cases by the shape of the skull and the presence of cerebellar signs
  Arachnoiditis
 	
Obstruction due to intracranial mass lesions
  Should always be considered in any child where head enlargement develops in late infancy or childhood
  Neoplasm, cysts
  – childhood tumours usually arise in the posterior cranial fossa and include medulloblastoma, astrocytoma and ependymoma
  – intracranial pressure develops early, due to their close proximity to the fourth ventricle
  – ataxia, incoordination nystagmus and papilloedema are suggestive of the diagnosis
  – differential diagnosis includes craniopharyngioma, gliomas, pinealomas and arachnoid cysts
  Haematoma
  Galanic vein aneurysm
 	
Ventricular inflammations (rare)
	Arnold–Chiari malformation
	  With myelomeningocele (type 2) (Fig. 59.3)
	  Without myelomeningocele (Type 1)
	  – consists of
	    • downward displacement and elongation of the hind brain
	    • herniation of the medulla, cerebellar vermis and inferior part of the fourth ventricle into the upper cervical canal
	  – CSF flow is impaired usually within the subarachnoid space
	  – hydrocephalus usually develops early in infancy
	  – frequently is associated with cranium bifidum, myelomeningocele and hydromyelia
	
	Encephalocele
	
	Meningeal adhesions
	  Postinflammatory
	  Posthaemorrhagic
	  – may be secondary to neonatal meningitis (postinflammatory adhesions) or intraventricular or subarachnoid haemorrhage
	  – hydrocephalus is common, and is usually communicating
	  – neurological deficit, developmental delay and seizures are usually the result of the infective process, but the hydrocephalus, if not relieved, will aggravate the brain injury
	
	Choriod plexus papilloma
	  A rare cause of hydrocephalus
	  Hydrocephalus is produced by excessive fluid secreted by the tumour, sometimes with obstruction to CSF flow
	  Recurrent haemorrhage from the tumour may play a role
	  Total excision of the tumour usually leads to a resolution of the hydrocephalic process

meningitis or an aneurysm of the vein of Galen may simulate intracranial neoplasms. The latter should be suspected if, in addition to hydrocephalus, a loud intracranial bruit, high output failure and vascular naevi are also present in the same patient.

Approach to clinical diagnosis

The clinical appraisal of the hydrocephalic child involves:
• the establishment of the diagnosis
• elucidation of the aetiology
• assessment of neurological and mental function
• a search for other associated malformations.

It is essential to determine the age and rapidity of onset hydrocephalus and its rate of progression. In most clinical situations, the child presents with a large head, which may already be apparent at birth or at a few months of age. Despite the obviously large head, many babies thrive and may develop normally apart from poor head control. Other infants with hydrocephalus, however, feed poorly, are irritable, vomit excessively and fail to gain weight. In infants with congenital hydrocephalus, the birth weight, nature of delivery and the neonatal course should be noted. In addition, enquiry as to whether there has been a similar illness in an older sibling or possible intrauterine infection is relevant.

Hydrocephalus which develops in an older and previously normal child suggests the possibility of a posterior fossa neoplasm. Because ventricular dilatation is generally subacute in children with cerebellar tumours, symptoms of raised intracranial pressure are often associated with changes in behaviour, a clumsy gait, abnormal articulation, tremors and incoordination. If elevation of ventricular pressure occurs abruptly, attacks of nausea, vomiting, head retraction and extensor spasms are prominent. In these very ill children, symptoms of intracranial hypertension may be obscured by those of the primary illness, such as cranial infection and haemorrhage. It is important in all cases to ascertain any neurological symptoms, determine the time of onset of head enlargement and assess the developmental progress of the child.

In children with myelomeningocele and shunted hydrocephalus, raised intracranial pressure is usually secondary to a blocked shunt. Children may present with features typical of a blocked shunt (irritability, headache, somnolence, vomiting, loss of consciousness) but may also present with atypical features such as seizures or unusual behaviours. Diagnosis requires exclusion of other underlying causes, and a high index of suspicion prompting the clinician to question shunt dysfunction.

Clinical example

William is an 11 year old boy with spina bifida and shunted hydrocephalus. During the course of the clinical consultation as part of long term follow up of his condition, he complained that he had been experiencing some right sided facial pain during the past 3 days. He had a decreased appetite, and his mother noted he had been confused about his daily routine, which surprised her.

On examination he had a flaccid lower limb paralysis and was wheelchair mobile. He had mild hyperreflexia in his upper limbs and nystagmus of gaze, all which were longstanding problems associated with his condition. His shunt appeared to empty, but was slow to refill. His fundi did not show evidence of papilloedema. There was no history of recent trauma or infection to explain his facial pain, and it was decided that he should have CT to exclude hydrocephalus as a cause. This revealed enlarged ventricles and he was taken to theatre that day by the neurosurgical team for revision of his shunt.

In this situation, the classical signs of raised intracranial pressure were not present, and diagnosis of shunt dysfunction required a high index of suspicion. This boy may well have progressed to developing further signs later but by then the risk of an adverse outcome would probably have increased.

Physical examination

Classically, hydrocephalus is recognised by a progressive increase in occipitofrontal head circumference out of proportion to other bodily dimensions. A single head circumference measurement that greatly exceeds the 97th percentile strongly suggests the existence of hydrocephalus. Where head enlargement is equivocal, and neurological abnormality is absent, serial head measurements will often indicate the need for further diagnostic studies. It must be emphasised that, once enlargement of the skull is clinically obvious, the ventricles are already grossly dilated and the cerebral cortex is thinned.

Clinical signs that frequently precede obvious enlargement of the head include:
- a large and bulging fontanelle
- thinning of the bones of the calvarium
- widening of the coronal, sagittal and lambdoidal sutures.

With advancing hydrocephalus:
- The scalp thins and becomes shiny and pale.
- There is upwards retraction of the eyelids.
- The eyes are fixed in a downward gaze (the 'setting sun' sign).
- The hair appears sparse.
- Superficial scalp veins become distended.
- The brow overhangs the small triangular face.

Despite the enormous head size, papilloedema is uncommon in congenital hydrocephalus. The shape of the skull should be noted. A large protruding occiput is typical of a Dandy–Walker cyst, while an asymmetrical head may be due to unilateral obstruction at the foramen of Monro. In addition, ausculation for cranial bruit should be performed over the eyeballs and over the calvarium.

Many mildly affected hydrocephalic children have remarkably normal development and minimal neurological deficit. Gross abnormalities in a child with mild hydrocephalus are usually related to the underlying disorder that caused the hydrocephalus. However, prolonged stretching and compression of neural structures will lead ultimately to profound neurological injury. Where the increase in intracranial pressure is rapid, and there has not been a compensatory increase in head size, the highly irritable child frequently gives a short, high pitched 'cerebral cry'. During these screaming episodes, decerebrate posturing may be evident. In the older child with 'arrested' hydrocephalus, it is important to evaluate the mental and psychological status. These children are frequently talkative, jovial and euphoric ('cocktail party syndrome') but their capacity for concentration, language comprehension and abstract thinking is often lacking. Manifestations of longstanding hydrocephalus include a variety of endocrinological and metabolic disorders, such as precocious puberty, diabetes insipidus and abnormal thermoregulation. Various anomalies, particularly neural tube defects, skeletal defects and cutaneous naevi, are known to coexist with obstructive hydrocephalus.

Investigations

The child's assessment, based on the history and examination, will often enable a diagnosis of hydrocephalus to be made with some degree of certainty. However, in all cases investigations are required to confirm the diagnosis, determine the extent of the disorder and, if possible, define the aetiology. Investigations are also of assistance in deciding the need or otherwise for active treatment and also as a means of assessing the success or otherwise of treatment. The plain skull X ray may be a useful initial investigation.

Ultrasound. The widespread use of ultrasound scanning (Fig. 59.1) has in recent times greatly facilitated the assessment of infants with suspected hydrocephalus. Real time ultrasound imaging through the open fontanelle provides a clear demonstration of the ventricles and may define other structural anomalies well. This non invasive risk-free investigation can be undertaken with little or no sedation, and can be repeated as often as required. When the fontanelle closes, satisfactory imaging can no longer be obtained. Ultrasound examination during pregnancy can indicate whether the fetus has hydrocephalus.

Computerised tomography. In the older child, and occasionally in infants where more detail is required, CT (Fig. 59.2) is the investigation of choice. This technique provides excellent detail of the intracranial anatomy and

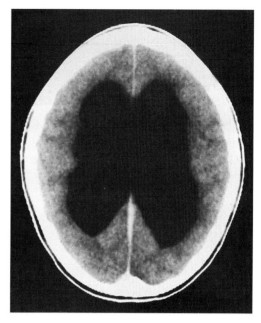

Fig. 59.2 CT demonstrating gross ventricular dilatation in hydrocephalus.

the images may be enhanced by the injection of contrast material. Many children can undergo CT without sedation, while others will require sedation or occasionally a general anaesthetic. The radiation involved in a single scan is of an acceptable degree, but a limitation should be placed on repeated studies.

Magnetic resonance imaging (Fig. 59.3). This investigation is rarely undertaken as a primary investigation, but

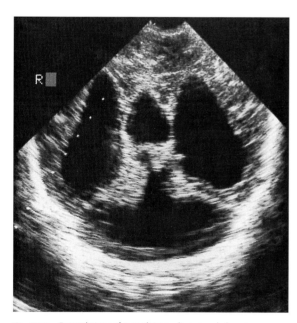

Fig. 59.1 Frontal view of a real time ultrasound showing markedly dilated ventricles on either side of a large posterior fossa cyst in a patient with Dandy–Walker malformation.

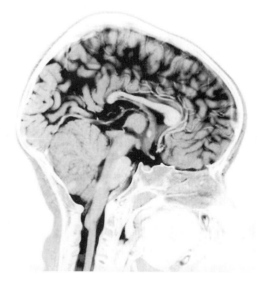

Fig. 59.3 MRI of a child with a spina bifida showing the Arnold–Chiari malformation. Note the herniation of the cerebellum into the upper cervical canal.

may be of value in defining the cause of the condition. Small tumours in the region of the aqueduct, causing obstruction to CSF flow, may not be visualised by CT but are clearly defined by an MRI study. Special techniques can visualise CSF flow patterns.

Treatment

The indications for treatment are based on a clear understanding of the natural history of the disorder. Three patterns may be described:
- The process continues, followed by neurological deterioration.
- The process progresses to a point, then stabilises ('compensated hydrocephalus')
- The process is temporary.

In the majority of patients, the ventricles will continue to enlarge and the overlying brain will become stretched, compressed and thinned. If the process starts in infancy before the skull bones have developed significant attachment to each other, massive head enlargement will result and under these circumstances significant brain injury will result. This type of progression will be detected by the presence and persistence of signs of raised pressure, an excessive rate of head growth and, less commonly, by the finding of neurological abnormality and developmental delay. Serial imaging will confirm progression of ventricular dilatation. In this group, treatment is essential if brain injury is to be avoided or minimised.

In a smaller number of patients limited enlargement of the ventricles will occur and then cease. The term 'compensated hydrocephalus' has been applied to this group. The ventricles remain somewhat larger than normal but there are no clear signs of raised intracranial pressure and brain function appears normal. The head may be large but the rate of growth will either be normal or only slightly excessive and serial images will show no significant alteration in ventricle size. With this pattern, decisions regarding treatment are less well defined. If the degree of dilatation is mild to moderate there is no good evidence that treatment will influence the outcome favourably. Under these circumstances frequent assessment is required to ensure that stability is maintained.

With the widespread use of head imaging techniques, it has become apparent that hydrocephalus may be a temporary state in certain circumstances. Posthaemorrhagic hydrocephalus in the low birth weight infant is often of this type, as is the disorder complicating certain forms of meningitis. In these patients it appears likely that the CSF pathways have regained their patency. These patients are usually defined by repeating imaging. Such studies would show reduction in size of ventricles to normal and this satisfactory state would be associated with the disappearance of all physical signs of progressive hydrocephalus. Obviously, no long term treatment is required

in this group, but intermittent removal of CSF by either a lumbar puncture or ventricular puncture may help resolve the process and prevent any excess ventricular dilatation during the period before effective CSF flow is established via normal pathways. On occasions, a reservoir may be inserted into a lateral ventricle to facilitate such intermittent removal. In addition, drugs which reduce CSF production, such as acetazolamide and isosorbide, have been used with the same intent.

Operative treatment

The definitive treatment of hydrocephalus is a surgical procedure. The usual method is by a shunt which diverts the CSF to some other site in the body. In some cases of non communicating hydrocephalus, ventriculostomy may successfully re-establish normal CSF pathways.

Ventriculoperitoneal shunt. This is the operation performed most frequently in paediatric patients with hydrocephalus. A Silastic catheter is placed in a lateral ventricle through a burr hole and the other end of the tube is passed subcutaneously to the abdomen and is then placed in the peritoneal cavity. A valve is interposed and an adequate length of tube is placed in the peritoneal cavity to allow for growth. The peritoneum absorbs CSF effectively.

Ventriculoatrial shunt. In this procedure the lower end of the shunt is passed via a neck vein to the right atrium. The catheter is designed so that CSF can pass from the catheter tip but blood cannot flow back into the lumen. The turbulent blood flow in the atrium prevents thrombus formation around the catheter. This operation is not undertaken often in childhood, as maintenance may involve the lengthening of the atrial catheter on several occasions.

Complications of ventricular shunts

The operation is generally well tolerated with infrequent early difficulties. Common complications include meningitis, ventriculitis and shunt obstruction.

The most common presentation of a child with a blocked shunt is that of a vague illness. Irritability and vomiting are frequent and headache may be present. The symptoms are very similar to those of many childhood illnesses and difficulties are often experienced in trying to decide if the symptoms are a consequence of shunt malfunction or an unrelated illness. Definite signs of raised intracranial pressure, if present, are of great assistance but are often not ascertained readily. Palpation of the shunt mechanism may also frequently be inconclusive.

The treatment of shunt obstruction is usually a simple procedure and involves the replacement of the defective component; however, a small number of patients suffer from repeated episodes of obstruction and management can be difficult and may involve many variations of shunt equipment and surgical technique.

Clinical example

Sara, a 6 year old child with a past history of having had a ventriculoperitoneal shunt inserted in infancy for congenital hydrocephalus, presented at the outpatient clinic for review, having missed a preceding planned attendance. Her mother stated that she was generally well but she was concerned about Sara's visual function. Sara insisted on sitting immediately adjacent to the television set and had been moved to the front of her class to enable her to see the blackboard.

When examined, she appeared to be generally well but head measurement indicated an excessive rate of growth. Her visual acuity was markedly diminished in each eye and fundoscopy revealed severe secondary optic atrophy. On palpation the shunt tubing was found to be disconnected and immediate CT showed very large ventricles. The shunt was revised immediately but unfortunately there was no improvement in her poor vision.

The shunt had obviously been malfunctioning for a prolonged period of time and had resulted in chronic raised intracranial pressure. She had not complained of any symptoms but the raised intracranial pressure produced marked optic atrophy during this time. If she had attended for the planned review it may well have been that the abnormality could have been recognised and corrected before visual deterioration had resulted.

Neural tube defects

The term neural tube defects (NTDs) refers to a group of malformations involving the brain and/or spinal cord in association with varying degrees of absence or malformation of the overlying tissues: meninges, bone, muscle and skin. *Myelomeningocele* (*myelo* meaning cord; *meninges*, coverings of the spinal cord; *cele*, sac) involves all the tissue layers, including the skin and bone, and is an outpouching of the spinal cord through the posterior bony vertebral column that has failed to form. *Meningocele* is an outpouching of the meninges or coverings of the spinal cord only, and not the cord itself. The term *spina bifida* refers to the normal bony projection over the spine being divided or 'bifid'. *Spina bifida occulta* is the failure of the formation of the posterior elements of the vertebrae, but without any outpouching of the meninges or spinal cord. It occurs in 5–10% of the normal population and is most often asymptomatic. The diagnosis is confirmed by X rays of the spine documenting the incomplete vertebral arch. Accompanying associated features may include dermal hyperpigmentation, a fatty swelling, a tuft of hair or a dermal sinus on the back. *Spina bifida cystica* refers to myelomeningocele and meningocele. Myelomeningocele is the much more serious and much commoner type of spina bifida cystica. *Spinal dysraphism*, which includes spina bifida occulta, meningocele and myelomeningocele, is part of the family of neural tube defects that encompasses abnormalities of the cranium and its contents (anencephaly, encephalocele and cranial meningocele) as well as abnormalities of the spine.

Incidence

The incidence has varied in different countries, with the highest rates being recorded in the past in Northern Ireland, the west of Scotland, and South Wales. In South Australia, the total incidence of neural tube defects during 1966–1991 was 2.01 per 1000 births, and the incidence of myelomeningocele was 0.97 per 1000 births, with no upward or downward trend. Despite the total incidence remaining stable, prenatal diagnosis and termination of pregnancy resulted in an 84% fall in the birth prevalence of all neural tube defects during the years studied. Screening by serum alphafetoprotein measurements or midtrimester ultrasonography, or both, detected over four fifths of cases in 1986–1991 in South Australia.

Recurrence risks in families have been documented extensively. Recurrence risk statistics suggest a polygenic or environmental aetiology. The risk of recurrence following the birth of the first child with a neural tube defect is approximately 4–8% or 1 in 25. The risk increases to at least 10% after the birth of two affected children.

Neural tube defects are found commonly in spontaneous first trimester miscarriages; they are more common in females and in lower socioeconomic groups and the incidence varies with different ethnic groups.

Embryology and pathogenesis

The neural tube is the embryological structure from which the brain and spinal cord develop. The human neural tube closes just before the 30th day postfertilisation and thus any influence affecting the closure of the neural tube must be present before this early stage of pregnancy. The typical motor, sensory and sphincter dysfunctions of spina bifida and myelodysplasia are the most evident clinical manifestations but represent only one aspect of this complex teratologic anomaly. There is a high incidence of gross and microscopic brainstem, cerebellar and cerebral malformations. The aetiology of neural tube defects is still debated. Polygenic inheritance and environmental and teratogenic factors have been implicated. It has been unequivocally demonstrated that vitamin supplementation with folic acid reduces the incidence of recurrence in high risk populations (Ch. 27). Dietary factors may therefore play a major part in low risk populations. Many other potential aetiological causes have also been examined during the last 20 years.

Antenatal diagnosis

The presence of abnormally high levels of alphafeto-protein in the amniotic fluid has a high correlation with myelomeningocele. Alphafetoprotein is a component of fetal CSF and it probably leaks into the amniotic fluid from the open neural rube defect. Closed lesions often do not cause an increased alphafetoprotein. The false positive rate for the determination of myelomeningocele is less than 0.5% and the false negative rate is 2%. Alphafetoprotein is synthesised by the yolk sac, hepatic cells and gastrointestinal tract of the fetus and normally is excreted in the amniotic fluid in fetal urine.

The detection rate for open neural tube defects using maternal serum screening is approximately 80%, with a low false positive rate. Ultrasonography can detect or confirm the extent of the neural tube defect.

Clinical features

Neural tube defects may be classified as in Table 59.2.

Table 59.2   Classification of neural tube defects

Anencephaly
>   At birth, presents as an opened, malformed skull and brain
>   Most babies are stillborn
>   No effective treatment is possible
>   Death usually occurs within hours or days

Cranium bifidum
>   **Cranial meningocele**
>>   The underlying brain is normal
>>   A meningeal sac protrudes through a skull defect

Encephalocele
>   A midline sac protrudes which may contain brain
>   Hydrocephalus is common

Spina bifida occulta
>   One or more vertebral arches are incomplete posteriorly but the overlying skin is intact; diagnosed incidentally, for example, as the result of an X ray of the spinal column during other investigations
>   Usually have a normal spinal cord; however, a number of abnormalities of the spinal cord have been described; ectodermal abnormalities may be associated
>>   a dermal pit
>>   a depression with a tuft of hair
>>   a fatty swelling (Fig. 59.4)
>   The ectodermal component
>>   may communicate with the dura
>>   may pose some risk of intraspinal infection (if associated with a dural sinus)
>>   the fatty swelling may be a lipomeningocele
>>   if present warrants full neurological examination

Spina bifida cystica
>   **Myelomeningocele** — (Fig. 59.5 and Fig. 59.6) in which vertebral column skin, meninges and spinal cord are involved
>   **Meningocele** — in which the spinal cord is not involved (Fig. 59.7)
>>   is almost always obvious at birth (most frequently, a midline sac protrudes through a spinal defect)
>>   may occur anywhere along the length of the spinal column
>>   the lumbar and lumbosacral regions are the most frequent anatomical levels
>>   abnormal spinal cord tissue and nerve roots may be readily apparent macroscopically
>>   there may be spinal abnormalities such as kyphosis at the site of the lesion
>   Functional deficits include
>>   paraplegia, with motor and sensory impairment
>>   hydrocephalus
>>   variable intellectual impairment
>>   neuropathic sphincter dysfunction

Sacral agenesis

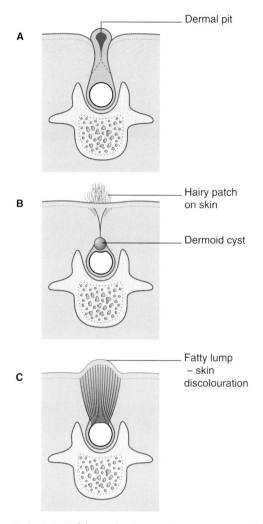

A — Dermal pit

B — Hairy patch on skin — Dermoid cyst

C — Fatty lump – skin discolouration

Fig. 59.4 Spina bifida occulta. **A** Dermal sinus. **B** Intraspinal cyst pressing on the cord. **C** Lipomatous mass infiltrating the cord elements.

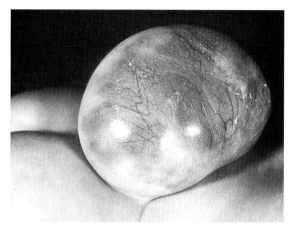

Fig. 59.5 A lumbosacral myelomeningocele.

Management of myelomeningocele

A team approach that includes the parents is essential for the proper management of myelomeningocele. An important factor compounding the disability is that the defect is apparent at birth. Information given to the parents and the manner in which it is conveyed will influence their reaction at this most vulnerable time and will affect the future of the child and the family. Medical specialists in this team include the neurosurgeon, orthopaedic surgeon and urologist. The medical team leader is most appropriately a paediatrician with special skills in the field of child development and rehabilitation. The team leader will coordinate the various activities to support the parents and child through the many problems, both physical and psychological, that invariably arise. The physiotherapist, occupational therapist, orthotist, psychologist and medical social worker, together with trained hospital and community based

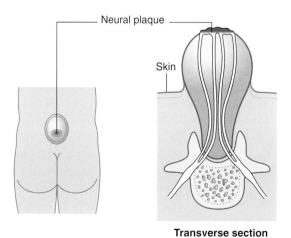

Neural plaque

Skin

Transverse section

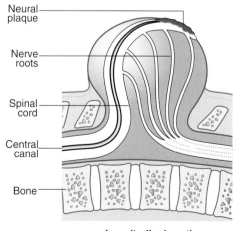

Neural plaque

Nerve roots

Spinal cord

Central canal

Bone

Longitudinal section

Fig. 59.6 Myelomeningocele: diagrammatic representation.

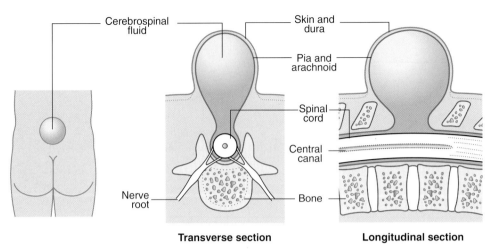

Fig. 59.7 Meningocele: diagrammatic representation.

nursing staff and teachers, are important members of this team. The team has three major goals:

- to promote good health in the short and long term
- to promote maximum function in the child so that, as nearly as possible, normal developmental sequences and timing can be followed to enable maximal independence for the child and family
- to promote good family functioning.

Specific problems in the management of the newborn with spina bifida

It is possible to predict with considerable accuracy the potential for future impairment in a number of areas. These include ambulation and subsequent mobility, likely bowel and bladder function, and hydrocephalus with its likely sequelae. It is much more difficult to predict the effects these impairments will have on the lifestyle of the individual and family. Also, it is possible to recognise early those lesions which are inoperable because of massive bony deformity and extensive skin loss which would prevent closure of the defect. The specific problems are as follows:

- Children with high lesions (thoracic and thoracolumbar), significant hydrocephalus at birth, major kyphosis or other significant problems (either congenital or acquired) have a significantly increased mortality in early life and substantial morbidity if they survive. In these circumstances, in discussion with the family, supportive care only may be recommended. If the infant survives the perinatal period, elective surgical care may be indicated. In the absence of such adverse factors in discussion with the family, early surgical repair/removal of the lesion is usually recommended.
- Careful serial evaluation of head circumference and ventricular size by ultrasound or CT will indicate if hydrocephalus is developing. Once it is established

that progressive hydrocephalus is present, a shunt procedure is recommended.

- Baseline orthopaedic, urology and neurosurgery assessments provide the basis for ongoing discussions with the family and management of the condition. Occasionally, active urological intervention is required for urinary retention.
- It is critical to begin to establish an empathetic, therapeutic relationship with the parents in the newborn period, forming the foundation for ongoing support throughout childhood.

Ongoing management issues

Management of physical disability and mobility. Physiotherapists play an essential role in reducing deformities and encouraging mobility. Foot deformities are common at birth, due to unopposed muscular activity in utero. Splinting and passive stretching are the mainstays of treatment in early life. Persistent foot deformities may require corrective surgery. Surgery also may be needed for dislocated hips, particularly if the child is likely to walk.

The outlook for walking depends on the level of the spinal cord lesion, intelligence and motivation. Most children with a lesion at L4 or lower will walk, with or without splints and crutches. Children with higher lesions may walk with orthotics in early childhood, but most will choose wheelchair mobility by mid to late childhood.

Spinal deformities. A significant percentage of children will develop scoliosis, and many of these will require spinal instrumentation. Spinal jackets are not well tolerated and have a very limited role in the management of paralytic scoliosis.

Neuropathic fracture. Fractures of the lower limbs are common in children with myelomeningocele due to disuse osteoporosis. Fractures may occur with minimal trauma. Encouraging children to walk, or stand in a standing frame, may improve the mineralisation of long bones and lessen the likelihood of spontaneous fractures.

Sensory deficit and skin care. Pressure ulcers or burns in anaesthetic areas are common. Parents are encouraged to check anaesthetic areas daily for the presence of pressure sores. Early recognition and treatment are essential to prevent long periods of morbidity and hospitalisation.

Neuropathic bladder. Almost all children with myelomeningocele have a neuropathic bladder. Failure to empty the bladder may lead to recurrent urinary tract infections, vesicoureteric reflux, renal calculi and hydronephrosis. Hypertension and renal failure may be seen in a small number of cases. Management of the neuropathic bladder is by clean intermittent catheterisation performed 4–5 times daily by the parents, and later by the child. This usually is commenced at around 3–4 years of age, or earlier if repeated urinary infections occur. Prophylactic antibiotics may be required for recurrent urinary infections. Bladder augmentation and/or artificial sphincter operations may be indicated if the clinical situation dictates. The use of anticholinergic medications to increase bladder capacity may be tried in the first instance. Regular assessment of renal function is essential throughout the person's life.

Neuropathic bowel. Most children have limited or absent rectal sensation and have little or no bowel control. Constipation with megacolon, faecal impaction and overflow incontinence is the major risk in spina bifida. Faecal softeners may be needed in infancy. Some children can attain continence simply by regular toileting, while others may need high fibre diets, faecal softeners, suppositories or microenemas. Aperients are avoided whenever possible. Refractory cases may require regular bowel washouts.

Sexual function. Many people with spina bifida achieve a satisfactory sexual relationship. In females, pregnancy has been achieved in many individuals. Predictably, there are a number of potential difficulties with pregnancy and confinement, urinary and spinal problems being particularly common. In males, the situation is more complex. Difficulties range from impotence to retrograde ejaculation and infertility. Sexual counselling is important in adolescence.

Tethered spinal cord. Following repair of a myelomeningocele, the lower end of the spinal cord may become tethered to the site of repair. As the child grows, this may cause progressive neurological deterioration in motor or sensory function, or in bladder control. Regular monitoring of the neurological state is essential, particularly during the rapidly growing phase. MRI is performed to demonstrate the tethering process. If the neurological deterioration is significant, consideration should be given to neurosurgical release of the tethered cord.

Arnold–Chiari malformation. This has been described earlier (Fig. 59.3). It is present in a significant number of children with myelomeningocele and is elegantly demonstrated by MRI. Symptoms are variable: they may be quite minor, for example strabismus, or mild difficulties with chewing and swallowing, or they may be severe, with laryngeal stridor and apnoeic spells. Life threatening episodes may necessitate neurosurgical intervention to decompress the posterior fossa.

Education. Children with myelomeningocele often have specific learning problems, requiring assistance at school. Overall intelligence generally is in the low average range, with a wide range of abilities. Verbal IQ is usually considerably higher than performance IQ. Difficulties with mathematical concepts are very common, as are problems with abstract reasoning. Many children have a poor attention span with distractibility. Problems with fine motor control and visual perceptual difficulties are present frequently. Most children with spina bifida attend normal schools, with varying levels of assistance from support teachers. Schools may require modification to provide access and suitable toilet arrangements.

Social and emotional adjustment and transition to adulthood. A child with a chronic disability places severe strains on the emotional and financial resources of a family. Members of the team must be alert to signs of distress, and be ready to provide the necessary support. During the teenage years, the usual problems of adolescence are superimposed on the difficulties associated with the disability, and these young people need sensitive counselling. For the families, parent groups provide valuable practical and emotional support.

There are now increasing numbers of young adults with spina bifida. A coordinated approach to management is still desirable, but more difficult to attain, because of the wish of the young people to be independent, and to break away from what they perceive as overprotection by the medical fraternity. Nevertheless, problems continue to occur, particularly pressure ulcers, shunt and urinary complications. In South Australia, the Spina Bifida Association employs two community nurses, who maintain close contact with all the adults with spina bifida and refer problems to appropriate agencies. This recent service has been invaluable in maintaining physical and emotional health among the group.

Prevention of neural tube defects

Neural tube defects (spina bifida, anencephaly and encephalocele) result from defective closure of the neural tube in early pregnancy. The human neural tube closes just before the 30th day postfertilisation and thus any influence affecting the closure of the neural tube must be present before this early stage of pregnancy. Primary prevention of this group of conditions may now be feasible. Research has suggested a relationship between maternal diet and the birth of an affected infant. Medical evidence has confirmed that folic acid (a water soluble vitamin found in many fruits, leafy green vegetables, wholegrain breads, cereals and legumes) may prevent the majority of neural tube defects (Ch. 27).

A randomised controlled clinical trial carried out by the Medical Research Council of the United Kingdom demonstrated a 72% reduction in risk of recurrence by periconceptional (that is, before and after conception) folic acid supplementation of 4 mg daily. Other epidemiological research, including research done in Australia, suggests that primary occurrences of neural tube defect births may also be prevented by folic acid either as a supplement or in the diet, and this has been confirmed in a randomised controlled trial from Hungary that found that a daily multivitamin supplement containing 0.8 mg folic acid was effective in reducing the occurrence of neural tube defects in first births.

The National Health and Medical Research Council of Australia has recommended the following.

All women planning a pregnancy or likely to become pregnant:

- should be offered advice about folate in the diet, and encouraged to increase their dietary intake of folate rich foods, particularly in the month before and in the first 3 months of pregnancy.

In addition:

Low risk women (no family history of neural tube defects, not on anticonvulsants):

- should be offered periconceptional folic acid supplementation (0.5 mg daily). Generally, periconceptional supplementation with other vitamins is not necessary. When supplements are used, the potential risks of vitamin overdose should be considered. In particular, large therapeutic doses of vitamin A may predispose to birth defects.

Women with a close family history of neural tube defects (for example, they or their partner has spina bifida, they have already had an affected child, they have a sibling or other close relative with a neural tube defect):

- should be referred for genetic counseling;
- should be advised to take periconceptional folic acid supplementation 5 mg daily; the 4 mg formulation is not available in Australia;

- should continue to be offered prenatal diagnosis with alphafetoprotein estimation and tertiary level ultrasound, by an operator experienced in anatomical scans, at 16–18 weeks gestation. Although the risk of recurrence is reduced significantly if folic acid supplementation is used appropriately, there is a residual risk of about 1% in women taking supplements who have had a previously affected infant.

Women on anticonvulsant drugs:

- should take folic acid supplementation only under the supervision of, and with close monitoring by their, physician;
- because of the increased risk of neural tube defects in the offspring of women taking some anticonvulsants (notably sodium valproate), these women also should be counselled and offered prenatal diagnosis.

Fortification of staple foods with folic acid

- Fortification of staple foods such as bread and cereals with folic acid, as is recommended in the USA and the UK, should be introduced in Australia.

Education, research and monitoring

- There should be education programmes, for health professionals and the public, on how to achieve adequate folate intake, with diet and supplementation to prevent neural tube defects.
- There should be continued research into the mechanisms of action of folic acid, and the minimum dose of folic acid required for prevention.
- Close monitoring of both the prevalence of neural tube defects (including terminations of pregnancy) and the increase in folate intake should be undertaken to evaluate the effectiveness of any health promotion campaigns.
- Further research should be monitored, and these recommendations reviewed in the light of any developments.

In Australia, health promotion campaigns have been undertaken to inform health professionals and women about folate and the prevention of neural tube defects. For example, folic acid (folate) in fruit and vegetables is easily destroyed by cooking and prolonged storage. It is wise to eat fruit and vegetables that are fresh and either raw or lightly cooked. For good health and enough folate per day, one would need to aim for at least two serves of fruit, five serves of vegetables and seven serves of bread and cereals every day. The safety of increased folate ingestion before and during early pregnancy appears to be confirmed. Furthermore, an intake of folate from fortified food is unlikely to be high enough to constitute a hazard for those people with untreated vitamin B_{12} deficiency.

Children with headaches

I. Wilkinson

Headache occurs in most children at some time. In a number of these, frequent headaches are a disabling problem. In one study in primary schools in Australia, 23% of parents believed that their children suffered from 'frequent headaches'.

Many processes result in headache. These will be considered in two major classes: 'cranial' headaches, where the cause of pain is a process directly involving the brain and associated structures, including meninges, cerebral blood vessels and scalp; and 'extracranial' headaches, where the primary cause is remote from the brain.

The actual mechanisms of headache are multiple, but it should be recognised that the brain itself is insensitive to pain. Some neurosurgical operations for intractable epilepsy are actually performed on the brain with the patient awake.

Structures that are sensitive to pain include:
- blood vessels
- meninges
- cranial nerves 5, 7, 9 and 10.

Pain is also generated from integumentary structures surrounding the skull including:
- skin
- muscle
- periosteum
- blood vessels.

This chapter will deal particularly with recurrent or chronic headaches and not with those that accompany acute events such as trauma, intracranial bleeds or infections of the nervous system.

Cranial causes

Migraine and stress or tension types are the most common of chronic or recurrent headaches with origins in and around the brain. The migraine subset is numerically the biggest in Australian children but in other parts of the world stress or tension headaches approach migraine in prevalence. This relates in part to the variability of diagnostic criteria that are used to define migraine, and this is discussed later. In reality, many headaches classified as 'stress' or 'tension' have an underlying migraine process, or alternatively start out as migraine headaches but, as a consequence of recurrent pain, disability and fear of the next headache, develop strong features suggesting that stress or tension is the primary cause.

Of the different headache types in children, migraine, because of its great prevalence and associated morbidity, will receive most attention in this discussion.

Migraine

Epidemiological features

- The commonest cause of recurrent headaches.
- Increasing prevalence. In a 1974 Finnish study using rigid criteria, 1.9% of children suffered from migraine headaches. In 1992 the study was repeated with the same criteria and the prevalence had increased to 5.7%. Other studies suggest up to 10% incidence.
- Leading cause of referrals to a child neurologist.
- More common in males before puberty, but in females after puberty.

Clinical manifestations

Childhood migraines result from the same process as those in adults, but clinical manifestations may be quite different. Some of these differences relate to the difficulty a child has in describing or explaining the features; for example, young children may not be able to describe throbbing, or lateralisation, or sensory associations.

'Classical' migraine (which is a relatively uncommon type of migraine even in adults) includes aura, or transitory neurological dysfunction, especially of the visual system, and may involve sophisticated hallucinations such as fortification spectra, which often precede the onset of headache and then disappear as the headache commences. This classic sequence may occur in older children and adolescents but often instead there is a description of sensory hallucination that commences with, or during, the headache. This may be a visual disturbance described in unsophisticated terms, such as 'flashing lights', 'seeing things double' or 'blurry like looking through a curtain', or something more complex and bizarre sounding and often very frightening. Such hallucinations include the appearance that objects are too big or too small, or that things moving in the environment appear to be going too fast or too slow. It is suggested that Lewis Carroll drew on personal migraine experiences when describing Alice's distorted body perception after she ate the magic substance.

Such hallucinations can involve the auditory process; for example, things sounding too loud or someone speaking too fast. At times the aura for a child defies description but may involve a sense of unreality or depersonalisation.

What can make the migraine process more difficult to unravel in a child is a not uncommon situation, where the actual sensory hallucination is not accompanied (during that event) by a headache. This is the referred to as migraine dissociée, and there is frequently more alarm and distress for a child or parent than when there is an accompanying headache.

Other variations from adult migraine involve the location of the pain. Whereas in adult migraine attacks the pain can often be lateralised (a true 'hemicrania' — the origin of the word migraine), this is frequently not the case in young children, who will simply point to their forehead (without lateralisation) as being the location. As the child grows older a description of pain that is unilateral and sometimes located in one or other temple becomes more common.

A description of the quality of the pain in migraine in children is often difficult for them. The pain tends to more of an aching type 'like a tummy ache' rather then sharp 'like a needle'. A combination of the two may be described. Further, in adults with pure migraine attacks it is frequent for the pain to be described as throbbing, implying involvement of vascular structures. Children with migraine may well experience throbbing pain but may not be able to describe it as such, although as the child becomes older, he or she may describe it as 'beating like a drum' or 'like a hammer'.

Although many adults do not acknowledge headaches as being migraine unless they are severe and resulting in cessation of usual activities, in children there can be a great range in the severity of migraine events, from the situation where the child is able to continue in school or at play, to the level where all activity must cease and the child retreats to bed in misery.

Adults with migraine attacks may not change greatly in external appearance but children are often extremely pale. Nausea and vomiting may occur in association with adult migraine, and not uncommonly continues and exacerbates the headache, resulting in treatment with an antiemetic. During the attack, abdominal pain, nausea and vomiting are extremely common in children but the sequence may be that a single vomit, often followed by a sleep, seems to terminate the attack.

Formulating rigid diagnostic criteria for childhood migraine has proven very controversial, and strict requirements for certain features to be present in combination before a diagnosis can be made may be counterproductive in clinical practice. In general, children with headaches with some of the previously mentioned features, occurring intermittently and with symptom-free periods, who are normal to neurological examination, may be considered to suffer from migraine.

The single feature that has caused most disagreement between those studying children with headaches and those studying adults is a requirement for the headache to be of a certain duration. A diagnosis of migraine in an adult has generally required, by International Headache Society criteria, a duration of at least 4 hours. Eventually it was conceded that childhood migraine attacks may last only 2 hours, but in reality the whole attack may be much briefer then this, even as short as half an hour at times.

Classic teaching about headaches due to tumours and other situations of raised intracranial pressure has been that they are present upon awakening, or actively cause the patient to waken. Although in reality this is not always the case, a contrast remains with childhood migraine, where the onset is most commonly later in the day, perhaps approaching midday or during the afternoon or evening.

Childhood migraine is a very cyclical condition. Patients may have a bout of recurrent headaches that lasts weeks or months, followed by a period of remission that may last a year or more, to be followed by another bout. Hot weather may be a factor in relapses.

Types of migraine

In the International Headache Society classification there are seven categories and ten subcategories of migraine. Precise classification is necessary in migraine research but is not always so important in clinical diagnosis and management, and there is often overlap between different types in children. To categorise according to the presence or absence of 'aura' in children can be very difficult. The 'aura', in children who can describe it, may often occur during the headache, and not precede it, and frequently involves some sense of disequilibrium, perhaps true vertigo. Visual auras are often basic and unsophisticated.

There are some conditions that are considered to be part of the migraine phenomenon, although appearing to have little relationship with adult migraine types:

- In infancy, paroxysmal torticollis, where the head becomes tilted strongly to one or either side for periods of hours or days, may be a precursor of migraine, although simultaneous headache may not be apparent. A similar process involving the trunk has been described. These infants have been demonstrated to be at greater risk of later developing migraine headaches.
- In early childhood, usually before the age of 5 years, some may experience recurrent episodes with sudden onset of true vertigo. These are extremely distressing, and cause the child to seek a cuddle, or lie on the ground to relieve the feeling of spinning. These events last a few minutes, sometimes hours, and may be associated with pallor, nausea and vomiting. In some

studies up to 80% of these children who are described as having benign paroxysmal vertigo subsequently develop migraine headaches.

- Unexplained attacks of vomiting, or abdominal pain, without associated headache may also be precursors of migraine. These attacks can be very puzzling diagnostically and often very debilitating, sometimes requiring intravenous fluids and hospitalisation. With the passage of time, headaches may become more of a feature of these attacks, which are labelled cyclical vomiting or abdominal migraine.
- Hemiplegic migraine may present with unilateral weakness, or unilateral sensory disturbance, and this often precedes the actual headache.
- Expressive or receptive language difficulties also may be a presenting feature of some attacks, with the headache not occurring till an hour or so later.
- In acute confusional migraine the patient is quite disoriented and distressed, with short term memory loss. This condition raises concerns about more sinister neurological processes, or drug intoxication, perhaps leading to invasive investigations. Again, the headache may not become apparent until later.

Aetiology

The basic mechanisms causing migraine in adults have been investigated extensively, and there has been controversy, contradiction and revision of theories as to causation. It is beyond the scope of this text to detail all the theories, but the two main schools postulate either:

- an initial central process involving neuronal pathways, or
- a peripheral process involving blood vessels.

Some researchers propose an interaction between these two as being the true basis.

At a chemical level both noradrenergic and serotonergic transmitter pathways are implicated, and this has relevance for drug therapy.

Genetic factors play a major role in childhood migraine. As many as 90% of children with migraine have a first degree relative with the condition. In some types, such as hemiplegic migraine, genetic loci have been found on particular chromosomes. In more common types of migraine it has been variously proposed that inheritance may be autosomal dominant, recessive, sex linked or polygenic.

Given that some children are at risk genetically to develop migraine, it is clear that there are provoking factors for individual attacks. These include head injuries, not necessarily severe ones. The head injury may be the commencing point for recurrent bouts of migraine headache, and this may have legal ramifications. Other provoking factors are:

- Intercurrent systemic infections, particularly with fever.
- Strenuous physical exercise.
- Hot weather.
- Dehydration.
- Worry and stress, either domestic, social or educational in origin. While these factors remain, they may greatly complicate treatment. The distinction from 'stress' or 'tension' headaches without an underlying migraine basis may be very difficult.
- Foodstuffs. This is a very controversial area, with evidence for and against. Citrus fruit, cheese, chocolate and processed meat have been implicated.
- Food additives, such as monosodium glutamate, sodium nitrite, benzoic acid, tartrazine.

Treatment

Treatment can be divided into the following tiers:
- avoidance of triggers
- non specific analgesia for attacks
- specific antimigraine medication for attacks
- prophylactic medication
- non medication treatments.

Avoiding triggers in childhood migraine can be difficult. In many they do not exist. Hot weather and exercise are common precipitants which are part of normal childhood exposures. Ensuring adequate hydration in the above situations may be helpful.

The role of restrictive diets is controversial. If it is evident that certain foodstuffs or drinks regularly provoke attacks then they should be avoided. Placing children on very limited diets is not only unpleasant and difficult to enforce, but may even have nutritional consequences.

The use of non specific analgesics in attacks is the simplest means of treatment. The most commonly used is paracetamol, best given in an initial dose of 20–30 mg/kg. Unfortunately children may not seek medication, or as a result of being at school may not be able to access medication, until the attack is advanced. The paracetamol may not be effective at this time, or may be vomited. There may be a role for rectal paracetamol in this situation.

A recent study has indicated that ibuprofen in a dose of 10 mg/kg may be more effective then paracetamol. Other non steroidal anti-inflammatory drugs may be helpful.

In recent years aspirin has been avoided in childhood because of concerns about its relationship with the Reye syndrome, a severe acute encephalopathy with potentially fatal outcome. Nevertheless, aspirin in doses of 15 mg/kg may be employed in older children with recurrent headaches.

The use of codeine and powerful narcotics in childhood headache is not usually necessary and is potentially hazardous, although restricted infrequent use of combinations of paracetamol and codeine in older children may be necessary and effective.

Ergotamine has long been a useful antimigraine drug in some adults. It has limited use in children because they delay seeking treatment and also because it is frequently ineffective or produces side effects such as vomiting and abdominal discomfort.

Triptans are a new generation of serotonin active drugs which abort migraine attacks. There have been limited trials in children, and triptans have not yet been accepted for childhood use in most countries. One trial in children found nasal sumatriptan to be effective, but administration by other routes has not been successful.

Prophylactic medications may be considered for frequent disabling attacks. What constitutes 'frequent' is arbitrary but more then two severe attacks per month may justify treatment. Controlled trials of prophylaxis in childhood migraine are confounded by the cyclical nature of childhood migraine and the tendency to remit spontaneously, as well as the high placebo response rate.

There are few controlled trials of prophylactic drugs in children but the following have been widely used in practice:

- Cyproheptadine, an antihistamine with serotonin blocking and calcium channel blocking properties. Side effects include drowsiness (which may be minimised with a single night-time dose regimen) and increased appetite. Effective doses range from 0.1 to 0.3 mg/kg per day, given either once or twice daily.
- Propranolol, a beta adrenergic blocking drug, also blocks release of serotonin from platelets. It is contraindicated in asthma. Doses range from 0.5 to 2.0 mg/kg per day, in two or three equal doses. Propranolol and similar drugs have been proven in adults, not children, but have been useful in the latter.
- Pizotifen, with antiserotonin and antihistamine properties, has side effects of increased appetite, weight gain and drowsiness. The latter may be avoided by a single night-time dose. Doses are limited by the single size pill format (0.5 mg) but range from one to three at night.
- Flunarizine, a calcium channel blocker, has been widely used in children in Europe but has restricted availability in Australia.
- Clonidine, a vasoactive drug, has been trialled in a range of conditions in children but lacks good evidence for use in migraine and has significant potential side effects.

Because of the high remission rates in children, prophylactic medications should not be used continuously for more than 6 months without attempting to wean children from them.

Non medication treatments may at times be successful, but again there is a paucity of controlled trials in children. Biofeedback and relaxation techniques have been used particularly in Europe and North America. Acupuncture has been proven successful in adults but is a potentially painful procedure. Homeopathic formulations are enjoying increased popularity in many conditions but lack evidence in childhood migraine. Chiropractic treatments are controversial, lack controlled trials and may be dangerous in young children.

Although discussion in this section has focused on migraine, the non specific medications and treatments cited may be useful in all headache types.

Prognosis

Childhood migraine is often cyclical, with bad bouts followed by prolonged remissions, sometimes followed by relapses in later childhood or adult life. Various studies have indicated an overall 30–40% 10 year remission rate. It is very common when taking a family history that parents, when pressed, remember childhood migraines long since in remission. Similarly, in apparent adult onset migraine, a long forgotten history of severe childhood headaches may be recalled eventually.

Other children, like adults, will have a history of infrequent migraines throughout their developing years.

> ### Clinical example
>
> Jason, who was 8 years old, presented in March with headaches that had occurred about twice a week for the previous 3 months, although he had had some following soccer last winter. They commenced after lunch at school, were frontal and throbbing and he looked very pale. Paracetamol sometimes helped him, but often he would vomit, go to sleep and then awake and eat his evening meal.
>
> His mother had a history of migraine. Neurological examination in Jason was normal. After daily treatment with cyproheptadine for 2 weeks his headaches ceased. The history is consistent with childhood migraine.

Stress and tension headaches

There is a broad spectrum of headache types in some way associated with emotional factors, perhaps more frequently seen in older children and adolescents. At one end is a small group where the symptoms of headaches may be used in a conscious and malingering way to avoid a situation. Examples include:

- the child who consistently develops a severe headache on a Monday morning in a setting of school difficulties
- the child who develops a severe headache when an unwelcome visit to a disliked non custodial parent is planned.

Further along the spectrum is the situation where the child is being exposed to a great deal of stress, often multifactorial, and this apparently constitutes the sole underlying aetiological basis for headaches. High parental expectations may be major factors here. It is a reality of modern urban life that children may be involved in a demanding combination of schooling, additional tutoring, competitive sport, training in the performing arts and so on to the point where their life allows for little relaxation or personal time.

In situations such as this, a pattern of headache may develop. The nature of this headache may differ from that of migraine. In migraine the headache does not occur daily, and indeed daily headaches by many definitions are not migraine. In addition, the quality of the headache may differ, for example they:

- may occur at all times and throughout the day
- cannot be localised or described in other than vague terms
- lack an association with pallor, nausea, vomiting, or disturbance of vision or balance.

For the clinician it may be frustratingly difficult to come to grips with the nature of these headaches.

Somewhere along this spectrum is the child who has a primary psychiatric disorder and in whom the symptom of headache may be part of a conversion reaction or a major psychosis.

Perhaps the more common situation is where the child with a past history of intermittent headaches sounding just like migraine, and a family history of this, experiences a crescendo effect, in which the headaches become daily, unremitting, but not always severe. Although daily headaches may be indicative of a more sinister process, such as raised intracranial pressure, this is not necessarily the case. In this group where the crescendo effect is seen, it may be that the exposure to frequent pain and the expectation of further severe pain results in secondary stress and anxiety, which in turn provokes further headaches, becoming a vicious cycle.

The sequence whereby individual stress events provoke a severe migraine attack is perhaps less frequently seen in children than in adults, but can still occur. Sometimes it is the 'let down' phenomenon following stress that provokes a headache.

In childhood headaches associated with emotional aetiologies there is usually no abnormality on neurological examination. The facial appearance can range from complete indifference through to one of intense anxiety.

Radiological investigations rarely contribute in any positive sense, but sometimes the performance of a normal brain scan in an extremely anxious patient may be the only way to allay anxiety, and enable successful treatment. On the other hand, where there is a conversion reaction it may produce a reinforcement that there really is an organic problem.

Treatment is often difficult. Where there appears to be an original underlying basis of migraine, treatment with adequate doses of analgesia, possibly non steroidal anti-inflammatory drugs, may be able to break the cycle. It may be prudent to commence migraine prophylaxis as well.

Where the headache appears to be further along the spectrum towards psychiatric disorders, then consultation with a child psychiatrist is strongly advised.

The tricyclic antidepressants may have a separate specific analgesic effect, and can be useful where an element of depression is a factor. Although monoamine oxidase inhibitors can also be useful in treating migraines in adults, the use of these in children may present dangers because of dietary interactions.

Caution must be exercised in drug treatment in this group of headaches, as it is common for such patients to finish up on combinations of medications in large doses, and may become dependent on these medications.

Several therapies may have a role here. These include:

- muscle relaxation
- stress avoidance
- biofeedback
- hypnosis
- acupuncture.

These therapies are used quite widely in other countries, but are often resource intensive.

Headaches due to raised intracranial pressure

The possibility of childhood headaches being caused by raised intracranial pressure, especially due to tumours, is often a cause for great concern in the treating physician, as well as the child and family. In reality only a very small number of childhood headaches are due to raised pressure. Even when there is pressure, the ability of the child's skull to expand may mitigate some of the effects.

Although headaches due to raised intracranial pressure have classically been described as worse in the morning upon awakening, or causing the patient to awaken, and associated with vomiting, this is not always the case.

Raised intracranial pressure can be a result of abnormal fluid collections, solid masses or vascular malformations. Interference with fluid dynamics without discrete collections can result in the condition of benign intracranial hypertension.

Fluid can collect abnormally either within ventricles, within the substance of the brain, or over the surfaces:

- Build up of fluid within the ventricles is referred to as hydrocephalus (Ch. 59). This often presents in infancy, and the ability of the skull to expand, coupled with the inability of the child to report the pain, may be the reason that headache is not a presenting feature. In older children, the onset of hydrocephalus is often associated with a mass lesion obstructing the intracerebral cerebrospinal fluid pathways, and this may result in major headaches.

- Intracranial abscesses are uncommon in children in Western society. Children with cystic fibrosis or cyanotic heart disease are at increased risk. Abscesses can develop by spread from infections of the paranasal sinuses. Headaches resulting from abscesses are associated with systemic manifestations such as fever, and tend to build up in severity over days or weeks.
- Arachnoid cysts occur in a number of different locations, often adjacent to the surface of the brain. They result from fluid collecting within a split arachnoid membrane, and may be asymptomatic, but can produce headaches.
- Fluid, including blood, can collect in the subdural or extradural spaces, often as a result of trauma. Accompanying headaches are often crescendo in frequency and severity, and may be associated with focal signs.
- Headaches due to tumours are most often due to mass effect, or obstruction of cerebrospinal fluid pathways, and are less likely to be due to direct local involvement of pain sensitive structures. Intracranial tumours in children are usually primary and are most frequently found in the posterior fossa, where they readily obstruct fluid pathways. It is not uncommon that there is a substantial delay in detection of the tumour in such headaches.
- Aneurysms are uncommon in children, but arteriovenous malformations or cavenous angiomas are found at this age. These may produce headache due to their size or obstruction of fluid pathways.

The signs associated with raised pressure often involve the eyes.

Papilloedema may take days to develop, even in the presence of grossly elevated pressure. Abnormalities of ocular movements, particularly failure of abduction with resultant convergent strabismus, or failure of upward gaze, can occur. Sluggish pupillary light reflexes may be found. Deep tendon reflexes are often brisk. There may be neck stiffness. Bradycardia and systemic hypertension are later effects.

Treatment of such headaches usually involves surgical approaches, either directly to the mass or to drain fluid from the ventricles or brain surface via a shunt. Oedema surrounding a mass may be treated with corticosteroids or osmotic diuretics, but these are temporary measures only.

Benign intracranial hypertension

This condition, also known as 'pseudo tumour cerebri' because the clinical feature can mimic a tumour, occurs in children and adults. It results from a build up in intracranial pressure, without a space occupying lesion, probably due to an imbalance between production and resorption of cerebrospinal fluid. It is potentially serious as it can eventually result in visual loss. There is often an association with adolescent females who are overweight but otherwise apparently healthy. This may have a hormonal basis.

Other proposed causes in individual cases include:
- recurrent middle ear infections, sometimes associated with mastoiditis, where the draining cerebral venous sinuses near the ear become obstructed
- head trauma
- oral contraceptives
- the use or withdrawal of corticosteroids
- excessive amounts of vitamin A
- tetracyclines
- growth hormone treatment.

In some cases a specific cause is not found.

The clinical features include:
- headache, which tends to be daily, often worse in the morning but not necessarily severe
- abnormalities of the eyes, most commonly papilloedema (which may be asymptomatic), and lateral rectus palsies due to pressure on the abducens nerves
- nausea and vomiting
- raised pressure at lumbar puncture, to figures of 20–40 cm of water or more
- normal laboratory findings in cerebrospinal fluid.

In the presence of papilloedema or other eye signs it is prudent to perform a structural study (computerised tomography or magnetic resonance imaging) before performing the lumbar puncture. A magnetic resonance venogram may be helpful in demonstrating obstructed venous sinuses.

Cerebral images are usually otherwise quite normal, without a space occupying lesion or dilatation of the ventricles. Even in the presence of a normal scan, it is reasonable to examine the cerebrospinal fluid for malignant cells, as in rare cases undifferentiated tumours can present with raised intracranial pressure in the presence of normal scans.

Treatment is varied but includes:
- Repeated lumbar punctures to remove fluid. This is quite traumatic and not always effective.
- Acetazolamide, which potentially reduces production of cerebrospinal fluid by interferring with the carbonic anhydrase enzymes; more powerful diuretics, such as frusemide, if acetazolamide fails.
- Steroids.
- Shunting procedures to remove fluid from the cranial cavity. These should be reserved for drug resistant cases.
- Decompression procedures on the optic nerves.
- Anticoagulation if there are thrombosed draining venous sinuses.

Patients must be seen by an ophthalmologist, to monitor visual function, as prolonged papilloedema can lead to optic nerve damage.

The prognosis for benign intracranial hypertension is generally good. The process, particularly where no underlying cause is demonstrated, often remits spontaneously.

> ### Clinical example
>
> Lisa, 14 years old, developed daily headaches. These were often present by the time she had breakfast, and were distressing but she could get to school most days. The pain continued throughout the day and was all over her head. She had noticed some visual difficulty. The problem started after she was placed on an oral contraceptive for dysmenorrhoea.
>
> On examination she was obese. There was papilloedema but no other neurological abnormality. Her blood pressure was normal. Cranial tomography was normal and a lumbar puncture resulted in the fluid pressure rising out of the top of the tube. The fluid was normal in the laboratory.
>
> She responded to cessation of the contraceptive and treatment with 250 mg acetazolamide each morning.
>
> The history is consistent with benign intracranial hypertension.

Seizure related headaches

In adults, severe headaches are common following a major seizure. In young children, postictal headaches tend to be less debilitating. Children may describe a headache during an actual epileptic event, while conscious. This is often associated with focal discharges, possibly from the temporal lobe, and may be only a brief event, not always associated with other clinical features. Electrical discharges in the occipital region may give visual hallucinations, vomiting, and pernicious headaches, not always associated with motor convulsions. This condition may be familial and often difficult to diagnose.

Extracranial causes

Headache is a frequent associate of systemic illness, without there being a primary pathological process in the nervous system:

- The most frequent association is with systemic febrile illnesses not directly involving the nervous system.
- Connective tissue disease, especially 'mixed connective tissue disease', may lead to vascular type headaches.
- Systemic hypertension is much less common in children, and hypertensive encephalopathy is not seen frequently. Nevertheless in persistent severe hypertension in children a major encephalopathy may develop, with headache, seizures and altered consciousness.

- Metabolic pathway disturbances such as urea cycle defects can produce headaches, especially during biochemical decompensation.
- Hypoglycaemia is a potent trigger for migraine, but can also result in non specific headaches, and may be a result of poor diabetic control.
- Hunger without demonstrable hypoglycaemia may also provoke headaches.
- Although controversial, allergic disorders may be associated with migraines and other headaches.
- Obstructive sleep apnoea and other sleep disorders may produce a clinical picture of daytime headaches and somnolence.

In these situations treatment of the underlying cause is preferable to symptomatic relief.

Overrated causes of childhood headaches

Children with recurrent headaches are frequently initially referred to optometrists or ophthalmologists. The basis for these headaches is often migraine.

Glaucoma (rarely seen in children) and iritis may product aching in and around the orbit. Convergence insufficiency and other ocular muscle imbalances are common findings in children. Headaches may be attributed to these problems, but the evidence is not convincing.

Minor refractive errors detected on examination, but with doubtful clinical relevance, may be blamed incorrectly as a cause of childhood headache. Spectacles or ocular movement exercises may result in apparent temporary relief of the headaches, but not infrequently they return.

Acute sinusitis is a potential cause of headache in children, often associated with other features such as fever, purulent nasal or postnasal discharge, local tenderness and puffiness around the eyes. The pain can be widespread in the skull, and the location can be confusing. This is a potentially dangerous condition, occasionally leading to intracranial abscesses.

More frequently seen is the situation where recurrent frontal migraine headaches are attributed to chronic sinusitis and referral for a radiographic series is the first investigation. These are frequently negative. With the increasing availability of computerised axial tomography and magnetic resonance imaging performed for other reasons, it is not uncommon that asymptomatic fluid collections are detected in paranasal sinuses, usually with no clinical consequences.

The frontal and other sinuses are not formed in early childhood, and may be not be capable of harbouring infections until the end of the first decade.

Headaches found in adults but not children

- Giant cell or temporal arteritis is a potentially serious cause of headaches in the elderly, and can lead to visual impairment or cerebrovascular accidents if not treated. Fortunately, it is not a condition of childhood.
- Acute angle closure glaucoma is another cause of pain in the ocular region. It is uncommon for this to occur in isolation in childhood.
- Cluster headaches are a condition of adult life and can result in some of the most severe headaches known. They can be very resistant to treatment. Although there are isolated reports, they are fortunately rarely seen in childhood.
- Headaches due to arthritic changes in the neck, often chronic disabling headaches, generally relate to long-standing degenerative processes and are not common in children.

Investigations

Childhood headaches are frequently overinvestigated. In general, blood investigations have little yield. Plain radiographs of the skull may demonstrate signs of chronically raised pressure, or sinusitis, but are of little use in most situations.

Computerised tomography is necessary only rarely but is most useful in hydrocephalus, other fluid collections and tumours, although it is not ideal for visualisation of the middle or posterior fossae. Magnetic resonance imaging is more likely to detect tumours and masses, particularly in the middle and posterior fossa. Magnetic resonance arteriography or venography are quite sensitive for detecting vascular abnormalities, and are relatively non invasive. Lumbar puncture is the diagnostic test for benign intracranial hypertension.

Specialist consultation is frequently more rewarding and less expensive then laboratory investigation.

PART 17   SELF-ASSESSMENT

Questions

1. **A 14 year old girl is brought to her general practitioner after having a brief seizure at home while watching television. She described feeling dizzy then things going black, prior to blacking out and being seen to stiffen and jerk briefly. She has a history of a similar seizure as a child after having her hand shut in a car door. Which of the following is true?**
   (A) An EEG should be arranged to clarify the nature of the attack
   (B) If epileptic, the warning symptoms would suggest partial seizure origin
   (C) Knowledge of the TV programme would further aid the diagnosis
   (D) Sodium valproate is the treatment of choice, given the tonic–clonic nature of the attack
   (E) Micturition would indicate the attack is a generalised tonic–clonic seizure

2. **Which of the following are true about febrile convulsions in infancy?**
   (A) Recurrence is likely if there is a family history of febrile convulsions
   (B) A family history of epilepsy suggests an underlying predisposition to epileptic seizures
   (C) The chance of later afebrile seizures is greater if there is evidence of developmental delay or the seizures are prolonged
   (D) The infant should be undressed, sponged and given paracetemol with first signs of a fever, to prevent further febrile convulsions
   (E) Meningitis should be suspected if repeated seizures occur in the emergency department

3. **An 8 year old boy is struggling at school and having episodes of staring, unresponsiveness and subsequent sleepiness. He has a past history of a prolonged, right sided febrile convulsion when aged 17 months, this was followed by several hours of right arm weakness. Hyperventilation in the clinic room did not induce an attack.**
   (A) Psychological assessment is warranted as the episodes may be simple inattention
   (B) Epilepsy is unlikely without provocation of attacks by hyperventilation
   (C) EEG and MRI will likely be recommended following neurological consultation
   (D) If complex partial seizures are the basis of the staring, treatment with carbamazepine will be indicated
   (E) Remission of seizures by puberty is expected

4. **John is the first child of unrelated parents. He was born at term following a normal pregnancy and**

birth. He presents at the age of 12 months as he is not yet sitting independently. John has begun to say 'Mum' and 'Dad' and is an interactive child. Physical examination reveals signs of spasticity in both lower limbs with increased deep tendon reflexes. Which of the following are correct?

(A) It is important to undertake a thorough assessment of his upper limb function

(B) Cerebral palsy is unlikely in view of the normal perinatal history

(C) The finding of periventricular leucomalacia on MRI brain scan points to a problem occurring in the early part of the third trimester of pregnancy

(D) Intelligence is likely to be normal but will require further assessment

(E) His inability to sit at 12 months means that his motor disorder is likely to be severe

5. Joe, aged 4 years, has severe cerebral palsy. He presents to the emergency department with a history of being irritable over the past few days, crying day and night. The parents have no idea why he might be so upset. Further questioning reveals that he has been vomiting about once a week, usually after meals. Physical examination is unremarkable but difficult in view of his irriatability. Which of the following are correct?

(A) Acute otitis media could explain his symptoms

(B) A normal temperature excludes infection

(C) A bone scan is not indicated as there is no history of trauma

(D) Oesophagitis and/or gastritis should be considered

(E) A dental opinion may be helpful

6. Mandy, age 3 years, began having multifocal myoclonic seizures 6 months ago, with epileptic discharges on EEG, and is being treated with sodium valproate and clonazepam. Before the onset of seizures there was mild delay in her language and fine motor development. In the last 2 weeks she has begun to fall over frequently, sometimes striking her face. She speaks less, is tremulous and has begun to drool saliva. Which of the following statements are correct?

(A) An EEG should be arranged promptly

(B) Such marked deterioration is unlikely to be due to her antiepileptic drugs

(C) Developmental stagnation and regression may occur in children with epilepsy in the absence of an identifiable underlying degenerative brain disorder

(D) An MRI brain scan is likely to provide a specific diagnosis to explain the recent deterioration

(E) Further investigation for a neurodegenerative disorder should be undertaken if she does not respond to changes in her antiepileptic drug regimen

7. A 15 year old female presents with a 3 day history of progressive inability to walk. She had a gastro-like illness approximately 10 days prior to the onset of her symptoms. She complains of severe back pain. Examination showed bilateral facial weakness, symmetric weakness in her limbs, worse in her lower extremities, with some proximal predilection. Reflexes were difficult to elicit. No sensory abnormalities were detected. She could take two steps with support. Which of the following is the most likely diagnosis?

(A) Botulism

(B) Polymyositis

(C) Myasthenia gravis

(D) Guillain–Barré syndrome

(E) Myelitis

8. A 7 year old male wakes one morning with severe leg pain, predominantly in the calf muscles, after an upper respiratory tract infection 4 days previously. He is unable to walk but is otherwise well. The casualty officer thinks that there is weakness distally and has difficulty obtaining reflexes. However, there is a lot of pain with the examination. The creatine kinase is 2000 IU/l (normal: 40–240 IU/l). Which of the following is the most likely diagnosis?

(A) Guillain–Barré syndrome

(B) Dermatomyositis

(C) Viral myositis

(D) Reactive arthritis

(E) Rhabdomyolysis

9. Marlene, a 3 month old infant, presents with a rapidly enlarging head and signs of raised intracranial pressure. Which of the following investigations would be appropriate initially?

(A) MRI

(B) CT

(C) Plain skull X ray

(D) Ultrasound

(E) Lumbar puncture

10. A complementary public health strategy is necessary for the prevention of neural tube defects because:

(A) Periconceptional 5 mg folic acid supplementation would be essential for all women

(B) Dietary intake of folate-rich foods may be sufficient without folic acid supplementation or fortification of staple foods

(C) Over 95% of infants with neural tube defects are born to women who have not previously had an affected pregnancy

(D) A large proportion of pregnancies are unplanned and many of those that are planned will occur in women not taking folic acid supplements

(E) Folate-rich foods and fortification of staple foods is preferable to the risks associated with folic acid supplementation in low risk women

11. **Which of the following are true in an infant or child with a significant neural tube defect?**
    (A) Following assessement of a newborn infant with myelomeningocele, early surgical repair of the spinal lesion is recommended
    (B) If hydrocephalus is present, a shunt is performed immediately
    (C) Clean intermittent catheterisation reduces the incidence of urinary infections
    (D) Constipation is avoided by the use of regular aperients in high doses
    (E) Surveillance of areas of insensate skin should occur daily to prevent the occurrence of pressure sores

12. **Fred, a 7 year old male, presents with a 2 month history of early morning headache, vomiting and increasingly unsteady gait. On examination, the significant findings were a wide based ataxic gait, horizontal nystagmus and severe bilateral papilloedema. What is the most likely diagnosis?**
    (A) Hydrocephalus due to an aqueduct stricture
    (B) A cerebellar tumour without hydrocephalus
    (C) Posthaemorrhagic hydrocephalus
    (D) A cerebellar tumour with hydrocephalus
    (E) Tuberculous meningitis

13. **In spina bifida cystica, which of the following clinical signs confirm that neural tissue is involved in the malformation?**
    (A) Paralysis of voluntary muscle groups
    (B) Sensory loss below the level of the lesion
    (C) Bladder paralysis
    (D) A patulous anus
    (E) Severe developmental delay

14. **In a patient with headaches due to benign intracranial hypertension, which of the following are true?**
    (A) CT of the brain usually shows dilated ventricles
    (B) Papilloedema is often detected
    (C) There is an association with females undergoing puberty
    (D) The condition may remit spontaneously
    (E) Ventriculoperitoneal shunts should be inserted as soon as possible after diagnosis

15. **In childhood migraine, which of the following are true?**
    (A) Many patients undergo spontaneous remission but will have a recurrence in later childhood or adulthood
    (B) Vomiting suggests the diagnosis of migraine is incorrect and that there may be an underlying tumour

(C) CT is a desirable early investigation
(D) The presence of headache on awakening is unusual during an attack
(E) Prophylactic medication should only be commenced if intermittent treatment is ineffective and attempts should be made to wean the patient off it after no more than 6 months of successful treatment

Answers and explanations

1. **(B)** and **(C)**. History is paramount to the correct diagnosis of episodic neurological phenomena. The TV programme could potentially have been something that might induce syncope in an adolescent, e.g. displaying a medical procedure or something horrific (A). In epileptic seizures, a warning or aura indicates focal seizure onset, in this case possibly in the visual cortex (B). EEG should not be performed when the diagnosis is uncertain (A) and treatment should not be commenced without a definite diagnosis (D). Micturition and convulsive features may occur with loss of consciousness in syncope, as is likely in this case (E).

2. **(A)**, **(B)**, **(C)** and **(E)**. Although (B) is correct, the chance of later seizures is still very small (<10%). Families should be reassured about the benign nature of febrile convulsions and given general advice about management of fevers and seizures, not made to have a 'fever phobia'.

3. **(A)**, **(C)** and **(D)**. The history is highly suggestive of complex partial seizures in temporal lobe epilepsy, with EEG being indicated to detect temporal lobe abnormalities, MRI necessary to look for an underlying lesion like hippocampal sclerosis, and treatment with carbamazepine being recommended. Hyperventilation typically induces absence seizures, although sleeping after staring episodes is not seen in absence seizures. Remission of seizures in the teens is typical of benign focal epilepsies, again the attacks not being typical of those seen in these syndromes.

4. The correct answers are **(A)**, **(C)** and **(D)**. It is important to assess upper limb function (A). This presentation could indicate a spinal lesion rather than cerebral palsy. Although further investigation is necessary, the presence of upper limb abnormalities is confirmatory evidence of spastic cerebral palsy. Many children with cerebral palsy have a normal perinatal history (B). Most cases of cerebral palsy are prenatal in origin. Periventricular leucomalacia can be found in children born at term and points to an earlier lesion (C). While intelligence is likely to be normal, assessment is difficult at this age and judgements should

never be made on limited information (D). A prognosis about the severity of the disability is impossible at a single assessment in such a young child (E). Studies have demonstrated that sitting independently by 2 years of age is strongly associated with the ability to walk.

5. The correct answers are **(A)**, **(D)** and **(E)**. Irritability is a common presentation in children with cerebral palsy. It is important to determine whether the onset is acute or chronic. Acute onset of irritability may be due to infection such as otitis media or urinary tract infection (A). Do not overlook the possibility of appendicitis. A normal temperature does not exclude infection (B). Some children with severe cerebral palsy develop subnormal temperatures with infection. Pathological fracture may occur with no known trauma and a bone scan is helpful (C). Oesophagitis and/or gastritis is a frequent cause of irritability in children with cerebral palsy (D). Dental problems are easily overlooked and can be a source of pain (E).

6. The correct answers are **(A)**, **(C)** and **(E)**. (A) An EEG is indicated to determine whether the regression is due to very frequent or continuous subtle seizure activity ('non convulsive status epilepticus') which may (C) be associated with regression in development, which sometimes persists after establishment of better seizure control, particularly in the Lennox–Gastaut syndrome (Ch. 56). (E) The differentiation between uncontrolled epilepsy, medication toxicity and an underlying degenerative disorder may be particularly challenging in this age group. In such a patient, careful examination of the optic fundi, electrophysiological examination of the visual system, and electron microscopy of skin or conjunctiva may lead to a diagnosis of one of a group of grey matter disorders collectively known as Batten disease. (B) Benzodiazepines such as clonazepam may increase secretions, leading to drooling as well as impaired coordination and behaviour change. Overdosing has occurred with the liquid preparation of this drug, when the dose, prescribed as a number of drops, is administered in error as that number of millilitres. (D) While an MRI scan may be of value in excluding a surgically treatable mass lesion, and may sometimes provide a clue to the presence of an underlying metabolic (e.g. mitochondrial) disorder, it is more likely to show a non specific abnormality such as cerebral atrophy, or a non progressive lesion such as cortical dysplasia.

7. Correct answer **(D)**. Guillain–Barré syndrome (GBS) is the most common acute neuropathy in clinical practice. Evidence suggests that it is immune mediated, although the exact pathogenic mechanisms have not been fully elucidated. As it is a 'syndrome', a variety of different mechanisms are likely to be involved in its pathogenesis. The annual incidence is in the range of 1–2 per 100 000 population or approximately half the incidence of multiple sclerosis or childhood brain tumours. The actual incidence may be higher as there is a spectrum of clinical severity, and some mildly affected individuals may not seek medical attention. GBS occurs across all age groups but is rare in individuals over 80 years of age or in children under 2 years of age. Most untreated patients begin recovery 2–4 weeks after progression of the weakness stops, but with treatment the onset of the recovery phase is usually earlier. Depending on how severely affected the patient was, recovery occurs over the ensuing weeks to months. The prognosis for recovery in GBS is good, with approximately 75% of patients recovering without significant neurological sequelae.

8. Answer **(C)**. Benign acute childhood myositis (BACM) is a recognisable syndrome first described in 1957. It is characterised by the sudden onset of calf pain and refusal to walk following a prodromal viral upper respiratory illness. There is often leucopenia and viral agents, particularly influenza B, have been isolated in many cases. The serum creatinine kinase (CPK) is usually elevated. Males are affected more commonly and it is followed by rapid recovery, usually within a week. It is rarely reported in adults. It is important to differentiate BACM from more serious causes of refusal to walk. Guillain–Barré syndrome is often considered but the presence of normal power and reflexes in the majority of cases combined with a markedly elevated CPK argues against this diagnosis. Children who are assessed are often thought to have muscle weakness, but rather than true weakness these children fail to generate power because of associated muscle pain. Acute rhabdomyolysis is a more serious differential diagnosis and can be caused by metabolic muscle disorders, exposure to toxins, or trauma, or it can be idiopathic. Idiopathic rhabdomyolysis is a rare condition that is associated with viral illness, elevated CPK levels and myoglobinuria and may lead to acute renal failure. Affected children tend to be younger than those with BACM; they are systemically unwell with the muscle pain occurring concurrently with other symptoms. The acute presentation of BACM would be unusual for dermatomyositis, particularly with the rapid improvement in symptoms without treatment. Reactive arthritis is commonly considered but the absence of true joint involvement with tenderness and pain in the gastrocnemius–soleus complex with a raised CPK level would mitigate against this diagnosis.

9. The correct answer is **(D)**. The initial investigation should be ultrasound imaging. This non invasive safe procedure requires no special preparation and demonstrates the intracranial anatomy well. An open fontanelle, a necessity for this technique, would be expected at this age. (B) CT or rarely (A) MRI may be required subsequently if more detail is needed. (C) and (E) There is little place for a plain skull X ray and a lumbar puncture runs the risk of causing deterioration.

10. (A) False. Periconceptional folic acid supplementation of 5 mg daily should only be necessary for women with a close family history of neural tube defects. As the safety of increased folate ingestion before and during pregnancy continues to be confirmed, there should not be a problem, however, if 5 mg daily was taken but it would not be essential. **(B)** True, but unlikely. The daily consumption of adequate amounts of folate-rich foods could be quite challenging compared with a simple solution of low dose folate supplementation and food fortification with folate. **(C)** True. This is the challenge for public health. **(D)** True. Also a challenge for public health. (E) False. Folic acid supplementation of 0.5 mg daily involves negligible risks. Thus, while folate-rich foods and food fortification with folate is very appropriate as a general public health strategy, the reason given is simply not correct. All three strategies — folate-rich foods, food fortification and folic acid supplementation — are indicated.

11. **(A)** True — in most cases. Early closure reduces the chance of infection developing in the lesion with ascending myelitis and possible worsening of the paralysis. In very unfavourable cases an expectant policy may be adopted, and delayed closure performed if the infant thrives. (B) False. This depends on the degree of hydrocephalus and the rate of progression. A few infants with severe hydrocephalus may need early shunting, otherwise careful observation over a few weeks will demonstrate whether the hydrocephalus is progressive. Some cases will arrest spontaneously. **(C)** True. Regular catheterisation keeps the bladder empty and reduces the likelihood of infection. Introduced infection may be minimised by care with hand and catheter washing. (D) False. Regular aperients should be avoided. Faecal softeners and dietary manipulation may be indicated to prevent constipation. **(E)** True. Pressure areas should be identified early so appropriate measures can be taken to prevent skin breakdown. The most important measure is to relieve pressure on the affected area.

12. The correct answer is **(D)**. This child has symptoms and signs of a cerebellar disturbance and raised intracranial pressure and this would make the most likely diagnosis a cerebellar tumour with associated hydrocephalus. (B) A cerebellar tumour not producing hydrocephalus would not cause signs of raised intracranial pressure, but simply a cerebellar disturbance. There is no history to suggest that this child could have suffered an intracranial haemorrhage to account for posthaemorrhagic hydrocephalus. (A) Hydrocephalus due to an aqueduct stricture would generally be of a slower onset in a child of this age and again have no features of a specific cerebellar disturbance. (C) The history is too short to be posthaemorrhagic hydrocephalus, which is a neonatal problem. (E) Tuberculous meningitis is unlikely to present in this manner and with such gross cerebellar disturbance.

13. The correct answers are **(A)**, **(B)**, **(C)** and **(D)**. Paralysis of voluntary muscle movement in the lower limbs is common in spina bifida and the degree of involvement can be used to assist in determining the level of the lesion (A). Sensory loss in dermatomes below the level of the lesion is also seen (B). Bladder sensation and control of the bladder outlet often is lost because of the spinal neural tissue involvement, with dribbling of urine and a distended palpable bladder or a small contracted bladder (C). Similarly, there may be a patulous anus with no anal sphincter function, and no anal reflex (D). Severe mental delay is not seen in all children with spina bifida (E). However, there is a high incidence of hydrocephalus, associated with a coexisting Arnold–Chiari malformation. This may lead to specific learning difficulties.

14. The correct answers are **(B)**, **(C)** and **(D)**. In this situation, CT is usually normal and there is no accumulation of fluid within the ventricles (A). (B) is true: papilloedema is a frequent manifestation. Lateral rectus or other ocular muscle palsies are also seen. Abnormal eye signs are present in 95% of patients. (C) is true. This is probably hormonally mediated. There is also an association with the use of oral contraceptives and corticosteroids. (D) also is true. This condition may respond to a range of treatments but many will resolve after a period of close observation, particularly of the visual acuity, without specific treatment. Loss of vision is the most severe outcome. (E) is false. Other treatments, including acetazolamide, other diuretics or corticosteroids, should be trialled first.

15. The correct answers are **(A)**, **(D)** and **(E)**. The condition is a very cyclical one in childhood and a cycle is often as short lived as a few months (A). (B) is false. Vomiting and abdominal pain are frequent concomitants of childhood migraine and may occur in the absence of headache at times. (C) also is false. The diagnosis is clinical. CT should be reserved for those with abnormal signs or unremitting headaches where no other cause, for example emotional, is

obvious. (D) is true. Headaches tend to develop later in the day. Persisting headaches on awakening raise concerns about increased intracranial pressure. (E) also is true. Prophylactic medications may have

side effects, for example increased appetite, drowsiness, and should not be used indiscriminately. As remission is common, courses should not be prolonged.

PART 17 FURTHER READING

American Academy of Pediatrics 1999 Folic acid for the prevention of neural tube defects. Pediatrics 104: 325–327

Australian and New Zealand Perinatal Societies 1995 The origins of cerebral palsy — a consensus statement. Medical Journal of Australia 162: 85–90

Bille B 1997 A 40-year follow-up of school children with migraine. Cephalgia 17: 488–491

Bodensteiner J B 1994 Congenital myopathies. Muscle Nerve 17: 131–144

Bruni O, Fabrizi P, Ottaviano S, Cortesi F, Giannotti F, Guidetti V 1997 Prevalence of sleep disorders in childhood and adolescence with headache: a case–control study. Cephalgia 17: 492–498

Bushby K M D 1999 Making sense of the limb-girdle muscular dystrophies. Brain 122:1403–1420

Cinciripini G, Donahue S, Borchert M 1998 Idiopathic intracranial hypertension in prepubertal pediatric patients: characteristics, treatment, and outcome. American Journal of Ophthalmology 127: 178–182

Crock P A, McKenzie J D, Nicoll A M et al 1998 Benign intracranial hypertension and recombinant growth hormone therapy in Australia and New Zealand. Acta Paediatrica 87: 381–386

Darras B T, Jones H R Jr 2000 Diagnosis of pediatric neuromuscular disorders in the era of DNA analysis. Pediatric Neurology 23: 289–300

De Vivo D C, Di Mauro S, Johnson W G, Rapin I, Stumpf D, Traeger E 1996 In: Rudolph A M (ed) Rudolf's pediatrics, 20th edn. Appleton & Lange, Stamford, CT, pp 2019–2061

Dormans J P, Pellegrino L 1998 Caring for children with cerebral palsy. A team approach. Paul H Brookes Publishing, Baltimore, MD

Dubowitz V 2000 Congenital muscular dystrophy: an expanding clinical syndrome. Annals of Neurology 47: 143–144

Engel J Jr, Pedley T A 1998 Epilepsy. A comprehensive textbook. Lippincott-Raven, Philadelphia

Garton H J, Kestle J R, Drake J M 2001 Predicting shunt failure on the basis of clinical symptoms and signs in children. Journal of Neurosurgery 94: 202–210

Kuban K C K, Leviton A 1994 Cerebral palsy (Review article). New England Journal of Medicine 330: 188–195

Gherpelli J, Nagae-Poetscher L, Souza A, et al 1998 Migraine in childhood and adolescence. A critical study of the diagnostic criteria and of the influence of age on clinical findings. Cephalgia 18: 333–341

Jones K J, Kim S S, North K N 1998 Abnormalities of dystrophin, the sarcoglycans, and laminin α2 in the muscular dystrophies. Journal of Medical Genetics 35: 379–386

Li B, Murray R, Heitlinger L, Robbins J, Hayes J 1999 Is cyclic vomiting syndrome related to migraine? Journal of Pediatrics 134: 567–572

Lyon G, Adams R D, Kolodny E H 1996 Neurology of hereditary metabolic diseases of children, 2nd edn. McGraw-Hill, New York

Mackay M T, Kornberg A J, Shield L K, Dennett X 1999 Benign acute childhood myositis: laboratory and clinical features. Neurology 53: 2127–2131

Moxley R T III 1997 Myotonic disorders in childhood: diagnosis and treatment. Journal of Child Neurology 12: 116–129

Northrup H, Volcik K A 2000 Spinal bifida and other neural tube defects. Current Problems in Pediatrics 30: 313–332

Pareyson D 1999 Charcot–Marie–Tooth disease and related neuropathies: molecular basis for distinction and diagnosis. Muscle Nerve 22: 1498–1509

Rosano A, Smithells D, Cacciani L et al 1999 Time trends in neural tube defects prevalence in relation to preventive strategies: an international study. Journal of Epidemiology and Community Health 53: 630–635

Saperstein D S, Katz J S, Amato A A, Barohn R J 2001 Clinical spectrum of chronic acquired demyelinating polyneuropathies. Muscle Nerve 24: 311–324

Schaumburg H H, Herskovitz S 2000 The weak child — a cautionary tale. New England Journal of Medicine 342: 127–129

Shillito P, Vincent A, Newsom-Davis J 1993 Congenital myasthenic syndromes. Neuromuscular Disorders 3: 183–190

Stanley F, Blair E, Alberman E 2000 Cerebral palsies: epidemiology and causal pathways. Clinics in Developmental Medicine No. 151. MacKeith Press, London

Strober J B, Tennekoon G I 1999 Progressive spinal muscular atrophies. Journal of Child Neurology 14: 91–695

Ueberall M, Wenzel D 1999 Intranasal sumatriptan for the acute treatment of migraine in children. Neurology 52: 1507–1510

Wyllie E 1997 The treatment of epilepsy: principles and practice, 2nd edn. Williams & Wilkins, Baltimore

Useful links

http://www.emedical.com.au (Australian doctors and pharmacy online: your questions answered)

http://www.epilepsy.org.uk/ (British Epilepsy Association)

http://www.epinet.org.au/ (Epilepsy Foundation of Victoria)

http://www.eqi.org.au/ (Queensland Epilepsy Foundation)

http://www.familyvillage.wisc.edu/specific.htm (Specific diagnoses card catalog: information about specific disabilities)

http://www.i-h-s.org (International Headache Society)

http://www.mda.org.au/ (The home of the Muscular Dystrophy Association)

http://www.mdausa.org/ (Another Muscular Dystrophy Association site)

http://www3.ncbi.nlm.nih.gov/Omim/searchomim.html (National Center for Biotechnical Information: mendelian inheritance in man)

http://www.neuro.wustl.edu/neuromuscular/ (Neuromuscular Disease Center, Washington University: disorders and syndromes)

http://www.parentdmd.org/ (Parent Project for muscular dystrophy)

http://www.rch.unimelb.edu.au/cep/ (Children's Epilepsy Program, Melbourne)

http://www.spinabifida.asn.au (Spina Bifida and Hydrocephalus Association of South Australia: news and information)

URINARY TRACT DISORDERS AND HYPERTENSION

61 Urinary tract infections and malformations

C. Jones

Urinary tract infections

Urinary tract infections are common febrile illnesses that affect infants and young children in particular. Urinary tract infection can cause septicaemia or chronic ill health with failure to thrive and is often an indication of underlying urinary tract malformation.

Epidemiology

Two per cent of boys and 8% of girls have a urinary tract infection by the age of 7 years; 75% of urinary tract infections occur under the age of 1 year in males and 50% under the age of 1 year in females. The incidence of neonatal urinary tract infection is 1.4/1000 children. In most series, boys having urinary tract infection outnumber girls in the first 3 months of life; after the age of 1 year, urinary tract infection is more common in girls. The incidence of urinary tract infection in uncircumcised boys is 4 times that in circumcised boys in the first 3 months of life.

Diagnosis

The frequency of symptoms of urinary tract infection in a recent series of 304 children less than 5 years of age presenting to a Sydney hospital emergency department is listed in Table 61.1. The presentation varies with age because of the developmental status of the child. While a wide range of symptoms can occur, an infant will have fever, vomiting or failure to thrive, reflecting the systemic response to infection at this age. The preschool child, who has usually achieved continence, will often show wetting or frequency, complain of generalised abdominal pain and sometimes indicate dysuria. The teenage girl will usually present with symptoms of cystitis: frequency, dysuria, stranguary and accurately localised pain. The symptoms of pyelonephritis at older ages will include loin pain and tenderness. At any age, symptoms of fever, vomiting and systemic unwellness occur with pyelonephritis.

Urinalysis is part of the physical examination of any child with a suspected urinary tract infection. Microscopy may reveal leucocytes and so called 'non glomerular' red cells (red cells that appear normally haemoglobinised, of even size and uniform shape under phase contrast microscopy) in freshly examined urine (although on standing for some hours in infected urine, red blood cells become crenated).

The most useful of the dipstick tests are for detecting nitrite and leucocytes in urine. The detection of haematuria is less specific and sensitive in the diagnosis of urinary tract infection. Table 61.2 shows that in the older child a negative dipstick test is useful in ruling out urinary tract infection, but that a positive result is less useful. Thus, tests for nitrite, leucocyte esterase or pyuria should not be used for the diagnosis of urinary tract infection.

Urinary nitrite tests are frequently used in monitoring the urine of children prone to recurrent urinary tract infection (for example, continent children with vesico-ureteric reflux). Nitrite testing of early morning urine on a weekly basis has been reported to detect urinary tract infection in asymptomatic children, enabling treatment to be initiated earlier than would otherwise occur.

The urine culture is the gold standard for diagnosis, but management decisions often have to made before the results are available.

Table 61.1 Frequency of symptoms in children under 5 years with symptomatic urinary tract infections. (From Craig et al, 1998)

Symptom	%
History of fever	79.6
Axillary temperature >37.5°C	59.5
Irritability	52.3
Anorexia	48.7
Malaise/lethargy	44.4
Vomiting	41.8
Diarrhoea	20.7
Dysuria	14.8
Offensive urine	13.2
Abdominal pain	13.2
Family member with past history of UTI[1]	11.2
Previous unexplained febrile episodes	10.5
Frequency	9.5
Urinary incontinence[2]	6.6
Macroscopic haematuria	6.6
Febrile convulsion	4.6

[1] First degree relative.
[2] Defined as a noticeable increase in the frequency of daytime wetting.

Table 61.2 Predictive value of urinary dipstick analysis in febrile children

Dipstick result		Age	Interpretation
Nitrite or leucocyte	+ve	<6 months	84% chance of UTI
	–ve	<6 months	95% no chance of UTI
	+ve	3 years	40% chance of UTI
	–ve	3 years	99% no chance of UTI
Nitrite and leucocyte	+ve	<6 months	89% chance of UTI
	–ve	<6 months	89% no chance of UTI
	+ve	3 years	49% chance of UTI
	–ve	3 years	99% no chance of UTI

The predictive value of dipstick analysis varies for children under 6 months old compared with children 3 years of age because the prevalence of urinary tract infection in a child with no obvious clinical site of infection is approximately 30% at 6 months and 5% at 3 years.

The four forms of urine collection are:
- paediatric bag
- suprapubic aspirate
- catheter specimen
- midstream collection.

The paediatric bag urine collection is useful in the infant or toddler who is at low risk for urinary tract infection (not febrile and no known urological abnormality). The periurethral area should be washed with soap and water before the urine sampling bag is applied. If the urinalysis is positive for nitrite or leucocytes or the child is to be treated with antibiotics, a suprapubic aspirate (SPA) or catheter specimen should be obtained for culture. The bag urine should only be sent for culture if the urinalysis is negative and the child is not treated with antibiotics. If the colony forming unit (CFU) count is greater than $10^8 l^{-1}$, the child should have a subsequent SPA or catheter urine culture. In practice, it is not unusual to have children referred in whom only bag urine has been obtained and who have subsequently had antibiotic treatment. This can result in unnecessary recall, delayed diagnosis and treatment, and unnecessary treatment, admission and radiological investigation.

The urine sample of choice in infants and toddlers who are unable to produce a midstream urine collection is an SPA. The potential problem of a dry tap can largely be eliminated by ultrasound scanning to ensure that there is urine in the bladder. Complications such as macroscopic haematuria or osteitis pubis are rare. Any CFU count greater $10^6 l^{-1}$ is significant. A urinary catheter sample has the advantage that urine can nearly always be obtained; the disadvantages are that the social acceptability of the test has diminished, patient resistance increases with age, and performance of the procedure where the foreskin is not retractable can be traumatic and give a contaminated result.

Midstream urine can be collected from a continent child (boys around 3 years, girls around $2\frac{1}{2}$ years). Younger children require the help of a parent. Where possible, the foreskin should be retracted. It is important to emphasise that the urine should be passed in a clear stream without stopping, and the sample container brought into the line of the stream to collect urine after the urethra has been washed clear of organisms by the first part of the stream. A CFU count of $10^7 l^{-1}$ is significant.

Microbiology

Escherichia coli accounts for 80–90% of pathogens isolated. *Proteus* species are the cause of infection in 30% of males over 1 year of age. Coagulase negative staphylococcus species are common in teenagers, and *Klebsiella* is frequent in the neonatal period. *Pseudomonas* species are frequently isolated in children with more complicated anatomical malformations, and in those children who have had surgical procedures, especially where foreign materials (such as urinary stents) have been left in situ. The enterococcus causes around 5% of urinary tract infections and is the most common organism found that is resistant to gentamicin. Approximately 5% of children will have two organisms isolated.

Initial management

Once the urine culture has been obtained a decision on acute management must be made. Intravenous therapy is required where the child is systemically unwell (dehydrated, signs of septic shock such as hypotension, tachycardia and decreased conscious state), where there is vomiting, so that oral medications will not be retained, and, in general, in the infant under the age of 6 months. In the child in whom an infection is likely on the basis of urinalysis and presentation, and the child is reasonably well (generally older and not vomiting), oral antibiotics may be commenced, with review once the culture is through in 24–48 hours. In the child in whom a urinary infection is a possibility and the child is not unwell then the results of the culture are obtained before starting treatment. The intravenous antibiotics and oral antibiotics used acutely are listed in Table 61.3. Intravenous antibiotics are usually ceased within 2–3 days once culture results have been obtained and the child has improved clinically. Acute treatment is completed with oral antibiotics, usually of 5 days duration.

Ongoing management: prophylactic antibiotics

After acute treatment the child is placed on prophylactic antibiotics given once each night. The antibiotics usually used for prophylaxis are listed in Table 61.3. These antibiotics are excreted in the urine, achieve high urinary

Table 61.3   Antibiotic treatment of urinary tract infection

Antibiotic and dose		Organisms sensitive[1] (%)
Acute		
Intravenous (sick, <6/12 months old, pyelonephritis)		
1. Benzyl penicillin	50 mg/kg (max. dose 3 g) 6 h	Covers enterccocus
	and	
2. Gentamicin	7.5 mg/kg (max. dose 360 mg)	95+
	<10 years, 6 mg/kg/24 h	
	>10 years, (max. dose 360 mg)	95+
	Monitoring: trough level <1 μg/ml	
	taken on 3rd day and serum creatinine 3rd day	
Oral		
Trimethroprim	4 mg/kg (max. dose 150 mg) 12 h	85+
	or	
Co-trimoxazole	(40/200 mg/5 ml)	85+
	0.5 ml/kg (max. dose 20 ml) 12 h	
	or	
Cephalexin	15 mg/kg	95
	(max. dose 500 mg) 8 h	
	or	
Augmentin[2]	10–25 mg/kg/8 h	95
Prophylactic		
Co-trimoxazole	(40/200 mg/5ml) 0.25 ml/kg/night	85+
Nitrofurantoin	1–2 mg/kg/night	85+
Cephalexin[3]	5 mg/kg/night	95+

[1]Percentage of bacteria causing urinary tract infection diagnosed in the emergency department of major Australian hospitals that are sensitive to antibiotics.
[2]Amoxycillin alone only covers 60% of organisms encountered, so Augmentin is preferred.
[3]The suspension forms of the cephalosporins and penicillins lose activity after a few weeks.

concentrations and are well tolerated over long periods of time without inducing excessive microbiological changes in the gut (leading to the emergence of resistant organisms or candidiasis).

Ongoing Management: investigations

Investigations are aimed at determining whether there are significant underlying urinary tract malformations. Nearly all centres perform a renal ultrasound. This enables the presence, site, size and shape of the kidneys to be determined. In the age group under 5 years, only 15% of abnormalities found on DMSA scan ('scars/dysplasia') will be seen on ultrasound examination. The ureters are not visualised unless enlarged. An idea of bladder function can be determined by measuring the postvoid residual volume (normally less than 20 ml in children under 7 years).

The radiological examination of the urethra and bladder, using a micturating cystourethrogram (MCU), is performed in nearly all centres as a routine on infants (less than 1 year of age) and some centres would routinely perform it on children up to the age of around 3 years. An MCU should be performed on any child who

has an abnormality on renal ultrasound (such as discrepant renal size, renal ectopia, pelvicalyceal dilatation, hydronephrosis or hydroureter).

Other investigations are performed for a specific indication. Nuclear medicine investigations with technetium-99 m labelled radioisotopes are useful for a number of purposes. These investigations carry radiation toxicity of less than a one tenth of a routine chest X-ray.

The **DTPA** radionuclide is injected intravenously, it is filtered by the glomerulus and then it is neither secreted nor absorbed by the tubule of the kidney. Like creatinine or inulin it can be used to obtain an accurate measure of the glomerular filtration rate.

The **Mag 3** scan has largely replaced the DTPA scan because, in addition to some glomerula filtration, the isotope is mainly secreted by the proximal tubular cells into the urine so that the signal to background ratio is higher than in the DTPA scan. This is particularly useful in children with renal impairment or infants in the first 3 months of life when the glomerular filtration rate is low. Both of these investigations are useful for diagnosing the presence of obstruction to urinary flow from the kidneys to the bladder, for determining the 'split' of kidney function (between the right and left kidneys), and for estimating overall renal function.

The **DMSA** radionuclide is filtered by the glomerulus and taken up by the proximal tubular cells. Scanning takes place when it has been taken up by these cells, which are in the renal cortex. Lack of uptake gives a defect on the scan and this can be due to either transient impairment of the tubular cell function (e.g. following acute inflammation with pyelonephritis for a period of up to 3–4 months) or absence of kidney tissue (renal 'scarring/dysplasia').

Delayed uptake of any of these three radionuclides may occur in conditions where perfusion to the kidney is abnormal (e.g. renal artery stenosis in a unilateral case or dehydration in a bilateral case).

Clinical example

Johnnie had a birth weight of 3.3 kg. He was breastfed and weighed 5.1 kg at 2 months of age. For the next month he put on no weight and his mother noted that he was irritable, fed poorly and had the occasional vomit. The family doctor took a bag sample of urine and found <$10^8 l^{-1}$ Gram negative colony forming units the next day on culture. The doctor arranged for a suprapubic aspirate of urine to be performed at the emergency department. This was done after a bladder scan showed a moderately full bladder. The child was admitted to hospital and received treatment with gentamicin and penicillin given intravenously for 48 hours before an *E.coli* sensitive to co-trimoxazole was identified. The infant was discharged to complete 3 days of oral co-trimoxazole therapy and then to commence night-time co-trimoxazole prophylactic antibiotic treatment. An MCU and renal ultrasound were performed in the next few days.

The ultrasound showed right sided hydronephrosis and hydroureter with a normal left kidney. The MCU showed a mild trabeculated bladder with right sided vesicoureteric reflux; the urethra was abnormal in appearance with some dilatation of the posterior urethra (Fig. 61.1). Prophylactic antibiotic treatment was continued and the child was referred to a paediatric urologist for cystoscopy and evaluation of the urethra.

The ongoing management depends on the results of investigations. A flow diagram of possibilities is shown in Figure 61.2.

Urinary tract infection and normal investigations

Antibiotics are stopped. If the child is completely asymptomatic, this author does not perform another urine culture at the end of treatment. If recurrent symptomatic infection occurs, the initial investigations are reviewed, the child is treated acutely, as outlined above, and, in the

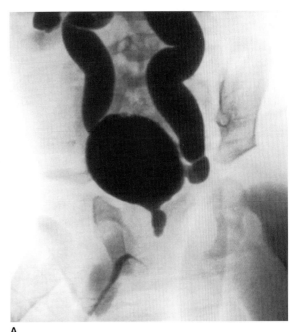

A

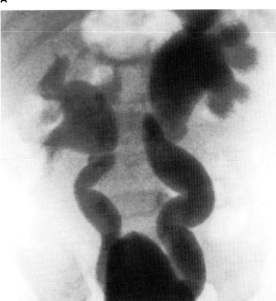

B

Fig. 61.1 **A** The MCU (from the clinical example) showing a dilated posterior urethra, mildly irregular appearance of the edge of the bladder (reflective and trabeculation) and bilateral vesicoureteric reflux into dilated tortuous ureters.
B Hydronephrosis with 'clubbing' of the calyces.

case of an infant, prophylactic antibiotics are continued for 3–6 months. In the case of an older child with recurrent infections and normal baseline investigations, the ultrasound would be repeated and an examination for constipation or a functional voiding disorder (daytime wetting) would be undertaken. Sexual activity should be considered in teenagers.

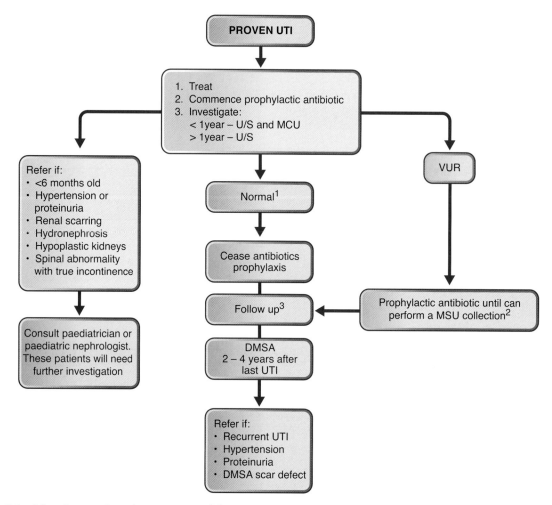

Fig. 61.2 A flow diagram of ongoing management following a proven urinary tract infection. U/S, ultrasound; MCU, micturating cystourethrogram; VUR, vesicoureteric reflux. A normal ultrasound does not exclude scarring. This age is chosen for convenience. Boys uncommonly get recurrent infections after 1 year, girls commonly have recurrent infection untill about 3 years. Follow up includes a yearly blood pressure check. The finding of a normal DMSA scan normalises the risk of developing hypertension.

Clinical example

Amy, a 14 year old girl, presented to her local doctor on three occasions over 6 months with culture proven urinary tract infections. There is no family history of urine infections, Amy has never had a urinary tract infection before, and there is no evidence of a wetting disorder. Further history reveals the onset of sexual activity at about the same time as the urinary tract infections started.

The girl is counselled regarding contraception and sexually transmitted diseases and and she and her parents are offered counselling regarding her sexual activity. She is advised to have a 300 ml glass of water with a citravescent sachet immediately prior to or just after sexual intercourse. However, 1 month later she represents with another urinary tract infection. She is now advised to take nitrofurantoin (100 mg capsule immediately after sexual intercourse). She is seen for review 3 and 6 months after this treatment, reports no further symptoms and remains compliant with the treatment. As she is readily changing sexual partners she is advised to continue on the treatment.

Asymptomatic infection

Up to 4% of adolescent girls have asymptomatic bacteriuria. A number of these children will have vesicoureteric reflux or reflux associated nephropathy (see below). There is no evidence treatment of asymptomatic bacteriuria is beneficial, and colonisation frequently recurs after treatment, sometimes with a more pathogenic symptomatic infection.

Vesicoureteric reflux (VUR)

This is a disorder in which urine passes in a retrograde direction from the bladder through the vesicoureteric junction (VUJ) into the ureter. It is a common disorder affecting 40% of children under 1 year of age who are investigated for a first urinary tract infection. The diagnosis is made on the basis of the finding on the MCU examination.

VUR is a familial trait affecting between 30 and 50% first degree relatives of index cases. This developmental abnormality is characterised by the distal end of the ureter running less obliquely through the wall of the bladder and having less muscle around it. In some cases, it is associated with renal malformation (variously referred to as renal scarring, dysplasia, reflux associated nephropathy), excessive dilatation and tortuosity of the ureter, occurrence on the contralateral side, abnormalities of bladder contraction and urinary tract infection.

The current primary treatment of VUR is prevention of symptomatic urinary tract infections using antibiotic prophylaxis with the drugs described previously (Table 61.3). This is continued until the child has passed the major risk period for developing urinary tract infections. Failure of prophylaxis (the occurrence of symptomatic urine infections) is the indication for antireflux surgery. Twenty per cent of children with reflux will have resolution occurring spontaneously each 3 year period, with less severe degrees of reflux resolving earlier than more severe degrees.

Reflux associated nephropathy

Once thought to be due to the combination of VUR and infection, this abnormality of the kidney is most often congenital in origin. The occurrence of acquired 'scarring' is a subject of controversy. It is found in approximately 10% of children with VUR. The importance of this lesion lies in the possibility of development of hypertension, which is rare in early childhood but occurs in up to 15% of cases by the age of 20 years. Bilateral extensive reflux associated nephropathy is a cause of renal failure occurring from mid childhood.

Posterior urethral valves

This abnormality is also referred to as congenital obstructive posterior urethral membranes (COPUMs). It affects males and causes obstruction to urine flow at the level of the posterior urethra. The bladder is often thick walled and trabeculated; there may be associated VUR with tortuous and dilated ureters draining grossly hydronephrotic kidneys. Antenatal ultrasound demonstrating hydronephrosis and megacystis is a common presentation, as is urinary infection in early infancy, but some children present later with dribbling and wetting.

Diagnosis is made on the urethrogram phase of the MCU and confirmation is obtained by cystoscopy. Treatment involves complex surgical procedures performed in the setting of a team approach to the patient, involving medical staff and continence physiotherapists. Preparation for end stage renal failure treatment is often necessary.

Neurogenic bladder

True neurogenic bladder is found in association with spina bifida and myelomeningocele or other spinal cord injury. Abnormalities of the spinal cord can often be demonstrated by ultrasound in the first months of life, but later magnetic resonance imaging is usually required.

The 'non neurogenic' neurogenic bladder is a term used when children have the clinical and investigation features of a neurogenic bladder but do not have demonstrable spinal pathology. Children with the latter present with urinary tract infections or wetting, when investigations may reveal a large or small trabeculated bladder with or without reflux and hydronephrosis. Urodynamic evaluation of the bladder reveals abnormal pressure volume characteristics, with abnormal bladder contraction.

Treatment involves manoeuvres aimed to keep the bladder empty so that high pressures which will damage the kidney are not generated. Clean intermittent catheterisation, vesicostomy or other drainage operations are frequently necessary. The bladder often requires enlargement to increase its storage capacity; this is performed by augmentation with bowel or redundant ureter.

Duplication

A kidney is said to be duplex if two separate collecting systems are identified. The ureters may join before entry into the bladder or they may have separate openings into the bladder. The upper pole ureter enters the urinary tract more distal to the lower pole ureter and may enter the urethra, giving rise to incontinence, or may be obstructed at its lower end (ureterocoele), in which case the upper pole of the kidney will be abnormal. The lower pole ureter often has vesicoureteric reflux.

Other causes of urinary obstruction

Pelviureteric junction obstruction. This is now most commonly diagnosed following the evaluation of hydronephrosis detected on antenatal scanning of the fetus. At least 9 out of 10 such cases will resolve spontaneously over the first year of life. Periodic renal ultrasound observation, sometimes supplemented by diuretic renography using DPTA or Mag 3 nuclear medicine imaging, is used to follow these infants. Pelviureteric junction obstruction may present in later childhood with renal colic and these cases usually require surgery.

Vesicoureteric junction obstruction. This often presents following investigation of urinary tract infection, with the ultrasound showing a dilated ureter, and nuclear medicine imaging showing delayed passage of urine from the ureter to the bladder with a widened ureteric image. Treatment is reimplantation of the ureter.

Renal calculi. These may present following urinary tract infection, in which case the calculus is usually a triple phosphate (magnesium, calcium and ammonium) stone and the infecting organisms often urea splitting (such as *Proteus mirabilis*), or renal colic. Other stones occasionally encountered are composed of cystine (autosomal recessive cystinuria), calcium oxalate, and uncommonly uric acid.

Antenatal renal abnormalities

The advent of almost routine antenatal scanning at 18 weeks gestation has led to the detection of approximately 1 in 200 infants having an increased renal pelvis diameter (greater than 4 mm at 18 weeks). The postnatal diagnoses are shown in Table 61.4.

Management

The antenatal ultrasound should be repeated in the third trimester of pregnancy. The presence of bilateral severe hydronephrosis with an enlarged bladder in the male infant suggests the diagnosis of posterior urethral valves. The presence of oligohydramnios suggests reduced urine output and this is associated with the development of pulmonary hypoplasia.

Table 61.4 Antenatal renal abnormalities: postnatal diagnoses

Diagnosis	%
Non refluxing non obstructive hydronephrosis	55
Vesicoureteric reflux	15
PUJ obstruction	5
Multicystic kidney	5
VUJ abnormalities	5
Duplex	5
Agenesis	5
Posturethral valves	2

After birth, the infant should be placed on prophylatic trimethoprim until the diagnosis is determined. If unwell or if significant severe abnormalities are suspected, imaging of the kidneys and urinary tract should be performed immediately. In contrast, if the baby is well and without severe urinary tract dilatation, a postnatal ultrasound is undertaken towards the end of the first week of life when the baby is well hydrated. Further investigations, usually looking for reflux or obstruction, are performed, depending upon the results of this ultrasound.

Cystic renal disease

Common forms of cystic renal disease and the modes of presentation are listed in Table 61.5.

Table 61.5 Forms and presentation of cystic renal disease

Cystic renal disease	Incidence	Genetics	Clinical features
Autosomal dominant polycystic kidney disease	1–2/1000 M = F	3 gene defects cause it; 50% risk in subsequent children	Usually discovered because of family history. Uncommon cause of hypertension or loin/abdominal discomfort in childhood. Progresses to renal failure later in life
Autosomal recessive kidney disease	1–2/10 000 births M = F	1 gene defect identified; 25% risk in subsequent pregnancies	Often present in infancy with enlarged kidneys, polycystic and olighydramnios which, in turn, is associated with pulmonary hypoplasia. Later, may get hypertension, renal impairment. Associated with hepatic fibrosis causing portal hypertension in mid childhood.
Cystic renal dysplasia	Common	Polygenic; low recurrence risk	Often asymptomatic. Associated with vesicoureteric reflux. May be bilateral.
Multicystic dysplastic kidney	Relatively uncommon	Unknown; low recurrence risk	Enlarged completely cystic non functioning kidney without blood flow. Contralateral kidney usually normal but may be associated with VUR or PUJ obstruction

Glomerulonephritis, related disorders and hypertension

J. R. Burke

Glomerulonephritis presents with various clinical manifestations; these are:
- nephrotic syndrome
- acute nephritis
- recurrent haematuria
- isolated proteinuria
- chronic renal failure.

Most forms of glomerulonephritis result from an immunologically mediated injury involving either deposition of circulating immune complexes in the glomerulus or a specific antibody to the glomerular basement membrane.

Nephrotic syndrome

Nephrotic syndrome is defined as:
- oedema
- proteinuria
- hypoalbuminaemia and
- hyperlipidaemia.

The annual incidence in children is approximately 2–4:100 000. The major pathological lesions in primary nephrotic syndrome are given in Table 62.1.

Minimal change nephrotic syndrome

Evidence now suggests that the aetiology of minimal change nephrotic syndrome is caused by an alteration in the glomerular anionic status. Sensitised lymphocytes secrete a number of lymphokines that alter the normal negatively charged sialoproteins on the glomerular basement membrane. Loss of membrane negative charge allows anionic proteins to leak across the basement membrane into Bowman's space. Light microscopy shows normal glomeruli but in some cases a mild increase in mesangial cells and mesangial matrix may occur.

Immunofluorescence is negative and electron microscopy shows fusion of foot processes.

Generalised oedema is the usual presenting symptom (Fig. 62.1). Minimal change lesion nephrotic syndrome comprises 80% of cases of nephrotic syndrome without significant constitutional disturbance in childhood and is more frequent in males than females, the majority presenting between ages 1 and 4 years. Renal biopsy is not initially indicated if clinical features suggest minimal change (Table 62.2).

Unless large pleural effusions, gross ascites or severe genital oedema are present, strict bed rest is not necessary and the child should be allowed normal ward activity. A high protein, low salt diet is encouraged. Fluid intake should not be restricted because of the risk of hypovolaemia and a free intake is encouraged. Prednisolone

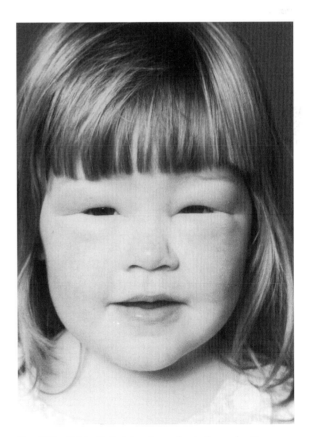

Fig. 62.1 Child with facial oedema due to the nephrotic syndrome.

Table 62.1 Classification of primary nephrotic syndrome

- Minimal change
- Focal segmental glomerulosclerosis
- Mesangial proliferative glomerulonephritis
- Membranoproliferative glomerulonephritis
- Membranous glomerulopathy
- Congenital nephrotic syndrome

Table 62.2 Clinical features of minimal change nephrotic syndrome

- Age 1–10 years
- Microscopic haematuria 30%
- Blood pressure normal
- Renal function normal
- Complements normal
- Selective index — low molecular weight protein urine loss

Clinical example

Sasha, a girl now aged 5 years, presented with nephrotic syndrome at 2 years. At presentation serum albumin was 18 g/l and 24 hour urine protein 1.5 g/l. Microurine showed 30 r.b.c./mm^3. Blood pressure and complement were normal. Prednisolone 60 mg/m^2/day induced remission in 12 days. In the next 2 years she had six relapses with upper respiratory tract infections and was then managed with prophylactic prednisolone and levamisole. In the last 12 months she had four further relapses, responding to prednisolone 60 mg/m^2/day. She is now cushingoid and height percentile has fallen from the 25th to below the 10th percentile. She is commencing a 10 week course of cyclophosphamide (2.5 mg/kg/day).

She has steroid dependent nephrotic syndrome with significant steroid side effects. Levamisole has not reduced her relapse rate.

2 mg/kg/day or 60 mg/m^2/day induces a remission in 90% of cases. The prednisolone dose is then reduced over 6 months, with later doses being given on alternate days to reduce side effects. If remission, as defined by complete loss of proteinuria, has not occurred by 4 weeks, the nephrotic syndrome is steroid resistant and a renal biopsy is then indicated to exclude other pathology, particularly focal segmental glomerulosclerosis.

Approximately 70% of children have relapses, which are more likely to occur in association with viral upper respiratory tract infections. These relapses may be prevented by prophylactic prednisolone 5–15 mg given on alternate days. Levamisole 2.5 mg/kg on alternate days is indicated when steroid side effects with multiple relapses become significant. Of children given cyclophosphamide, 50% have no further relapses and most of the rest have substantially fewer episodes of nephrotic relapse. Cyclosporin also reduces the frequency of relapses, but does not give longlasting remission (Table 62.3).

The major complications of the nephrotic syndrome are infections, hypovolaemia and thromboembolism. Both Gram positive and Gram negative organisms cause peritonitis and septicaemia. The susceptibility to infections is related to loss of opsonins and immunoglobulins in the urine. If the patient develops a serious infection, the initial antibiotic treatment should cover both Gram positive and Gram negative organisms until cultures and sensitivity results are available. Hypovolaemia, which occurs in 5%, should be suspected if such a child develops oliguria (< 100 ml per day), abdominal pain, tachycardia or postural hypotension. This complication is confirmed by a high haematocrit and a low urine sodium (< 10 mmol/l). Hypovolaemia is due to loss of plasma water into the tissues with a consequent fall in the circulating blood volume. The preferred treatment is intravenous 20% albumin (1 g/kg over 3–6 hours). Albumin infusions may need to be repeated, according to response.

At the end of each infusion intravenous frusemide (2 mg/kg) is given.

A hypercoagulable state exists for a number of reasons. These include haemoconcentration and loss of antithrombin III in the urine. Renal vein thrombosis and pulmonary embolism are relatively rare occurrences which require prompt treatment with anticoagulants. The avoidance of bed rest and the treatment of hypovolaemia probably account for the decreasing incidence of these complications.

Approximately 90% of children with relapsing nephrotic syndrome cease relapsing by 16 years of age. Even those children who continue to relapse into adult life usually remain steroid sensitive. It is very rare for a child with a steroid sensitive minimal change lesion nephrotic syndrome to progress to chronic renal failure. The 20 year mortality has now decreased from 60% to less than 5% since the introduction of antibiotics and corticosteroids. The morbidity and mortality should continue to decrease with adequate management of complications and avoidance of excess immunosuppression.

Focal segmental glomerulosclerosis

This glomerulopathy comprises 5–10% of children with nephrotic syndrome. The presentation is often similar to a minimal change lesion but with steroid resistance. Renal biopsy (Fig. 62.2) shows segmental sclerosis or hyalinosis with other glomeruli completely sclerosed or normal. Immunofluorescence shows IgM and IgG in the affected segmental lesions.

The majority of children with this lesion are resistant to steroids, cyclophosphamide and cyclosporin. Those children who remain nephrotic require treatment with diuretics (frusemide, spironolactone), mild fluid restriction and a low salt diet. Approximately 60% progress to

Table 62.3 Drug therapy for relapsing minimal change

- Prednisolone
- Levamisole
- Cyclophosphamide
- Cyclosporin

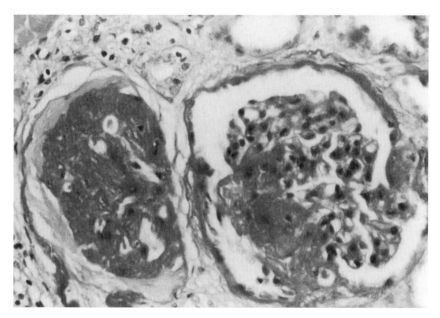

Fig. 62.2 Segmental and global sclerosis (PAS ×500).

end stage renal failure over 10 years. This glomerulopathy has a 30% recurrence risk in a transplanted kidney and in some cases plasmapheresis is beneficial.

Congenital nephrotic syndrome

Nephrotic syndrome in the first 3 months of life is most common in Finland, where the pathology is described as microcystic disease. Other types with minimal lesion histology, diffuse mesangial sclerosis or congenital syphilis are seen occasionally. The Finnish types are now seen in descendants of other European communities and the condition is inherited in an autosomal recessive fashion. The gene is localised to chromosone 19q13.1 and encodes a transmembrane protein, called nephrin, which appears to be expressed in glomerular podocytes. Oedema is noted in the first weeks of life, with placentomegaly and prematurity being common precursors. There is no specific treatment, but transplantation can be performed without recurrence of the glomerulopathy.

Glomerulonephritis

Acute glomerulonephritis is defined as:
- haematuria
- proteinuria
- oedema
- hypertension and
- renal insufficiency.

This acute onset is seen usually in poststreptococcal glomerulonephritis. Other forms of glomerulonephritis (Table 62.4) in childhood have a less severe onset.

Table 62.4   Causes of acute nephritis

- Postinfectious glomerulonephritis
- Henoch–Schönlein purpura
- IgA nephropathy
- Alport syndrome
- Lupus erythematosus
- Membranoproliferative glomerulonephritis

Poststreptococcal glomerulonephritis

This disorder follows 2–3 weeks after group A haemolytic streptococcal throat or skin infection. Circulating antigen–antibody complexes form in the blood and deposit in glomeruli with activation of the complement system. The pathological appearance consists of proliferation of mesangial and endothelial cells with neutrophil infiltration (Fig. 62.3). Crescents may be present. Immunofluorescence shows IgG and C3 and electron dense deposits are demonstrated by electron microscopy.

The usual presentation is a child, usually of school age, with macroscopic haematuria, oedema or headache caused by hypertension. Lassitude, fever and loin pain also may be present. Physical examination may reveal hypertension, papilloedema, facial and leg oedema. On laboratory investigation urinalysis shows red blood cell casts and dysmorphic red cells. Serum urea, creatinine and potassium concentrations are often elevated. Mild normocytic normochromic anaemia is common and indicates haemodilution is present.

The antistreptolysin O titre (ASOT) and antistreptococcal DNAase B are elevated in 90% of cases.

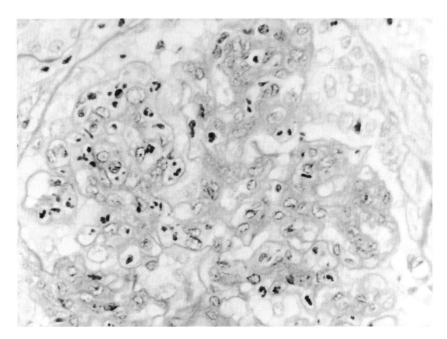

Fig. 62.3 Mesangial proliferation and neutrophil infiltration in poststreptococcal glomerulonephritis (PAS ×800).

Complement activation may occur via both classical and alternative pathways. Serum levels of C3 complement are low and return to normal within 6–12 weeks. Complement C4 may be low in the early stages of the disease.

Careful management of the acute renal failure, and especially of the hypertension, is the basis of treatment in this condition. Salt and water accumulation, with suppression of plasma renin, is the major cause of hypertension. Mild hypertension is best managed with frusemide 2–4 mg/kg/day and fluid restriction. Moderate to severe hypertension requires management with oral captopril, nifedipine or prazosin. Parenteral hydralazine, diazoxide and nitroprusside are rarely required. Beta blockers should be avoided in the presence of pulmonary oedema. Bed rest is necessary only when the blood pressure is elevated. A course of oral penicillin for 10 days eradicates any existing streptococcal infection but does not alter the natural history of this condition. When renal insufficiency is present the diet consists of restricted protein (1 g/kg/day) and low salt and potassium intake.

The major *complications* of acute post streptococcal glomerulonephritis are hypertensive encephalopathy, left ventricular failure and acute renal failure. Hypertensive convulsions are often associated with papilloedema and a temporary cortical blindness. This complication is best treated by parenteral diazoxide 2–5 mg/kg followed by oral medication.

Acute heart failure is related to hypertension and fluid overload. Severe fluid restriction, high dose frusemide administration and adequate control of hypertension are then necessary.

The period of oliguria lasts up to 10 days and dialysis is indicated in cases where the blood urea rises above 50–60 mmol/l, or when hyperkalaemia or pulmonary oedema are not controlled by intravenous frusemide and fluid restriction. Dialysis should be performed only in a centre with the appropriate expertise. The long term prognosis is excellent, with only 1% developing chronic renal failure. Microscopic haematuria may continue for 2 years, but proteinuria should clear within 6 months. Renal biopsy is not indicated unless there is uncertainty of diagnosis with the initial investigations or the period of oliguria lasts longer than 3 weeks.

Other infectious agents including viral and bacterial organisms rarely can produce an illness similar to post-streptococcal nephritis. These organisms include staphylococcus and pneumococcus, echo, coxsackie and Epstein–Barr viruses.

Henoch–Schönlein purpura

This disease is a vasculitic illness predominantly involving small vessels in the skin, large joints and gastrointestinal tract (Ch. 54). The illness is preceded by upper respiratory tract infection in 30–50% of patients. These children present with a petechial or purpuric rash, abdominal pain and arthritis. A mild nephritis is seen in 50–70% of cases, manifest usually by microscopic haematuria and proteinuria. Rarely blood pressure and serum creatinine are elevated. Renal histology shows a proliferative glomerulonephritis with IgA in the mesangium. The prognosis is good, with less than 5% developing chronic renal failure.

IgA (Berger) disease

This glomerulopathy is present in 50% of children who have recurrent episodes of macroscopic haematuria. The episodes of haematuria often occur simultaneously with intercurrent viral infections and flank pain. Other presentations include abnormal urinalysis on medical examination and rarely chronic renal failure in childhood. The histology of focal proliferative glomerulonephritis with IgA in the mesangium is similar to that of Henoch–Schönlein purpura (Fig. 62.4). Very few children develop chronic renal failure, as the disorder is more common in adults.

Alport syndrome

This is a familial disorder in production of type IV collagen and is inherited as an X linked dominant or autosomal dominant condition. Males are affected more severely than females. In males this disorder presents in the first 10 years of life with haematuria and proteinuria. Renal histology shows a proliferative glomerulonephritis, with typical changes in the basement membrane of splitting of the internal elastic lamina found on electron microscopy. Renal failure develops in the teenage years.

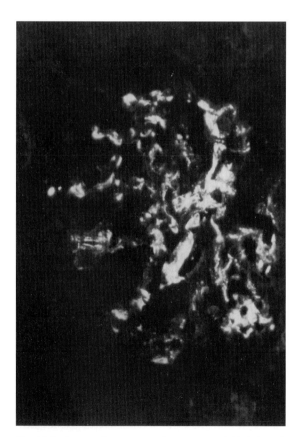

Fig. 62.4 Immunofluorescence shows mesangial IgA deposits (×600).

High tone nerve deafness and eye abnormalities are the other features of the syndrome.

Lupus erythematosus

Systemic lupus erythematosus (SLE) in childhood is seen more in females in the later childhood years. Facial rash, arthritis and fever are common presenting symptoms. Renal biopsy is indicated if haematuria and proteinuria are present. Serum C3 complement is usually low. This disorder is discussed further in Chapter 44. The type of glomerulonephritis in SLE can vary from a mild focal proliferative glomerulonephritis to a diffuse crescentic glomerulonephritis with associated membranous features. The treatment includes prednisolone, azathioprine, cyclophosphamide and mycophenolate. The amount of immunosuppression is dependent on the severity of renal impairment, proteinuria and type of renal histology.

Benign microscopic haematuria

In every 200 children, one has intermittent microscopic haematuria as an incidental finding on urinalysis. This condition is usually benign providing there is no infection or proteinuria, renal function is normal and no structural abnormality is present on ultrasonography. Renal biopsy sometimes shows thinning of basement membrane on electron microscopy (thin membrane disease). Often inheritance is in an autosomal dominant fashion.

Postural proteinuria

Intermittent or orthostatic proteinuria occurs in 10% of children. Testing with albustix or protein: creatinine ratio shows a normal amount of urinary protein in the early morning and increased protein during the day. The 24 hour protein estimation can sometimes be as high as 300–400 mg/day. This phenomenon is benign, but proteinuria in an overnight urine specimen will usually require biopsy to determine the cause.

Haemolytic uraemic syndrome (HUS)

Haemolytic uraemic syndrome is characterised by the triad of:
- microangiopathic haemolytic anaemia
- thrombocytopenia and
- acute renal insufficiency.

It is a major cause of acute renal failure in childhood. It has been broadly classified into two groups: the typical or epidemic form, also known as diarrhoea associated (D+) HUS; the atypical or sporadic form, diarrhoea negative (D–) HUS.

This disorder is more common under the age of 3 years. Usually it follows a mild gastroenteritis, but the diarrhoea is often blood stained. Over the next few days, the child becomes pale, oliguric and unwell. Examination of the blood film shows fragmented red blood cells and thrombocytopenia. Urinalysis reveals haematuria and proteinuria. The serum creatinine is usually elevated and hypertension is often severe.

Pathogenesis is related to a verotoxin for *Escherichia coli* (0157) crossing the damaged mucosa and adhering to endothelial cells in arterioles, with consequent swelling and widening of the subendothelial space with fibrin deposition. Atypical cases may follow pneumococcal pneumonia in which neuramidase causes T cell activation.

Dialysis is often necessary in the management of acute renal failure. Management is complex and should only be undertaken by an expert in paediatric renal disease; 90% of children make a complete recovery. Bad prognostic signs are oliguria lasting more than 2 weeks, cerebral involvement and age of onset over 5 years.

Chronic renal failure

> ### Clinical example
>
> Thomas aged 30 months has chronic renal failure from birth from urethral valves and dysplastic kidneys. He has poor appetite and required nasal gastric feeding from 3 months. X ray of the wrist at 18 months shows rickets requiring additional dosage of calcitriol. At 24 months he developed anaemia (Hb 9.5 g/l) and commenced subcutaenous erythropoietin twice weekly. He has grown 2 cm in the last 12 months. Investigations now show Hb 11.3 g/l, serum sodium 136 mmol/l, potassium 6.5 mmol/l, urea 42 mmol/l, creatinine 0.65 mmol/l, calcium 2.4 mmol/l, phosphate 2.4 mmol/l, alkaline phosphatase 850 u/l. Parathormone is elevated.
> He has now reached end stage renal failure and will commence peritoneal dialysis. Growth hormone is indicated for growth failure. He will continue calcium carbonate at meal times in addition to calcitriol for renal oesteodystropy and erythropoietin for anaemia.

- The incidence of chronic renal failure in children is 2–4 per million total population per year. The commonest causes include:
- chronic glomerulonephritis
- reflux nephropathy
- obstructive uropathy and
- medullary cystic disease.

Identification of structural renal abnormalities by obstetric ultrasound and early investigation of urinary tract infections may decrease the incidence of renal failure in the future.

The principles of management are as follows:
- Control of hypertension.
- Adequate nutrition. Growth becomes impaired when the glomerular filtration rate is less than 25% of normal/1.73 m^2. With this degree of renal impairment, hyperfiltration can produce further sclerosis of the remaining functioning glomeruli. A low protein diet (0.8–1.5 g/kg/day) with low phosphate and adequate calorie intake may delay the progression of renal failure. Salt and fluid intake will vary with the type of renal disease.
- Prevention of renal osteodystrophy. Hyperphosphataemia should be vigorously treated with a low phosphate diet and dietary phosphate binders (calcium carbonate or aluminium hydroxide) in an attempt to prevent secondary hyperparathyroidism. Vitamin D supplementation with calcitriol (1,25-dihydroxycholecalciferol) is given in early renal failure to prevent rickets.
- Administration of alkali to control acidosis (2–3 mmol/kg/day).
- Anaemia is corrected by erythropoietin. This is administered subcutaneously 1–2 times each week. Iron supplementation is often necessary.
- Growth retardation is improved by growth hormone. Resistance to growth hormone is caused by low insulin-like growth factor levels.

Dialysis and transplantation are now standard for young children with end stage renal failure. Under the first year of age there are considerable technical, ethical and psychological problems. Young children tolerate continuous cyclic peritoneal dialysis (CCPD) better than haemodialysis. Both cadaver and live related transplants are performed in children with good results. Approximately 80% of children survive for at least 10–15 years after entering dialysis/transplant programmes.

Hypertension

The recording of blood pressure should be part of the normal examination in children. The blood pressure cuff should cover two thirds of the upper arm, as a smaller cuff will often lead to a falsely high reading. The child should be still and not crying. Using sphygmomanometry, the diastolic component is probably best recorded by the fifth Korotkoff sound, but if difficulties arise in obtaining an accurate recording a machine using oscillometric techniques should be used.

Normal blood pressure for children varies with age (Fig. 62.5). A child should not be regarded as being hypertensive unless three recordings give levels above the 95th percentile for that age group. In borderline hypertension oscillometric 24 hour ambulatory blood

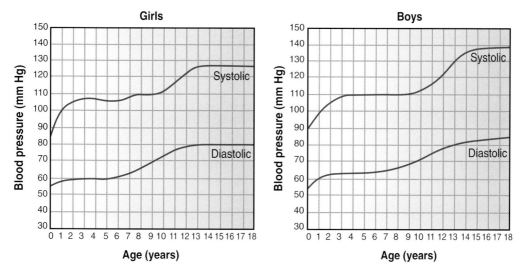

Fig. 62.5   Normal values (means) for systolic and diastolic blood pressure in **A** girls and **B** boys from 0 to 18 years.

pressure recordings are useful to distinguish constant blood pressure elevation from 'white coat hypertension'.

The major causes of hypertension are given in Table 62.5. Renal disease accounts for approximately 80% of cases.

The investigation of hypertension should commence with a good history and examination. Symptoms of chronic renal disease include polyuria and polydipsia, urinary tract infections and headaches. History should include neonatal umbilical artery catheterisation. Hypertension in a parent or an early stroke in a relative may be a pointer to essential hypertension. Physical examination may assist in making a specific diagnosis, for example, a palpable renal mass, pigmentation, delayed femoral pulses and renal artery bruits.

Initial screening investigations will include examination of the urine for erythrocytes, proteinuria or infection, and estimation of serum creatinine and electrolyte levels.

An ultrasound and DMSA scan of the kidneys will reveal scarring from reflux nephropathy. A DTPA or Mag 3 renal scan will exclude an obstructive uropathy, and with captopril is useful in renal artery stenosis. If renal artery stenosis is suspected, further investigations with Doppler ultrasound, renal angiogram and renal vein renin ratio are necessary. In acute nephritis elevated ASOT and depressed C3 complement levels will establish a diagnosis of acute poststreptococcal glomerulonephritis. Estimation of urinary and plasma catecholamines could be a delayed investigation unless a phaeochromocytoma or neuroblastoma is suspected clinically, as the incidence of phaeochromocytoma in childhood hypertension is only 1%. If a rare form of adrenogenital syndrome (11-hydroxylase or 17-hydroxylase deficiency) or familial hyperaldosteronism is suspected, serum aldosterone: renin ratio, plasma and urine steroid analyses are performed.

Treatment of hypertension depends on the severity, presence of symptoms and underlying cause. Severe hypertension is present if examination of the fundi, or chest X ray and echocardiogram are abnormal. In the acute hypertensive emergency situation, drugs with a rapid onset of action are needed (Table 62.6).

Table 62.5   Causes of hypertension

- Renal
  - Acute glomerulonephritis
  - Chronic glomerulonephritis
  - Reflux nephropathy
  - Obstructive uropathy
  - Haemolytic uraemic syndrome
  - Polycystic kidneys
- Coarctation of aorta
- Renal artery stenosis
- Phaeochromocytoma
- Adrenogenital syndrome
- Familial hyperaldosteronism
- Essential

Table 62.6   Drug therapy of hypertensive emergency

• Hydralazine	0.1–0.5 mg/kg i.v. or i.m. q. 4–6 h
• Diazoxide	2–5 mg/kg i.v.
• Nifedipine	0.5–1 mg/kg oral 12 h
• Captopril	0.2–0.5 mg/kg oral q. 8–12 h
• Minoxidil	0.1–0.5 mg/kg oral 12 h
• Sodium nitroprusside	0.5–10 mcg/kg/min i.v. infusion
• Frusemide	2 mg/kg i.v. q. 12 h
• Labetolol	1–3 mg/kg/h i.v.

Clinical example

Sally, aged 6 years, had a blood pressure recording of 140/100 mmHg at the time of tonsillectomy. Urine analysis, renal function and renal ultrasound were normal; an echocardiogram showed left ventricular hypertropy; a Mag 3 scan showed left kidney contributed 44% and right kidney 56% of total function; a renal angiogram showed a midaortic syndrome with bilateral renal artery stenosis from fibromuscular hyperplasia.

Her blood pressure was controlled with metoprolol 7.5 mg daily and amlodipine 5 mg daily. Left balloon angioplasty to 3–4 mm has been performed and she is awaiting a similar procedure on the right renal artery.

In essential hypertension, advice on a low salt diet, weight reduction and exercise may assist reduction in blood pressure. Intervention techniques such as transluminal angioplasty for renal artery stenosis, resection of coarctation of the aorta, and nephrectomy for a small scarred kidney may cure a small percentage of children.

The drug treatment of chronic hypertension is similar to that of adult patients; drugs used include:

- converting enzyme inhibitiors (captopril, perindopril)
- calcium channel inhibitors (nifedipine, amlodipine)
- beta adrenergic blockers (atenolol, metoprolol)
- vasodilators (hydralazine, prazosin)
- diuretics (hydrochlorothiazide, frusemide).

PART 18   SELF-ASSESSMENT

Questions

1. **A 5 month old boy presents with fever and vomiting. Bag urine testing shows a negative nitrite test, a negative test for leucocyte esterase and a negative test for blood. Which of the following statements are true?**
   (A) A urinary tract infection can be excluded
   (B) A suprapubic aspirate or catheter collection of urine for culture should be collected if there are no clearcut signs of a non urinary tract infection
   (C) If there are no clinical signs of non urinary tract infection, the boy has a high chance of having a urinary infection
   (D) If appropriate urine cultures are not taken and the child is treated, then the child should at least have a renal ultrasound examination
   (E) After clinically responding to an appropriate course of antibiotics, prophylactic antibiotics should be commenced

2. **Which of the following statements are correct? Regarding urinary infection and vesicoureteric reflux in infants and children:**
   (A) Girls are more likely to develop urinary infection than boys throughout childhood
   (B) Vesicoureteric reflux is present in <10% of children who are investigated following an episode of urinary infection
   (C) The majority of children with vesicoureteric reflux require surgical correction
   (D) Children with vesicoureteric reflux and urinary infection should be treated with prophylactic antibiotics, at least through infancy

3. **Tom, a 6 year old boy, presents with an upper respiratory tract infection. Urine analysis is positive blood on haemostix. Microurine on three occasions over 4 months shows 20–50 r.b.c./mm³. Serum creatinine is 0.05 mmol/l, 24 urine protein is 50 mg. Complement C_3 is normal. Blood pressure is 80/60 mmHg. Which of the following statements is correct?**
   (A) He has poststreptococal glomerulonephritis
   (B) Benign microscopic haematuria is likely
   (C) Prophylatic penicillin is indicated
   (D) Renal biopsy may show thin membrane disease
   (E) Microscopic haematuria may be present in other family members

4. **Susan, a 7 year old Aboriginal girl, presents with macroscopic haematuria. She has mild leg oedema. Blood pressure is 130/90 mmHg. Serum sodium is 131 mmol/l, potassium 6.5 mmol/l, creatinine 0.15 mmol/l, albuminin 27 g/l. C3 complement is low and C4 is normal. Microurine shows greater than 1000 r.b.c./mm³ and 4+ protein. Which of the following statements is correct?**
   (A) She has minimal change nephrotic syndrome
   (B) Blood pressure is mildly elevated and does not require specific treatment
   (C) She has a 30% chance of progressing to chronic renal failure
   (D) Microscopic haematuria may persist for 6–12 months
   (E) Complement level returns to normal in 10 weeks

5. **Damion, a 10 year old boy, presents with lassitude. He has a history of a urinary tract infection at 12 months. Blood pressure is 125/85 mmHg. Height is 125 cm (< 3rd percentile). Serum sodium**

is 135 mmol/l, potassium 5.8 mmol/l, CO_2 18 mmol/l, urea 20 mmol/l, creatinine 0.25 mmol/l, calcium 2.1 mmol/l, phosphate 2.4 mmol/l. 24 hour urine protein is 850 mg, microurine shows 20 w.b.c./mm^3, 0 r.b.c./mm^3 and sterile culture. Ultrasound of the kidneys shows scarring to the right upper and the left lower poles. Micturating cystogram shows bilateral grade 3 reflux. Which of the following statements is correct?

(A) Mag 3 renal scan would assist in diagnosis

(B) The presence of proteinuria is a bad prognostic feature

(C) Bilateral ureteric reimplantation is indicated.

(D) A low protein diet would slow the progress of chronic renal failure

(E) Growth hormone is likely to improve his final height

Answers and explanations

1. From Table 61.2, the boy has an 89% chance of not having a urinary tract infection. Thus a urinary tract infection cannot be excluded (A). A collection of urine that will definitely prove or exclude a urinary tract infection should be taken, thus (B) is true. The boy has presented with typical symptoms of urinary tract infection and urinary tract infection is common at this age. Thus (C) is true. Also, (D) is true because the child will have a high chance of having an underlying urinary malformation. Prophylactic antibiotics should be used until investigations (renal ultrasound and MCU in this case) have defined the urinary tract anatomy. Thus (E) is true.

2. The correct answer is (D). (A) Up to the age of 3 months, boys are more likely to develop urinary infections than girls, but beyond this age girls are more likely to develop urinary infections. (B) Vesicoureteric reflux is found in 40% of children under the age of 1 year who present with a first urinary tract infection. (C) While there is some difference in the indications for antireflux surgery amongst different centres, relatively few children with reflux are ever considered for antireflux surgery. Antireflux surgery does not decrease the incidence of urinary tract infection but may decrease the incidence of pyelonephritis. (D) Prophylactic antibiotics should be used in infancy and usually until the child is continent.

3. The correct answers are (B), (D) and (E). His most likely diagnosis is benign microscopic haematuria — thin membrane disease (B), (D). Poststreptococcal glomerulonephritis usually occurs 2–3 weeks after an upper respiratory tract infection and has a low complement (A). There is no evidence that prophylactic penicillin improves the prognosis, which is usually very good (C). The condition is often an autosomal dominant disorder (E).

4. The correct answers are (D) and (E). This girl has nephritic nephrotic syndrome from poststreptococcal glomerulonephritis. Minimal change nephrotic syndrome is not associated with macroscopic haematuria, hypertension or impaired renal function (A). Her blood pressure is significantly elevated for a girl of her age and requires initial treatment with frusemide and fluid restriction (B). Prognosis for poststreptococcal nephritis is excellent, with 98% full recovery (C). Microscopic haematuria often persists for 6–12 months (D). Low complement returns to normal after 8–12 weeks but may persist in membanoproliferative nephritis (E).

5. The correct answers are (B) and (E). He has chronic renal failure from reflux nephropathy. A DMSA renal scan demonstrates renal scarring, and Mag 3 obstruction (A). Significant proteinuria indicates hyperfiltration damage and subsequent progression to end stage renal failure (B). Ureteric reimplantation would not improve prognosis and is only indicated if there are recurrent urinary tract infections (C). There is little evidence that a low protein diet slows the progression of renal failure (D). Growth failure caused by chronic renal failure is improved by growth hormone (E).

PART 18   FURTHER READING

Barratt T M, Avner E D, Harmon W E 1999 Pediatric nephrology. Lippincott, Williams and Wilkins, Baltimore

Chandler W L, Jelacic B S, Boster D R et al 2002 Prothrombotic coagulation abnormalities preceding the hemolytic–uremic syndrome. New England Journal of Medicine 346: 23–32

Craig J C, Irwig L M, Knight J F et al 1998 Symptomatic urinary tract infections in pre-school Australian children. Journal of Paediatric Child Health 34: 154–159

Haffner D, Schaefer F, Nissel R et al 2000 Effect of growth hormone treatment on the adult height of children with chronic renal failure. New England Journal of Medicine 343: 923–930

Hanson S, Jodal U 1999 Urinary tract infection. In: Barratt T M, Avner E D, Harmon W E (eds) Paediatric nephrology. Lippincott, Williams and Wilkins, Baltimore, 835–850

Hodson E, Knight J S, Willis N S, Craig J 2000 Corticosteroid therapy in nephrotic syndrome: a metanalysis of randomised controlled trials. Archives of Disease in Childhood 83: 45–51

Hogg R J, Portman R J, Milliner B et al 2000 Evaluation and management of proteinuria and nephrotic syndrome in children. Pediatrics 105: 1242–1249

Hruska K 2000 Pathophysiology of renal osteodystrophy. Pediatric Nephrology 14: 636–640

Kashtan C E 2000 Alport syndromes: phenotypic heterogenicity of progressive hereditary nephritis. Pediatric Nephrology 14: 502–512

McIlroy P J, Abbott G D, Anderson N G et al 2000 Outcome of primary vesicoureteric reflux detected following fetal renal pelvic dilation. Journal of Paediatric Child Health 36: 569–573

McTaggart S J, Gelati S, Walker R G et al 2000 Evaluation and long term outcome of paediatric renovascular hypertension. Pediatric Nephrology 14: 1022–1029

Martinelli R, Okumura A S, Pereira L et al 2001 Primary focal segmental glomerulosclerosis in children: prognostic features. Pediatric Nephrology 16: 658–661

Soergel M, Kirschstein M, Busch C et al 1997 Oscillometric twenty-four hour ambulatory blood pressure values in healthy children and adolescents: a multicenter trial including 1141 subjects. Journal of Pediatrics 130: 178–183

Streeton C L, Hanna J N, Messer R D 1995 An epidemic of acute post streptococcal glomerulonephritis amongst aboriginal children. Journal of Pediatrics and Child Health 31: 245–248

Useful links

http://www.cari.kidney.org.au (Caring for Australians with Renal Impairment: newsletters, guidelines and other information)

http://www.kidneyatlas.org (Online edition of Atlas of Diseases of the Kidney, Shrier R W (ed), Blackwell)

http://www.kidney.org.au (Australian Kidney Foundation: fact-sheets, study reviews, information)

ENDOCRINE DISORDERS

Growth and variations in growth

J. Batch

Growth may be defined as the proliferation of cells and the accompanying synthesis of cellular and extracellular protein and other macromolecules. Growth is a multifactorial process and is influenced by the interplay of genetic, nutritional, hormonal, psychosocial and other factors, including the general health of a child. As such, growth mirrors the psychosocial and physical wellbeing of a child and adolescent.

Growth is the process which is unique to paediatric and adolescent medicine and distinguishes it from all other branches of clinical medicine. The study of normal and abnormal growth is facilitated by a knowledge of the effects of physiological and pathological processes on growth and development at the different stages of life. The three major determinants of growth are:

- genetic factors
- nutritional factors
- hormonal factors.

Genetic factors

The genetic background of individuals is the basis for the major determinant of growth potential: tall parents do tend to have tall children, while short parents have short children. Although children's heights at maturity resemble those of their parents, little is known about the exact location of the individual height controlling genes, how many genes are involved or how they direct cellular growth. Major genetic disturbances such as occur with chromosomal abnormalities are often reflected in growth patterns. For example, with loss of a sex chromosome in 45,XO Turner syndrome as shown in Figure 63.1, adult stature is severely compromised. Other less severe chromosomal abnormalities also may result in abnormalities in stature.

Many inherited genetic conditions can also result in growth disturbance. The most striking of these are the skeletal dysplasias, which often follow an autosomal dominant mode of inheritance. The classic example of a skeletal dysplasia is achondroplasia, which is described in Chapter 29. Chromosomes may also influence tall stature, as seen in the case of an individual with an extra sex chromosome, for example Klinefelter syndrome XXY, which frequently leads to an adult height above that anticipated from the family pattern.

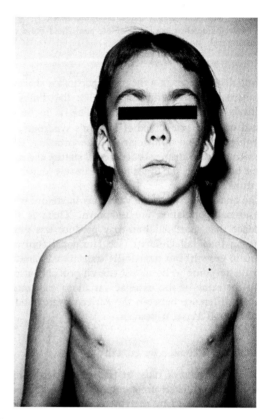

Fig. 63.1 Turner syndrome. Note webbing of the neck and the broadly spaced nipples.

Nutritional factors

Nutrition is the second most important factor determining normal growth in childhood and adolescence. In a global sense, malnutrition is the world's primary cause of poor growth. Both under- and overnutrition may have long-lasting effects on growth patterns. Undernutrition, particularly if it occurs in utero or at significant postnatal periods, may affect both the weight and height growth patterns and also the development of body organs. In utero, undernutrition has also been associated with increased long term risks of cardiovascular morbidity and mortality in children who are born small for dates. Undernutrition later in life is complicated by the interaction between the quality and the quantity of the diet and the duration of dietary inadequacy.

Emotional deprivation also has a profound influence on the growth process and may interact with provision of food. Furthermore, the mechanism of poor growth in many chronic illnesses of childhood is at least in part due to undernutrition or to nutritional influences on the balance of hormones and growth factors. Overnutrition may lead to obesity with advanced linear growth and early pubertal maturation. Overnutrition at a time when linear growth is declining in late adolescence may lead to lifelong obesity with the attendant risks of hypertension, insulin resistance and the development of type II diabetes.

Hormonal factors

Those of significance in growth are:
- growth hormone
- thyroid hormone
- testosterone and adrenal androgens
- oestrogens

Growth hormone–insulin like growth factor 1 axis

The major hormonal influence involved in growth regulation at all ages is the growth hormone–insulin like growth factor 1 axis (GH–IGF-I). Growth hormone is secreted by the anterior pituitary gland in a pulsatile pattern. Major peaks of secretion occur particularly at night. Growth hormone is bound to a specific growth hormone binding protein and subsequently acts on a broad range of tissues via cell surface receptors, resulting in a range of metabolic and growth related effects. Many of these effects are mediated via IGF-I, which is produced by the liver and many other tissues (Fig. 63.2). The secreted IGF-I then acts either locally on adjacent tissues (paracrine action) or via endocrine mechanisms (that is, via the circulation). IGF-I levels are age dependent, being low in the fetus, rising through infancy and childhood, peaking during puberty and then falling to adult levels. IGF-I is very sensitive to nutritional status and in itself is of limited diagnostic value in the assessment of short stature. It circulates bound to one of its six major binding proteins (IGFBPs 1 to 6).

Thyroid hormone

Thyroxine is very important for postnatal growth. Children with untreated hypothyroidism show both profound mental and growth retardation, with very delayed bony development. In many developed countries, neonatal thyroid screening programmes have been set up and treatment of congenital hypothyroidism ensures normal growth and intellectual development.

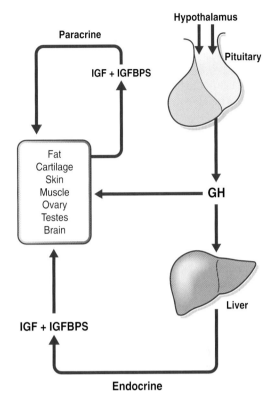

Fig. 63.2 A model showing the factors regulating pituitary growth hormone (GH) release and its targets in specific tissues as well as the liver, inducing release of insulin-like growth factor I (IGF-I) and its binding proteins (IGFBPs).

Testosterone and adrenal androgens

These hormones are anabolic and growth promoting. In males, testosterone and growth hormone act synergistically to promote the adolescent growth spurt. Excess androgens in childhood due to exogenous treatment, arising from adrenal enzyme disorders (congenital adrenal hyperplasia), precocious puberty or tumours will rapidly cause bone age advancement and may limit the potential for final height.

Oestrogens

Oestrogens in small doses may synergise with growth hormone to cause growth promotion. In higher doses, oestrogens will inhibit growth and promote early fusion of the bony epiphyses.

Phases of growth

There are three main phases of growth: fetal and childhood growth, and the pubertal growth spurt.

Fetal growth

Fetal growth is the most rapid phase of growth. Fetal growth is characterised by rapid differentiation of body organs, while late fetal growth involves continued rapid enlargement in tissues and organs and growth in length. The most rapid linear growth velocity of all ages occurs in the weeks before birth. Factors controlling fetal growth include placental supply of nutrients and oxygen and a range of local growth factors including insulin-like growth factors (IGFs). Pituitary growth hormone probably plays a relatively small part in this phase of growth, while thyroxine is involved in brain and bone growth in the fetus. Pituitary gonadotrophins (luteinising hormone (LH), follicle stimulating hormone (FSH)) regulate testicular testosterone synthesis in the male fetus, which is essential for normal growth of the male phallus. Thus a male infant with hypopituitarism may have a micropenis at birth.

Childhood growth

During the first years of life, linear growth velocity is still very rapid (on average 8–12 cm/year), but plateaus through childhood to an average of approximately 5 cm/year. The growth velocity immediately before the prepubertal growth spurt may be lower than this and represents a transient phase of poor growth. If the onset of the pubertal growth spurt is delayed then this phase of poor growth may be prolonged. During the childhood growth phase the limbs grow faster than the trunk, so that the ratio of the upper to lower body segments (divided at the pubic symphysis) diminishes from approximately 1.7:1 during infancy to 1:1 by age 10. It may fall to around 0.8 by mid puberty. The span–height ratio remains unchanged at approximately 1:1.

Factors controlling this phase of growth include genetic determinants, nutrition, absence of chronic disease and hormones, the most important of which are growth hormone and thyroxine.

Pubertal growth spurt

Puberty is associated with the onset of sex hormone production in boys and girls under the influence of pulsatile release of gonadotrophins (FSH/LH) from the pituitary gland. The earliest sign of puberty in boys, usually occurring at an average age of 11 years, is testicular enlargement (volume greater than 3–4 ml measured with an orchidometer). Penile and scrotal growth follow, with development of pubic and axillary hair in response to testosterone synthesis. In girls, ovarian oestrogen secretion leads to the earliest pubertal sign of breast development at an average age of 10.5–11 years, followed by pubic and axillary hair growth in response to adrenal and ovarian androgens. In boys, testosterone also leads to muscle growth, while in girls, oestrogens cause pelvic broadening and fat redistribution, leading to a female body shape. In both sexes, the onset of puberty is followed by a peak linear growth velocity, at an average age of 12.5 years in girls and 14.5 years in boys.

The hormonal events of puberty include an increase in the amplitude of growth hormone pulses, probably due to sex hormone effects. IGF-I levels rise during puberty in association with the high growth hormone levels. The sex hormones (testosterone or oestrogens) also appear to have direct effects at the skeletal growth plate, ultimately leading to fusion of the bony epiphyses and cessation of growth at an average age of 15 years in girls and 17 years in boys. The pubertal growth spurt may be influenced by genetic factors and also may be affected adversely by poor nutrition or chronic disease, both of which can cause pubertal delay.

Assessment of growth

Percentile charts

Any doctor who deals with children must have a working knowledge of normal variations in growth and development and must be able to use a percentile chart. The childhood and pubertal growth patterns can be appreciated by examining growth charts, including linear height and weight charts (Fig. 63.3) as well as height velocity charts, indicating annual rate of growth (Fig. 63.4).

These charts demonstrate the range of normal growth, expressed either as percentiles or as standard deviations (SD) from the mean for age. The percentile curves are derived from the overall distribution (bell shaped curve) of the data. The median or mid point is the 50th percentile and the normal range of average height or weight on the charts falls between the 3rd and 97th percentiles (Fig. 63.3). The median or 50th percentile indicates that 50% of the measurements of a normal group of children are above and 50% below that point. The range between the 3rd to 97th (or −2 SD to +2 SD) includes 94% of all normal children. It must be realised that there will be 3 normal children in every 100 who will be at or below the 3rd centile and 3 in every 100 who will be at or above the 97th centile.

Assessment of growth velocity (Fig. 63.4) is of far greater clinical significance than single measurements of height, and should be based on sequential measurements taken at 3-monthly intervals over a period of 6–12 months. When measured over this time period, a normal child will tend to follow the same height percentile. A child with an organic or endocrine disease will tend to deviate away from the percentile line and may move downwards across percentile lines. Thus serial measurement of children is the key to the assessment of their growth status.

Boys: 2 to 18 years height percentile

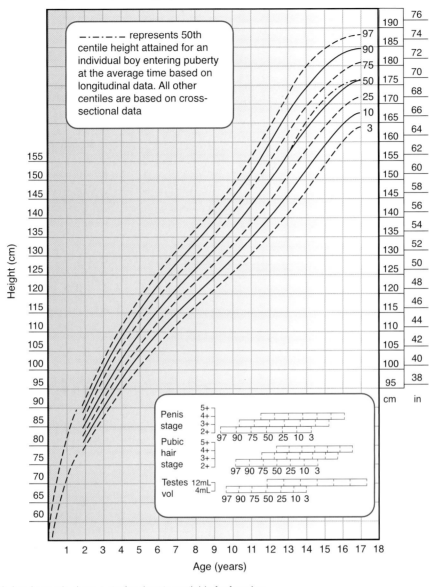

Fig. 63.3 Male height centile chart. A similar chart is available for females.

Bone age

Bone age is an index of physiological maturity, indicating the state of bony epiphysial maturation. A bone age is obtained by performing an X ray of the left wrist and hand and is interpreted according to an atlas of age and sex specific standards. The bone age indicates the average age of children at a similar stage of bony maturation and is a guide to the remaining growth potential of the child. In normal children the bone age can be delayed up to 2 years behind the chronological age, but is rarely advanced a year beyond the chronological age.

Height age

Height age is the age at which a child's current height would represent the 50th percentile. This means that the height age indicates the average age of children of a similar height.

Mid parental height

The mid parental height (MPH), also known as the target height, allows the height of any individual child to be considered in relation to the heights of his/her biological

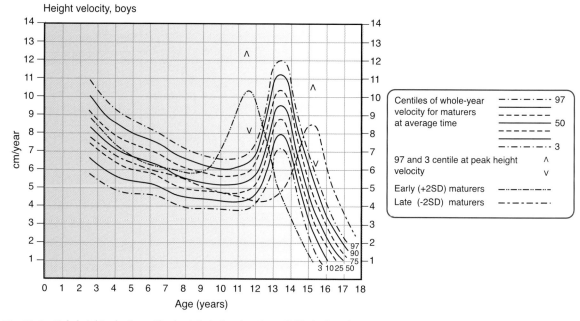

Fig. 63.4 Male height velocity centile chart. A similar chart is available for females.

parents. The midparental height can be calculated using the following formulae:

For boys: MPH = (father's height + [mother's height + 13])/2 ± 7.5 cm

For girls: MPH = (mother's height + [father's height − 13])/2 ± 6 cm

A child should not be assumed to be short 'because he/she has a short family', unless the actual height of the child has been plotted on the growth chart and found to be consistent with the mid parental height outlined above.

Short stature

The management of a child with short stature requires consideration of a number of issues. It is important to realise that the majority of short children will have no pathology, but will be either following a familial pattern or have a variant of normal growth. The main causes of short stature in order of frequency of diagnosis are summarised in Table 63.1 which demonstrates that endocrine causes of short stature are the least common.

Variations from normal

Familial (genetic) short stature

- These children will be growing on the 3rd centile or below but parallel to the 3rd centile.
- The growth rate is usually normal.

Table 63.1 Causes of short stature

Genetic/familial short stature
Constitutional delay
Intrauterine growth retardation
Chronic illness — malnutrition
Skeletal dysplasia
Iatrogenic (steroids/irradiation)
Chromosomal abnormality/syndrome
Psychosocial
Endocrine

- The adult height percentiles of both parents should be plotted on the child's growth chart to assess whether the child's height is appropriate for the heights of the parents.
- Pubertal development usually occurs at the appropriate time.
- Markers of physical maturation such as bone age tend to be consistent with chronological age.

Constitutional delay in growth and pubertal development

- A very common variation of growth and leads to short stature during childhood with a height prognosis consistent with the mid parental height expectation.
- Usually affects boys far more commonly than girls.
- Often a family history of a parent, being short as a child, with delayed puberty and eventual catch up to peers.

- Are the so called 'slow growers and late bloomers'. The typical growth pattern shows a growth rate which is mostly normal except for a period of 6–12 months in the first 2 years of life, when the growth rate falls transiently.
- The nadir in the growth velocity prior to puberty may be exaggerated, with the delayed appearance of pubertal development.
- Markers of physical maturation such as bone age are delayed and are consistent with the height age, indicating a true constitutional delay in growth.
- The delay in puberty and associated delay in closure of bony epiphyses means that both the pubertal growth

spurt and the completion of growth will be slowed according to the delay in bone age.
- These children (most often boys) tend to grow into their late teenage years or early twenties.

The remaining causes of short stature are all pathological causes. The differences in growth patterns between genetic short stature, constitutional delay and pathological short stature are summarised in Figure 63.5. The relationship between chronological age, bony age and height age for common growth abnormalities is summarised in Table 63.2.

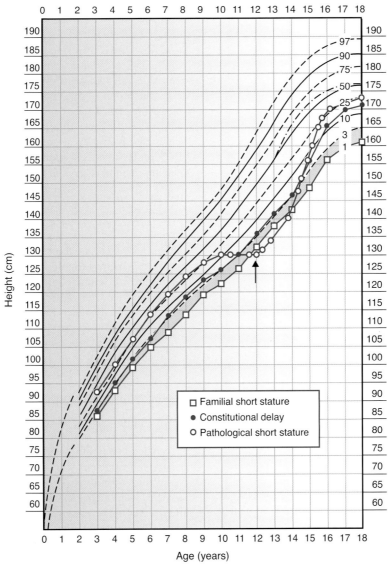

Fig. 63.5 The typical growth patterns and height outcomes for familial short stature, constitutional delay and pathological short stature are illustrated on the percentile chart. The arrow indicates detection of the cause of the pathological growth pattern and commencement of appropriate therapy, thus allowing catch up growth.

Table 63.2 The relationship between chronological age, bone age and height age for common growth problems

Growth problem	Chronological age (CA) (years)	Height age (HA)	Bone age (BA)
Genetic short stature	10	HA < CA	BA = CA
Constitutional delay	10	HA < CA	BA < CA BA = HA
Delayed puberty	15	HA < CA	BA < CA
Precocious puberty	6	HA > CA	BA > CA

Clinical example

Rosie presented at age 11 years for assessment of her short stature. Both she and her parents were concerned about her growth as she seemed to be significantly shorter than most of her cousins and friends. On further questioning it was elicited that Rosie had always been one of the short children in her class at school. Rosie had no significant past medical history. Her mother was 152 cm (5 ft) and her father was 160 cm (5 ft 3 in), that is, both parents were of short adult stature.

Review of previous growth records revealed that Rosie had always been on or just below the 3rd height centile. General physical examination showed that Rosie was completely normal and was in early puberty with stage 2 breast and pubic hair development. She had normal body proportions for age. A bone age examination showed a bone age of 11 years.

The diagnosis for Rosie's growth pattern was familial short stature. Both Rosie and her parents asked if any treatment could be given to make her grow faster. Unfortunately no treatment, including growth hormone, has the ability to alter the final height in familial short stature. Both Rosie and her parents were reassured that she was a completely normal girl and would end up with a final height consistent with the mid parental height.

Pathological causes

Intrauterine growth retardation

This results in growth retarded babies of appropriate gestational age. Major causes include a variety of genetic disorders primarily affecting the fetus. An abnormal intrauterine environment due to maternal illness, placental insufficiency or intrauterine infection may also lead to poor fetal growth. If the insult to the fetus occurs early in gestation, cell number is reduced and the potential for catch up is diminished.

Chronic disease

- A major cause of growth failure.
- Usually associated with a similar fall off in weight velocity.
- Chronic infections may also present as failure to grow and gain weight.
- A hormone or endocrine problem is unlikely to be the cause of poor growth if both the weight and height are affected.
- Nutritional insufficiency may contribute to the growth failure of chronic disease due to inadequate or inappropriate intake, poor absorption or impaired or excessive tissue utilisation.

Skeletal disorders

Skeletal disorders are usually familial, involving intrinsic cartilage or bone defects. Examples include achondroplasia (the classic dwarf), other milder bony dysplasias (particularly hypochondroplasia) and the mucopolysaccharidoses. The major distinctive features of all of these disorders is body segment disproportion; that is, increased upper to lower body segment ratios. Limbs are usually short, leading to a reduced span–height ratio. Weight gain is usually normal. These disorders in their mild form are relatively common and often overlooked. More information is given in Chapter 29.

Iatrogenic

Iatrogenic causes include corticosteroid excess seen in children with steroid treated chronic illnesses, such as severe asthma, juvenile arthritis and nephrotic syndrome. Marked growth failure is associated with weight gain. Irradiation to the head and spine may result in hypothalamic–pituitary dysfunction and poor spinal growth, which may lead to poor growth of the trunk with increased span–height ratio and a reduced upper to lower body segment ratio.

Chromosomal abnormalities and syndromes

Turner syndrome and its variants is the most common chromosomal cause of short stature. This condition must be excluded in any girl with short stature as the typical phenotypic features may not be seen, particularly in the mosaic forms of Turner syndrome. The most common associated abnormality is ovarian dysgenesis resulting in failed pubertal development in 95% of cases. Other commonly seen features include a webbed neck (Fig. 63.1), small ears, increased carrying angle, coarctation of the aorta, horseshoe kidney, dysplastic nails and recurrent otitis media. All or none of these dysmorphic and clinical features may be present. The full range of features is summarised in Table 63.3.

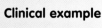

Clinical example

Brendan was a 15 year old boy with short stature. He was said to be of average height as an infant and young child, but from the age of 7–8 years had grown slowly. Brendan had a normal pregnancy and neonatal history. His only medical problem was asthma, which he had first developed at the age of 4 years. Over the years he has been admitted to hospital on numerous occasions with exacerbations of his asthma, including an intensive care admission when he was 9 years of age. Over the preceding 5 years, Brendan had been treated with daily inhaled corticosteroids (fluticasone dipropionate 1000 μg/day) and Ventolin every 4 hours as required. He had also had frequent courses of oral prednisolone for 3–5 days, particularly during the winter months. Brendan's physical examination demonstrated that his height was on the 10th percentile and his weight on the 25th percentile for age. He was not cushingoid and had evidence of chronic asthma, i.e. chest hyperinflation and a Harrison sulcus. He was completely prepubertal. The rest of his examination was normal.

The most likely explanation for Brendan's growth problem is a combination of growth suppression from moderately severe asthma and the effects of both the inhaled and intermittent oral corticosteroids. The growth suppression has also been compounded by delayed puberty, also a frequent accompaniment of poorly controlled asthma and high dose inhaled corticosteroids.

Table 63.3   Features of Turner syndrome

General
Short stature
Developed puberty
Amenorrhoea

Lymphatic abnormalities
Neck webbing
Low posterior hairline
Lymphoedema
Nail convexity/dysplasia

Skeletal abnormalities
Micrognathia
High arch palate
Short fourth/fifth metacarpals
Increased carrying angles
Madelung deformity
Kyphoscoliosis
Broad chest
Abnormal upper/lower body segment ratio

Metabolic
Thyroiditis
Carbohydrate intolerance

Miscellaneous
Recurrent middle ear infections
Decreased hearing
Cardiac: coarctation or aortic stenosis (bicuspid aortic valve)
Renal anomaly
Naevi

Other chromosomal disorders are less common causes of short stature. Common dysmorphic syndromes presenting with short stature include Noonan syndrome, intrauterine growth retardation (Russell–Silver dwarfism) and Aarskog syndrome. Further details of these conditions are found in Chapter 29.

Psychosocial

Psychosocial causes of short stature cover the spectrum from severe deprivation to overt abuse, and may be associated with nutritional deficiencies. Fall off in weight gain is usually as striking as failure of linear growth.

Clinical example

Hayley presented at 7 years and 9 months for assessment of short stature. At birth, she was of average birth weight and length but from the age of 4–5 years it was noted that she seemed to be growing at a slower rate than her cousins and friends at kindergarten and school. Hayley's past medical history included repair of a coarctation of the aorta detected in the neonatal period. Additionally, she had had problems from the age of 2 years with recurrent otitis media requiring insertion of grommets. Further history revealed that Hayley was otherwise a healthy girl who had parents of average height. There was no significant family history.

Physical examination confirmed that Hayley was indeed less than the 3rd height centile, and her weight was on the 25th centile for age. There were no dysmorphic features and no other abnormal physical findings. Examination of previous growth records showed that at 3 years of age Hayley had been just under the 3rd height centile and had been at that point from birth. Her current height was 8 cm less than the 3rd centile for age.

Investigations for short stature showed that Hayley had normal haematology and biochemistry results and was euthyroid. Her bone age was delayed 2 years behind her actual age. A chromosome analysis was performed and showed that she had an abnormal karyotype, 46,X,i(X)(q10). In every cell examined there was one X isochromosome, resulting in monosomy for the X short arm region. This is a variant karyotype associated with Turner syndrome, of which short stature and coarctation are some of the known clinical features.

The diagnosis for Hayley's short stature therefore was Turner syndrome, which would not have been diagnosed unless a chromosome analysis had been performed.

Hayley was commenced on growth hormone treatment with subcutaneous injections given 6 days per week. With this treatment her growth rate improved markedly. When she reaches adolescence it will be necessary to give her supplemental oestrogen treatment to bring about pubertal development and to help augment her growth. Fertility is likely to be a problem in the long term for Hayley and in time these issues will need to be discussed with her and her family.

Endocrine

Endocrine causes of short stature are the least common pathological cause and include hypothyroidism, growth hormone deficiency (possibly associated with other pituitary hormone deficiencies), Cushing syndrome (hypercortisolism) and adrenal insufficiency. In all of these cases the fall off in linear growth exceeds the fall in weight gain.

Assessment

Issues to determine

- Is he/she short?
- Is he/she growing slowly (could this be pathological)?
- What is the underlying cause?
- What is the adult height prognosis?
- How is he/she coping with the short stature?
- Is any specific therapy warranted?
- Is any supportive therapy indicated?

The approach to the assessment of short stature should include history, examination, investigations if necessary, therapy and follow up.

History

- What is the height compared to peers? How long has he/she been short? Who is concerned about the short stature and is there teasing at school? What is the school performance?
- What are the birth details and past medical history? Was there unexplained neonatal hypoglycaemia (suggesting pituitary hormone deficiency) or early illnesses? Determine the dental and milestone development, specific disease symptoms and nutritional status. Has puberty commenced? Are previous growth measurements available (child health record or measurements from local doctor or school)?
- What are the heights and ages of pubertal onset of the parents and siblings? Is there a family history of specific diseases?

Examination

- Accurate height and weight (using a reliable measuring device, particularly for height); body proportions (span, upper and lower segments).
- Assessment of pubertal status. Pubertal stages for boys and girls are summarised in Table 63.4. The characteristic pubertal changes in males and females are illustrated in Figures 63.6 and 63.7. Further issues regarding puberty will be considered later in this chapter.
- General physical examination including evidence of chronic disease, nutritional state and dysmorphic features suggesting a syndrome.

Table 63.4 Stages of puberty

Males: genital (penis) development

Stage 1	Preadolescent, testes, scrotum and penis are of about the same size and proportion as in early childhood
Stage 2	Enlargement of scrotum and testes. Skin of scrotum reddens and changes in texture. Little or no enlargement of penis at this stage
Stage 3	Enlargement of the penis, which occurs at first mainly in length. Further growth of the testes and scrotum
Stage 4	Increased size of penis with growth in breadth and development of glans. Testes and scrotum larger; scrotal skin darkened
Stage 5	Genitalia adult in size and shape

Females: breast development

Stage 1	Preadolescent: elevation of papilla only
Stage 2	Breast bud stage: elevation of breast and papilla as small mound. Enlargement of areola diameter
Stage 3	Further enlargement and elevation of breast and areola, with no separation of their contours
Stage 4	Projection of areola and papilla to form a secondary mound above the level of the breast
Stage 5	Mature stage: projection of papilla only, due to recession of the areola to the general contour of the breast

Both sexes: pubic hair

Stage 1	Preadolescent: the vellus over the pubes is not further developed than that over the abdominal wall, that is, no pubic hair
Stage 2	Sparse growth of long, slightly pigmented downy hair, straight or slightly curled at the base of the penis in boys, or chiefly along labia in girls
Stage 3	Considerably darker, coarser and more curled. The hair spreads sparsely over the junction of the pubes
Stage 4	Hair now adult in type, but area covered is still considerably smaller than in adult. No spread to the medial surface of thighs
Stage 5	Adult in quantity and type with distribution of the horizontal (or classic 'feminine') pattern. Spread to medial surface of thighs but not up linea alba or elsewhere above the base of the inverse triangle (spread up linea alba occurs late and is rated stage 6)

- Any sign of goitre or clinical signs of hypothyroidism, including dry hair and skin, bradycardia and delayed reflexes.
- Evidence of 'midline brain development syndromes' which may result in hypopituitarism. This includes cleft palate, single central incisor and small male genitalia (associated with gonadotrophin deficiency in utero). The combination of neonatal hypoglycaemia and small genitalia suggests hypopituitarism.
- Examination of visual fields and optic fundi to exclude the possibility of a pituitary lesion, in particular craniopharyngioma.

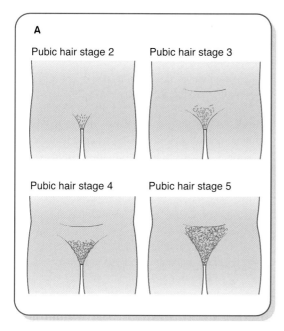

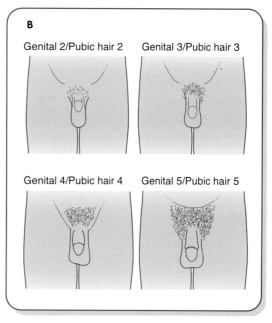

Fig. 63.6 **A** Pubertal pubic hair changes in the female, and **B** pubertal genital and pubic hair changes in the male. A more detailed explanation is given in Table 63.4.

Management

The single most important aspect of the management of short stature is to plot the current and previous heights and weights and parental heights on a percentile chart in order to answer the following questions:
- Is the child short and below the 3rd height centile? Is this appropriate for mid parental height?
- Is the child growing slowly and is there evidence that the height is falling across the percentile lines? This can be further plotted on a height velocity chart (Figure 63.4).

A velocity below the 25th centile for bone age is potentially abnormal in a short child. A reliable height velocity requires at least 6 months of growth data, and preferably 12 months with consistent measurements at 3–4 monthly intervals over that time. Examination of the growth data plus the points obtained in history and examination should allow distinction between a variation of normal or a pathological cause of short stature.

Investigations

Investigations should be performed if there is any evidence of specific chronic disease, a suggestion of chromosomal abnormality or if the growth velocity is subnormal. The following investigations may be performed:
- bone age X ray
- full blood count and ESR
- urea, creatinine and electrolytes
- urinalysis ± microscopy and culture
- calcium and phosphate
- thyroid function tests
- chromosomes (girls only)
- ± endomysial antibodies (exclude coeliac disease).

It is important to note that all girls with unexplained short stature should have a karyotype performed to exclude the possibility of Turner syndrome.

If puberty is markedly delayed it may be worthwhile measuring gonadotrophins (FSH/LH) and testosterone or oestradiol.

These investigations provide a screen for underlying chronic disease, infection or nutritional deficiency as well as hypothyroidism and Turner syndrome. Other investigations may be indicated by specific physical findings. In a child with unexplained combined weight and height fall off, a malabsorptive disorder should be excluded and consideration should be given to measuring endomysial antibodies as a possible indicator of the presence of coeliac disease. If these are elevated, a small bowel biopsy may be necessary.

Investigation for growth hormone deficiency

Growth hormone deficiency may be suggested by association with midline defects or if other pituitary hormone deficiencies, including hypothyroidism or gonadotrophin deficiency, are present. The presence of biochemical growth hormone deficiency suggests a need for CNS imaging and biochemical testing for other pituitary

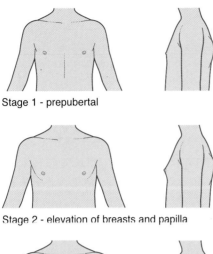

Stage 1 - prepubertal

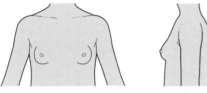

Stage 2 - elevation of breasts and papilla

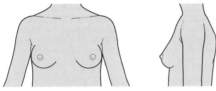

Stage 3 - further enlargement and elevation of breast and areola but no separation of contour

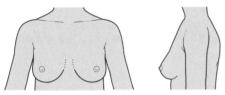

Stage 4 - areola and papilla form a secondary mound above level of the breast

Stage 5 - areola recedes to the general contour of the breast

Fig. 63.7 Pubertal breast changes in the female. A more detailed explanation is given in Table 63.4.

deficits. Specific underlying causes of growth hormone deficiency include idiopathic (most common), pituitary or hypothalamic tumours/structural abnormalities, cranial irradiation and genetic growth hormone deficiency. Specific tests to determine the presence of growth hormone deficiency include:

- Physiological tests of growth hormone sufficiency, including:
  - Exercise growth hormone (GH) tests: performed in the fasting state on a bicycle ergometer with blood for GH levels taken pre- and 30 minutes post exercise. This is a screening test with 20% of normal children failing to reach cut off levels.
  - Overnight sleep studies of growth hormone secretion.
- Measurement of IGF-I and IGFBP-3 levels. This test is being advocated for screening for GH deficiency prior to proceeding to more involved pharmacological tests. As yet the data are not sufficiently reliable to recommend that these tests be performed as a single diagnostic entity in a clinical setting. They may however be useful when considered in combination with other clinical information and growth hormone tests.
- Pharmacological tests of growth hormone sufficiency, including:
  - glucagon stimulation test
  - arginine–insulin hypoglycaemia test
  - clonidine stimulation test.

Although no one test is superior to another, the glucagon stimulation test is at present the preferred pharmacological test of GH secretion. The glucagon stimulation test also provides information about the adrenocorticotrophin–cortisol axis. The arginine–insulin hypoglycaemia test is used rarely as hypoglycaemia is an obligate part of this test and potentially dangerous.

For the purposes of defining GH deficiency and assessing eligibility for hGH as a pharmaceutical benefit in Australia, biochemical growth hormone deficiency is defined as failure to achieve a peak serum GH concentration of > 10 mU/l in response to two stimulation tests, at least one of which would be a pharmacological test, or in response to one test in the presence of other evidence suggestive of GH deficiency such as structural CNS abnormalities or low plasma IGF-I and IGFBP-3 levels.

Treatment

Short stature is considered by some children and their families to be a physical and psychosocial disability. Extreme short stature certainly can be considered as a handicap both in a social and medical sense. Many paediatricians and paediatric endocrinologists consider that if the estimated final height of a female will be less than 152.4 cm (5 ft) or a male less than 162.6 cm (5 ft 4 in), then consideration should be given to the use of a growth promoting agent. The major growth promoting agent used in the treatment of short stature is biosynthetic growth hormone. Biosynthetic growth hormone has been available commercially in Australia since 1985. In 1988, the 'Guidelines for the Use of Growth Hormone in Australia' were liberalised, allowing the use of growth hormone in short children who are growing poorly but who are not growth hormone deficient.

Clinical example

Luke, a 6 week old male infant, presented for assessment of persisting jaundice. He was the first child of unrelated parents. The pregnancy was uncomplicated and he was born at term via a normal vaginal delivery with a birth weight of 3250 g. He was in good condition at birth with Apgars of 9[1], 10[5]. At 24 hours of age he was hypoglycaemic with blood sugar levels (BSLs) of 1.6 and 1.2 mmol/l. The hypoglycaemia persisted despite frequent feeds and required an intravenous dextrose infusion in addition to normal breast feeds to maintain adequate BSLs. At 48 hours of age he was noted to be jaundiced and required phototherapy for 24 hours. By day 5 he was feeding well, his neonatal screening test had been performed and he was discharged. When reviewed by his general practitioner at 6 weeks of age Luke was still jaundiced. Physical examination was normal with no other evidence of liver disease or congenital infection; however, the baby's penis was small for age.

Investigations showed a conjugated hyperbilirubinaemia, with mildly elevated liver transaminases. Thyroid function tests showed a low FT_4 and low TSH, and a morning cortisol level as very low at 10 mmol/l. Testing of blood sugars prior to feeds and after a 6 hour fast demonstrated that there was no evidence of persisting hypoglycaemia. A provisional diagnosis of congenital hypopituitarism was made. Evidence to support this diagnosis included micropenis (due to absence of in utero gonadotrophins (LH/FSH) and GH), neonatal hypoglycaemia (due to absent GH and ACTH), secondary (pituitary) hypothyroidism (TSH deficiency), low morning cortisol (ACTH deficiency) and conjugated hyperbilirubinaemia. The neonatal screen detects only primary (i.e. thyroid abnormalty) hypothyroidism as the screening test is based on detection of elevated TSH levels. Thus cases of secondary (pituitary) and tertiary (hypothalamic) hypothyroidism will not be detected.

Following treatment with thyroxine and oral hydrocortisone replacement Luke's jaundice resolved. Supplemental intramuscular testosterone injections during the first 3 months were given to increase the size of Luke's penis. Continuing management of this infant will involve monitoring of the baby's linear growth and weight gain, with adjustment of thyroxine and hydrocortisone doses as necessary. It is likely that this infant is growth hormone deficient and will manifest growth failure. MRI of the pituitary should be performed to detect structural pituitary abnormalitiy. Subcutaneous hGH treatment will be required in time to maintain normal growth, and further hormonal treatment at the time of puberty will be necessary.

The Commonwealth Department of Health and Family Services has provided guidelines for the use of growth hormone in Australia. These can be summarised as follows:

A child must have abnormally short stature (height less than the 1st percentile) with an abnormally low growth rate, measured over a minimum period of 1 year at intervals of not greater than 6 months. The child should be growing at a height velocity below the 25th centile for skeletal age and sex.

Variations to these guidelines exist for particular groups of patients with Turner syndrome, growth hormone deficiency, combined growth hormone deficiency and precocious puberty, chronic renal insufficiency and those patients with growth retardation secondary to an intracranial lesion or cranial irradiation.

Growth hormone treatment has been shown to be of benefit in the following conditions:
- growth hormone deficiency
- Turner syndrome (final height can be improved by up to 8–10 cm)
- growth retardation secondary to renal insufficiency.

Despite extensive clinical trials in Australia and worldwide, results of growth hormone therapy for short stature associated with constitutional delay, intrauterine growth retardation, glucocorticoid induced growth failure, chromosomal and genetic disorders and skeletal dysplasias have been disappointing. Although the definite indications for growth hormone treatment of short stature are limited, any child who is short and growing slowly with a poor ultimate height prognosis should be referred for assessment. After assessment it may be appropriate to offer the child a trial of growth hormone therapy.

Epidemiological studies have recently reported that serum IGF-I levels in the upper normal range may be associated with an increased risk of prostate, breast and colon cancer in non growth hormone treated adults. However, a cause and effect relationship between cancer risk and IGF-I has not been established. Whether there is any implication of this observation for growth hormone treated children remains to be established. IGF-I levels during growth hormone treatment should be maintained within the appropriate age and gender matched reference range.

Other specific agents used in the treatment of short stature associated with constitutional delay have included oxandrolone (a biosynthetic testosterone analogue) and low dose oral testosterone preparations.

Growth hormone can be administered only by subcutaneous injections, usually given 6–7 days per week. Despite the availability of biosynthetic growth hormone, the annual cost of growth hormone therapy remains very high. Growth hormone should therefore only be used for children who have short stature and who could potentially benefit from the therapy.

Psychological support and counselling

Psychological support and counselling is undoubtedly the most important part of the management of short stature and can be provided by either health professionals or lay support groups. Often reassurance regarding the normality of the child and the reassurance of a reasonable height prognosis is all that is required. If the height prognosis is poor, then counselling and support should be used in conjunction with growth promoting agents. Families should be advised to encourage self-esteem in the child by promoting the child's strengths, for example, sporting, musical or academic, rather than concentrating on the perceived limitations imposed by short stature. Lay support groups associated with growth hormone deficiency or Turner syndrome are now quite common in most large cities, and have active programmes for children and their families. On occasions it may be necessary to seek formal psychological or psychiatric help for a child or family who are very distressed by the problem of short stature.

Tall stature

Tall stature is a relatively infrequent problem compared with the number of children who present because of short stature. In general, very few tall children have an organic disease process as a basis for their disease. The most common reason for tall stature is genetic tall stature. Compared to 20 years ago, relatively few teenagers and their parents are concerned about tall stature as it is now more socially acceptable for girls to be tall. However, girls may be presented for assessment of their final height if it is thought that they will be in excess of 178 cm (5 ft 10 in). A final height of 183 cm (6 ft) may be acceptable for a girl if her parents and other siblings are also tall. As with short stature, there is no clear demarcation between normal and tall stature. A child whose height is above the 97th percentile for age should be considered tall.

Causes

- Familial or normal variant
- Precocious puberty
- Syndromes: Marfan, Klinefelter, triple X, homocystinuria, Sotos
- Endocrine causes: hyperthyroidism and pituitary gigantism.

Familial/normal variant tall stature

Most tall children are normal in all respects and their height is genetically determined. Some children with early but otherwise normal pubertal development (8–10 years in girls, 10–12 years in boys) will appear tall in relation to their peers and family during adolescence, but will have a predicted final height within the accepted normal range. These early developers have an advanced bone age and are at the opposite end of the spectrum to the short children with delayed maturation, who have delayed puberty but who will also reach a normal adult height commensurate with their mid parental height.

Precocious puberty

Precocious puberty is defined as pubertal development at less than 8 years of age in girls and less than 9.5 years in boys. Because of rapid acceleration of bone maturation and early epiphysial closure, many children with precocious puberty are excessively tall in early to mid childhood but finish up as relatively short adults (Fig. 63.8). It is important to recognise precocious puberty, as treatment can be given to switch off the premature activation of the hypothalamic–pituitary–gonadal axis. It is also important to sort out whether the appearance of precocious puberty may be due to an aberrant source of androgen or oestrogen production, such as an adrenal or ovarian tumour. Occasionally the appearance of precocious puberty may be due to iatrogenic causes, such as oestrogen cream application or excessive administration of anabolic steroids to improve appetite and growth.

Syndromes causing tall stature

Marfan syndrome may present with the classical picture of arachnodactyly, ligamentous laxity, chest deformity, cardiac abnormalities, high arched palate and subluxation of the lenses. Often, however, one sees tall thin children with some marfanoid features who are difficult to classify. Children with homocystinuria have a marfanoid phenotype but are retarded intellectually. Homocystinuria may be diagnosed by a study of urinary and serum amino acids. Tall girls with intellectual retardation should also be screened for the triple X syndrome, and tall boys with disorders of pubertal maturation, with small testes, gynaecomastia and sometimes behavioural disturbance, should have chromosomal analysis. They may have either XYY syndrome or Klinefelter syndrome (XXY).

Endocrine causes of tall stature

Hyperthyroidism is relatively uncommon in childhood and is an infrequent cause of tall stature. The clinical features of hyperthyroidism are discussed in Chapter 64. Pituitary gigantism is extremely rare but should be suspected if the history and examination suggest pituitary involvement in association with tall stature. Children with pituitary gigantism will have an abnormally rapid growth rate as well as tall stature, in contrast to genetically tall children who grow above but parallel to the 97th centile but have a normal growth velocity.

Approach to diagnosis and treatment

The approach to diagnosis in a tall child consists of a full history, including a history of family heights and pubertal maturation patterns. In addition, it is important to ascertain whether there are associated abnormalities or

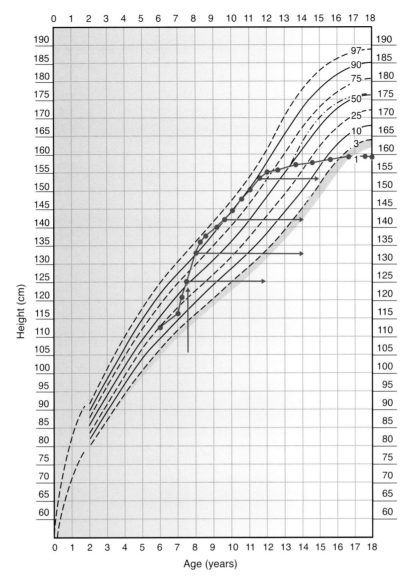

Fig. 63.8 The typical growth pattern and outcome of precocious puberty. The vertical arrow indicates commencement of specific therapy to halt/slow down the precocious puberty. The horizontal arrows indicate the degree of bone age at the given chronological ages, advancement (for example bone age 12 years at chronological age 7.5 years) ultimately leading to premature fusion of the epiphyses and early cessation of growth.

developmental delay which may suggest one of the chromosomal or syndromal disorders causing tall stature.

A full physical examination is essential, with emphasis on accurate height measurement, body build, limb proportions and pubertal status. Neurological assessment should include fundoscopy, assessment of visual fields and intellectual function and should determine any evidence of hyperthyroidism.

In most instances a tall child will in fact have a normal growth velocity above but parallel to the 97th centile. An accurate height measurement and bone age assessment by an experienced radiologist or paediatric endocrinologist will enable an adult height prediction to be made.

Frequently this is found to be at or below 178 cm (5 ft 10 in) for a girl or 193 cm (6 ft 4 in) for a boy and no further action is necessary. If the final height prediction for a girl is excessive then it may be possible to treat her with high dose oestrogen therapy to accelerate puberty and cause earlier fusion of the epiphyses; however, this treatment can have side effects and should only be given by a paediatric endocrinologist skilled in its use, after discussion of the risks and likely duration of treatment with the girl and her parents. For boys, high dose testosterone therapy can be given to try to limit final height; however, this treatment is less successful than high dose oestrogen therapy for tall girls. Somatostatin, which blocks the release of growth hormone and other hormones, has also been used in the management of tall stature.

Variations of pubertal development

Early normal puberty

In many countries, including Australia, children appear to be going through puberty at an age which is much younger than children in previous generations. This is called the secular trend in growth and development. The earlier age of puberty is probably due to effects of improved nutrition and living circumstances and absence of chronic disease. This seems to be particularly true for girls, with many girls showing early signs of breast development just before 8 years of age and starting to have menstrual periods while still in primary school. In most cases this early puberty is just a variation of normal. After assessment by a specialist, no specific treatment is usually required. The girl and her family need to have the situation explained. Enlisting the help of the teacher is also very helpful.

Delayed puberty

Delayed puberty is very common and occurs in approximately 2% of the adolescent population. Delayed puberty is defined as the absence of pubertal changes over the age of 14 years for girls and over the age of 14–15 years for boys. In general, adolescents have a heightened awareness of body image and are often preoccupied with the normality or otherwise of their pubertal development. Boys in particular may suffer major psychological effects resulting from delayed puberty as they may experience bullying, may be left out of sporting teams and may be less generally able to compete with their peers due to poor muscular development. The most common causes of delayed puberty are familial or constitutional delay in puberty for which there is often a family history, particularly in the father of a teenage boy. Puberty may also be delayed in the presence of any chronic illness of childhood or adolescence. The causes of delayed puberty are usually considered on the basis of the serum gonadotrophins (LH/FSH) and are outlined in Table 63.5.

Diagnosis and management

Assessment of delayed puberty requires a complete history, including a family history of pubertal maturation patterns. Also, it is important to look carefully for the possibility of occult chronic disease, such as inflammatory bowel disease, which may become apparent initially as a delay in the onset of puberty. If the history is suggestive of familial or constitutional delayed puberty, and this is confirmed by physical examination, no further investigation may be

Table 63.5 Causes of delayed puberty

Associated with normal or low serum gonadotrophins

Constitutional delay	Usually familial: associated with slow growth and a delayed bone age
Chronic illness	Poor nutrition, for example, cystic fibrosis, juvenile arthritis, inflammatory bowel disease
Endocrine causes	Hypopituitarism, isolated gonadotrophin deficiency, Kallmann syndrome, hypothyroidism, hyperprolactinaemia

Associated with elevated serum gonadotrophins*

Gonadal dysgenesis	Turner syndrome, Klinefelter syndrome, Noonan syndrome
Anorchia	
Gonadal damage, vascular events	Vascular damage, irradiation, infection (mumps), torsion or autoimmune disease

*This usually signifies primary gonadal dysfunction.

necessary. If the diagnosis is not clear, then the following investigations may need to be performed:

- full blood count and ESR
- urea/creatinine and electrolytes
- liver function tests
- thyroid function tests
- chromosomes
- bone age X ray
- serum FSH and LH, testosterone or oestradiol
- serum prolactin
- ± growth hormone studies.

Treatment

Indications for treatment of delayed puberty are primarily psychological. Induction of pubertal development in boys through the judicious use of intramuscular or oral testosterone preparations may be very useful in alleviating the psychological stress caused by delayed puberty. Recent research also suggests that treatment of delayed puberty is important, as puberty is the time when peak bone mass is accumulated. Failure to achieve peak bone mass in adolescence may place individuals at risk of osteoporosis in adult life. Treatment of delayed puberty should only be carried out by paediatricians and endocrinologists experienced in this area as excessive administration of sex steroids can adversely accelerate bony epiphysial maturation and affect long term height outcome.

Psychological support and counselling

Psychological support and counselling is an extremely important part of the management of pubertal delay, and in some instances may be all that is required while waiting for the onset of spontaneous pubertal development. It is very important to reassure the adolescent and his/her family that he/she is normal and that appropriate pubertal and sexual development will occur or can be relatively easily assisted with hormonal intervention. Such reassurance and support can profoundly improve an adolescent's self-esteem and can help reverse problems such as truanting from school, oppositional behaviour and bullying.

Clinical example

Gavin was a 14 year old boy who had been truanting from school. On further questioning, it emerged that he was being teased about his lack of pubertal development and had been bullied by some of the bigger, more muscular boys at school. Gavin had also recently been left out of the football team, a sport at which he previously excelled.

Further history revealed that Gavin was a healthy boy who had no physical complaints. Review of previous growth records showed that he was growing quite steadily along the 3rd centile throughout childhood but during the past 2 years he had fallen below the 3rd height centile (Fig. 63.9). Gavin's father, who was very worried about the situation, admitted that as a teenager he had had a similar problem at school and could remember being much slower than his peers to go through puberty. In fact he remembered still growing after he was 20 years old. Gavin's physical examination confirmed that he was entirely prepubertal. The rest of his physical examination was completely normal.

The most likely diagnosis was familial delayed puberty, and because of the psychological problems being caused for Gavin by this, he was given a course of intramuscular testosterone treatment. Following this, he had a growth spurt, development of some pubic hair and genital enlargement and also began to gain weight and become more muscular.

Six months after the initial presentation, Gavin continued to grow with further pubertal development without the need for ongoing testosterone treatment (Fig.63.9). He was very pleased with his progress, was no longer truanting from school and was back in the football team. Gavin's case is typical of the problems faced by boys with simple familial delayed puberty and is a very common pubertal problem.

Precocious puberty

Precocious puberty is a rare problem and occurs much less frequently than delayed puberty. Precocious puberty is defined as pubertal development before age 8 years in girls and 9.5 years in boys. True or central precocious puberty is associated with raised gonadotrophins. True precocious puberty is much more common in girls than boys, and girls are less likely to have an identifiable underlying pathological cause than boys. Girls with this disorder will have accelerated growth and development of both breasts and pubic hair. Boys with true precocious puberty have evidence of enlargement of both testes as well as accelerated linear and genital growth and pubic hair development. The most common cause of central precocious puberty is a hypothalamic harmartoma, but many tumours involving the hypothalamic–pituitary area can be associated with an increased prevalence of precocious puberty.

Gonadotrophin independent (pseudo) precocious puberty may be seen with congenital adrenal hyperplasia, adrenal, testicular or ovarian neoplasms and tumours that secrete non pituitary gonadotrophin such as chorionic gonadotrophin. The McCune–Albright syndrome is also a cause of gonadotrophin independent precocious puberty.

If precocious puberty is suspected, referral should be made to a paediatric endocrinologist who will organise appropriate investigations, which will include measurement of serum FSH and LH, testosterone or oestradiol, dynamic tests of gonadotrophin secretion such as luteinising hormone releasing hormone (LHRH) testing, bone age assessment and cerebral imaging including CT and/or MRI head scanning. Treatment of precocious puberty should be managed by a paediatric endocrinologist experienced in this area. Treatment options include LHRH superagonists, medroxyprogesterone acetate or cyproterone acetate. Indications for treatment for precocious puberty will include factors such as the age of the child and the rate of progression of the pubertal development.

Conditions resembling precocious puberty

Premature thelarche

Isolated breast development, either unilateral or bilateral, is relatively common in girls under than 2 years of age and may occur at any time throughout childhood. By definition, premature thelarche has no other features of precocious puberty. All cases should be referred for assessment by a paediatrician or endocrinologist; however, in most cases observation and follow up is all that is required.

Premature adrenarche

The appearance of isolated pubic hair development under the age of 8 years in a girl may occur as a variant of normal, but may also be associated with an adrenal disorder such as a non classical form of congenital adrenal hyperplasia. Careful assessment for any associated signs of virilisation, such as clitoral enlargement, hirsutism or acne, should be performed. The appearance of pubic hair in a boy before the age of 9 years rarely occurs as a normal variant and should always be investigated. In all cases of premature pubic hair development, referral should be made to a paediatrician or paediatric endocrinologist so that appropriate investigation of adrenal androgens can be performed.

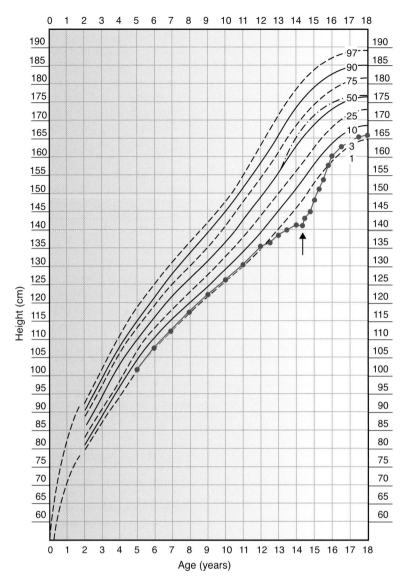

Fig. 63.9 The typical growth pattern of a boy with short stature and familial delayed puberty. The vertical arrow indicates the point at which a short course of testosterone therapy was given with a resulting growth spurt, onset of pubertal development and resumption of normal growth.

Isolated premature menarche

At the beginning of normal puberty in a girl, the small amounts of oestrogen made by the ovary switch 'on and off'. If enough lining of the womb is made with each 'switch on', there may be a small vaginal bleed when the 'switch off' occurs. This may happen several months in a row, then disappears as total oestrogen increases and normal puberty progresses. It is a normal variant and usually needs no treatment. Before the diagnosis of

premature menarche is accepted, all other causes of premature oestrogen secretion and/or any local casues of vaginal bleeding must be eliminated by the specialist.

Pubertal gynaecomastia

Gynaecomastia is a very common finding in adolescent boys, occurring in 40–70% of 14 year olds. In most instances the breast development is minor, transient and regresses. Rare causes of marked pubertal gynaecomastia

Clinical example

Sally was a 6.5 year old girl brought to her general practitioner by her mother, who was very concerned that Sally was going into early puberty. Sally had always been a big child, with height and weight on the 97th percentile for age since infancy. These growth parameters were consistent with the midparental height expectations. She was other wise a very healthy child, with no significant past medical history, She was not taking any medications and was not having any health food preparations or tonics.

From the age of 6, Sally's mother had noticed that Sally had developed a few pubic and axillary hairs and that she often had adult type body odour. In fact Sally had started using an underarm deodorant regularly, as the other children had told her she had 'BO'. Sally had also developed some whiteheads and blackheads on her face and was becoming quite self-conscious. Sally's mother was very concerned that Sally would soon begin to have menstrual periods when she would be far too young to cope.

Physical examination showed that Sally was a tall girl whose height and weight remained on the 97th percentile for age. She had stage 2 pubic hair and a few axillary hairs bilaterally. There was no breast development. She had some facial seborrhoea with whiteheads and blackheads. The rest of the general physical examination was normal.

The provisional diagnosis was premature adrenarche. Investigations, including bone age, adrenal androgens, gonadotrophins and oestradiol, were consistent with the diagnosis. Sally's mother was reassured that Sally did not have true precocious puberty. Simple measures such as deodorant and regular astringent facewashes were recommended and Sally was also reassured that she was completely normal. During subsequent follow up Sally had the onset of breast development, a pubertal growth spurt and menarche at an appropriate time.

include Klinefelter syndrome, adrenal and gonadal tumours, and drugs such as cimetidine, digoxin, spirono-lactone and marijuana use. If significant breast enlargement is causing psychosocial difficulties it may be necessary to refer a teenage boy to a plastic surgeon for consideration for subareolar mastectomy. Hormonal therapy does not influence the natural history of pubertal gynecomastia.

Asymmetrical breast development

Asymmetrical breast development can occur in both males and females. In males, it is clearly a variant of pubertal gynaecomastia. In females, breast development can be asymmetrical at the beginning of breast budding or subsequently through breast development. The degree of asymmetry can be quite marked. Consideration should be given to the possibility of an underlying chest wall or pectoral muscle abnormality and examination should be conducted appropriately. However, in most cases asymmetrical breast development is just a physiological variant of puberty.

In rare cases, an underlying vascular abnormality or lipoma may cause one breast to appear larger than the other. This can usually be readily determined by a physical examination and confirmed by ultrasound. Reassurance and monitoring are all that are usually required. For self-esteem and cosmetic reasons, advice should be given to teenage girls about temporary use of breast prostheses or even shoulder pads to equalise the breast form. Most girls cope with the situation by wearing loose fitting garments and T shirts over swimwear. In most situations, the asymmetry resolves with full pubertal development. On rare occasions, however, referral to a reconstructive surgeon for breast reduction or augmentation may need to be considered.

Thyroid disorders in childhood and adolescence

F. Cameron

Normal thyroid function throughout infancy, childhood and adolescence is essential for a normal developmental and physiological outcome. Thyroid disease is one of the most common groups of endocrine disorders in childhood and adolescence, with approximately 1–2% of all children having a thyroid disorder at some time. Therefore, knowledge of thyroid disease and its management is fundamental to paediatric medicine.

Thyroid physiology

The thyroid gland removes iodide from the blood stream, combines it with tyrosine and releases iodinated tyrosine to the peripheral tissues. The thyroid gland is able to trap iodide and synthesize iodothyronine from 70 days gestation. Release of thyroxine, however, does not occur until 18–20 weeks gestation. Thyroid gland growth is regulated by thyroid stimulating hormone (TSH), released from the anterior pituitary gland, which is in turn regulated by thyrotropin regulating hormone (TRH), released from the hypothalamus. These regulating hormones are in turn controlled by negative feedback from triiodothyronine (T_3), the active metabolite of the major thyroid hormone thyroxine (or tetra-iodothyronine, T_4).

The thyroid gland is extremely effective at trapping serum iodide, with a concentration gradient from thyroid to serum of 30–40. This gradient increases in times of iodide deficiency. Once trapped, iodide is oxidised to iodine and organification occurs. Organification is the iodination of thyroglobulin-bound tyrosyl residues to form monoiodiotyrosine (MIT) and diiodiotyrosine (DIT). Organification and iodide oxidation (to iodine) are catalysed by thyroid peroxidase. Thyroid peroxidase couples the iodotyrosines to form iodothyronines within the thyroglobulin molecule, resulting in T_4 and T_3. In the absence of iodine deficiency the T_4 to T_3 synthesis ratio is 10–20:1. In adults, the release rate of T_4 to T_3 is 3:1. Once released, both hormones bind to thyroxine binding globulin (TBG). Eighty per cent of circulating T_3 results from deiodinatination of T_4 in peripheral tissues. Thyroid hormones bind to a nuclear receptor. T_3 binds to this receptor with 10 times the affinity of T_4. Once bound, thyroid hormones regulate gene transcription, increasing cytoplasmic proteins which stimulate mitochondrial activity, thus increasing metabolic rate.

Disorders of thyroid function in childhood can be divided into the following categories:
- hypothyroidism
- hyperthyroidism
- thyroid masses.

Hypothyroidism

Congenital

Screening for congenital hypothyroidism has been performed in most developed countries for the last 15–20 years. In Australia, screening for congenital hypothyroidism, phenylketonuria and cystic fibrosis occurs on day 3–5 of life. Due to such screening the clinical picture of 'cretinism' is now thankfully rarely seen.

Incidence

One in 3000–5000 with some geographic variation.

Aetiology

Seventy-five per cent are due to dysgenesis (agenesis, ectopia), 10% to dyshormonogenesis (often autosomal recessive, Pendred syndrome = peroxidase deficiency associated with sensorineural deafness), 5% to hypothalamic–pituitary deficiency (secondary or tertiary hypothyroidism) and 10% to transient hypothyroidism (iodine exposure, maternal antithyroid antibodies, etc.).

Clinical picture

Often subclinical and detected on routine screening. Jaundice, dry skin, hoarse cry, puffy face, prominent tongue, listless, umbilical herniae, hypothermia, bradycardia, failure to thrive.

Investigation results

Unconjugated hyperbilirubinaemia (due to glucronyl transferase deficiency), elevated TSH detected on heel-prick drop of blood collected on filter paper day 3–5 (except in secondary or tertiary disease).

Management

Confirmatory investigations: repeat T_4 and TSH; thyroid scan (showing absent, lingual or increased uptake of radioisotope), X ray distal femoral epiphysis (absence implying prolonged/prenatal hypothyroidism), assessment and imaging of pituitary gland if indicated; commencement of therapy (thyroxine replacement at 8–10 μg/kg/day).

Prognosis

Normal intellectual and physical development if treatment is commenced promptly and monitored closely. Overtreatment may result in craniosynostosis.

Acquired

Hypothyroidism in the child or adolescent is relatively uncommon. In iodine sufficient regions of the world the most common cause is autoimmune thyroiditis. Accordingly, acquired hypothyroidism is seen twice as commonly in females than in males, usually manifesting in early puberty.

Prevalence

Between the ages of 1 and 18 years the prevalence is 1.2%. Rare prior to 4 years of age.

Aetiology

The causes in order of frequency are as follows: primary hypothyroidism — chronic lymphocytic, autoimmune (Hashimoto) thyroiditis, late appearing congenital dyshormonogenesis, exogenous factors (high dose iodine exposure (Wolff-Chaikoff effect), radiation) and severe iodine deficiency; and secondary/tertiary hypothyroidism — congenital and acquired hypopituitarism.

Clinical picture

The most common presentation is growth retardation and goitre. In addition, the triad of short stature, obesity and mental dullness indicates hypothyroidism until proven otherwise. Growth impairment usually mainly affects the limbs so that body proportions predominantly remain infantile. Other features include hypothermia, bradycardia, slow reflex relaxation, constipation, dry hair and skin, pallor, facial puffiness ('myxoedema') and dental delay. The onset is often insidious, with delays of up to 4–5 years being reported between onset of growth retardation and diagnosis of hypothyroidism. While delayed puberty usually occurs, some cases of precocious puberty have been reported.

Autoimmune thyroiditis may be associated with other autoimmune disease (autoimmune polyglandular syndromes) such as type 1 diabetes, autoimmune adrenalitis (Addison disease), vitiligo and pernicious anaemia. Occasionally, autoimmune hypothyroidism can be preceded by a period of transient hyperthyroidism.

Investigation results

Goitre (detected either clinically or sonographically) is common. Low circulating T_4 and (usually) high circulating TSH. Delayed bone age. Positive thyroid autoantibodies (in autoimmune thyroiditis). Patchy uptake of isotope on thyroid scan (in autoimmune thyroiditis). Hypothalamic or pituitary anomalies seen on CT or MRI (in tertiary or secondary disease).

Management

Replacement thyroxine (usually 50–100 μg/day in a single dose). Appropriate individual dose is determined by measuring serum TSH at 2+ weeks after commencing therapy.

Prognosis

Severely hypothyroid children often show dramatic clinical changes with treatment. These include: weight loss, rapid growth, loss of primary teeth, some transient hair loss and increased energy/alertness. The long-term neurodevelopmental outcome is good, given that the rapid growth phase of the brain in the first 2 years of life has usually been protected. Despite short term rapid catch up growth, restoration of full growth potential often does not occur due to rapid advancement of bone age in the first 18 months of treatment. Long term treatment is usually required.

Hyperthyroidism

Congenital

This is always due to maternal thyrotoxicosis and is a rare clinical event. However, if unrecognised and untreated, neonatal hyperthyroidism may be fatal.

Incidence

Maternal thyrotoxicosis is uncommon (1–2 cases per 1000 pregnancies). Neonatal disease occurs in 1 per 70 cases of pregnancies affected by thyrotoxicosis.

Aetiology

Neonatal hyperthyroidism is the result of the transplacental passage of TSH receptor stimulating antibodies from a mother with either active or inactive Graves disease. Measurement of maternal antibody status, rather than thyroxine levels, is predictive of the likelihood of neonatal hyperthyroidism.

Clinical picture

Neonates may present with any of the following; irritability, poor weight gain, tachycardia, cardiac arrythmias, flushing, hypertension, goitre, exomphalos, jaundice and hepatosplenomegaly. While presentation soon after birth is more common, if the mother has been taking antithyroid drugs, presentation may be delayed until day 8–9 after birth, when the antithyroid medication has been eliminated from the neonate's circulation.

Investigation results

High circulating T_4 or T_3 levels and low TSH levels in neonatal blood sample.

Management

Immediately after diagnosis, sedation and treatment with either beta blockade or digoxin may be required. Subsequent treatment with antithyroid medication (carbimazole, methimazole or propylthiouracil) is usually required. A therapeutic response should be seen within 24–36 hours after commencing treatment.

Prognosis

Mortality rates of up to 25% have been reported. The half-life of thyroid stimulating antibodies in the fetal circulation is approximately 12 days; however, the clinical course may extend for a period of up to 12 weeks.

Acquired

Hyperthyroidism in childhood and adolescence is less common than either euthyroid goitre or hypothyroidism. As with acquired hypothyroidism, it is most commonly due to autoimmune disease and is usually seen in young adolescent females.

Incidence

Females are affected 6–8 times more commonly than males. Some ethnic groups (such as Asian females) have a greater reported incidence of autoimmune hyperthyroidism.

Aetiology

Autoimmune hyperthyroidism (Graves disease) is the most common form of acquired hyperthyroidism in childhood and adolescence. Less frequent causes include the acute toxic phase of autoimmune hypothyroidism (Hashimoto disease) and a toxic thyroid nodule (rare). There is often a family history of autoimmune thyroid disease (either Graves or Hashimoto diseases). The primary defect is the presence of stimulating autoantibodies (thyroid receptor antibodies) which mimic the action of TSH. Overstimulation of the TSH receptor leads to thyroid growth and excess thyroxine production. There is often an associated ophthalmopathy due to the deposition of proteoglycans in the extraocular muscles and retro-orbital spaces.

Clinical picture

The clinical features of hyperthyroidism result from sympathetic drive causing a hypermetabolic state. Many of the florid signs of thyrotoxicosis that are seen in adults are less pronounced in children. Symptoms include deteriorating school performance, weakness/fatigue, restlessness/sleeplessness, polyuria, hunger, heat intolerance, excessive sweating, anxiety and diarrhoea and weight loss. Clinical signs include: goitre or localised thyroid mass, tremor, tachycardia and brisk reflexes. Approximately 30% of children will have associated proptosis and other signs of thyroidal ophthalmopathy (lid lag, lid retraction and ophthalmoplegia).

Investigation results

Suppressed serum TSH levels associated with elevated T_4 or T_3 levels. Elevated levels of thyroid autoantibodies (TRH antibodies positive in Graves disease). Advanced bone age and sonographic evidence of thyromegaly. Generalised and localised increased uptake of isotope is seen in Grave disease and toxic adenoma, respectively.

Management

In the setting of autoimmune hyperthyroidism there are three treatment options. The first of these, antithyroid medication, is the most commonly used. Carbimazole and methimazole have traditionally been used most commonly in Australia and Europe, whereas propylthiouracil has been more commonly used in North America. Both types of medication, block organification and are similarly efficacious with comparable side effect profiles. Beta blockade (with propranolol) may also be used in the first 2–4 weeks of therapy to gain symptom control. This is contraindicated in children who suffer from asthma. Treatment with organification blocking drugs is continued for 2 years in the first instance. Other treatment options include thyroidectomy (subtotal or total) and radioactive iodine. In the setting of toxic adenoma surgery is usually the preferred treatment option.

Prognosis

After 2 years of medical therapy approximately 20–50% of patients can be expected to enter spontaneous remission, with resolution of thyroid autoantibody status. Among those patients who do not remit spontaneously, long term drug therapy is both safe and effective. In the advent of poor compliance with medical therapy, lack of control or increasing thyromegaly, a second treatment option — surgical subtotal or complete thyroidectomy — is considered. This results in 20% of patients becoming euthyroid, 50% of patients becoming hypothyroid and 30% of patients becoming thyrotoxic in the long term. Other paediatric and adult centres use a third treatment option, that of radioactive iodine. This treatment results in total thyroid ablation and requires subsequent lifelong thyroxine replacement therapy.

Clinical example

Tina, aged 15, has noticed increasing anxiety levels recently. She is quite bright academically and has set high standards for herself at school. Her parents are concerned that her anxiety is associated with some recent difficulties in concentrating during classes. Her teachers complain that she 'fidgets' all the time and is quite restless. Despite a healthy appetite ('she eats more than anyone else in the family') Tina has been losing weight and has frequent loose bowel actions. Her mother also reports that, despite it being winter, Tina refuses to wear appropriate cold weather clothing, preferring a T-shirt most of the time.

On examination, Tina appears quite anxious and has very prominent eyes (proptosis). She has difficulty in sitting still on the examination couch and squirms around quite a lot. Her resting pulse is 110 and she has a fine tremor when her hands are held out. Her palms are very sweaty. She has a firm, smooth goitre with an audible bruit. Her reflexes are very brisk and she has difficulty standing from a squatting position.

A provisional diagnosis of Graves disease is made. This is confirmed by finding that her serum TSH levels are unrecordably low in the face of a T_4 level of 52 nmol/l (high). Her anti-TSH receptor antibody titre is elevated. A thyroid ultrasound demonstrated a uniformly enlarged thyroid with no focal changes.

Tina was commenced initially on both carbimazole and propranolol. Her symptoms had largely abated within 3 weeks and her propranolol was ceased at this time. Ophthamological review confirmed the presence of proptosis, with no other thyroidal eye signs being present. Over the following year Tina's goitre diminished in size; however, her proptosis remained unchanged. She was initially treated with carbimazole for 2 years. At this time she was still TSH receptor antibody positive and it was decided to continue treatment for a further 2 years.

Thyroid masses

Goitre

The commonest cause of goitre on a worldwide basis remains iodine deficiency. In developed countries this had become rare, until recent times, with the iodination of table salt and some infant milks. Recently, iodine deficiency has been reported again in Australian populations, presumably due to low salt diets encouraged for cardiovascular health reasons.

Incidence

Goitres or diffuse enlargement of the thyroid gland occur in 4–5% of all children. They are more common in girls during puberty and are often not detected.

Aetiology

In Australia the main causes in order of frequency are: Hashimoto thyroiditis (majority are euthyroid), Graves disease, mild dyshormonogenesis, tumour (benign/malignant), acute/subacute thyroiditis and iodine deficiency. Foods that inhibit thyroxine synthesis and can lead to goitre (goitrogens) include cabbage, soybeans and cassava.

Clinical picture

Most often the goitre is asymptomatic, frequently detected on routine examination. Thyroid hypo- or hyperfunction will present with signs and symptoms discussed above. Occasionally pressure symptoms related to the enlarged thyroid (dysphagia, stridor or neck discomfort) may be the presenting feature. Thyroidal tenderness is seen in acute/subacute thyroiditis. Regional lymphadenopathy associated with a goitre or thyroid nodule is suggestive of malignancy and is an ominous sign.

Investigation results

Sonography, serum thyroid function tests and serum thyroid antibody levels will distinguish most causes of goitre. Fasting urinary iodine levels will also help to define iodine status. Thyroid scanning will show increased uptake with mild dyshormonogenesis and patchy distribution in Hashimoto thyroiditis.

Management

Smoothly enlarged goitres with normal thyroid function can be managed simply by observation and iodine supplementation if required. Goitres with functional consequences will require either thyroxine supplementation or suppressive medication.

Prognosis

This depends on the cause of the goitre. As most cases of asymptomatic goitre result in no disturbance of thyroid function, the prognosis is usually good.

Thyroid nodules

Nodules within the thyroid gland are palpable, localised swellings. They may be single or multiple. The Chernobyl nuclear reactor disaster in 1986 led to a markedly increased incidence of benign and malignant thyroid nodules in children from the surrounding iodine deficient areas.

Incidence

Less than 2% of children have thyroid nodules. Of these, approximately 2% are malignant. If the nodule is single the risk of malignancy increases to 30–40%.

Aetiology

Benign nodules include cysts, cystic adenomas and variations of Hashimoto thyroiditis. Malignant nodules are carcinomas and occur in the following order: papillary/mixed, follicular, medullary and anaplastic. In one series of children with thyroid cancers reported in the 1950s, 80% had a history of having received head/neck radiotherapy. Recently, however, head/neck irradiation is now less commonly used and the aetiology of most thyroid cancers remains obscure. Medullary carcinomas may be sporadic, familial (autosomal dominant mode of inheritance) or part of a multiple endocrine neoplasia (MEN2) complex. Patients with MEN2 have been found to have mutations in the RET proto-oncogene.

Clinical picture

The most common presentation is the lobular, irregular thyroid gland seen in Hasimoto thyroiditis. Nodules are usually asymptomatic and detected upon routine examination. Rarely, nodules may be hyperfunctional ('toxic adenoma'). Medullary carcinomas may be associated with phaeochromocytoma (in later life) and parathyroid hyperplasia (MEN2A), or multiple mucosal neuromas, Marfan-like habitus and phaeochromocytoma (MEN2B). It is very rare for a child with MEN2 to present with clinical disease. They are usually detected as part of a kindred subjected to genetic screening.

Investigations

Nodules may be detected both sonographically and by thyroid scanning. The finding of multiple hot nodules associated with positive thyroid antibody titres and/or disturbed thyroid function is against a diagnosis of malignancy. Alternatively, a single cold nodule with or without serum calcitonin levels (associated with medullary carcinomas) is suggestive of malignancy. Fine needle aspiration is not widely used in the diagnosis of thyroid nodules in children.

Management

If there is any doubt as to the nature of any thyroid nodule it is appropriate to proceed to open biopsy. Solitary benign nodules are usually excised. Papillary thyroid cancers are treated with total thyroid excision, with subsequent radioactive iodine therapy if metatstases are thought to be present. Medullary thyroid cancers are unresponsive to radioactive iodine and early total thyroidectomy remains the treatment of choice. In individuals with RET proto-oncogene mutations from families with a strong history of medullary carcinomas, prophylactic thyroidectomy is considered.

Prognosis

Most thyroid nodules are benign and have an excellent prognosis. In the case of papillary carcinomas, serial thyroid scans for the first 3 years after surgery will detect any residual thyroid tissue or tumour recurrence. In patients suffering from medullary carcinomas, serial measures of serum calcitonin levels are the monitoring strategy of choice.

In summary, disorders of the thyroid gland can have many manifestations: hypofunction, hyperfunction, pressure symptoms and incidental tumours. Given the importance of normal thyroid function for both neurological and physical development, and the potential for malignancy in thyroid nodules, a clinical awareness of potential thyroid problems in paediatrics is essential. Once detected, most thyroid problems can be successfully managed, with excellent clinical outcomes.

65 The child with genital abnormalities

U. Kuhnle

Genital abnormalities at birth are estimated to be present in 1 out of 100 children; the incidence of severe abnormalities or intersexuality is estimated to be 1 in 6900 live births. The major difference from congenital malformations of other organ systems such as facial abnormalities like cleft lip and palate, is that the appearance of the external genitalia determines the social sex which is announced at birth. In the absence of 'normal' development of the external genitalia, definitive gender assignment and its announcement have to be postponed. Postponement of sex assignment causes tremendous stress and insecurity to the parents.

To reduce parental stress, sex assignment should be as early as possible and should not be delayed more than 1–2 weeks. Most diagnostic procedures, for example steroid hormone determinations and chromosomal and/or molecular genetic analysis, can be achieved within this time frame. To delay legal registration for 2–4 weeks is possible in most countries.

Normal sexual differentiation

Normal sexual differentiation is a complex process which starts at conception with the presence of either an X or a Y chromosome. During the first 4–5 weeks of gestation primordial cells migrate into the genital ridge and induce the development of the indifferent gonad, which is initially indistinguishable in both sexes. Further differentiation into an ovary is dependent on the contribution of two intact X chromosomes, whereas a gene located on the short arm of the Y chromosome, the SRY gene, is required for the development of the testis.

During the indifferent stage of development in both sexes, two pairs of genital ducts, the müllerian and wolffian ducts, are present; these will further differentiate under the influence of gonadal hormones.

Development of the ovary and female genitalia

In the presence of two X chromosomes ovarian development commences slowly and primordial follicles containing oogonia can be seen at 16 weeks gestation. Before birth many oogonia degenerate but 1 or 2 million continue to develop into oocytes. Degeneration is increased when only one X chromosome is present, as in patients with Turner syndrome. While the ovary is capable of oestrogen synthesis, it contributes little or nothing to the high circulating maternal hormone levels present during pregnancy.

The development of female external genitalia does not require the presence of gonadal hormones. The growth of the genital tubercle decreases and forms the clitoris; the urogenital folds and labioscrotal folds form the labia minora and majora, respectively.

The wolffian ducts regress and in the absence of müllerian inhibiting factor the müllerian ducts develop into a uterus, whereas the vagina develops from the urogenital sinus. The development of the internal and external genitalia in the female is completed by 12 weeks gestation.

Development of the testis and male genitalia

Development of the testis is initiated by the SRY gene, a transcription factor located on the short arm of the Y chromosome. In addition, a variety of other autosomal genes are necessary for the development of a normal testis but these are also involved in the development of other organ systems. A summary of these genes and their role in organ development is given in Table 65.1.

The testis consists of a dense tunica albuginea, the rete testis and the seminiferous tubules, which give rise

Table 65.1 Genes involved in gonadal development and malformations associated with mutations other than gonadal dysgenesis

Gene	Chromosome	Associated malformations
WT-1	11p13	Wilms tumour, nephropathy, gonadoblastoma
LIM-1	11p12–13	Unknown
SF-1 (FTZF1)	9q33	Adrenal insufficiency
SRY	Yp11.3	None
DAX-1	Xp21	Duplication: gonadal dysgenesis in males. Mutation: adrenal insufficiency
SOX-1	17q24.3–25.1	Campomelic dysplasia
DMRT1/ DMRT2	9p24.3	Renal malformation, mental retardation

Table 65.2 Clinical and laboratory findings compared to the aetiology of the major causes of ambiguous genitalia

Aetiology	Disorder	Phenotype	Chromosomes	Associated problems	Laboratory tests
Gonadal abnormality	Gonadal dysgenesis	Female	XY XO/XY	See Table 65.2 Dysmorphic features	Laparotomy Gonadal biopsy Molecular genetics
Gonadal abnormality	True hermaphroditism	Ambiguous	XX,XY Mosaicism	Gonadal malignancies	Gonadal biopsy
Defective testosterone biosynthesis	Deficiency of: 17/20 lyase 17β HSD 5α reductase	Ambiguous	XY	None	Testosterone Dihydrotestosterone hCG stimulation Molecular genetics
Aromatase deficiency	Deficiency of: P$_{450}$ aromatase	Ambiguous Male	XX XY	None	Testosterone Oestradiol Molecular genetics
Receptor defect	Complete or partial androgen insensitivity	Female or ambiguous	XY	None	Testosterone Molecular genetics
Receptor defect	LH receptor defect	Female or ambiguous	XY	None	LH, FSH Testosterone hCG stimulation Molecular genetics
Congenital adrenal hyperplasia	Deficiency of: 21 hydroxylase 11β hydroxylase	Ambiguous Male	XX XX XY	Salt loss Skin pigmentation Hypertension	17 OHP Molecular genetics

to the interstitial cells of Leydig, secreting testosterone, and the Sertoli cells, secreting müllerian inhibiting factor. Normal development of male genitalia depends on the secretion of these two hormones.

The androgen, testosterone, stimulates the wolffian ducts to differentiate into male internal genitalia, namely the epididymis, vas deferens and ejaculatory ducts, and the external genitalia to masculinise. For further virilisation of the external genitalia testosterone is reduced to dihydrotestosterone. Under the influence of the androgens the phallus enlarges and the genital tubercle elongates to form the glans penis, whereas the labioscrotal folds grow and fuse to form the scrotal sac. The line of fusion is visible as the scrotal raphe. In complete masculinised males the urethra opens at the tip of the penis. Hypospadias describes a condition in which, depending on the severity, the urethra opens somewhere along the shaft of the phallus, along the scrotal raphe or on the perineum.

The müllerian inhibiting factor inhibits the development of the female internal ducts and hence the development of a uterus and the upper portion of the vagina. As in the female, the entire process of differentiation is completed during the 12th week of fetal development. A deficiency of any of the two testicular hormones prior to the 12th week of gestation leads to incomplete male sexual development.

Abnormal development of the genitalia

The difference between male and female external genitalia is the result of androgenic hormones secreted by the fetal testis. The ovaries do not contribute to sex differentiation. In normal sexual development the chromosomal sex corresponds to the appearance of the internal and external sex, while in abnormal sexual development there is a discrepancy between the chromosomes and the genitalia, with the development of various degrees of intersexuality (Table 65.1).

Abnormal sexual development in the female

Female fetuses exposed to high androgens during the sensitive first 12 weeks of gestation develop abnormalities of the external genitalia to varying degrees, while the development of the internal genitalia, namely the ovaries and uterus, are androgen independent and develop normally (Fig 65.2).

The most common cause of abnormal genitalia in genetic females is congenital adrenal hyperplasia. This term refers to a family of inherited disorders of adrenal steroidogenesis caused by an enzymatic deficiency of one of the five steps involved in cortisol synthesis, the most

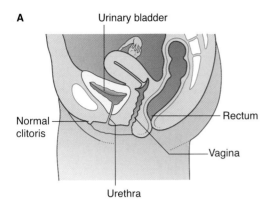

A

Urinary bladder

Normal clitoris

Rectum

Vagina

Urethra

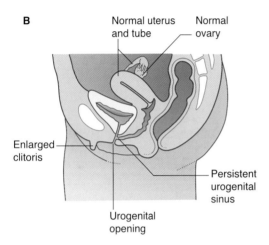

B

Normal uterus and tube

Normal ovary

Enlarged clitoris

Persistent urogenital sinus

Urogenital opening

Fig. 65.1 Schematic illustration of normal and ambiguous female genitalia as in congenital adrenal hyperplasia. Note the urogenital sinus leading to a single opening and the enlarged clitoris induced by androgens. (Adapted from Moore and Persaud, 1993.)

common being a defect in the 21 hydoxylase enzyme system. All other causes of androgen excess in female infants are extremely rare.

Sexual development in the female fetus might be abnormal due to:

- the presence of a testis, resulting in true hermaphroditism
- defective adrenal steroidogenesis with increased adrenal androgen secretion, as in congenital adrenal hyperplasia (CAH)
- aromatase deficiency in the fetus and/or the placenta (defective conversion of testosterone to oestradiol)
- exogenous androgens:
  — virilising disease in the mother
  — virilising drugs ingested by the mother.

True hermaphroditism

True hermaphroditism describes a condition where testis and ovaries are present in the same individual. The presentation at birth depends upon the amount of testosterone

> ### Clinical example
>
> Alpay, a Turkish boy, the first child born to a young consanguineous couple, was brought to the emergency department at the age of 14 days. He had started to vomit during the morning and refused to feed. On examination he was clearly dehydrated but there were no other abnormalities. Vital signs were stable but the blood pressure was 85/45 and his heart rate 140/min. His birth weight had been 3.4 kg; his actual weight was 2.9 kg.
>
> Pyloric stenosis was considered initially but he was found to be severly acidotic with a pH of 7.15 and a base deficit of 18 mmol/l. His electrolytes showed a serum sodium of 120 mmol/l and a potassium level of 7.9 mmol/l. Congenital adrenal hyperplasia was suspected and he was started on intravenous rehydration and responded well to hydrocortisone i.v. and oral fludrocortisone. His plasma 17 hydroxyprogesterone was found to be grossly elevated, which confirmed the diagnosis. The parents were counselled and the genetic implications discussed.

secreted. The most frequent karyotype is 46,XX (70%) and familial cases are common. The most extreme cases are 46,XX males, with no ovarian tissue detectable. Sex assignment depends upon the degree of virilisation. When testicular tissue is removed, female fertility is possible; male fertility has never been proven. True hermaphroditism can also be caused by sex chromosomal mosaicism or rarely in 46,XY individuals.

Congenital adrenal hyperplasia

Congenital adrenal hyperplasia refers to a series of disorders caused by an enzymatic deficiency in the adrenal steroidogenic pathway, the most common (90% of all

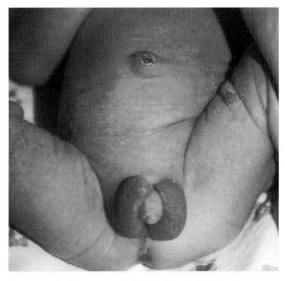

Fig. 65.2 Ambiguous genitalia of a female infant with congenital adrenal hyperplasia associated with salt wasting.

cases with congenital adrenal hyperplasia) being a defect in the P_{450} cytochrome enzyme, 21 hydroxylase. It is important to realize that this form of congenital adrenal hyperplasia can be associated with life threatening salt wasting due to an aldosterone synthesis defect, present in 60% of cases. Therefore this diagnosis has to be anticipated and looked for in all virilised female newborns. Overstimulation of the adrenals with pituitary adrenocorticotrophin (ACTH) leads to increased synthesis of androgens which are not 21-hydroxylated. Increased androgen synthesis during fetal life causes virilisation of the external genitalia of affected females; however, the differentiation of the internal female organs, i.e. ovaries, fallopian tubes and uterus, are unaffected and develop normally (Figs. 65.1 and 65.2).

In affected male infants, the 21 hydroxylase deficiency does not cause genital abnormalities at birth, but a salt losing crisis in early infancy or precocious puberty later in childhood are suspicous and should initiate workup for congenital adrenal hyperplasia. Since male infants are often diagnosed late or even missed, screening tests for congenital adrenal hyperplasia have been introduced into neonatal screening programmes in some countries.

Abnormal development of male genitalia

The complexity of the development of male genitalia and the need for various hormones to be synthesised and to act via specific hormone receptors allow errors at various stages of sexual development. The clinical and biochemical pattern is often characteristic and diagnostic.

Sexual development in the male fetus might be abnormal due to:
- abnormal differentiation of the testis → gonadal dysgenesis
- luteinising hormone (LH) receptor defects:
  — loss of function → Leydig cell agenesis → testosterone deficiency → incomplete sexual male differentiation;
  — gain of function → constitutive activation of the LH receptor → normal male phenotype but early precocious puberty
- deficiency of, or insensitivity to, antimüllerian hormone: persistent müllerian duct syndrome
- enzymatic defects of testosterone synthesis
- 5-alpha reductase deficiency
- androgen receptor defects → complete (testicular feminisation syndrome) or incomplete androgen insensitivity.

Gonadal dysgenesis

Female external and internal genitalia in 46,XY children can be due to gonadal dysgenesis and is then described as sex reversal. Dysgenetic gonads are caused by mutations in sex determining genes (Table 65.2) and are frequently associated with gonadal tumours such as gonadoblastomas or dysgerminomas; therefore these gonads have to be removed early.

Complete or partial androgen insensitivity

The gene for the androgen receptor is located on the X chromosome and mutations cause insensitivity to the action of androgens. Depending on the degree of loss of function of this receptor the external genitalia in genetic males are either unambigous female in complete androgen insensitivity (CAIS) or associated with various degrees of hypospadias in partial androgen insensitivity (PAIS).

In complete androgen insensitivity internal genitalia are always male, i.e. there is no uterus, although a small vagina is usually present. The diagnosis may be made unexpectedly when testes are found during surgery for inguinal hernia in a phenotypic girl. Testosterone synthesis is normal and often elevated. The disorder is transmitted by female carriers; other family members may be affected. Sex assignment depends upon the degree of virilisation but has to be female in complete androgen insensitivity, as no further virilisation will take place during puberty.

Clinical example

Benedict, a 10 month old boy, was brought to a paediatric surgeon for the correction of penoscrotal hypospadias. A karyotype at birth had been done and shown normal 46,XY chromosomes. On examination of his genitalia there was a single orifice at the base of the phallus, the scrotum was bifid, but there were two well developed gonads in the scrotal sac, with a volume of 3 ml each. There was no history of neonatal problems. The family history revealed that the mother's brother had had unilateral undescended testis and had developed gynaecomastia during puberty, which was corrected surgically. There were two adult cousins from a maternal aunt who had been operated during infancy for penile hypospadias (second degree hypospadias) and both had also developed gynaecomastia during puberty. One of them had fathered two children.

Investigations showed unmeasurably low baseline testosterone and gonadotrophins. Molecular genetic analysis of the androgen receptor gene revealed a point mutation in the hormone binding domain, causing incomplete virilisation. In addition, all three adult males had the identical mutation but highly elevated baseline testosterone levels. They had undergone normal pubertal development. It was very helpful for the parents of our patient to see that the future development of their son would be normal. Hypospadias repair is scheduled at a chronological age of 3–4 years.

Chromosomal disorders

Numeric aberrations of the sex chromosomes are not always associated with abnormal genitalia at birth. In all cases, however, gonadal development will be disturbed resulting in disturbed, pubertal development and decreased fertility or infertility.

The most frequent disorders associated with sex chromosomal abnormalities are:
- Turner syndrome (45,XO)
- Klinefelter syndrome (47,XXY)
- Mixed gonadal dysgenesis (XO/XY)
- Chromosomal mosaicism, for example XX/XY

Turner and Klinefelter syndromes

These are relative frequent causes of dysgenetic gonadal development; however the external genitalia are female or male, respectively, without abnormalities. Pubertal development is disturbed and infertility is the rule, but female fertility is preserved in about 3% of patients with Turner syndrome. Sex hormone replacement should be started around puberty to initiate pubertal development; and gynaecomastia, common in Klinefelter syndrome, needs surgical correction.

Mixed gonadal dysgenesis

This refers to a chromosomal pattern of 46,XY/45,XO with streak gonads on one side and a testis on the other side. Since malignancies are common, the gonads have to be either removed or regularly (i.e. twice yearly) monitored with palpation and ultrasound.

Genital malformations unrelated to androgen deficiency or excess

An isolated, enlarged clitoris at birth can be associated with a variety of tumours, such as lipomas, lymphangiomas (Fig. 65.3) and gliomas, the last of which might be the first manifestation of neurofibromatosis. Congenital absence of the clitoris or phallus is extremely rare and probably due to inadequate ectodermal and mesodermal interactions of the genital tubercle.

Diagnostic workup

History

- The most important part is the family history, in particular whether there are other children with similar disorders among siblings or first degree relatives. Note that all forms of congenital adrenal hyperplasia and testosterone biosynthesis defects are transmitted as autosomal recessive traits, while androgen receptor

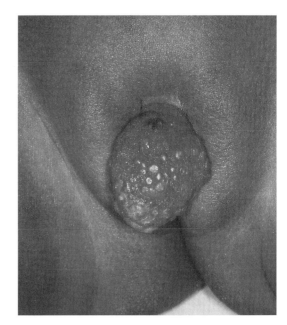

Fig. 65.3 Clitoromegaly due to a lymphangioma.

defects are linked to the X chromosome and are transmitted via healthy carrier mothers.
- Are the parents consanguineous?
- Did the mother take virilising drugs during pregnancy?

Clinical examination

- Is it possible to feel any gonads; is it possible to identify a uterus, either by ultrasound or rectal examination?
- Are there associated malformations?
- How is the clinical condition of the child? Are there signs of dehydration? Is there lack of weight gain or loss of weight? Is there increased skin pigmentation?

Laboratory evaluation

- Monitor electrolytes and blood glucose.
- Request urgent hormone analysis for 17 hydroxy-progesterone.
- Request an urgent karyotype.
- Collect a 24 hour urine specimen for sodium excretion to determine salt loss and for evaluation of steroid excretion; the latter is useful for the determination of all forms of congenital adrenal hyperplasia
- In 46,XY individuals testicular function can be evaluated by measuring testosterone levels before and 72 hours after a single intramuscular injection of 5000 IU human chorionic gonadotrophin (hCG).
- An exaggerated increase of LH and follicle stimulating hormone (FSH) 30 minutes after stimulation with a single dose of 0.1 mg luteinising hormone releasing hormone (LHRH) indicates dysgenetic gonads.

Management

In the management of children with genital abnormalities three important points must be considered:
- reduce parental stress.
- decide sex assignment.
- avoid a salt losing crisis in congenital adrenal hyperplasia.

Reduce parental stress

The parents should be shown the infant's genitalia so they can see for themselves that there is a problem. It should be clearly stated that this problem can be solved and that a rapid decision will be reached. The parents need reassurance that the child will grow up as a boy or a girl and not as something in between. The medical and nursing staff involved in the parents' care need to be instructed and the problems arising should be discussed. Avoid conflicting information!

Sex assignment

This should be possible within the first few days of life, after the following information has been obtained:
- Does the child have congenital adrenal hyperplasia?
- What gonads does the child have? Are they dysgenetic?
- Is there a uterus?

Virilised girls with congenital adrenal hyperplasia should be raised as girls, as fertility can be achieved. Children with complete androgen insensitivity are phenotypically females and cannot respond to androgens. They have to be raised as girls; however, they will be infertile.

While it had formerly been thought easier for an under-virilised boy to live as a girl, rather than as a boy with a small phallus which might function poorly despite corrective surgical procedures, recent case reports and patient support groups have challenged this hypothesis. Affected individuals feel that the decisions made by doctors and parents in early infancy were premature and irreversible operative procedures had been performed without the patients' own informed consent. This criticism has led to considerable insecurity on the part of pediatricians and surgeons in charge of children with genital abnormalities. The present author feels strongly that, while a decision regarding the sex of rearing has to be made, corrective surgery should be delayed if possible until the child can give his or her own consent.

Treatment of micropenis

Severe micropenis, that is a penile length at birth below 2 cm, can be treated with low dose testosterone. Percentile curves for penis length for the different age groups are available and low dose testosterone treatment can be repeated if penile length is again below the third percentile for age. Careful monitoring is necessary to avoid overtreatment and systemic effects such as premature bone age maturation.

Congenital adrenal hyperplasia

When congenital adrenal hyperplasia is suspected it should be possible to confirm the diagnosis within 24 hours. The following management is suggested:
- Intravenous fluid and electrolyte replacement.
- Prevention of hypoglycaemia.
- Hydrocortisone in a dose of 15–25 mg/m^2 body surface area/day.
- 9-alpha fludrocortisone 0.05–0.2 mg/day. Steroid therapy will be required for life.
- Referral to an experienced paediatric surgeon.
- Genetic counselling. CAH is inherited as an autosomal recessive trait.

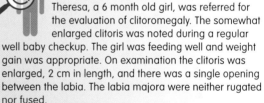

Clinical example

Theresa, a 6 month old girl, was referred for the evaluation of clitoromegaly. The somewhat enlarged clitoris was noted during a regular well baby checkup. The girl was feeding well and weight gain was appropriate. On examination the clitoris was enlarged, 2 cm in length, and there was a single opening between the labia. The labia majora were neither rugated nor fused.

Congenital adrenal hyperplasia was suspected and 17 hydroxyprogesterone was found to be highly elevated. Electrolytes and blood glucose were normal, no renal salt loss could be found in a spontaneous urine sample and the simple virilising form of the 21-hydroxylase deficiency was confirmed. When taking the family history it was found that the girl had a 4 year old brother who was growing and developing well. On investigation, this boy was also shown to suffer the 21 hydroxylase deficiency. His height was on the 75th percentile for his age, but bone age was advanced and corresponded to 7 year old boys. There was no pubic hair, but his phallus was well developed. Testicular volume was 2 ml. Both siblings were started on hydrocortisone replacement therapy. There is hope that the final adult height in the boy will not be compromised significantly, as his epiphyseal maturation is not yet too advanced. The prognosis for the girl, however, is better. Theresa was referred to a paediatric surgeon, and corrective surgery planned for the age of 5 years, before she starts school. Prior to surgery, radiological examination of the lower genital tract will be scheduled to determine the size of the vagina and urogenital sinus.

Prevention of genital malformations in CAH

In pregnancies at risk for congenital adrenal hyperplasia one can offer the mother treatment with dexamethasone, which has been shown to reduce genital virilisation in affected girls. This therapy has to be initiated as soon as the pregnancy is suspected and confirmed. Prenatal diagnosis of CAH can be made in chorionic villous biopsy at around 9 weeks of gestation. If CAH can be excluded or the fetus is shown to be a male, treatment is stopped. This therapy is effective, although side effects in the mother, such as weight gain, depression, skin changes, gestational diabetes and hypertension may complicate the pregnancy.

Childhood diabetes 66

J. Couper

Diabetes mellitus

Diabetes mellitus is caused by a deficiency in insulin production or in the action of insulin. It is the second most common chronic disease of childhood and is responsible for considerable morbidity due to acute metabolic derangements and long term microvascular and macrovascular complications. In childhood the majority of diabetes is type 1 diabetes (previously known as insulin dependent diabetes). However, with the increasing incidence of type 2 diabetes in childhood in North America, it is likely this will be the trend in Australia and New Zealand, especially in Aboriginal and Polynesian populations.

The prevalence of type 1 diabetes mellitus in Australia is approximately 1 in 750 for children under the age of 15 years, with an annual incidence of 12–13 per 100 000 population. This is similar to incidences reported for New Zealand, USA and the UK. In Asia the incidence is very low, whereas in parts of Scandinavia it exceeds 30 per 100 000. The reasons for these variations are presumed to be both genetic and environmental. The sex ratio in diabetes is equal. Diabetes is uncommon in infancy. In childhood the incidence shows two peaks, at ages 4–6 years and 10–14 years.

Pathogenesis of type 1 diabetes

There are two major factors that contribute to the pathogenesis of diabetes:
- genetic predisposition
- environmental triggers.

Autoimmune destruction of beta cells

Type 1 diabetes is caused by autoimmune destruction of the beta cells (insulin producing cells) of the islets of Langerhans. T cell infiltration of the islets and circulating autoantibodies precede the development of diabetes for months to years. Target antigens are insulin, glutamic acid decarboxylase and a tyrosine phosphatase. This preclinical phase, when blood glucose is normal and circulating antibodies are present, provides clues to the possibility of preventing or postponing the onset of clinical diabetes. There is an increased frequency of certain HLA types (HLA DR3/DQ2 and DR4/DQ8) in children with diabetes. The HLA genes are located on chromosome 6 and encode HLA molecules on the beta cells.

Environmental factors that are potential candidates to initiate autoimmunity or act as progression factors are viruses (particularly enteroviruses) and dietary factors (particularly cow's milk protein). However, only congenital rubella is a proven environmental trigger and this is a rare cause of type 1 diabetes.

Metabolic effects of insulin

Insulin is the hormone of energy storage and anabolism. It allows glucose to enter cells to be stored as glycogen in the liver and muscle, and as tryglyceride in fat. Insulin deficiency prevents glycogen and tryglyceride storage and causes their breakdown as well as that of protein. In addition, insulin deficiency promotes hepatic gluconeogenesis. The combined effects of glycogen breakdown, enhanced gluconeogenesis and failure of glucose entry into cells results in a rise in blood glucose. When the blood glucose exceeds approximately 10 mmol/l, the renal threshold is exceeded and glycosuria occurs. The osmotic effect of the glycosuria causes polyuria and dehydration. The breakdown of triglyceride (lipolysis) releases free fatty acids into the circulation. In the liver these are converted to ketoacids (ketogenesis). In insulin deficiency, not only is ketogenesis marked but peripheral use of ketoacids is diminished. This results in a rapid accumulation of these organic acids with eventual development of ketoacidosis.

When the autoimmune process has destroyed approximately 90% of the beta cell mass, persistent hyperglycaemia indicates the onset of clinical diabetes. Symptoms are usually present 2–6 weeks before the diagnosis is made; however, a child with a suspected diagnosis of diabetes should be investigated immediately. As the insulin deficiency proceeds, diabetic ketosis and then ketoacidosis develop and, if not treated, result in death. Ketoacidosis causes vomiting and later rapid deep breathing (Kussmaul respiration). The hyperventilation is an attempt by the body to compensate for the metabolic acidosis by removing carbon dioxide. Chemical breakdown of acetoacetic acid in the body yields acetone, which can be detected on the patient's breath. Breakdown of fat and protein and dehydration lead to weight loss. Abdominal pain mimicking an acute surgical abdomen may occur. Dehydration (shock) occurs because of continuing massive urinary losses caused by the osmotic diuresis. The acidosis, dehydration and changes in plasma osmolality cause initial irritability, confusion, drowsiness and eventual coma. Because immune function becomes compromised in diabetes, the possibility of serious infection should always be considered, although is rarely present. A summary of the clinical features and useful investigations at the time of presentation of type 1 diabetes is presented in Table 66.1.

Table 66.1 Type 1 diabetes: clinical features at presentation and useful investigations at diagnosis

Clinical presentation
Polyuria and polydipsia
Enuresis and nocturia
Weight loss and fatigue
Thrush
Vomiting (with increasing ketosis)
Kussmaul breathing and coma (with increasing acidosis)

Investigations
Urinalysis for glucose and ketones
Random blood glucose (postprandial)
Blood electrolytes and acid–base when unwell
Blood or other cultures and blood count (if infection suspected)
Islet antibodies and fasting C peptide (if type 2 diabetes suspected)

Differential diagnoses

The diagnosis of type 1 diabetes in childhood is not usually difficult, providing the physician is aware that this condition occurs even in the very young. The most common misdiagnoses are to mistake:

- polyuria for a urinary tract infection
- the overbreathing of metabolic acidosis for a respiratory tract infection or asthma
- vomiting and abdominal pain for gastroenteritis or an acute abdomen.

Children with intercurrent infections, acute asthma or hypernatraemic dehydration may have transient hyperglycaemia and glycosuria that resolves with the intercurrent illness. Only very rarely do these children develop type 1 diabetes. Islet autoantibodies can be tested to determine whether there is an increased risk of the child developing type 1 diabetes.

Treatment of diabetic ketoacidosis

The aims of therapy are:

- Emergency fluid replacement (10–20 ml/kg/h), using volume expanders, if shock is present so that the circulation is restored.
- Correction of dehydration slowly over 24–48 hours, using normal (isotonic or 0.9%) saline.
- Replacement of electrolyte losses and slow correction of acidosis. Supplemental potassium of 40–60 mmol/l in intravenous fluids is required to maintain normal serum potassium levels once insulin therapy has begun. Higher levels of supplementation will require ECG monitoring.
- Correction of the insulin deficiency, with an infusion of soluble insulin.

Treatment should be undertaken only in a centre equipped with paediatric intensive care facilities: the child may need to be transported there by an expert retrieval team. Frequent biochemical monitoring of the blood glucose, electrolytes and blood gases is required. The initial rate of insulin infusion of 0.1 unit/kg/h is adjusted to produce a fall in the blood glucose level of 5 mmol/h. More rapid reductions in the blood glucose level and/or a fall in serum sodium concentration alter the plasma osmolality too quickly and increase the risks of life threatening cerebral oedema.

When urinary ketones disappear, subcutaneous insulin is begun with regular food intake. Most children are stabilised on two to three daily injections of short and intermediate acting insulins. Within days to weeks of the introduction of insulin therapy, some recovery of the remaining viable beta cells may occur. During this period of partial remission (also known as the 'honeymoon' phase), insulin requirements may diminish. This phase may last for weeks or months, but as the underlying autoimmune destruction of beta cells is still in progress, more complete insulin deficiency occurs, so that blood glucose levels and insulin requirements rise permanently.

Management

Aims of management

Type 1 diabetes is a lifelong disorder. By definition, insulin treatment is necessary and at present can only be given by injection. The long term aims are for the child to have normal physical and emotional development, to lead a fulfilling life, with as little restriction on lifestyle and occupation as possible, and to minimise the risk of long term microvascular and macrovascular complications.

Management principles

The attainment of these aims depends largely on maintaining good diabetic (metabolic) control. This is difficult to achieve and is especially difficult in the under 5 year age group and for the adolescent. The aim is to keep the blood glucose levels as close to normal as possible pre- and postprandially. To measure the blood glucose, a spring loaded lancet is used to prick a finger, the blood is placed on a reagent strip and the glucose can be measured accurately by a variety of meters designed for home use. Most children measure their blood glucose two to three times a day. The key elements in achieving stability in the blood glucose levels are:

- insulin
- diet
- exercise.

Insulin

Insulin therapy is individualised. Generally prepubertal children require 0.8–1 unit per kilogram body weight per day, given as 2–4 subcutaneous injections daily. This requirement increases with more variability during puberty. Preschool children may be very sensitive to short acting insulin and therefore receive predominantly intermediate acting insulin. More intensive regimens using bolus doses of short acting insulin before meals and an intermediate or longer acting insulin before bed, or insulin pump regimens (basal insulin infusion subcutaneously and bolus doses of insulin with meals and snacks), are especially suitable for the adolescent needing more flexibility in the treatment schedule. These regimens may also improve metabolic control, provided compliance is excellent and there is accompanying blood glucose monitoring.

The dose of insulin is adjusted according to blood glucose measurements, anticipated diet and exercise. Glycosylated haemoglobin (HbA_{1C}) levels indicate the level of control during the preceding 6–8 weeks and often provide the most meaningful guide when blood glucose levels are erratic. The target range for blood glucose levels is generally 4–8 mmol/l but may need to be higher in preschool children or children with a history of recurrent severe hypoglycaemia.

Diet

Food raises the blood glucose level and this must be balanced by the glucose lowering effect of insulin and exercise. This balance is best achieved by having the diabetic diet supply a consistent quantity of carbohydrate each day and for the carbohydrate to be distributed as three major meals (breakfast, lunch, dinner) and three snacks (morning tea, afternoon tea and supper); however, toddlers will usually have a grazing pattern of food intake and older adolescents may not need three snacks per day.

The diabetic diet is relatively high in complex carbohydrates, low in simple carbohydrates (sugar) and low in saturated fats. It provides 50–55% of the kilojoules as complex carbohydrates, 30–35% as fat and 15% as protein. Dietitians frequently use the glycaemic index of foods to guide the child and family to appropriate food choices. The glycaemic index is a classification of foods based on their postprandial blood glucose response and, as such, is a more predictable guide than merely measuring the carbohydrate content of foods. The diet must be adequate nutritionally for normal growth and must be acceptable and satisfying to the child. Individual and changing food plans are essential if the diet is to be adhered to. It is also necessary to account for pre-existing family and cultural traditions. Frequent review by an experienced dietitian is necessary to cope with changing requirements as the child grows. Extra food usually needs to be taken with exercise to prevent hypoglycaemia.

Exercise

Exercise increases the uptake of glucose by the exercising muscles and lowers the blood glucose level. This effect is seen only if the diabetes is in good control and adequate serum levels of insulin are present (exercise undertaken during poor control and with low insulin levels may paradoxically raise the blood glucose levels). To combat the hypoglycaemic effect of exercise, the child should eat extra food, which should contain both rapidly absorbed carbohydrate and more complex carbohydrate for more prolonged absorption. Regular exercise schedules in the older child may be better managed by a small reduction in the preceding insulin dose. Exercise should be encouraged on a regular basis. Exercise does not, per se, improve metabolic control in children, but it may do so indirectly in some individuals by improving wellbeing and self-esteem.

Outpatient management

For most children with diabetes, the initial hospitalisation at diagnosis for stabilisation and education is their only hospital admission. Children who are well may be discharged early and complete the full education programme provided by the diabetes educator and dietitian as an outpatient, provided there are adequate resources for this and no contraindications exist, such as severe parental distress or communication difficulties. Follow up visits are usually every 3 months once the child is stabilised; the following are assessed:

- general wellbeing
- history of hypoglycaemic episodes
- home blood glucose monitoring
- insulin schedule
- food plan
- school progress and absenteeism
- height
- weight
- injection sites
- size of the thyroid gland
- presence of skin infections.

The blood glucose profile is examined in the logbook kept by the patient, or is downloaded from the patient's blood glucose monitor, and the adequacy of the dietary and insulin regimen is assessed. The physician has available several biochemical parameters that indicate the degree of glycaemic control. The glycosylated haemoglobin (also called HbA$_{1C}$ or fast haemoglobin) measures the degree of glycosylation of haemoglobin, while the serum fructosamine measures the extent of non enzymatic glycosylation of serum proteins. These parameters thus give an indication of the glycaemic control over the life span of the red cells (120 days) and the serum proteins (3 weeks). HbA$_{1C}$ levels can be measured in capillary blood within minutes in the outpatient clinic setting, which is ideal. With the combined efforts of the parents, the child and the diabetes management team (physician, dietitian, diabetes educator, social worker and psychologist) most children grow and develop normally, achieve their educational potential and have a satisfying childhood and adolescence.

Long term microvascular and macrovascular complications

These are:
- nephropathy
- retinopathy
- neuropathy
- cardiovascular disease
- peripheral vascular disease.

It is extremely rare for children and adolescents to show clinical signs of these complications, but subclinical signs can be detected, particularly from adolescence onwards. These form the basis of complication screening programmes. It is recommended that, from 5 years duration of type 1 diabetes, the patient has an annual review including:

- measurement of resting blood pressure
- assessment of urinary albumin excretion, either by an overnight urine collection or an early morning sample
- fundoscopy on dilated pupils by an ophthalmologist.

Serum lipids also are relevant, particularly when there is a family history of a lipid disorder or of premature cardiovascular disease. The major risk factors for the development of complications are:
- metabolic control
- duration of type 1 diabetes
- smoking
- hypertension.

The patient can be encouraged that any improvement in their metabolic control, even if it is still not ideal, will reduce their risk of developing complications.

Special problems in management

Hypoglycaemia

For parents, the occurrence of severe hypoglycaemia in their child (loss of consciousness or a convulsion) is one of the most distressing aspects of diabetes management. Usually no long term harmful effects result from a severe hypoglycaemic episode. However, the concern remains of possible cerebral damage in the very young child, or in the adolescent with a cocktail of other drugs such as alcohol, and the possible development of hypoglycaemic unawareness with recurrent episodes of hypoglycaemia. Minor hypoglycaemic episodes are very frequent and reflect the difficulties in achieving stable control with current insulin delivery regimens, particularly as an improving HbA$_{1c}$ increases the risk of hypoglycaemia. All patients with type 1 diabetes should carry some rapidly absorbable carbohydrate (for example, glucose tablets or jelly beans) for immediate treatment of hypoglycaemic symptoms.

Hypoglycaemia may occur if the insulin dose is excessive, if insufficient food is eaten or if extra exercise is undertaken. Severe hypoglycaemia is most common during the night when the glucose threshold for counterregulatory hormone responses is lower.

The clinical features of hypoglycaemia can be divided into:
- stimulation of the sympathetic nervous system: anxiety, palpitations, tachycardia, pallor, perspiration
- headaches and abdominal pain
- effects on the central nervous system: lethargy, dizziness, ataxia, weakness, confusion, personality changes, visual disturbance, unconsciousness, localised and generalised convulsions.

These clinical features appear rapidly in a previously well child, and there is no difficulty in differentiating hypoglycaemic coma from the coma of diabetic ketoacidosis.

The emergency treatment for the unconscious hypoglycaemic child is to lie him or her on their side and check the airway. Oral fluids must not be given. Intramuscular or subcutaneous glucagon (0.5 mg for children under 5 years of age and 1 mg for older children and adults) or intravenous glucose (2.5 ml of 20% dextrose per kilogram of body weight) is administered. All families with a diabetic child should have glucagon at home and should be able to give it intramuscularly or subcutaneously; absorption is rapid by either route. The response to therapy is seen within minutes. For the less severely affected child, so called mild hypoglycaemia can be treated with oral glucose, for example, half a glass of sugar containing non diet lemonade or jelly beans. On improvement after the emergency treatment, the child should receive some food containing complex carbohydrate to ensure that the glucose levels are maintained.

Management of sick days

Children with well controlled diabetes are no more prone to infections than the non diabetic child. When these occur, however, special problems arise. The stress of the infection, especially if associated with fever, causes a temporary insulin resistance and more insulin is required. Blood glucose tends to rise despite a poor oral intake. Ketonuria may occur. This is a sign of significant insulin deficiency allowing fat to be broken down and converted into ketoacids. If untreated, diabetic ketoacidosis could develop. Parents are taught to measure blood glucose levels frequently, monitor the presence of ketonuria (with reagent strips) and give frequent small doses (10–20% of daily requirements) of short acting insulin every 3–4 hours until the diabetes is stabilised again. Generally regular phone contact with the diabetes consultant or educator will keep the child out of hospital, except when vomiting and ketosis complicates home management.

Growth and delayed puberty

Because insulin is the principal hormone of energy storage and anabolism, growth disturbances occur if diabetes control is poor. The Mauriac syndrome is an extreme example of this, with short stature and hepatic enlargement due to fatty infiltration of the liver. The growth of a diabetic child should be charted on a growth chart at each clinic visit. Similarly, chronic poor control delays entry into puberty. The possibility of Hashimoto thyroiditis, coeliac disease or, less commonly, adrenal insufficiency should also be considered because of their association with type 1 diabetes : many clinics routinely screen for thyroid function and coeliac disease.

Psychological stresses

Major problems arise with diabetic control in the presence of psychological stresses. Easily identifiable acute stresses such as school examinations usually do not cause significant problems. However, family conflicts, parental separation, teenage rebellion and other emotional problems may cause a more profound instability and psychological counselling or formal psychotherapy may be required for the child and the whole family.

The relevance of psychological well being to good diabetes control is of such importance that the social worker or psychologist is an integral part of the management team. Most units also have patient and parent support groups. Diabetes camps may also nurture self-esteem and confidence.

Adherence

Excellent diabetes control in childhood and adolescence is difficult in the best of circumstances. It becomes impossible when the child or the family become non compliant with diet, monitoring or injections of insulin. Refusal to perform blood tests and to conform to the prescribed diet are not unusual periodically and represent a normal rebellion against the never ending discipline that characterises diabetes management. The commonest cause of recurrent diabetic ketoacidosis and chronic poor metabolic control in adolescence is insulin omission. Patience and counselling are necessary, especially in adolescence, when normal risk taking behaviour and growing independence do not combine well with diabetes. The adolescent and family should not be made to feel guilty when diabetes control is less than ideal. It is often useful for the doctor to consider how well she or he would have coped with the diabetes regimen during adolescence.

Clinical example

Jane, a 12 year old girl with a 5 year history of diabetes, has had three episodes of diabetic ketoacidosis in 3 months. Her blood glucose logbook showed all the values to be 4–8 mmol/l but a glycosylated haemoglobin level (HbA_{1C}) was 11.1% (normal range 4–6%). Her insulin dose was 0.9 units/kg/day and it was apparent that the blood glucose levels were spurious. Admission to hospital for stabilisation confirmed elevated blood glucose levels. Management included appropriate increases in the insulin dose, education and counselling. The diabetic ketoacidosis did not recur.

Sometimes it is necessary for someone else (for example, the parents or a community nurse) to temporarily take over responsibility for the insulin injection when there is a serious problem with insulin omission.

Factors limiting management

- Family functioning.
- Hypoglycaemia.
- Adherence and psychological stresses (particularly in adolescence).

Future directions

Families frequently ask about research advances and it is important that they have access to up to date information through regular seminars and reliable web sites. New synthetic insulin analogues provide a better range of very short, short, intermediate and long acting insulins. Inhaled insulin is under investigation. Specific immunotherapy of the autoimmune process is being trialed in subjects with preclinical diabetes in an attempt to prevent or postpone diabetes. The early introduction of angiotensin converting enzyme inhibitors, in patients with persistent microalbuminuria before blood pressure rises, delays the onset of chronic renal failure. Novel approaches to preventing complications include targeting the intracellular mechanisms by which glucose is toxic, for example, inhibitors of protein kinase C and agents that interfere with the accumulation of advanced glycation end products. Transplantation of isolated islets of Langerhans in adults has shown recent promise with new and less beta cell toxic immunosuppressive drugs. Transplantation of the whole pancreas is being undertaken successfully in conjunction with renal transplantation. Prevention of rejection of the transplant requires lifelong immunosuppression and donors of the pancreatic graft are not plentiful. However, research is addressing pig islets for transplantation and the possibility of genetically engineering cells such as hepatocytes to produce insulin.

Type 2 diabetes

The true incidence of type 2 diabetes is not known, as, unlike type 1 diabetes, patients maybe asymptomatic. Characteristics of type 2 diabetes at diagnosis are shown in Table 66.2.

The distinction between type 1 and type 2 diabetes in childhood may be difficult to make on clinical grounds alone (for example, many children with type 1 diabetes are overweight and have a family history of type 2 diabetes). Therefore measurement of C peptide (a measure of endogenous insulin) and islet antibodies is usually necessary to confirm the diagnosis. The distinction is important, as patients with type 2 diabetes are treated with a weight reducing diabetes diet and oral hypoglycaemics as first line measures. Insulin may still be required, especially during intercurrent acute infections when ketoacidosis can occur. Screening for microvascular and macrovascular complications should begin from the time of diagnosis in type 2 diabetes. There is an association between hyperandrogenism in adolescence and type 2 diabetes.

Table 66.2 Characteristics of type 2 diabetes at diagnosis

- Obesity
- Acanthosis nigricans
- Family history of type 2 diabetes
- Absence of ketosis (although ketosis and ketoacidosis can occur in type 2 diabetes in childhood)
- Raised C peptide/insulin levels
- Absence of islet antibodies
- Microvascular complications, hypertension and lipid abnormalities may be present
- Hyperandrogenism maybe present
- More common in Aboriginal and Polynesian populations

Bone mineral disorders

C. Jones

Hypocalcaemia, rickets and hypercalcaemia are the most common manifestation of disorders of calcium, phosphate and vitamin D metabolism. Disorders of magnesium metabolism are rare but share many features of calcium disorders.

Calcium, magnesium and phosphorus (Table 67.1)

Calcium and phosphate form the major structural components of bone in the form of hydroxyapatite. The majority of magnesium is also found in bones. A large proportion of each mineral in bone is freely exchangeable with the extracellular fluid (ECF). Calcium and phosphate ions, under normal circumstances, are present in supersaturated solution. A rise in phosphate will lead to the deposition of more calcium phosphate into bone as hydroxyapatite and cause hypocalcaemia. The distribution of calcium and phosphate between bone and the ECF is determined by hormonal regulation of the concentrations of these minerals. The most important hormones are 1,25-dihydroxyvitamin D_3 (activated vitamin D) and parathyroid hormone (PTH). The actions of these hormones are summarised in Figure 67.1.

The ionised ECF forms of calcium and magnesium are responsible for physiological effect. The ionised form of calcium should be measured to confirm that abnormalities in concentration are present because the equilibrium between the ionised and protein bound forms can change. For instance, an increase of 0.1 pH unit decreases the

Table 67.1   Distribution, serum concentrations, dietary requirements and sources of calcium, magnesium and phosphate

	Calcium	Magnesium	Phosphorus
Body distribution (%)			
Bone[1]	99	60	80
Intracellular	—	40	20
Serum status (%)			
Ionised[2]	46	55	85
Complexed	14	25	5
Protein bound	40	20	10
Serum levels (mmol/l)			
Cord blood[3]	2.4	0.7	1.6
Neonatal	2.1–2.7	0.75–1.1	2.0–3.3
Adult	2.2–2.6	0.75–1.1	1.0–1.3[4]
Dietary intake RDI[5] (mg/day)			
0.6 months	300	40	150
6–12 months	550	60	300
1–10 years	800	100	800
11–18 years	1200	200	1200
Milk content (mg/l)			
Human	300–500	40	100–300
Cow	1500	130	1000
Other food sources	Tinned fish, dairy products	Green vegetables, seeds, nuts	Meats, dairy products

RDI, recommended dietary intake.
[1]Ionic exchange occurs readily between extracellular fluid (ECF) and bone, enabling ECF concentrations to be kept fairly constant.
[2]The ionised form of phosphorus at pH 7.4 is HPO_4^{2-} (70%) and $H_2PO_4^-$ (20%).
[3]Cord blood concentrations are higher than maternal blood concentrations, indicating active transport mechanisms are involved in transplacental transfer. Parathyroid hormone related peptide (PTHRP) is probably involved in these processes.
[4]Levels of phosphate slowly decline during childhood and reach adult levels on completion of bone growth.

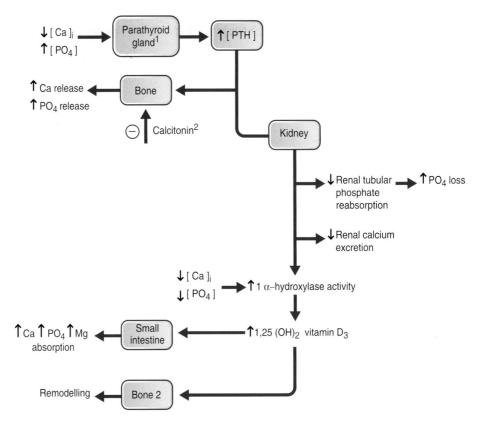

1. Calcium sensitive receptors on the parathyroid cells lead to PTH production increasing with a rise and decreasing with a fall in ionized calcium concentrations.

2. Calcitonin is a hormone produced in the medullary (parafollicular) cells of the thyroid gland in response to an increase in calcium concentrations. It inhibits reabsorption of bone.

Fig. 67.1 Hormonal control of calcium, magnesium and phosphate.

ionised calcium by 10%. Hypoalbuminaemia reduces total serum calcium but not the ionised calcium concentration because 90% of bound calcium is bound to albumin.

> ### Clinical example
>
> Kylie, a 6 year old girl, has nephritis with a metabolic acidosis (pH 7.32, [HCO3⁻] = 15 mmol/l, P_{CO_2} 30 mmHg). She has an albumin of 20 g/l, the serum total $[Ca^{2+}]$ = 1.0 mmol/l and serum [phosphate] = 3.6 mmol/l. Is it safe to correct the acidosis with i.v. NaHCO₃? From Table 67.1, if the serum albumin was normal, 46% of the total serum Ca^{2+} would be ionised. However, the serum albumin concentration is reduced by 50%, thus the amount of calcium bound to albumin will be reduced by 50% (the proportion of total calcium bound to albumin will be reduced to approximately 20%), leaving the ionised proportion of total serum calcium increased from the normal 46% to approximately 66% = 0.66 mmol/l. Increasing the pH to 7.4 could reduce the ionised portion and precipitate overt symptoms of hypocalcaemia. Thus, the calcium concentration should be corrected before giving NaHCO₃.

Hypocalcaemia

In the neonatal period hypocalcaemia is a total serum calcium concentration below 1.8 mmol/l (ionised calcium 1.0 mmol/l). Beyond this age, a total plasma calcium below 2.1 mmol/l (ionised calcium 1.2 mmol/l) constitutes hypocalcaemia. Clinical signs usually only occur with total serum calcium below 2 mmol/l (ionised calcium 0.75 mmol/l), although some patients will tolerate much lower levels and remain asymptomatic. The signs of hypocalcaemia are due to neuromuscular excitability. Jitteriness, apnoea, laryngeal spasm and convulsions are frequent in infants. Tetany, carpopedal spasm and the Chovstek and Trousseau signs are seen mainly in older children. Intracerebral calcification and cataracts are complications.

Patients who have hypocalcaemic symptoms that are not the result of hyperphosphataemia should be treated with intravenous calcium. A dose of 12 mmol/m² over a period of 3 hours can be given, and can be expected to increase the serum calcium by 0.5–1 mmol/l. Serum magnesium should also be checked, as hypomagnesaemia may lead to a refractory type of hypocalcaemia.

The causes of hypocalcaemia are listed in Table 67.2.

Early neonatal hypocalcaemia is common in premature infants and infants of diabetic mothers. In premature infants it is possibly due to interruption of the maternofetal calcium transfer; the signs are seen within hours of birth, become most severe about 48 hours after birth and then improve spontaneously. It can be aggravated by early phosphate-rich formula feeding or hypoxic–ischaemic injury.

Late neonatal hypocalcaemia usually presents as tetany after the first few days of life. The main cause is transient hypoparathyroidism, as demonstrated by high plasma phosphate and low serum PTH concentrations in the face of hypocalcaemia. Treatment may involve a calcium infusion, calcitriol, oral calcium supplementation and a low phosphate formula. The infant can be weaned from this treatment after a few weeks. Persistence of the hypocalcaemia beyond this time should prompt a search for other causes of hypoparathyroidism such as DiGeorge syndrome (aplasia of the parathyroids, thymic aplasia with T cell immunodeficiency and cardiovascular abnormalities), hypomagnesaemia or idiopathic congenital hypoparathyroidism. An abnormality of the calcium sensing receptor on the parathyroid cells (an activating mutation decreasing PTH release) is also a cause. Treatment is based on the use of calcitriol, often in combination with phosphate restriction.

Late onset hypoparathyroidism may occur with destructive injury of the parathyroids (copper deposition in Wilson disease, iron deposition in haemosiderosis) or autoimmune type I polyglandular syndrome). In this latter condition, children, usually girls, present with tetany or convulsions and may have candidiasis and adrenal insufficiency, or other autoimmune disorders such as alopecia, malabsorption, thyroiditis and diabetes. Pseudohypoparathyroidism is due to end organ resistance to PTH and blood levels of PTH are high. Mental deficiency and skeletal abnormalities (particularly a short fourth metacarpal) may be associated. Treatment is the same for hypoparathyroidism.

Hyperphosphataemia can cause hypocalcaemia acutely (as seen in tumour lysis syndrome, where cell death following the initiation of chemotherapy for bulky tumours results in the release of phosphate). Acute renal failure with retention of phosphate is associated with hypocalcaemia. The primary treatment in these conditions is to reduce serum phosphate concentrations through dietary restriction of phosphate, the use of phosphate binders (such as calcium carbonate) and dialysis. Rickets due to vitamin D deficiency or disorders of vitamin D metabolism can cause hypocalcaemia (see below)

Clinical example

Kylie has hypocalcaemia associated with a raised serum phosphate. How should the hypocalcaemia be managed? The administration of intravenous calcium would result in metastatic deposition of calcium phosphate, as the solubility product of calcium phosphate, was exceeded. The calcification would occur in blood vessels and soft tissues. Such an approach might, in fact, be necessary if Kylie had symptomatic hypocalcaemia (convulsions) but it would be preferable to lower the serum phosphate first. This can be achieved by implementing a low phosphate diet, administering oral phosphate binders (such as calcium carbonate), which bind the phosphate in the gut (the calcium complexes the phosphate). It would be uncommon to use dialysis or haemofiltration, but these treatments would also lower serum phosphate concentrations.

Table 67.2   Causes of hypocalcaemia

- Pseudohypocalcaemia
    Hypoalbuminaemia

- Vitamin D associated
    Nutritional deficiency
    Disorders of vitamin D metabolism
- Parathyroid hormone associated
    Hypoparathyroidism
      idiopathic
      transient neonatal
      autoimmune polyglandular disease
      calcium sensing receptor activating mutations or
        antibodies
      hypomagnesaemia
      destructive lesions of the glands
      hypoplasia — DiGeorge syndrome
    PTH receptor defect — pseudohypoparathyroidism

- Hyperphosphataemia
    Tumour lysis
    Renal failure

- Pancreatitis

- Medical treatment associated
    Large blood transfusion/exchange transfusion

Rickets

Rickets is impaired mineralisation of osteoid tissue in the growing child. The mineralisation defect affects the epiphysial growth plates, where cartilage cells proliferate, and unmineralised osteoid tissue accumulates, resulting in widening metaphyses, weak bones and development of deformity, particularly in the weight bearing bones. In established bones there is continued bone resorption but failure of mineralisation results in soft, rarefied bones (this is osteomalacia, which is the same disease as rickets, in the adult).

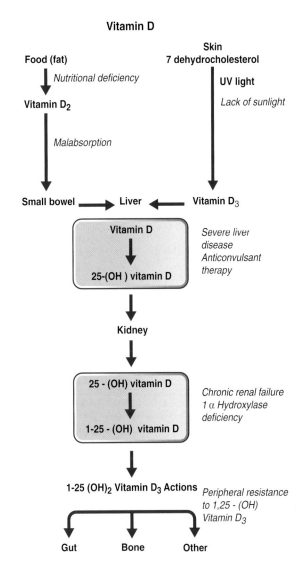

Fig. 67.2 Vitamin D metabolism and rickets.

pigmented skin combined with a range of social factors, including poor housing, lack of adequate infant welfare services for non English speaking migrants and unusual feeding patterns, have combined to make rickets more prevalent.

Malabsorption associated with gastrointestinal, hepatic or pancreatic disease can cause vitamin D deficiency. In approximately 50% of cases hypocalcaemia is present at the time of diagnosis. Severe liver disease and prolonged use of anticonvulsant therapy with diphenylhydantoin or phenobarbitone (through an increased hepatic turnover of vitamin D) can cause rickets.

1α-Hydroxylase deficiency (type 1 vitamin D dependent rickets, characterised by normal or high 25-dihydroxy-vitamin D_3 levels and low 1,25-dihydroxyvitamin D_3 levels) and peripheral resistance to 1,25-dihydroxyvitamin D_3 (type II vitamin D dependent rickets, characterised by high concentrations of 1,25-dihydroxyvitamin D_3) present as severe hypocalcaemic vitamin D deficiency that fails to respond to treatment with vitamin D.

The clinical features of these forms of rickets are quite variable: young children may present with tetany and convulsions; older children incidentally when a chest X ray is performed for an intercurrent chest infection. Early signs in nutritional rickets include weakness of the outer table of the skull (craniotabes), thickening of the costochondral junctions (the 'rachitic rosary') and widening of the wrists and ankles. Later, asymmetry of the head with delayed closure of the arterior fontanelle, frontal and occipital bossing of the skull, development of a Harrison groove, scoliosis and lumbar lordosis, delayed dentition and bowing and bending of the legs develop. Muscular weakness, ligament laxity and fractures are common.

The radiology of the ends of long bones is characteristic, showing widening of the space between metaphysis and epiphysis (Fig. 67.3). The metaphyseal ends of the long bones are widened and appear cupped and frayed. The biochemical changes are a normal or a low serum calcium, a low serum phosphate, a high serum alkaline phosphatase and a high PTH.

Treatment of nutritional vitamin D deficiency is with oral vitamin D at a dose of 3000–5000 units per day for 6 weeks. Radiological improvement is usually apparent within 4 weeks. Some cases are refractory and require longer treatment periods. If there is no response then tests for 1α-hydroxylase deficiency, peripheral resistance to 1,25-dihydroxyvitamin D_3 or hypophosphataemic rickets should be undertaken.

Hypophosphataemic rickets

X-linked dominant hypophosphataemic (vitamin D resistant) rickets is caused by failure of phosphate reabsorption in the renal tubule and lack of an appropriate increase in 1α-hydroxylase activity (low phosphate

Causes of rickets are deficiency of the effect of vitamin D and phosphate depletion. Figure 67.2 outlines the causes of vitamin D deficiency and abnormal metabolism of vitamin D in relation to the physiological production of the active product, 1,25-dihydroxyvitamin D_3.

The recommended dietary intake of vitamin D is 400 international units per day. With exposure to a small amount of afternoon sunlight, vitamin D supplementation is unnecessary. Breast milk contains 20–50 IU/l, yet rickets is uncommon in breastfed infants in the first year of life, provided the mother does not have osteomalacia. Most commercial milk formulas have 400 IU/l of vitamin D.

In the last 20 years, the incidence of vitamin D deficiency has increased in Australia. This increase has been seen in the children of migrants from the Middle East, southern Europe and Asia, especially where the mother wears a hejab. Reduced sunlight and darkly

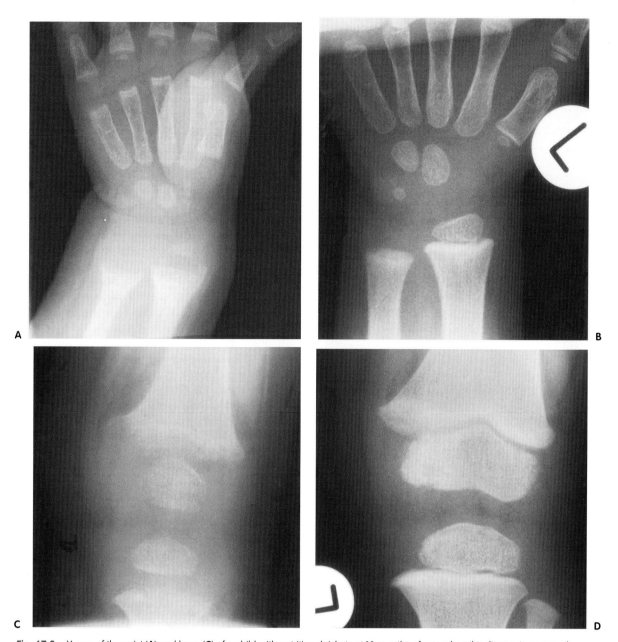

Fig. 67.3 X rays of the wrist (**A**) and knee (**C**) of a child with nutritional rickets at 18 months of age when the diagnosis was made, and 8 months later (**B, D**) after treatment was finished.

concentrations normally increase the activity of this enzyme, which produces 1,25-dihydroxyvitamin D_3). In 50% of cases it is familial; the rest of the cases are due to new mutations. Clinically, the rickets affects the lower limbs predominantly, and investigations show the calcium and PTH concentrations are normal, while the phosphate concentration is quite low. Males are more severely affected than females. Treatment consists of dietary phosphate supplementation and calcitriol.

Chronic phosphate deficiency (e.g. renal Fanconi syndrome, dietary phosphate deficiency) from any cause will result in rickets.

Renal osteodystrophy

This condition predictably occurs when the glomerular filtration rate in chronic renal failure decreases to less than 25% of normal. It occurs as a result of a combination of events, including an increase in plasma phosphate and decreased 1α-hydroxylation of 25-hydroxyvitamin D_3 in the kidney, leading to a fall in 1,25-dihydroxyvitamin D_3 production. This leads to hypocalcaemia and an increase in PTH. The combination of rickets and secondary hyperparathyroidism can result in gross skeletal deformation. Treatment consists of a graded range of measures beginning with dietary phosphate restriction, use of phosphate binders (calcium carbonate) and addition of calcitriol.

Hypercalcaemia

Hypercalcaemia is a total serum calcium above 2.7 mmol/l (ionised calcium >1.3 mmol/l). Symptoms of hypercalcaemia include nausea and vomiting, polyuria and polydipsia, hypertension and failure to thrive. Hypercalciuria may cause nephrocalcinosis and urinary calculi.

A list of causes of hypercalcaemia is given in Table 67.3. Most of these are rare. Primary hyperparathyroidism occurs with some frequency in the second decade of life and is due to hyperplasia or adenoma of the parathyroid glands. It may occur as part of the multiple endocrine neoplasia syndromes (type I hyperparathyroidism associated with prolactinoma or gastrinoma; type II with hyperfunction of the adrenal, parathyroid and medullary cells of the thyroid). Investigations reveal high PTH concentrations, and X ray appearances include subperiosteal resorption of bone (particularly the phalanges), 'salt and pepper' appearance of the cranium and cyst formation in long bones. Treatment of symptomatic disease usually involves subtotal parathyroidectomy.

Familial hypocalciuric hypercalcaemia is an autosomal dominant and usually asymptomatic condition caused by an inactivating mutation of the parathyroid calcium sensing receptor.

Idiopathic hypercalcaemia of infancy is a condition in which there is increased absorption of dietary calcium. The condition usually resolves by the end of the first year of life. Occasionally it is associated with cardiovascular abnormalities (supravalvular aortic stenosis) and dysmorphic facial features (Williams syndrome). The genetic defect for Williams syndrome involves the elastin gene and many cases can be diagnosed using fluorescent in situ hybridisation (FISH) studies.

Treatment is directed at the cause of the hypercalcaemia. Severe symptoms may necessitate initiation of a diuresis using sodium chloride infusion, dietary phosphate supplements to bind calcium, glucocorticoids to reduce intestinal calcium absorption, and bisphosphonates to prevent calcium release from bone. A low calcium milk formula is used to treat idiopathic hypercalcaemia of infancy.

Hypercalciuria

The normal upper limit of urinary calcium excretion is 0.15 mmol/kg/day or <0.7 mmol per mmol creatinine. Hypercalcaemia usually causes hypercalciuria (Table 67.3), with the notable exception of familial hypocalciuric hypercalcaemia. Normocalcaemic hypercalciuria is caused by frusemide or corticosteroid therapy, immobilisation of limb fractures, distal renal tubular acidosis and some rare syndromes.

Idiopathic hypercalciuria is common and appears to be an autosomal dominant condition with incomplete penetrance. On a calcium rich or calcium sufficient diet there is intestinal hyperabsorption of calcium and the PTH and 1,25-dihydroxyvitamin D concentrations are normal. On a lower calcium diet, 'renal' loss of calcium occurs and higher levels of PTH and 1,25-dihydroxyvitamin D are found. Excessive bone resorption occurs in some patients and can cause osteoporosis. Thus, the therapeutic safety of a low calcium diet is limited because of the risks of development of osteoporosis. Hypercalciuria can cause nephrocalcinosis (Fig. 67.4) and urinary calculi. Where treatment is necessary, thiazide diuretics have proven useful.

Osteoporosis

Osteoporosis is decreased mineral content of the skeleton. Measurement of bone mineral density has improved over the last decade with the use of dual energy X ray absorptiometry (DEXA). However, DEXA must be carefully interpreted with regard to the size of the bone where measurements are taken and the age of the patient, especially with regard to pubertal development of the child. Osteoporosis is only apparent radiologically when approximately half of the bone mineral content has been lost. Causes of osteoporosis are given in Table 67.4.

Idiopathic juvenile osteoporosis is a rare condition that occurs in mid childhood with gross demineralisation

---

Table 67.3 Causes of hypercalcaemia

- Vitamin D excess
  - Iatrogenic
  - Ectopic production — sarcoidosis, tuberculosis, lymphoma

- Parathyroid hormone excess
  - Primary hyperparathyroidism
    - multiple endocrine neoplasia (MEN) syndromes
  - Familial hypocalciuric hypercalcaemia
  - Abnormalities related to PTH receptor or PTH related peptide (PTHRP)

- Idiopathic hypercalcaemia of infancy
  - Williams syndrome

- Other
  - Bone disease, trauma and immobilisation
  - Thyrotoxicosis and hypothyroidism
  - Neonatal fat necrosis

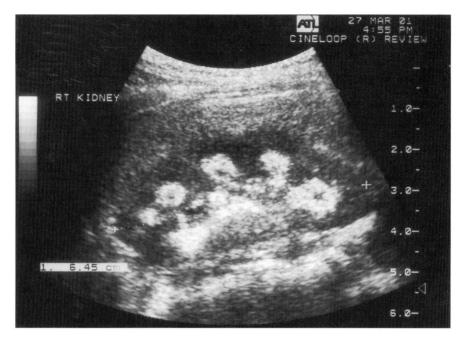

Fig. 67.4 Renal ultrasound showing nephrocalcinosis of the medullary pyramids in a 4 year old child with idiopathic nephrocalcinosis.

Table 67.4   Causes of osteoporosis

- Calcium deficiency
    Nutritional
    Malabsorption

- Malignancy
    Leukaemia

- Glucocorticoid excess
    Iatrogenic
    Cushing disease

- Homocystinuria

- Osteogenesis imperfecta

- Immobilisation

- Idiopathic juvenile osteoporosis (neonatal form)

of the skeleton that can result in extensive fractures (particularly vertebral crush fractures). The disease remits spontaneously with the onset of puberty.

Osteopetrosis

Osteopetrosis is a rare familial disorder of the skeleton in which there is a defect in bone and cartilage resorption and hence of bone remodelling. This leads to a dense but brittle type of bone, which fractures easily. Infants usually present early in life with a severe leuco-erythroblastic anaemia, symptoms of compression of cranial nerves (particularly optic atrophy leading to blindness) and marked hepatosplenomegaly. The bones show a characteristic dense and poorly modelled X ray appearance.

Magnesium disorders

Causes of hypomagnesaemia are given in Table 67.5. The symptoms of hypomagnesaemia resemble those of hypocalcaemia, with increased neuromuscular irritability. Severe hypomagnesaemia interferes with the release of PTH and consequently hypomagnesaemia and hypocalcaemia often coexist.

Hypermagnesaemia occurs rarely in the absence of renal failure. The exception is the neonate born prematurely to a mother given magnesium sulphate for pre-eclampsia.

Table 67.5   Causes of hypomagnesaemia and hypermagnesaemia

Hypomagnesaemia
Malabsorption, prolonged intravenous therapy
Diuretic therapy
Renal tubular acidosis
Hereditary disorders of renal tubular reabsorption

Hypermagnesaemia
Neonate of mother given $MgSO_4$ for pre-eclampsia
Medications containing magnesium given to patients with
    renal failure

Questions

1. **A 14 year old boy is being teased because he appears to be growing poorly and all the other boys are overtaking him. He has always been at the small end of the class for height, but this has become worse over the last 18 months. He is completely well and has had no significant past illnesses. His older brother and father had a similar experience. The general practitioner assesses him and finds that his height is on the 3rd percentile and that he is prepubertal. His current height is on the 50th percentile for a 10 year old and his bone age is 10.5 years.**
   (A) The most likely diagnosis is constitutional delay of growth and puberty
   (B) Prognosis for his final height is consistent with the midparental height expectation
   (C) Hormonal treatment in this condition is never appropriate as this is a variation of normal growth
   (D) This condition occurs more often in girls than boys
   (E) Reassurance of normality and pubertal induction with testosterone may be the treatment of choice

2. **In pubertal gynaecomastia:**
   (A) Most breast development is minor, transient and regresses
   (B) Hormone treatment to reverse the breast development is effective
   (C) Breast development is always symmetrical
   (D) Subareolar mastectomy is frequently required
   (E) Exclusion of underlying endocrine abnormality is required in all cases

3. **In premature thelarche:**
   (A) Unilateral breast development may occur
   (B) There is no associated growth spurt
   (C) Pubic and axillary hair development is frequently present
   (D) Extensive endocrine investigation must always be performed
   (E) There is an increased risk of breast malignancy in later life

4. **In delayed puberty:**
   (A) The most common causes are familial delayed puberty and constitutional delay of growth and puberty
   (B) Chronic illness and treatments for the illness may delay pubertal development

(C) Bone age is usually delayed, indicating that growth potential is available
   (D) Hormone treatment should not be given as this will definitely reduce final height potential
   (E) Girls usually have more psychological distress from delayed puberty than boys

5. **True or false? Congenital hypothyroidism:**
   (A) Has an incidence of around 1 in 3500 live births
   (B) Is usually due to thyroid enzyme defects (dyshormonogenesis)
   (C) Will usually lead to permanent brain damage if untreated by age 2–3 months
   (D) Is usually diagnosed by amniocentesis
   (E) May be diagnosed in the absence of obvious signs

6. **True or false? Acquired hypothyroidism in childhood:**
   (A) Is usually due to iodine deficiency
   (B) Is often associated with thyroid autoantibodies
   (C) Leads to delayed bone growth and maturation
   (D) Has a poor prognosis for intellectual function
   (E) Is treated with 50–100 µg thyroxine daily

7. **True or false? Goitres in childhood and adolescence:**
   (A) Are usually associated with malignancy
   (B) Are often due to Hashimoto thyroiditis
   (C) May be associated with hyperthyroidism
   (D) Will require biopsy if associated with isolated nodules
   (E) Are more common in boys

8. **True or false? Thyrotoxicosis in childhood and adolescence:**
   (A) Is usually due to a solitary hot nodule
   (B) May present with choreiform movements and anxiety symptoms
   (C) Is an autoantibody disorder
   (D) Is best treated with antithyroid drugs
   (E) Remits in less than 10% of cases

9. **A newborn was found to have a small phallus with a marked chordee and a single opening at the base. There are no gonads palpable in the scrotum. Which is the first differential diagnosis to be considered?**
   (A) True hermaphroditism
   (B) Pure gonadal dysgenesis
   (C) Congenital adrenal hyperplasia
   (D) Turner syndrome
   (E) Androgen insensitivity syndrome

10. Which of the following disorders causing genital abnormalities are inherited as an autosomal recessive trait?
(A) Congenital adrenal hyperplasia due to a 21-hydroxylase deficiency
(B) Partial androgen insensitivity
(C) Klinefelter syndrome
(D) Mixed gonadal dysgenesis
(E) 5α-reductase deficiency

11. Which of the following disorders causing abnormal sexual differentiation are associated with infertility?
(A) Complete androgen insensitivity
(B) True hermaphroditism
(C) Congenital adrenal hyerplasia due to a 21-hydroxylase defect
(D) Gonadal dysgenesis
(E) Turner syndrome

12. In pure gonadal dysgenesis, the following is true:
(A) The gonads are usually palpable in the inguinal canal
(B) The external phenotype is female
(C) Internal genitalia are male
(D) Short stature is common
(E) Female fertility can be achieved

13. A child of 8 years has glycosuria without ketonuria during an acute asthmatic attack. Random blood glucose levels are 14 mmol/1 and 9 mmol/1. The following are useful investigations:
(A) Further random (fasting and postprandial) blood glucose levels
(B) Oral glucose tolerance test
(C) Pancreatic islet cell autoantibodies
(D) HLA typing
(E) HbA$_{1C}$ level

14. In insulin dependent diabetes mellitus (IDDM):
(A) Children who are recently diagnosed may have increased insulin needs or even become insulin dependent for a period of time after initial diagnosis and initial insulin therapy
(B) Insulin requirements decrease at the time of puberty
(C) Most children will require insulin at least twice daily
(D) An illness with fever and anorexia will lead to a decrease in insulin requirements
(E) There is a strong family association with adult onset diabetes

15. During adolescence:
(A) Insulin omission is the major cause of diabetic ketoacidosis
(B) Requirements of insulin remain at 1.0 unit/kg/day
(C) Subclinical diabetic complications are seen frequently
(D) Severe hypoglycaemia is more common than in adult life
(E) HbAlc levels frequently rise

16. In a 6 month old child with recurrent hypoglycaemic convulsions occurring in the early hours of the morning, which of the following statements apply?
(A) The most diagnostic blood sample is the one collected at the time of hypoglycaemia
(B) If nesidioblastosis is found to be the cause, then 95% pancreatectomy may be necessary
(C) Growth hormone and cortisol deficiency can be excluded on the history
(D) Hypoglycaemia is defined as a blood glucose of less than 2.2 mmol/1

17. Adam, a 6 year old boy recently diagnosed with Burkitt lymphoma, has had induction chemotherapy. The next day he is noted to be twitchy. Investigations show a total serum calcium of 1.2 mmol/l, phosphorus of 3.8 mmol/l and a serum albumin of 32 g/l. What would you do?
(A) Ignore the serum calcium because the result is due to a low serum albumin
(B) Give intravenous calcium to prevent Adam having a convulsion
(C) Measure Adam's renal function tests and uric acid and prepare for dialysis
(D) Administer oral calcium carbonate
(E) Ensure Adam is on low phosphate diet

Answers and explanations

1. The correct answers are **(A)**, **(B)** and **(C)**. Constitutional delay is a variation of normal growth with a strong familial predisposition. It is a very uncommon problem in girls. The indication for treatment is usually psychological distress caused by the short stature and delayed puberty and associated bullying and exclusion from sporting teams. Even without treatment, normal growth and pubertal development will occur in time, with final height being consistent with midparental height expectations.

2. The only correct answer is **(A)**. Pubertal gynaecomastia is a very common condition in males and usually requires no investigation or specific treatment. It is usually transient and regresses spontaneously over time.

3. The correct answers are **(A)** and **(B)**. Isolated breast development, either unilateral or bilateral, may occur at < 2 years of age or at any time before puberty. No other features of puberty including a growth spurt should be present. After assessment by a paediatrician, investigations may not be necessary. There is no reported increased incidence of malignancy or fertility problems in adult life.

4. The correct answers are **(A)**, **(B)** and **(C)**. Delayed puberty occurs commonly and may be due to familial factors, constitutional delay or chronic illness and associated treatment. Hormone deficiencies causing delayed puberty are uncommon. Bone age is usually delayed and judicious use of sex steroids to induce pubertal development may alleviate psychological distress while maintaining growth potential. This treatment is more often used for boys, as the degree of psychological distress is usually greater in boys than girls.

5. **(A)** True. (B) False. It is usually due to maldevelopment of the thyroid gland. **(C)** True. (D) False. It is diagnosed by neonatal screening. **(E)** True.

6. (A) False. It is usually an autoimmune disorder. **(B)** True. **(C)** True. Thyroid autoantibodies are usually present and bone and growth maturation are delayed. **(D)** True. (E) False.

7. (A) False. **(B)** True. **(C)** True. **(D)** True. (E) False.

8. (A) False. **(B)** True. **(C)** True. **(D)** True. (E) False — the correct answer is 50%.

9. The correct answer is **(C)**. While in (A), (B) and (D) there is also no gonad palpable, congenital adrenal hyperplasia has to be excluded first, as these children are threatened by a salt losing crisis.

10. **(A)** and **(E)** are true. (B) is inherited as an X chromosome linked trait; (D) and (C) are chromosomal disorders and not familial.

11. The correct answers are **(A)** and **(D)**. In true hermaphroditism, congenital adrenal hyperplasia and a certain percentage of patients with Turner syndrome female fertility may be possible.

12. The true answers are **(B)** and **(D)**. The gonads are streaks and attached to the uterus; that is, the internal genitalia are female but the patients are infertile due to streak gonads. Short stature is common in patients with 45,XO gonadal dysgenesis (Turner syndrome) but not in 46,XY gonadal dysgenesis.

13. **(A)** True. (B) False. This is not necessary to make the diagnosis of insulin dependent diabetes. **(C)** True. These will indicate whether the child has an increased risk of diabetes. (D) False. **(E)** True. This will indicate whether high blood glucose levels precede the asthma attack.

14. The correct answer is **(C)**. Insulin requirements often decrease for a period of time after initial presentation in IDDM in childhood (A). This is sometimes called the 'honeymoon period'. However, eventual insulin dependence always occurs, usually within weeks. At puberty there is an increased need for insulin because of rapid growth and increased secretion of growth hormone and sex hormones (B). Insulin is almost always required twice daily for adequate control of IDDM (C). During illness, there is an increased demand for insulin with the increased metabolic demands and there is a relative insulin resistance: illness leads to ketoacidosis and insulin is needed for control (D). Although there are some potential genetic markers for increased risk of IDDM, there are no indications that there is a strong family association with adult onset diabetes (E).

15. **(A)** True. (B) False. Insulin requirements increase to above 1.0 unit/kg/day. (C) False. **(D)** True. **(E)** True.

16. **(A)** True. **(B)** True. (C) False. (D) False.

17. The correct answers are **(C)**, **(D)** and **(E)**. The serum albumin is not low enough to account for the very low calcium concentration, and symptoms consistent with hypocalcaemia are present (A). Administering intravenous calcium will cause metastatic calcification and only transiently increase the serum calcium. It is not indicated in the absence of more severe symptoms (B). The likely cause of the hypocalcaemia and hyperphosphataemia is tumour lysis syndrome. It is likely the uric acid concentration in serum is elevated and that a degree of renal failure is present. It would be appropriate to make sure that dialysis facilities were available if needed (although this would not be usual). Calcium carbonate would decrease further absorption of phosphate from the diet. Similarly a low phosphate diet would help, although these latter measures will take some days to have effect (C), (D) and (E).

PART 19 FURTHER READING

Ahmed S F, Chemg A, Dovey L et al 2000 Phenotypic features, androgen receptor binding, and mutational analysis in 278 clinical cases reported as androgen insensitivity syndrome. Journal of Clinical Endocrinology and Metabolism 85: 658–665

American Academy of Pediatrics 2000 Evaluation of the newborn with developmental anomalies of the external genitalia. Pediatrics 106: 138–142

Anon 2000 Type 2 diabetes in children and adolescents. Diabetes Care 23: 381–389

Argente J 1999 Diagnosis of late puberty. Hormone Research 51: 95–100

Australasian Paediatric Endocrine Group 1996 Handbook on diabetes (Silink M (ed.). Government Printing Service (obtainable via The Children's Hospital, Westmead, Australia)

Cheetham T D, Hughes I A, Barnes N D, Wraight E P 1998 Treatment of hyperthyroidism in young people. Archives of Disease in Childhood 78: 207–209

Dattani M T, Robinson I C 2000 The molecular basis for developmental disorders of the pituitary gland in man. Clinical Genetics 67: 337–346

Eastman C J 1999 Where has all our iodine gone? Medical Journal of Australia 171: 455–456

Fisher D A 2000 The importance of early management in optimizing IQ in infants with congenital hypothyroidism. Journal of Pediatrics 136: 273–274

Francis I 1991 Newborn screening in Australia and New Zealand 1984–1990. Human Genetics Society of Australasia/Australian College of Paediatrics Committee on Newborn Metabolic Screening. Medical Journal of Australia 155: 821–823

Hausler G 1998 Growth hormone therapy in patients with Turner syndrome. Hormone Research 49: 62–66

Havercamp F, Eiholzer U, Ranke M B, Noeker M 2000 Symptomatic versus substitution growth hormone therapy in short children: from auxology towards a comprehensive multi-dimensional assessment of short stature and related interventions. Journal of Pediatric Endocrinology and Metabolism 13: 403–408

Houchin L D, Rogoal A D 1998 Androgen therapy in children with constitutional delay of puberty: the case for aggressive therapy. Baillière's Clinical Endocrinology and Metabolism 12: 427–450

Langman C B 1999 Disorders of phosphorus, calcium, and vitamin D. In: Barratt T M, Avner E D, Harmon W E (eds) Paediatric nephrology. Lippincott, Williams & Wilkins, Baltimore, 529–544

Lerman S E, McAleer I M, Kaplan G W 2000 Sex assignment in cases of ambiguous genitalia and its outcome. Urology 55: 8–12

Ong Y C, Wong H B, Adaikan G, Yong E L 1999 Directed pharmacological therapy of ambiguous genitalia due to an androgen receptor gene mutation. Lancet 354: 1444–1445

Reiner W G 1999 Assignment of sex in neonates with ambiguous genitalia. Current Opinions in Pediatrics 11: 363–365

Rogol A D, Clark P A, Roemmich JN 2000 Growth and pubertal development in children and adolescents: effects of diet and physical activity. American Journal of Clinical Nutrition 72: 521S–528S

Sherman L D 1997 Diagnosis and management of ambiguous genitalia. Indian Journal of Pediatrics 64: 195–203

White P C, Speiser P W 2000 Congenital adrenal hyperplasia due to 21-hydroxylase deficiency. Endocrine Reviews 21: 245–291

Wilson J D 1999 The role of androgens in male gender role behaviour. Endocrine Reviews 20: 726–737

Useful links

http://www.cgf.org.uk/ (Child Growth Foundation)

http://www.cmhc.com/factsfam/puberty.htm (Puberty: general information for families)

http://www.diabetes.org (American Diabetes Association)

http://www.genetic.org/hgf/ (Human Growth Foundation)

http://www.idf.org (International Diabetes Federation)

http://www.isha.org/index.html (Iowa speech–language hearing association)

http://www.jdrf.org (Juvenile Diabetes Research Foundation)

http://www.joslin.org (Joslin Diabetes Center)

http://www.magicfoundation.org.cpp.html (The Magic Foundation: precocious puberty)

http://www.magicfoundation.org/ghd.html (The Magic Foundation: growth)

http://www.nih.gov/nichd/ (National Institutes of Health: relevant pages)

http://www.rch.unimelb.edu.au/CAH (Centre for Adolescent Health)

http://www.rch.unimelb.edu.au/hormone (Centre for Hormone Research)

http://www.rch.unimelb.ede.au/publications/CAIS.html (Booklet on complete androgen insensitivity syndrome)

PART 20

DISORDERS OF THE GASTROINTESTINAL TRACT AND HEPATIC DISORDERS

Abdominal pain and vomiting in children

S. W. Beasley

Acute abdominal pain and vomiting are common symptoms in children, and a frequent reason for children to be taken to the doctor. Their causes are many and diverse; those which require surgery must be distinguished from those with a medical origin. While there is considerable overlap of age in many disorders (for example, gastro-oesophageal reflux), other conditions only occur within a specific age range; for example, pyloric stenosis is not seen after the age of 3 months.

Abdominal pain in the first 3 months of life

Abdominal pain without other symptoms is unusual in early infancy. Severe pain may be accompanied by vomiting, abdominal distension, constipation or other features, in which situation it is more likely to have a surgical cause, for example, malrotation with volvulus.

'Infantile colic' is an extremely common condition that usually commences in the first few weeks of life. The cause is poorly understood. The infant:

- has attacks of screaming
- draws up the legs
- is unable to be comforted.

Vomiting is absent, bowel actions are passed normally, and the infant is otherwise thriving well. There is no evidence of a strangulated inguinal hernia. The colic almost invariably disappears by the fourth month of age; until then, treatment is supportive. In some infants, apparent colic may be due to oesophagitis from gastro-oesophageal reflux or to hunger in inadequately breastfed babies. Crying babies may cause stress in the family, which in turn increases the irritability. In a vulnerable or unstable family situation this may place the infant at risk of abuse.

Abdominal pain later in the first year

The main surgical cause of abdominal pain between 3 and 12 months of age is intussusception. Vomiting is a frequent accompanying feature, such that when the colicky abdominal pain is not pronounced, intussusception must be distinguished from other causes of vomiting in this age group (see below).

Intussusception

In intussusception, the distal ileum (the intussusceptum) telescopes into adjoining distal bowel (the intussuscipiens), resulting in intestinal obstruction. It can occur at any age, but is most likely in the infant between 3 and 18 months who suddenly develops screaming attacks of pain with vomiting. During each episode of pain the infant becomes pale and may draw up the legs.

The spasms of pain tend to last 2–3 minutes and occur at intervals of about 10–20 minutes, although after a while the pain becomes more persistent. Vomiting is an early symptom. The passage of a few loose stools early on represents evacuation of the bowel distal to the obstruction. The small volume and limited duration of loose stools in intussusception helps differentiate it from acute gastroenteritis. Congestion of the intussusceptum may lead to the passage of bloodstained or 'red currant' stools. Many infants with intussusception present with little more than pallor, lethargy and vomiting and may have little evidence of abdominal pain. Should these symptoms be ignored, the infant may progress to develop signs of septicaemia or shock.

The infant with intussusception is pale, lethargic, anxious and unwell. A vague mass may be felt in the right or left upper quadrants of the abdomen, but once abdominal distension has developed, the mass becomes obscure and difficult to palpate. The apex of the intussusceptum may be palpable on rectal examination in a few, and the examining glove may be bloodstained. A plain X ray of the abdomen will often be normal, but may show an unusual bowel gas distribution or features of bowel obstruction. Ultrasound examination may be helpful in making the diagnosis. Where intussusception is suspected clinically, a gas or barium enema must be performed unless the child has peritonitis. The enema will demonstrate the position of the apex of the intussusception.

Treatment

Gas enema reduction is the treatment of choice, and is successful in 80–90% of patients (Fig. 68.1). If gas enema facilities are not available, a barium enema under continuous fluoroscopic control is a less effective but satisfactory alternative. Peritonitis and septicaemia, which suggest the presence of dead bowel, are the only contraindications to attempted enema reduction. A

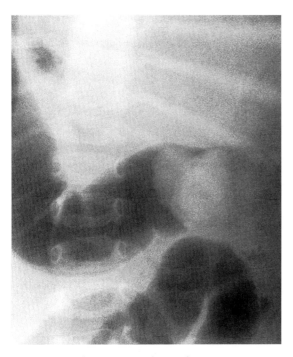

Fig. 68.1 X ray demonstration of apex of intussusception during reduction using a gas enema.

dehydrated child should have intravenous fluid resuscitation and be wrapped in warm blankets before commencing an enema reduction. The success of enema reduction is recognised when there is sudden or rapid flow of gas or barium into the ileum. If partial reduction is achieved, and the child remains in good clinical condition, a further enema should be attempted after several hours (so called 'delayed repeat enema'), and in about half of these patients it will be successful. Recurrence of intussusception occurs in about 9% of children after enema reduction, usually within days. Surgery is reserved for:

- those in whom enema reduction has failed
- those who have clinical evidence of necrotic bowel, such as peritonitis and septicaemia
- those in whom there is evidence of pathological lesions at the lead point.

Differential diagnosis

Gastroenteritis is often confused with intussusception, but becomes obvious on clinical grounds by the volume and persistence of the fluid stools. The plain radiological appearance of the abdomen may be similar in both conditions. Where doubt persists, a gas or barium enema is indicated. Other causes of intestinal obstruction include volvulus secondary to malrotation, a band from a Meckel diverticulum, a duplication cyst or a strangulated inguinal hernia. Examination of the groin will detect the irreducible tender lump of a strangulated hernia.

Acute abdominal pain in older children

Children often present with abdominal pain, and in most no specific cause is found. Constipation and mesenteric adenitis are probably the most common non surgical identifiable causes.

Acute appendicitis

Appendicitis may occur at any age, although it is rare under 5 years of age. Early diagnosis is difficult in the young child (under 5 years) and in the mentally retarded child; the majority of these children have established peritonitis or an appendix abscess at presentation. Delays in the diagnosis of acute appendicitis in childhood is related in part to its variable symptomatology. For example, there may be few complaints of pain, vomiting may be absent, and diarrhoea may be a misleading feature.

Nevertheless, the most important and consistent feature is localised abdominal pain. The pain may be intermittent and colicky initially, or situated in the epigastrium or periumbilical region, but soon shifts to the right iliac fossa. Constant pain which is worse with movement is the result of peritoneal irritation ('peritonism'). Vomiting occurs in the majority of children, and some may pass a loose stool. The temperature is usually normal or slightly elevated, but occasionally may be in excess of 38°C.

Physical examination of the abdomen should be directed at showing that movement of adjacent peritoneal surfaces causes pain. The child's cooperation makes assessment easier, and repeated examination of the abdomen may be required to make the diagnosis. A child with appendicitis usually will exhibit tenderness and guarding localised to the right iliac fossa. Gentle palpation and percussion tenderness, performed while observing the child's face, will provide the most reliable evidence of abdominal tenderness and involuntary guarding. Rebound tenderness is an unreliable sign in children, and attempts to elicit the sign may cause unnecessary pain and destroy the child's confidence in the doctor. Rectal examination is only indicated if a pelvic appendix or pelvic collection is suspected, and should not be performed if examination of the ventral abdominal wall has already enabled a confident diagnosis of acute appendicitis to be made. Bowel sounds may be normal or reduced, and contribute little to the diagnosis.

Peritonitis should be suspected when the child is acutely ill with abdominal pain and fever, and is reluctant to move. On examination, there will be generalised abdominal tenderness and guarding.

Laboratory studies and radiology are rarely helpful in making the diagnosis. However, the urine should be checked routinely.

Differential diagnosis

Mesenteric adenitis is the most difficult disorder to distinguish from acute appendicitis. In general, localisation of pain and tenderness is variable and less specific, and the temperature may be higher. Guarding is rarely present in mesenteric lymphadenitis.

Other conditions that may mimic acute appendicitis are relatively uncommon. Meckel diverticulitis has symptoms identical to those of appendicitis, such that differentiation is possible only at laparotomy. Pain in the right iliac fossa may represent radiation from torsion of the right testis or a strangulated inguinal hernia, and highlights the importance of examination of the genitalia in all boys with lower abdominal symptoms. Acute abdominal pain may occur with renal colic, pyelonephritis, and, at times, in acute glomerulonephritis. Pain and tenderness is usually referred to the loin. Urine analysis and radiology will confirm the diagnosis. In Henoch–Schönlein purpura, the abdominal pain is often severe and colicky, and may be accompanied by vomiting. The characteristic skin lesions over the buttock and legs may be inconspicuous or absent when the child is first examined.

In the appropriate ethnic group, sickle cell anaemia is a prominent cause of acute abdominal pain, and should be considered in a pale child with splenomegaly.

Children with cystic fibrosis frequently experience episodes of abdominal pain from faecal impaction (called 'meconium ileus equivalent'), a well known manifestation of this disease. The symptoms resolve following a bowel washout.

It is unusual for constipation in an otherwise normal child to produce sufficient abdominal pain to suggest a surgical emergency. A plain X ray of the abdomen will demonstrate the extent of faecal accumulation (Fig. 68.2).

Less common causes of abdominal pain include urinary tract infection, haemolytic uraemic syndrome and

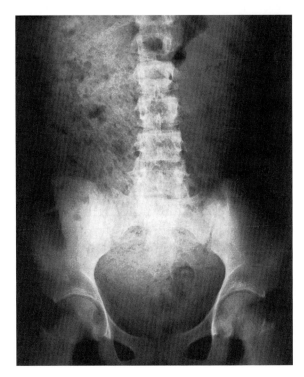

Fig. 68.2 Plain X ray of the abdomen demonstrating gross faecal overload in a child with severe constipation causing abdominal pain. The child also had soiling of his underwear.

diabetes. Acute hepatitis, cholecystitis and pancreatitis, although all rare in childhood, may also cause abdominal pain. In pancreatitis, vomiting is prominent, and epigastric tenderness with guarding may be marked. These children often look ill and obtunded. Pancreatitis may follow a blunt injury to the abdomen, for example a handlebar injury, and later may produce a pancreatic pseudocyst (a pseudocyst becomes apparent weeks after the injury). The diagnosis is suggested by estimation of the plasma or urinary amylase or plasma lipase, and is confirmed with CT. The management of acute pancreatitis involves correction of shock, intravenous fluid administration, nasogastric suction to keep the stomach empty, and analgesia.

Right lower lobe pneumonia may masquerade as appendicitis. The child is usually febrile, with an increased respiratory rate, and has a cough. Signs of pneumonia may be difficult to elicit clinically, so that a chest X ray will be required.

A general summary of disorders associated with abdominal pain is listed in Table 68.1.

Peptic ulceration

The abdominal pain of peptic ulceration is epigastric and usually is unrelated to meals. Nausea and vomiting may occur. Haematemesis and melaena suggest the diagnosis; alternatively it may be made following investigation of iron deficiency anaemia.

Table 68.1 Causes of abdominal pain in childhood

Common
Appendicitis
Mesenteric adenitis
Constipation
Intussusception
Urinary tract infection
Torsion of the testis

Uncommon
Volvulus secondary to malrotation
Meckel diverticulitis
Renal colic
Pyelonephritis
Acute glomerulonephritis
Glandular fever
Drug ingestion
   For example: salicylates, non steroidal anti-inflammatory
   drugs, corticosteroids, some antibiotics, imipramine,
   phenytoin, iron preparations
Peptic ulceration
Reflux oesophagitis

Rare
Sickle cell anaemia
Henoch—Schönlein purpura
Pancreatitis
Cholecystitis
Acute hepatitis
Diabetes mellitus
Haemolytic uraemic syndrome
Inflammatory bowel disease, for example Crohn disease

Acute gastritis and acute duodenitis produce abdominal pain with epigastric tenderness. A positive hydrogen breath test is suggestive of *Helicobacter pylori* infection. Culture of biopsy specimens taken during endoscopic examination of the upper gastrointestinal tract will confirm *H. pylori* (Ch. 71). Treatment with ampicillin, metronidazole or tripotassium dicitrabismuthate (De-Nol) usually is successful, but relapses are common.

Reflux oesophagitis

Gastro-oesophageal reflux is common in infancy but usually resolves with growth. Sometimes it may persist into later childhood, with symptoms of belching, acid eructation and intermittent vomiting. Substernal and epigastric pain suggest reflux oesophagitis. Oesophageal pH monitoring measures lower oesophageal pH over a period of 24 hours and can establish the relationship of reflux to symptoms (Ch. 71). Oesophagoscopy and biopsy confirm oesophagitis. Initial management may involve the administration of H_2 receptor antagonists, but where non operative measures fail, or an oesophageal stricture is present, surgical correction of the reflux by fundoplication may be indicated.

Recurrent abdominal pain in children

A child with recurrent bouts of abdominal pain may cause great anxiety to parents and doctors alike. Many appear to suffer from recurrent bouts of appendicitis, and a few have had an appendicectomy. The clinical example is illustrative of this syndrome.

Clinical example

Thomas, aged 7 years, was brought in by his mother, who stated that for the last 2 months he had had severe bouts of abdominal pain. The attacks occurred at any time, but were more frequent at breakfast time. He was never awakened at night by them. Vomiting was not a feature, and his bowels had been regular. The pain usually was localised to the periumbilical region, and usually lasted less than 1 hour. His parents felt he was pale and had a poor appetite. Clinically, he looked pale and anxious, but was of normal height and weight. Physical examination was otherwise unremarkable. The urine was clear. Further questioning elicited the fact that the bouts of abdominal pain had occurred periodically since the age of 3 years.

Doctors will be impressed by the concern exhibited by parents of these children, who vividly describe the severe pain the child experiences and the degree of pallor; the disparity between the parents' description and the physical findings is marked. Investigation almost invariably produces negative results. Enquiry into the personality of the child and into the home situation may reveal that the child is highly strung, anxious, timid or apprehensive, and has problems with eating; but often episodes may occur for no apparent reason. Sometimes the episode of pain appears to be related to stress within the family. A diagnosis of non organic recurrent abdominal pain can be made only after careful appraisal of the child in relation to the environment, and when physical examination is normal. Further investigation is required when the abdominal pain is associated with abdominal tenderness or distension, bile stained vomiting, persistent diarrhoea, fever, weight loss or urinary symptoms. Investigation may include full blood examination and ESR, radiological and endoscopic studies of the gastrointestinal tract, and specific investigations for malabsorption and inflammatory bowel disease. The urine should be examined. If the vomitus is bile stained, malrotation with volvulus should be excluded by an urgent barium meal.

The general status of the patient must be assessed. Retardation of height and growth may occur in chronic inflammatory bowel disease, malabsorption syndromes and tuberculosis. Pallor may be associated with anaemia, or conditions such as lead poisoning, sickle cell anaemia and other haemolytic diseases.

Management

This is often difficult, but the mere uncovering of the personality of the child and the family situation may be therapeutic. Parents must realise that the problem has been taken seriously by the doctor, and the doctor must understand the parents' perception of the abdominal pain. With this knowledge and the negative physical findings, reassurance can be given more positively. Once parents are convinced that there is no significant organic basis to the recurrent abdominal pain they are usually much relieved. The child should be encouraged in all activities and self-esteem improved. Recurrent pain tends to disappear by the age of 12 years, but in females may recur at the time of menarche. However, some children with recurrent pain in childhood present in adult life with bowel problems and neurotic behaviour.

Vomiting in the neonatal period

Neonates frequently vomit small amounts of mucus and blood swallowed during labour. This vomiting usually clears spontaneously within 24 hours. If not, gastric lavage with normal saline will usually relieve it.

In the early weeks of life, many normal newborn babies regurgitate after feeds. The cause of this 'spitting up' or 'possetting' is not clear, but is presumably related to gastro-oesophageal reflux.

Cerebral hypoxia

There is often a history of fetal distress during labour and asphyxia at birth requiring resuscitation. Following this, some infants remain lethargic and feed poorly, while others may be abnormally wide awake, excessively irritable and cry frequently. The cry may be high pitched and associated with intermittent twitching and hypertonia; there is head retraction and the thumbs are adducted across the palms with flexion of the fingers. The Moro reflex may be exaggerated, but in severe cerebral anoxia it may be lost. The fontanelle tension is not increased initially unless there has been cerebral haemorrhage, but within 24 hours cerebral oedema occurs and causes a rise in the fontanelle tension. In cerebral anoxia the vomiting occurs before or after feeding, and may be forceful.

Treatment

Cerebral haemorrhage is shown on ultrasonography, which may also demonstrate cerebral oedema. Treatment is symptomatic: sedation with diazepam 0.1–0.3 mg/kg i.v., or phenobarbitone 2 mg/kg i.m., may be required. The pulse, temperature, state of consciousness and the degree of dehydration should be monitored. Aspiration of vomitus is potentially dangerous. Oral fluids are given in small volume and are offered frequently. An intravenous infusion may be necessary, but fluid requirements on the first day of life are only 60 ml/kg. This amount increases gradually each day until the end of the first week, when they reach 150 ml/kg. Frequent blood glucose estimations will detect hypoglycaemia early, before it exacerbates the cerebral disturbance and accentuates the vomiting.

Subdural haematoma

With the current high standard of obstetrics, a subdural haematoma is now rare in the neonatal period. In about 50% of infants, vomiting is the only symptom. In others, vomiting is accompanied by developmental delay, convulsions, an expanding head and retinal haemorrhages. The diagnosis is confirmed on ultrasonography and CT. A subdural haematoma during childhood must alert the clinician to the possibility of child abuse.

Hypoglycaemia

Vomiting may be the only symptom of hypoglycaemia in the neonatal period. It is more common in 'small for dates' babies and in infants of diabetic mothers, but may be seen in any stressful situation in the neonatal period, including low birth weight, neonatal meningitis, septicaemia and severe rhesus isoimmunisation. Symptomatic hypoglycaemia does not usually occur with a blood glucose in excess of 2 mmol/l.

Systemic infection

Vomiting is one of the many non specific signs of infection in the neonate. Thus, unexplained vomiting should be an indication to culture the blood, urine and CSF. Urine will usually be obtained by suprapubic aspiration in this age group.

Bowel obstruction

In duodenal obstruction, vomiting appears early and is bile stained because the site of the obstruction is almost always at the second part of the duodenum, just distal to the ampulla of Vater. In duodenal atresia, there may be other abnormalities such as Down syndrome and imperforate anus. The bile stained vomiting commences from birth. The diagnosis is made on plain X ray of the abdomen (Ch. 36). Where there is bowel obstruction beyond the duodenum (for example, small bowel atresia, Hirschsprung disease and meconium ileus), vomiting commences slightly later and is associated with increasing abdominal distension (Ch. 36). A strangulated inguinal hernia may cause a bowel obstruction when a loop of ileum becomes trapped within the hernial sac at the external inguinal ring. The diagnosis becomes evident when a tender irreducible lump is observed in the groin (Ch. 26).

Malrotation with volvulus

Volvulus in a neonate or infant with malrotation causes a high bowel obstruction and produces bile stained vomiting. The volvulus may cut off the blood supply to the midgut and lead to small bowel infarction, septicaemia and death if not treated promptly. Any infant with bile stained vomiting, otherwise unexplained, should be assumed to have malrotation with volvulus until proven otherwise. A barium meal will confirm the diagnosis. An urgent laparotomy is required to untwist the bowel (Fig. 68.3) and to perform a Ladd procedure to broaden the mesentery of the small bowel: this will prevent subsequent volvulus.

Renal disease

In the neonatal period, urinary infection and renal insufficiency may present with vomiting and poor weight gain, reflecting an underlying urinary tract abnormality. Initial urological investigation will include urine culture, renal ultrasonography, micturating cystourethrography and estimation of electrolytes, urea and creatinine. Renal tubular lesions occasionally present in the neonatal period with vomiting.

Adrenal insufficiency

In congenital adrenal hyperplasia, there is deficiency of the enzyme 21 hydroxylase (Ch. 65), which presents with ambiguous genitalia in the female. If this is not recog-

nised, it may present (as in the male) early in the second week of life with unexplained vomiting, dehydration and collapse. If the adrenal insufficiency is of the salt losing type, the diagnosis is further suspected by finding low levels of sodium and elevated levels of potassium in the serum, and is confirmed by appropriate hormonal studies.

Inborn metabolic errors

Although individually rare, there are a number of inborn errors involving, separately, amino acid, carbohydrate and organic acid metabolism. Most are inherited recessively, and a number can now be treated. Frequently, the presentation is with unexplained vomiting, lethargy, collapse, seizures and coma (Ch. 31).

Vomiting in infancy

Vomiting is a common non specific symptom in infancy, and disease of almost every system may present with vomiting.

Infection

Vomiting is frequently in response to infections such as tonsillitis, otitis media, pneumonia, meningitis and urinary tract infection. Physical examination will exclude many of these, but early signs may be minimal in meningitis and pneumonia, such that a lumbar puncture and

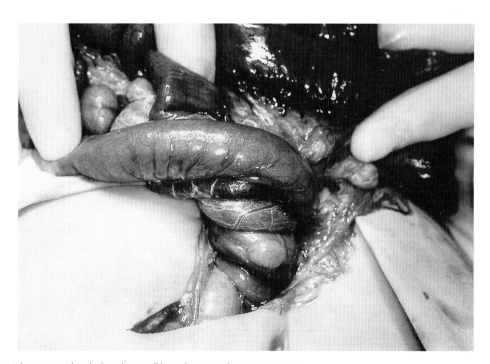

Fig. 68.3 Malrotation with volvulus: the small bowel is twisted on its mesentery.

chest X ray will be required if these are suspected. In infants with urinary tract infection, dysuria, frequency of passing urine and loin pain cannot be relied upon for diagnosis, and the urine must always be examined. When infection is controlled, the urinary tract should be imaged to exclude underlying structural abnormalities.

Lesions of the gastrointestinal tract

Conditions which produce vomiting in infancy are different from those seen in the neonatal period, except for duodenal obstruction from volvulus complicating malrotation, and gastro-oesophageal reflux. Failure to recognise malrotation with volvulus may result in infarction of the entire midgut (Ch. 36). Bowel trapped in a strangulated inguinal hernia in an infant will also produce vomiting. The diagnosis can be made easily if the inguinal orifices are examined (Ch. 26).

Gastro-oesophageal reflux

This is the most common cause of vomiting in infancy. The vomiting may commence soon after birth, or be delayed a few weeks. After a feed, a small amount is regurgitated and may continue until the next feed. At times, the vomiting is forceful. The vomitus may contain altered blood but is not bile stained. These infants usually thrive well and are rarely distressed by the vomiting. Physical examination reveals no abnormality. The diagnosis is made from the history and, if necessary, can be confirmed by barium swallow, when barium is seen to reflux from the stomach back into the oesophagus. In practice, the main use of barium studies is to exclude a hiatus hernia or other gastrointestinal cause of vomiting. Continuous 24 hour oesophageal pH monitoring appears to be a more sensitive method of detecting gastro-oesophageal reflux, but is only available in specialised centres. Radioisotope studies may demonstrate aspiration.

The natural history of gastro-oesophageal reflux is of spontaneous improvement, with resolution by the end of the first year of life (Ch. 71). In a few infants, ulceration of the lower end of the oesophagus from acid regurgitation may result in repeated haematemesis, oesophageal stricture or anaemia. Occasionally, the child may fail to thrive or suffer repeated aspiration of gastric contents. The symptoms of hiatus hernia are similar to those of gastro-oesophageal reflux. The management of gastro-oesophageal reflux is discussed in Chapter 71.

Rumination

In this syndrome, the infant consciously regurgitates and chews food which has already been swallowed. Some infants initiate vomiting by inserting their fingers into their mouths. Many of these infants are overactive and some may be emotionally deprived.

Pyloric stenosis

This is one of the most dramatic causes of vomiting in infancy. Typically, the onset is sudden, between the second and sixth week of life. Males are affected five times more often than females, and there is a definite familial incidence. Before the onset of vomiting, these infants fed well and were thriving. The vomiting is forceful and rapidly becomes projectile. The infant loses weight and becomes dehydrated. Despite vomiting, these infants remain hungry and are keen to feed immediately after vomiting. The vomitus is not bile stained, but may contain altered blood. The diagnosis is made clinically by feeling the thickened pylorus ('pyloric tumour') in the midline in the epigastrium between the rectus abdominis muscles or in the angle between the right rectus and the liver edge. The pyloric tumour is palpable as a hard mobile mass about the size of a small pebble. Peristaltic waves passing from the left costal margin to the right hypochondrium ('golf ball waves') may be visible long after the last feed. Palpation of the tumour is sufficient to establish the diagnosis. Pyloric stenosis can also be shown on ultrasonography (which reveals a thickened pylorus) and barium meal (which shows delayed gastric emptying and a narrow pyloric canal). These infants develop a hypokalaemic, hypochloraemic metabolic alkalosis which, together with dehydration, must be corrected before surgery. Pyloromyotomy is curative (Fig. 68.4).

Gastroenteritis

Vomiting in association with fluid stools is suggestive of gastroenteritis, particularly if the stools contain mucus or blood. However, these features may be seen in a variety of other medical and surgical disorders, which include intussusception and appendicitis. The diagnosis and management of gastroenteritis is discussed in Chapter 69.

Malabsorption

In the majority of malabsorption syndromes vomiting is not a feature. At times, in the more severe cases of coeliac disease (gluten enteropathy, Chapter 70) vomiting may be prominent. A gluten free diet rapidly reverses the clinical features of this disorder.

Intussusception

Vomiting commences early in intussusception and is the most consistent symptom. The general features, diagnosis and treatment are discussed in more detail above.

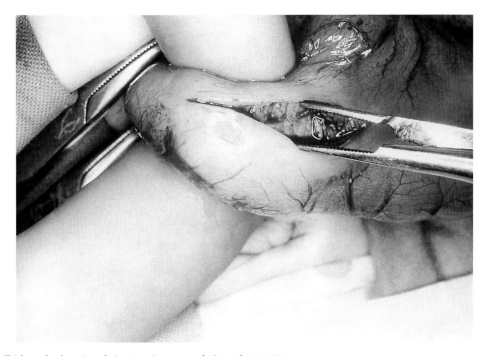

Fig. 68.4 Thickened pylorus in pyloric stenosis as seen during pyloromyotomy.

Clinical example

Bruce was a healthy 5 month old baby boy until 24 hours prior to admission, when he commenced vomiting, refused feeds, was lethargic and had marked pallor. His mother had noted that at times he appeared to be in pain. There was an impression of a slightly tender mass in the right upper quadrant. There was no blood rectally. A provisional diagnosis of intussusception was made, and at gas enema an intussusception in the mid transverse colon was encountered. This was reduced, with rapid relief of symptoms. He was observed overnight before being discharged the next morning.

Strangulated inguinal hernia

Strangulation of an inguinal hernia is common in infants and young children. All irreducible inguinal hernias should be assumed to be strangulated. In practice, the vast majority of so called irreducible hernias can be reduced manually by skilled hands (Ch. 26).

Vomiting in older children

Vomiting in older children is usually associated with infection, particularly viral or bacterial infection of the respiratory and gastrointestinal tracts. Nevertheless, there are some other less frequent but important causes of vomiting.

The possibility of an intracranial neoplasm should always be considered in a child with unexplained vomiting. There may be signs of increased intracranial pressure with midline cerebellar tumours, tumours involving the fourth ventricle, and tumours involving the pons or medulla. Initially, vomiting tends to occur in the morning before breakfast. There may be remissions for several days, but the vomiting invariably returns.

Migraine

In the older child, the association of severe paroxysmal frontal headache with pallor and vomiting is suggestive of migraine (Ch. 60). A positive family history is common. Transient loss of vision, transient hemiparesis, cerebellar ataxia or ophthalmoplegia may be evident. In some children migraine is precipitated by minor trauma. In the younger child, attacks of pallor or vomiting may be the only symptom. The diagnosis of migraine is made on clinical history, but where it is difficult to exclude an intracranial space occupying lesion clinically, cerebral CT may be required.

Acute appendicitis and peritonitis

In acute appendicitis in childhood, vomiting is a frequent early symptom, but usually is preceded by pain. The general features of appendicitis are described above.

In the young child (under 5 years), vomiting with or without diarrhoea may be the only obvious symptom. Physical examination in this age group can be difficult and unreliable; the child will prefer to lie still, as movement causes pain. This pain and the fear of its exacerbation by palpation may make the child appear uncooperative. It is only by repeated examination of the abdomen and an ongoing high index of suspicion that the diagnosis will be made before widespread peritonitis has developed.

Poisoning

Vomiting and respiratory and circulatory collapse in a previously well child should raise the possibility of poisoning (Ch. 21). Non accidental poisoning is becoming more frequent, and the age incidence of children attempting suicide is decreasing. A history of family discord and emotional problems in the child is not always volunteered at the onset of symptoms.

Psychological causes of vomiting

Psychogenic vomiting may occur in any age group. It is often associated with attempts to forcefeed a toddler or a schoolchild, after punishment, and as an attempt to avoid situations perceived as threatening, such as going to preschool or school. Almost any stressful situation may precipitate vomiting in a tense or anxious child. The absence of abnormal physical signs will be a feature.

Cyclical vomiting

Cyclical vomiting is a syndrome of persistent periodic vomiting of childhood. The severity varies, but ketosis and metabolic acidosis may develop rapidly. The aetiology is unknown and attacks usually cease spontaneously. Children with cyclical vomiting are often tense and anxious and may develop migraine or psychosomatic disease later in life. Recurring episodes of volvulus from malrotation, and metabolic disease should be excluded before labelling these children as having cyclical vomiting.

The child with diarrhoea 69

M. Oliver

Diarrhoea is defined as a measured stool volume greater than 10 ml/kg/day. Both the consistency of the stool (loose or watery) and frequency (usually at least three stools in a 24 hour period) are important defining features of diarrhoea. Acute diarrhoea lasts less than 10 days and has a major impact on both fluid and electrolyte status, while chronic diarrhoea suggests that the symptom is present for more than 2–3 weeks and can have a significant effect on the nutritional state of a child. The basic pathological mechanisms causing diarrhoea include osmotic, secretory and inflammatory processes (Table 69.1). Often more than one mechanism may operate simultaneously to cause diarrhoea.

Acute gastroenteritis

Aetiology

- Rotavirus infection (Fig. 69.1) is the most common cause of acute gastroenteritis in children under 5 years of age in developed countries, causing 40–50% of cases where hospital admission is required. It accounts for more severe episodes in infants in developing countries than any other single pathogen; it is more likely to cause dehydration, and is associated with a higher mortality than other agents. The mucosal damage it causes (Fig. 69.2), and hence the need for structural repair, has considerable nutritional implications for malnourished children. Asymptomatic reinfection can occur several times each year and helps maintain lifetime immunity.
- Enteric adenoviruses (types 40 and 41) cause 7–17% of cases requiring admission to hospital, and several other virus candidate pathogens have been recognised, such as calicivirus, coronavirus and other small viruses.

- Bacteria cause fewer episodes than viruses in developed countries. *Campylobacter jejuni* is responsible for 5–10% of cases. *Salmonella* spp., *Shigella* spp., and various types of *Escherichia coli* each account for a small percentage. In developing countries, *E. coli* (enterotoxigenic, enteropathogenic and enteroinvasive) and *Shigella* are especially important: *E. coli* because of the huge number of episodes it causes, and *Shigella* because it causes prolonged debilitating illness, and antibiotic resistant strains are emerging.
- *Giardia lamblia* rarely causes acute dehydrating diarrhoea, but another parasite, *Cryptosporidium*, is now known to cause 1–4% of cases of acute diarrhoea in infants admitted to hospital.

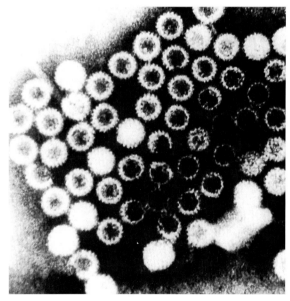

Fig. 69.1 The rotavirus (electron micrograph).

Table 69.1	Classification of diarrhoea		
	Osmotic	**Secretory**	**Inflammatory**
Clinical features	Ceases when enteral feeding is ceased	Continues when enteral feeding is ceased	Presence of blood and mucus in the faeces
Stool volume	<200 ml/day	>200 ml/day	Variable, usually <200 ml/day
Faecal sodium	<60 mosmol/l	>90 mosmol/l	Variable

675

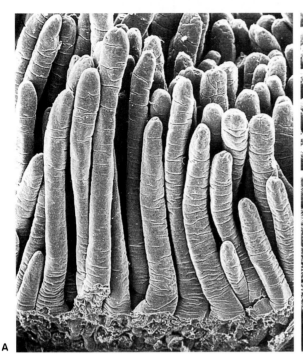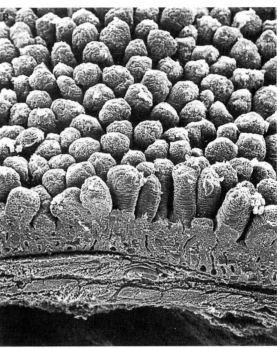

A   B

Fig. 69.2 Scanning electron microscope appearances of **A** normal, and **B** rotavirus infected calf jejunum. Villi are short, the epithelium is damaged and crypts are deep. (Courtesy of D. G. A. Hall, Institute for Animal Health, Compton, UK. From Walker et al 1991, with permission.)

Clinical features

- Symptoms of acute gastroenteritis include vomiting, fever and watery diarrhoea (up to 10–20 stools daily).
- Blood, mucus and the passage of small frequent bowel actions accompanied by abdominal pain suggests a diagnosis of bacterial gastroenteritis.
- Acute gastroenteritis is a diagnosis of exclusion. A few loose stools and vomiting does not necessarily equate with the diagnosis. There are several systemic disorders and surgical emergencies that can cause 'parenteral diarrhoea' and mimic infective gastro-enteritis (Table 69.2).

Management

Once the diagnosis of acute gastroenteritis is made on thorough clinical history and physical examination, the next step is to assess the degree of dehydration and insti-tute an appropriate plan for rehydration. This should be combined with nutritional support that aids the patient during the recovery phase.

Dehydration

- This risk is related to the child's age, with young infants being at greatest risk. This is because infants less than 1 year of age have a high surface area:body volume ratio, resulting in increased insensible fluid

Table 69.2   Different diagnosis of acute diarrhoea and vomiting in infants and children

Enteric infection
Rotavirus
Other viruses
Bacterial
   Salmonella spp.
   Shigella spp.
   Escherichia coli
   Campylobacter jeiuni
Protozoa
   Cryptosporidium
   Giardia lamblia
   Entamoeba histolytica
Food poisoning
   Staphylococcal toxin

Systemic infection
Urinary tract infection
Pneumonia
Septicaemia

Surgical condition
Appendicitis
Intussusception
Partial bowel obstruction
Hirschsprung disease

Other
Diabetes mellitus
Antibiotic diarrhoea
Haemolytic uraemic syndrome

loss. They also have a tendency to more severe vomiting and diarrhoea compared with older children and adults.

- Fluid loss is usually assessed on the basis of per cent body weight loss. Physical signs of dehydration are not usually apparent until 4% of body weight is lost.
- The signs of dehydration traditionally described are outlined in Table 69.3. However, three signs discriminate adequately between dehydration and adequate hydration: deep breathing, decreased skin turgor and poor peripheral perfusion.

Electrolyte loss

- This is usually isotonic (water and electrolytes being lost in equal amounts). Hypertonic hypernatraemic dehydration (fluid loss > electrolyte loss) occurs in 5–10% of cases of acute gastroenteritis, and hypotonic hyponatraemic dehydration (electrolyte loss > fluid loss) can occur if the colon (a major site of sodium reabsorption) is out of circuit, e.g. short gut syndrome.
- If corrected too rapidly, hypernatraemic dehydration will result in convulsions due to rapid shifts of water into cells. Hyponatraemic dehydration can also cause significant neurological morbidity and mortality, and, in contrast to the hypernatraemic state, requires vigorous replacement of sodium.

Table 69.4	Suitable fluids for the non dehydrated child
Solution	Dilution
Carbonated beverages (not low calorie)	1 in 4 with warm water to remove bubbles
Unsweetened frutit juice	1 in 4 with tap water
Fruit juice drinks	1 in 4 with tap water
Glucose	2 teaspoons in 240 ml boiled water

Each of these fluids has an osmolality of less than 200 mmol/kg water and sugar content below 200 mmol/l.

Rehydration guidelines

No dehydration

- Use of suitable fluids includes those outlined in Tables 69.4 and 69.5.
- Nutritional intake should not be modified, but extra fluid to keep up with ongoing losses outlined above should be continued (5–6 ml/kg/hour).

Mild to moderate dehydration

- Oral rehydration solution (ORS) is the cornerstone of successful rehydration, and is recommended globally for the management of acute diarrhoea.
- The success of ORS is based on the basic observation that intestinal sodium transport is enhanced by glucose transport in the small intestine, and that this sodium coupled mechanism for glucose transport remains intact during acute gastroenteritis.
- To facilitate optimal absorption of sodium glucose and water, the sodium and glucose must be in the range recommended (Table 69.5).
- Rehydration should take place over 4–6 hours and can be given orally, or if either vomiting or fluid refusal is a problem, a nasogastric tube may be used to achieve a steady infusion of fluid.

Table 69.3	Assessment of dehydration

Mild
≤ 5% body weight loss
Decreased peripheral perfusion*
Thirsty, alert, restless
Deep acidotic breathing*

Moderate
6–9% body weight loss
Thirsty, restless, lethargic but irritable
Rapid pulse, normal blood pressure
Sunken eyes, sunken fontanelle
Dry mucous membranes, absent tears
Pinched skin retracts slowly (1–2 seconds)*

Severe
10% or more body weight loss
General appearance
   Infants: drowsy, limp, cold sweaty, cyanotic limbs, comatose
   Older children: apprehensive, cold, sweaty, cyanotic limbs
Rapid feeble pulse, low blood pressure
Sunken eyes and fontanelle
Pinched skin retracts slowly (> 2 seconds)*

*These are the only signs proven to discriminate between hydration and dehydration.

Table 69.5 Oral rehydration preparations available in Australia

	Na	K	Cl	Citrate	Glucose (%)
WHO	90	20	80	10	2.0
Recommended for Australia	50–60	20	40–80	10	2.0
Gastrolyte	80	20	60	10	1.8
Repalyte	60	20	60	10	1.8

Concentration expressed as mmol/l of made up solution (except glucose %).

Table 69.6   An infant of 10 kg estimated at 7.5% dehydration has fluid requirements equal to:

Maintenance 100 × 10 kg	=	1000 ml
Deficit 7.5% of 10 kg	=	750 kg

Total	=	1750 ml

Using oral rehydration the deficit can be replaced in 6 hours rather than 24 hours, so in the above example the infant would be offered fluid as follows:

First 6 hours

Deficit	=	750 ml
Maintenance 6/24 of 1000	=	250 ml

Total	=	1000 ml (170 ml/hour)

Next 18 hours

Maintenance 18/24 of 1000	=	750 ml (45 ml/hour)

Another simple method which gives about the right answer is to calculate the fluid deficit, double it, and give that volume over 6–12 hours.

- Volume required for rehydration = estimated deficit and maintenance; maintenance for:
  — 1–3 months of age   = 120 ml/kg/24 hours
  — 3–12 months of age   = 100 ml/kg/24 hours
  — 12 months onwards   = 80 ml/kg/24 hours.
  (see Tables 69.6 and 69. 7).

Severe dehydration (10% plus)
- Circulatory insufficiency is present and intravenous therapy is required. The usual requirement is to fill the vascular compartment quickly to restore circulation. This will require rapid rehydration, often using boluses of normal saline by intravenous or intraosseous infusion.
- Once dehydration is corrected and normal organ perfusion is restored, ORS can be used in conjunction with intravenous fluids. The latter is rarely required for longer than 24 hours.
- Clinical observations must be highlighted: this allows the physician to reassess the patient's state of hydration and also helps confirm the diagnosis of acute gastroenteritis.

Table 69.7   A 10 kg child with 15% dehydration and shock

- Total fluid deficit = 10 kg × 15% = 1.5 l = 1500 ml
- Assume a total of 40 ml/kg (400 ml) normal saline needed to restore circulation
- Remaining deficit = 1500 – 400 = 1100 ml
- Maintenance fluid requirement is 100 ml/kg/day = 10 × 100 = 1000 ml
- Fluid in next 24 hours = remaining deficit + maintenance = 1100 + 1000 = 2100 ml = 90 ml/hour
- Therefore, give 400 ml normal saline quickly, then 90 ml/hour of 5% dextrose in N/4 saline with KCl 40 mmol/l for the next 24 hours

---

- All patients with dehydration require regular checks on pulse, temperature and respiration, and strict fluid balance charts must be kept. The child should be weighed on admission and, in severe cases, after 6 hours and 24 hours, with an increase in weight being a reliable sign of rehydration. However, in some patients weight may not fall even in the presence of severe dehydration, especially if the child has an ileus, so other signs of dehydration must be sought.

Recommendations on nutritional management

- Breastfeeding should continue through rehydration and maintenance phases of treatment, and formula feeds need to be restarted after rehydration.
- Use of special formulas or diluted formulas is unjustified.

Pharmacotherapy

- Infants and children with acute gastroenteritis should not be treated with antidiarrhoeal agents.
- Antibiotic treatment may be indicated in *Salmonella* spp. gastroenteritis in the very young (<3 months), those who are immunocompromised or those who are systemically unwell. It may also be indicated in *C. jejuni* infection in compromised hosts and *Yersinia enterocolitica* in children with sickle cell disease.
- Pathogens for which antibacterial therapy is always indicated include *Shigella* spp. *and Giardia lamblia.*

Complications of acute gastroenteritis

Febrile convulsions

- These are generally uncommon, but rotavirus infection can cause fevers as high as 39–40°C.

Sugar malabsorption

- Is more common in infants less than 6 months of age and is recognised by the persistent nature of the diarrhoea when nutrition is reintroduced.
- Stools are often watery, frothy and tend to excoriate the buttocks. If sugar intolerance is suspected, the napkin should be lined with thin plastic material, or a rectal examination should be performed and the fluid stool collected and tested for reducing substances. It is pointless to test solid stool material.
- To test for lactose intolerance, mix 5 drops of liquid stool with 10 drops of water and add a Clinitest tablet. A positive test of >0.5% indicates lactose or glucose malabsorption, but not sucrose, which is not a reducing sugar.

- Diarrhoea due to lactose malabsorption resolves rapidly on a lactose-free diet, which should be continued for approximately 4 weeks.
- A very small proportion of infants continue to have diarrhoea despite the exclusion of lactose and sucrose. Under these circumstances, a carbohydrate-free feed is given, with glucose and fructose (different transport mechanisms across the enterocyte) added to tolerance.

Prevention of acute gastroenteritis

- Enteral immunoglobulin in the form of hyperimmune bovine antirotavirus colostrum has been shown to reduce the duration and severity of rotavirus diarrhoea. However, due to its expense, it is not routinely used and is reserved to treat immunocompromised children with a prolonged rotavirus illness.
- Vaccines against typhoid and cholera infection are available, but are not required in developed countries.
- A rotavirus vaccine, composed of rotaviruses derived from animals that are genetically engineered to carry human rotaviral genes, has been developed. The vaccine was recommended by the American Academy of Pediatrics in 1999. Unfortunately after it had been licensed, reports of intussusception occurring 3–7 days after the first dose were received. As a result of this, the vaccine has been withdrawn. Other strategies for vaccination are currently under assessment in Melbourne and other centres.

> ### Clinical example
>
> Stacey, a previously well 15 month old infant, suddenly became unwell, refused feeds, developed a temperature of 39°C and subsequently passed five loose bowel actions in 6 hours. She appeared to be having bouts of abdominal pain. On the second day, a few flecks of blood were noted in the stools. Her weight was 11.8 kg, compared with 12.5 kg 2 weeks previously. A provisional diagnosis of acute bacterial gastroenteritis was made.
>
> She was treated with oral rehydration solution and solids. Her temperature gradually settled over 4 days and her stools were normal after 1 week. *C. jejuni* was grown from two of three stool samples.

Chronic diarrhoea

This is defined as the presence of diarrhoea for more than 2–3 weeks. It can follow a bout of acute gastroenteritis, but usually begins insidiously.

Many causes of chronic diarrhoea are associated with malabsorption of nutrients and are dealt with in detail in Chapter 70. Only chronic non specific diarrhoea, postinfective diarrhoea, sucrase-isomaltase deficiency and inflammatory bowel disease will be discussed in this chapter.

An approach to diagnosis

- Answers to a small number of key questions will usually get very close to a definitive diagnosis. Figure 69.3

1. EXCLUDE RETENTION WITH OVERFLOW

2. IS THERE FAILURE TO THRIVE?

| YES | ALWAYS investigate |
| NO | Sometimes investigate
Time is on your side. |

3. IS STOOL VOLUME INCREASED?

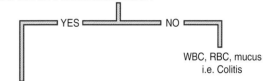

4. IS THERE FAT MALABSORPTION?

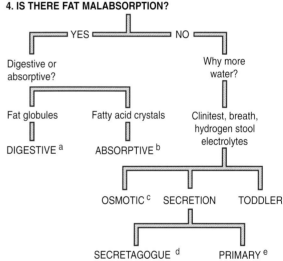

5. IS THERE PROTEIN LOSING ENTEROPATHY?

Raised alpha -1-AT clearance [f]

a. Digestive pancreatic insufficiency (confirmed by low trypsin) liver disease obvious)

b. Absorptive mucosal damage: coeliac disease, giardias, protein hypersensitivity, IBD. lymphatic block: lymphangiectasis.

c. Osmotic disaccharidase defieciency monosaccharide transport: glucose-galatose transport overload: high sugar fluids, fruits, sorbitol

d. Secretagogue bacterial toxin *(C. difficile)* deconjugated bile salts

e. Primary transport defect (rare) chlorideorrhoea

f. Protein losing enteropathy lymphangiectasia, polyposis

Fig. 69.3 Investigation of chronic diarrhoea.

outlines a suggested scheme. Performance of simple stool tests is all that is necessary to guide selection of the appropriate definitive tests. Many of the specific causes are discussed in Chapter 70. Others are dealt with here.

Chronic non specific diarrhoea

- Is seen in children between the ages of 12 months and 4 years and current scientific evidence suggests that disturbed intestinal motility is pivotal in the pathogenesis of this condition.
- The history is one of frequent, poorly formed and slightly offensive stools. Food material is often recognised in the stool, suggesting rapid gastrointestinal transit. The condition often resolves spontaneously at about 3–4 years of age.
- The child is usually active, with unimpaired growth, appetite is normal, and there is a history of increased fluid intake. Further questioning about diet often reveals a high intake of fruit juices and cordial.
- The cornerstone of successful treatment includes restriction of fruit juice in the diet, normalising fluid intake and (re-) introduction of wholemeal and other dietary fibres which add bulk to the stool.
- It has also been suggested that many of these children are on a relatively low fat diet, and normalising fat content acts to slow proximal gastrointestinal transit and improve symptoms.

Postinfective diarrhoea

- This is defined as the persistence of diarrhoea and failure to gain weight for more than 7 days after hospital admission for gastroenteritis.
- It is generally due to a sugar intolerance, which can be confirmed on the basis of stool analysis for reducing sugars and will resolve with elimination of the sugar from the diet.
- Other causes include cow's milk protein hypersensitivity or a persistent gastrointestinal infection.

Sucrase–isomaltase deficiency

- This is an uncommon inherited disorder (autosomal recessive), with symptoms beginning after sucrose is introduced into the diet.
- Symptoms consist of watery diarrhoea and abdominal distension. Growth is usually normal.
- Diagnosis is dependent on a positive breath hydrogen test using sucrose as the test sugar. Alternatively a small bowel biopsy containing very low isomaltase and sucrase levels will establish the diagnosis.
- Management is based on dietary restriction of sucrose.

Chronic inflammatory bowel disease (IBD)

The incidence of Crohn disease (CD) has increased annually; that of ulcerative colitis (UC) has shown an annual fluctuation without an upward trend. Current opinion regarding the cause of IBD favours the hypothesis that these two conditions result from an interaction between immunological, genetic and environmental factors.

Crohn disease can present in several ways:
- Extraintestinal signs of growth retardation, including anorexia, fatigue, delayed puberty, erythema nodosum, arthritis, clubbing or hepatitis.
- Gastric and intestinal symptoms, including nausea, vomiting, abdominal pain and diarrhoea.
- Colonic involvement, including bloody diarrhoea, perianal skin tags and fissures.

Children with UC will usually present with lower abdominal pain, diarrhoea and rectal bleeding; additionally:
- Systemic symptoms are less marked.
- The child can develop arthritis, which usually correlates with disease activity.
- Pyoderma gangrenosum occurs more commonly in UC.
- The child can develop chronic hepatitis.

Children may experience the same symptoms, clinical presentations, complications and response to treatment as adults with IBD. This chapter will highlight some of the features of IBD that have particular importance in the paediatric patient.

Investigation

Several laboratory tests will point to a diagnosis of IBD; however, endoscopy is the gold standard. Gastroscopy and colonoscopy (with ileoscopy) is essential, taking biopsies at all levels of the gut, whether or not there is macroscopic disease. Biopsies from a normal appearing stomach or duodenum may contain granulomas, making the diagnosis clear. Pathological alterations above the ileum exclude the diagnosis of UC. A barium meal or a labelled white cell scan can be helpful in assessing the area of the gut that is involved in CD.

Treatment

Enteral therapy

- Provides a similar remission rate to corticosteroids in the treatment of childhood CD (not UC) and improves growth and inflammatory markers.

- Probably exerts its beneficial effects by alterations in gut flora, enterocyte nutrition and modulation of endogenous growth factors.
- Chronic supplementary enteral therapy reduces relapse rates in CD but not UC.
- Often utilises polymeric and elemental feeds, which are probably equally effective but are not generally palatable and may require nasogastric infusion. All other oral intake is ceased during this treatment, which usually lasts 6–8 weeks.

Corticosteroids

- Are used in the dose range of 1–2 mg/kg of prednisolone for moderate to severe UC or CD, usually for a 2–3 month period with a gradual dose reduction.
- Can adversely affect growth and has many unpleasant cosmetic and systemic side effects.
- Can have a significant effect on bone mineral density and lead to osteoporosis later in life.
- Newer corticosteroids, such as budesonide, have fewer side effects and are particularly useful for ileal and right-sided colonic disease.
- Steroid enemas are helpful in the management of lower colonic inflammation in both CD and UC.

Other pharmacological treatments

- Aminosalicylates can be used in both an oral and topical form to manage colitis in both CD and UC. This is often used in mild UC to achieve remission and in both UC and Crohn colitis as maintenance therapy.
- Azathioprine is often used in children with both UC and CD if they are steroid dependent, but will take 6–8 weeks to be clinically effective.
- Medications such as tacrolimus, cyclosporin and methotrexate may be used in the most severe disease; however, the effectiveness of such agents has only been assessed in open labelled studies.
- Antitumour necrosis factor α has shown promising results in the management of adults with severe CD, but has been used sparingly in children. Side effects such as severe allergic reactions and the possible development of lymphoproliferative disorders are a major concern.

Surgery

- Is usually indicated in children with CD who have growth failure, and who have not responded to pharmacological or nutritional therapies. This usually applies to an area of localised disease.
- Appropriately timed surgery in children with CD may accelerate growth and advance puberty.
- Colectomy is rarely required in children with UC unless toxic megacolon is present.

Cancer risk

- Is greatest in children with UC, particularly those with pancolitis for more than 10 years and who also have coexisting sclerosing cholangitis.
- Observed accumulative incidences range from 5 to 10% after 20 years disease duration and 12 to 20% after 30 years. This infers that a person with UC has roughly a 12% chance of developing colorectal cancer between 10 and 15 years after the onset of the IBD.
- To avoid colonic cancer, patients with longstanding extensive colitis face either prophylactic colectomy or regular surveillance colonoscopy. Neither option is perfect; a more reliable, cheaper process of screening needs to be found.
- This general approach also applies to children and adults with extensive and longstanding colonic CD.

Clinical example

Renee presented at the age of 12 years with a 6 month history of recurrent abdominal pain, poor appetite and weight loss of 2 kg. Her stools had been loose at times, but they contained no blood. Abdominal examination was normal. An anal skin tag was present. Blood tests revealed an iron deficiency anaemia (Hb 101 g/l) and an ESR of 55 mm. Stool microscopy showed white cells and mucus, but cultures were negative.

At colonoscopy, patchy colitis with rectal sparing and ileitis was found. Barium meal and follow through confirmed ileal involvement, but was otherwise normal.

Her Crohn's disease was treated initially with high dose steroids, then later with sulphasalazine, with a good clinical response.

Chronic diarrhoea and malabsorption

E. O'Loughlin

Malabsorption is not a clinical entity. It can be defined as the failure to absorb nutrients. A wide range of intestinal, pancreatic and hepatic disorders can be associated with malabsorption. To understand how one approaches the problem of malabsorption in the clinical setting, an understanding of the normal physiology of nutrient digestion and salt, water and macronutrient and micronutrient absorption is essential. This information is available in general physiology texts.

Diagnostic approach

A large number of children have loose stools without having underlying gastrointestinal disease. In young children this is called 'toddlers' diarrhoea'. A major clinical challenge is to differentiate well children with loose stools from children who have gastrointestinal disease. The diagnosis of the majority of children with malabsorption can be established with thorough clinical assessment, stool examination and simple ancillary tests.

Clinical assessment

Initial assessment can reveal whether a child is ill. If so, immediate evaluation will be required. In the well child, a 'wait and see approach' may be more rewarding than immediate investigation.

Malabsorption does not present as malabsorption per se. Rather, individuals with malabsorption can present with a wide array of symptoms and physical signs (Table 70.1). Diarrhoea is the most common presentation and may be accompanied by loss of appetite, decreased physical activity, lethargy and growth failure. Children with coeliac disease may have decreased appetite, and are often cranky and irritable. In contrast, children with pancreatic insufficiency often develop a voracious appetite. In children with failure to thrive, a detailed dietary history is required. Occasionally, parents manipulate the child's diet in an attempt to control the diarrhoea, which can lead to significant dietary insufficiency with attendant weight loss. Assessment of the age of introduction of various foods into the diet may give insight to the underlying diagnosis. Onset of symptoms 3–6 months after the introduction of wheat products suggests the possibility of coeliac disease. Onset shortly after introduction of cow's milk suggests cow's milk protein intolerance. History of overseas travel

Table 70.1   Some symptoms and signs of nutrient deficiencies

Protein	
Growth failure	
Muscle wasting	
Hypoproteinaemic oedema	
Fat	
Weight loss	
Muscle wasting	
Manifestation of deficiency of vitamins A, D, E, K	
Carbohydrate	
Weight loss	
Salt/water	
Electrolyte disturbances	
Growth failure (chronic salt deficiency)	
Dehydration (acute loss)	
Vitamins	
A	Night blindness
	Skin rash
	Dry eyes (xerophthalmia)
D	Rickets
	Hypocalcaemia
K	Bruising (coagulation defects)
E	Anaemia
	Peripheral neuropathy
B_{12}	Megaloblastic anaemia
	Irritability
	Hypotonia
	Peripheral neuropathy
Folate	Megaloblastic anaemia
	Irritablility
Minerals	
Iron	
Microcytic anaemia	
Delayed development	
Calcium	
Rickets	
Irritability	
Seizures	
Zinc	
Diarrhoea	
Skin rash (mouth, perineum, fingers and toes)	
Poor growth	

is important, as some unusual infections, such as amoebic dysentery can cause chronic bloody diarrhoea.

The nature of the loose stool is important to ascertain as it provides important clues to the pathophysiology and thus aetiology. Diarrhoea can be thought of in terms of fatty stools (steatorrhoea), watery diarrhoea (osmotic due to carbohydrate malabsorption or secretory) and bloody diarrhoea. Table 70.2 provides a differential diagnosis of chronic diarrhoea and malabsorption categorised by the nature of the stool.

Assessment of general health is important, as many gastrointestinal disorders exhibit extraintestinal manifestations. Cystic fibrosis (Ch. 50), Shwachman syndrome and immunodeficiency disorders (Ch. 43) are associated with infections, particularly sinopulmonary infections. Delayed pubertal development can accompany many chronic disorders but is particularly prevalent in Crohn disease (Ch. 69).

Family history may be of note. Cystic fibrosis, primary disaccharidase deficiencies and abetalipoproteinaemia are recessively inherited. Coeliac disease and inflammatory bowel disease are more frequently observed in first degree relatives.

Physical examination includes assessment of growth, nutritional status and pubertal development. Plotting percentile charts is mandatory. A child who is growing normally is unlikely to be suffering from serious gastrointestinal disease. Plotting longitudinal measurements, if available, is very important as it may give clues to the onset of disease and could indicate the diagnosis. Other physical signs of malabsorption and specific nutritional deficiencies include: loss of muscle bulk and subcutaneous fat; peripheral oedema (hypoproteinaemia); bruising (vitamin K deficiency); glossitis and angular stomatitis (iron deficiency); finger clubbing (cystic fibrosis, Crohn disease, coeliac disease); skin rashes in coeliac disease (dermatitis herpetiformis) and inflammatory bowel disease (erythema nodosum, pyoderma gangrenosum); and specific skin disorders associated with zinc, vitamin A and essential fatty acid deficiencies (Fig. 70.1). Rickets (vitamin D deficiency) is very uncommon in sunny climates, even in conditions with severe steatorrhoea. It is important to examine carefully as there are many extraintestinal manifestations of gastrointestinal disease and malnutrition.

Stool examination

Stool examination is very simple and provides very important information. The presence of numerous white and red cells indicates colitis. This is usually due to bacterial or parasitic infection, to chronic inflammatory disorders of the large bowel, or milk protein intolerance when identified in infants. Leucocytes are not increased in the stool of individuals with small bowel or pancreatic disease. Cysts of parasites such as *Giardia lamblia* indicate giardiasis.

Table 70.2 Differential diagnosis of chronic diarrhoea and malabsorption categorised according to type of stool

Steatorrhoea
Pancreatic insufficiency
  Cystic fibrosis
  Shwachman syndrome
  Chronic pancreatitis
  Malnutrition (developing world)
  Isolated lipase deficiency
Inadequate bile salt concentration
  Biliary atresia
  Cholestatic syndromes
    Congenital
    Acquired
  End stage liver disease
  Bacterial overgrowth syndrome
  Bile salt malabsorption (ileal resection)
Inadequate absorptive surface
  Coeliac disease
  Surgical resection (short gut syndrome)
  Milk protein intolerance
  Immunodeficiency
Enterocyte defect
  Abetalipoproteinaemia
Defective lymphatic drainage
  Intestinal lymphangiectasia
  Constrictive pericarditis

Watery diarrhoea
Osmotic
Disaccharidase deficiency
  Lactase
  Sucrase–isomaltase
Glucose–galactose malabsorption
Excessive intake
  Sorbitol
  Fructose

Abnormal water and electrolyte transport
Congenital electrolyte transporter defects
  Congenital chloride diarrhoea
  Congenital sodium diarrhoea
Infection
Mucosal disease
  Coeliac disease
  Milk protein intolerance
  Inflammatory conditions (inflammatory bowel disease)
  Immunodeficiency disorders
  Autoimmune enteropathy
Bile salt malabsorption
  Congenital
  Ileal resection
Bacterial overgrowth syndromes
  Gastrointestinal motility disorders
  Anatomical (blind loop)

Bloody diarrhoea
Infection
  Bacterial
  Parasitic
Idiopathic inflammatory bowel disease
  Crohn disease
  Ulcerative colitis
Milk protein intolerance

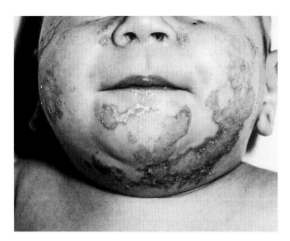

Fig. 70.1 Exfoliative rash of zinc deficiency.

Oil droplets seen on stool microscopy are always abnormal outside the newborn period and usually indicate fat maldigestion, as occurs with pancreatic insufficiency, for example in cystic fibrosis. Mucosal disease, such as coeliac disease, in general does not interfere with fat digestion because pancreatic function is usually normal. Mucosal disease interferes with the absorption of triglyceride products. These products are observed as fatty acid crystals on polarising microscopy.

The presence of carbohydrate in the stool can be detected with Clinitest tablets. This is a commercially available bedside test in which the reaction between stool sugars such as lactose causes a colour change when added to the tablets. Greater than 500 mg/dl indicates carbohydrate malabsorption. Measurement of stool electrolytes and osmolality in the stool water is also a very useful test. When the sum of the stool electrolytes, that is sodium + potassium + chloride + bicarbonate, equals measured osmolality, a secretory diarrhoea is present. If the sum of the electrolytes is substantially less than the measured osmolality (>100 mosmol/l) this indicates an osmotic diarrhoea.

Malabsorption with chronic diarrhoea

Diarrhoea is the most common presentation of malabsorption. Diarrhoea can be defined as increased frequency, fluidity and volume of stool. The following discussion will provide a systematic approach to the child with malabsorption and diarrhoea based on the type of stool, that is:

- fatty
- watery or
- bloody.

Some illustrative cases will be provided.

Fatty diarrhoea (steatorrhoea)

Clinical example

Mary is 9 months old. She presented with poor weight gain, chronic diarrhoea and a history of recurrent respiratory illnesses, including one admission at age 3 months with 'bronchiolitis'. Loose stools are found each time her nappy is changed. On occasion mother has noted oil drops in the stool. Despite the poor weight gain, Mary has an excellent appetite and is described as a voracious eater. She consumes a mixed diet, including infant formula, appropriate for age. Cereal was introduced at age 6 months. Mother also commented that she tasted salty when she kissed her.

On examination, Mary was found to be a thin wasted girl. Her height was on the 50th percentile and her weight was less than the 3rd pecentile. She had mild finger clubbing, peripheral oedema, pallor of the tongue and palmar creases but no signs of chronic liver disease. There was no abdominal distension of note, although she had a fine scaling rash over her trunk. Respiratory examination was normal. No other abnormal physical signs were present.

Results of investigations included Hb 85 g/l (normal range, 110–140) with a normocytic normochromic film, normal white cell count and differential; albumin 24 g/l (normal range, 34–44) and normal liver function tests. Stool microscopy revealed copious fat droplets. Three day faecal fat excretion estimation demonstrated an output of 35% of ingested fat (normal <7% of intake).

Mary's diarrhoea was due to fat malabsorption, as evidenced by her mother's observation of fat droplets in the stool.

Mary's sweat test demonstrated a sweat chloride of 80 mmol/l (a result of >60 mmol/l is diagnostic of cystic fibrosis). Genetic testing indicated that she was homozygous ΔF508 (the commonest mutation), consistent with her relatively severe symptoms. Introduction of pancreatic exocrine replacement therapy, a high fat diet and vitamin supplements alleviated her diarrhoea and eventually corrected her failure to thrive, anaemia and skin rash.

The differential diagnosis of fat malabsorption is quite wide ranging (Table 70.2); however, if one understands the normal physiology of fat digestion and absorption, the differential diagnosis is much less daunting. Conditions which cause steatorrhoea can also be associated with protein maldigestion and/or malabsorption, although symptoms most commonly relate to the malabsorption of fat. The presence of fat in the stool is also more readily observed than protein.

Fat and protein digestion and absorption

Ingested fat in the form of triglycerides, cholesterol and phospholipids is, to a large extent, digested in the lumen of the small intestine and absorbed in the jejunum. This requires bile salts, which form micelles and solubilise the fat; pancreatic enzymes, such as lipase and colipase, which digest the fat; and an intact intestinal mucosa, which is required for absorption of the products of digestion. Following digestion in the micelles, breakdown products diffuse across the enterocyte apical membrane and are reconstituted in the cell into chylomicrons. These are small packets of triglyceride, phospholipid and cholesterol which associate with carrier proteins, such as beta lipoprotein, essential for cellular trafficking of the chylomicrons. After the chylomicrons are reconstituted they exit the mucosa into the lymphatic system and subsequently pass into the systemic circulation. Some small chain triglycerides can bypass this system and enter the portal venous system directly.

Protein digestion begins in the stomach by the action of pepsin and acid. However, most protein hydrolysis occurs in the lumen of the jejunum by action of pancreatic proteases. These are secreted as inactive precursors. Chymotrypsin is converted to trypsin by the action of the small intestinal enzyme enterokinase. Activated trypsin further activates chymotrypsin and other proteases, such as carboxypeptidase. The products of protein hydrolysis are amino acids and oligopeptides. The latter are further hydrolysed to mono-, di- and tripeptides by brush border hydrolyases and are absorbed by specific membrane transporters. Di- and tripeptides undergo hydrolysis to amino acids in the cytoplasm of the enterocyte. Isolated protein maldigestion/malabsorption is extremely rare. It usually occurs in association with malabsorption of other macronutrients.

Fat malabsorption

Diseases of the pancreas and the small intestine are the usual causes of steatorrhoea in children. Chronic liver disease may cause steatorrhoea, but this is in the setting of severe and obvious liver disease (such as the patient who is cirrhotic and jaundiced) and is not usually a diagnostic problem.

Steatorrhoea causes bulky stools and can lead to other nutritional deficits. Fat is responsible for approximately 40% of caloric intake in the Western diet. Thus fat malabsorption can lead to failure to thrive due to an energy deficient diet. Some vitamins are fat soluble and require normal fat digestion for their absorption. These include A,D, E and K. Thus patients with steatorrhoea may also develop signs of fat soluble vitamin deficiency, as described above. Essential fatty acids such as arachidonic acid are also malabsorbed in patients with pancreatic malabsorption. A scaling skin rash is one physical manifestation of essential fatty acid deficiency.

Pancreatic and intestinal diseases associated with fat malabsorption can also result in protein and carbohydrate maldigestion/malabsorption. Thus it is not uncommon to find a mixed picture of malabsorption. Protein maldigestion/malabsorption results in hypoproteinaemia. The main physical manifestations are growth failure, peripheral oedema and ascites.

Pancreatic disease

Cystic fibrosis (Ch. 50)

Cystic fibrosis (CF):
- is the commonest cause of pancreatic malabsorption in the Caucasian population
- incidence in the population is approximately 1 per 2000
- is an inborn error in epithelial chloride secretion (cystic fibrosis transmembrane conductance regulator (CFTR)).

Organs affected include:
- gastrointestinal tract and liver
- sinopulmonary tract
- pancreas
- exocrine portion of the sweat glands
- vas deferens
- sweat duct (CFTR absorbs rather than secretes chloride in this organ).

Because of the fluid and salt transport defects, patients with CF produce more viscous secretions in lung, gut, pancreas and vas deferens, leading to:
- chronic suppurative lung disease
- nasal polyps
- pancreatic insufficiency
- intussusception
- meconium ileus and distal intestinal obstruction syndrome
- infertility
- elevated sweat sodium and chloride, which can lead to heat prostration in warmer climates.

Chronic liver disease will develop in 10–15% of children with CF.

Malabsorption in CF frequently results in malnutrition and there may be symptoms and signs of specific nutrient deficits such as hypoalbuminaemic oedema, night blindness due to vitamin A deficiency or skin rash due to essential fatty acid deficiency. Median life expectancy is 30 years, with death usually from respiratory failure or haemorrhage from portal hypertension and oesophageal varices.

Many mutations have been identified in the CFTR. Depending on what part of the channel the mutation affects, the phenotype can vary from mild to severe disease. Individuals with milder mutations have milder lung disease and do not usually have malabsorption, as pancreatic function is normal.

Newborn screening:
- can detect CF in the neonatal period
- involves measurement of immunoreactive trypsinogen and/or CFTR mutations

• is the commonest mode of presentation when it is performed.

In children with the severe phenotype who are missed by screening, or in countries where screening is not performed, presentation is usually in the first year with chronic diarrhoea and failure to thrive, with or without respiratory symptoms. In milder phenotypes, patients may not present until adult life with respiratory disease or infertility.

Diagnosic investigations for CF are:
• elevated sweat sodium and chloride ('sweat test') — simplest and cheapest
• CFTR mutation analysis.

Treatment is usually undertaken in a tertiary referral multidisciplinary clinic and involves:
• Physiotherapy, inhalation therapy and antibiotics for chest disease.
• Pancreatic enzyme supplements and nutritional support.
• Specific therapy may be required for the other intestinal/liver complications.

Shwachman syndrome

The features of Shwachman syndrome are:
• agenesis of the pancreatic acinus
• short stature
• dysplasia of the metaphysis of the long bones
• cyclical neutropenia.

There is no specific diagnostic test; treatment includes pancreatic exocrine replacement and treatment of infections.

Chronic pancreatitis

Causes of chronic pancreatitis include:
• protein energy malnutrition
• hereditary pancreatitis (rare)
• idiopathic fibrosing pancreatitis (rare).

Small bowel disease

Coeliac disease (gluten enteropathy)

Coeliac disease is a disorder characterised by intestinal injury induced by the cereal protein gluten. Gluten is a glycoprotein found in wheat, barley and rye and, to a lesser extent, oats. In susceptible individuals, the ingestion of gluten induces a cell mediated injury of the intestinal mucosa resulting in severe villous atrophy, crypt hyperplasia and infiltration of the epithelium with lymphocytes (intraepithelial lymphocytes). In Western countries, the incidence of coeliac disease in the general population may be as high as 1 in 70, although not all affected individuals develop the classical manifestations of coeliac disease.

Modes of presentation include:
• 'Classical' coeliac disease (Fig. 70.2)
— between 9 and 18 months of age
— anorexia, weight loss, abdominal distension and wasting
— chronic diarrhoea with or without:
iron deficiency anaemia,
hypoproteinaemic oedema
fat soluble vitamin deficiency.
• The older child with:
— growth failure
— chronic diarrhoea
— iron deficiency.
• Positive antibody screening (now the commonest form of assessment leading to diagnosis). Examples of antibodies used to screen when there is suspicion of coeliac disease include:
— antigliadin
— anti endomysial
— antitissue transglutaminase antibodies.

Antiendomysial and antitissue transglutaminase antibodies have sensitivity and specificity of greater than 95%. However, it is important to note that these are screening tests only.

The following are important points in the approach to the diagnosis of coeliac disease in childhood:
• Small bowel biopsy is mandatory for the diagnosis (Fig. 70.3).
• Small bowel biopsy should be performed while the patient is on an unrestricted diet.
• There is no place for an empirical trial of a gluten-free diet.
• Definitive diagnosis is important, as treatment is a life-long gluten-free diet.

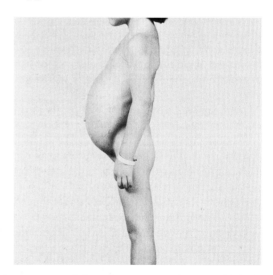

Fig. 70.2 Typical physical appearance of a young child with coeliac disease. Note the protuberant abdomen, buttock and shoulder girdle wasting and oedema of the lower limbs. Courtesy of Professor K. Gaskin.

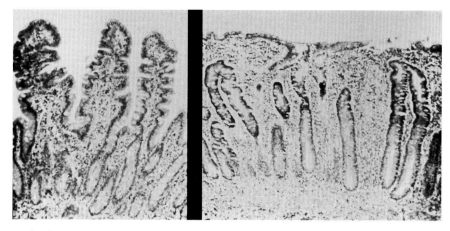

Fig. 70.3   Micrographs of normal intestine (left) demonstrating normal crypt villus structure, and coeliac disease (right) with marked crypt hyperplasia and villous atrophy.

A second biopsy can be undertaken to establish that the intestine has returned to normal on a restricted diet. If there is doubt about the diagnosis, a subsequent gluten challenge with repeat biopsy can be undertaken.

Enterocyte defect

Abetalipoproteinaemia is a recessively inherited defect in chylomicron assembly. Patients develop steatorrhoea early in life with:
- fat soluble vitamin deficiencies
- low serum cholesterol and triglycerides.

Small bowel biopsy reveals fat laden enterocytes.

Impaired lymphatic drainage

Obstructed lymphatics drainage prevents chylomicrons from migrating from the gut to the systemic circulation. The main cause is intestinal lymphangiectasia. This can lead to:
- fat malabsorption
- low serum cholesterol and triglycerides
- hypoproteinaemia and lymphopenia (loss of lymph into gut lumen)
- abnormal mucosal biopsy.

Other causes of reduced mucosal surface and reduced contact time

Miscellaneous inflammatory and surgical conditions can lead to loss of absorptive surface or reduced contact between chyme and the mucosa. Such conditions include:
- milk protein intolerance (severe)
- infections such as rotavirus infection
- severe immunodeficiency disorders
- autoimmune enteropathy

- short gut syndrome (surgical removal)
- motility disorders causing very rapid intestinal transit.

Watery diarrhoea

> **Clinical example**
>
> George is 9 years old. He presented with a 6 month history of intermittent bloating, abdominal pain and diarrhoea up to 6–7 times per day. He had lost 1 kg in weight in the past 2 months. He reported that dairy products such as milk and icecream made his symptoms worse. He had no past history of significant illness. George is the oldest son of Greek migrants. His mother reported that she cannot drink milk as it make her feel sick.
>
> On examination he was well looking. His weight was on the 50th percentile and his height was on the 10th percentile. There was no abdominal distension, organomegaly, signs of chronic liver disease or evidence of nutritional deficiency such as anaemia or peripheral oedema. Examination of his anus did not reveal any evidence of perianal disease.
>
> Investigations included a normal full blood count, differential white cell count and ESR. C reactive protein was <1 g/l. Lactose breath hydrogen measurement following oral ingestion of 50 g of lactose increased 100 parts per million above baseline levels within 60 minutes of ingestion of lactose (normal rise < 20 parts per million), indicating lactose intolerance.
>
> George was diagnosed as having lactose intolerance. His history suggests ontogenic lactase deficiency. This was confirmed by small bowel biopsy, which demonstrated normal morphology, and disaccharidase measurement, which revealed very low lactase activity but normal sucrase and maltase activities. Treatment is a low lactose diet.

Carbohydrate digestion and absorption

Dietary carbohydrates are primarily starch (polysaccharides, amylose and amylopectin), disaccharides (sucrose, in table sugar; lactose, in milk) and some monosaccharides such as fructose.

Starch polymers are large molecules composed of long chains of glucose. These chains are broken down by the action of salivary and pancreatic amylase which release a disaccharide (amylose), trisaccharide (maltotriose) and a series of branched oligosaccharides (alpha limit dextrins). These molecules are further digested by the brush border enzymes, sucrase-isomaltase and glucoamylase, to the monosaccharide glucose.

The disaccharides sucrose and lactose are metabolised by disaccharidases on the intestinal brush border. Sucrase breaks sucrose down to glucose and fructose and lactase breaks down lactose into glucose and galactose. Glucose and galactose are absorbed by the enterocyte sodium–glucose cotransporter (SGLT), which absorbs the monosaccharides in an energy dependent fashion. Fructose is absorbed by facilitated diffusion (non energy dependent) by the transporter termed GLUT-5.

Carbohydrate malabsorption

The presence of non absorbed osmotically active nutrients in the gut lumen results in osmotic retardation of water absorption, leading to watery diarrhoea. This is referred to as osmotic diarrhoea. Osmotically active compounds are usually low molecular weight compounds such as monosaccharides and disaccharides. Osmotic diarrhoea is usually due to maldigestion and/or malabsorption of carbohydrates but can be caused by the ingestion of laxatives such as sorbitol or $MgCl_2$. Unabsorbed carbohydrate present in the lumen of the large bowel is fermented to short chain fatty acids such as butyrate. This results in a highly acidic stool, which can cause perianal excoriation. The colon can absorb the anionic forms of these acids in exchange for bicarbonate, causing a mild hyperchloraemic acidosis.

While stating the obvious, it is important to appreciate that one cannot malabsorb a nutrient which has not been ingested. Thus it is useful to obtain a dietary history in patients suspected of osmotic diarrhoea. One needs to ascertain the nature of the carbohydrates being ingested, and in some instances the age of introduction of the carbohydrate, which can then be compared with the age of onset of symptoms. For example, the onset of osmotic diarrhoea commensurate with the introduction of fruit into the diet suggests the diagnosis of congenital sucrase-isomaltase deficiency.

Disaccharidase deficiencies and monosaccharide malabsorption

Congenital

Ontogenic lactase deficiency:
- occurs in most of the non Caucasian population of the world
- is dominantly inherited
- is physiological (due to the disappearance of lactase)
- presents in late childhood.

Ingesting lactose causes diarrhoea, bloating, excessive flatus and weight loss. Treatment is a low lactose diet.

Congenital sucrase–isomaltase deficiency is caused by inactivating mutations in the sucrase–isomaltase gene. These mutations:
- are recessively inherited
- lead to similar symptoms as for lactase deficiency with the ingestion of sucrose
- cause onset of symptoms at the time of weaning when fruit is introduced to the diet.

Treatment is a low sucrose diet.

Congenital monosaccharide malabsorption refers to defective glucose/galactose malabsorption. Features are:
- mutations in SGLT1
- recessively inherited
- present in the neonatal period.

Treatment is substitution of fructose for glucose–galactose.

Acquired

Except for ontogenic lactase deficiency, acquired disorders are much more common than inherited deficiencies. Lactase is more susceptible to injury than sucrase.

Causes of disaccharidase deficiencies include:
- viral gastroenteritis
- coeliac disease
- chronic giardiasis
- milk protein enteropathy
- small bowel bacterial overgrowth syndrome
- immunodeficiency disorders
- autoimmune enteropathy.

Monosaccharide transporters are less susceptible to injury because, unlike disaccharidase enzymes, they are deeply embedded in the brush border membrane. However, severe enteropathies can occasionally result in monosaccharide malabsorption. Examples include:
- congenital villous atrophy (which presents in newborns)
- severe postinfectious enteritis
- milk protein intolerance
- autoimmune enteropathy.

Monosaccharide malabsorption is life threatening and requires a level of care found only in tertiary paediatric centres. The treatment is to remove the offending carbohydrate from the diet and substitute an alternative. In acquired disorders, treatment may also be required for the primary mucosal disease.

Disorders of fluid and electrolyte transport

In the normal child approximately 5 litres (depending on size!) of fluid and electrolytes enters the upper gastrointestinal tract per day. One litre is ingested and the remaining volume is from normal secretions into the lumen. The majority of this fluid is absorbed before reaching the colon. Stool weights range from 75 to 150 g per day, of which approximately 75% is water. Small increases in stool water, as little as 30–40 ml/day are enough to produce diarrhoea.

Water is absorbed by osmosis through paracellular pathways in the mucosa. Electrolytes are absorbed by a variety of active transport or passive transport processes. Anions such as chloride and bicarbonate can be absorbed or actively secreted. This varies according to the region of small or large intestine. Regulation of gastrointestinal fluid and electrolyte transport is closely integrated by humoral and neural factors involved in fluid and electrolyte homeostasis. Abnormal fluid and electrolyte transport can be due to inherited defects in specific electrolyte transporters, but more commonly it is due to mucosal damage or inflammation.

Congenital

Congenital sodium diarrhoea and congenital chloride diarrhoea are rare inherited disorders of Na/H exchange and Cl/HCO exchange, respectively. They cause:
- diarrhoea in utero which results in polyhydramnios
- profuse diarrhoea, obvious from birth
- systemic electrolyte disturbances.

Acquired

Isolated water and salt malabsorption is very rare in childhood in the developed world. However, defective salt and water transport can contribute to diarrhoea in:
- disorders which damage or inflame the mucosa of small or large intestine
- bile salt malabsorption (bile acids irritate the colonic mucosa and act as potent stimulants of secretion).

Excessive salt and water loss in the stool may lead to dehydration and electrolyte disturbances. Treatment may require salt and water replacement in addition to treatment of the underlying disease.

Bloody diarrhoea

Chronic bloody diarrhoea is usually caused by inflammatory disorders of the colon such as:
- milk colitis in infants
- infections such as bacteria or parasites
- inflammatory bowel disease in older children. The two major forms are:
  — ulcerative colitis
  — Crohn disease

Blood is not always obvious in the stool. However, the presence of leucocytes on stool microscopy (Fig. 70.4) indicates the presence of colitis. Malabsorption of fluid and electrolytes by the inflamed colonic mucosa is a major factor contributing to diarrhoea. Malabsorption of nutrients is uncommon in milk colitis and inflammatory bowel disease. In contrast, excessive blood and protein loss from the inflamed intestinal mucosa can cause iron deficiency anaemia and hypoproteinaemic oedema. This is called protein losing enteropathy.

Nutrient malabsorption with little or no diarrhoea

Children present with symptoms and signs of nutrient deficiency with little or no accompanying diarrhoea. This is often due to dietary insufficiency, e.g. inadequate iron intake, but sometimes it can be due to malabsorption of the specific nutrient.

Vitamin B$_{12}$

Vitamin B$_{12}$ is ingested in animal protein and is liberated by pepsin in the stomach. In the stomach, the free vitamin B$_{12}$ binds to a binding protein (R protein) which has greater affinity for the vitamin than intrinsic factor (carrier protein). Intrinsic factor is produced by epithelial cells in the gastric mucosa. The vitamin B$_{12}$–R protein complex moves to the duodenum where trypsin cleaves the complex, releasing free vitamin B$_{12}$, which then binds to intrinsic factor. The intrinsic factor-vitamin B$_{12}$ complex moves to the ileum where it is absorbed into the enterocytes by carrier mediated transport. On entry into the enterocyte, vitamin B$_{12}$ is separated from intrinsic factor and subsequently exits the enterocyte into the circulation bound to transcobalamin, which carries the vitamin to sites distant from the intestine.

Both congenital and acquired disorders can lead to vitamin B$_{12}$ malabsorption.

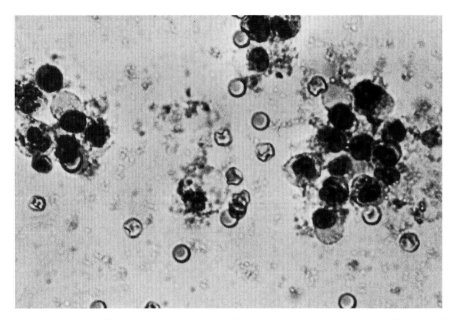

Fig. 70.4 Microscopic appearance of leucocytes in a stool smear. The large dark structures are polymorphonuclear leucocytes; the small round objects are red blood cells.

Clinical example

John is 9 months old. He presented with a 6 week history of poor weight gain, irritability and pallor. His mother was also concerned about his development. He was able to sit but could not pull himself to standing. His language had not progressed from babbling, which was in stark contrast to his older sibling who had several single words at this age. He had a poor appetite but no diarrhoea. He was originally breast fed and his mother ingested a normal diet during pregnancy and lactation.

On examination he was a pale irritable boy. He had moderate abdominal distension but no organomegaly. He could sit up unsupported but was mildly hypotonic and would not weight bear. There were no focal neurological signs.

Investigation results included: Hb of 65 g/l (normal 120–150) with a megaloblastic blood film, serum B_{12} 50 pmol/l (normal 120–600) and red blood cell folate 350 nmol/l (normal 200–1000). A Shilling test revealed urinary excretion of ingested radioactive vitamin B_{12} (after parenteral administration of a non radioactive flushing dose of 1 mg vitamin B_{12}) of 1% (normal > 8%), with no enhancement of urinary excretion with the addition of intrinsic factor.

John's Shilling test suggested a defect in the ileal vitamin B_{12} transporter, as the test was abnormal and did not recover with the addition of intrinsic factor. His age of presentation and lack of prior intestinal surgery suggest a congenital defect. His symptoms and megaloblastic anaemia corrected with administration of parenteral vitamin B_{12}.

Congenital disorders

Congenital defects in:
- ileal vitamin B_{12} transporter
- intrinsic factor
- transcobalamin

can lead to vitamin B_{12} malabsorption and deficiency. This usually presents in the second 6 months of life after the vitamin B_{12} accumulated during intrauterine life is exhausted.

Symptoms are due to megaloblastic anaemia and the central nervous system effects of deficiency. Babies born to vegan mothers (who ingest no animal product and thus can themselves be vitamin B_{12} deficient) and weaned on to a vegan diet can present with a similar picture, although usually in the first 6 months, as they are deficient from birth. Dietary history is important to differentiate between dietary deficiency and malabsorption.

Acquired disorders

Acquired disorders that lead to B_{12} malabsorption are:
- surgical resection of the ileum
- atrophic gastritis
- gastric surgery
- autoimmune pernicious anaemia (blocking antibodies to intrinsic factor)
- pancreatic insufficiency (failure to hydrolyse vitamin B_{12}–R protein)

- small bowel bacterial overgrowth (competition for vitamin B_{12} by bacteria).

Iron

Iron absorption occurs in the duodenum and proximal jejunum. An apical enterocyte carrier called the divalent metal cation transporter mediates uptake into the enterocyte. Iron is exported to the circulation via a basolateral process which has not yet been fully defined. In non breastfed children, only 5–10% of dietary iron is absorbed. The efficiency of iron absorption is greater in breastfed infants because the iron carrier, transferrin, is present in breast milk. Iron absorption is finely regulated at the level of the enterocyte so that absorption does not exceed requirements. Excessive iron accumulation can lead to multiple organ damage (haemochromatosis).

Iron deficiency is the commonest nutritional deficiency in humans and is usually due to:

- inadequate dietary intake
- excessive gastrointestinal blood loss (bleeding lesions or inflammation).

Inherited defects in iron uptake mechanisms leading to iron deficiency not responsive to oral iron have been described but have not yet been delineated at the molecular or genetic level.

Acquired disorders

Iron deficiency anaemia can occasionally be the primary presenting feature of small intestinal disease such as:

- coeliac disease
- milk protein intolerance
- Crohn disease.

Miscellaneous nutrients

Calcium. Calcium absorption occurs in the duodenum and proximal jejunum and is largely under the regulation of vitamin D:

- Hypocalcaemia can be associated with a wide variety of digestive disorders affecting intestinal calcium uptake or the biosynthesis and availability of Vitamin D (Ch. 67).
- It commonly presents with tetany of the fingers and occasionally seizures.

Zinc. Zinc is absorbed by the small intestine. Zinc deficiency can be due to:

- low breast milk zinc levels in solely breastfed infants
- an inherited defect in zinc absorption (acrodermatitis enteropathica)
- conditions associated with steatorrhoea
- intestinal inflammatory disorders.

Zinc deficiency can cause diarrhoea but the most dramatic manifestation is an erythematous scaly rash on the finger tips and around the perineum and mouth (Fig. 70.1).

Magnesium. Magnesium is absorbed in the proximal small intestine. Magnesium malabsorption leading to deficiency can be:

- inherited (primary hypomagnesaemia)
- secondary to other conditions leading to malabsorption.

Hypomagnesaemia causes similar symptoms to calcium deficiency.

Isolated protein malabsorption. Enterokinase deficiency:

- is a very rare disorder
- presents with diarrhoea, growth failure and severe hypoproteinaemia.

Amino acids. Defective amino acid absorption due to mutations in amino acid transporters can occur in:

- Hartnup disease
- cystinuria
- lysinuric protein intolerance.

These defects are rare disorders affecting amino acid transport in gut and kidney and in other organs in the last case. They do not have gastrointestinal symptoms and there are no nutritional consequences because of compensatory absorptive mechanisms for peptide and amino acid absorption.

Summary of the diagnostic approach to suspected malabsorption

Initial clinical assessment and stool examination will suggest the diagnosis in most children. Stool microscopy and measurement of stool reducing substances can be performed in the clinician's office and are readily available 'bedside' tests. If the diagnosis is not immediately obvious, the clinician will be in a position to investigate a limited differential list with simple and well directed diagnostic tests.

In patients with steatorrhoea the following will be useful but are not necessarily indicated for each patient:

- full blood count and differential white cell count
- serum triglycerides/cholesterol
- sweat test
- small bowel biopsy
- X ray of long bones.

In patients with carbohydrate maldigestion/ malabsorption the following might be indicated:

- breath hydrogen testing: challenge with the carbohydrate of interest (for example, lactose)

- small bowel biopsy/mucosal disaccharidase activities
- occasionally with monosaccharide malabsorption — inpatient dietary manipulation with close observation of stool output.

In patients with bloody diarrhoea (if stool cultures negative for pathogens) consider:
- gastroscopy and colonoscopy
- biopsy of small bowel and colon
- sometimes radiology looking for inflammatory bowel disease in jejunum/ileum.

Sometimes highly specialised investigations will be required to establish the diagnosis of some disorders:
- Measurement of micronutrients such as iron, zinc and calcium for suspected deficiency.
- Schilling test is required for the workup of vitamin B_{12} deficiency. Abnormally low urinary excretion of the ingested radioactive vitamin B_{12} indicates vitamin B_{12} malabsorption.
- Schilling test can be used to assess patients with bile salt malabsorption due to ileal resection.
- Specialised breath tests are used in the workup of bacterial overgrowth syndrome.
- Immunoglobulins and B and T cell subset determination for detection of immunodeficiency disorders.

Key learning points:

- Diagnosis is not by exclusion.
- A through history, physical examination and stool examination will suggest the diagnosis in most disorders.
- simple well directed investigations usually confirm the clinical diagnosis.
- there is no such thing as a 'malabsorption workup'.

Gastro-oesophageal reflux, and *Helicobacter pylori*

G. Davidson

This chapter introduces gastro-oesophageal reflux, a very common clinical problem in infants and children, and an infectious agent which colonises the stomach in more than 50% of the world's population. *Helicobacter pylori* is acquired in childhood but its disease manifestations usually do not occur until adulthood. It is also possible there may be a relationship between the two and this will be discussed.

Gastro-oesophageal reflux

Gastro-oesophageal reflux (GOR) can be defined as the spontaneous or involuntary passage of gastric content into the oesophagus. The origin of the gastric content can vary and includes saliva, ingested food and fluid, gastric secretions, and pancreatic or biliary secretions that have first been refluxed into the stomach (duodenogastric reflux). The difference between physiological reflux and gastro-oesophageal reflux disease (GORD) is often blurred by the anxiety engendered in parents, particularly first time parents, by symptoms such as vomiting and irritability. These symptoms, which often peak at 3–4 months of age, rarely lead to GORD and it is important to manage conservatively, particularly in an otherwise normal infant, so as not to label the condition as a disease state when in fact it is not. It is important to realise that about half of 3–4 month old infants will regurgitate or will occasionally vomit.

Pathophysiology (Table 71.1)

The main barrier to GOR is the pressure gradient across the lower oesophageal sphincter (LOS) which is formed by the intrinsic LOS (thickened smooth muscle of the lower oesophagus) and the extrinsic striated muscle of the crural diaphragm. Both components work together to generate LOS pressure, which can be measured by intraluminal manometry. The current understanding of LOS function suggests that a LOS pressure, of 5–10 mmHg above intragastric pressure is sufficient to maintain an antireflux barrier. Sphincter incompetence as a pathological mechanism for GORD is extremely unlikely. Transient lower oesophageal sphincter relaxation (TLOSR) is the major mechanism responsible for GOR in infants children and adults. A TLOSR is defined as an abrupt decrease in LOS pressure unrelated to swallowing

Table 71.1 Pathophysiological mechanisms of gastro-oesophageal reflux in infants, children and adolescents

- Delayed volume clearance
  - — Impaired primary or secondary peristalsis
  - — Reduced pressure wave amplitude

- Increased occurrence of GOR:
  - — Transient LOS relaxation
  - — Straining
  - — LOS sphincter hypotonia
  - — LOS pressure drift
- Delayed gastric emptying

Modified from Davidson GP, Omari TI 2001 Current Gastroenterology Reports 3: 257–262.

or oesophageal body peristalsis. TLOSRs are significantly longer in duration than swallow related sphincter relaxation and also have a lower nadir pressure. It is unclear at present whether GORD in children is characterised by either a higher rate of TLOSR or a greater incidence of GOR episodes during TLOSRs. Both have been noted in adults.

Abdominal straining

Abdominal straining which occurs frequently in infants probably exacerbates GOR only when there is simultaneous TLOSR, because both LOS tone and the crural diaphragm are inhibited. The neuroregulation of TLOSR is controlled via a vagovagal reflex. The afferent arm of the reflex is initiated by mechanoreceptors in the wall of the proximal stomach, and the efferent arm via a brainstem pattern generator. The presynaptic neurotransmitter is acetylcholine and the postsynaptic neurotransmitter is nitric oxide. Feeding is a potent stimulus for TLOSRs, evidenced by the fact that, in children with GORD, TLOSRs increase from 4 per hour in the fasting state to 8 per hour in the fed state.

Oesophageal body peristalsis

Assessment of oesophageal volume clearance is difficult because of the lack of defined motility criteria. Primary oesophageal body peristalsis following a swallow facilitates clearance. Secondary peristalsis is initiated by an abrupt sustained increase in intraoesophageal pressure that accompanies a reflux episode. The frequency of swallowing and type of pressure wave sequence propagated determine the effectiveness of volume clearance. While severe GORD with reflux oesophagitis is associated with a 30–50% decrease in pressure wave amplitude, this in itself may not impair bolus clearance.

Gastric emptying

The role of gastric emptying in the pathophysiology of GORD is not clear. Delayed gastric emptying may exacerbate GOR by prolonging gastric distension and increasing the frequency of TLOSR. However, attempts to correlate gastric emptying with acid GOR have been unsuccessful. While the final answer to this question awaits the development of more sophisticated investigative techniques, there are some children at the severe end of the GORD spectrum in whom delayed gastric emptying may be an issue, especially those with neurological or respiratory disease.

Clinical manifestations

There are many causes of regurgitation and vomiting in infants and children, both within the gastrointestinal tract and external to it. The more common causes are outlined in Table 71.2.

Regurgitation can be defined as effortless spilling of gastric content that is usually benign. Vomiting, on the other hand, is a forceful emptying of gastric content that should always be explained. The content of the vomitus is important because of the likely cause, as is the age at onset. Bile staining implies small bowel obstruction and should be examined immediately. Blood staining implies ulceration or gastritis.

Table 71.3 highlights the symptoms suggestive of GORD in infants and children. Symptoms do vary according to age. Infants more frequently regurgitate but can also have reflux related behaviours, which include apparent discomfort, yawning, stretching, stridor or mouthing. More serious complications include apnoea, acute life threatening events and recurrent chest disease secondary to aspiration.

Older children, usually over the age of 4 years, can describe common symptoms such as heartburn, chest pain and a sick or sour taste in the mouth, implying refluxate. Some younger children may complain of a hot feeling in the abdomen or throat.

GORD is a common problem in neurologically impaired children and, while regurgitation is the most likely symptom, problems such as recurrent chest disease, feeding difficulties and food refusal, anaemia, weight loss and behavioural changes can all masquerade as manifestations of GORD.

Table 71.2 Common causes of regurgitation and vomiting in infants and children

Gastrointestinal tract
Oesophagus
  Achalasia
  GOR
  Foreign body
  Congenital defects
Stomach
  Pyloric stenosis
  Peptic ulcer disease/gastritis
Duodenum
  Malrotation
  Duodenal ulcer
  Superior mesenteric artery syndrome
Small intestine/colon
  Infectious diarrhoea
  Intussusception
  Soy cow's milk protein intolerance
  Meconium ileus
  Inflammatory bowel disease
  Appendicitis
Other organs
  Hepatitis
  Gallbladder disease
  Pancreatitis

Extraintestinal disorders
Generalised sepsis
Rumination
Intoxications
Intracranial lesions, e.g. tumour, hydrocephalus
Adrenal insufficiency
Metabolic disorders

Diagnostic tests

There is no single test for the diagnosis of GOR. In most cases of physiological GOR diagnostic tests are not needed. If there are symptoms or signs of pathological reflux, such as pain, growth failure or respiratory symptoms, then further testing is required. The test used will depend on the age of the child, the type of tests available and the type and severity of symptoms. The most commonly used tests are outlined in Table 71.4.

Barium oesophagram

Most commonly used but least sensitive for the diagnosis of GOR. Useful for detecting structural abnormalities such as pyloric stenosis, malrotation and strictures, and may be useful to assess swallowing function or aspiration. Most useful in children with persistent vomiting.

Radionuclide scintigraphy

Radioactive 99Tc-sulphur colloid is added to an age appropriate meal and can be used as a direct measure of

Table 71.3   Symptoms suggestive of gastro-oesophageal reflux disease in infants and children

	Infants	Children
Vomiting		
Gastrointestinal	Feeding difficulties	Waterbrash
	Failure to thrive	Nausea
	Malnutrition	Dysphagia
	Cow's milk protein intolerance	
Respiratory	Cough, stridor	Chronic cough
	Cyanotic episodes	Aspiration pneumonia
	Bronchopulmonary dysplasia	Bronchiectasis
	Apnoea	
	Acute life threatening events	
Acid reflux		
Gastrointestinal	Apnoea, cyanotic episodes	Heartburn
	Colic, irritability	Oesophageal obstruction
	Sleep disturbance	Dysphagia, odynophagia
	Flexion patterns after feeds	Night walking
	Hiccoughs	Haematemesis
	Iron deficiency anaemia	Hoarseness
		Iron deficiency
Respiratory	Apnoea, cyanotic episodes	Chronic cough, asthma
	Stridor	
Neurobehavioural	Sandifer syndrome	
	Seizure-like events (?infantile spasms)	

Table 71.4   Commonly used diagnostic tests for GORD

- Barium oesophagram
- Radionuclide scintigraphy (milk scan)
- Upper gastrointestinal endoscopy and biopsies
- 24 hour intraoesophageal pH monitoring
- Oesophageal manometry

reflux. It can also be used to evaluate gastric emptying and to document aspiration due to reflux.

Upper gastrointestinal endoscopy and biopsies

Endoscopic examination of the upper gastrointestinal tract is indicated in GOR with complications such as chest or epigastric pain, heartburn, haematemesis or persistent unexplained iron deficiency.

Unlike adult medicine, oesophageal biopsies form an important part of the diagnostic strategy in GORD in children. They can support a reflux aetiology and exclude other less common causes of oesophagitis, such as cytomegalovirus and herpes simplex virus infections, candidiasis, Crohn disease or eosinophilic oesophagitis.

Twenty four hour intraoesophageal pH monitoring

This provides the most reliable assessment of oesophageal acid exposure. In the majority of infants with GOR, this test is not required and it should only be carried out if it will alter diagnosis, treatment or outcome. Current indications for its use are outlined in Table 71.5. While it can be considered to be the gold standard for determining whether GOR occurs or not, it is not the gold standard for determining whether GOR is causing symptoms or disease.

This is not a simple test and should be carried out in a specialist centre, as many factors need to be considered, including pretest preparation, medication, positioning, symptom assessment and analysis of results.

Oesophageal manometry

This is rarely needed clinically in the diagnosis of GOR in children but may be useful prior to fundoplication in children with a suspected motility disorder.

Diagnostic approach to GORD (Fig. 71.1)

The diagnostic approach depends largely on the severity of symptoms and the presence or absence of complications. In the otherwise healthy infant whose main symptoms are vomiting or regurgitation, parental reassurance is all that is required.

If symptoms persist despite simple therapy, a barium oesophagram should be carried out to exclude anatomical abnormalities.

Infants presenting with acid reflux related symptoms suggestive of oesophagitis require endoscopy and biopsies. In infants with atypical symptoms, the approach is more difficult but initially aspiration needs to be

Table 71.5   Current indications for 24 hour intraoesophageal pH monitoring

- Diagnose occult reflux in:
  - Unexplained recurrent pneumonia
  - Patients with bradycardia, apnoea
  - Non gastrointestinal symptoms caused by reflux, such as stridor, laryngeal symptoms, atypical chest pain, severe irritability
- Assessment of adequacy of medical therapy in cases of severe intractable GORD

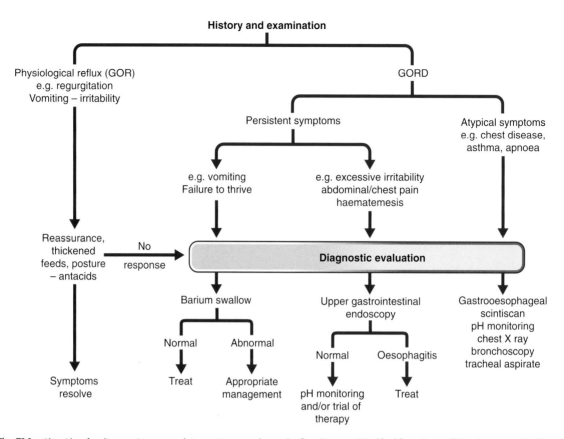

Fig. 71.1 Algorithm for diagnostic approach to gastro-oesophageal reflux disease. (Modified from Youssef NN, Orenstein SR. Clinical Perspectives in Gastroenterology Jan/Feb 2001: 11–17.)

Clinical example

Sophie, the 7 month old daughter of Greek parents, presented with a history of recurrent haematemesis, with bright and altered blood noted in regurgitated fluid and also dark stains on bibs and pillow. She was generally quite happy and thriving, although clinically a little pale. She did not have any evidence of abdominal tenderness.

In view of the recurrent bleeding and the possibility of oesophagitis or gastritis, an upper gastrointestinal endoscopy was carried out; this showed macroscopically an ulcerative oesophagitis but normal stomach and duodenum. She was treated with omeprazole 10 mg b.d. and after 4 weeks the bleeding had stopped clinically and the spilling had also decreased. A repeat endoscopy 8 weeks later showed macroscopic healing but still histological evidence of moderate oesophagitis. Sophie remained on omeprazole for a further 4 months, but following a trial off therapy her symptoms recurred and she underwent a Nissen fundoplication. When reviewed at age 2 years she was well and asymptomatic.

detect evidence of GOR but this does not prove the association. Presence of pepsin in a tracheal aspirate taken at bronchoscopy may be a useful adjunct but as yet remains unproven.

Treatment approach (Table 71.6)

The ideal therapy would include the use of a drug which specifically reduces the frequency of TLOSRs, but this is considered. Barium oesophagram, chest X ray and a gastro-oesophageal scintiscan may provide support for this diagnosis. Ambulatory 24 hour pH monitoring may

Table 71.6 Treatment approach to GORD

- General
  - Reassurance
  - Positioning
  - Thickened feeds

- Drug therapy
  - Acid suppression
  - Antacids
  - H_2 receptor antagonists
  - Proton pump inhibitors

- Continuous nasogastric feeds

- Surgery

currently not available. The prokinetic agent cisapride will not be discussed as it is no longer recommended for GORD due to cardiac toxicity.

General measures

These include reassurance, positioning and thickening feeds. The importance of reassurance in relation to the otherwise healthy infant cannot be overstated in order to avoid numerous dietary changes, unnecessary investigations and multiple drug therapies that are often recommended by others or are tried by parents. The only posture proven to be effective scientifically is the prone position, but the increased risk of sudden infant death syndrome (Ch. 13) has made this recommendation untenable. Feed thickening has been shown to reduce symptoms and there are now commercially available infant formulae which contain thickening compounds. The risk is that the attenuation of overt symptoms may mask complications of GORD.

Acid suppression

This is effective in reduction of symptoms due to acid irritation of the oesophagus: Acid suppressing agents are:

- Antacids. In infants with mild symptoms suggestive of heartburn such as irritability between feeds, a trial of 0.5–1 ml/kg/dose 3–6 times a day may be worthwhile. If this is not effective, do not persist with antacids.
- H_2 receptor antagonists. Ranitidine has proved the most effective, in doses often higher than used in adults. The dose recommended is 3 mg/kg three times a day.
- Proton pump inhibitors. These are the most potent acid suppressing agents and are used if acid related symptoms fail to respond to other therapies. They are often used as first line treatment where more complete acid suppression is required, for example in chronic respiratory disease, neurologically disabled children, and repaired tracheo-oesophageal fistula. Omeprazole has been most extensively studied and is used in doses ranging from 0.7 to 3.3 mg/kg/day.

Continuous feeding

Children with intractable vomiting and growth failure may respond to continuous nasogastric tube or gastrostomy feeding with catch up growth, and surgery may be avoided.

Surgery

The Nissen fundoplication is the most common surgical procedure and the indications are shown in Table 71.7. It can now be carried out laparoscopically in children. This may work, not by acting as a valve or increasing LOS pressure but by decreasing TLOSRs due to reduction in

Table 71.7   Indications for anti-reflux surgery in children

Absolute
Acute life threatening event or chronic lung disease due to aspiration
Severely neurologically impaired children
Continuing severe oesophagitis or oesophageal ulceration despite adequate therapy
Oesophageal stricture secondary to GOR
Intractable vomiting with growth failure secondary to GOR

Relative
Persistent symptoms with oesophagitis or growth failure
Severe asthma or respiratory disease unresponsive to therapy

the fundal surface area. Fundal distension is an important trigger for TLOSRs. This option needs very careful consideration in children because of the risk of complications and failure of effectiveness of surgery.

Summary

It is important to realise that only a small percentage of children with GOR go on to develop GORD. For most infants, symptoms resolve completely before age 2 years, and the majority show resolution by 12 months. It is equally important that those with continuing symptoms are recognised and treated effectively.

Helicobacter pylori infection in children

Helicobacter pylori is the commonest bacterial pathogen in humans, infecting more than 50% of the world's population. This infection (initially called *Campylobacter pylori*) was first described by Warren and Marshall in Perth, Australia in 1982, when they cultured the organism from the gastric antrum of adults with peptic ulcer disease. *H. pylori* as a paediatric infection is usually acquired in the first 2 years of life but the disease consequences rarely arise in childhood. In 1999, the North American Society for Pediatric Gastroenterology and Nutrition convened an expert group to develop evidence based guidelines on *H. pylori* infection in children to address the issues of diagnostic tests, when testing is indicated, treatment indications and appropriate therapeutic regimens.

Epidemiology

In developing countries, up to 80% of children are infected by age 2 years, with a lower prevalence in breastfed infants. A similar pattern is seen in children in lower socioeconomic groups in developed countries. In developed countries, only 10% of all children are infected by age 10 years. The route of transmission is probably similar to other enteric pathogens, being faecal–oral, oral–oral or gastric–oral. *H. pylori* has been detected in vomitus, saliva, faeces and on children's dummies, and also in contaminated water and food prepared with contaminated water. The house fly has also been implicated as a vector. The spread of infection within families is most likely from infected mother to child, although there is some evidence of sibling to sibling spread. Risk factors for *H pylori* infection in children are shown in Table 71.8.

The natural history of *H. pylori* infection in childhood remains obscure. A significant finding has been spontaneous clearing and reacquisition of gastric infections in preschool children, as spontaneous eradication does not appear to occur in adults.

H. pylori **associated disease**

General

In the past, gastric and duodenal ulcers in children have been described as primary or secondary. Secondary ulcers, which are more common in younger children (<10 years) are caused by systemic stresses, such as trauma, burns, septic shock, corticosteroids or non steroidal anti-inflammatory drugs. Primary ulcers, which usually occur in older children, give rise to symptoms similar to adults, with epigastric nocturnal abdominal pain and vomiting and often a positive family history of peptic ulceration. It is now clear in this group that the disease is due to *H. pylori* infection of gastric mucosa.

All H. pylori strains produce urease, which is thought to be important in the inflammatory reaction in the stomach and also in maintaining the ideal submucous environment for the organism. The urease reaction is also exploited in a number of diagnostic tests.

Genetic analysis of *H. pylori* has demonstrated strains with certain virulence factors, for example, vacuolating cytotoxin (Vac A), and cytotoxin associated genes (cag A, cag E). In adult ulcer disease there is a correlation between cag A positivity and peptic ulcer, but this is less clear in children. Recently a study has shown a strong correlation between disease severity and the cag E genotype in children.

Table 71.8	Risk factors for *H. pylori* infection
• Poor socioeconomic status
• Household crowding
• Ethnicity
• Migration from high prevalence areas
• Infected parent, particularly mother
• Contaminated water

Gastrointestinal infection (Table 71.9)

Gastritis. *H. pylori* colonisation of gastric mucosa in children is almost always associated with gastritis, which resolves with eradication of the organism. Endoscopy can be negative and biopsy is essential for diagnosis, although on occasions nodular antral hyperplasia can be seen and is diagnostic of infection.

Duodenal ulcer. *H. pylori* gastritis is found in 90% of children with duodenal ulcers. Ulcers heal faster if anti *H. pylori* therapy is given, compared with suppression alone. Importantly, ulcers do not recur if the infection is successfully eradicated.

Gastric ulcers. *H. pylori* infection as a cause of gastric ulcers is much less common in children than adults, probably reflecting the fact that the majority are secondary to systemic causes.

Gastric adenocarcinoma. The epidemiological association between *H. pylori* infection and gastric cancer has been judged by the WHO as sufficiently strong for it to classify *H. pylori* as the first bacterium to be a human carcinogen. *H. pylori* induced gastric cancer has not been reported in children.

Gastric lymphoma and MALT lymphoma. Seroepidemiological studies support an association between long standing *H. pylori* infection and lymphoma and mucosal associated lymphoid type (MALT) lymphomas. Eradication of *H. pylori* has resulted in regression of MALT lymphoma in some cases. Both these tumours are rare in children.

Recurrent abdominal pain In adults, a link between non ulcer dyspepsia (possibly the equivalent of recurrent abdominal pain in childhood) and *H. pylori* has been suggested by a recent meta-analysis of a large number of controlled studies in adults. A comparable study in children with recurrent abdominal pain does not support an association. The major problem with studies in children is the lack of a standardised validated reproducible

---

Table 71.9	Consequences of *H. pylori* Infection

Gastrointestinal
Gastritis
Duodenal ulcer
Gastric ulcer
Gastric adenocarcinoma
Gastric lymphoma and MALT lymphoma
Recurrent abdominal pain

Extragastric
Gastro-oesophageal reflux
Iron deficiency anaemia
Short stature

symptom assessment instrument. It is possible that there is a subset of children in whom *H. pylori* induced gastritis is responsible for recurrent abdominal pain, but more information is required.

Extragastric disease

Gastro-oesophageal reflux. It is postulated that certain *H. pylori* strains cause decreased acid production and atrophic gastritis, and that with eradication of *H. pylori* acid rebound occurs, causing GOR disease. This is still a controversial area in adults and there is very little supporting evidence in children.

Iron deficiency/growth stunting. Iron deficiency has been described in growth retarded adolescents with *H. pylori* infection. Eradication of *H. pylori* infection corrected the deficiency and led to growth improvement.

Diagnostic tests (Table 71.10)

The ideal test for *H. pylori* infection does not exist, but it should be non or minimally invasive, accurate, inexpensive, readily available and able to discriminate between past and present infection.

Endoscopy and biopsy is the only method that can provide evidence of disease activity such as gastritis or an ulcer. Urease testing of biopsy material gives indirect identification of infection but has only a 50% positive predictive value in children.

The urea breath test is currently the best non invasive test. It has a greater than 95% positive and negative predictive value for *H. pylori* infection. The principle of the test is outlined in Figure 71.2. Urea can be labelled with either radioactive ^{14}C or stable isotope ^{13}C. In children and women of child bearing age ^{13}C-urea is recommended.

Serology, while commercially available, is frequently unreliable and cannot distinguish between past and present infection. All the other non invasive tests are still under trial or are not sufficiently sensitive.

The aim of testing is not to detect the presence of infection but to find the cause of clinical symptoms, and

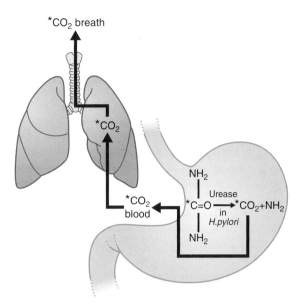

Fig. 71.2 The principle of the $^{13/14}$C-urea breath test.

therefore the important question is who should be tested (Table 71.11).

Treatment

The discovery of *H. pylori* as the cause of primary peptic ulceration and gastric ulcers has changed their management, as eradication of the organism cures the disease and prevents recurrence. If endoscopy is indicated to investigate organic disease and *H. pylori* is found, the child should receive treatment (Table 71.12); however, if no ulcer is found the patient/parents should be informed that *H. pylori* eradication may not relieve the symptoms.

Table 71.11 Those who should be tested for *H. pylori* infection

Yes
Endoscopic/radiologically proven gastric or duodenal ulcers
Confirmation of eradication of *H. pylori* infection

No
Recurrent abdominal pain without ulcer disease
Asymptomatic children
Children in families with history of gastric cancer of ulcer
disease

Table 71.10 Diagnostic Tests for *H. pylori*

Endoscopic
Biopsy and histology
Rapid urease test
Bacterial culture

Indirect tests
Serum antibody (IgA, IgG)
Saliva antibody
Urine antibody
Stool culture/stool antigen
Urea breath test

Table 71.12 Who should be treated for *H. pylori* infection

- Histologically proven infection with gastrointestinal symptoms
- Duodenal/gastric ulcers
- Lymphoma
- Atrophic gastritis with intestinal metaplasia

Clinical example

A 10 year old Vietnamese child, Than, who has resided in Australia since birth, presents with a long history of recurrent epigastric pain that wakes him from his sleep at night. His appetite is described as poor. There is a family history of peptic ulcer disease. Examination reveals a thin child on the 3rd percentile for weight and 25th centile for height. Epigastric tenderness was present. The signs and symptoms suggested peptic ulcer disease and at endoscopy antral nodular hyperplastic gastritis was noted, as well as an ulcer in the first part of the duodenum. Histology showed evidence of *H. pylori* infection. Treatment with triple therapy (clarithromycin, amoxycillin and omeprazole) for 1 week led to resolution of symptoms within 4 weeks. Six weeks after stopping therapy a ^{13}C-urea breath test was carried out and was negative, confirming eradication. At review 12 months later Than was well and his height and weight were on the 25th percentile.

The traditional treatments do not eradicate *H. pylori* infection and current treatment in children advocates a combined regimen using two antibiotics and a proton pump inhibitor, based on adult treatment regimens. At present there are no published peer reviewed controlled studies of treatment regimens in children.

The currently recommended first line treatment is a combination of a proton pump inhibitor, clarithromycin and amoxycillin twice daily for 7 days. Metronidazole can be substituted for either amoxycillin or clarithromycin but there is a high resistance to this drug and its use may lead to treatment failure. Failure of eradication leads to the use of second line options, which usually include bismuth subsalicylate in a triple or quadruple therapy regimen.

The burden of illness caused by *H. pylori* is considerable, making the development of a prophylactic vaccine to prevent infection or a therapeutic vaccine to eliminate existing infection desirable but to date no vaccine is available.

Liver diseases in childhood 72

D. Forbes

Compared with many other childhood problems, liver disease is infrequent beyond the newborn period; however, it is important because early recognition and diagnosis can be critical to the outcome of some disorders, and because chronic liver disease carries a high burden of disability for children and their families.

The liver has a central role in:
- intermediary metabolism and homeostasis
- synthesis of proteins
- bile acid metabolism
- bilirubin metabolism (uptake, conjugation and excretion)
- detoxification reactions.

Liver disease disturbs these processes, resulting in one or more of the following problems:
- abnormalities of liver size and consistency (an enlarged or firm liver)
- jaundice
- hepatitis (jaundice and/or elevation of liver transaminases)
- liver failure:
  — failure of synthetic function (bleeding or oedema)
  — failure of detoxification and waste elimination (encephalopathy)
- obstruction to blood flow through the portal system (portal hypertension).

Features that help us understand the nature of liver problems include:
- dark urine (excretion of bilirubin and urobilinogen in urine)
- pale stools (with biliary obstruction or severe impairment of hepatic function)
- tender liver (liver capsule stretched)
- hard liver (chronic liver disease with cirrhosis)
- splenic enlargement (in portal hypertension)
- bruising and bleeding (failure of synthesis of coagulant proteins)
- oedema and ascites (failure of albumin synthesis).

Liver size is proportional to body weight (rather than height), and increases during childhood. The physical findings of liver examination and the landmarks of the liver change during childhood. Liver size is best determined by percussing the upper border of the liver, usually at the fifth intercostal space in the midclavicular line anteriorly, and gently palpating up from the right lower quadrant to determine the liver edge, and then measuring the 'span' between the upper and lower borders in the midclavicular line.

Table 72.1 Liver span (cm) during childhood

Age	Mean	Range
Birth	5.5	4–7
1 year	6	5.5–7
2 years	6.5	6–8
3 years	7	6–9
4 years	7.5	6–9
5 years	8	6–9
12 years	9	7–11

Overly firm palpation may make it difficult to palpate the liver edge. The normal liver span at different ages is shown in Table 72.1. During infancy the liver usually is palpable 2–4 cm below the costal margin. Variants in liver shape that make the liver seem enlarged include a prominent Riedel lobe, felt well below the right costal margin, and a prominent left lobe of liver felt in the epigastrium. The normal liver is soft and the surface is smooth and yielding. The consistency of the liver frequently changes when it is abnormal, generally becoming harder.

The liver enlarges through the accumulation of additional tissue or fluid because of:
- inflammation
- infiltration
- storage
- congestion.

Causes of liver enlargement are shown in Table 72.2.

Jaundice

Jaundice occurs because of failure of the liver to excrete the bilirubin load owing to:
- excess bilirubin load due to haemolysis
- deficiency of conjugating enzymes
- secretory defect
- obstruction of the biliary tree
- damage to liver cells with leakage of bilirubin into the circulation.

Jaundice in infancy

Jaundice is very common in newborn infants. Up to 50% of Caucasian babies will become jaundiced, and even

Table 72.2	Causes of hepatomegaly

Inflammation
Infectious hepatitis
Autoimmune hepatitis
Drug reactions

Infiltration
Primary neoplastic liver cancers
Primary non neoplastic liver cancers
Secondary liver cancers: leukaemia, lymphoma, neuroblastoma

Storage
Glycogen storage disorders
Lipid storage disorders
Steatohepatitis: obesity, steroids, diabetes mellitus, starvation

Vascular congestion
Congestive heart failure
Pericardial disease
Hepatic vein thrombosis

higher proportions of Asian babies may be jaundiced in the first weeks of life.

Physiological jaundice usually develops after the first 24 hours of life and by the fourth day of life and resolves by 10–14 days of age. It is discussed in Chapter 33. Jaundice requires further investigation when it:
- develops within the first 24 hours of life
- is severe
- is associated with fever or other symptoms of systemic illness
- persists beyond the first 2 weeks of life.

The first step is to differentiate between conjugated and unconjugated hyperbilirubinaemia by measuring the total bilirubin level and the conjugated fraction. Most newborn babies will have unconjugated hyperbilirubinaemia. Non physiological causes of an elevation of unconjugated bilirubin include:
- breast milk jaundice
- haemolysis
- duodenal atresia
- pyloric stenosis
- hypothyroidism
- conjugating enzyme deficiency syndromes.

Breast milk jaundice. Elevation of unconjugated bilirubin associated with breast feeding is common, occurring once in every 50–200 breastfed infants. It is a benign disorder recognised by:
- jaundice persisting beyond 2 weeks of life
- a thriving healthy baby
- no evidence of other disease
- resolution of jaundice with temporary interruption of breast feeding.

Conjugated hyperbilirubinaemia occurs with
- obstruction to bile flow in intrahepatic or extrahepatic ducts
- liver cell damage (hepatitis).

It is considered to be present if greater than 20% of the total bilirubin level is conjugated. It may develop soon after birth, but may also manifest later in infancy after dietary change exposes a metabolic defect. Every infant with jaundice persisting beyond the first 2 weeks of life should have the conjugated fraction of their bilirubin determined.

Bile duct obstruction and hepatitis in this age group are difficult to differentiate because of overlap of the disease processes and clinical features. It is useful, however, to attempt to differentiate these clinical syndromes and identify infants who have treatable disease: obstruction of the large ducts, infections and metabolic diseases. Early recognition and treatment is necessary for satisfactory outcome of these diseases. The clinical approach requires recognition of features suggesting neonatal hepatitis or bile duct obstruction (Table 72.3) and the application of general and then specific tests leading to a diagnosis.

Tests used to distinguish biliary obstruction from neonatal hepatitis include:
- ultrasound examination of the biliary tree to identify dilatation of extrahepatic ducts
- iminodiacetic acid isotope scanning to demonstrate bile flow or obstruction
- liver biopsy to identify characteristic features of hepatitis or cholestasis syndromes
- operative cholangiogram to document the patency of extrahepatic biliary structures.

Most of the identifiable causes of neonatal hepatitis syndrome and cholestatic syndromes are rare (Table 72.4). The major clinical issue is differentiation of idiopathic neonatal hepatitis from biliary atresia.

The outcome for neonatal hepatitis syndromes varies greatly, depending upon the specific cause. Idiopathic neonatal hepatitis and many infections have a good prognosis for spontaneous and complete recovery. Extrahepatic biliary atresia is treated surgically. Infants with biliary

Table 72.3	Clinical features of biliary obstruction and neonatal hepatitis syndromes	
	Neonatal hepatitis	Biliary obstruction
Growth	Often impaired	Usually normal
Wellbeing	Often sickly	Usually well
Pale stools	Variable	Usual
Dysmorphic features	Common	May occur
Synthetic function	Often impaired	Preserved until late
Hypoglycaemia	Common	Uncommon

Table 72.4   Causes of conjugated hyperbilirubinaemia in infancy

Biliary obstruction syndromes in infancy
Surgical obstruction of large extrahepatic ducts
Choledochal cyst
Extrahepatic biliary atresia
Spontaneous perforation of the common bile duct
Paucity of intrahepatic ducts
  Alagille syndrome
  Non syndromic paucity of intrahepatic ducts

Neonatal hepatitis syndromes in infancy
Infections
  Bacterial
    Listeria
    Escherichia coli
    Syphilis
  Protozoan
    Toxoplasmosis
  Viral
    Cytomegalovirus
    Rubella
    Parvovirus
    Herpesvirus
    Coxsackie virus
    Echovirus family
    Hepatitis B virus
Metabolic disorders
  α-1-Antitrypsin deficiency
  Cystic fibrosis
  Carbohydrate metabolic defects
    Galactosaemia
    Fructosaemia
    Glycogen storage disorder type IV
  Amino acid metabolic defects
    Tyrosinaemia
  Lipid metabolic defects
    Cholesterol ester storage disease
    Wolman disease
    Gaucher disease
    Niemann–Pick disease
  Disorders of bile acid metabolism
Endocrine disorders
  Hypopituitarism
  Hypothyroidism
Chromosomal disorders
Toxic disorders
  Parenteral nutrition
Idiopathic neonatal hepatitis

Clinical example

Sarah was a healthy fullterm breastfed infant who was jaundiced at the third day of life, but completely recovered by the eighth day of life. She gained weight normally. She again became jaundiced at 4 weeks of age. The jaundice increased and she started passing dark urine and had intermittent but increasingly pale stools. When seen at 7 weeks of age she looked healthy but was deeply jaundiced. Her liver was firm and had a span of 7 cm. Blood tests revealed that her bilirubin was elevated at 240 μmol/l with a conjugated fraction of 190 μmol/l, her alanine aminotransferase was 210 μmol/l, her gamma glutamyl transpeptidase was 148 μmol/l and albumin 30 g/l. At ultrasound it was not possible to visualise the gallbladder or the common bile duct. A liver biopsy demonstrated bilirubin plugs, and bile duct proliferation together with inflammation of the hepatic parenchyma. A radioisotope DESIDA scan showed no excretion.

These findings were suggestive of biliary atresia and so an operative cholangiogram was undertaken, with injection of contrast into the small atretic gallbladder found at laparotomy. This showed some dilatation of intrahepatic biliary ducts but no excretion of contrast via the common bile duct. The surgeon therefore proceeded to a portoenterostomy (Kasai procedure). Within a week of surgery Sarah had some pigmented stools, indicating that some biliary flow had been established.

usually have a conjugated hyperbilirubinaemia, and often manifest all the features of liver failure: jaundice, bleeding, oedema and encephalopathy (drowsiness, irritability, deteriorating mental function, convulsions). They require urgent assessment, and frequently urgent treatment is provided on the basis of a presumed diagnosis, pending confirmation by specific tests.

Jaundice in older children

Jaundice occurs in children because of:
• hepatitis (liver inflammation)
• biliary duct obstruction.

Table 72.5   The acutely ill jaundiced baby

Infections	Metabolic disorders
E. coli bacteraemia	Mitochondrial disorders
Echovirus	Galactosaemia
Coxsackie virus	α-1-Antitrypsin deficiency
Cytomegalovirus	Organic acidaemias
Adenovirus	Tyrosinaemia
Herpes simplex virus	Urea cycle defects
Parvovirus	Fatty acid oxidation defect
	Reye syndrome
	Neonatal iron storage disorder

atresia who are treated within the first 60 days of life have a much greater potential for establishing bile flow and restoring liver function than infants who are treated after this time. Late treatment frequently results in biliary cirrhosis and progressive liver failure.

The acutely ill, jaundiced infant should be considered differently from infants with biliary duct obstruction or neonatal hepatitis syndromes, as these babies are likely to have a metabolic defect or an infection (Table 72.5). They

Most older children who develop hepatitis have an infectious illness, but autoimmune and metabolic disorders may also be the cause (Table 72.6).

The apparent length of history of jaundice or other symptoms is often not a reliable guide to the duration of liver disease, and children with a short history may in fact have longstanding liver problems. Because of limited opportunities for effective treatment of some liver disease it is very important to establish a diagnosis for all children who develop hepatitis.

Chronic liver disease should be suspected in any child who has persistent elevation of liver enzymes 3 months or more after a presumed acute infection. Hepatitis in these circumstances is likely to be associated with progressive liver damage.

Chronic liver disease is identified by clinical features in both history and examination:

History

- Recurrent hepatitis
- Prolonged jaundice
- Lethargy
- Anorexia
- Bruising
- Pruritus
- Poor growth.

Examination

- Muscle wasting
- Poor growth

Table 72.6 Hepatitis in older children

Infections
Hepatitis A
Hepatitis B
Hepatitis C
Hepatitis D (Delta agent: coinfection with hepatitis B)
Hepatitis E
Hepatitis G
Infectious mononucleosis/Epstein–Barr virus
Cytomegalovirus
Herpesvirus
Parvovirus

Autoimmune disease
Autoimmune hepatitis
Sclerosing cholangitis

Metabolic disease
α-1-Antitrypsin deficiency
Hereditary fructose intolerance
Tyrosinaemia
Wilson disease
Cystic fibrosis
Reye syndrome

- Clubbing
- Spider naevi
- Oedema
- Hard liver
- Splenomegaly
- Ascites.

Evidence of liver fibrosis and cirrhosis may be documented on ultrasound, and confirmed with liver biopsy and histology.

The clinical features of infectious hepatitis depend upon the age of the child, as well as the specific infectious agent. Younger children may remain asymptomatic despite evidence of significant hepatitis, but as children get older they are more likely to have symptoms of nausea, lethargy, fever, vomiting and abdominal pain. A small proportion of children with hepatitis from any cause may develop rapidly progressive, severe hepatitis, known as fulminant hepatitis, which will result in some deaths.

In Australia and New Zealand most children with acute hepatitis will have an acute viral infection. Typically they are jaundiced, have a tender enlarged liver and variable splenic enlargement. They have elevation of their liver transaminase enzymes (alanine aminotransferase, aspartate aminotransferase) and gamma glutamyl transpeptidase, and elevation of serum bilirubin (usually). The urine contains bilirubin and urobilinogen.

Hepatitis A

The commonest cause of hepatitis, hepatitis A typically:
- is spread by orofaecal transmission
- has an incubation period of around 30 days
- causes an acute illness with malaise, nausea, vomiting and diarrhoea
- is associated with examination findings of jaundice, dark urine and an enlarged, tender liver.

Hepatitis A virus excretion in faeces occurs prior to the onset of jaundice. Complete recovery from infection is usual, although a small proportion of children will develop fulminant hepatitis. Immunity develops following infection, and may be stimulated in unexposed individuals with hepatitis A vaccine, an inactivated virus vaccine. Recent infection can be confirmed by a rise in antihepatitis A virus IgM antibody, and immunity by the presence of specific IgG antibodies.

Hepatitis B

Infection with hepatitis A virus (HBV) is a worldwide problem that is more frequent among socially disadvantaged groups and those Australian and New Zealand children who come from Pacific Island, Asian and African backgrounds. Transmission occurs via body fluids, and vertical transmission from mother to baby readily occurs.

Hepatitis B infection can result in an acute hepatitis, but the majority of acute infections are asymptomatic.

HBV is a DNA-containing hepadnavirus with distinct surface and core proteins which act as antigens. Infection is confirmed by the presence in serum of these antigens. Antibody to these proteins indicates development of immunity. HBV surface antigen (HBsAg) is the first antigen detectable after exposure and persists until recovery occurs. HBV e antigen (HBeAg) also appears in the acute phase of the infection and is indicative of a high viral load and high infectivity (up to 80% of infants of HbeAg positive mothers will acquire hepatitis B infection). The response of the infected host is initially an anticore antibody (HbcAb), and subsequently HbeAb and HbsAb.

Chronic HBV infection is most likely to occur with perinatal infection. Infection is usually not recognised at the time, and may only be identified when the child is found to have elevated liver enzymes at a later date. It may also present as an arteritis, arthritis or nephritis. It carries increased risks of cirrhosis and hepatocellular carcinoma later in life.

Passive immunisation against hepatitis B using immunoglobulin rich in antihepatitis B antibodies should be initiated at the time of exposure (such as at birth). Active immunisation should be undertaken in all high risk groups. HBV immunisation has recently become a part of routine immunisation programmes in Australia (Ch. 8).

Treatment of chronic HBV infection is indicated in children with persistent elevation of liver enzymes, carriage of HBV antigens and DNA, and who have biopsy evidence of chronic hepatitis. Treatment is undertaken with alpha interferon or lamivudine for 4–6 months.

> ### Clinical example
>
> Claire is a 4 year old girl, adopted in Korea in infancy. She is well but during a recent febrile illness she had elevation of her transaminases and was subsequently found to be positive for HBsAg and HBeAg. Physical examination was normal. She was not immunised against hepatitis B in the newborn period. Claire is a chronic, asymptomatic carrier of hepatitis B, almost certainly infected in the perinatal period, and is at risk of chronic hepatitis and hepatocellular carcinoma. Hepatitis B can be transmitted to other children and so immunisation of all children in her school group is encouraged.

Hepatitis C

The hepatitis C virus (HCV) is an RNA containing virus that often causes chronic infection. Children acquire HCV infection via blood transfusions, from their mother at or around birth, and in a number from other as yet unknown sources. Children who have received multiple blood product infusions because of thalassaemia, cancer or haemophilia are at increased risk of HCV infection. Shared needles are an important source of infection in drug using populations. A high proportion of infected children will develop chronic liver disease. HCV infection should be suspected in high risk individuals who have elevated transaminases, and can be confirmed by detection of HCV antibody or HCV RNA. Children who have progressive liver disease may be treated with alpha interferon, although the best approach to treatment is still not known.

Hepatitis D

This is a 'superinfection' which occurs in association with HBV and is likely to be recognised as very severe or aggressive hepatitis B infection.

Hepatitis E

This infection resembles hepatitis A, but usually affects adolescents and adults rather than children. Serological tests for hepatitis E are not routinely available in Australia.

Autoimmune hepatitis

This can occur at any age, although it is more likely to occur in the older child and adolescent than in infancy, and can be confined to the liver or be part of a systemic autoimmune illness. It may be triggered by viral infections, or drugs, but commonly has no identifiable

> ### Clinical example
>
> Elizabeth is an 8 year old girl who was seen by her general practitioner because of recurrent hives. She was found to have elevated immunoglobulin concentrations, and then elevation of her transaminases (alanine aminotransferase 320 units/l and aspartate aminotransferase 250 units/l). Screening for α-1-antitrypsin deficiency, Wilson disease, hepatitis B and C was negative, but she had elevated anti-liver–kidney microsomal antibody. A liver biopsy showed evidence of active inflammation with piecemeal necrosis, and fibrosis. A diagnosis of autoimmune hepatitis was made and she was commenced on prednisolone, 2 mg/kg/day, which was tapered to a lower dose over 3 months. There was an initial decrease in the levels of transaminases, but these rebounded when the steroid dose was decreased. Azathioprine 1 mg/kg/day was added to her therapy, with subsequent normalisation of transaminases. A follow up liver biopsy showed a marked decrease in the inflammatory infiltrate and no progression of fibrosis. Attempts at withdrawing therapy after 2 years resulted in an increase in liver transaminases.

antecedents. Girls are affected more commonly than boys. The onset is frequently insidious, and often comes to light with vague non specific symptoms or with elevated liver enzymes. Different types can be identified, based upon the pattern of auto antibodies:

- type 1: antinuclear antibody and antismooth muscle antibody
- type 2: anti-liver–kidney microsomal antibody
- type 3: anti-soluble liver antigen antibody.

Treatment involves immunosuppression, usually with steroids and another immunomodulator, such as azathioprine or cyclosporin, often for prolonged periods of time. Liver transplantation is utilised in children with progressive, chronic liver disease that results in liver failure.

α-1-Antitrypsin deficiency

This disorder is commonly identified as a cause of neonatal hepatitis, but may present at any stage of life with elevated liver enzymes, jaundice or advanced liver disease. It is due to a gene mutation that results in dysfunctional protease inhibitors in the liver and lung, leading to hepatitis and emphysema. Associated hepatitis eventually leads to cirrhosis.

Clinical example

Samuel became jaundiced at about 4 weeks of age. He was otherwise well, was breastfeeding and was gaining weight. His stools were normally pigmented, but he had dark urine. His bilirubin was 180 μmol/l with a conjugated fraction of 120 μmol/l. His alanine aminotransferase was 260 units/l. Because he had a conjugated hyperbilirubinaemia with evidence of hepatitis he had serological testing for viral infections (negative), urine testing for non glucose reducing sugars (negative, making galactosaemia unlikely), a urine microscopy and culture, measurement of serum α-1-antitrypsin (very low) and Pi type (ZZ). An ultrasound of his biliary tree showed normal gallbladder and no evidence of duct dilatation. A liver biopsy revealed a giant cell hepatitis with accumulation of bilirubin plugs within bile ducts and accumulation of α-1-antitrypsin granules within the liver cells. A diagnosis of neonatal hepatitis due to α-1-antitrypsin deficiency was established. He was commenced on ursodeoxycholic acid to promote bile flow, plus the fat soluble vitamins A, E and K. His jaundice gradually cleared and he grew satisfactorily during early childhood, although his transaminases never returned to normal. In middle childhood he developed easy bruising and prolongation of his prothrombin time, hypoalbuminaemia, muscle wasting and oedema. He received a liver transplant when he was aged 8 years, and remains well, although on long term immunosuppression.

Wilson disease

This disease arises due to failure of copper excretion into the bile, secondary to a defect in a transport protein. The disorder leads to accumulation of copper in the liver, brain, kidneys and bone. Liver disease typically becomes apparent in late childhood as hepatitis, portal hypertension or liver failure. Patients usually have so called Kayser–Fleischer rings of copper accumulation in the peripheral cornea by the time they manifest liver disease. Diagnosis is established by demonstrating low plasma caeruloplasmin (a copper containing protein), increased urinary copper excretion and increased liver copper. Although this disorder is uncommon, recognition of Wilson disease is important because it is a treatable cause of chronic liver disease and will often present in childhood. Treatment is with a low copper diet and long term penicillamine, which increases the urinary excretion of copper.

Hepatitis, or liver inflammation, is typically recognised because of the development of jaundice, but asymptomatic children may be found to have elevated liver enzymes, and can have any of the disease processes discussed above.

It is important to remember that jaundice in older children may also be due to obstruction of biliary ducts due to:

- a choledochal cyst
- congenital abnormalities of the biliary tree
- gallstones
- parasites.

These children may have features of hepatitis, but may also present with pale stools, dark urine and abdominal pain. They need assessment with liver biochemistry to determine whether they have elevation of alkaline phosphatase and gamma glutamyl transpeptidase out of proportion to elevation of their transamimases. Imaging with ultrasound, computed tomography or magnetic resonance imaging is necessary to define the anatomy of the biliary ducts.

Liver failure

This is the end result of failure of the metabolic and synthetic functions of the liver. The clinical features of liver failure are relatively common for all causes at different ages. Jaundice may not be seen until late in the course of liver failure. The earliest evidence is usually failing production of the vitamin K dependent clotting factors resulting in prolongation of the prothrombin time and, eventually, easy bruising and bleeding. Oedema due to hypoalbuminaemia is generally a late feature of liver disease. Encephalopathy is a late effect of failure of elimination of neurotoxic factors. It may be subtle initially, with drowsiness and then later confusion and tremor.

Portal hypertension

Portal hypertension develops because of increased resistance to blood flow through the portal venous system, resulting in distension of the portal vasculature and oesophageal, gastric or perianal varices, splenic enlargement, neutropenia and thrombocytopenia. Portal hypertension occurs with liver disease with cirrhosis, but, in up to one third of cases, with portal vein obstruction in the absence of liver disease. These cases probably arise after neonatal portal venous thrombosis. Portal hypertension should be suspected in children with splenomegaly, especially if associated with thrombocytopenia, and in any child who has a significant haematemesis. Uncomplicated portal hypertension does not require intervention, but children should be kept under surveillance, and should avoid aspirin or other factors likely to increase the risk of bleeding. Underlying liver disease should be treated in those children who have cirrhosis.

Variceal haemorrhage is a medical emergency treated with resuscitation and then control of haemorrhage by decreasing portal blood flow with vasopressin or octreotide or with local compression. Endoscopic injection or banding of varices is frequently required to control bleeding and prevent further bleeding. Following variceal bleeding, consideration should be given to lowering portal blood pressure with propranolol or by the surgical creation of a 'shunt'.

Treatment

Treatment of chronic liver disease is aimed at anticipating and treating the complications of malnutrition and deficiency of energy and fat soluble vitamins, failure of protein synthesis, portal hypertension and encephalopathy for as long as possible. This involves treatment of the following components:

- malnutrition
  - increased dietary energy with food and special supplements
  - supplementation with vitamins A, D, E and K
- ascites
  - diuretics such as spironolactone or frusemide
  - albumen infusions
- portal hypertension
  - monitoring of white blood cells and platelets
  - lowering of portal blood pressure with beta blockers.

Liver transplantation is life saving in children with acute or chronic, irreversible end stage liver failure, evidenced by coagulopathy, hypoalbuminaemia, encephalopathy and variceal haemorrhage. The commonest problems leading to paediatric liver transplantation are biliary atresia, α-1-antitrypsin deficiency and other rarer metabolic disorders, chronic autoimmune hepatitis and fulminant hepatitis secondary to paracetamol toxicity, or infections. Three quarters of children undergoing liver transplantation will survive at least 4 years, the majority leading healthy lives. They generally need to take immunosuppressive therapy for life.

PART 20   SELF-ASSESSMENT

Questions

1. **James, a 3 month old infant, presents with vomiting since the first week of life. The vomiting occurs daily, is usually small in amount, but occasionally is projectile. Physical examination reveals a happy infant who is thriving well. The breathing is noisy and an occasional cough is heard. You would:**
   (A) Palpate for a pyloric tumour and, if no tumour was felt, order a barium study
   (B) Order a barium study to diagnose gastro-oesophageal reflux
   (C) Nurse the infant with the head elevated to 60° and thicken the feed
   (D) Obtain a chest X-ray

2. **Tracey had features of Down syndrome at birth, which was uncomplicated. At 12 hours, she had several vomits which stained the clothing a green colour. On examination, features of Down syndrome were present; the abdomen was not distended, the anus was normal and meconium had been passed. You would:**
   (A) Pass a gastric tube and lavage the stomach with normal saline
   (B) Reassure the nursery staff that vomiting is common at this period of life and continue to feed the infant
   (C) Order a plain radiograph of the abdomen
   (D) Take cultures of blood, urine and CSF

3. **David, a 2 week old infant, is brought to your general practice consulting rooms by his mother, who is concerned that, having been completely well until this morning, he commenced bile stained vomiting. He has been alert and examination of his abdomen is unremarkable. There is no diarrhoea. You would:**

(A) Get his mother to check his hernial orifices when the vomiting recurs to exclude a strangulated hernia

(B) Arrange an urgent barium meal

(C) Review him the following day, if the vomiting persists or if he develops diarrhoea

(D) Perform a lumbar puncture to exclude meningitis

4. **In children with acute gastroenteritis:**
   (A) Antibiotics should always be prescribed if Salmonella is found on faecal culture
   (B) Rehydration should always take place gradually over 24 hours
   (C) Isotonic is more common than hyponatraemic or hypernatraemic dehydration
   (D) Antidiarrhoeal agents aid recovery
   (E) Who are moderately dehydrated, intake of nutrient (milk or solids) should be delayed for 24 hours allowing the gut to recover from the infection

5. **Chronic non specific diarrhoea of early childhood:**
   (A) Should always be investigated
   (B) Is usually self-limited, with improvement of the symptom at age 4–5 years
   (C) Is associated with sucrase–isomaltase deficiency
   (D) Is due to a dysmotility of the gut
   (E) Can improve with normalising fat content in the diet

6. **In children:**
   (A) Crohn disease is more common than ulcerative colitis
   (B) Colonic Crohn disease is not associated with an increased incidence of malignancy
   (C) Elemental and polymeric feeds improve symptoms of ulcerative colitis
   (D) Surgery for Crohn disease should be avoided prior to puberty
   (E) Chronic mouth ulcers may be a mode of presentation

7. **Which of the following statements regarding GOR in infants is/are correct?**
   (A) Colic occurring mainly in the evening is a frequent symptom of GOR
   (B) Curdled milk in the vomitus is a sign of gastric hyperacidity
   (C) Irritability in young infants is usually due to oesophagitis
   (D) Regurgitation without weight loss is present in at least one third of healthy infants
   (E) Iron deficiency is often present in infants with GORD

8. **Which of the following management strategies is the most appropriate in a vomiting infant?**
   (A) Positioning the infant in a seated position for 1 hour after feeds

(B) Thickening of feeds either with rice cereal or a commercial thickened formula

(C) A trial of acid suppressant therapy with ranitidine, an H_2 receptor antagonist

(D) A trial of soy formula for several months

(E) A trial of a prokinetic drug such as cisapride or metoclopramide

9. **Of the diagnostic tests available to detect *H. pylori* infection in children, which one of the following is the most appropriate?**
   (A) Serology
   (B) ^{13}C-urea breath test
   (C) Upper gastrointestinal endoscopy and biopsy
   (D) Culture of gastric biopsy material
   (E) Stool culture

10. **Emma is a 3 week old female infant, the first born child of healthy Caucasian Australian parents. She became jaundiced on the third day of life. This was initially mild but increased progressively, except for two periods of 48 hours when her breastfeeding was interrupted. She has pigmented stools and dark urine. In the last 24 hours she has become lethargic and has lost interest in feeding. Examination reveals her to be moderately jaundiced. She is irritable. Her liver is easily palpated and has a span of 7 cm. You measure her bilirubin and find that it is elevated at 240 μmol/l, with a conjugated fraction of 90 μmol/l.**
    (A) The most likely diagnosis is biliary atresia
    (B) The most likely diagnosis is congenital hypothyroidism
    (C) You would arrange for urgent testing of the urine for reducing sugars
    (D) Breastfeeding should be ceased and antibiotics commenced

11. **John is a 9 year old boy who developed an acute illness with nausea and vomiting. He had been previously well, has had no overseas travel, but was camping with friends a month before his illness. Because he was still feeling unwell after 6 weeks you assess his liver biochemistry, which reveals an alanine aminotransferase of 110 IU/L. His physical examination is normal.**
    (A) It is reasonable to assume that he had hepatitis A, acquired while camping, and to await his recovery
    (B) You would order serological tests for hepatitis A, B and C
    (C) This illness could be due to glandular fever
    (D) If your serological testing was negative you would consider referral to an ophthalmologist

12. **Tommy is a healthy 4 year old boy, normal on physical examination, who has hepatitis B serology assessed prior to immunisation. He is HBsAg,**

HBeAg and HBcAb positive, is negative for anti-HBs, and has normal hepatic transaminase levels. His mother has a past history of intravenous drug use. Which of the following are corrrect?

(A) He has chronic hepatitis B infection and should be treated for chronic hepatitis

(B) He should be excluded from school until he clears the virus

(C) Because he has cAb present he does not pose any risk to his classmates at school

(D) Passive immunisation at birth may have prevented this problem

(E) Only persons in immediate personal contact with him require immunisation

Answers and explanations

1. The correct answers are **(C)** and **(D)**. (C) The history is consistent with a diagnosis of gastro-oesophageal reflux. Posture and thickening the fluids is the treatment of choice. (D) A chest X ray may indicate aspiration pneumonia, particularly if cough and wheeze are associated with feeding. (A) Infants with pyloric stenosis fail to thrive, lose weight and have projectile vomiting. Infants almost never reach the age of 3 months without surgical correction. (B) The diagnosis of gastro-oesophageal reflux is made on the clinical history. Occasionally, it is confirmed by barium studies, but the value of barium studies is to exclude other causes of vomiting.

2. The correct answer is **(C)**. (B) The green colour indicates the vomiting was bile stained. Bile stained vomiting must always be taken seriously. (C) A plain upright X ray of the abdomen will demonstrate duodenal obstruction (the double bubble) which is strongly suggestive of duodenal atresia, a well known association of Down syndrome. (A) Gastritis, for which gastric lavage may be useful, tends to follow complicated labours when meconium may be swallowed and inhaled. This is not appropriate here, as an initial step. (D) In an uncomplicated labour infection is uncommon at the age of 12 hours and blood, urine and CSF cultures would not be indicated as an initial step in management here.

3. The correct answer is **(B)**. (B) Sudden onset of bile stained vomiting in an otherwise well infant must be assumed to be due to malrotation with volvulus until confirmed or excluded on a barium study. (A) It is correct that he should be checked for a strangulated inguinal hernia but, in this situation, pain and irritability are the usual first symptoms. Vomiting tends to be seen later, and the diagnosis should be obvious on inspection. (C) To wait until abdominal signs of peritonitis have developed could result in the demise of the infant. (D) If the child has volvulus, there will be no 'following day'; an otherwise well child is less likely to have meningitis.

4. **(C)** is the correct answer. Antibiotics should be used to treat typhoid fever, which is rare is Australia, or if a non typhoid species causes illness in an immuno-compromised child, osteomyelitis, meningitis or sepsis as a result of the infection, and in infants who are less than 3 months of age. Rehydration needs to take place over 4–6 hours in most cases of dehydration, except for hypernatraemic dehydration, where the rehydration phase is more gradual, as a sudden fall of serum sodium can be associated with seizures and neurological dysfunction. Isotonic dehydration is much more common than hyponatraemia and hypernatraemia. Antidiarrhoeals are never indicated in the treatment of gastroenteritis in children and in fact are dangerous, as these drugs can result in ileus with significant third space fluid losses. It is now recommended that nutrient intake begins as soon as rehydration is completed, as it has been shown to shorten the duration of illness.

5. The correct answers are **(B)**, **(D)** and **(E)**. Chronic non specific diarrhoea is a self-limiting condition and usually does not require further investigation unless the child is not thriving or there is a history suggestive of lactose or sucrose intolerance. It has been suggested that fructose, which is present in fruit juice, can make symptoms worse and may be related to poor absorption of fructose. Sucrose malabsorption is a different entity and is due to an inherited defect in the expression of sucrase–isomaltase in the small bowel. There is a moderate amount of circumstantial evidence suggesting that this form of diarrhoea is due to a dysmotility syndrome. Normalising fat, fibre and fluid intake can be helpful in decreasing the severity of the diarrhoea.

6. **(A)** and **(E)** are the correct answers. The incidence of Crohn disease is 3–4 times as common as ulcerative colitis. Colonic Crohn disease is associated with an increased risk of developing a local malignancy. Elemental or polymeric feeds have been shown to be at least as successful in inducing a remission as steroids in children with predominantly small intestinal Crohn disease. There is little evidence to suggest that it is useful in the treatment of ulcerative colitis. Resection of localised medically resistant Crohn disease prior to puberty will often stimulate growth. Mouth ulcers, anal skin tags and general malaise may be the only early symptoms of Crohn disease.

7. The correct answer is **(D)**. Simple regurgitation is very common in young infants in the first 3–4 months of life. It often becomes more apparent in the third or fourth week of life when feed volumes start to

increase. It is a benign symptom generally and management should be explanation and reassurance. Colic is very common, occurring in 40–50% of infants in the first 3 months of life, and is rarely a symptom of GOR (A). It is probably a normal developmental condition, as most infants have wakeful periods of up to 3 hours a day but it is often misinterpreted by young parents as being abnormal. Again, reassurance and explanation is the answer. Curdled milk is commonly noted in vomitus and only indicates that the normal process of digestion is occurring in the stomach (B). It also indicates that the vomiting is unlikely to be due to oesophageal obstruction. Irritability in young infants is rarely due to oesophagitis (C). Studies have shown that it is probably related in less than 5% of cases. GOR with oesophagitis rarely presents as iron deficiency unless there is significant ulceration, which is very uncommon in infants (E). The commonest cause of iron deficiency is nutritional inadequacy.

8. The correct answer is (B). If the infant continues to regurgitate or occasionally vomit and is growing well, a trial of formula thickening is worthwhile (B). This has been shown in clinical trials to reduce the symptoms of vomiting and regurgitation, increase calorie intake and reduce irritability and poor feeding. Like other forms of therapy, if it has made no difference after several weeks the child should be returned to its usual formula. The best position for infants with vomiting is the prone position (A). This now cannot be recommended because of the risk of SIDS. Other positions have not been shown to be of benefit. The American Academy of Pediatrics have recommended the prone position for infants with proven GORD, as it not only decreases reflux but also improves gastric emptying, decreases aspiration, energy expenditure and crying time. Avoidance of soft bedding materials and mattresses is also recommended. The Division of Paediatrics of the RACP has not supported this statement. Both the supine position and the seated position should be avoided as much as possible as they provoke reflux. Acid suppressant therapy is only indicated in children with symptoms suggestive of oesophagitis or those with atypical symptoms proven to be associated with acid reflux (C). In children with GORD, proton pump inhibitors have been shown to reduce regurgitation and vomiting because of their significant effect on meal stimulated acid secretion and resultant gastric volume decrease. There is evidence in some families with a history of allergy that cow's milk protein intolerance may contribute to symptoms. If this is suspected a 2 week trial of an elemental formula may be worth trying. If the infant is being breast fed then a trial of elimination of cow's milk from the mother's

diet for a similar period may be worthwhile. The use of a soy formula for a diagnostic test is not helpful (D), as there is a high frequency of soy protein intolerance in cow's milk intolerant infants. The evidence for the use of cisapride in GOR even prior to the problem of cardiac toxicity being recognised was overestimated. While it may have a role in certain children with evidence of delayed gastric emptying, it is no longer available for use in GOR (E). Other prokinetic agents such as metoclopramide have a low efficacy-to-adverse reaction ratio with a high incidence of extrapyramidal side effects.

9. The correct answer is (C). Upper gastrointestinal endoscopy and biopsy provide the most complete information on the disease process compared with other diagnostic tests (C). It is the only method by which biopsies can be obtained and at the same time allows other causes of organic disease to be diagnosed, such as eosinophilic oesophagitis/gastroduodenitis, coeliac disease, giardiasis and other enteropathies. Gastric biopsies can also be cultured for *H. pylori* and, if required, tested for antibiotic sensitivity, allowing more targeted therapy. The most important step in this process is the justification for endoscopy. Symptoms should be investigated only when they are severe enough to justify the risks of therapy. If *H. pylori* is found in this situation then it should be eradicated, as infected persons have a 10–15% lifetime risk of development of *H pylori* associated serious organic disease. Serology is not a reliable test for diagnosis and treatment of *H. pylori* infection (A). Most commercial kits have not been validated in children and thus can be very insensitive. Serology also does not distinguish between actual and previous infection because the antibody titre decreases very slowly after cure. The ^{13}C-urea breath test is a reliable diagnostic tool but there is still a need for further evaluation, particularly in young children. This test seems better placed to monitor eradication, as, while it may detect infection, it does not provide the information needed regarding other organic disease (B). Culture of gastric biopsy material requires an upper gastrointestinal endoscopy (D). Culture is an important component of this investigation. Stool culture of *H. pylori* is possible and may be a useful tool in the future, as may stool antigen detection, but at this stage not enough information is available to recommend it (E).

10. Answers (C) and (D) are correct. This infant has a conjugated hyperbilirubinaemia, making hypothyroidism unlikely (B). While biliary atresia (A) is a possible diagnosis, Emma is ill with lethargy, irritability and poor feeding, suggestive of sepsis, a common complication of galactosaemia. The presence of non glucose reducing sugars in the urine

(C) would be consistent with the diagnosis of galactosaemia, which can be confirmed by measuring red cell galactose phosphate uridyl transferase. Galactosaemia is due to a congenital metabolic defect in the enzyme(s) responsible for the metabolism of galactose, a monosaccharide derived from milk. Toxic products accumulate, causing liver disease, neurological disease, cataracts and neutrophil function abnormalities. This last complication increases the risks of bacterial sepsis, and a number of infants will present with Gram negative sepsis. Initial treatment comprises withdrawal of breastfeeding (and other mammalian milks), and initiation of antibiotics because of presumed sepsis (D). Long term treatment is avoidance of milk and galactose-containing vegetables.

11. Answers **(B)**, **(C)** and **(D)** are correct. The 1 month between the time of camping and the onset of symptoms is shorter than the usual incubation period for hepatitis A (A). Even if the time were more consistent, it is not appropriate to make assumptions about the cause of hepatitis. It is important that all children with clinical or biochemical hepatitis are followed to full recovery and reasonable efforts should be made to define a cause for the hepatitis. It is appropriate to undertake serological testing for hepatitis A, B and C (B), Epstein–Barr virus (C) and cytomegalovirus (C). If these are negative then other causes of hepatitis such as α-1-antitrypsin deficiency, Wilson disease and autoimmune hepatitis should be considered and tested for. Kayser–Fleischer rings may be seen with slit lamp examination of the eyes (D). In Wilson disease it is important to initiate treatment with a low copper diet and penicillamine as soon as possible.

12. The corrrect answer is **(D)**. Tommy is a chronic carrier of the hepatitis B virus, but does not have evidence of chronic hepatitis (A). His family history, the presence of HbcAb and his normal transaminases are in keeping with perinatal acquisition of infection. He has the potential to transmit the virus to other children, but should not be excluded from school (B, C). Only 10–15% of chronic carriers will clear hepatitis B virus. He has long term risks of chronic hepatitis and hepatocellular carcinoma. Passive immunisation with HB immunoglobulin (D) followed by hepatitis B vaccine will dramatically reduce the risk of acquisition of hepatitis B infection. All unimmunised schoolchildren should complete hepatitis B immunisation (E).

PART 20   FURTHER READING

Bai J C 1998 Malabsorption syndromes. Digestion 59: 530–546

Davidson G P, Omari T I 2000 Reflux in children. Baillière's Clinical Gastroenterology 14: 839–855

Drumm B, Koletzko S, Oderda G 2000 *Helicobacter pylori* infection in children: a consensus statement. Journal of Pediatric Gastroenterology and Nutrition 30: 207

Gold B D, Colletti R B, Abbott M et al 2000 *Helicobacter pylori* infection in children: recommendations for diagnosis and treatment. Journal of Pediatric Gastroenterology and Nutrition 31: 490–497

Kagnoff M F 1992 Celiac disease. A gastrointestinal disease with environmental, genetic and immunologic components. Gastroenterology Clinics of North America 21: 405–425

Kelly D A 1999 Disease of the liver and biliary system in children. Blackwell Science, Oxford

Murphy M S 1998 Guidelines for managing acute gastroenteritis based on a systematic review of published research. Archives of Disease in Childhood 79: 279–284

Nelson S P, Chen E H, Syniar G M et al 2000 Prevalence of symptoms of gastroesophageal reflux during childhood: a pediatric practice-based survey. Archives of Pediatric and Adolescent Medicine 154: 150–154

North American Society for Pediatric Gastroenterology and Nutrition 2001 Guidelines for evaluation and treatment of gastroesophageal reflux in infants and children. Recommendations of the North American Society for Pediatric Gastroenterology and Nutrition. Journal of Pediatric Gastroenterology and Nutrition 32(Supplement 2): S1–S31

Orenstein S R 2000 Update on gastroesophageal reflux and respiratory disease in children. Canadian Journal of Gastroenterology 14: 131–135

Phillips S 1972 Diarrhoea — a current view of the pathophysiology. Gastroenterology: 63: 495–518

Schuppan D 2000 Current concepts of celiac disease pathogenesis. Gastroenterology 119: 234–242

Suchy F J, Sokol R J, Balistreri W F 2001 Liver disease in children. Lippincott, Williams and Wilkins, Philapelphia

Torres J, Perez-Perez G, Goodman K J et al 2000 A comprehensive review of the natural history of *Helicobacter pylori* infection in children. Archives of Medical Research 31: 431–469

Walker W A, Durie P R, Hamilton J R, Walker-Smith J A, Watkins J B 2000 Pediatric gastrointestinal disease: physiology, diagnosis and management. BC Decker, Philadelphia

Walker-Smith J A et al 1997 Medical position paper. Guidelines prepared by the ESPGAN working group on acute diarrhoea. Recommendations for feeding in childhood gastroenteritis. Journal of Pediatric Gastroenterology and Nutrition 24: 619–620

Welsh M J, Smith A E 1993 Molecular mechanisms of CFTR chloride channel dysfunction in cystic fibrosis. Cell 73: 1251–1254

Wolf A D, Lavine J E 2000 Hepatomegaly in neonates and children. Pediatrics in Review 21:303–310

Zevering Y 2001 Vaccine against *Helicobacter pylori*? Annals of Medicine 33:156–166

Useful links

http://www.aap.org/policy/01207.html (American Academy of Pediatrics: prevention of hepatitis A infection guidelines)

http://www.aap.org/policy/re9733.html (American Academy of Pediatrics: abstract on hepatitis C infection)

http://www.childliverdisease.org/ (Child Liver Disease Foundation website)

http://www.liverfoundation.org/html/livheal.dir/livheal.htm (American Liver Foundation website)

SKIN DISORDERS

Skin disorders in infancy and childhood

M. Rogers

Neonatal conditions

Pustular lesions in the neonate

There are many conditions which present in the neonatal period with pustules or pustule like lesions. Some of these are benign and transient and of no systemic significance; however, many potentially serious infections can present with similar pustular lesions and it is vital to exclude infection in any pustular eruption in a neonate.

Sterile benign transient pustular disorders
(Fig. 73.1)

- *Toxic erythema of the newborn.* Widespread red macules each surmounted by a papule or pustule; onset in the first 2 days of life and disappear by the end of the first week.
- *Transient neonatal pustular dermatosis.* Onset at birth of flaccid pustules which dry out in 48 hours, leaving postinflammatory hyperpigmentation in dark skinned infants.
- *Infantile acropustulosis.* Crops of spontaneously resolving pustules on the hands and feet during the first few months or life.

- *Eosinophilic pustular folliculitis of the scalp.* Recurrent groups of pustules on a red base on the scalp and later occasionally elsewhere.
- *Pustular miliaria or sweat duct occlusion rash.* Short-lived pustules in among more typical red papules of miliaria, occurring particularly on the face, scalp and upper trunk.

Benign transient lesions simulating pustules

- *Milia.* Firm white papules especially on the face, which extrude in early weeks of life.
- *Sebaceous hyperplasia.* Yellow papules on the nose, resolve in early weeks.

Infective disorders presenting with pustules

- Staphylococcal infection
  — Folliculitis
  — Impetigo
- Candida
- Herpes simplex
- Varicella

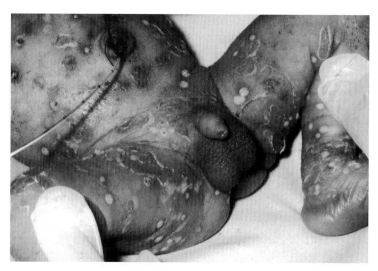

Fig. 73.1 Transient neonatal pustulosis.

Rare disorder presenting with pustules

Incontinentia pigmenti. A linear arrangement of pustules and blisters, particularly on the limbs; important associations are seizures and cataracts.

Blistering lesions in the neonate

There is some overlap between pustular and blistering disorders in the neonatal period. Several conditions may present with blisters and then become pustular.

Infections

- Herpes simplex
- Bullous impetigo
- Staphylococcal scalded skin syndrome
- Congenital syphilis.

Other

- *Zinc deficiency.* Blistered and crusted lesions around mouth, nose and in napkin area.
- *Epidermolysis bullosa.* Blistering in areas of trauma.
- *Bullous ichthyosis.* Blisters on the basis of a bright red skin; skin thickens in early days.
- *Bullous mastocytosis.* Blisters on the background of a leathery skin with a peau d'orange appearance.
- *Langerhans cell histiocytosis.* Vesicles and purpuric crusted lesions; a serious disease.
- *Incontinentia pigmenti.* A linear arrangement of blisters.

The red, scaly neonate or young infant

A number of important conditions can present with diffuse redness and variable scaliness in the neonate; affected infants often have major problems with temperature regulation and fluid balance and may seriously fail to thrive:

- *Seborrhoeic dermatitis.* Dull red erythema with a greasy yellow scale involving particularly the scalp, centrofacial area and all flexures. The scale may be absent in the flexures and secondary monilia is common. Usually asymptomatic and self-limiting after the early months of life. Responds to weak steroids and antimonilial agents.
- *Atopic dermatitis.* Rarely this condition presents in very early infancy with a widespread red scaly and itchy rash. These patients often have food allergies and will go on to difficult long term disease.
- *Ichthyoses* (Fig. 73.2). Some of these conditions present with the child covered in a shiny red membrane which peels off in the early weeks of life to leave a red scaly skin. Some commence with a dramatic degree of redness and scale, without the membrane.
- *Immunodeficiencies.* Patients with severe combined immunodeficiency and other immunodeficiencies may present with a widespread red scaly rash in the neonatal period or early infancy. In some cases this represents a congenital graft versus host disease.
- *Staphylococcal scalded skin syndrome.* The child is initially bright red and then blisters appear, initially involving the face and flexures and then widespread; these subsequently dry up into scaly crusts.

Birthmarks and other naevoid conditions

Pigmented birthmarks

Congenital melanocytic naevi (Fig. 73.3)

These occur at birth as raised verrucous or lobulated lesions of varying shades of brown to black, sometimes with blue or pink components, with an irregular margin and often growing long dark hairs. They may become increasingly lobulated and hairy with time. Giant sized lesions may produce considerable redundancy of skin and often occur in a 'garment' distribution on the trunk

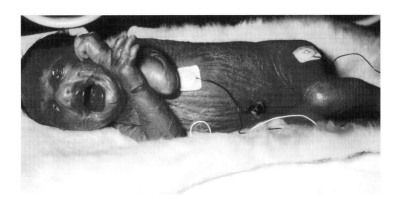

Fig. 73.2 Neonate with congenital ichthyosis covered in tight, thick, red membrane.

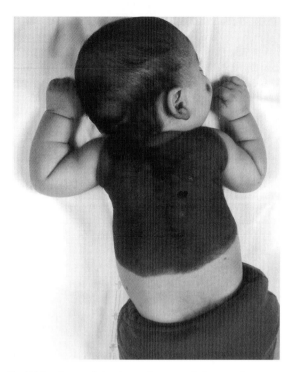

Fig. 73.3 Congenital melanocytic naevus in 'garment' distribution on the back.

occur particularly on the lumbosacral area, although the shoulders, upper back and occasionally other areas may be involved. They are found in over 80% of Oriental and black infants and in up to 10% of white infants, particularly those of Mediterranean origin. They usually fade considerably by puberty, but may remain unaltered through life.

Naevus of Ota

This is a patchy blue-grey discoloration of the skin of the face, particularly on the cheek, periorbital area and brow. It is usually unilateral and often there is a similar pigmentation of the sclera of the ipsilateral eye. It is most common in Oriental individuals and is present at birth in over 50% of cases. It is a permanent lesion. An associated sensorineural deafness has been reported, and very rarely these lesions may be complicated in adult life by development of malignant melanoma.

Epidermal naevi

Epidermal naevi (Fig. 73.4) arise from the basal layer of the embryonic epidermis, which gives rise to skin

and adjacent limbs. In patients with large naevi an eruption of smaller, but essentially similar lesions may occur during the first few years of life. Malignancy in giant naevi can occur in childhood and the incidence over a lifetime is possibly of the order of 2%. In medium and small lesions the risk is much lower and any development of malignancy is always postpubertal.

Naevoid hyperpigmentation

These are flat areas of pigmented skin, obvious at or very soon after birth. They occur in characteristic patterns — either segmental, or whorled and streaky following the lines of Blaschko, which define the tracks of clones of genetically identical cells and are now recognised as genetic mosaic patterns. They may have smooth or irregular edges and are various shades of brown in colour and may occur anywhere on the trunk, limbs or face. They usually occur as isolated phenomena but may be associated, as part of certain mosaic phenotypes, with neurological, skeletal and other abnormalities. An important differential diagnosis is the café au lait spots of neurofibromatosis, which are rarely present at birth and which continue to increase in number.

Mongolian spot

These are flat blue or slate-grey lesions with poorly defined margins. They may be single or multiple and

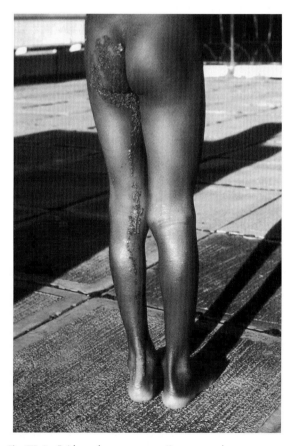

Fig. 73.4 Epidermal naevus presenting as a scaly verrucous line on the leg.

appendages as well as keratinocytes. These naevi have been conventionally classified, according to the tissue of origin, into keratinocytic, sebaceous and follicular types. They can involve any area of skin. They may be present at birth or appear in the first few years of life; they may simply grow with the patient or can extend well beyond their original distribution. On the scalp and face the naevi have a yellowish colour, due to prominent sebaceous glands, and present as a hairless, often linear plaque, usually flat in infancy and childhood and becoming verrucous at puberty.

Lesions elsewhere are usually dark brown but are occasionally paler than the normal skin. They occur as single or multiple warty plaques or lines, often arranged in a linear or swirled pattern. It is now clear that the linear and swirled patterns taken by epidermal naevi follow the lines of Blaschko, and that all epidermal naevi can be explained on the basis of genetic mosaicism, with each type of naevus representing the cutaneous manifestation of a different mosaic phenotype. In most patients the naevus is the only detectable manifestation but in some patients there are associated abnormalities in other organ systems, particularly skeletal, neurological and ocular. Skeletal abnormalities occur particularly with naevi of keratinocytic type on the limbs, and neurological and ocular abnormalities with naevi of sebaceous type on the head.

Vascular birthmarks

These can be divided into:
- haemangiomas, which are proliferative vascular tumours
- vascular malformations, which represent fixed collections of dilated abnormal vessels.

Haemangiomas

Haemangiomas usually appear just after birth, undergo a fast growth phase and then, over a long period, tend to spontaneous resolution. It is now clear that haemangiomas, whether superficially or deeply located in the skin, have the same structure, being composed in the early stage of proliferating masses of endothelial cells with occasional lumina, and later, as they resolve, of large endothelial lined spaces. The terms capillary, cavernous and capillary-cavernous are misleading and should be abandoned in favour of the simple term haemangioma.

Superficial haemangiomas (Fig. 73.5). These are not usually present at birth but appear in the first weeks of life as an area of pallor, followed by a telangiectatic patch. They then grow rapidly into a lobulated, well demarcated, bright red tumour. Rapid growth continues over the first 6 months of life; the growth rate then slows and further growth after 10 months is unusual. After a

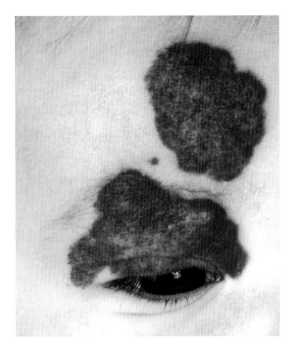

Fig. 73.5 Superficial haemangioma, threatening closure of the eye.

stationary phase, signs of involution begin, with the appearance of grey areas which enlarge and coalesce. The tumour becomes softer and less bulky and then disappears in 90% of cases by 9 years of age.

Deeper haemangiomas (Fig. 73.6). These may occur alone or beneath a superficial lesion (Fig. 73.7). The overlying skin is normal or bluish in colour. As they resolve, they soften and shrink and complete disappearance occurs in many cases.

Complications
- Incomplete resolution — redundant tissue, residual telangiectasia, scarring following ulceration.
- Ulceration — full thickness tissue loss on 'edge structures' (lip, lid, ala), inevitable scarring, cicatricial ectropion from scarring of eyelids, cicatricial alopecia.

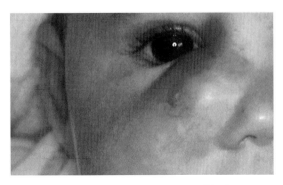

Fig. 73.6 Deep haemangioma presenting as bluish tumour.

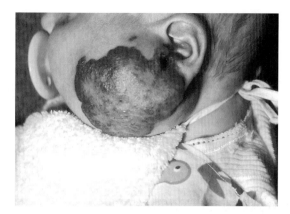

Fig. 73.7 Combined superficial and deep haemangioma.

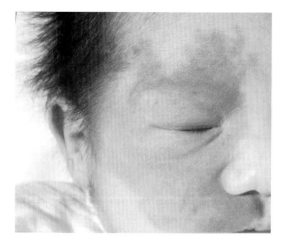

Fig. 73.8 Capillary malformation on the face, involving the brow, which suggests the possibility of the Sturge–Weber syndrome.

• Obstruction — of eye producing amblyopia, of nose leading to difficulty in breathing during feeding, of lip leading to problems with sucking, of larynx (a 'beard' distribution haemangioma is a marker for possible laryngeal involvement).

Management. Simple observation and reassurance while awaiting natural resolution is the ideal approach for most haemangiomas. Indications for active intervention are an alarming growth rate, threatening ulceration in areas where serious complications could ensue, interference with vital structures and severe bleeding. Oral corticosteroids will slow the growth of potentially dangerous or cosmetically serious lesions.

Vascular malformations

These are collections of dilated abnormal vessels divided according to the vessels of origin. The most appropriate terminology refers to the component vessels and many outdated terms can be abandoned:

• *Capillary malformation* (port wine stain, Fig. 73.8) — flat purple stain, most commonly on the face but may occur anywhere.
• *Venous malformation* (varix) — bluish tumour, empties with pressure and when elevated; fills when dependent; phleboliths may develop within it.
• *Lymphatic malformation* (lymphangioma, cystic hygroma) — macrocystic deep lesions present as skin coloured tumours, often with bruising; superficial lesions present as groups of haemorrhagic vesicles or warty lesions.
• *Arteriovenous malformation* — skin coloured lump which enlarges, becomes painful and may bleed at puberty.
• *Other mixed malformations*

All vascular malformations are present at birth and grow only in proportion to the growth of the child. They show no tendency to involution.

Moles (acquired melanocytic naevi)

These usually first appear after the age of 1 year and increase in number throughout childhood. They commence as brown or black macules, some of which become raised and enlarge laterally as they develop. They are usually of uniform colour and well circumscribed. The risk of melanoma arising from acquired melanocytic naevi is very low (less than 0.1%): melanoma almost never occurs in childhood so their prophylactic removal in young patients is not justified.

Halo naevi

A depigmented halo may occur around a melanocytic naevus; the lesion may appear inflamed and often disappears, leaving a white spot which may eventually repigment. This is a completely benign change.

Dysplastic or atypical naevi

A subtype of acquired melanocytic naevi with characteristic clinicopathological features and a marker for an increased risk of developing malignant melanoma. They differ from more typical moles by being larger (more than 5 mm diameter), having irregular and indistinct margins and irregular tan brown coloration, often with an erythematous component. They are predominantly macular, sometimes with a central elevated portion. They may appear in childhood as small, typical appearing naevi which after puberty develop the atypical features. Characteristic dysplastic naevi may appear on the scalp in childhood. The final confirmation is based on the finding of some or all of a constellation of histopathological features. Patients with multiple dysplastic naevi should be observed frequently and monitored with serial photography. Any such naevus showing significant alteration should be removed immediately.

Cutaneous infections and infestations

Mollusca contagiosa

This is a poxvirus infection that is rare under 1 year of age and occurs particularly in the 2–5 year age group. The spread of lesions is enhanced in warm water and outbreaks occur among children who swim together or share baths or spas. Further spread of mollusca in the individual is also encouraged by being in warm water.

Clinical features

- Typical lesions are spherical and pearly white with a central umbilication, but they may vary from tiny, 1 mm papules to large nodules over 1 cm in diameter. They occur on any part of the skin surface, with common sites being the axillae and sides of the trunk, the lower abdomen and the anogenital area. Rarely they occur on the eyelids, where they may cause conjunctivitis and punctate keratitis.
- A secondary eczema often occurs around lesions, particularly in atopic children, and scratching of this spreads the mollusca. Hundreds of lesions may be present in an individual patient.
- Secondary bacterial infection may occur, producing crusting, redness and pus formation. However, these same changes may be seen during spontaneous resolution, which occurs in most within several months, leaving normal skin or small varicella-like scars.

Management

- Each lesion lasts for only weeks, and if the child is kept out of heated pools and spas and has showers rather than baths at home the proliferation is curbed and the numbers of lesions usually decreases quickly. If these measures are rigidly adhered to, treatment is rarely required.
- Mollusca are surprisingly resistant to chemical therapies.
- The most definitive treatment is deroofing of the lesion with a large cutting edged needle and wiping out the contents. The lesion itself is virtually anaesthetic and this procedure can be performed almost painlessly with large lesions where the needle can be introduced into the molluscum without penetrating the surrounding or underlying skin.
- With multiple small lesions in a young child spontaneous resolution should be awaited, but if the lesions are troublesome due to site, surrounding eczema or

frequent secondary infection, removal under nitrous oxide sedation, or if absolutely necessary general anaesthetic, may be considered.

Warts

These are benign tumours caused by infection with a variety of papilloma viruses of the papova group:
- The common wart (verruca vulgaris) occurs particularly on hands, knees and elbows.
- Plane or flat warts, 1–3-mm pink or brown barely raised papules, occur on the face and often spread along scratch marks or cuts.
- Plantar warts occur particularly over pressure points on the soles and can be differentiated from calluses by a loss of skin markings over the skin surface. Warts at mucocutaneous junctions often have a filiform or fronded appearance.
- Anogenital warts may be acquired from maternal infection during delivery, but their presence should always raise the suspicion of sexual abuse.

Management

Various forms of treatment are available: they depend on the area, the type of wart and the age of the patient. Because spontaneous disappearance is common, aggressive treatment is often inappropriate. These include:
- Keratolytic wart paints (for example salicylic acid, lactic acid and collodion) — for common warts and plantar warts.
- Retinoic acid preparations — for facial plane warts.
- Podophyllotoxin and imiquimod — for anogenital warts, used under strict supervision.
- A 20% formalin solution — for plantar warts, combined with serial paring.
- Cautery or diathermy — useful for lesions on the lips or anogenital area but elsewhere recurrence is fairly frequent following their use and there is also a risk of producing a painful scar, particularly over the joints of digits or on the palms or soles.
- Liquid nitrogen cryotherapy — is a successful method of dealing with common warts and is useful for older children.
- Oral cimetidine — has recently been demonstrated to be a useful treatment in some cases of multiple refractory warts.

Dermatological presentations of herpes simplex

Herpes simplex virus (HSV) infections are extremely common in children, and serological studies confirm that more than 90% of the population have been infected by the time of reaching adulthood. The commonest type is

HSV1, although HSV2 is more important in adulthood, being the cause of genital herpes. Several distinct presentations are recognised in childhood.

Intrauterine herpes simplex

- Cutaneous lesions include blisters and erosions, sometimes in a dermatomal distribution, and irregular, often linear scars.
- Other features are microcephaly, short digits, cardiac abnormalities and a variety of ocular abnormalities.

Neonatal herpes simplex

- This is a potentially devastating infection usually contracted from infected vaginal secretions (HSV2) during delivery; however, intrauterine and postnatal infection may occur.
- The skin lesions are grouped blisters, localised initially on the presenting part, usually the head, with the onset usually between the fourth and eighth days of life. The eruption may become widespread, with individual lesions a few millimetres across coalescing to produce large erosions.
- A rapid immunofluorescence test on material from the blister base enables a diagnosis within a few hours.
- Assess immediately for the presence of and extent of other organ involvement, of which the most potentially devastating is neurological.
- Regard any blisters in the neonate as herpes until proven otherwise.
- Immediate treatment with intravenous acyclovir is indicated.

Primary herpetic gingivostomatitis

The child is systemically unwell with a high fever and there is severe swelling, erosion and bleeding of the gums and the anterior part of the buccal mucosa. Spread to the lips and the facial skin often occurs. There may be considerable soft tissue swelling and prominent lymphadenopathy.

Primary cutaneous herpes simplex

- Can occur anywhere on the body, depending on the source of infection; painful grouped blisters or pustules on an erythematous base which soon break to produce erosions or crusted lesions.
- Often there is local swelling and regional lymphadenopathy and the child may be febrile.
- When a primary lesion occurs on the thick skin of a finger, the blisters do not break easily and intact, grouped pustules last for several days, producing an appearance suggestive of a bacterial infection. If the lesion is opened, pus does not come out freely and, of course, the result of a bacterial culture is negative.

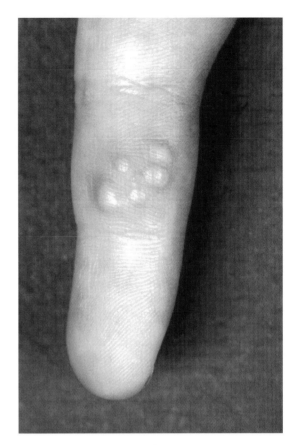

Fig. 73.9 Herpes simplex on a finger, presenting as intact pustules.

- When primary herpes simplex occurs in the napkin area it presents as a severe erosive napkin rash. This is usually contracted from a herpes lesion on the lip of a carer, directly or via the hands, but occasionally occurs as a result of sexual abuse.

Recurrent cutaneous herpes simplex

- Recurrent herpes simplex of the face, particularly around the lips (herpes labialis), is common in childhood. As in adults, various factors, including fever and sun exposure, may reactivate the virus.
- Recurrent herpes on a finger, presenting as longlasting intact pustules (Fig. 73.9), is often mistaken for a recurrent bacterial infection; the chance of a bacterial infection recurring in exactly the same site would be very low indeed and this story should always suggest herpes simplex.

Disseminated herpes simplex (eczema herpeticum)

This occurs as a complication of atopic eczema and in immunosuppressed patients (Fig. 73.10). It may originate from a primary or recurrent infection or from external

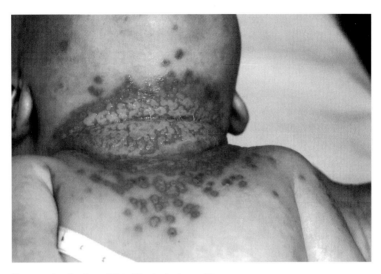

Fig. 73.10 Disseminated herpes simplex in a child with atopic dermatitis.

reinfection. Spread is both on the surface of the skin and also by haematogenous dissemination. The lesions are vesicles or pustules 2–4 mm across which may spread with alarming rapidity and have a tendency to coalescence to produce geographic shaped erosions with scalloped edges. If there are more than very few lesions the patient should be hospitalised. Topical agents should be avoided as their application may spread the virus. Secondary bacterial infection should be treated with oral antibiotics and saline or tap water packs used to relieve discomfort and dry out the lesions. In severe cases systemic acyclovir is indicated.

Indolent ulceration in the immunosuppressed patient

An unusual presentation of herpes simplex in immuno-suppressed patients is as a chronic, slowly growing ulcer,

often with rather overhanging edges. The outline is usually irregular, reminiscent of the geographic shapes produced by coalescing lesions in the more typical forms of herpes simplex. It requires systemic antiviral therapy.

Impetigo

Impetigo is a bacterial infection caused by *Staphylococcus aureus,* group A *Streptococcus* or a com-bination of these organisms; it occurs in two forms, bullous and non bullous (or crusted).

Clinical features

- Bullous impetigo (Fig. 73.11) is always due to staphy-lococci. Blisters arise on previously normal skin and increase rapidly in size and number, soon rupturing to

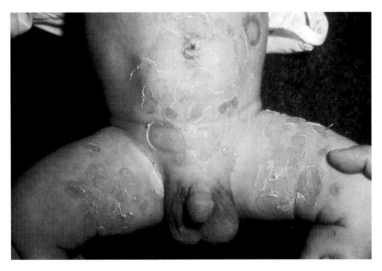

Fig. 73.11 Bullous impetigo in a neonate.

produce superficial erosions with a peripheral brown crust. The erosions continue to expand, sometimes clearing centrally to produce annular lesions.

- Non bullous impetigo may be due to either organism or to a combination. The lesions begin with a small transient vesicle on an erythematous base. The serum exuding from the ruptured vesicle produces a thick soft yellow crust, below which there is a moist superficial erosion.
- Impetigo is often superimposed on other skin diseases such as insect bites, scabies, pediculosis and atopic eczema.
- Staphylococcal impetigo does not scar but deep streptococcal lesions may. Postinflammatory pigmentation can occur, particularly in dark skinned patients.

Management

- Saline bathing may be used to dry out the lesions.
- A swab for culture and sensitivity testing should always be taken.
- Topical mupirocin may be successful for localised early disease.
- In general, oral antibiotics should be used. Because of the rarity in most areas of pure streptococcal impetigo, a penicillinase resistant penicillin or erythromycin are the treatments of choice while awaiting culture results.
- If a group A *Streptococcus* is isolated the patient should be watched for 8 weeks for signs of glomerulonephritis.

Staphylococcal scalded skin syndrome (SSSS)

SSSS (Fig. 73.12) is a widespread blistering disease caused by an epidermolytic toxin produced by certain strains of *Staphylococcus aureus,* most often of phage group 2, types 70/71 or 51 but occasionally of phage group 1. This toxin produces a superficial splitting of the skin, with the level of split being high in the epidermis. Clinical disease occurs when there is sufficient toxin load produced from an infection with these organisms.

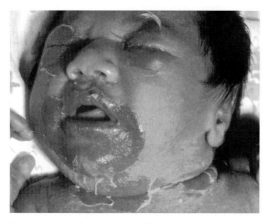

Fig. 73.12 Staphylococcal scalded skin syndrome in a neonate.

Clinical features

- The commonest sites of infection are the umbilicus (in neonates), the nose, nasopharynx or throat, the conjuctiva and deep wounds.
- The condition commences with a macular erythema, initially on the face and in the major flexures and then becoming generalised. The skin is exquisitely tender and the child draws back from contact. After 2 days flaccid bullae develop and the skin wrinkles and shears off. The exfoliation is most marked in the groin, neck fold and around the mouth and may involve the entire body surface but mucosae remain uninvolved.
- The child is usually febrile but because of the superficial level of the split, fluid loss is rarely significant. The erosions crust and dry and heal with desquamation over the next 4–8 days leaving no sequelae.
- Cultures from skin and blister fluid are usually negative. Cultures should be obtained from any area of obvious infection but, if none is apparent, from nasopharynx and throat.

Management

- Nurse the child naked on a non stick material and handle as little as possible.
- Avoid topical agents in the early stages.
- A penicillinase resistant penicillin is the treatment of choice and is usually given intravenously.
- Analgesia is often necessary in the early stages.
- Emollients are useful once the skin dries and desquamation commences.

Boils (furuncles)

Boils are cutaneous abscesses centred around hair follicles, caused by certain species of coagulase-positive *Staphylococcus aureus*.

Clinical features

- Local predisposing factors are cutaneous injury, friction and sweating.
- Episodes are often recurrent and many patients with recurrences are found to carry furuncle producing strains of *Staphylococcus aureus* in nostrils, axilla or groin or to have close contact with someone who does.

Management

- Early lesions should be treated with warm compresses and oral penicillinase resistant penicillins. Erythromycin may be used in patients allergic to the preferred antibiotics.

- For older lesions which have matured and pointed, incision and drainage may occasionally be indicated in conjunction with the use of antibiotics.
- Chronic and recurrent furunculosis should be treated with a course of antibiotics of several weeks duration. While the patient is on antibiotics, all clothing, towels and bed linen which has contacted the affected areas should be washed in hot water. Attempts should be made to deal with the carrier state in the patient and/or close contacts. Washing of the groin, axilla and hands with an antiseptic soap can help, as can topical nasal antibiotics such as mupurocin. Oral rifampicin has also been successful in reducing carriage but should not be used alone because of the rapid development of resistance.

Streptococcal perianal disease

This is a distinctive perianal eruption due to group A beta haemolytic *Streptococcus* (GABHS).

- Peak incidence is in children 3–4 years of age but it may occur in infants.
- A likely mode of transmission is digital contamination from an infected oropharynx, although symptoms of pharyngitis are rarely present.
- The child complains of pain on defecation and often refuses to open the bowels.
- Bright blood is frequently seen on the stool. A bright pink erythema extends from the anal rim, which is often fissured and macerated, 2–3 cm out from the anus; the skin is tender but not indurated.
- Lymphangitis and lymphadenopathy are absent.
- There may be an associated GABHS balanitis or vulvovaginitis.
- Diagnosis is established by culture, on blood agar, of GABHS from a swab of the perianal skin.
- The treatment of choice is oral penicillin V 50 mg/kg/day in four divided doses, combined with the use of topical mupurocin twice a day. Recurrences are very frequent without this combined therapy, which should be continued for 10 days. Erythromycin is appropriate in penicillin allergic patients.

Tinea

This is an infection due to dermatophyte fungi: the source of the fungus is an animal (for example, dog, cat, guinea pig, cattle), the soil or another human. Tinea occurs on any part of the skin surface and can involve hair and nails.

Clinical features and diagnosis

- Classical features of tinea on the general body skin are itch, erythema studded with papules or pustules, annular or geographical lesions ('ringworm') with a tendency to central clearing and a superficial scale (Fig. 73.13).

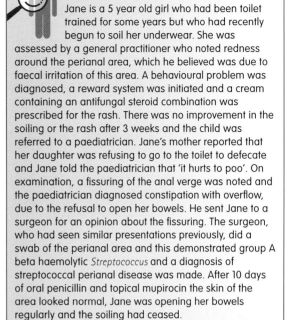

Clinical example

Jane is a 5 year old girl who had been toilet trained for some years but who had recently begun to soil her underwear. She was assessed by a general practitioner who noted redness around the perianal area, which he believed was due to faecal irritation of this area. A behavioural problem was diagnosed, a reward system was initiated and a cream containing an antifungal steroid combination was prescribed for the rash. There was no improvement in the soiling or the rash after 3 weeks and the child was referred to a paediatrician. Jane's mother reported that her daughter was refusing to go to the toilet to defecate and Jane told the paediatrician that 'it hurts to poo'. On examination, a fissuring of the anal verge was noted and the paediatrician diagnosed constipation with overflow, due to the refusal to open her bowels. He sent Jane to a surgeon for an opinion about the fissuring. The surgeon, who had seen similar presentations previously, did a swab of the perianal area and this demonstrated group A beta haemolytic *Streptococcus* and a diagnosis of streptococcal perianal disease was made. After 10 days of oral penicillin and topical mupirocin the skin of the area looked normal, Jane was opening her bowels regularly and the soiling had ceased.

- Tinea is often unilateral and always asymmetrical, whereas eczema and psoriasis, which it may resemble, are often symmetrical in distribution.
- Between the toes maceration with a thick white scale is the main finding and an annular lesion may extend onto the dorsum of the foot.
- Nail tinea produces a white discoloration and crumbling of the nail plate with an accumulation of subungual debris. On the soles there are deep seated blisters or pustules which dry to produce brown crusts.
- On the scalp there is a characteristic combination of alopecia and inflammation with the hair loss being due to breaking of the hair shafts. Depending on the pattern of hair invasion by the fungus, the hairs are either broken off flush with the scalp or at lengths of up to 2–3 mm, but in an individual case all the hairs break at the same length. The inflammation varies from mild erythema and a fine dandruff-like scale to a pustular carbuncle-like lesion (kerion).
- A Wood light (an ultraviolet lamp) is useful in the diagnosis of some varieties of scalp tinea, with the infected hairs fluorescing bright green. Other varieties of scalp tinea produce no typical fluorescence and the Wood light has no place in the diagnosis of tinea on the skin surface.
- The diagnosis of tinea is confirmed by scraping hairs or scales on to a slide, adding 20% potassium hydroxide and examining the specimen microscopically.

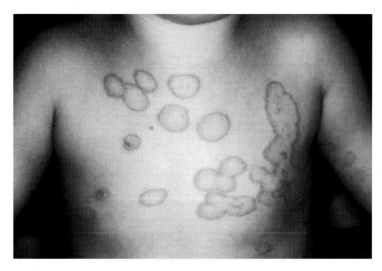

Fig. 73.13 Annular lesions of tinea.

Septate branching hyphae are seen in skin scales and spores are found in hair. The fungus can be cultured on appropriate media.

Management

- Topical antifungals may be satisfactory for small localised patches of tinea on the skin.
- Oral griseofulvin is the treatment of choice for long-standing or severe cutaneous tinea and hair tinea. This fat soluble drug is best taken after meals, preferably with a glass of milk. In general a 3 month course is used.
- Nail tinea is particularly resistant to treatment and may require other antifungals such as terbinafine.

Tinea versicolor

This is an infection with *Pityrosporum* species which are part of the normal skin flora. It occurs mainly in tropical and temperate zones and usually affects adolescents and young adults.

Clinical features and diagnosis

- Presents as well demarcated, asymptomatic or slightly itchy macules with a fine branny scale which is often only obvious on light scratching of the lesions. Primary macules 1–10 mm in diameter coalesce into larger patches.
- Lesions occur in two colours — red-brown, especially in the fair skinned, and hypopigmented in darker skinned children. In a partially tanned individual, lesions of both colours may he found.

- The hypopigmented form must be differentiated from vitiligo, where the depigmentation is total and scale is absent, and pityriasis alba, where lesions are less well demarcated and some erythema may be seen.
- In young children it often presents with only facial lesions and almost invariably a parent or older relative will have tinea versicolor in the typical distribution.
- Diagnosis is confirmed by microscopic examination of skin scrapings to which 20% potassium hydroxide has been added. Grape-like clusters of spores and short fragments of thick mycelia are seen.

Management

- Untreated, the condition is persistent, although some improvement may occur in winter.
- The treatment of choice is with topical imidazole creams.
- With the depigmented form, therapy deals with the scale but sun exposure is required for full repigmentation.
- Rarely in severe disease in adolescents a short course of oral ketoconazole is required

Scabies (Fig. 73.14)

This is due to *Sarcoptes scabei,* an eight legged, oval shaped mite less than 0.5 mm in length. The disease is transmitted by close physical contact, with transmission by fomites being exceptional. A small number of mites burrow into the skin in certain sites, particularly between the fingers, the ulnar border of the hand, around the wrists and elbows, the anterior axillary fold, nipples and penis and, in infants, the palms and soles.

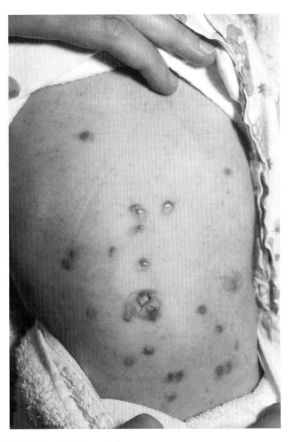

Fig. 73.14 Scabies nodules.

which can be mastered with practice. A burrow, which may be softened by the application of 20% potassium hydroxide, is scraped and the material smeared on a slide for microscopic examination. Burrows may be more easily identified by rubbing a thick black marking pen over suspicious areas and wiping with an alcohol swab, leaving a burrow outlined with ink.

> ### Clinical example
>
> Jordan, a 1 year old Samoan boy, presented with large pustules on his soles and areas of weeping and crusting. He was miserable and febrile and his feet were obviously painful. Impetigo was suspected. A swab from the pustules grows group A beta haemolytic *Streptococcus* and after 5 days of penicillin treatment Jordan was well and the pustules had disappeared. The crusting and weeping remained and were diagnosed as eczema and treated with topical steroid with good effect. As the eczema cleared, small vesicles and curved lines were seen on the soles. Careful examination demonstrated similar lesions on the palms and between the fingers and there were also several nodules found on the penis and in the axillary folds. There were a few excoriated papules on the abdomen. One of the curved lines was scraped and mites were demonstrated, finally confirming a diagnosis of scabies.

Clinical features and diagnosis

- The pathognomonic primary lesion, a typical burrow, is rarely seen. It is a 2–3 mm long curved grey line with a vesicle at the anterior end.
- Other lesions which mark the sites of burrows are small blisters or papules, larger blisters on the palms and soles of infants, scratch marks, secondary eczema and secondary bacterial infection.
- Eczema or impetigo in the target areas for scabies should always raise suspicion of this disease, as should blisters on the palms and soles of infants.
- Often more prominent than the evidence of burrows is the so called secondary eruption of scabies. This presents as multiple, very pruritic, urticarial papules which are soon excoriated. They occur particularly on the abdomen, thighs and buttocks.
- Large inflammatory nodules may form part of the secondary eruption, occurring particularly on covered areas, especially on axillae, scrotum, penis and buttocks. They may, however, be very widespread, producing diagnostic difficulties. They may persist for months after effective scabies treatment.
- The diagnosis of scabies is usually a clinical one but can be confirmed by demonstration of the mite, an art

Management

- The patient and all close contacts should be treated simultaneously.
- 5% Permethrin cream is the treatment of choice and should be applied to all body surfaces from the neck down and left on overnight. A repeat application should be administered after 1 week.
- In extremely young infants 6% precipitated sulphur is preferred.
- Bedclothes and clothing should be washed in the normal way with no disinfection required.
- An irritant dermatitis may follow scabies treatment, particularly in atopic children, and may require emollients and topical steroids once the miticide therapy is fully completed.
- Persistent nodules may respond to topical corticosteroids but a coal tar solution painted on is preferable for the very resistant ones.

Pediculosis

Human lice are six legged insects without wings, grey in colour or brown-red when engorged with blood. The body louse and the head louse have a thin body 2–4 mm long and three similar pairs of legs; the pubic louse is wider and shorter and the second and third pair of legs are larger than the first, producing a crab-like appearance. The ova (nits) appear as oval grey-white 0.5 mm specks, attached by a firm chitin ring to hairs or clothes.

Pediculosis capitis (head lice)

This is a common infestation, often occurring in epidemics in schools. The occipital area of the scalp is preferentially involved and may be the only site affected. The condition is itchy, leading to scratching with excoriations and also eczematisation and secondary infection which may mask the underlying infestation. Permethrin shampoos are effective pediculicides but may not destroy ova and a repeat application after a few days is recommended to kill further hatched lice. Removal of nit cases with a fine comb is easier if the chitin is softened by a prior application of vinegar.

Pediculosis corporis (body lice)

This is rare in children except in severely overcrowded conditions with poor hygiene. The organism infests bedding and clothing and the nits are not found on the human host. The lice hatch with body warmth and puncture the skin, producing very itchy, small, red papules with haemorrhagic puncta. Spots of dried blood may be found on the clothing and bed linen. Treatment is directed towards removal of the organisms from materials with hot water laundering and hot ironing or the use of a hot electric dryer.

Pediculosis pubis (pubic lice, crab lice)

This is mainly an adult disease. The pubic louse has as its normal habitat the anogenital area but in children it is particularly seen on the eyelashes. Eyelash infestation in children may occur from innocent close contact with an affected adult but the possibility of sexual abuse must always be considered. Pediculosis of the eyelashes is best treated with petroleum jelly applied thickly twice a day for a week.

Arthropod bites

Patients with arthropod bites present to a dermatologist in two situations: the severe local allergic reaction and the more chronic hypersensitivity condition called 'papular urticaria'. The arthropods most encountered are mosquitos, sand flies, fleas and grass mites. The distribution of the bites helps to suggest the causative agent.

Severe local reactions

- Include blisters, purpura and cellulitis and lymphangitis even in the absence of infection.
- As the lesions are extremely itchy, scratching occurs, leading to secondary eczematisation and secondary infection.

Papular urticaria

- A very common condition in children, particularly between 10 months and 4 years.
- In a child who has been sensitised by previous exposure the bite produces an itchy urticarial (hive-like) wheal which is succeeded by a firm itchy papule which lasts for many days.
- The wheal and papule usually show a central punctum and the papule may be surmounted by a tiny blister.
- The persistence and severity of the condition are explained by the fact that new bites by the same species will often cause a recrudescence of activity in resolving lesions.
- Secondary infection and eczematisation from scratching also contribute to the chronicity of the condition, which may plague the child through an entire summer.
- Management involves avoidance of insect attack, with the use of insect repellents, insecticides, protective clothing and changes in activities, which clearly are difficult in an active child. Wrapping the affected areas in wet dressings overnight as soon as new bites occur is helpful in reducing the itch and preventing scratching which leads to the secondary eczema and infection. Topical corticosteroids will improve the secondary eczema and have some effect in dampening the severity of the actual bite reaction but must not be used for prolonged periods. Oral antibiotics are required if there is significant secondary infection.

Forms of dermatitis

Atopic dermatitis (atopic eczema)

Atopy is a genetically determined disorder with an increased tendency to form IgE antibody to inhalants and foods and increased susceptibility to asthma, allergic rhinitis and atopic eczema (Ch. 42). This eczema may begin at any age but 75% of patients show the first signs by 6 months.

Clinical features

The characteristic clinical features are a generalised dryness and a tendency to lichenification or thickening of the skin, pruritus and excoriations and patches of acute, subacute or chronic eczema. Involvement of the whole cutaneous surface may occur but the predominant areas are the face in infants, extensor aspects of the limbs as the child begins to crawl and the limb flexures in older children. In severe cases the whole skin may be erythematous and in these patients white dermographism is often a prominent feature: this indicates that the condition is likely to be unstable and difficult.

Complications

Patients with atopic eczema may develop secondary bacterial infection that presents either as yellow crusting impetigo or folliculitis, or simply as worsening eczema. Mollusca contagiosa are common and atopic patients are at risk of developing severe widespread herpes simplex infections. The usual childhood immunisations are quite safe.

Management

Explanation and education. The most important aspect of the management of atopic eczema is explanation of the condition to the patient or, more commonly, his or her parents. The family should understand that the child has been born with an inherently dry, irritable skin and that this will be a lifelong tendency. While the skin does become more stable with time, it will always require extra care as without it eczema may ensue at any age. It is essential to talk in terms of control rather than cure, otherwise the family search for an end point after which care will no longer be required and this is an unrealistic expectation. The condition should be explained as a multifactorial disorder as it must be appreciated that just as there is no 'cure', there is no single 'cause'.

Avoidance of irritants. Factors which will often irritate the atopic skin should be discussed. Woollen material in direct contact with the skin is a major irritant; apart from the child's own clothing it is important to remember the parent's clothing, carpets, blankets, stroller and car seat covers, furniture and toys. Shiny nylon materials and some acrylics irritate but cotton-polyester mixtures are usually well tolerated. Sand contact is often troublesome, especially with prolonged close contact as in playing in a sandpit. Chlorinated water may aggravate but this is variable. Soap in excess and bubble baths overdry the skin, and many perfumed and 'medicated' products, disinfectants and strong cleansers cause irritation.

Dealing with dryness. Bath oils and oatmeal containing products are useful and prevent the defatting of the skin that bathing can induce. It is essential to find a suitable moisturiser which can be applied all over twice a day, whether or not there is active eczema. Glycerine 10% in sorbolene cream is useful in many cases but more or less greasy preparations are available to suit individual patients and climatic conditions. Urea containing products sting broken skin and are unsuitable in these children.

Topical corticosteroids. These are an essential part of treatment. In general ointment bases are preferred because they are more emollient than cream bases. Nothing stronger than 1% hydrocortisone should be used on the face or in the axillae or groin. Medium strength fluorinated corticosteroids are usually adequate for lesions on the trunk and limbs; the stronger preparations are rarely required. These preparations are best used three times a day and, of course, ceased as soon as the eczema is clear.

Wet dressings. There are useful in severe widespread eczema. A water based emollient is applied all over; a corticosteroid cream (rather than ointment in this case because cream is more water miscible) is applied to the areas of active eczema; sheeting soaked in tap water is applied and bandaged on with a crepe bandage and a net material is used to hold the dressings in place. The procedure is repeated three times a day. These dressings cool the skin down, reduce itching, physically prevent scratching, increase the hydration of the skin and enhance the penetration of topical steroids. This treatment is usually effective in clearing the eczema in 3 or 4 days. If dressings are required for longer periods the corticosteroid should be used only once a day. Particular care should be taken with infants.

Systemic therapy. If significant bacterial infection occurs a swab should be taken and oral antibiotics used. Nocturnal sedation is often valuable during severe episodes but daytime sedation should be avoided; antihistamines are the preferred sedatives. While they may be essential for associated diseases, oral corticosteroids should never be instituted for the eczema itself; a severe rebound can occur on their withdrawal and after several courses the eczema can become very unstable. A number of non sedating antihistamines may be helpful in very unstable difficult cases.

Dietary manipulation. No alteration should be made to the patient's diet unless the atopic eczema has failed to respond to conventional therapy properly carried out. There is only a small group of patients with unstable eczema with an associated urticarial element in whom dietary factors are of major significance; skin prick tests are useful in this group to give a guide for dietary manipulation, which should be instituted only by those with a full understanding of the nutritional requirements of young children.

Dust mite allergy. This is important in a selected group of patients. In these children the eczema is usually particularly troublesome on the face and neck. The family should be given details of dust mite reduction strategies.

Discoid eczema

- In children this is often a manifestation of a combined atopic and psoriatic diathesis.
- Well defined patches of acute eczema occur in a strikingly symmetrical distribution. In infants the commonest sites are the upper back and the tops of the shoulders; in older patients the extensor aspects of the limbs are particularly involved. The lesions may be very thick and exudative and they are very itchy.

- Discoid eczema should be distinguished from tinea and impetigo, which are less symmetrical, and classical psoriasis, which is rarely moist.
- Management involves emollients and topical steroids as for atopic dermatitis, with the continued use of emollient helping to prevent recurrences.

Pityriasis alba

This condition probably represents a very mild eczema, which, however, produces a striking postinflammatory depigmentation. The condition is more common in atopics, and occasionally some areas will show erythema and more definite eczematous changes:

- Appears as poorly defined, slightly scaly, hypopigmented patches occurring particularly on the face and the upper arms.
- The mild irritation and signs of mild eczema respond to emollients and weak topical corticosteroids but the hypopigmentation may be very persistent and require sun exposure over a prolonged period before repigmentation is complete.
- The condition should be differentiated from vitiligo, where there is total depigmentation and no scale, and from tinea versicolor, which is rare on the face, has very well demarcated lesions and has a very fine branny scale.

Contact allergic dermatitis from plants
(Fig. 73.15)

- The commonest causative agents in Australia are rhus and a variety of grevilleas, including Robyn Gordon, Ned Kelly and Hookerana.
- The dermatitis is usually very severe and blistering often occurs.

Clinical example

Harry, aged 4, presented with a swelling and redness around one eye. It was diagnosed by the ophthalmology registrar as preseptal orbital cellulitis, the child was admitted to hospital and intravenous antibiotics were started. It was remarked that a lack of fever and pain was unusual in a child with cellulitis. The next day the area was more swollen and some blistering had occurred. Harry was noted also to have multiple linear blistered red lesions on his arm. Harry's mother told the registrar that Harry's best friend from the preschool had similar lesions on the arms and face, which had been diagnosed by a dermatologist as a plant contact dermatitis. The history obtained was that the preschool garden had been landscaped by parents over the previous weekend and the two children carried Robyn Gordon grevilleas in the car for planting. Harry's antibiotics were ceased and he was discharged from hospital on a 5 day course of oral steroids. The swelling resolved in 2 days and in 6 days all the rash had disappeared. The following weekend the Robyn Gordon grevilleas were removed from the preschool.

- It often occurs in a streaky pattern where the plant has brushed against the skin
- Initially there may be much oedema, especially on the face, and cellulitis is often suspected; however, the child is afebrile and the area is itchy rather than painful.
- The condition may be spread beyond areas of initial contact due to retention of allergen on clothing and under the nails.
- A strong topical steroid may be adequate for localised areas but a short course of oral steroids is usually indicated. Low and medium strength topical corticosteroids are usually ineffective.

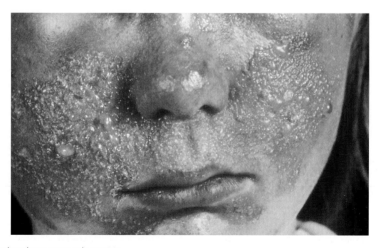

Fig. 73.15 Acute vesicular plant contact dermatitis.

Napkin rashes

Common causes

- *Seborrhoeic dermatitis*. Presents as a dull red rash covering most of the napkin area, sometimes with a greasy yellow scale, although this is characteristically absent in this moist area.
- *Monilia*. Manifested as a thick white material deep in the folds and as small annular lesions with an overhanging white macerated scale at their margin.
- *Irritant dermatitis from urine and faeces*. Irritant dermatitis due to urine affects mainly the convex surfaces, with relative sparing of the flexures; irritation due to faeces particularly affects the natal cleft. Napkin dermatitis is rarely caused by irritant or allergic reactions to laundering products.
- *Miliaria*. Sweat duct occlusion may occur alone or in combination with other elements, particularly in children wearing plastic overpants. This presents as small red papules which are very transient so the pattern varies considerably from hour to hour.

Variants of common types

- *Gluteal granuloma*s. Occur on top of a pre-existing napkin rash as purplish nodules which tend to be oval in shape, following the lines of the skin folds.
- *Erosive napkin rash*. Occurs in the perianal and natal cleft area and usually follows a period of diarrhoea. It is seen in infants with lactose intolerance.
- *Ulcerated nodules*. Most often occur in the vulval area in a situation of a constant urinary leak in the presence of major congenital anomalies.
- *'Frog plaster' napkin rash*. Due to the accumulation of faeces, and to a lesser extent, urine under the plaster used in cases of developmental dysplasia of the hip and is usually of a mixed erosive and ulcerated nodule type.

Rarer causes

- *Psoriasis* (Fig. 73.16). Produces a bright red, glazed, clearly marginated napkin rash. This may develop into the condition called 'napkin psoriasis'. A few small scaly spots occur on the trunk above the psoriatic napkin rash, followed by a sudden explosion of typical psoriatic lesions on scalp, face and all over the trunk. The infant is well and the condition is usually asymptomatic. The eruption is self limiting in a few weeks.
- *Impetigo.* Presents as small pus filled blisters which quickly rupture and expand into large superficial erosions, usually asymptomatic.
- *Herpes simplex*. Punched out 3–8 mm individual erosions that coalesce to form geographic shaped lesions; considerable swelling is usually seen and there is associated lymphadenopathy and fever.

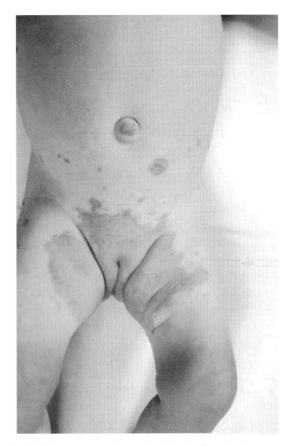

Fig. 73.16 Psoriatic napkin rash with early dissemination.

- *Staphylococcal scalded skin syndrome*. May present in the napkin area with a very painful bright red rash with superficial blistering.
- *Kawasaki disease*. Often presents in the napkin area with a tender red scaly rash in a febrile child.
- *Langerhans cell histiocytosis*. Produces a severe napkin rash with a brownish scale, erosions and purpuric spots.
- *Zinc deficiency*. Produces a well marginated shiny rash rather similar to psoriasis, but with a characteristic dark peripheral scale. Similar lesions are present around the mouth and nose.

Psoriasis

Psoriasis is a hereditary disease: it is probably an autosomal dominant condition with variable penetrance. It commences by the age of 15 years in 30% of patients. It may present in the typical adult form of large erythematous plaques, with a thick silvery white scale, predominantly on the knees, elbows, buttocks and scalp, but certain differences are seen in childhood disease:

- Plaques are usually smaller and with a finer scale (Fig. 73.17).

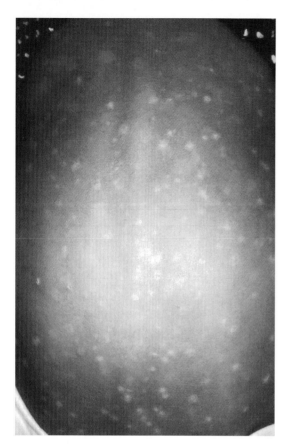

Fig. 73.17 Small plaque psoriasis leaving a striking hypopigmentation.

- A particularly common presentation is acute guttate psoriasis with the eruption of tiny papules in a widespread distribution. The eruption is often preceded by an intercurrent illness, particularly a streptococcal throat infection.
- The face and intertriginous sites, such as retroauricular areas, axillae, groin, genital and perianal area, are commonly affected in children.
- Children presenting with vulvitis, balanitis and perianal itching may be found to have psoriasis. In these areas the typical scale is absent and the condition presents as a glazed erythema, often with fissuring.
- Nail involvement is usually absent or minimal with minor pitting.
- Pustular psoriasis and psoriatic arthropathy are extremely rare in children.
- There is a particular type of well marginated, bright red napkin rash, described above, which is a marker for psoriasis.
- Many therapies used in adults are inappropriate in children. In general psoriasis in children is better treated with tars than topical corticosteroids. No treatment can alter the course of the condition.

Photosensitivity

Photosensitivity may be manifested by exaggerated sunburn or another rash appearing in a light exposed area. There are many causes and some are briefly reviewed here:

- Phytophotodermatitis — contact with a phototoxic agent (for example lime juice, perfumes) followed by sun exposure causes an exaggerated sunburn reaction.
- Drug reactions — rare in children.
- Polymorphous light reaction — may produce recurring erythematous, itchy vesicles and papules on the cheeks, ears, side of the neck and exposed limbs. The onset of the eruption may be delayed 1–2 days after sun exposure, but the distribution of the lesions and history of exacerbation in the summer months are typical.
- Solar urticaria — a very transient urticarial rash appearing immediately after sun exposure.
- Connective tissue diseases
  - Lupus erythematosus
  - Dermatomyositis.
- Porphyrias
  - Erythropoietic protoporphyria
  - Congenital erythropoietic porphyria.
- Other genetic disorders leading to increased sun sensitivity
  - Albinism
  - Xeroderma pigmentosum
  - Bloom syndrome
  - Rothmund–Thomson syndrome.

Hair loss in children

There are two major types of hair loss (alopecia): diffuse and patchy. The commonest cause of localised alopecia is telogen effluvium, and the main causes of patchy alopecia are tinea, alopecia areata and trichotillomania.

Diffuse alopecia

- Telogen effluvium — high fever causes a large number of hairs to enter the resting or telogen stage of the hair cycle prematurely; 2–3 months later these inevitably fall. The hairs have a club shaped end visible as a white dot with the naked eye. New hairs immediately appear in the empty follicles. The condition may continue for several months but is fully reversible.
- Some other causes
  - Drugs
  - Malnutrition
  - Iron deficiency
  - Various aminoacidurias
  - Hereditary hair shaft abnormality syndromes
  - Congenital atrichia
  - Alopecia as a part of other genetic syndromes.

Patchy alopecia

- Tinea — combination of inflammation of varying degree and broken hairs.
- Alopecia areata — autoimmune disease with areas of total hair loss and no obvious inflammation; there may be some short so-called 'exclamation mark hairs' at the edges.

- Trichotillomania — hair twisting or plucking. Hairs broken at different lengths, usually no inflammation.
- Some other causes
  - Traction: from tight hair styles
  - Infections: boils, erysipelas, herpes simplex, herpes zoster, tick bites
  - Localised scleroderma.

Systemic implications of skin disease in children

R. Phillips

Virtually all systemic diseases lead to skin changes sooner or later. This chapter focuses on skin changes in children that require examination and/or investigation for systemic problems.

Vesicular, bullous or pustular rashes

Vesicles and pustules are considered together in this section as there is substantial clinical overlap. Vesicles from any cause usually become pustular in a couple of days.

In the neonatal period, pustules may be part of several transient dermatological conditions (Ch. 73) but pustules or vesicles may be a marker of serious underlying illness, even in the absence of fever and lethargy. Consider:

- Infection, either congenital or acquired. *Herpes simplex* virus (Ch. 73), *Varicella*, *Listeria*, *Staphylococcus*, *Streptococcus*, *Haemophilus*, *Neisseria* or *Candida* species may be present.
- Neutropenia from any cause. Superficial bacterial pustules may be the only sign of congenital neutropenia.
- Incontinentia pigmenti. This disease is X linked and fatal in male fetuses. Girls present with lesions distributed in linear patterns following the lines of Blaschko (not dermatomal lines; Fig. 74.1). Lesions evolve through vesicular and warty phases to eventually leave permanent hyperpigmented streaks. Seizures and developmental, ocular and dental problems may occur.

At any age, consider:
- Langerhans cell histiocytosis.
- Drug reactions. These can manifest as phototoxic or photosensitive reactions (Ch. 73) or bullous drug reactions. Stevens–Johnson syndrome presents with mucocutaneous erosions and blistering in association with erythematous or purpuric macules, lethargy, fever, lymphadenopathy, and conjunctivitis, occasionally leading to death or blindness. Most cases are secondary to medications, often non steroidal anti-inflammatory drugs.
- Dermatitis herpetiformis. This may present in older children as itchy papules or vesicles, often on extensor surfaces. Most patients have gluten enteropathy (coeliac disease) and may have abdominal discomfort, diarrhoea or anaemia.

Acneiform rashes

Some degree of acne is occasionally seen on the face in infancy and is common on the face and upper trunk during puberty. Comedonal acne may be the first sign of puberty. Acne, particularly if severe, can lead to significant depression in adolescents and is a risk factor for suicide. Both the depression and the acne need to be recognised and treated. Acne that is atypical in age of onset, distribution, morphology or severity may be associated with systemic disease. Consider:

- Glucocorticoid excess, either exogenous or endogenous. This can give a monomorphic acneiform rash on the face and trunk (Fig. 74.2). Other cushingoid stigmata are usually present.
- Androgen excess. Other features depend on the age and sex of the child and in younger children include accelerated growth, body odour, pubic hair, clitoromegaly (but not breast development) and penile (but not testicular) enlargement. In teenage females, polycystic ovary syndrome is commonly the cause.
- Precocious puberty.
- Medications. In postpubertal children, antiepileptic medications, especially phenytoin and phenobarbitone, may induce acne.

Chronic erosions or ulcers

Several primary skin conditions can cause chronic erosions or ulcers in children, including itchy conditions such as scabies and papular urticaria. Also consider:

- Immunodeficiencies. Recurrent boils can be seen in chronic granulomatous disease and hyper IgE syndrome. Poor wound healing is a feature of leucocyte adhesion defects.
- Skin fragility syndromes. In junctional and dystrophic forms of epidermolysis bullosa, chronic ulcers related to minimal skin trauma may be seen in association with failure to thrive, anaemia and gastrointestinal tract involvement.
- Porphyria. Several enzyme defects in haem metabolism are associated with chronic erosive lesions, photosensitivity and hyperpigmentation. Episodes of acute pain or neurological dysfunction are rarely seen in childhood porphyrias.

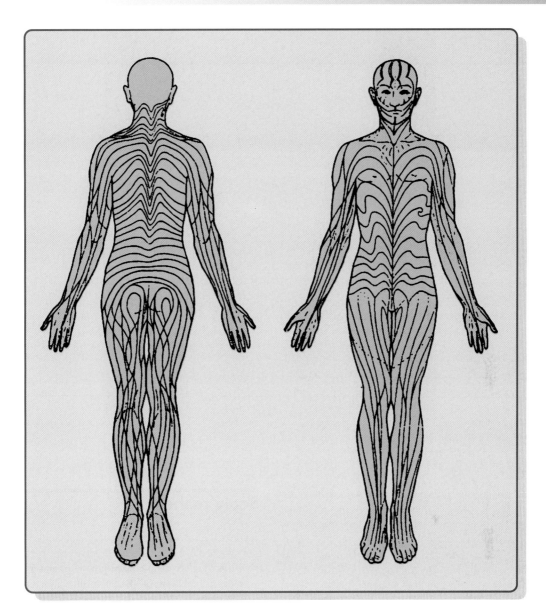

Fig. 74.1 Lines of Blaschko.

Recurrent mouth ulcers

These are generally due to aphthous stomatitis. Such ulcers are usually small and resolve in a few days. Recurrent mouth ulcers can also be seen in:

- Iron, folate or vitamin B_{12} deficiency.
- Gastrointestinal disorders. Coeliac disease, Crohn disease and ulcerative colitis are all associated with mouth ulceration. Recurrent abdominal pain, intermittent diarrhoea and failure to thrive may be present.
- Connective tissue disorders. Patients with Behçet disease usually present in late childhood with ulcers at one site (mouth or genitals) and it may be many years before a second site is involved. Systemic lupus

erythematosus and juvenile rheumatoid arthritis may cause recurrent mouth ulcers.

- Immunodeficiency states, HIV infection.
- Malignancy. Lymphoma and histiocytosis can present with non-healing mouth ulcers.

Papular rashes

Papules or nodules may occur in a number of disorders, including acute rheumatic fever, juvenile chronic arthritis, systemic lupus erythematosus and neurofibromatosis, but are rarely the presenting feature. Erythematous

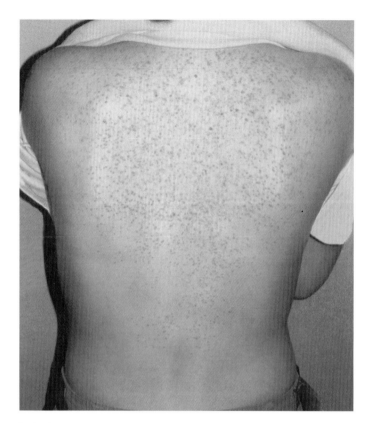

Fig. 74.2 Steroid acne on the back.

papules, often itchy, scaly or purpuric, may be widespread in acute Langerhans cell histiocytosis. Severe, recalcitrant 'cradle cap' or weeping intertriginous lesions may also be present, along with single or multiple bone lesions, mucosal ulceration and involvement of other organs. In neonates, Langerhans cell histiocytosis may present as a few nodules, classically with a raised border and central necrosis. This congenital self-healing form usually shows complete regression within months but visceral involvement may occur.

In children, yellow papules are commonly xanthogranulomas. These are often isolated lesions that resolve within a few years and are not associated with lipid disorders. Multiple eruptive xanthomas, tuberous xanthomas (usually distributed over the elbows, knuckles, buttocks, knees and heels) and tendinous xanthomas (usually on tendons around the elbow, wrist, hand or ankle) are associated with elevated cholesterol levels. Consider:

- Primary hyperlipoproteinaemias. Skin lesions may present between 5 and 15 years of age, sometimes as tendinitis or tenosynovitis. Look for signs of atherosclerotic disease, and a family history of high cholesterol, early myocardial infarcts or strokes.
- Secondary hypercholesterolaemia. This can occur in hypothyroidism, biliary cirrhosis, diabetes mellitus, glycogen storage disease and nephrotic syndrome.

Scaly rashes

Ichthyosis refers to generalised scaly skin. Some ichthyoses only affect the skin but several involve other organs:

- X linked ichthyosis. This is quite common but may be undiagnosed. A fine scaling at birth is later replaced by larger brown scales. Diagnosis is confirmed by enzyme analysis. Boys with X linked ichthyosis need to be monitored for hypogonadism, cryptorchidism, anosmia, short stature and mental retardation. Female carriers may have obstetric difficulties.
- In Sjögren–Larsson syndrome, a yellow-brown lichenified appearance is present in infancy. This evolves into a more florid scaling with a symmetric spastic paralysis and mental retardation.
- In some trichothiodystrophies, ichthyosis is associated with brittle hair and mental and growth retardation.
- Several ichthyoses are linked with deafness, cataracts or other eye problems. Mild, generalized scaling may be the first feature in later onset Refsum disease, before development of multiple visual problems, deafness and neuropathy.

Ectodermal dysplasias are a heterogeneous group of conditions characterised by congenital, non progressive abnormalities of hair, teeth, nails and sweat glands. The skin is dry and may be hyperpigmented. Deficient sweating may cause overheating in summer. Teeth are often poorly developed or absent. Cleft lip and palate, limb abnormalities and mucous retention in the upper airway and ear may be present.

Eczematous rashes

Atopic eczema is common and in most cases can be readily controlled with minimal sequelae (Ch. 73). However, a few children have chronic and severe disease requiring frequent, time consuming applications of topical medicines and wet dressings. These children may have recurrent infections, particularly with *Staphylococcus aureus* and Herpes simplex virus. There may be failure to thrive. Severe psychosocial, behavioural and marital problems are common in these severely affected children, although often hidden from medical staff. These problems need to be identified and addressed.

Eczematous skin lesions can also be associated with:

- Immunodeficiency syndromes. Thrombocytopenia, immunodeficiency and eczema are seen in Wiskott–Aldrich syndrome. Failure to thrive, recurrent infections, diarrhoea or haematological abnormalities may suggest this or other immunodeficiencies that are variably associated with eczema.
- Multiple food allergies with consequent dietary restrictions and secondary nutritional and psychosocial problems.
- Metabolic or nutritional disorders. Phenylketonuria often presents with eczema. Less typical eczematous lesions, more prominent in periorificial areas, are seen in biotin, essential fatty acid and zinc deficiency syndromes. Malnutrition and organoacidaemias, e.g. methylmalonicacidaemia, can result in similar lesions.

Erythematous rashes

Neonatal erythroderma

Erythroderma (inflammation of almost all the skin surface) in the neonatal period requires close monitoring and early investigation to identify the underlying cause. Eczema rarely presents as erythroderma. Exclude staphylococcal toxin mediated infections and congenital candidiasis. Metabolic causes include inherited carboxylase deficiencies and essential fatty acid deficiency secondary to any severe malabsorption, and can be associated with severe acidosis and coma. Omenn syndrome, (familial reticuloendotheliosis with eosinophilia), maternal graft versus host disease and other severe immunodeficiencies can present as erythroderma. Drug reactions are an unlikely cause at this age. Some variants of ichthyosis can present as erythroderma and may be associated with multiple infections, failure to thrive, or cataracts.

Annular rashes

Annular lesions are ring shaped with relatively normal skin centrally. Such lesions are typical of tinea corporis, urticaria and granuloma annulare but may require investigation for neonatal lupus (look for heart block and maternal antinuclear antibodies), rheumatic fever, syphilis and Lyme disease.

Erythema nodosum

Erythema nodosum can occur at any age and presents initially as subcutaneous erythematous lesions mainly on the anterior lower legs. It may be idiopathic or associated with chronic streptococcal disease, pulmonary or other tuberculosis, Crohn disease, chronic gastrointestinal infections, sarcoidosis and *Mycoplasma* infection. It may also be secondary to a number of drugs.

Urticaria

Urticaria describes circular erythematous macules or swellings, often with central pallor that appear, migrate and disappear over minutes or hours. It is common. Usually no cause is found but recurrent or chronic urticaria may be related to underlying inflammatory conditions such as systemic lupus erythematosus, juvenile chronic arthritis, other vasculitic diseases and parasitic infection. In a child who is very unwell, consider Kawasaki disease.

Generalised erythematous rashes

Erythematous rashes with fever are common in children. Many widespread childhood viruses may be accompanied by an erythematous rash. Occasionally the clinical pattern is distinctive and a confident diagnosis can be made. Usually the diagnosis cannot be made clinically. If the diagnosis is not clear, decide if the child is significantly unwell. Any signs of decreased responsiveness, lethargy or shock may require urgent investigation for causes such as septicaemia and Kawasaki disease. In otherwise well children, consider whether the rash may be a drug reaction. If any relatives may be at risk (e.g. immunosuppressed siblings, pregnant women), serological and virological testing to identify a cause may be appropriate. Usually, no investigation is needed:

- The skin lesions of systemic lupus erythematosus include a characteristic butterfly distribution over both cheeks and the base of the nose. Patchy lesions may also present over the ears, neck and less commonly the limbs. In acute systemic lupus erythematosus, erythematous macules are also seen about the nail beds, on the tips of the fingers, the toes, and on the palms of the hands and soles of the feet.
- An erythematous maculopapular rash is often seen in the systemic form of juvenile chronic arthritis. This rash usually has a salmon pink colour, and tends to come and go, being particularly evident at the time when the fever is at its height. It may be urticarial.
- The lesions of Henoch–Schönlein purpura may be erythematous and urticarial rather than purpuric.
- An erythematous rash which is distributed over the extensor surfaces of the joints, particularly over the knuckles, elbows and knees, is characteristic of dermatomyositis. In addition, most children with this disorder show a violaceous facial rash and periorbital oedema.
- An erythematous rash accompanied by oedema of the palms and soles is often prominent in Kawasaki disease. Other early features include prolonged high fever, conjunctivitis, redness, swelling or ulceration of mucosal surfaces and enlargement of lymph nodes. Desquamation of the hands and feet is a later finding.

Purpuric rashes

Most children presenting with fever and petechiae (pinpoint purpura) but who are otherwise well have an enteroviral infection without other findings. However, purpuric rashes are associated with several life-threatening diseases. They require urgent assessment.

Neonatal purpura

Purpuric rashes in the neonatal period may be an early presentation of any cause of childhood purpura (see below). In addition, consider:

- congenital infection including rubella, cytomegalovirus, toxoplasmosis, and herpes simplex
- haemolytic disease of the newborn
- malignancy, including neuroblastoma, Langerhans cell histiocytosis and leukaemia
- iatrogenic injury, including birth trauma, extravasation of drugs and arterial injury during catheterisation.

Childhood purpura

Purpuric rashes in childhood are usually secondary to vascular dysfunction rather than a low platelet count. Consider:

- Septicaemia. An unwell febrile child with purpura should be treated for meningococcal septicaemia without waiting for the results of investigations. Septicaemia from *Haemophilus influenzae*, streptococci, staphylococci and some Gram negative organisms may cause purpura. Less extensive, but diagnostically useful, are the purpuric lesions of subacute bacterial endocarditis, typhus and typhoid fever. Purpura may also occur in certain viral haemorrhagic fevers.
- Coagulation disorders. There may be a history of joint pain or swelling, or bleeding from other sites.
- Henoch–Schönlein purpura. This is quite common in childhood. Purpuric lesions on the legs and buttocks may be the only finding in Henoch–Schönlein purpura or there may be associated abdominal pain, arthritis or renal involvement. Children with Henoch–Schönlein purpura should be monitored for months for the development of nephritis.
- Other vasculitic diseases.
- Glucocorticoid excess.
- Any cause of abnormal skin elasticity.
- Scurvy. Irritability, bone pain, gum sponginess and bleeding may be present. Wrist X rays are diagnostic.
- Child abuse. Bruises of different ages and at unusual sites may be seen.
- Trauma.

Childhood purpura with thrombocytopenia

Purpura in association with a low platelet count is often associated with bruising and signs of bleeding elsewhere. Idiopathic thrombocytopenic purpura is the most common cause. Children need to be examined and investigated for leukaemia, pancytopenia, splenomegaly and drug induced thrombocytopenia or aplastic anaemia (chloramphenicol, antithyroid medications).

Haemangiomas and vascular malformations

Haemangiomas and vascular malformations are discussed in Chapter 73. They are often isolated lesions but may be part of systemic disease. Consider:

- Ocular and intracranial involvement. Children with haemangiomas or vascular malformations around the eye should be screened for glaucoma and other eye abnormalities. Children with capillary malformations involving the region of the first or second division of the trigeminal nerve may also have intracranial involvement and develop epilepsy, strokes, hemiplegia or mental retardation (Sturge–Weber syndrome).
- Occult spinal abnormalities.
- Intestinal lesions. Multiple cutaneous and visceral vascular lesions occur in blue rubber bleb syndrome and may cause intestinal bleeding. Telangiectases in hereditary haemorrhagic telangiectasia usually appear on the face, mouth and nose. Nose bleeds become frequent in late childhood and gastrointestinal bleeding occurs in adult life.
- Overgrowth syndromes. Extensive vascular malformations can be associated with limb overgrowth and other organ involvement in Klippel–Trénauney and Proteus syndromes.
- Cutis marmorata telangiectatica congenita. Reticulated, vascular lesions on the skin may be associated with asymmetric limb growth (sometimes distant from the skin involvement) and glaucoma.
- Coagulopathy (Kasabach–Merritt syndrome). This occurs with rare subtypes of haemangioma. Rapid enlargement of the haemangioma accompanies purpura and bleeding, thrombocytopenia and disseminated intravascular coagulation.
- Fabry disease. Angiokeratomas (flat or raised, slightly warty, telangiectatic or vascular lesions) appear on the lower trunk, pelvis and thighs. There may be limb pain or paraesthesia, or corneal opacities. Renal, cardiac and central nervous system problems occur later.
- Fucosidosis. Severely affected children die early. In mild cases, children may present with angiokeratomas and anhidrosis in later childhood. Look for coarse facies, developmental delay and growth retardation.

- Telangiectasia ataxia. Some degree of ataxia is usually present by the time conjunctival telangiectases are noted.

Lumbosacral birthmarks

Congenital lesions over the lumbosacral area may be associated with occult spinal abnormalities such as a tethered cord. These spinal anomalies may not cause problems until later in childhood when they can present insidiously with irreversible bladder, bowel or limb dysfunction. These problems can be prevented by early MRI screening and surgical correction. Congenital lesions that have been associated with underlying spinal problems include haemangiomas, capillary malformations, lipomas, dimples, sinuses and hairy patches.

Hypopigmented lesions

Generalised hypopigmentation

Generalised hypopigmentation, blonde hair and grey-blue eyes are seen in several genodermatoses involving chromosomes 11 or 15. The clinical presentations vary from mild to complete loss of pigmentation and individuals may go undiagnosed unless compared to their siblings and parents. Early diagnosis and investigation is important to ensure early ophthalmological intervention and rigorous sun protection. Look for:

- Poor vision, photophobia and nystagmus. Type 1 oculocutaneous albinism usually results in more severe disease than type 2.
- Bleeding diathesis, due to a platelet defect in Hermansky–Pudlak syndrome.
- Recurrent infections in Chediak–Higashi syndrome.
- Mental retardation, obesity. Both Angelman and Prader–Willi syndromes can present with albinism.

Localised hypopigmentation

Localised patches of hypopigmented skin or hair may be due to piebaldism, pityriasis versicolor (usually in adolescence), pityriasis alba (usually in mid childhood), previous inflammation and vitiligo. Also consider:

- Endocrinopathies. Vitiligo in children is weakly associated with other endocrine conditions. Children with vitiligo should be reviewed for features of diabetes and thyroid dysfunction.
- Tuberosclerosis. Hypopigmented patches may be the first sign of tuberosclerosis. These patches can be regular or irregular in shape. An isolated hypopigmented patch in a young child is far more likely to be a simple achromic naevus than to be part of tuberosclerosis, but multiple hypopigmented patches

increase the likelihood of tuberosclerosis. Look also for forehead plaques (pink, initially flat but later slightly raised) and shagreen patches (rough, slightly thickened skin usually over the back). Other skin findings such as periungual fibromas and facial angiofibromas usually appear in older children. The diagnosis of tuberosclerosis may require imaging of eyes, brain, heart and kidneys and investigation of relatives.

- Streaks, lines and whorls of hyper- or hypopigmentation that may be present from birth. These patterns reflect mosaicism. Usually these children are otherwise normal but a wide range of associated abnormalities in other systems have been reported. Apart from audiological and ophthalmological examination, investigations are not required unless suggested by clinical findings but these children should be reviewed until settled in school.
- Leprosy. Focal pale patches may be the only marker of leprosy in an individual from an endemic area.

Hyperpigmented lesions

Generalised hyperpigmentation

Generalised darkening of the skin is often most obvious on the palmar creases, linea alba and areola. It is uncommon in childhood. Consider:

- Endocrine disease. Addison disease, Cushing syndrome of pituitary origin, exogenous ACTH administration and acromegaly can all cause hyperpigmentation.
- Renal failure may cause greying of the skin.
- Haemochromatosis. In children, this is usually secondary to transfusions.

- Photosensitivity.
- Lipoidoses. A yellow-brown darkening of skin, most prominent in sun exposed areas, can occur in the Niemann–Pick diseases. Look for waxy indurated skin, purpura, hepatosplenomegaly and neurological deterioration. Although a similar colour can be seen in adult onset Gaucher disease, it is not a feature of the earlier onset forms.

Localised hyperpigmentation

Many normal children have one or two well defined pigmented macules, generally not present at birth but appearing in the early years. In a child with pigmented macular lesions, consider:

- Neurofibromatosis. Five or more café au lait spots greater than 0.5 cm in diameter are strong evidence for neurofibromatosis. Examine for other features (axillary 'freckling'; Fig. 74.3), pigmented or thickened skin over plexiform neurofibromas, iris pigmentation, optic tumours, skeletal abnormalities, short stature, skin neurofibromas, macrocephaly and learning difficulties). The diagnosis may be uncertain early in life. Regular follow up is needed including assessment of intellectual progress. Apart from audiological and ophthalmological examination, investigations are not required unless suggested by clinical findings.
- McCune–Albright syndrome. Macules are often large and may stop at the midline. Look for fibrous dysplasia, sexual precocity and mental retardation.
- Incontinentia pigmenti. If the earlier phases have occurred in utero, hyperpigmented streaks may be present at birth.

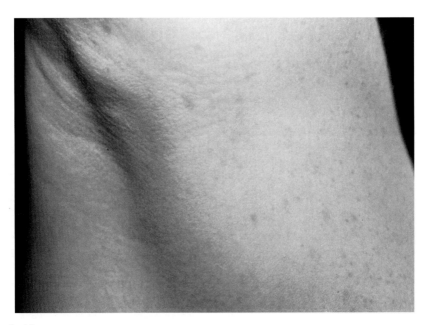

Fig. 74.3 Axillary freckling.

- Peutz–Jeghers syndrome. Small pigmented macules present on the lips and mucosa from birth are associated with intestinal polyposis. Care must be taken when assessing any episodes of abdominal pain as these children are at higher risk of intussusception and collapse.
- Naevoid hyperpigmentation (see localised hypopigmentation above).
- Pellagra. Hyperpigmentation and erythema on sun exposed areas, cheilitis, perineal inflammation and diarrhoea may be seen.

If areas of hyperpigmentation are roughened, raised, depressed or warty, consider:
- Congenital pigmented naevi. Depending on their site and size, infants with congenital pigmented naevi over the posterior scalp or spine may require imaging to look for meningeal involvement, obstructive hydrocephalus, cerebellar malformation or tethered cord.
- Genodermatoses such as dyskeratosis congenita. Congenital nail dystrophy, pancytopenia, skeletal and eye anomalies may be present.
- Necrobiosis lipoidica. Atrophic pigmented patches on the lower legs may be the first sign of diabetes in childhood.
- Acanthosis nigricans. Rough 'dirty' skin on the neck or axillary folds is associated with obesity, polycystic ovary syndrome, other insulin resistance syndromes and hypothyroidism.

Skin texture

Lax, hyperextensible skin is seen in Ehlers–Danlos syndromes. There may be bruising, scarring at sites of minor trauma, joint hyperextensibility and arthritis, and recurrent urinary infections.

Unusually firm skin is an early feature of systemic sclerosis. In children, there is usually widespread skin involvement. The Raynaud phenomenon may be present, and involvement of lungs, heart, kidneys and gastrointestinal tract usually occurs within a few years.

Waxy indurated skin may accompany neurological degeneration and hepatosplenomegaly in type A Niemann–Pick disease.

Anogenital rashes

Common causes of anogenital rashes include irritant napkin dermatitis, seborrhoeic dermatitis and yeast infection. These usually settle rapidly with treatment. More resistant rashes may be due to psoriasis or perianal streptococcal infection, but also consider:

- Langerhans cell histiocytosis. This may present in infancy as a chronic inguinal rash, often erosive and unresponsive to treatment. A scaly, papular eruption on the scalp or trunk may appear. Petechiae, purpura, fever, diarrhoea or hepatosplenomegaly may be present.
- Nutritional deficiencies. Anogenital lesions are an early and prominent manifestation of zinc deficiency. Look for perioral and acral rashes, alopecia, diarrhoea and failure to thrive. Serum zinc levels do not correlate well with body zinc status. Biotin and essential fatty acid deficiency syndromes can give a similar picture.
- Malabsorption. Both an intractable irritant napkin dermatitis and secondary nutritional deficiencies may contribute to anogenital rashes in malabsorptive conditions.
- Congenital syphilis. Perianal erosions and moist warty lesions may be seen in early infancy, with erythema on the palms and soles, fever, failure to thrive and hepatosplenomegaly.
- Human immunodeficiency virus can present as severe, erosive napkin dermatitis which may be secondarily infected.
- Family factors. Irritant or traumatic anogenital rashes may be seen in circumstances of suboptimal care, emotional abuse or physical abuse.

Hair problems

Hair loss

See Ch.73

Hypertrichosis

Generalised hypertrichosis (increased hair in all areas) may be an isolated finding or may be related to:
- inherited syndromes, including Hurler and De Lange syndromes
- medications, especially minoxidil, phenytoin and cyclosporin
- gastrointestinal disease, including coeliac disease
- hypothyroidism
- Porphyria; look for photosensitivity and blisters.

Hirsutism

Increased pubic or axillary hair in young children may be due to adrenal, gonadal or central nervous system disease and requires investigation. Hirsutism in adolescent females may be an isolated finding or may be seen with obesity and amenorrhea in polycystic ovary syndrome. Cushing syndrome, mild congenital adrenal hyperplasia, virilising adrenal and ovarian tumours and thyroid dysfunction may cause hirsutism.

PART 21　SELF-ASSESSMENT

Questions

1. **Regarding allergic contact dermatitis due to plants:**
   (A) The condition responds quickly to moderate strength topical steroid therapy
   (B) Lesions are often linear in distribution
   (C) Grevilleas are a major cause of the condition
   (D) Blistering is rare

2. **Regarding streptococcal perianal disease:**
   (A) The erythema rarely extends more than 3 cm from the anal area
   (B) Bleeding on defecation is a common symptom
   (C) The condition is more painful than itchy
   (D) Recurrence is rare after 5 days of oral penicillin

3. **Regarding childhood psoriasis:**
   (A) As with adults, large plaques are the commonest lesions
   (B) As with adults, facial involvement is rare
   (C) Annular lesions are more common than in adult disease
   (D) Rebound following the use of topical steroids is a major problem

4. **The following are true/false:**
   (A) Erythroderma in a 1 week old baby is likely to be due to atopic eczema
   (B) Annular erythematous lesions in a neonate are likely to settle and do not require investigation
   (C) A 9 year old girl who develops obvious facial comedonal acne and no other signs of puberty does not require hormonal investigation
   (D) A child presents with a prominent vascular malformation over the lumbosacral area. Imaging of the spine is not necessary provided the child's growth and development are reviewed during preschool years

Answers and explanations

1. The correct answers are **(B)** and **(C)**. This condition usually requires oral steroids or at least a strong topical agent (A). A linear distribution is common, due to brushing against leaves or flowers of the causative plant (B). The commonest causative plants are rhus (now designated a noxious weed) and certain types of grevillea (C), which are still very popular plants. The condition manifests as a very acute dermatitis and blisters often occur (D).

2. The correct answers are **(A)**, **(B)**, and **(C)**. This condition is usually limited to the immediate perianal area (A). Because of the fissuring in the area, bright blood is often found on the stool or toilet paper (B). This is an extremely painful condition and children often withhold faeces because of the discomfort associated with defecation (C). The condition is very likely to recur unless 10 days of penicillin and a topical antibiotic are used (D).

3. The correct answers are **(C)** and **(D)**. In children smaller plaques and tiny guttate lesions are more common than large plaques (A). Facial involvement is much more common in children than in adults (B). An annular configuration is common in both plaque and pustular psoriasis in children (C). In general, tars are preferred to steroids in childhood psoriasis because of the tendency to rebound following cessation of the latter (D).

4. **(C)** is true, provided no other concerns are raised by the history and examination. (A) is false. Eczema is an uncommon cause of erythroderma. Investigate for infections, metabolic disorders, immunodeficiencies and other causes. (B) is false. Neonatal lupus is associated with complete heart block in many babies, and other causes of annular lesions may also require investigation and treatment. (D) is false. A tethered cord may present in late childhood with insidious development of bladder, bowel and limb problems that may be irreversible.

PART 21 FURTHER READING

Callahan E F, Adal K A, Tomecki K J 2000 Cutaneous (non-HIV) infections. Dermatologic Clinics 18: 497–508

Diaz L A, Giudice G J 2000 End of the century overview of skin blisters. Archives of Dermatology 136: 106–112

Metry D W, Hebert A A 2000 Benign cutaneous vascular tumors of infancy: when to worry, what to do. Archives of Dermatology 136: 905–914

Nichol N H 2000 Managing atopic dermatitis in children and adults. Nurse Practitioner 25: 58–59, 63–64, 69–70, 80–81

Raimer S S 2000 Managing pediatric atopic dermatitis. Clinical Pediatrics 39: 1–14

Raimer S S 2000 New and emerging therapies in pediatric dermatology. Dermatologic Clinics 18: 73–78

Sidbury R, Hanifin J M 2000 Old, new and emerging therapies for atopic dermatitis. Dermatologic Clinics 18: 1–11

Tyring S K, Carlton S S, Evans T 1998 Herpes. Atypical clinical manifestations. Dermatologic Clinics 16: 783–788

Wyatt A J, Hansen R C 2000 Pediatric skin tumors. Pediatric Clinics of North America 47: 937–963

Useful links

http://www.aad.org/patient_intro.html (American Academy of Dermatology patient information)

http://www.childrenshospital.org/vascularanomalies/vascanom.html (Boston Children's Hospital Vascular Anomalies Centre)

http://www.dermis.net/index_e.htm (Dermatology online atlas)

http://www.dermnet.org.nz/index.html (New Zealand Dermatological Society website)

http://www.eczema-assn.org (National Eczema Association for Education and Science)

http://www.skincarephysicians.com/eczemanet (Eczema net)

PART 22

ENT, EYE AND DENTAL DISORDERS

75 Ear, nose and throat and head and neck surgery problems

B. Benjamin

Paediatric ear, nose and throat disorders cover a wide field of congenital and acquired diseases of the ear, nose and paranasal sinuses, oral cavity, tongue, pharynx, larynx, tracheobronchial tree and oesophagus. They include craniofacial abnormalities, tumours and cysts of the head and neck, deafness, speech, language and communication problems. This chapter covers only common disorders.

The ear

The external auditory canal and the tympanic membrane are usually inspected (if necessary and if possible after removal of wax) using a handheld, battery operated otoscope or a Seigle magnifying pneumatic speculum. An ENT specialist uses a slim short telescope or a microscope for more detailed examination.

The external ear

Congenital abnormalities

Differences in the shape of the pinna are common — small ears, large ears, accessory skin tags and unusual configuration of the helix and antihelix — but usually no treatment is needed except for unsightly protruding ears which can be corrected surgically. Major abnormalities of the external canal such as stenosis or atresia are sometimes associated with small malformed pinnae, abnormalities of the ossicles and possibly hypoplastic inner ear abnormalities with consequent major hearing problems. When these anomalies affect both ears, hearing aids or reconstructive surgical procedures may be necessary.

Otitis externa

Swimming in contaminated or heavily chlorinated water predisposes the delicate skin lining the ear canal to infection with bacteria or fungi. Otitis externa causes itch, soreness, discharge and partial deafness. Treatment includes removal of debris by swabbing and/or syringing followed by careful drying and regular administration of appropriate antibiotic/steroid drops. Water in the ear should be avoided.

Severe pain and exquisite tenderness indicate acute localised or acute diffuse infection requiring systemic antibiotics, especially when there is surrounding cellulitis, lymphadenitis or generalised toxicity. ENT referral and hospitalisation may be required in severe or intractable cases.

Wax

Black, brown, yellow or pale wax is a mixture of sebaceous material and ceruminous gland secretion combined with desquamated epithelium. Although normally removed by the self-cleaning chewing movement of the temporomandibular joint and evaporation, wax occasionally accumulates to occlude the canal, causing a hearing loss and a sensation of blockage. Obsessive parental attempts to 'clean' normal wax with cotton buds or a matchstick or repeated daily insertion of a hearing aid mould may cause impaction of the wax, requiring removal by syringing or use of special blunt probes and suction by an ENT specialist. Sometimes, in obstinate cases, wax must be removed under general anaesthesia with the aid of an operating microscope.

Foreign bodies

Foreign bodies such as beads, pips, pieces of paper, insects, etc. sometimes become lodged in the external auditory canal where they cause discomfort, pain and partial deafness. Occasionally they are discovered by chance. If attempts at careful extraction using a syringe or small grasping forceps are unsuccessful in a young or fractious child, referral to a specialist is indicated for removal, if necessary under general anaesthesia. Rough or ill judged attempts at removal may cause damage to the tympanic membrane or the middle ear ossicles.

Injury of the tympanic membrane

Indirect trauma such as a slap or blow to the ear, a blast injury or impact with water can compress the column of air in the ear canal and rupture the tympanic membrane. Direct trauma may be caused by a cotton bud, hairpin or by incorrect syringing technique. There is pain, bleeding, deafness and some initial unsteadiness. On inspection, bleeding or a tear may be visible. The ear should not be cleaned and no drops should be given. Antibiotics are usually given to prevent infection. Almost all traumatic injuries will heal within a month or two; if not, a graft may eventually be necessary.

The middle ear

This air containing, irregular shaped, bony cavity is lined by mucous membrane and includes the mastoid air cells posteriorly and the eustachian tube anteromedially. The latter opens and closes on swallowing, yawning and blowing the nose and has an active mucociliary lining to cleanse, ventilate and maintain air pressure in the middle ear. Motion of the tympanic membrane and the lever action of the three small articulated ossicles create an efficient transducer mechanism to transfer sound energy at the air–water interface. As the footplate of the stapes moves rapidly in the oval window, vibrations in air become wave motion in the perilymph fluid of the inner ear.

Acute suppurative otitis media (ASOM)

> **Clinical example**
>
> Emma, aged 3 years 8 months, complained of a 'sore' ear late in the afternoon, refused her dinner and later developed distressing pain and a fever of 39.4°C. The family doctor found a crying, upset, vomiting child and an agitated mother. Otoscopy showed a red, bulging tympanic membrane on the left and a thickened, pink membrane on the right. The advice was bed rest, fluids as tolerated, paracetamol, amoxicillin and a progress examination next day.
> Note that ASOM causes severe pain, often worse in the evening. Both ears and the upper respiratory tract must be examined.

Acute secretory suppurative otitis media is due to infection of part or all of the mucoperiosteum that lines the spaces of the middle ear. The diagnosis can be verified only by examination of the tympanic membrane.

It is much more common in infants and children than in adults, with a peak incidence under 2 years of age and again between 5 and 7 years. It is more common in winter and where there is overcrowding and malnutrition. About 50% of children will have experienced an attack before the age of 2 years and about 75% by the age of 3 years. This high incidence is apparently due to an immature immune response and increased frequency of upper respiratory tract infections in this age group.

Many factors predispose to middle ear infection:
- Pre-existing middle ear effusion or 'glue ear'.
- Infants and small children have a short, wide, straight eustachian tube, the dynamic protective function of which is less effective in minimising middle ear contamination from the nasopharynx than the mature adult eustachian tube.
- Nasopharyngeal disease, such as seen with acute or chronic upper respiratory tract infection, enlarged infected adenoids and (to a lesser extent) tonsils or rhinosinusitis can act as a focus of infection.
- Coexistent chronic middle ear disease such as chronic otitis media or a pre-existing tympanic membrane perforation.
- Cleft palate or repaired cleft palate or other rarer craniofacial structural abnormality affects the normal opening by the palate muscles and the normal closure by the spring action of the cartilagenous portion of the eustachian tube.
- Contamination of the nasopharynx in babies being bottle fed in the recumbent position or in infants who are vomiting.
- Attendance at preschool or kindergarten with exposure to pathogens.
- Parental cigarette smoking.
- Deficiency of surface tension lowering substance, surfactant, in the tube.
- Abnormality of mucociliary action affecting the normal cleansing mechanism.
- Immunodeficiency syndromes.

In ASOM, the pathological sequence of events in the air spaces and mucosa of the middle ear proceeds rapidly with oedema, hyperaemia and exudate into the middle ear, more often than not following a head cold or upper respiratory tract infection. Inflammatory swelling occludes the eustachian tube. The serous fluid becomes purulent after secondary bacterial infection and causes bulging of the pain sensitive tympanic membrane. The body's natural defences, with or without assistance from antibiotics, usually achieve resolution. If not, the tympanic membrane continues to bulge, forming an area of ischaemic necrosis which ultimately ruptures.

The microbiology of ASOM primarily involves bacteria but in 5–10% viruses may play a role, usually paving the way for secondary bacterial invasion. Common organisms include *Streptococcus pneumoniae*, *Strep. pyogenes*, *Branhamella catarrhalis*, *Haemophilus influenzae* (especially in younger children), *Staphylococcus aureus* and some Gram negative or mixed infections. About 30–40% of aspirates will yield no pathogen.

The clinical features of ASOM vary with the age of the child, the efficiency of the host defence and the effectiveness of treatment. Severe, throbbing pain in one or both ears is the commonest feature. There may be minor earache for an hour or two or a fulminating febrile illness with acute pain. These symptoms are often worse in the evening or at night when the child is lying down. Infants may present with fever, attempts to pull at the affected ear, irritability, vomiting and abdominal pain. Rupture of the tympanic membrane, with blood stained then purulent discharge, relieves the pain and allows a culture and sensitivity to be obtained. If perforation occurs it usually heals within a few weeks.

The diagnosis is confirmed by the appearance of the tympanic membrane; however, many sick, irritable infants and smaller children are difficult, if not impossible, to examine so in some cases a clinical diagnosis is made and treatment is commenced without visualisation of the tympanic membrane.

The progression of ASOM can be divided into four stages:
1. Eustachian tube obstruction with a stuffy, blocked feeling of discomfort in the ear and a slightly retracted, pink tympanic membrane.
2. Early infection with increasing earache, fever, and redness due to some mucoid or purulent material behind the tympanic membrane.
3. Suppurative stage with severe local pain, constitutional symptoms and purulent exudate under pressure, bulging the tympanic membrane which develops a yellowish colour with ischaemic necrosis prior to rupture.
4. Resolution stage with dramatic lessening of pain and improvement of the tympanic membrane.

Treatment usually requires bed rest, adequate fluid intake, antipyretics and sufficient analgesic medication. Sometimes local warmth is helpful.

Although there is discussion about whether antibiotics are given too freely, many experienced physicians believe they limit the disease, control pain and minimise possible complications. Others suggest that antibiotics should be withheld pending further observation and given to those not recovering in 24–48 hours. As a first line treatment amoxycillin for 5–10 days is the drug of choice and is generally well tolerated. Erythromycin, sulphamethoxazole: trimethoprim or cefaclor are alternatives. Very occasionally a resistant or complicated infection requires myringotomy. Severe, otherwise uncontrolled infections require intravenous treatment in hospital.

There are no data to support the use of decongestants or antihistamines; in fact there is some evidence that they may be harmful. Topical antibiotic drops have no place in the treatment of acute suppurative otitis media.

The untoward sequelae of otitis media include:
- Incomplete resolution with persistence of effusion ('glue ear').
- Rarely, a ruptured tympanic membrane that will not heal. The chronic perforation will require grafting.
- Acute mastoiditis or its complications are still seen despite the use of antibiotics and present usually as a subperiosteal abscess behind the ear.

- Labyrinthitis with severe vertigo and vomiting.
- Intracranial complications include lateral venous sinus thrombosis, extradural or subdural abscess, meningitis, cortical thrombophlebitis and intracerebral or intracerebellar abscess.

Remember that otitis media has not been 'cured' until both the appearance of the tympanic membrane and the hearing have returned to normal.

Glue ear or otitis media with effusion (OME)

> ### Clinical example
>
> John's mother was called to the school because he complained of earache and the teacher observed that he was not hearing well. She stated that her 6 year old son had suffered four attacks of 'ear abscess' in the last 10 months. On examination, both tympanic membranes were dull and dilated vessels were seen to be running in a radial fashion. The tympanogram was 'flat'. Referral to an ENT surgeon for treatment of glue ears was arranged. In fact, David had probably had OME for 10 months. Parents may be unaware of the hearing loss in OME. Variable deafness and ear infections almost always indicate OME.

A confusion of names has been applied to 'glue ear', but otitis media with effusion (OME) or secretory otitis media are those used most often. It is a common cause of repeated earaches, fluctuating mild to moderate conduction deafness and educational impairment.

The aetiology is uncertain but the ventilation, drainage and clearing mechanism of the eustachian tube is abnormal. Organisms similar to those found in ASOM can be cultured in 30–50% of cases — the effusion apparently follows incomplete resolution of ASOM. A mucoid, non purulent effusion, containing leucocytes, dead or live bacteria, serum protein and mucus, accumulates in the middle ear. The effusion may be thin, thick, gelatinous or, in advanced cases, even 'rubbery'. The middle ear mucosa becomes oedematous and granular in appearance. Microscopically, the goblet cells and mucous glands increase dramatically in number and small cysts filled with watery or inspissated mucus can be seen in the thickened subepithelial layer, which is infiltrated by chronic inflammatory cells

The clinical features of OME are common up to 8 or 10 years of age, are usually seen first in winter and are sometimes variable and unpredictable. Symptoms often follow a viral upper respiratory tract infection or incompletely resolved ASOM. Because at first there may be no symptoms it may remain unrecognised. Earache and deafness are the two important features.

Earache presents in two ways. Firstly, as a flareup during an acute respiratory infection there may be typical ASOM with severe pain. Secondly, repeated 'small' earaches, lasting for minutes rather than hours, may wake the child at night or occur at school and settle quickly.

Deafness is often suspected by the parents or teacher or may be discovered at a routine screening hearing test. School performance is often affected: 'doesn't pay attention', 'can do better' or 'not concentrating' are frequent remarks. Non specific symptoms include poor school achievement, decreased learning skills, interference with language development, an adverse affect on emotional growth, irritability and personality changes. The child may be at an educational disadvantage. A few children become clumsy if their balance is mildly affected. Infants may be irritable, crying or constantly unsettled at night.

Recognition of physical signs in the tympanic membrane is often difficult for the inexperienced: a good pneumatic otoscope with magnification is invaluable. The common physical signs include:
- Yellow or amber appearance.
- Vascular dilatation, which is easier to see with magnification.
- Thickening and dullness of the tympanic membrane.
- Indrawing of the tympanic membrane, giving a concave appearance so that the handle of the malleus appears short.
- In advanced cases there may be atelectasis in the middle ear with atrophy and thinning of the tympanic membrane.

Sluggish or poor movement of the tympanic membrane detected using a pneumatic otoscope is a most important physical sign. The thicker the fluid, the less the 'bounce'. In children old enough to perform a pure tone audiogram (Fig. 75.1) a mild to moderate conduction deafness will be detected. Impedance tympanometry tests the bounce of the tympanic membrane and typically shows a 'flat' curve.

Management. In many children OME will resolve without treatment over weeks or months; however referral for specialist assessment is indicated:
- when infants and toddlers are persistently irritable, sleep poorly at night and rub or pull at their ears
- when older children have repeated earaches and/or persistent hearing loss.

There is no evidence that antibiotics, antihistamines, decongestants, mucolytics or antiallergy treatment have any significant beneficial effect.

In some cases, after adequate observation indicates that the effusion has been present for 3 months or more, myringotomy, suction removal of the fluid and insertion of tympanostomy tubes for middle ear ventilation/ drainage is indicated. The tube remains in the tympanic membrane, functioning as a 'temporary' artificial eustachian tube providing sustained middle ear ventilation, discouraging recurrent effusions and promoting recovery, usually without any complications. The tube is extruded after 6–12 months but the effusion can recur. Insertion of the tubes may need to be repeated if the symptoms warrant it. In some children, predisposing causes such as infection and hypertrophy of the adenoids or upper respiratory tract mucosal disease or rhinosinusitis need treatment.

If untreated, the long term irreversible complications of OME include atrophic thinning of the tympanic membrane, atelectasis of the middle ear space, damage to the middle ear mucosa, adhesive otitis media, retraction pockets, avascular necrosis of the incus and stapes, tympanosclerosis, cholesteatoma and cholesterol granuloma.

Chronic suppurative otitis media (CSOM)

The tympanic membrane is perforated. The patient complains of partial deafness and painless, recurrent or persistent discharge.

There are two types of CSOM:
- Mucoperiosteal disease with a central perforation from pinhole size up to complete destruction of the tympanic membrane. The basic middle ear disease is chronic, persistent or intermittent infection with a purulent, sometimes profuse, discharge due to infection of the mucoperiostium of the middle ear space. For this reason it is often called tubotympanic disease. Because complications are rare this is known as a 'safe' ear.

A clean, dry, chronic, central perforation, whether large or small, is suitable for tympanoplasty, using fascia or perichondrium, usually waiting until the child is 7 or 8 years old. Grafting is successful in about 95%, prevents recurrent infections causing further damage, restores hearing and allows swimming without the risk of infection.

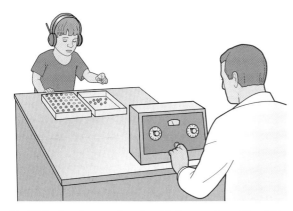

Fig. 75.1 Pure tone audiometry at 3–4 years of age. The child drops a coloured bead into the box when a sound is heard. A reasonably reliable pure tone audiogram can be obtained.

- Bony disease with a small marginal perforation at the superior bony edge of the tympanic membrane is usually associated with cholesteatoma and chronic, often smelly discharge. Complications are likely — an 'unsafe' ear.

A cholesteatoma is not a tumour but is a very slowly enlarging, pearl-like pocket of misplaced squamous epithelium accompanied by enzymatic destruction of the surrounding bone and ossicles. It is sometimes called atticoantral disease because of its position high in the middle ear. Mucoperiosteal infection is usually controlled by repeated dry mopping or suction cleaning of the ear and use of appropriate topical antibiotic drops. Water must not get into the ear. The common organisms are *Pseudomonas aeruginosa*, *Bacillus proteus* and *Escherichia coli*. Therefore a chronic or intermittently discharging ear must not be neglected. Cholesteatoma and bony disease usually requires surgical mastoidectomy to remove the disease, combined with tympanoplasty to repair the tympanic membrane and reconstruct the ossicular chain to preserve hearing.

The complications of cholesteatoma include erosion and destruction of the ossicles, osteitis, petrositis, mastoiditis, labyrinthitis, facial nerve paralysis, thrombosis of the sigmoid venous sinus, meningitis, extradural, subdural or cerebral abscess and septicaemia. Some of these complications are life threatening.

Deafness

The accurate assessment of the type, degree and cause of deafness is essential for optimum treatment.

The type of hearing loss is usually described according to the site of pathology:

- *'Conductive' deafness*. Sound vibrations are not conducted normally via the ear canal (for example, obstructing wax), the tympanic membrane (for example, perforation) or the ossicles (for example, congenital malformation). Conduction deafness is usually treatable.
- *'Sensorineural' deafness*. There is malfunction of the sensory (cochlear) components (for example, rubella deafness) or the neural (retrocochlear) components (for example, acoustic neuroma). Sensorineural deafness is often congenital, may be acquired and cannot be cured. If severe enough, sensorineural deafness requires a hearing aid for amplification, or consideration for cochlear implant.

Hearing loss is commonly suspected by the child's mother (Fig. 75.2). The degree is assessed by audiological methods according to age:

- In infants days or weeks old, the normal but non quantitative response to a sudden loud sound is the 'blink' or 'startle' reaction (Fig. 75.3). This test is best done with the infant lightly asleep.

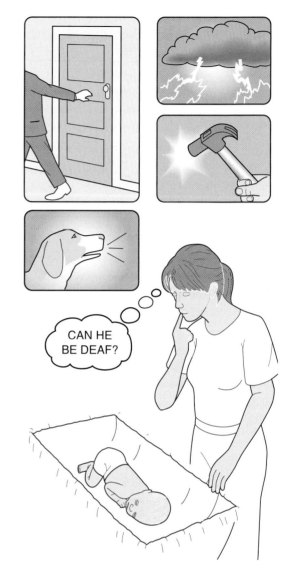

Fig. 75.2 Parents often suspect deafness if the baby consistently fails to respond to loud sounds and 'sleeps peacefully'. Their suspicion of deafness should be investigated.

- In special units, computerised electrophysiological tests are available to record small electrical changes evoked in the inner ear during transmission of acoustic signals. An accurate measure of function in the brainstem and the ear can be provided by electrocochleography and auditory brainstem tests in infants and children, including those with behavioural problems or multiple handicaps.
- In babies from 4 months of age, normal head turning responses (Fig. 75.4) are elicited towards the side of a sound stimulus, which can be varied from a soft whisper to the jingle of keys or the crumple of paper. An approximate, clinical quantitative estimate of hearing can be obtained.

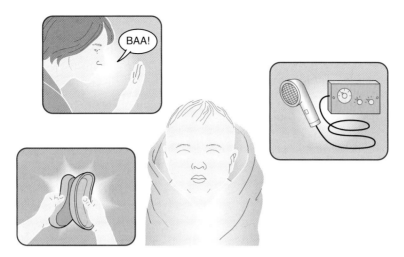

Fig. 75.3 There are a number of tests for screening the hearing of newborn babies. The normal response to a sudden loud sound (80–90 dB) is a 'blink' or 'startle' reaction. This test is best done with the infant lightly asleep.

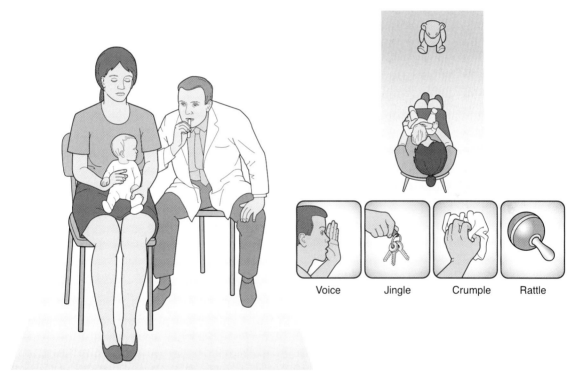

Voice Jingle Crumple Rattle

Fig. 75.4 Most babies over the age of 4 or 5 months are able to turn to a noise from an unseen source, so that each ear can be tested. The intensity of the sound may be varied to estimate the level at which response occurs.

- Older toddlers can be assessed in specialised paediatric units by behavioural methods, observing the child's reaction to ambient sounds or by conditioning them to respond to a puppet or peep show — known as condition oriented response (COR) audiometry.
- Children of 3 or 4 years of age or older can usually cooperate so that a quantitative pure tone threshold audiogram (Fig. 75.1) can be obtained for different frequencies for both air conduction and bone conduction.

The cause of deafness determines the need for treatment. The many causes of conduction deafness each need specific attention; for example:

- removal of wax

- operation for congenital external ear canal atresia
- myringoplasty for tympanic membrane perforation
- ventilating tube for persistent otitis media with effusion
- reconstruction of congenital ossicular chain abnormality.

Approximately 1 baby in 1000 is born with severe deafness and approximately 1 in 1000 infants become deaf before they have developed speech. In many cases the cause of sensorineural deafness is difficult to determine. The known causes can be considered in four groups, as follow.

Prenatal hereditary deafness

Transmitted by a dominant gene in 10%. If one parent carries the gene, up to 50% of children will be affected. There is a recessive gene in 90%, and in this situation both parents must carry the gene and 25% of children will be affected. Consanguinity increases recessive transmission. There is, therefore, sometimes a positive family history of deafness. There are many hereditary syndromes with hearing loss as a feature. Some examples include:

- Waardenburg syndrome — epicanthic folds, different coloured irises, white forelock
- Usher syndrome — retinitis pigmentosa, epilepsy
- Pendred syndrome — sporadic thyroid disease
- Alport syndrome — progressive renal disease
- Hurler syndrome — gargoylism
- Fanconi syndrome — anaemia, skin pigmentation, skeletal deformities, mental retardation.

Prenatal acquired deafness

Damage in the first trimester can affect the developing cochlea. Detailed radiological imaging will define the Michel deformity, which is total absence, and the Mondini deformity, which is partial maldevelopment of the bony cochlea. The Scheibe deformity has a normal bony cochlea but damaged hair cells in the organ of Corti. Causes of prenatal acquired deafness include maternal infection such as rubella, cytomegalovirus, toxoplasmosis, herpes and congenital syphilis. Drugs which are ototoxic to the embryo include aminoglycosides, loop diuretics, quinine and thalidomide.

Perinatal acquired deafness

Causes include prematurity, prolonged or difficult labour, hypoxia, Rh incompatibility, kernicterus, ototoxins, infectious diseases and others.

Deafness in infancy and childhood

The common causes of acquired deafness at this age are mumps, measles, meningitis, traumatic fracture of the petrous bone through the inner ear or acoustic nerve and patent cochlear aqueduct. Fortunately in these cases, if only one ear is affected, the handicap is not as devastating as with bilateral deafness.

Treatment of sensorineural deafness

Most deaf children have normal intellectual capacity and some usable residual inner ear function. The diagnosis must be made early and the child fitted with hearing aids or be considered for a cochlear implant. He or she should receive early and continued auditory training. Many such deaf children learn to understand the spoken word, to develop intelligible speech and play an active role in society. However, the hearing of speech sounds does not guarantee normal understanding, as amplification may be accompanied by distortion and decreased intelligibility. Thus general practitioners, paediatricians and otologists have an enormous responsibility to take the mother's suspicion of deafness seriously and arrange prompt investigation and assessment. Early diagnosis is the key to optimal outcome.

The nose

Congenital conditions

Many congenital anomalies affect the nasal structures:
- Craniofacial and external nasal malformations.
- Cleft lip, palate and face clefts.
- Haemangioma and vascular malformations.
- Dermoid, encephalocoele, nasolacrimal duct cyst and other rare masses.
- Bilateral congenital choanal atresia poses the greatest threat to life because neonates, being obligate nose breathers, develop increasing cyanosis and even fatal asphyxia when their nasal airways are completely obstructed. However, if the baby cries and takes a breath through the mouth the obstruction is momentarily relieved until the mouth closes. Choanal atresia can be confirmed by failure to pass a 3 mm diameter plastic catheter through the nose into the oropharynx. The airway can be maintained using a Guedel oral airway or an endotracheal tube pending CT assessment and surgical correction.
- Unilateral choanal atresia presents as persistent glairy discharge later in life.

Acute rhinosinusitis

Acute infective rhinosinusitis presents with purulent nasal discharge, nasal obstruction, pain and tenderness over the involved sinuses, and general malaise. The acute episode often follows an upper respiratory tract infection, swimming or diving and usually affects the maxillary sinuses, and in older children the ethmoid sinuses. Plain X rays and CT are required only in difficult cases. Treatment is symptomatic, using decongestant nasal drops or oral decongestants and paracetamol. Antibiotics are given in severe, persistent, recurrent or complicated cases. Amoxycillin for 7–10 days to cover the common upper respiratory tract pathogens is the drug of first choice. In penicillin hypersensitive patients use cefaclor, erythromycin or doxycycline (not in children under 8 years).

Infective rhinosinusitis in infants and children usually responds to medical treatment. Surgical drainage may be necessary for chronic disease or acute complications such as subperiostial abscess, periorbital cellulitis, osteomyelitis or intracranial spread.

Chronic rhinosinusitis

Chronic rhinitis often has an allergic basis, with secondary bacterial infection being common. In younger children it is aggravated by, or inseparable from, hypertrophy and infection of the adenoids. Swollen turbinates cause intermittent or persistent nasal stuffiness and catarrhal discharge. Therapy with antihistamines and pseudoephedrine may be helpful but symptoms are more often controlled with regular use of intranasal metered aerosol steroid spray. Nasal allergy, often with hay fever or asthma (Chs 42, 45, 47) may be traced to specific allergens, which should be avoided where possible. Desensitisation can be considered in older children. In severe, persistent cases cautery, laser or surgical reduction of the inferior turbinates may provide substantial relief. Nasal polyps in children strongly suggest cystic fibrosis.

Nasopharyngeal tumours and cysts

Antrochoanal polyp, dermoid cyst, meningoencephalocoele, glioma and chordoma are rare benign conditions. Nasopharyngeal angiofibroma is an uncommon locally destructive, non metastasising very vascular tumour, occurring mostly in adolescent boys. It usually presents as frequent, often severe, epistaxes and nasal obstruction. Treatment is surgical removal after embolisation of the feeding vessels, although some advocate radical radiotherapy. Rhabdomyosarcoma or lymphosarcoma are rare malignant nasopharyngeal tumours.

Trauma

Fracture or dislocation deformity of the external nose and nasal septum sometimes occurs during a difficult birth or after forceps delivery. The degree of displacement and nasal obstruction are occasionally severe enough to require correction in the neonatal period. Injuries of the

Clinical example

Benjamin, aged 9, was struck on the nose by the seat of a swing while he was playing in the park. His nose bled, appeared 'crooked' and became swollen. He was taken to the casualty department, where the ENT registrar confirmed traumatic fracture of the nasal bones by clinical examination. Corrective surgery was arranged for later in the week.

Bruising and swelling will rapidly hide the deformity. Careful palpation usually confirms the displacement without the need for X ray.

nose, nasal bones and nasal septum occur commonly when toddlers fall during vigorous play and in older children during contact sports. Depressed, displaced nasal bones require correction within 10 days. Haematoma of the nasal septum should be drained and treated with antibiotics to minimise development of a septal abscess, which destroys cartilage and can lead to a saddle-nose deformity.

Foreign bodies

Unilateral purulent, sometimes blood stained nasal discharge in a young child suggests the presence of a foreign body, such as a bead, eraser, piece of vegetable, etc., until proven otherwise. Unreactive inorganic objects may remain undetected for months or years. The most dangerous foreign body is an alkaline battery which emits a small current and leaks its caustic contents, rapidly causing local tissue necrosis; it must be treated as an emergency. Removal may require general anaesthesia.

Epistaxis

Bleeding from a prominent vessel on the anterior nasal septum (Little's area) is common and is sometimes frightening for parents. It may be aggravated by accidental trauma, nose picking, nose blowing and infection. Occasionally epistaxis may be the presentation of a blood dyscrasia or a nasopharyngeal angiofibroma. First aid is to apply constant pressure to the side of the nose with a cold face cloth for at least 5 minutes. Packing with ribbon gauze controls many persistent cases. If the bleeding continues and the vessel can be identified, it can be thermally or chemically cauterised using topical anaesthesia in older cooperative children or under general anaesthesia in others.

The oropharynx

Acute sore throat is a symptom common to both acute tonsillitis and acute pharyngitis. The former has inflammation mainly confined to the tonsils, and the latter has more widespread inflammation involving the mucous membrane of the pharynx. For the most part the symptoms and local signs accompanying acute sore throat correlate poorly with the presumed causative (or later proven) aetiological microorganism. Differentiation may be easy, for example, in coryza there is initially a burning sensation above the palate, then fever, nasal obstruction, nasal discharge and sore throat with generalised inflammation of the mucous membranes. In approximately 50% of patients with acute sore throat beta haemolytic streptococci can be isolated by surface throat culture; it seems reasonable to assume a cause and effect relationship. In fact this organism is more likely to be pathogenic when there are also local clinical findings of intense cellulitis of the uvula and soft palate and haemorrhagic palatal petechiae. Remember that 10–20% of otherwise normal children may be carriers of beta haemolytic streptococci. What then is acute tonsillitis?

Acute tonsillitis has been defined clinically not only as a condition with inflammation mostly confined to the tonsils but the clinical features also include acute sore throat, fever, difficulty in swallowing, enlarged tender regional cervical lymph nodes, halitosis and constitutional symptoms such as lethargy, nausea and vomiting. Sometimes there is abdominal pain. Examination can show various appearances:

- Red mucosa over the tonsils and oedematous, generalised inflammation (parenchymatous tonsillitis).
- Yellowish-white exudate in the crypts of the tonsils (follicular tonsillitis).
- The crypts become filled with 'debris', an exudate of desquamated epithelium and pus.
- Coalescence of these follicles can form a thin white non confluent patchy membrane which peels away without bleeding (membranous tonsillitis).
- The typical redness, oedema and purulent secretion (exudative tonsillitis). Note that this appearance is not necessarily diagnostic of streptococcal infection.

Acute sore throat is one of the commonest complaints seen in general practice and can be caused by viral, bacterial, fungal or other infectious microorganisms (Ch. 45). It is occasionally a manifestation of a serious systemic disease. A useful classification of causes includes:

- Acute viral pharyngitis. Examples are coryza, influenza, parainfluenza, the viral exanthemas and infections with coxsackie viruses (herpangina), the ECHO virus group and many others.
- Acute tonsillitis, often due to *beta haemolytic streptococcus* but occasionally other bacterial organisms in immunocompromised patients. It seems also that adenoviruses and Epstein–Barr viruses may lie dormant in tonsils for years and be activated by non specific environmental factors such as fever, chilling and stress.
- Infectious mononucleosis (glandular fever), caused by the Epstein–Barr virus, has many manifestations (Ch. 37). Acute sore throat is consistently a prominent feature.
- Thrush, due to *Candida albicans* and predisposed to by diabetes, general debility, immunosuppression, nutritional deficiency and disturbances in the normal flora due to prolonged administration of antimicrobial agents.
- Vincent angina (also known as ulceromembranous gingivostomatitis), caused by a combination of the normal spirochaetes of the mouth and an anaerobic fusiform bacillus, often in injured necrotic tissue of the gums which provides the necessary anaerobic environment.
- Diphtheria. A sore throat is part of the much more serious systemic toxic illness.
- Aphthous stomatitis. The ulcers are usually in the mucosa of the gingiva or the anterior part of the oral cavity, but when they occur in the soft palate or the fauces the patient complains of sore throat.
- Patients with acute leukaemia, agranulocytosis, aplastic anaemia or HIV infection may present with an acute sore throat.

Approximately 50% of cases of acute sore throat are eventually proven to be bacterial. Pending the result of culture it would seem prudent to immediately treat with an antibiotic those children who are extremely ill or toxic, and to await the result of culture in other children.

Clinical example

The family doctor saw Andrew, a 7 year old boy who had had a sore throat, difficulty in swallowing and fever for 2 days. The appearance in the throat was described as 'tonsillitis'. An antibiotic was prescribed but when he was no better 3 days later it was changed to a different antibiotic. Again Andrew was no better and in addition was complaining of feeling weak, with aching in the muscles and headache. Careful examination 8 days after the illness commenced revealed tender, enlarged lymph nodes in the neck, axilla and inguinal region. His spleen was enlarged and tender. Blood tests were diagnostic of infectious mononucleosis.

An atypical sore throat needs caution about the diagnosis. Infectious mononucleosis is a systemic illness whose principal features are sore throat, fever, cervical (often generalised) lymphadenopathy and a feeling of malaise. Many organs in the body can be affected with protean manifestations. Antibiotics have no therapeutic value.

Indications for tonsillectomy and adenoidectomy

There is now reliable information to prove that the frequency of throat infections is reduced in selected patients undergoing these procedures. Operation is clearly indicated in a small number of children. There may be disagreement about the operation in individual cases and at times a second opinion may be in the best interests of the patient.

Indications for tonsillectomy

- Repeated attacks of acute tonsillitis: at least three documented attacks a year for 2 years or more, making a minimum of 6 attacks in two years.
- Chronic or acute on chronic upper airway obstruction caused by enlarged lymphoid tissue. There may be an obstructive sleep pattern, even apnoea. Some cases with severe obstruction develop cardiac changes and cor pulmonale.
- Chronic tonsillitis. This usually applies to older children and adults.
- Peritonsillar abscess (quinsy). Two or more attacks are a definite indication for tonsillectomy.
- Biopsy excision for suspected new growth.

Indications for adenoidectomy

- Enlargement causing severe nasal obstruction and breathing discomfort.
- Persistent discharge of infected mucopurulent material caused by large and infected adenoids.
- Possible benefit in repeated acute or chronic ear disease.

The tonsils and adenoids are often removed in a single, combined operation but there are clear indications for tonsillectomy alone or adenoidectomy alone. There is now greater awareness of the incidence and severity of obstructive sleep problems which occur in an age range from 6 months to 10 years of age.

Contraindications to tonsillectomy and adenoidectomy

- Lack of staff or facilities to recognise and manage the potential complications.
- Recent respiratory tract infection, within the previous 2 weeks.
- Systemic disorder, such as poorly controlled diabetes.
- Bleeding disorder.
- Pharyngeal insufficiency, such as repaired cleft palate, submucous cleft palate or paralysis or paresis of the palate and so-called 'short' palate. Adenoidectomy may cause or worsen escape of air through the nose (hypernasality), making speech difficult to understand.

Injuries of the tongue and oropharynx

Children with, for example, a pencil in the mouth may fall and injure the soft palate, tonsils or pharyngeal wall. At other times it is not uncommon for teeth to lacerate the tongue and cause considerable bleeding. It is usually necessary to suture only the most severe of these injuries.

The larynx and trachea

Features of upper airway disease include:
- Stridor: a prominent, audible manifestation of upper airway obstruction caused by turbulent airflow through a narrowed airway, usually the larynx or sometimes the trachea. It is most often inspiratory, sometimes expiratory and occasionally both.
- Other signs of partial or severe airway obstruction: tachypnoea, chest retraction.
- Cyanotic or apnoeic attacks.
- Husky, weak or absent cry.
- Repeated aspiration.
- Recurrent or atypical croup.
- Features of weakness, compression or stenosis of the trachea and/or bronchi.

Suzanna, a 7 week old baby with intermittent 'noisy breathing' for 3 or 4 weeks, was brought to the family doctor because the noise was getting worse and had become more worrying for her parents. There had been no cyanotic or apnoeic episodes, the cry was normal, she was otherwise progressing well and was gaining weight normally. Chest X ray was normal. She was seen by a paediatrician who found no abnormality other than the stridor and referred her to a paediatric ENT surgeon. At laryngobronchoscopy under general anaesthesia the characteristic supraglottic changes of laryngomalacia were seen but there was no other abnormality of the upper aerodigestive tract. The parents were reassured there was no serious disease, there was no relationship to 'cot death' and that, with time, the stridor would resolve without treatment.

The descriptive terms 'congenital laryngeal stridor' and 'infantile stridor' are not diagnoses. This baby could have had a serious problem, such as an enlarging cyst, subglottic stenosis, subglottic haemangioma, vascular compression of the trachea, mediastinal tumour or developmental cyst or other rare conditions. Imaging and endoscopy will lead to a definitive diagnosis.

Laryngomalacia

This is a common cause of stridor in infants (Ch. 46). It is also appropriately called 'floppy larynx', both names implying collapse of the supraglottic tissues during inspiration. The cause is unknown. The features are intermittent inspiratory stridor, signs of upper airway obstruction, a normal cry and general health which is usually (but not always) normal. The features are often alarming to parents. As the condition is usually self-limiting there is seldom need for treatment once a certain diagnosis has been established to differentiate laryngomalacia from the many other causes of stridor in infants. Occasionally severe cases warrant laser removal of part of the redundant, floppy, supraglottic tissues.

Congenital and acquired subglottic stenosis

The reported incidence of subglottic stenosis has increased, partly because of improved survival of premature babies who have been treated by prolonged intubation and partly because of more accurate diagnosis. Severe cases require tracheotomy and later repair by rib graft laryngotracheoplasty or even cricotracheal resection.

Vocal cord paralysis

Unilateral paralysis causes few symptoms in infants and children. Bilateral vocal cord paralysis is the cause of stridor in about 10% of infants with airway obstruction and is associated with a central nervous system anomaly (for example, Arnold–Chiari malformation) in many cases. Tracheotomy is usually, but not always, required for bilateral paralysis.

Other causes of stridor

Laryngeal web, laryngeal atresia and laryngeal cleft are uncommon anomalies. Cysts causing clinical features include retention cysts, congenital cysts and cystic hygroma. Subglottic haemangioma is the commonest laryngeal tumour in infants and presents with inspiratory stridor in the first 6–8 weeks. The clinical features of tracheal obstruction are caused by tracheomalacia, tracheal compression by a vascular ring or other anomalies or congenital tracheal stenosis.

Investigations include X rays, CT, contrast oesophagogram and ultrasound of the neck or mediastinum. Flexible laryngoscopy and direct laryngoscopy, bronchoscopy and possibly oesophagoscopy under general anaesthesia ultimately establish a firm diagnosis.

Acute inflammatory airway obstruction

Acute infectious diseases of the upper respiratory tract which cause airway obstruction fall into two groups:
- *Oropharynx.* Acute bacterial or viral infection with obstructive hypertrophy of the tonsils and adenoids; infectious mononucleosis causing obstructive enlargement of the tonsils and adenoids; peritonsillar abscess;

retropharyngeal or parapharyngeal abscess and Ludwig angina.
- *Larynx and trachea.* Acute laryngotracheobronchitis or croup; spasmodic croup; bacterial tracheitis; acute supraglottitis or epiglottitis (with a frighteningly rapid onset) and diphtheria. Some cases (especially patients with acute supraglottitis, epiglottitis or diphtheria) have critical, life threatening airway obstruction, a situation which requires immediate recognition and transfer to a paediatric hospital for relief of airway obstruction, if necessary by endotracheal intubation or tracheotomy, and intensive care management.

Important advances in treatment of these diseases include more effective antibiotics, diphtheria immunisation. diphtheria antitoxin, the use of racemic adrenaline (epinephrine) for croup, steroids for croup, and the Hib vaccine, which has dramatically reduced the incidence of *H. influenzae* supraglottitis and epiglottitis, and the use of intubation in place of tracheotomy.

Multiple respiratory papillomas

Papillomas are the most common benign growths in the larynx. Human papillomavirus (HPV) type 6, type 11 and occasionally type 16 cause papillomas in the respiratory tract, most often in the mucosa of the larynx. About two thirds of patients are younger than 15 years and one third older than 15 years, with the highest incidence before the age of 5 years. There is a tendency for recurrence after removal, although sometimes unexpected spontaneous improvement can occur. In infants, large obstructing masses may threaten life. There is a strong association between recurrent respiratory papillomas in infants and children and maternal condylomata acuminata or genital warts, but transmission of HPV during passage through the birth canal is unlikely, as some infants have papillomas already in their larynx at birth.

Growth may be slow and persistent or irregular and unpredictable. The commonest presentation is change in the cry or voice, sometimes with increasing airway obstruction, and often an erroneous diagnosis of asthma, laryngitis, bronchitis or croup has been made. Therefore persistent or progressive huskiness in an infant or child should suggest the possibility of papillomas. The mainstay of treatment is repeated removal at microlaryngeal surgery under general anaesthesia, using forceps or the carbon dioxide laser, which is a precise modality attended by minimal bleeding, causing little pain and limited local scarring. Many adjunctive treatments have been tried because of frustration and recurrence of the tumour, but none of these have proven beneficial over the long term. There is no tendency for regression or disappearance at puberty, as was formerly thought.

Ingested and inhaled foreign bodies

Clinical example

Cuthbert, aged 2 years and 6 months, ran to his mother in great distress, gasping for breath, coughing and crying. She rushed him to the nearby emergency department. The respiratory distress had lessened but pulse oximetry showed only 90% saturation. There was a wheeze and decreased air entry on the right side. An expiratory chest X ray showed air trapping on the same side with shift of the mediastinum to the left. He was observed in the high dependency ward until an impacted peanut was removed from the right main bronchus under general anaesthesia 90 minutes later. He made an uneventful recovery thereafter.

With inhalation of foreign bodies into major airways, if death does not occur in the first few minutes after inhalation, the situation usually improves but the implications remain serious. In this case the peanut, acting as a ball valve in the right main bronchus, let air into that side, but as the bronchus narrowed during expiration air was trapped in the lung.

Foreign bodies in the pharynx and oesophagus

Children often swallow foreign bodies. Sharp objects such as fishbones can impact in the tonsils, base of tongue or pyriform fossa. More often objects such as coins, buttons, lumps of meat or vegetable, plastic or pins lodge somewhere in the oesophagus, usually at the upper end but occasionally at a site of pathological narrowing (stenosis). Some show on X ray but, ultimately, if an impacted foreign body is suspected, oesophagoscopy is necessary. Remember most small smooth objects will pass through the oesophagus and the gastrointestinal tract and be recovered in the stools; however, ingestion of a small alkaline button battery is extremely destructive of surrounding tissue and must be treated as an acute emergency to prevent perforation of the oesophagus and mediastinitis.

Foreign bodies in the larynx and tracheobronchial tree

The highest incidence of inhaled foreign bodies is in the 2nd and 3rd years of life and about 60% of deaths occur in children less than 4 years of age. Occasionally they lodge in the larynx or subglottic region but more often in one or other main bronchus. Diagnosis is made by awareness of the possibility and from a history of inhalation of a foreign body (a history of possble inhalation is present in about 65% of cases).

Clinical presentation may be:

- Immediate, with sudden coughing, choking, gasping, spasm and cyanosis; yet, fortunately, few deaths occur in this stage.
- Delayed, with wheeze, chronic cough, atypical pneumonia, and chest X ray changes (but about 20% show no abnormality). The foreign body may be found days, weeks or even months later.
- Symptomless. Although most foreign bodies will ultimately cause symptoms, occasionally some are found by chance on a chest X ray or at endoscopy.

Only 5 or 10% of ingested foreign bodies impact in the larynx or subglottic region and then stridor, laryngospasm, dyspnoea, a husky voice, inspiratory wheeze or repeated atypical croup dominate the clinical picture. If death does not occur in the first few minutes after the foreign body is inhaled, the prognosis is good if the patient is promptly transported by road or air ambulance to a major paediatric unit where experienced personnel and adequate instruments are available. Ill advised attempts at bronchoscopic diagnosis or removal by inexperienced surgeons or anaesthetists often worsen the situation.

Two thirds of inhaled foreign bodies are nuts. Parents should be made aware that children under 4 years of age should be denied access to nuts, especially peanuts, in the hope that aspiration accidents will be minimised.

Eye disorders in childhood

J. E. Elder

A systematic approach to children's eye disease allows rapid determination of the correct diagnosis or initiation of appropriate further investigation.

Visual development

A rapid sequence of anatomical and functional changes in the visual apparatus enables vision to develop from a very low level after birth to near adult levels by 12–18 months of age. At birth an infant has visual acuity of approximately 6/120 and by 12 months this has improved to about 6/12. This rapid development is the result of retinal maturation, myelination of the visual pathways, the ability to accommodate (change the focal length of the eye) and maturation within the visual cortex. The first three of these processes (retinal maturation, myelination and accommodation) are complete by 4–6 months of age. The maturation of the visual cortex occurs more gradually, over a 6–8 year period, with the most rapid phase being in the first 2 years. It is this gradual cortical maturation that permits the development of amblyopia, which is one of the commonest ophthalmic abnormalities of childhood (see Amblyopia below).

Measurement of vision in children

Measurement of visual acuity in preverbal children presents a challenge. Asking the parent 'Does your child see well?' or 'How well do you think your child sees?' often gives a useful insight into an infant's visual function. If a parent expresses concern about an infant's vision, take note, as this concern is often well founded.

An understanding of normal visual behaviour is vital to estimating visual function in infancy. At birth, when alert an infant should be able to fix on a face briefly. By 6 weeks of age most infants smile in a visually responsive fashion to a face. At this age the infant will also be able to follow a face or light through an arc of 90°. By 6 months of age an infant can reach for a small object and actively follow objects in the visual environment. At 12 months of age a child should be able to reach and pick up tiny objects such as hundreds-and-thousands ('sprinkles').

More formal assessment of visual acuity becomes possible with the development of language. Children with specific language delay or more general intellectual delay will have difficulty with these tests of visual acuity. Picture naming tests can be done by children between 2 and 3 years of age. Single letter matching tests are within the abilities of most 3–4 year olds. The standard Snellen chart test is often not performed well until the child is between 5 and 6 years of age. The vision should be tested for each eye individually. As with all testing in children, patience and an encouraging manner are vital to obtain the best results. Repeat the test on another occasion if the test results seem inaccurate.

The notation for documenting visual acuity is the Snellen fraction, for example, 6/6. Most visual acuity tests use standard distances of 3 or 6 metres between subject and chart. If the vision is poor the subject should be brought closer to the chart. The vision then may be recorded as 2/18 or 1/60, etc. depending on how close the subject is to the chart and which line is read.

What level of vision is abnormal? (Or, when to refer!)

This depends on the age of the child. An infant who is not fixing and following by 3–4 months, or reaching for small objects and tracking objects in the visual environment by 8–12 months, deserves further examination and investigation.

If the child is able to do a more formal test of acuity, a difference between the two eyes of two or more lines (that is 6/6 and 6/12) indicates the need for further assessment. In children less than 3 years of age vision of 6/18 or less in either eye should prompt referral and in children older than 3 years 6/12 is an acceptable cut-off for referral.

Assessment of a child with a possible eye problem

History

Prematurity, perinatal difficulties (for example, birth asphyxia), significant syndromes (for example, Down syndrome) and other sensory impairment (for example, deafness) are associated with an increased risk of eye disease. Developmental delay often interferes with assessment of visual acuity, especially if language or intellect is affected. Common childhood eye problems such as strabismus and refractive errors have a clearly identified familial tendency, although the precise genetics are not well understood. Finally, the parents' perception of a child's visual function is important, particularly if there is concern that the vision is poor.

Examination

In keeping with paediatrics in general, observation without approaching or touching a child often supplies a great deal of information. By observation it is possible to rapidly determine an infant's use of vision. Does the child smile at a face? Is the child looking around the room? If something moves, does the child look to it? If there is a noise, does the child look to the source of the noise? A blind child will become still and will often drop the head down while using hearing to further localise the source of the sound, but will not look towards this source.

Most eyelid, eyelash and ocular surface abnormalities can be detected readily by simple observation. Many intraocular abnormalities can be detected by examination of the 'red reflex'. This is the red to orange colour seen within the pupil when the line of illumination and observation are approximately coaxial (that is, the same). This situation is most easily obtained by observing the child's eye with a direct ophthalmoscope from a distance of about 1 metre. It is then easy to compare the reflexes for the two eyes and the child is not threatened by the examiner getting too close. A dull or absent red reflex indicates an opacity, such as a cataract, in the normally clear media of the eye. A white reflex results from an abnormally pale reflecting surface within the eye, such as a white retinal tumour (retinoblastoma). While these intraocular disorders are rare, they are important in terms of the severe effect on vision or threat to life.

Misalignment of the eyes

Strabismus or squint is common in childhood and accurate assessment to confirm or refute the presence of misalignment is an important skill for anyone who deals with children.

Observation will confirm the presence of large angle strabismus. However, a broad nasal bridge or prominent epicanthic folds will mimic milder degrees of strabismus, especially in younger infants. This situation is known as pseudostrabismus (Fig. 76.1). The epicanthic folds cover the sclera on the medial aspect of the globe while the lateral sclera is easily visible. This creates the appearance of misalignment, particularly when the child looks laterally. Examining the symmetry of corneal light reflections will help to avoid being misled by pseudostrabismus.

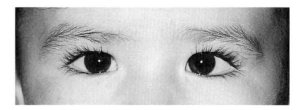

Fig. 76.1 This infant has prominent epicanthic folds giving rise to the appearance of misaligned eyes. This is pseudostrabismus. Note that the corneal light reflections are symmetrical. Cover testing failed to reveal misalignment of either eye.

The cover test is by far the most reliable method of detecting strabismus. The cover test is done by first getting the child to fix on an object while the observer determines which eye appears to be misaligned. The eye that appears to be fixing on the object (and not misaligned) is then covered while the apparently misaligned eye is observed. If strabismus is present a corrective movement of the misaligned eye will be seen as this eye takes up fixation on the object of regard (Fig. 76.2). If no movement is seen then the eye is uncovered. The cover test is then repeated but the other eye is covered this time and the eye which is not covered is again observed for a corrective movement and, if present, strabismus is confirmed. The test can be repeated as many times as necessary. If no movement is seen following repeated covering of either eye, then no strabismus is present. Care must be taken to let the child fix with both eyes open before covering either eye, otherwise normal binocular control may be prevented and a small latent squint (phoria) may be detected. Latent squints are normal variants and of no significance.

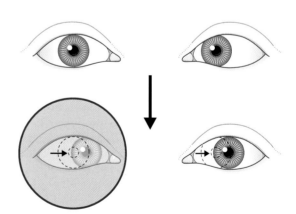

Fig. 76.2 Cover test. First the child's attention is attracted with a toy (top). Then the eye which appears to be looking directly at the toy is covered and the other eye is observed for a refixation movement (bottom). If there is a convergent squint there will be an outward movement of the uncovered eye (pictured) and if there is a divergent squint there will be an inward movement of the eye. If no movement is detected, the test should be repeated but covering the other eye first.

Common eye problems in childhood

Amblyopia

Amblyopia in childhood is reduction of visual acuity secondary to some functional abnormality of the eye or eyes. Provided it is detected early enough, amblyopia is treatable. Amblyopia is the cortical response to abnormal input from the eyes. While the visual cortex is still developing, amblyopia is potentially reversible. Conversely if the amblyopia is not treated before visual cortex maturation (about 7 years of age), it is not reversible later in life. Detection of amblyopia is one of the major reasons for routine visual screening in childhood.

Common causes of amblyopia are strabismus and refractive errors. Refractive errors cause a poorly focused image to form on the retina and thus a poor quality image to be transmitted to the cortex. Such input does not stimulate normal cortical development and amblyopia results. Strabismic (misaligned) eyes are not necessarily out of focus; however, if the cortex 'paid attention' to the image from each eye diplopia would result, as each eye is sending a different view of the world. In children the immature visual cortex is capable of ignoring the image from one eye. If this situation is allowed to persist the cortex may completely ignore or suppress the input from a deviating eye and amblyopia will result.

Treatment of amblyopia involves correcting any focusing errors with appropriate spectacles and forcing the brain to use the amblyopic eye by depriving the brain of clear input from the better seeing eye, most commonly with a patch. Unfortunately, simply realigning strabismic eyes is not enough to overcome amblyopia secondary to strabismus.

Strabismus

A squint or misaligned eye is important to detect as it is frequently associated with amblyopia. Most childhood strabismus is the result of cortical central nervous system (CNS) abnormalities in eye movement control; less commonly it is the result of cranial nerve lesions or extraocular muscle disease. In most children this CNS abnormality in eye movement control is an isolated abnormality with no other associated neurological or intellectual problems. However, children with widespread CNS abnormalities have an increased risk of developing strabismus. Down syndrome is a good example of this, with an approximately tenfold increase in the risk of developing strabismus.

The diagnosis of strabismus is outlined above and detailed consideration of the therapy of strabismus is beyond the scope of this chapter. The following is a brief description of the commoner patterns of strabismus seen in childhood and an outline of management.

Infantile esotropia

This is a large angle convergent squint seen before 6 months of age. Strabismic amblyopia is common in infantile esotropia, but refractive errors are rare. Patching followed by surgery is the most common initial treatment. Children with infantile esotropia need to be followed up throughout childhood, as about one third need more than one operation and amblyopia can occur following apparently successful initial treatment.

Intermittent divergent strabismus

This occurs from 18 months of age onwards. It is often more noticeable on distance fixation and may be associated with closure of the deviating eye, especially in bright light. Amblyopia is uncommon, as the deviation is intermittent and presumably when the eyes are straight normal visual development proceeds. In some cases the divergence becomes more constant and in such situations surgery may be undertaken to improve alignment.

Accommodative esotropia

This occurs in children who are excessively longsighted (hypermetropic). To overcome hypermetropia and focus a clear image on the retina, accommodative effort is used. Accommodation consists of the combination of changing focal length of the lens and converging the eyes (so that both are directed at the nearer object of regard). Thus in children with excessive hypermetropia there is increased focusing and at times excessive convergence; that is, a convergent squint (esotropia) appears as a result of the increased accommodative effort used by these children. Accommodative esotropia can be completely or partially corrected by prescribing glasses that compensate for the appropriate amount of hypermetropia. Amblyopia is often seen in association with accommodative esotropia and requires treatment. If glasses only partly correct the esotropia, surgery may be indicated to obtain optimal alignment.

Refractive problems

Refractive problems are the result of defects in the focusing components of the eye. These defects include abnormality of corneal curvature (a frequent cause of astigmatism) and abnormalities of lens power and axial length of the eye (which may result in hypermetropia or myopia). Children will rarely complain of poor vision related to refractive error, rather they readily accept the vision they have and get on with life. Children with high myopia will often manifest myopic behaviour (they will go very close to objects to look at them). Different refraction in either eye will often result in amblyopia because one eye generally will have a clearer image than the other and thus enable better cortical development for that eye.

Routine screening of visual acuity is the only reliable way of detecting the majority of refractive errors in children. In many countries there are both preschool and school entry tests of visual acuity for this reason. Such screening testing needs to be reliable, available to all of the target population, and followed up with appropriate intervention when defects are identified. As cortical maturation of vision occurs at about 7 years of age, screening should ideally commence in 3–4 year olds, before any amblyopia becomes difficult to reverse.

If a refractive error is suspected in a young child because of strabismus or poor visual acuity, then accurate and objective testing with cycloplegic retinoscopy is required. This involves dilating the pupils and temporarily paralysing the ciliary muscle with cycloplegic drops (for example, cyclopentolate 1.0%). Refractive errors can then be determined by retinoscopy. If a child is prescribed glasses, these should be worn the majority of the time.

Watery and sticky eyes

This occurs commonly in infancy as the result of congenital nasolacrimal duct obstruction. About 10% of newborn infants have obstructed nasolacrimal ducts. This will present as a watery and sticky eye in the first 1–2 weeks of life. Despite the persistent discharge the eye is generally not red or inflamed. An inflamed eye suggests an alternative diagnosis such as infective conjunctivitis. If the obstruction persists, the lower lid will often become red and sometimes slightly scaly as a result of the skin being constantly moist.

The differential diagnosis includes trauma, conjunctivitis and infantile glaucoma. These conditions are all described below.

Most congenital nasolacrimal duct obstructions resolve spontaneously. Approximately 95% of cases have resolved by the time of the first birthday, with most doing so in the first 6 months. In persistent cases probing under a general anaesthetic is recommended after 1 year of age.

Trauma

Trauma to the eye can take many forms. Physical trauma to the eye and surrounding structures may be blunt or sharp. Trauma can also result from radiation (thermal and electromagnetic) and chemical agents.

Direct blunt trauma to the eye may disrupt iris blood vessels, causing bleeding in the anterior chamber of the eye (hyphema), tear the iris, dislocate the lens, rupture the choroid and rarely rupture the eye wall (sclera) if the force is sufficient. Simple inspection of the eye will reveal most of these injuries and choroid and globe rupture may be suspected on the basis of the nature of the injury and associated poor vision. Referral to an ophthalmologist is necessary in these cases for confirmation of the injury and further management.

Sharp trauma may result from tiny objects such as a subtarsal foreign body causing a corneal abrasion, to fingernail scratches through to penetration of the eye by sharp objects such as a scissors blade or dart. Surface trauma can be diagnosed easily with the help of fluorescein staining and a cobalt blue light. Areas of epithelial abrasion will fluoresce green. If a round ulcer and/or vertical linear abrasions are seen, suspect a subtarsal foreign body and the upper lid should be everted. If identified, most subtarsal foreign bodies can be removed with a moistened cotton bud. Superficial trauma is treated with antibiotic ointment and a patch and daily review until any epithelial defect (ulcer or abrasion) is healed.

If the wall of the eye (cornea or sclera) has been penetrated, intraocular contents may prolapse out through the wound, the iris and pupil may appear distorted or the anterior chamber may be shallower than normal. Any suspected penetration of the eye must be referred to an ophthalmologist for further investigation and management. The eye should be protected with a cone which does not exert any pressure on the eye. If vomiting is likely or occurs an antiemetic should be given to prevent further prolapse of intraocular tissue.

Thermal injuries to the eye itself are rare, as in most burn situations the eyelids are firmly closed and thus protect the eye. Facial burns may cause scarring which interferes with lid function, leading to exposure and drying of the eye's surface. If a primary thermal injury to the eye is suspected, fluorescein dye should be used to detect any ulceration. If ulceration is found, treatment is with antibiotic ointment and a patch.

Radiation injuries to the eye are rare in childhood and most are the result of intentional irradiation as part of medical therapy for facial and ocular neoplasia. Typical injuries are cataract, dry eye syndrome, radiation retinopathy and optic neuropathy. These changes are seen some considerable time after the irradiation.

Chemical burns to the eye are unusual in childhood but potentially are very serious, especially if the chemical is alkaline. Many domestic cleaning agents are alkaline. Strong alkali will denature and dissolve protein and penetrate deeply into the surface of the eye. Acids tend to coagulate surface structures and this often prevents deeper penetration of the acidic chemical into the eye. Immediate first aid should consist of copious irrigation with water at the site of the accident and this should be continued for at least 10 minutes. Following adequate irrigation all chemical burns of the eye should be referred to an ophthalmologist.

Conjunctivitis

Conjunctivitis may result from infective, allergic or chemical agents interacting with the conjunctiva. Symptoms are itch, pain and irritation or a gritty sensation. Signs are epiphora (watering), discharge and erythema of conjunctiva and lids. The relative prominence of different symptoms and signs varies with the cause of the conjunctivitis (Table 76.1).

Conjunctivitis occurring in the first few days of life is generally bacterial and frequently is acquired from the birth canal. *Neisseria gonorrhoeae* and *Chlamydia trachomatis* both cause a conjunctivitis with copious discharge and marked erythema in the neonatal period, termed ophthalmia neonatorum. Gonococcal conjunctivitis is serious because of the risk of spontaneous perforation of the cornea and resultant loss of vision and also the risk of more generalised sepsis. Chlamydial conjunctivitis is significant because of the risk of more generalised chlamydial sepsis. For accurate and prompt diagnosis of these infections microbiological diagnosis and systemic as well as topical antibiotic therapy is needed. For culture, conjunctival swabs should be directly inoculated onto culture medium plates and conjunctival scrapings for Gram staining and immunofluorescent staining should be taken.

Bacterial conjunctivitis occurring outside the first few days of life in children is usually the result of relatively innocuous organisms (for example, *Staphylococcus* spp. and *Haemophilus* spp.) Microbiological investigation is not usually indicated and a broad spectrum topical antibiotic should be prescribed (such as neomycin/polymyxin or chloramphenicol). Recently, concern has been raised about topical chloramphenicol preparations because of a perceived risk of secondary agranulocytosis. It is the author's belief that this risk is extremely low but does exist.

Viral conjunctivitis is relatively common at all ages and clinically may be very difficult to differentiate from bacterial conjunctivitis. The discharge may be somewhat less with viral conjunctivitis. If the aetiology is uncertain, topical antibiotics as for bacterial conjunctivitis should be used.

Allergic conjunctivitis is common in children of all age groups and has itch as its most prominent symptom. House dust mite, grass and other plant pollens are common allergens that precipitate allergic conjunctivitis. Therapy depends on the severity of the symptoms. If mild, cold compresses may be all that is needed. For more severe symptoms soothing topical astringent agents that include a topical antihistamine are helpful. In more persistent and severe cases topical sodium cromogylcate and steroid preparations may be indicated. Topical steroid should be used with the supervision of an ophthalmologist because of the risk of significant side effects, including cataract and glaucoma.

Clinical example

A 4 year old boy presented with a 12 hour history of a red and watery eye. He complained of pain and his parents had not observed any discharge. Examination revealed a red eye with no obvious trauma or foreign body on the surface of the eye. Fluorescein staining demonstrated a round ulcer on the upper part of the cornea. On everting the upper eyelid a small foreign body was found and was removed with a moistened cotton bud. The ulcer was treated with antibiotic ointment and a pad and healed in 1 day.

Lid infections

These are common in children and most arise in the skin appendages of the eyelids (lash follicles and meibomian glands). Infection of a lash follicle is called a stye (or hordeolum externum) and acute infection of a meibomian gland is known as hordeolum internum. Unless there is significant secondary erythema of the surrounding lid, topical and systemic antibiotics are not indicated. Occasionally severe preseptal cellulitis will follow a focal lid infection and systemic (often intravenous) antibiotics will then be needed for treatment.

More chronic inflammation of a meibomian gland is known as a chalazion. This is generally the result of sterile chemical inflammation rather than infection and occurs when the contents of a meibomian gland escape

Table 76.1 Signs and symptoms of conjunctivitis. The descriptions in this table are intended to be a guide; there may be considerable variation and overlap in the signs and symptoms of conjunctivitis due to different causes

Cause of conjunctivitis	Symptoms	Signs
Viral	Moderate discomfort	Moderate epiphora Mild discharge Mild to moderate erythema
Bacterial	Moderate to severe discomfort	Moderate epiphora Copious discharge Moderate to severe erythema
Allergic	Itch often prominent	Mild to moderate epiphora Stringy discharge Mild erythema
Chemical	Pain intense	Severe epiphora Mild discharge Moderate to severe erythema

into the lid following blockage of the opening of the gland at the lid margin. A chalazion will appear as a lump in the substance of the lid and is often not particularly inflamed in appearance. Topical antibiotics seldom hasten resolution. Warm compresses may give symptomatic relief and help drainage. Chalazia may persist for many months. Some will discharge through the conjunctiva or the skin. On occasions surgical drainage is indicated for a persistently inflamed and large chalazion.

Ptosis

Ptosis, also called blepharoptosis, is a droopy upper eyelid and results from innervational or muscular defects of the levator superioris or Muller muscles. Innervational defects include third cranial nerve palsy, Horner syndrome (sympathetic nervous system) and myasthenia gravis. Congenital ptosis is the commonest muscle defect causing ptosis in children. Ptosis will cause visual defects when the lid is so low that it occludes the visual axis or if it induces astigmatism by altering the corneal curvature. Ptosis is also a cosmetic concern in that it may make an affected child look sleepy or dull. Surgical correction is possible in most cases.

Learning difficulties

Learning difficulties are common in school age children and it is commonly assumed that there may be a visual abnormality that contributes to or even causes the learning difficulty. This assumption is ill founded and arises because vision is so obviously involved with activities such as reading and writing. Children with learning difficulties are no more or less likely to have visual problems than children without evidence of learning problems. Rather than expending effort on therapies for perceived ocular abnormalities, parents should be encouraged to take an educational approach to their child's learning difficulties.

Visual handicap

Visual handicap in childhood may be the result of ocular and/or cortical visual abnormalities and may be associated with other abnormalities; for example, deafness, motor defects, intellectual defects, and so on. Intervention and support for a particular child needs to be planned after a thorough assessment of the child's visual and associated handicaps. From a purely visual point of view, interventions may include mobility training, low vision aids, such as magnifiers and closed circuit television, and training in alternative means of communication, such as 'reading' braille and using a computer to write.

The presence of additional handicap such as deafness or an intellectual deficit compounds the situation and necessitates skilled intervention over many years to achieve optimal outcomes.

Rare but important eye problems in childhood

These are mentioned briefly because prompt recognition enables early treatment and optimal outcomes.

Poor vision in infancy

This first comes to attention when a child fails to achieve normal milestones of visual development (see Measurement of vision in children, above). If the cause of severe visual impairment is within the eye, sensory nystagmus will develop at about 3–4 months of age. This nystagmus is often slow and somewhat pendular rather than jerky in appearance. Severe visual loss secondary to CNS abnormality does not cause nystagmus. Causes of poor vision in infancy include:
- cataracts
- congenital retinal dystrophy
- albinism
- retinal colobomas
- infantile glaucoma
- retinoblastoma
- delayed visual maturation
- cortical visual impairment.

Prompt recognition is vital as there may be a treatable cause (for example, cataracts) and, even if no treatment is possible, early and appropriate intervention minimises the negative effects of severe visual impairment on general development.

Cataract

A cataract is any opacity within the lens. Bilateral congenital cataracts will often cause poor vision in infancy, while unilateral congenital cataract may go unrecognised, as one eye has normal vision. Both bilateral and unilateral congenital cataracts are treatable if diagnosed early. Cataracts are detected readily by inspection of the red reflex with the direct ophthalmoscope.

There are numerous causes of congenital cataracts, including: hereditary (dominant, recessive and X linked); metabolic (for example, galactosaemia); association with systemic syndromes (for example, Down syndrome), and congenital infection (for example, rubella embryopathy). Many, especially unilateral cataracts, are idiopathic.

Retinoblastoma

This is a rare childhood cancer arising within the retina. Sporadic and hereditary forms are recognised. The sporadic form is the result of two separate mutations which negate the action of the retinoblastoma gene (Rb gene) within a single retinoblast cell, and thus is always unilateral. The hereditary form arises when the first of these two mutations occurs in one Rb gene within a germ cell (most often a sperm). The second mutation occurs within the retinoblast. As all retinoblasts descended from an affected germ cell have the first mutation by chance, more than one retinoblastoma will usually develop and hence the hereditary form is often, but not always, bilateral.

Retinoblastoma most often presents with leukocoria (white pupillary reflection; the white tumour is seen immediately behind the lens), strabismus, poor vision, or a known family history of retinoblastoma. Prompt recognition is vital as early treatment will increase the possibility of preserving vision and life. With current treatments the 5 year survival of this childhood cancer is about 98%.

Glaucoma

Glaucoma in infancy presents with a cloudy and enlarged cornea with associated epiphora (watery eye) and photophobia. It may be unilateral or bilateral and is usually an isolated ocular abnormality. If unrecognised it will result in severe and untreatable visual loss over weeks to months. Prompt diagnosis allows surgical treatment which controls the glaucoma in the majority of cases.

Colobomas

These defects result from failure of complete fusion of the embryonic fissure of the developing eye between the fourth and sixth week of gestation. If the optic nerve or macula area of the retina is involved then vision will be significantly affected. An iris coloboma may or may not be present in association with a visually more important posterior pole colobomas. Colobomas are not treatable.

The eye in paediatric systemic disease

The following is a brief account of the common ocular features of some paediatric systemic diseases.

Extreme prematurity

Marked prematurity gives rise to eye problems by interfering with the orderly development of retinal blood vessels. This disorder is known as retinopathy of prematurity (ROP). Mild ROP is seen in 30–50% of infants weighing less than 1250 g at birth and then regresses without ill effect on vision. In some infants the ROP progresses and a fibrovascular proliferation develops within the eye which detaches the retina, with resultant loss of vision.

Excess oxygen administration to premature infants has been known to be a potent cause of severe ROP since the 1950s. Curtailment of oxygen use to amounts sufficient to limit respiratory and neurological sequelae has greatly reduced the incidence of blinding ROP but has not completely prevented it. In general it is the sicker and smaller infants that are still at risk of severe ROP.

Screening of at risk infants (birth weight < 1250 g) by an ophthalmologist enables detection of significant ROP before retinal detachment occurs. Retinal ablation with laser or cryotherapy will then greatly reduce the risk of the development of retinal detachment.

Juvenile chronic arthritis

Childhood chronic arthritis gives rise to inflammation of the iris (iritis or anterior uveitis) in some affected children. Those at particular risk are young girls with oligoarticular juvenile chronic arthritis who are antinuclear antibody positive. The iritis that occurs in these children is painless and chronic and will, if untreated, often cause cataract and glaucoma. Periodic assessment by an ophthalmologist will detect early iritis and permit treatment to minimise the risk of visual loss.

Down syndrome

Down syndrome is associated with an approximately tenfold increase in the risk of developing eye problems during childhood when compared with the normal incidence. The eye problems are the same as for any child. An increased index of suspicion for eye problems should be maintained for individuals with Down syndrome.

Physical child abuse

Non accidental injury may involve the eye. Direct trauma to the eye or eyelids will generally be obvious on inspection. Violent shaking of a small child is often associated with the development of retinal haemorrhages and a severe closed brain injury. Although not pathognomonic for child abuse, the presence of retinal haemorrhage is highly suggestive of abuse in cases of unexplained severe brain injury in a young child.

Diabetes mellitus

Diabetes mellitus is common in childhood. Fortunately the duration of diabetes in children is often insufficient for there to be much risk of the development of eye complications. Screening for eye complications should begin at about puberty and occur 2 yearly thereafter if the examination is normal. Significant retinal abnormalities are seen in a small number of diabetic children in mid to late adolescence, particularly if the disease was of early onset and control has been poor.

Tooth and oral problems

R. K. Hall

Teeth consist of a crown and a root, which is held in the alveolar bone of the maxilla or mandible by the periodontal membrane. The crown consists of a cap of enamel which covers an inner structure of dentine and dental pulp, while the root dentine and pulp are covered by cementum, which is a bone like substance. The primary (deciduous) dentition consists of 20 teeth: 4 incisors, 2 cuspids (canines) and 4 molars in each jaw. The permanent dentition has 32 teeth: 4 incisors, 2 cuspids, 4 premolars and 6 molars in each jaw.

The mouth of the newborn child

The mouth of the normal newborn baby has well developed alveolar ridges with obvious bulges of tooth buds in both maxilla and mandible. The crest of the ridge anteriorly is initially a thin fibrous band with the maxillary labial frenulum crossing this and attaching into the incisive papilla. The palate is broad and flat and the alveolar ridges posteriorly are flattened.

Abnormalities or variations of normal development

Natal and neonatal teeth

- Present 1:3000 births, or erupt in the neonatal period — usually in the mandibular incisor region.
- In infants with cleft lip and palate commonly occur high in the cleft.
- Most are prematurely erupted normal primary teeth, but some are 'supernumerary' teeth.
- Rarely interfere with breast feeding (nipple trauma).
- Removal (using topical local anaesthesia and a haemostat) only indicated for extreme maternal anxiety (of possible dislodgement and aspiration during feeding — but no report of this eventuality).
- X rays not necessary as the decision to remove a natal tooth is made solely on clinical grounds.

Congenital epulis

- A benign pedunculated soft tissue tumour on the alveolar ridge, present at birth.
- Composed of sheets of granular cells.
- Management is by careful surgical excision.
- Does not recur.

Oral alveolar developmental cysts (Bohn nodules)

- Multiple 1–5 mm creamy nodules on the outer surface of the alveolar ridges (normally shed *in utero*).
- Composed of epithelial remnants.
- Sometimes mistaken for prematurely erupting teeth.
- Similar nodules, found along the palatal midline, are known as Epstein's pearls.
- No treatment indicated for any of these nodules or cysts as contents discharge spontaneously by 3rd month.

Palatal odontogenic hamartoma

- Unilateral or bilateral 3–5 mm dome like swellings adjacent to the midline of the palate behind the incisive papilla.
- Contain odontogenic epithelium or a developing tooth (demonstrated on occlusal radiograph).
- Appear from 8–12 months of age.
- Managed by elective surgical excision under general anaesthesia (can be deferred to 12 months of age).

Eruption cyst and eruption haematoma

- A blue or clear swelling overlying the crown of an erupting tooth, most frequently in the incisor region of the maxilla.
- Eruption is slightly delayed and discomfort or pain may occur.
- Management is by parental paracetamol administration at night and before meals. Surgical intervention is contraindicated.

During tooth eruption, as blood vessels separate over the erupting tooth, blood may enter the loose tissue over the crown (between fusing oral and dental epithelia), forming an eruption cyst; should tissue fluid and serum escape but some blood remains the anomaly is referred to as an eruption haematoma.

Melanotic neuroectodermal tumour of infancy (MNTI)

- Very rare solid benign but locally invasive blue-black pigmented tumour.
- Cells of neural crest origin (two cell types: neuroblasts and black pigment cells).

- Tumour cells associated with each primary tooth in one jaw quadrant.
- Commences *in utero* and always presents before 3 months age.
- Management by careful surgical excision, and removal of associated teeth; does not recur if completely removed.
- CT essential to locate all individual tumour deposits.

This tumour should not be confused with an eruption cyst or haematoma. It is the only oral lesion which can appear blue-black in this region at this age.

Normal tooth development

The initiation of tooth development is from cells of the oral ectoderm which form the dental lamina, together with mesodermal cells which migrate from the neural crest. Tooth buds and their dental papillae develop from ectodermal thickenings of this lamina and condensation of the subadjacent mesoderm under the control of genes EGF and BMP-4. Morphogenesis is controlled by genes which include Lef-1, MSX-1, Pax-9, Shh and FGF.

The key times of tooth formation are:
- Epithelial dental lamina formed by 38th day *in utero.*
- Tooth buds commence formation from incisor region backwards to the molar region on 49th day *in utero.*
- Calcification of the organic matrix commences 2 weeks after the beginning of tooth matrix formation.

Abnormalities of tooth development

Developmental defects of enamel

Disturbance of the metabolism, or death of the sensitive enamel forming cell (ameloblast), will leave a permanent developmental defect in and on the erupted tooth enamel surface as loss of tooth substance (hypoplasia) or an internal (subsurface) defect within the enamel (opacity defect). By using published tables (or diagrams) of normal tooth development, enamel defects can frequently be clearly related chronologically to:
- prenatal events (usually occurring between the 3rd and 7th month *in utero*), such as maternal rubella virus or cytomegalovirus (CMV) infection, maternal syphilis and pregnancy toxaemia
- natal events; may be prematurity, hypoxia and hyperbilirubinaemia
- postnatal events; measles virus infection, gastrointestinal disease, hypoparathyroidism and administration of tetracycline are some of the over 100 possible aetiological factors capable of inducing developmental defects of tooth enamel.

These defects will be found symmetrically and developmentally chronologically distributed on areas of the tooth crown which were at that particular developmental stage at the time of insult (Fig. 77.1). When isolated defects occur in developing permanent teeth they are usually due to infection or trauma of the primary precursor tooth. An isolated, circular, hypoplastic defect, usually of the mandibular cuspids bilaterally, is the earliest tooth defect recorded in prehistoric populations — its aetiology is still being debated.

Fluorosis

High serum levels of fluoride can produce a developmental abnormality of enamel maturation known as fluorosis. Mild cases appear clinically as usually a white flecking or linear opacity of the enamel. Mild fluorosis is sometimes difficult to distinguish from enamel opacity defects arising from other causes. The recommended fluoride supplement dosage in children's toothpaste has been reduced with the aim of preventing even mild fluorosis, while retaining fluoride's caries preventive effect.

Genetic defect of tooth enamel: amelogenesis imperfecta (AI)

Amelogenesis imperfecta is a generalised non chronologically distributed defect of tooth enamel affecting all teeth of both primary and permanent dentitions. AI may be

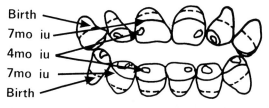

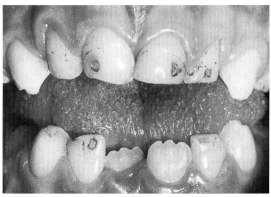

Fig. 77.1 Developmental defects of primary tooth enamel at 4 months *in utero* (iu), 7 months *in utero*, and birth stages of tooth development.

inherited as an autosomal dominant, autosomal recessive or X linked trait. A mutation in the amelogenin gene AMELX has been shown to be responsible for the defect in cases with X linked inheritance. It may be either an isolated defect or be associated with other disorders, for example pseudohypoparathyroidism and epidermolysis bullosa, and occurs as a main feature of certain rare syndromes such as AI-nephrocalcinosis syndrome, Kohlschutter syndrome and trichodento-osseous syndrome.

Clinical use of developmental defects of enamel in paediatric diagnosis

Knowledge of the aetiology of developmental defects of enamel is of importance both diagnostically and to explain their apparent cause to parents. Should enamel defects be present, these must be due either to a genetic defect or to a significant metabolic disturbance prenatally, neonatally or postnatally (the exact time of occurrence developmentally can be determined by the position of the defects on the teeth).

It is also well documented that 62% of very low birth weight and 27% of low birth weight premature infants have developmental defects of primary tooth enamel (compared with 13% of normal birth weight fullterm infants).

> ### Clinical example
>
> Miranda, now aged 2 years, was born normally at term with a normal birth weight. Since then she has demonstrated slow developmental milestones and mild hemiplegia with no obvious cause. Dental examination revealed a caries free primary dentition, which, however, had chronologically distributed enamel hypoplastic (developmental) defects, affecting the teeth at the 4–7 months in utero stage of development. On questioning, her mother could not recall any major abnormal event during pregnancy; however, the grandmother had recorded in her diary the dates when her daughter had a severe viral infection and was in bed for several days (and she had gone to look after her).
>
> Antibodies to CMV were detected on testing. CMV was the presumptive cause of the enamel defects and possibly also of the mild neurological defect and hemiplegia. This diagnosis helped early planning for future assessment and care. The tooth enamel defects can be enamel bond sealed to reduce plaque retention and prevent dental caries. Good oral hygiene care initially by the parents will be essential.

Genetic defects of tooth dentine: dentinogenesis imperfecta (DI)

This abnormality, which, due to the pathological changes in the dentine gives teeth the optical appearance of opalescence or an amber colour, may occur as an isolated genetically inherited disorder or as one feature in Sillence types IB, IC, III and IVB osteogenesis imperfecta. (In the other Sillence types of osteogenesis imperfecta, the teeth appear clinically normal but all have ultrastructural defects of the dentine).

Genetic defects of tooth form and number

In certain genetic disorders, the structure of teeth and other tissues of ectodermal origin, such as skin, hair and nails, is disturbed in a consistent and characteristic way. The most common of these conditions is hypohidrotic ectodermal dysplasia, where many teeth are congenitally missing and those present occur in unusual positions and with abnormal crown form. Anterior teeth present have a strange conical extremely pointed form.

Multiple additional (supernumerary) teeth occur in cleidocranial dysplasia and Gardner syndrome. Single supernumerary teeth are common in the incisor region, especially in cleft lip and palate. Fused or geminated teeth and abnormal tooth forms (odontomes) are quite common.

Abnormalities of oral soft tissues

Tongue tie (abnormal lingual frenulum)

Parents and medical practitioners are often concerned about this problem. Interference with speech or swallowing occurs only in the most severe cases, where the tongue cannot be protruded and 'grooves' when this is attempted. Under these circumstances lingual frenectomy should be carried out carefully by an expert in surgery in this area.

Abnormal maxillary labial frenulum

The upper labial frenum may be broad and large and separate the upper incisor teeth. Surgical frenectomy is not indicated unless the frenulum is still attached to the incisive papilla by strong fibres which prevent physiological closure of the space between the incisors, and then not usually before the permanent cuspids have erupted at 9–10 years of age.

Multiple abnormal frenula

Multiple soft tissue bands occur in all four quadrants in the genetic disorder of oral–facial–digital syndrome in association with a bifid or trifid cleft tongue and sublingual hamartomas.

Tooth eruption and teething

Primary tooth eruption occurs symmetrically at specific times and depends upon genetic factors and the health and physical developmental age of the child. Eruption commences with the lower incisors at 6 months of age and by 12 months of age all eight primary incisors are present; the first molars erupt at 8 months and the full primary dentition of 20 teeth is present by 30 months of age (the lower teeth preceding the upper, and at most a few weeks separating left and right sides).

Teething symptoms which are maximal a week before tooth eruption include irritability, increased salivation and alveolar mucosal erythema. Other symptoms such as transient mild diarrhoea, anal and facial rashes and slight fever are frequent at the time of eruption, but may be coincidental.

There is a wide range in times, 8–12 months or longer, at which the first primary tooth erupts, but eruption can be delayed much longer in chronic illness, Down syndrome, hypothyroidism and a number of rare conditions. Failure of incisor teeth to erupt by 12 months of age or any wide departure from symmetric eruption is an indication for early referral to a paediatric dentist.

Shedding of primary teeth and permanent tooth eruption

At 6 years of age the primary lower incisors shed following resorption of their roots by the erupting permanent central incisors. The mandibular permanent incisors erupt, followed closely (often unnoticed) by the first permanent molars, then the maxillary central incisors. For some time after eruption the anterior teeth may appear crowded or rotated (because of the discrepancy between tooth and jaw size) until maximum face and jaw width is reached at 9 years of age. The full permanent dentition (less the third molars) is normally established by 13 years of age.

Early childhood dental caries

Dental caries, although a declining disease in most developed countries (mainly due to the use of fluoride containing toothpaste), is still a world problem. It results from the effect of acids, produced by the action of bacterial enzymes on fermentable carbohydrates and sugars (mainly sucrose) in the mouth, on tooth enamel (Fig. 77.2). Acid dissolution of the enamel is followed by the ingress of oral cariogenic bacteria, producing progressive demineralizatrion and proteolysis of the dentine.

Dental caries, even in fluoridated areas is a particular problem in infancy and early childhood (from 12 months to 3 or 4 years of age). Why does early childhood caries occur? The different clinical patterns of caries resulting from infant feeding and nursing practices common in all sections of the community regardless of economic or social factors are illustrated in Figure 77.3.

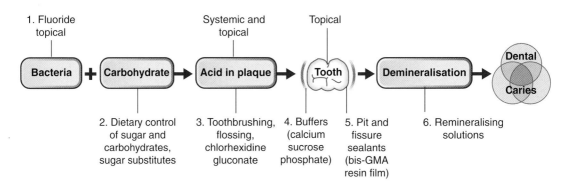

Fig. 77.2 Dental caries and possible preventive techniques.

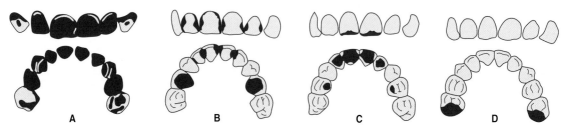

Fig. 77.3 **A** Pacifier or dummy caries. **B** Nursing bottle caries. **C** High frequency breastfeeding caries. **D** Operculum caries.

Dummy (pacifier) caries (Fig. 77.3A) occurs with the frequent use of a pacifier or dummy dipped in a sweetening agent, most often honey, molasses, jam or glycerine. Severe destruction of all upper primary teeth, lower molars and canines can occur, as the dummy bulb is soft and spreads over all the molar teeth.

Nursing bottle caries (Fig. 773.3B) results from the undesirable habit of high frequency bottle feeding during the day and of leaving a nursing bottle of milk or fruit juice with a sleeping baby. The remaining bottle contents continually bathe the teeth, resulting in enamel decalcification and dental caries. During sleep the salivary flow (which buffers the acid produced) is reduced and the salivary composition changes. The four maxillary incisors and first molars are the main teeth affected because of the shape of the bottle teat, which also spreads laterally in the mouth during sucking. Correct infant feeding practice is recommended, with weaning from bottle to cup feeding after 12 months of age, 'mothering' during feeding, and removing the nursing bottle once a baby has fallen asleep.

High frequency 'at will' breastfeeding caries (Fig. 77.3C) can occur when a mother encourages frequent 'at will' suckling (more than 40 separate daytime suckling periods are commonly recorded in such cases; these babies usually sleep in the same bed as the mother, suckling 'at will' during the night). The palatal surfaces of the maxillary incisors are primarily affected, as they are almost continually in a decalcifying environment beneath a milk bathed nipple. The palatal surfaces break down, leaving a ragged notch on the incisal edge. If 'at will' breastfeeding continues beyond 18 months, the palatal surface of the maxillary first molars may be affected. The smaller number of teeth affected is because of the smaller size of the human nipple in comparison to the bottle teat or dummy.

The family medical practitioner, infant welfare nurse and paediatrician can do much to intercept and help prevent this problem by guiding mothers to adopt sound infant feeding practices. Management of such extensive dental caries at this young age requires care by a paediatric dentist, who will need to use intubation general anaesthesia in an appropriate paediatric hospital setting for a procedure lasting 1–2 hours.

Persistent operculum caries (Fig. 77.3D). Slow eruption of the second primary molar, with its deep occlusal pits and grooves, results in the persistence of a flap of gum tissue (the operculum) over the posterior of the erupting tooth, providing an ideal nidus for the accumulation of cariogenic bacteria. This may be a factor in children who have had a period of chronic illness or slowing of growth at this time (2–3 years of age).

Clinical example

Jimmy, aged 3 years and 6 months, presented with his mother because he had been crying when he ate or drank at the day care centre. Recently his mother had noticed that he sometimes cried at night too and that he had a chipped front tooth, although he had never fallen over. On being asked about his health and feeding during infancy, his mother acknowledged that he still regularly took his bottle of milk to bed at night to help him go to sleep. His mother said that she sometimes put a little of his favourite chocolate powder in the milk and did take the bottle away some hours later when she went to bed herself. She mentioned that he saw the heart doctor at the children's hospital because he had a 'hole in the heart' and she had been told that he would need an antibiotic if he 'had to have his teeth out'.

Oral and dental examination revealed that he had early childhood dental caries due to the persistent use, especially at night, of the feeding bottle of sweetened milk. The pattern of the extensive carious lesions, which involved the incisor and cuspid teeth in both upper and lower jaws, also the palatal surfaces of the upper first molars with even some white areas of early enamel demineralisation on the recently erupted second molars, was typical of prolonged 'at will' nursing bottle caries. The caries of the first molars was advanced, the extent of the enamel loss indicating likely involvement of the tooth pulp, also suspected from the history of pain on eating (fortunately he had not yet experienced spontaneous pain at night, which would have predicted pulpitis or pulp necrosis).

Management required early treatment to relieve pain and eliminate infection, using general anaesthesia (because of his age and the extent of the treatment to be carried out) administered by a paediatric anaesthetist in the children's hospital, with an appropriate antibiotic cover of amoxycillin given at the time of anaesthetic induction. Teeth which could be saved were restored but several teeth were unrestorable and had to be extracted.

Close cooperation was required between the paediatric dentist and paediatrician to help Jimmy's mother to understand the problem without inducing feelings of guilt and to cease the problem without inducing feelings of guilt and to cease the practice of giving him the bottle, especially at night in bed.

Prevention of dental caries

The following preventive measures (Fig. 77.2) have been developed to counteract the various phases of the caries process:

- Fluorides act mainly topically, but when given systemically during tooth formation alter tooth morphology and crystal structure, rendering the tooth enamel more resistant to acid dissolution. Fluorides also inhibit oral bacterial enzyme systems, which convert sugar into acids in plaque and interfere with

Table 77.1 Recommended fluoride supplement dosage (National Health and Medical Research Council, with comments after Hall 1994).

Natural fluoride in drinking water	Age and daily supplement recommended (2.2 mg sodium fluoride is equal to 1 mg fluoride ion (F)).		
	6 months–2 years	2–3 years	3–13 years
<0.3 parts per million (p.p.m)	0.25 mgF	0.5 mgF	1.0 mgF

Fluoride supplements should only be used where the natural fluoride content of the water supply is less than 0.3 mg/l (check with local dentist or local water supply authority).
Note: 'tank water' may contain 0.14 p.p.m fluoride (0.094–0.38 p.p.m) (galvanised iron tanks) or 0.58 p.p.m (0.10–2.30 p.p.m fluoride) (concrete tubs).
For fully breastfed babies: 0.25 mgF in orange juice or water daily from 6 months of age at latest for duration of breastfeeding.

bacterial reproduction, inhibit storage of intracellular polysaccharides, reduce the tendency of the enamel surface to absorb proteins and favour remineralisation. Fluoride supplement should be prescribed for all children in areas with less than the optimum 0.7 parts per million (p.p.m.) fluoride in their water supply. Table 77.1 gives the currently recommended dietary fluoride supplement dosage.

- Dietary modification aimed at the reduction of refined carbohydrates and sucrose containing drinks.
- Plaque removal by correct toothbrushing, flossing, and the use of chlorhexidine gluconate mouthrinse or brush-on gel.
- Buffering of acid formed using calcium sucrose phosphate-containing food products.
- Fissure sealing by the application of photocured Bis-GMA resin film to seal developmental pits and fissures.
- Remineralisation of small areas of enamel decalcification.

Dental abscess and cellulitis

Dental abscess occurs following necrosis of the dental pulp, from untreated or inadequately treated dental caries or dental trauma, the necrosed dental pulp becoming colonised by bacteria of systemic or oral origin. An acute dental abscess may become chronic, and acute flare up of a chronic abscess (granuloma) may sometimes follow a blow to the tooth or jaw. In the primary dentition an abscess is usually superficial, pointing beneath the labial or buccal oral mucoperiosteum (grandmother's 'gum-boil'). Untreated, these become chronic: a fistula forming discharging pus, or cyst formation may occur. In the permanent dentition, pus may perforate the bone, usually buccally, subperiosteally, then into the soft tissues of the face, along tissue planes as a sinus, finally perforating the facial skin, forming a fistula. This will self-heal following antibiotic therapy and removal of the tooth which is the source of the infection, and should not be excised.

Cellulitis is common and serious, with infection from an acute abscess spreading to the deeper submandibular, infraorbital or facial soft tissue planes and lymph nodes. Cellulitis occurs most commonly with an abscessed permanent tooth, due to the more deeply placed roots. High dose antibiotic therapy should be promptly instituted and intravenous antibiotic will be required for severe cellulitis, together with surgical drainage in severe submandibular cellulitis. The involved tooth should be extracted immediately antibiotic control is established (usually within 24 hours). Delay can lead, in the extreme case, to mediastinitis or cavernous sinus thrombosis.

Osteomyelitis of the maxilla and mandible

Osteomyelitis of the jaws in children is rare apart from neonatal maxillary osteomyelitis, when the infection spreads rapidly, involving developing tooth germs. Osteomyelitis of the mandibular condyle can occur in the neonatal period or infancy, secondary to septicaemia (especially due to *Staphylococcus aureus*), producing rapid destruction of the growing cartilaginous condyloid process and leading to bony ankylosis or severe disruption of the temporomandibular joint, and later severe progressive growth disturbance of the mandible.

Osteomyelitis of the maxilla or mandible in later childhood occurs only rarely, and usually in the immunocompromised patient, from local or systemic infection.

Oral soft tissue infections and ulceration

- *Marginal gingivitis* in children is due to irritation of the soft tissue attachment by plaque adherent to tooth surfaces.
- *Primary (and later recurrent) herpetic gingivostomatitis* is by far the most common oral infection in children (Ch. 37).
- *Thrush (acute pseudomembranous candidiasis)* is the first oral infection most infants will experience and is the most common mucosal fungal infection in children. Immunologically compromised children are at high risk of candidiasis (and also of recurrent herpetic gingivostomatitis). The condition of *chronic mucocutaneous candidiasis* involves nails as well as oral and other mucous membranes. *Angular cheilosis* is another chronic atrophic monilial infection which is not uncommon in children, especially those with hypohidrotic ectodermal dysplasia.
- *Oral mucosal lesions in childhood leukaemia* are mostly due to the complications of treatment (immunosuppression). Leukaemic cell infiltration is only rarely present. Mucositis, drug induced ulceration, oral gingival bleeding, neutropenic ulceration, herpetic gingivostomatitis, candidiasis and viral, bacterial and fungal infections can all be prevented or minimised by strict attention to oral hygiene and by using chlorhexidine gluconate and nystatin mouthwashes, and acyclovir prophylactically.
- *Graft versus host disease* may occur in children who have received **bone marrow transplants**.
- *Drug-related gingival overgrowth* occurs in cardiac, liver and renal transplant patients receiving cyclosporin A and/or nifedipine.
- *Oral features of HIV infection (AIDS)* in children are persistent oral candidiasis and recurrent herpetic gingivostomatitis (in addition to the general clinical features of AIDS in children).
- *Aphthous ulcers* are non infective, extremely painful ulcers, occurring most commonly on the labial and buccal mucosa and tongue borders. A prodromal burning sensation precedes breakdown of an initially white papule to form an ulcer with a crateriform base which heals slowly over 8–10 days. Aphthous ulcers may be of minor or major type and are usually associated with stress, but the cause is unknown. Secondary infection can occur if the mouth is not kept clean. Chlorhexidine gluconate or tetracycline or combination mouthrinses and careful toothbrushing help relieve pain and control secondary infection.
- *Oral features of Crohn disease* are those of *orofacial granulomatosis (OFG)* and can frequently be diagnostic. They consist of:
  — marked lip enlargement, together with enlargement of the buccal mucosa
  — alveolar mucosal erythematous granulomatosis in the incisor and cuspid region of the maxilla
  — Large, linear ulceration in the buccal sulci posteriorly.
    These oral findings can occur on their own or together with anal fissuring, genital swelling and gastrointestinal changes.
- Palatal and sometimes buccal ulcerative lesions present in all jaw quadrants adjacent to primary molar teeth which are mobile are the typical oral lesions of *Langerhans cell histiocytosis.* Detected and diagnosed early, these lesions and the disease respond in most cases to chemotherapy.

Enlargement of the gingival tissues

- Most often due to *gingivitis with periodontal disease* producing inflammation and oedema.
- *Phenytoin overgrowth of the gingivae* occurs in epileptic children medicated with phenytoin for seizure control. Part of the enlargement is inflammatory, and a high standard of oral hygiene and the use of chlorhexidine gluconate brush-on gel will therefore reduce the inflammation, and hence the enlargement. The enlargement disappears 3 months after ceasing the drug administration in most children.
- *Hereditary gingival fibromatosis* is an autosomal dominant inherited condition with dense, firm, general enlargement of the gingival tissue.
- *Cyclosporin gingival overgrowth* occurs in children who have been given cyclosporin with organ transplantation; it causes a similar but distinctive enlargement of gingival tissues.
- *Nifedipine gingival overgrowth* also occurs in transplant patients given nifedipine to counteract the hypertensive effect of ciclosporin or when nifedipine is used alone.
- *Mucopolysaccharidosis gingival enlargement* is present in certain of the mucopolysaccharidoses (Hurler (I–H), Hunter (IIA and B) and Maroteaux–Lamy (VIA and B) syndromes). The enlargement may be huge, also involves the tooth follicle and prevents or delays eruption.

Trauma to the teeth and oral soft tissues

Clinical example

Sally, aged 8 years, was playing on her big sister's new bicycle when the wheel hit a brick on the ground and she fell off over the handlebars onto her face. There was a good deal of blood and she had knocked out a front tooth. Her upper lip rapidly became swollen but there was no laceration. Her other front tooth was a little displaced and her lateral incisors slightly mobile. Sally's mother was a school teacher and had learnt the correct first aid for this situation; holding the tooth by the crown she gently rinsed off the loose dirt under running tap water and then placed the tooth in a plastic container of milk.

Sally's mother was, however, not sufficiently confident to replace the tooth and so she bundled Sally into the car and took her to the local children's hospital, arriving there within half an hour of the injury. After triage, the casualty officer rang the dentist 'on call' for assistance. He advised immediate reimplantation of the tooth after careful irrigation of the root with saline. After irrigation of the socket and gentle replacement of the tooth (with the curved surface to the front), a tetanus booster dose was given and amoxycillin prescribed for 5 days.

When the dentist arrived, a flexible bonded splint was constructed across the anterior teeth to remain for 6 days, and following the reimplantation (and repositioning of the other central incisor) the teeth were radiographed to ensure that no alveolar bone fracture was present or root fracture of the other loosened tooth. These teeth will be monitored carefully by clinical appearance, mobility, and with vitality tests and radiographs at frequent intervals for possible root resorption and ankylosis; the reimplanted tooth will need pulp removal and endodontic treatment within 10 days.

Managed ideally in this way there should be a 90% chance of success, as the tooth with its vital periodontal root membrane was adequately stored in milk, was not allowed to dry out, was reimplanted within a reasonable time and there was no alveolar bone fracture

Causes of dental and orofacial injuries in children

One of every three children is likely to suffer an injury to a primary or permanent tooth. As with all trauma, boys suffer twice as often as girls. The teeth most frequently injured are the more prominent maxillary central incisors. Dental injuries may involve actual fracture of the tooth crown and/or root, concussion, or partial/total displacement of a tooth from its socket.

In infants and very young children dental injuries are usually the result of a fall while crawling or learning to walk — sometimes with an object in the mouth. Tongue and frenulum lacerations and displacement of teeth are the most common injuries. Dog bites are most frequent at this age and cause severe soft tissue injury.

Orofacial injuries from child maltreatment are most frequent in the preschool age group. At preschool and school ages, falls in playgrounds and injuries from play equipment, especially swings, are most common; later falls from bicycles, sporting injuries and motor vehicle accidents, as pedestrians, passengers or cyclists, become more frequent causes of injury.

Injuries to the teeth may occur from 'head drop' in children with epilepsy and cerebral palsy.

Certain special causes or types of orofacial trauma in children

Child maltreatment

Orofacial trauma is present in 50% of reported cases of child abuse. Bruising of lips and alveolar mucosa, avulsion of mucoperiosteum and teeth, alveolar bone fractures, finger and bite marks on face and neck are all frequent signs of child abuse. These result from slapping, punching, hand over mouth, forcible feeding with spoon or fork, and forcible intrusion or removal of a feeding bottle, dummy or toy from the mouth. Sexual abuse of children may also cause oral bruising and palatal contusion. Oral signs should not be neglected when considering the possibility of child abuse.

Sublingual Riga–Fédé ulceration

Riga–Fédé ulceration is most common in mentally retarded and cerebral palsied children who continually rub the tongue backward and forward over the sharp edges of the lower incisor teeth. A small composite bonded or cast splint covering the incisors allows the ulcer to heal.

Neuropathological chewing trauma in comatose children

Self-trauma injury of tongue, lips and teeth occurs frequently in comatose children due to neuropathological chewing activity. A cast silver splint with a bite block on the molar teeth cemented to the lower teeth is the most positive long term way to prevent trauma and also provides oral access for oral suction and nursing care. At times a lip buffer, mouthguard, screen or even an orthodontic 'Nuk' pacifier will prevent injury if movements are not too vigorous.

Reimplantation of an avulsed permanent tooth: the most important dental injury

- Ideally this should be accomplished within 10 minutes and a flexible splint applied by a dentist for 6 days.
- If immediate replacement is not possible, the tooth should be stored in milk or wrapped in plastic film (to keep the root membrane moist until the tooth can be reimplanted); the tooth should only be handled by the crown.
- Reimplantation should be within 2 hours to minimize root resorption which follows drying or damage of the root membrane.
- Tooth root and socket may be irrigated with saline before reimplantation (but the tooth must not be stored in tap water).
- Reimplantation must be accompanied by tetanus prophylaxis and antibiotic therapy.
- Dental follow up for endodontic therapy within 10 days is essential.

The most misdiagnosed orofacial injuries in children

- Mucoperiosteal avulsion injuries (which require immediate repair under general anaesthesia).
- Mandibular subcondylar fractures and intra-articular temporomandibular joint injuries (which are managed conservatively).

Fractures of the mandible and maxilla will not be further considered here and the reader is referred to Chapter 13 of *Maxillofacial Injuries* by Rowe & Williams.

Cleft lip and palate management

The paediatric dentist, orthodontist, prosthodontist and maxillofacial surgeon, as well as the family general practitioner, are essential dental members of the cleft palate team. Management of the newborn baby with a cleft lip and/or palate may involve treatment with a small plate or adhesive strip across the lip prior to lip repair, to mould the palatal segments and control the otherwise unrestrained premaxillary growth. Later treatment will include a bone graft to the cleft in the alveolus at 9 years of age, to unite the maxillary segments and permit permanent cuspid tooth eruption, facilitating orthodontic correction of the teeth and finally, cosmetic prosthodontic restoration of residual dental irregularities and of the missing lateral incisor tooth, possibly using a single-tooth, osseo-integrated implant.

Dental care of the handicapped child

Preventive dental care is of the utmost importance for the handicapped child, and parents or health care workers may need to learn special techniques and use special brushes to help clean the teeth. If cooperation or control of movement for treatment cannot be achieved, general anaesthesia will usually be necessary. Orthodontic treatment is rarely successful for handicapped children, but in the few cases where cooperation can be achieved it has become possible. Special appliances can be made which may assist with salivary control.

Adolescent temporomandibular disorder

Recurring pain in the face, head or temporomandibular joints is most common in adolescent girls and frequently has an emotional basis. Pain due to spasm of masticatory, neck and facial muscles leads to limitation and disturbance of balanced jaw movement, with audible clicking and pain in the joints.

Management is by:
- sensitive elicitation of the aetiology and counselling aimed at the underlying initiating problem
- relief of pain with a potent analgesic such as Mersyndol
- breaking the anxiety–muscle tension–pain cycle using relaxation techniques, and if necessary a tranquilliser such as diazepam
- use of a lower bite plate, which may provide some relief by reducing pressure on the temporomandibular joint. (However, dental malocclusion is rarely a factor in children and adolescents.)

Questions

1. **Which statements are correct? A foreign body in the auditory canal:**
   (A) Can be removed by syringing (except with a perforated tympanic membrane)
   (B) Can be extracted using small grasping forceps
   (C) Should always be removed under general anaesthesia

2. **Which factors predispose to acute suppurative otitis media?**
   (A) Pre-existing effusion in the middle ear space
   (B) Cleft palate
   (C) Teething
   (D) Immune deficiency

3. **Which features occur in a child with 'glue ear'?**
   (A) Persistent but variable hearing loss
   (B) Attacks of giddiness
   (C) Repeated earache
   (D) Persistent discharge

4. **Tympanostomy tube insertion should be considered for 'glue ear' after:**
   (A) 1 month
   (B) 3 months
   (C) 6 months

5. **Which of the following are true?**
   (A) Pain is the most consistent feature of acute suppurative otitis media
   (B) A middle ear abscess (ASOM) that progresses to rupture the tympanic membrane seldom heals
   (C) There is always a perforation of the tympanic membrane with chronic suppurative otitis media
   (D) Infants' hearing cannot be tested until 12 months of age

6. **What is the most likely serious cause of complete obstruction of the nasal airways in a newborn child?**
   (A) Encephalocoele
   (B) Cleft palate
   (C) Bilateral choanal atresia
   (D) Vascular formation

7. **Should antibiotics be given for acute sinusitis?**
   (A) No
   (B) In some circumstances
   (C) Yes

8. **Are haemolytic streptococci the cause of acute tonsillitis?**
   (A) Always
   (B) Never
   (C) Often

9. **Which of the following cause stridor?**
   (A) Bilateral vocal cord paralysis
   (B) Laryngomalacia
   (C) Subglottic haemangioma
   (D) Vascular compression of the trachea
   (E) Glottic web

10. **Which features occur in 'delayed' presentation of an inhaled foreign body?**
    (A) Wheeze, cough
    (B) Choking, cyanosis
    (C) Chest X ray changes

11. **Treatment for amblyopia**
    (A) Is rarely successful and is a waste of time
    (B) May involve penalisation of the better seeing eye to 'force' the brain to use the amblyopic eye
    (C) Should be commenced as soon as amblyopia is suspected
    (D) Should not be commenced until the age of 5 years

12. **Sally, aged 6 months, had a persistent discharge from both eyes since leaving the nursery. One eye cleared at 4 months, but the other persists despite treatment with local antibiotics. The conjunctiva is not inflamed. The most likely diagnosis is nasolacrimal duct obstruction. You would recommend the parents to:**
    (A) Arrange to have a probing performed before it is too late
    (B) Wait until 12 months of age before considering undertaking a probing
    (C) Treat the discharge with a broad spectrum systemic antibiotic
    (D) Keep the eye free of discharge with regular bathing and minimize the use of topical antibiotics

13. **A 2 month old baby presents with a 1 week history of a watery left eye and there is no obvious discharge from the eye. This infant could have:**
    (A) Ophthalmia neonatorum and needs immediate microbiological investigation and admission for systemic antibiotics
    (B) A blocked nasolacrimal duct and should be admitted for urgent probing
    (C) Infantile glaucoma and needs urgent referral to an ophthalmologist for confirmation of the diagnosis and definitive surgical treatment
    (D) Allergic conjunctivitis and should be treated with cold compresses
    (E) A foreign body with corneal ulcer and needs antibiotic eye drops

14. **The parents of a 2 year old girl are concerned that her right eye has been deviating inwards for 3 months. Your examination using the cover test confirms a right convergent squint. You suggest to the parents:**
    - (A) Further treatment is unnecessary at this age and their daughter should be seen again in 1 year
    - (B) This girl should be referred to an ophthalmologist for examination (including funduscopy and refraction) and further definitive management
    - (C) This child is highly likely to have a retinoblastoma and needs urgent assessment
    - (D) This child will almost certainly need an operation to straighten the eye and this should be arranged as soon as possible
    - (E) This child may have amblyopia and may need glasses, and further assessment is needed

15. **Broken down, chipped and discoloured teeth in an otherwise well 3 year old child may be due to:**
    - (A) Enamel hypoplasia
    - (B) 'Nursing bottle' caries
    - (C) 'High frequency at will breastfeeding' caries
    - (D) 'Dummy' caries
    - (E) Trauma following a fall

16. **An unwell, febrile, 9 year old boy presents with a red swollen face over the right mandible and slight trismus. He had severe toothache 2 weeks ago and saw a dentist who said that he needed a filling in his six year old molar. How would you manage this boy?**
    - (A) Prescribe an antibiotic and plan to review him in 1 week
    - (B) Admit him to hospital under a surgical unit for intravenous antibiotic therapy and surgical drainage
    - (C) Telephone his dentist (or the appropriate emergency dental or children's hospital service) and arrange for him to be seen by a dentist immediately
    - (D) Tell him to see his dentist again as soon as possible

17. **A girl, 7 years of age, presents with a very swollen upper lip and reddening of the oral mucosa in the upper incisor region. She has just recovered from some nasty large ulcers in her cheeks. On questioning, you find that she has at times had some bleeding from her bowel and still has a small, red fissure behind her anus. Which of the following conditions would you consider in differential diagnosis?**
    - (A) Recurrent herpetic gingivostomatitis
    - (B) A dental abscess from a traumatised incisor tooth
    - (C) Orofacial granulomatosis, possibly as a component of Crohn disease
    - (D) Leukaemia

Answers and explanations

1. The correct answers are **(A)** and **(B)**. In a cooperative child the foreign body can usually be removed without general anaesthetic (C).

2. The correct answers are **(A)**, **(B)** and **(D)**. There is no evidence that teething (C) influences otitis media, although both occur at about the same age.

3. **(A)** and **(C)** are true. (B) Occasionally children are a little clumsy if the inner ear is affected. (D) There can be no discharge while the tympanic membrane remains intact.

4. The correct answer is **(B)** — with significant symptoms and no signs of natural resolution.

5. The correct answers are **(A)** and **(C)**. Most children with ASOM have significant pain and require analgesia (A). Rupture of the tympanic membrane in ASOM is usually followed by healing within 2 weeks (B). Perforation of the tympanic membrane occurs in chronic suppurative otitis media both with mucoperiosteal disease and with bony disease (C). Simple clinical tests of hearing in infancy include the 'blink' and 'startle' and the head turning responses (D). Quantitative electrophysiological tests are available.

6. The correct answer is **(C)**. Total obstruction of the nasal airways due to bilateral choanal atresia can lead to fatal asphyxiation. The other conditions are unlikely to lead to complete bilateral nasal airway obstruction in the newborn, even if they involve the nasal airway.

7. The correct answer is **(B)**. Antibiotics are worthwhile for severe or recurrent sinusitis and must be given (usually intravenously) for complications.

8. The correct answer is **(C)**. Streptococci can be cultured from the mucosal surface of the tonsils in about 50% of cases. Few other bacteria cause tonsillitis.

9. The correct answers are **(A)**, **(B)**, **(C)**, **(D)** and **(E)**. All of these congenital abnormalities can cause airway obstruction and stridor.

10. The correct answers are **(A)** and **(C)**. Choking and cyanosis are often prominent when the foreign body is first inhaled (B). There are changes in the chest X ray in about 80% of cases.

11. **(A)** Is incorrect as, provided therapy is started early, amblyopia is often reversible. **(B)** This is correct. Glasses may also be used to correct associated refractive errors. **(C)** Correct. The earlier amblyopia therapy is commenced the more likely it is to be successful. (D) Incorrect (see above).

12. **(B)** and **(D)** are correct. (A) Probing is rarely indicated before 12 months of age. **(B)** This is reasonable advice because of a good prospect of spontaneous resolution by 12 months of age. (C) The discharge associated with nasolacrimal obstruction is rarely due to infection and thus antibiotics (systemic or topical) are rarely indicated. **(D)** Correct. Bathing is generally all that is required to keep the eye clean.

13. **(C)** is correct. (A) Ophthalmia neonatorum presents within 1 week of birth. (B) A blocked tear duct usually has discharge as well as epiphora and the history is of discharge and epiphora from a week or two of age. **(C)** This is possible and if further examination reveals an enlarged and cloudy cornea this diagnosis should be strongly suspected and urgent assessment by an ophthalmologist arranged. (D) This diagnosis is very unusual at 2 months of age. **(E)** This is possible but would need to be confirmed by fluorescein staining of the cornea to confirm the ulcer, followed by removal of the foreign body.

14. **(B)** and **(E)** are correct. (A) Wrong! Further assessment to exclude serious abnormalities within the deviating eye is mandatory, as well as appropriate treatment for the squint and any associated amblyopia. **(B)** Correct. You should check the red reflex before referring to an ophthalmologist. If an abnormality of the red reflex is found, the referral should be urgent. (C) This child could have a retinoblastoma but this not highly likely as retinoblastoma is a rare cause of strabismus. (D) Incorrect. This child may require an operation, but treatment of any refractive error and amblyopia will be needed before considering an operation. **(E)** Correct.

15. **All of the answers (A–E) could produce this appearance** and referral to a general dentist or paediatric dentist is essential for correct diagnosis and management. In (A) the discoloration is not usually a feature and the tooth enamel defects are smooth and symmetric (rather than chipped). In (B), (C) and (D) there is characteristic cavitation with yellow/ brown discoloration of the exposed dentine. Once the enamel breaks down the edges are chipped. The lesions may or may not be symmetric. In (E) the chipping and discoloration would be restricted to one or two damaged teeth; such fractures frequently involve one or both angles of the teeth. Discoloration, if present, is of a grey/brown/purple colour due to blood breakdown products which have seeped into the dentine.

16. Answer **(C)** is correct. The only appropriate management is to refer to a dentist or emergency dental service where he will be fully examined and assessed, an orthopantomogram taken, an antibiotic prescribed and arrangements made to extract the tooth within 24 hours once the infection is responding to the antibiotic. Should the assessment be that he requires hospitalization and intravenous antibiotics, it is preferable that the dentist makes that decision. Should the cellulitis spread across across the midline and the trismus become complete, external submental drainage may be required, but this is the extreme situation and only arises when the correct management has not been instituted early. Antibiotic therapy alone will not eliminate the infection: extraction of the tooth (or, in a suitable case, endodontic treatment of the tooth) is also necessary. External facial drainage should never be undertaken — only submental drainage. (In the absence of any dental cause, supramandibular, or more rarely, facial lymph node abscess and cellulitis will be the likely diagnosis.)

17. Answer **(C)** is correct. The swollen lip and reddened labial mucosa are two characteristic features of orofacial granulomatosis and are very often coexistent or predictive signs of juvenile Crohn disease; the existence of gastrointestinal bleeding and an anal fissure make Crohn disease an even more likely diagnosis. Referral to a paediatric gastroenterologist is essential for endoscopic examination and bowel biopsy; these can be performed at the same time as an oral lip or mucosal biopsy. Oral ulceration and thickening of cheek mucosa may also occur, as may swelling of the genitalia, particularly in males. Despite positive oral and anal biopsies the gut may appear clinically normal and biopsies may also be negative. In such cases the question arises as to whether to institute systemic therapy or to attempt to control the local lesions. The child must be kept under regular gastro-enterological and paediatric dental review as Crohn disease may develop many years after the initial signs. (A) Recurrent herpetic gingivostomatitis could produce some of the same features but this possible diagnosis shuld be simple to eliminate. (B) A dental abscess could produce a reddened gum and a swollen lip, but the other features would not be present and there would be a history of trauma some time previously. Regarding (D), leukaemic cell infiltration could produce a reddened area of gingiva and mucosa anteriorly, but the history would be known and the girl would be very unwell.

PART 22   FURTHER READING

Andreasen J O, Andreasen F M 1994 Textbook and colour atlas of traumatic injuries of the teeth, 3rd edn. Munksgaard, Copenhagen

Beasley S 1993 Paediatric diagnosis. Chapman and Hall, London

Brook I 2001 Sinusitis — overcoming bacterial resistance. International Journal of Pediatric Otorhinolaryngology 58: 27–36

Burton M 2000 Hall and Coleman's diseases of the nose, throat and ear, and head and neck. Churchill Livingstone, Edinburgh

Cameron A, Widmer R 1997 Handbook of paediatric dentistry. Mosby-Wolfe, London

Daya H 2000 Paediatric vocal cord paralysis. A long-term retrospective study. Archives of Otolaryngology — Head and Neck Surgery 126: 21–25

Hall R K 1994 Paediatric orofacial medicine and pathology. Chapman and Hall, London

Isenberg S J 1994 The eye in infancy, 2nd edn. Mosby, St Louis

Moore A 2000 Fundamentals of clinical ophthalmology: paediatric ophthalmology. BMJ Books, London

Taylor D 1997 Pediatric ophthalmology, 2nd edn. Blackwell Scientific, Boston

Welbury R R 1997 Paediatric dentistry. Oxford University Press, Oxford

Wright K W, Spiegel PH 1999 The requisites in ophthalmology, pediatric ophthalmology and strabismus. Harcourt, St Louis

Useful links

http://www.bcm.edu/oto/othersa.html (Otolaryngology resources on the internet)

http://www.bite-it.helsinki.fi/toothexp (Gene expression in the tooth)

http;//www.entnet.org/aspo/ (American Society of Pediatric Otolaryngology)

http://www.kids.ent.com (Paediatric ear, nose and throat page for parents)

PART 23

PAEDIATRICS IN THE FUTURE

In many of the world's countries, childhood mortality rates are lower than at any other time in history. Standards of living for many are higher than ever before. Life expectancy has increased, while fertility rates are falling and family sizes are smaller. Relative household incomes have increased. New technological advances have altered the ways in which we communicate, and have increased the horizons of medical diagnosis and intervention. Such improvements in the health and standard of living of children in developed countries have not been paralleled in the developing world, and the inequalities between children being raised on different parts of our planet are greater than ever.

What will the next 10–15 years provide for the health and wellbeing of children? Childhood is a period of physical, developmental, and emotional growth. Health and wellbeing for all children results from a complex mix of genetic, environmental, sociological and political factors. Any attempt to improve the future health and wellbeing of children must consider these.

Global health for children: the need for change

Major needs remain to be addressed for a very large proportion of the world's children. These include poverty, adequate nutrition, hygiene, access to health facilities, the effects of war, vaccine preventable diseases, family disruption, and commercial and personal exploitation of children.

Poverty

Many of the world's children live in conditions of abject poverty. This is represented by the inability of children and their families to have their basic needs of shelter, water, food and sanitation met.

Adequate nutrition

At a time of greater capacity for food production than at any period in history, it is of major concern that commercial and political concerns prevent the equitable provision of food to many of the world's disadvantaged societies.

Hygiene

Safe drinking water is a continuing major need for many children, as is effective sanitation. In many parts of the world, infective diseases causing early childhood death are the result of non existent basic public health hygiene programmes.

Access to health facilities

Major improvement in access to affordable health care facilities is needed in many parts of the world. Appropriate and affordable use of antibiotics is a priority in treating infections. Prevention of nutritional disorders requires the attention of health professionals in developing countries. Accessible immunisation services are needed.

War

Children are the greatest victims of any armed conflict. Disruption of society, infrastructure, families and food supplies in times of conflict have major effects on children. War results in displacement and dislocation of families, loss of caregivers, malnutrition, increased prevalence of infectious disease, loss of educational facilities, physical injury, and major psychological damage to children.

Vaccine preventable diseases

One of the great public health advances of the last century has been the development of vaccines that prevent life threatening disease in early life. Smallpox has been eradicated, poliomyelitis is no longer seen in most of the world, infections such as tetanus and diphtheria are rare, and measles is becoming uncommon in the developing world. However, significant numbers of the world's children still have no or limited access to community based immunisation programmes.

Family disruption

Families have become smaller, and often are more isolated within communities as the extended family unit structure has changed. In developed countries, divorce rates have increased, as has the number of single caregiver family units. In many countries, especially in the developing world, HIV infection leading to loss of parents and other adult caregivers from AIDS has left children orphaned and isolated.

Commercial and personal exploitation of children

The inappropriate and sometimes enforced use of children in the labour force continues in many countries in the world. Sexual exploitation of children continues in most societies.

The approaches to the above needs for children must be at a societal, governmental and global organisational level. The United Nations, World Health Organization, UNICEF, the World Trade organisations and worldwide financial institutions are important instruments for change on behalf of children and their families.

Future medical developments relevant to the health of children

Table 78.1 lists other potential future developments in child health, with an emphasis on prevention of health abnormalities, diagnostic approaches, and treatment possibilities if there is a health abnormality. The major areas of impact will be in prenatal life, physical health during growth and development, and intellectual and psychological wellbeing.

Prenatal life

Prenatal wellbeing depends on genetic factors, maternal health and intrauterine nutrition. Many health disorders of adult life now are recognised as having their origins in fetal life. In vitro fertilisation techniques for genetic selection are providing ethical challenges in relation to our ability to select for or alter genetic factors impacting on later growth and development. High resolution imaging will enable early detection of fetal structural abnormalities, and also will allow functional studies of the fetus in the near future. A widening range of 'minimally invasive' surgical techniques is being developed for fetal surgery.

Physical health in childhood

The major emphasis for the health and wellbeing of individual children in developed countries in the next 10–15 years will be on disease prevention and early detection of health abnormalities. Early screening for detection of congenital disorders with significant childhood morbidity and mortality will develop further. Genetic techniques for screening for cystic fibrosis have been the major example in the last decade. These techniques will be expanded to other disorders, and the challenge will be early detection of susceptibility to disorders, such as atopy and cancer, that have a complex genetic and environmental aetiology. There will be developments in the corrective treatment of specific

Table 78.1   Future developments in child health

	Prevention	Diagnosis	Treatment
Prenatal wellbeing	• Improved nutrition • Vitamin supplements • Drug avoidance programmes • Carrier screening	• Genetic screening of fetal cells in maternal blood • High resolution imaging • Invasive physiological monitoring	• Fetal surgery • Transplacental medication • Improved high risk pregnancy services
Physical wellbeing	• Avoidance of war • Accident prevention • Reduction of pollution • Enhanced immunisation • Improved nutrition • Neonatal screening for monogenic and polygenic disorders	• Genetic and molecular diagnosis, e.g. for susceptibility to asthma, cancer, mental retardation • High resolution imaging • Rapid microbiological diagnosis using molecular techniques	• Enzyme replacement therapy • Targeted therapy, e.g. cancers • Gene therapy • Improved organ transplantation
Intellectual and psychological wellbeing	• Safe environments • Avoidance of poverty • Avoidance of family breakdown • Avoidance of violence • Rewarding employment	• Improved analyses of intellectual function by functional imaging • Improved psychometric testing instruments • Molecular genetic tests for specific learning difficulties	• Target educational programmes • Improved family support programmes • Rational drug therapies

genetic disorders, such as storage diseases and disorders of the haematological system, by gene therapy or gene product therapy.

Clearer understandings of the interplay of genetic and environmental factors in the pathophysiological pathways leading to developmental disabilities such as cerebral palsy should lead to new strategies for prevention.

On a more universal basis, the greatest developments in child health will be the production of effective vaccines against important bacterial, viral, protozoal and parasitic infections. Effective vaccines for prevention of some pneumococcal and meningococcal strains in childhood are already available, but at a cost that is prohibitive for children in most countries of the world. Effective and universally available vaccines against rotavirus, respiratory syncytial virus, influenza viruses and parainfluenza viruses will become available and will change significantly the pattern of use of acute health services by children.

Increased physical safety measures for children will lead to further decreases in death and disability from road trauma and accidents in the home.

It will become possible to detect speech and hearing deficits earlier in life, with better outcomes from earlier interventions. Later visual impairment arising from nutritional or infective disorders in early life will become preventable.

Intellectual and psychological wellbeing

In all societies, the developmental and psychological health and wellbeing of children needs further resources. The change in physical health needs for children arising from avoidance of some genetic disorders and infectious diseases will allow a reallocation of public expenditure to developmental, educational and psychological needs. In developed countries, many of the needs for children that now demand attention from paediatricians are in relation to actual or perceived learning difficulties. Improved assessment and screening tools will allow earlier and more precise definition of learning disorders, with more directed use of learning supports. Mental health issues will become even more prominent, with high rates of depression, youth suicide and behavioural disorders requiring professional expertise and public health measures.

Changes in the way medicine is practised

The great increase in the use of information technology, particularly the internet, is already changing the role of health professionals. Families now have easy access to a wide variety of sources of information, of varying quality, about their child's health or medical problems. They may even be able to access individual opinions from international experts, or others claiming to be experts. Their child's own doctor will become only one source of advice. Health professionals need to be able to manage this change in their role, to embrace the new technologies and use them positively to the advantage of their own patients and the wider childhood community.

The last decade has seen a big increase in the community's use of complementary and alternative medicines. In Australia, the community now spends more on these therapies than on medicines prescribed under the Pharmaceutical Benefits Scheme. These therapies are being widely used in children. It is likely that some forms of alternative therapy are good, with important potential roles in health care. Some will be ineffective but harmless, while others will be dangerous. We can no longer afford to dismiss these as 'fringe' therapies, but rather we need to understand what is being used and why, and examine them for potential benefits and risks, including the risks of interactions with our own 'conventional' therapies.

The future

The challenges and opportunities for improving the health and wellbeing of children are exciting. Many of the needs are global: it is important to keep these overall needs of children in perspective as we consider the technological advances occurring in medicine highlighted in the media. Health professionals must be strong in their advocacy for children as we move to the future.

Index

793

813